Maudsley

精神科处方指南

The Maudsley®
Prescribing Guidelines in Psychiatry

第 14 版

原著 David M. Taylor
Thomas R. E. Barnes
Allan H. Young

主译 司天梅

人民卫生出版社
·北 京·

图书在版编目（CIP）数据

Maudsley 精神科处方指南 /（英）大卫·M. 泰勒
（David M. Taylor），（英）托马斯·R. E. 巴恩斯
（Thomas R. E. Barnes），（英）艾伦·H. 杨
（Allan H. Young）原著；司天梅主译. -- 北京：人民
卫生出版社，2024.10
ISBN 978-7-117-35581-0

Ⅰ.①M… Ⅱ.①大… ②托… ③艾… ④司… Ⅲ.①
精神病 – 处方 – 指南 Ⅳ.①R749.05–62

中国国家版本馆 CIP 数据核字（2023）第 214688 号

人卫智网	www.ipmph.com	医学教育、学术、考试、健康， 购书智慧智能综合服务平台
人卫官网	www.pmph.com	人卫官方资讯发布平台

图字：01-2021-7484 号

Maudsley 精神科处方指南
Maudsley Jingshenke Chufang Zhinan

主　　译：	司天梅	
出版发行：	人民卫生出版社（中继线 010-59780011）	
地　　址：	北京市朝阳区潘家园南里 19 号	
邮　　编：	100021	
E - mail：	pmph @ pmph.com	
购书热线：	010-59787592　010-59787584　010-65264830	
印　　刷：	河北宝昌佳彩印刷有限公司	
经　　销：	新华书店	
开　　本：	787 × 1092　1/16　印张：55	
字　　数：	1338 千字	
版　　次：	2024 年 10 月第 1 版	
印　　次：	2024 年 11 月第 1 次印刷	
标准书号：	ISBN 978-7-117-35581-0	
定　　价：	198.00 元	

打击盗版举报电话：010-59787491　E-mail: WQ @ pmph.com
质量问题联系电话：010-59787234　E-mail: zhiliang @ pmph.com
数字融合服务电话：4001118166　E-mail: zengzhi @ pmph.com

Maudsley
精神科处方指南

The Maudsley®
Prescribing Guidelines in Psychiatry

第 14 版

原　著　David M. Taylor　Thomas R. E. Barnes　Allan H. Young

主　译　司天梅

译　者（以姓氏笔画为序）

王华丽	北京大学第六医院	李清伟	同济大学附属同济医院
方贻儒	上海交通大学医学院附属精神卫生中心	吴仁容	中南大学湘雅二医院精神卫生研究所
孔庆梅	北京大学第六医院	张　燕	中南大学湘雅二医院精神卫生研究所
司天梅	北京大学第六医院		
司昱琪	上海交通大学医学院附属精神卫生中心	张雨龙	安徽医科大学
		岳伟华	北京大学第六医院
刘寰忠	安徽医科大学附属巢湖医院	赵　敏	上海交通大学医学院附属精神卫生中心
苏允爱	北京大学第六医院		

审　校　田成华　北京大学第六医院

翻译秘书　郭春梅　北京大学第六医院　　孙雅馨　北京大学第六医院

人民卫生出版社
·北京·

Maudsley 指南的系列丛书还包括：

The Maudsley Practice Guidelines for Physical Health Conditions in Psychiatry
David Taylor，Fiona Gaughran，Toby Pillinger
《Maudsley 精神科躯体健康实践指南》

The Maudsley Guidelines on Advanced Prescribing in Psychosis
Paul Morrison，David Taylor，Phillip McGuire
《Maudsley 精神病处方实用指南》
主译：司天梅　人民卫生出版社(2022)

《Maudsley 精神科处方指南》
使用注意事项

本书旨在为临床医师在日常或少见的临床情形中,处方精神药物时提供实用的建议。本书包含的建议综合了文献综述、临床经验和专家贡献。我们并不认为这些建议必须是"正确的",或者比其他专业团体或特别兴趣小组的指南更值得重视。但是我们希望能提供一本有助于确保精神科安全、有效和经济用药的指南。我们也希望能明确提示用在指南中的信息来源。请注意,这里的很多推荐意见可能超出药物在英国或其他国家所批准的适应证。此外,还需注意,虽然我们努力确保所引用的剂量正确,但临床医师需要在开具处方前始终查阅法定文本。《Maudsley 精神科处方指南》的使用者也应牢记在心,本书内容是基于 2021 年 3 月我们能获取到的信息。随着研究的进行和新文献的发表,这里的很多建议可能会过时。

对于任何伤害、损失或损害,无论其原因如何,我们均不承担任何责任。

所含药物的注意事项

《Maudsley 精神科处方指南》可用于英国以外的其他国家。因此,在这版《Maudsley 精神科处方指南》中,包括 2021 年 3 月份以前广泛用在西方国家的药物,也包括一些未在英国上市的药物,如依匹哌唑、去甲文拉法辛、匹莫范色林和维拉唑酮。此外,许多老一代药物或未广泛使用的药物(如:左甲丙嗪、哌噻嗪、马普替林、佐替平、口服洛沙平等),在撰写本文时,基于这些药物尚未广泛使用,仅被简单提及或未被列入。

贡献者的利益冲突

《Maudsley 精神科处方指南》的大多数贡献者曾接受过制药企业的资助,用于研究、咨询或讲座。读者应该意识到,这些关系不可避免地影响了对药物选择或偏好等问题的看法。因此,我们不能保证这里提供的指导不受制药行业的间接影响,但希望用大量的文献证据来支持所持的每个观点,以此来减轻这种风险。关于直接影响,任何制药公司都不得查看或评论《Maudsley 精神科处方指南》的任何初稿或清样,也不得对任何主题、建议或指导提出纳入或忽略的要求。因此,《Maudsley 精神科处方指南》的编写独立于制药工业之外。

中文版序

《Maudsley 精神科处方指南》的第 12 版，在由司天梅教授带领团队翻译成中文出版的时候，我应邀写了如下的文字，算作推荐：

Henry Maudsley 在捐出靠自己私人行医赚到的 3 万英镑，建立一个新的精神病院时，向伦敦市政府提出了他的附加条件：一定要专注于急性和早期精神病而非慢性精神病的治疗；设立门诊；要有教学和研究功能。1923 年，Maudsley 医院作为精神病院正式开业，次年其附设的医学院开始招收研究生，并于 1948 年在洛克菲勒基金会的支持下改建为伦敦精神病学研究所，现在仍然是英国唯一的精神科研究生培训机构。

"把科学研究与临床实践结合起来"是 Maudsley 建院时的使命。为这一使命背书的，除了 Maudsley 医院一直是精神病学研究新进展的弄潮儿以外，还有持续不断再版的 Maudsley 系列丛书，包括这一本已经是第 12 版的《Maudsley 精神科处方指南》。

我当住院医师时，作为翻译人员接待过美国的一个精神科医师代表团。一个团员送了我一本用过的外文书，就是《Maudsley 精神科处方指南》，我记不得是第几版，但是应该是我个人拥有的第一本原版外文书。美国人一向自视颇高，但是肯"屈尊"去用这本指南，也间接说明了这本书在世界范围内的权威性。我注意到前言中编者不无得意地提到"第 11 版在其他国家的销量高于英国，而且至少被翻译为 10 种语言版本"。据我所知，这是这一处方指南第一次用中文出版。

翻译精神药理学的著作是既劳神费力、又不讨好的工作。既要注意其科学上的严谨性，也要照顾对临床医师的可读性。本书的译者均是国内著名的精神病学专家，而且有着丰富的翻译经验。感谢他们又为我们奉上了一本临床精神药理学的好书。对于本书的编著者和翻译者的最好回报，就是认真读，努力做，让更多的中国精神障碍患者得到恰当的治疗。

此书由人民卫生出版社在 2017 年出版发行后，好评如潮。不少精神科临床工作者都将其视为案头宝典，碰到问题随查随用。这也正体现了本书的价值：从内容到编排，作者都在实用性上下足了功夫。随后原著又出了第 13 版，译者团队不断收到同步更新中文版的呼吁。司天梅教授认为这一版内容变化不大，并未仓促动手。2021 年，《Maudsley 精神科处方指南》出了第 14 版，我们一方面感叹原编著者团队的勤勉，能够在 6 年之间做了两版的更新，也钦佩司天梅教授的果断决策，着力组织一干人马在较短时间内高质量地完成了翻译工作。这一版无论从内容还是编排上都做了相当大的改动，从第 12 版的 8 章，扩充到 14 章，同时这些章节被整合到 4 个部分中，既强化了章节间的逻辑联系，又改善了阅读体验。虽然主编团队更换了两人，但其实用性的风格仍然得以保留，如各章的小标题切中一个临床应用场景，正文中有大量的表格、流程图和小结,书末的索引,等等,都可以让忙碌的临床医师快速找到自己的治疗答案。而简洁清晰的文字表达,也会让医师在闲暇时仔细阅读,做到"知其然,知其所以然"。我相信即使没有我的大力推荐,这本书也会成为受临床医师追捧的工具书。我也特别希望在不断借鉴国外先进精神科治疗经验的同时,中国的临床精神药理工作者也能有自己风格的类似著作问世。

于 欣 教授

北京大学第六医院

2024 年 8 月

译者序

非常高兴《Maudsley 精神科处方指南》(第 14 版)译著在各位同道的共同努力下,完成翻译和校对,即将出版。《Maudsley 精神科处方指南》是由伦敦国王学院精神病学研究所编写并出版的系列丛书之一,本书主要针对精神医学临床实践中遇到的治疗问题,推荐建立在循证医学基础上的处理原则和指导意见,充分体现了其"把科学研究与临床实践结合起来"的宗旨,非常适合临床医师使用。在过去近 30 年间,伦敦国王学院精神病学研究院的作者们根据全球精神药理和药物治疗学领域的最新研究进展和证据积累,每两年进行一次修订和完善。2015 年 5 月,在获得该书作者伦敦国王学院临床治疗学和药理学、病理学系主任 David Taylor 教授同意后,我们联合上海精神卫生中心的赵敏教授、黄继忠教授、方贻儒教授、李华芳教授,上海同济医学院的李清伟副教授,湘雅二院的吴仁容副教授、张燕副教授,北京大学第六医院郭延庆副教授和苏允爱研究员,首次将《Maudsley 精神科处方指南》(第 12 版)的中文版权引进中国,由北京大学第六医院田成华主任医师负责全书的校对,该书出版后获得了我国精神科临床同道们的一致认可和好评,针对每个临床问题简明清晰、规范合理、可操作性强的指导推荐,也成为精神科住院医师不可或缺的临床技能提升指导书籍。

近 4 年来,借助于新型研究技术的推广应用,精神病学学科和诊疗经历了快速发展。今年《Maudsley 精神科处方指南》(第 14 版)出版发行,相比于第 12 版,《Maudsley 精神科处方指南》(第 14 版)补充了新型的治疗技术和手段,丰富了特殊人群精神障碍的处置原则和推荐意见,完善了以提高患者生命质量和社会功能为目标的治疗理念,内容从第 12 版的 8 个章节,增加到第 14 版的 14 个章节。我也非常荣幸能继续和上海精神卫生中心的赵敏教授、方贻儒教授、司昱琪副教授,上海同济医学院的李清伟主任医师,湘雅二院的吴仁容教授、张燕教授,北京大学第六医院苏允爱研究员合作翻译本书。同时,我也非常高兴北京大学第六医院的岳伟华、孔庆梅和王华丽教授、安徽医科大学附属巢湖医院的刘寰忠和安徽医科大学的张雨龙教授参与到翻译团队中,北京大学第六医院的田成华主任医师继续负责本书的审校工作。他们都是国内颇有成就的临床精神病学家或精神药理学家,他们深厚的专业知识和科学严谨的学术态度保证了本书的翻译质量。郭春梅和孙雅馨医师担任翻译秘书,负责和各位译者沟通协调、标注索引和缩略词等。和第 12 版的翻译过程一样,每一章都邀请了临床一线的青年医师,请他们提出意见和问题,担任审校的田成华医师对每一个意见和问题都给予了认真的反馈和修改,保证了本书的高质量翻译,非常感谢这些医师们给予的宝贵建议。

我们真诚希望《Maudsley精神科处方指南》(第14版)能够继续成为精神科及其他相关临床学科的医师、护士和临床药师得力的指导用书。由于本书内容庞杂,翻译者和校对者精力和能力均有限,书中难免有些不足之处,敬请大家批评指正,在此表示感谢。再次衷心感谢所有参与本书翻译、校对和协调工作的各位专家,为我们能够给临床医师提供有益的治疗指导参考用书感到欣慰!

司天梅
北京大学第六医院
2024年8月

《Maudsley 精神科处方指南》(第 14 版)是在新型冠状病毒大流行这一特殊情况下完成编写的。新型冠状病毒在全球的大流行彻底改变了数十亿人的生活和工作方式,我们大多数人现在都亲身或间接地熟悉了与 COVID-19 相关的、严重躯体病症的这种体验。

那些从事医疗保健工作的人员尤其受到严重的影响,他们冒着被感染的风险照顾那些罹患该病的人群。在这种环境下,写书的优先级,如果有排序的话则降到极低。正因为处于这种背景下,我向在如此具有挑战性的情境下为本版《Maudsley 精神科处方指南》做出贡献的所有人致以无限诚挚的感谢!

当然,在大流行期间,心理健康问题并未消失,对精神疾病的最佳治疗仍然是至关重要的,并且这一目标在应对大流行所致的心理健康问题时更为突出。

本版《Maudsley 精神科处方指南》进行了彻底更新,包含自 2017 年以来发表的有影响力的研究以及此后上市的所有主要精神药物。此版《Maudsley 精神科处方指南》的内容也进行了一定程度的扩展,如新增了激越谵妄患者的治疗管理、生命晚期精神疾病患者的用药、抗精神病药的静脉注射剂型、氯氮平的肌内注射剂型和按周口服的五氟利多。与之前的版本一样,《Maudsley 精神科处方指南》(第 14 版)的宗旨依然是立足于全球范围内应用,同时保留了对英国实践的略有侧重。

我要特别向 Siobhan Gee 致敬,她精心准备了大量氯氮平使用相关的资料和证据;向 Mark Horowitz 表示敬意,他提供了以循证为基础、以患者为中心的精神药物停药指导;向 Delia Bishara 表示敬意,她近乎独自完成了老年精神障碍患者治疗的章节;向 Ian Osborne 表示敬意,他对多个主题均有重要的贡献。感谢 Emily Finch,组织编写了最近十版《Maudsley 精神科处方指南》的增补章节,尤其值得肯定。最后,我要感谢我的助手 Ivana Clark,她耐心地协调本版《Maudsley 精神科处方指南》的出版工作,并对细节极其地关注。

David M. Taylor
2021 年 3 月于伦敦

致谢

感谢下列人员对《Maudsley 精神科处方指南》(*The Maudsley® Prescribing Guidelines in Psychiatry*)(第 14 版)做出的贡献：

Alice Debelle
Andrea Danese
Andrew Wilcock
Annabel Price
Anne Connolly
Bruce Clark
Claire Wilson
Colin Drummond
Daniel Harwood
David Mirfin
Deborah Robson
Delia Bishara
Derek Tracy
Ebenezer Oloyede
Elizabeth Naomi Smith
Emily Finch
Emmert Roberts
Eromona Whiskey
Francis Keaney
Frank Besag
Gabriel Ruane
Georgina Boon
Hubertus Himmerich
Ian Osborne
Irene Guerrini
Iris Rathwell
Ivana Clark
James Stone

Jane Marshall
Janet Treasure
Jemma Theivendran
Jonathan Rogers
Justin Sauer
Kalliopi Vallianatou
Kwame Peprah
Louise Howard
Luke Baker
Luke Jelen
Marinos Kyriakopoulos
Mark Horowitz
Max Henderson
Mike Kelleher
Nicola Funnell
Nicola Kalk
Nilou Nourishad
Oluwakemi Oduniyi
Paramala Santosh
Paul Gringras
Paul Moran
Petrina Douglas-Hall
Sameer Jauhar
Shubhra Mace
Siobhan Gee
Sotiris Posporelis
Stephanie J Lewis
Stephen Barclay

缩略语

缩写	英文全文	中文全文
AACAP	American Academy of Child and Adolescent Psychiatry	美国儿童和青少年精神病学学会
ACE	angiotensin converting enzyme	血管紧张素转换酶
ACh	Acetylcholine	乙酰胆碱
AchE	Acetylcholinesterase	乙酰胆碱酯酶
AchE-I	acetylcholinesterase inhibitor	乙酰胆碱酯酶
ACR	Albumin：creatinine ratio	白蛋白肌酐比值
AD	Alzheimer's disease	阿尔茨海默病
ADAS-cog	Alzheimer's Disease Assessment Scale-cognitive subscale	阿尔茨海默病评估量表 - 认知量表
ADH	alcohol dehydrogenase	乙醇脱氢酶
ADHD	attention deficit hyperactivity disorder	注意缺陷多动障碍
ADIS	Anxiety Disorders Interview Schedule	焦虑障碍访谈表
ADL	activities of daily living	日常生活能力量表
ADR	Adverse drug reaction	药物不良反应
AF	atrial fibrillation	心房颤动
AIDS	Acquired immune deficiency syndrome	获得性免疫缺陷综合征
AIMS	Abnormal Involuntary Momement Scale	异常不自主运动量表
ALP	alkaline phosphatase	碱性磷酸酶
ALT	alanine transaminase/aminotransferase	丙氨酸转氨酶
ANC	Absolute neutrophil count	中性粒细胞绝对值
ANNSERS	Antipsychotic Non-Neurological Side-Effects Rating Scale	抗精神病药的非神经系统不良反应量表

APA	American Psychological Association	美国心理学协会
ARB	angiotensin Ⅱ receptor blocker	血管紧张素Ⅱ受体拮抗剂
ASD	autism spectrum disorders	孤独症谱系障碍
ASEX	Arizona Sexual Experience Scale	亚利桑那性体验量表
AST	aspartate aminotransferase	天冬氨酸转氨酶
AUDIT	Alcohol Use Disorders Identification Test	酒精使用障碍筛查测验
BAC	blood alcohol concentration	血液酒精浓度
BAP	British Association for Psychopharmacology	英国精神药理协会
BBB	blood-brain barrier	血-脑屏障
bd	*bis die*(twice a day)	每日两次
BDD	body dysmorphic disorder	躯体变形障碍
BDI	Beck Depression Inventory	贝克抑郁问卷
BDNF	brain-derived neurotrophic factor	脑源性神经营养因子
BED	binge eating disorder	暴食障碍
BEN	benign ethnic neutropenia	良性种族性中性粒细胞减少症
BMI	body mass index	体重指数
BN	bulimia nervosa	神经性厌食
BP	blood pressure	血压
BPD	borderline personality disorder	边缘型人格障碍
BPSD	behavioural and psychological symptoms of dementia	痴呆的行为和心理症状
BuChE	Butyrylcholinesterase	丁酰胆碱酯酶
CAM	Confusion Assessment Method	谵妄评定法
CAMS	Childhood Anxiety Multimodal Study	儿童焦虑多模式研究
CATIE	Clinical Antipsychotic Trials of Intervention Effectiveness	临床抗精神病药干预有效性试验
CBT	cognitive behavioural therapy	认知行为治疗
CBZ	Carbamazepine	卡马西平
CDRS	Children's Depression Rating Scale	儿童抑郁量表
CDT	Carbohydrate-deficient transferrin	缺糖转铁蛋白
CES-D	Center for Epidemiological Studies Depression Scale	流调用抑郁自评量表

CGAS	Children's Global Assessment Scale	儿童总体评定量表
CGI	Clinical Global Impression Scales	临床总体印象量表
CI	confidence interval	置信区间
CIBIC-Plus	Clinician's Interview-Based Impression of Change	基于医师访谈的改变印象
CIGH	clozapine-induced gastrointestinal hypomotility	氯氮平导致的胃肠动力不足
CIWA-Ar	Clinical Institute Withdrawal Assessment of Alcohol scale revised	临床戒断反应评估量表修订版
CK	creatine kinase	肌酸激酶
CKD	chronic kidney disease	慢性肾病
CKD-EPI	Chronic Kidney Disease Epidemiology Collaboration	慢性肾病流行病学合作
CNS	central nervous system	中枢神经系统
COMT	catechol-O-methyltransferase	儿茶酚氧位甲基转移酶
COPD	chronic obstructive pulmonary disease	慢性阻塞性肺疾病
COX	cyclo-oxygenase	环氧化酶
CPK	creatinine phosphokinase	肌酸磷酸激酶
CPP	child-parent psychotherapy	亲子心理治疗
CPSS	Child PTSD Symptom Scale	儿童创伤后应激障碍症状量表
CrCl	creatinine clearance	肌酐清除率
CREB	cAMP response element-binding protein	环磷腺苷反应元件结合蛋白
CRP	C-reactive protein	C 反应蛋白
CT	complementary therapy	辅助疗法
CUtLASS	Cost Utility of the latest Antipsychotic Drugs in Schizophrenia Study	最新抗精神病药在精神分裂症研究中的成本效用
CVA	cerebrovascular accident	脑血管事件
CY-BOCS	Children's Yale-Brown Obsessive Compulsive Scale	儿童耶鲁布朗强迫量表
CYP	cytochrome P	细胞色素 P
DAI	drug attitude inventory	服药态度问卷
DESS	Discontinuation-Emergent Signs and Symptoms scale	停药出现的体征和症状量表

DEXA	dual-energy X-ray absorptiometry	双能 X 线吸收测量法
DHEA	Dehydroepiandrosterone	脱氢表雄酮
DIVA	Diagnostic Interview for DSM-Ⅳ ADHD	DSM-Ⅳ中 ADHD 的诊断性访谈
DLB	dementia with Lewy bodies	路易体痴呆
DMDD	disruptive mood dysregulation disorder	破坏性心境失调障碍
DOAC	direct-acting oral anticoagulant	直接作用的口服抗凝药
DoLS	Depriveation of Liberty Safeguards	约束性保护
DSM	*Diagnostic and Statistical Manual of Mental Disorders*	《精神疾病诊断和统计手册》
DVLA	Drivers and Vehicle Licensing Agency	交通管理局
EAD	early after depolarization	后早期去极化
ECG	Electrocardiogram	心电图
ECT	electroconvulsive therapy	电抽搐治疗
EDTA	ethylenediaminetetraacetic acid	乙二胺四乙酸
EEG	Electroencephalography	脑电图
eGFR	estimated glomerular filtration rate	肾小球滤过率估计值
EMDR	eye movement desensitization and reprocessing	眼动脱敏和再处理
EOSS	early-onset schizophrenia-spectrum	早发精神分裂症谱系障碍
EPA	eicosapentanoic acid	二十碳五烯酸
EPS	extrapyramidal side-effects	锥体外系不良反应
ER	extended release	缓释剂
ERK	extracellular signal-regulated kinase	细胞外信号调节激酶
ERP	exposure and response prevention	暴露反应预防疗法
ES	effect size	效应值
ESR	erythrocyte sedimentation rate	红细胞沉降率
FBC	full blood count	全血细胞计数
FDA	Food and Drug Administration（USA）	食品药品管理局
FGA	first-generation antipsychotics	第一代抗精神病药
FPG	fasting plasma glucose	空腹血糖
FTI	Fatal Toxicity Index	致死性中毒指数
GABA	gamma-aminobutyric acid	γ-氨基丁酸

GASS	Glasgow Antipsychotic Side-effect Scale	格拉斯哥抗精神病药不良反应量表
GBL	gamma-butaryl-lactone	γ- 丁内酯
G-CSF	granulocyte colony-stimulating factor	粒细胞集落刺激因子
GFR	glomerular filtration rate	肾小球滤过率
GGT	gamma-glutamyl transferase	谷氨酰转肽酶
GHB	gamma-hydroxybutyrate	γ- 羟基丁酸
GI	Gastrointestinal	胃肠的
GM-CSF	granulocyte-macrophage colony-stimulating factor	粒 - 巨噬细胞集落刺激因子
GSK3	glycogen synthase kinase 3	糖原合成激酶 3
HADS	Hospital Anxiety and Depression Scale	医院焦虑抑郁量表
HAMA	Hamilton Anxiety Rating Scale	汉密尔顿焦虑量表
HAND	HIV-associated neurocognitive disorders	HIV 相关神经认知障碍
HD	Huntington's disease	亨廷顿病
HDL	high-density lipoprotein	高密度脂蛋白
HDRS	Hamilton Depression Rating Scale	汉密尔顿抑郁量表
HIV	human immune deficiency virus	人类免疫缺陷病毒
5-HMT	5-hydroxy-methyl-tolterodine	5- 羟 - 甲基 - 托特罗定
HPA	hypothalamic-pituitary-adrenal	下丘脑 - 垂体 - 肾上腺
HR	hazard ratio	危险比
IADL	instrumental activities of daily living	工具性日常生活活动
ICD	International Classification of Diseases	国际疾病分类
ICH	intracerebral haemorrhage	脑出血
IFG	impaired fasting glucose	空腹血糖异常
IG	intra-gastric	胃内
IJ	intra-jejunal	空肠内
IM	intramuscular	肌内
IMCA	independent mental capacity advocate	独立精神能力倡导
IMHP	intramuscular high potency	肌内注射高效价
INR	international normalised ratio	国际标准化比值
IR	immediate release	速释剂
IV	intravenous	静脉注射

IVHP	intravenous high potency	静脉注射高效价
Kiddie-SADS	Kiddie-Schedule for Affective Disorders and Schizophrenia	Kiddie 情感障碍和精神分裂症问卷
LAI	long-acting injection	长效针剂
LDL	low-density lipoprotein	低密度脂蛋白
LFTs	liver function tests	肝功能化验
LIGIB	lower gastrointestinal bleeding	下消化道出血
LSD	lysergic acid diethylamide	麦角酸二乙酰胺
MADRS	Montgomery-Asberg Depression Rating Scale	蒙哥马利抑郁量表
mane	Morning	早晨
MAOI	monoamine oxidase inhibitor	单胺氧化酶抑制剂
MARS	Medication Adherence Rating Scale	服药依从性评定量表
MASC	Multidimensional Anxiety Scale for Children	儿科多维焦虑量表
MCA	Mental Capacity Act	心智能力法案
MCI	mild cognitive impairment	轻度认知损害
MDA	3,4-methylynedioxyam-phetamine	3,4- 亚甲二氧基苯丙胺
MDMA	3,4-methylynedioxymetham-phetamine	3,4- 甲基炔二氧基甲胺
MDRD	Modification of Diet in Renal Disease	肾脏疾病饮食调整
MHRA	Medicines and Healthcare Products Regulatory Authority	药物和保健产品管理部门
MI	myocardial infarction	心肌梗死
MMSE	Mini Mental State Examination	简易精神状态检查
MR	modified release	控释剂
MS	mood stabilisers/multiple sclerosis	心境稳定剂 / 多发性硬化
NAS	neonatal abstinence syndrome	新生儿戒断综合征
NICE	National Institute for Health and Clinical Excellence	英国卫生与临床优化研究所
NMDA	N-methyl-D-aspartate	N- 甲基 -D- 天冬氨酸
NMS	neuroleptic malignant syndrome	神经阻滞剂恶性综合征
NNH	number needed to harm	致成伤害需治疗人数

NNT	number needed to treat	需治疗人数
nocte	at night	夜间
NPI	neuropsychiatric inventory	神经精神症状问卷
NRT	nicotine replacement therapy	尼古丁替代治疗
NSAID	non-steroidal anti-inflammatory drug	非甾体抗炎药
NVC	neurovascular coupling	神经血管耦合
OCD	obsessive compulsive disorder	强迫症
od	*omni die*(once a day)	每天 1 次
OD	Overdose	过量
OGTT	oral glucose tolerance test	口服葡萄糖糖耐量试验
OOWS	Objective Opiate Withdrawal Scale	客观阿片类物质戒断量表
OST	opioid substitution treatment	阿片替代治疗
PANDAS	Paediatric Autoimmune Neuropsychiatric Disorder Associated with Streptococcus	链球菌感染相关儿童自身免疫神经精神疾病
PANS	Paediatric Acute-onset Neuropsychiatric Syndrome	儿童急性神经精神综合征
PANSS	Positive and Negative Syndrome Scale	阳性与阴性症状量表
PBA	pseudobulbar affect	假性延髓情绪(强哭强笑症)
PCP	Phencyclidine	苯环己哌啶
PD	Parkinson's disease	帕金森病
PDD	pervasive development disorders	广泛性发育障碍
PDD-NOS	pervasive development disorders-not otherwise specified	广泛性发育障碍,未在他处注明的
P-gp	P-glycoprotein	P- 糖蛋白
PHQ-9	Patient Health Questionnaire-9	患者健康问卷 -9
PICU	psychiatric intensive care unit	精神科重症监护病房
PLC	pathological laughter and crying	病理性笑哭
PLWH	people living with HIV	HIV 病毒感染者
PMR	post-mortem redistribution	死后药物再分布
po	*per os*(by mouth)	口服
POMH-UK	Prescribing Observatory for Mental Health	精神卫生处方监测站

PPH	post-partum haemorrhage	产后出血
PPI	proton pump inhibitor	质子泵抑制剂
prn	*pro re nata*（as required）	按需
PT	prothrombin time	凝血酶原时间
PTSD	post-traumatic stress disorder	创伤后应激障碍
qds	*quarter die sumendum*（four times a day）	每天 4 次
OTc	QT interval adjusted for heart rate	校正后 Q-T 间期
RC	responsible clinician	责任医师
RCADS	Revised Children's Anxiety and Depression Scale	儿童焦虑抑郁量表修订版
RCT	randomised controlled trial	随机对照试验
RID	relative infant dose	相对婴儿剂量
RIMA	reversible inhibitor of monoamine oxidase A	单胺氧化酶 A 可逆性抑制剂
RLAI	risperidone long-acting injection	利培酮长效针剂
ROMI	Rating of Medication Influences scale	药物影响量表
RPG	random plasma glucose	随机血浆葡萄糖
RR	relative risk	相对风险
RRBI	restricted repetitive behaviours and interests	限制性重复行为和兴趣
RT	rapid tranquillisation	快速镇静
RTA	road traffic accident	道路交通事故
rTMS	repetitive transcranial magnetic stimulation	重复经颅磁刺激
RUPP	Research Units on Paediatric Psychopharmacology	儿童精神药理学研究小组
RYGB	Roux-en-Y gastric bypass	鲁克斯恩 -Y 胃旁路术
SADQ	Severity of Alcohol Dependence Questionnaire	酒依赖严重程度问卷
SAWS	Short Alcohol Withdrawal Scale	简明酒精戒断量表
SCARED	Screen for Child Anxiety and Related Emotional Disorders	儿童焦虑及相关情绪障碍筛查表
SCIRS	Severe Cognitive Impairment Rating Scale	严重认知障碍评定量表
SCRA	synthetic cannabinoid receptor agonist	合成大麻素受体激动剂
SGA	second-generation antipsychotics	第二代抗精神病药

SIADH	syndrome of inappropriate antidiuretic hormone	抗利尿激素分泌过多综合征
SIB	severe impairment battery	严重损害成套问卷
SJW	St John's wort	圣约翰草
SLE	systemic lupus erythematosus	系统性红斑狼疮
SNRI	selective noradrenaline reuptake inhibitor	选择性去甲肾上腺素再摄取抑制剂
SOAD	second opinion appointed doctor	第二意见指定医师
SPC	summary of product characteristics	产品特点总结
SPECT	single photon emission computed tomography	单光子发射计算机断层成像术
SROM	slow release oral morphine	口服缓释吗啡
SS	steady state	稳态
SSRI	selective serotonin reuptake inhibitor	选择性 5- 羟色胺再摄取抑制剂
STAR*D	Sequenced Treatment Alternatives to Relieve Depression Study	抑郁症的序贯治疗研究
STS	selegiline transdermal system	司立吉林透皮贴剂
TADS	Treatment of Adolescents with Depression study	青少年抑郁症治疗研究
TCA	tricyclic antidepressant	三环类抗抑郁药
TD	tardive dyskinesia	迟发性运动障碍
tds	ter die sumendum (three times a day)	每天 3 次
TEAM	treatment of early age mania	早发躁狂治疗
TF-CBT	trauma-focused cognitive behavioural therapy	聚焦创伤的认知行为疗法
TFT	thyroid function test	甲状腺功能化验
THC/CBD	tetrahydrocannabinol/cannabidiol	四氢大麻醇 / 大麻二酚
TIA	transient ischaemic attack	短暂性脑缺血发作
TMS	transcranial magnetic stimulation	经颅磁刺激
TORDIA	Treatment of Resistant Depression in Adolescence	青少年难治性抑郁症治疗研究
TPR	temperature, pulse, respiration	体温、脉搏、呼吸
TRS	treatment-resistant schizophrenia	难治性精神分裂症

TS	Tourette's syndrome	抽动秽语综合征
U&Es	urea and electrolytes	尿素和电解质
UGIB	upper gastrointestinal bleeding	上消化道出血
UGT	UDP-glucuronosyl transferase	尿苷二磷酸葡萄糖醛酸转移酶
VaD	vascular dementia	血管性痴呆
VNS	vagal nerve stimulation	迷走神经刺激
VTE	venous thromboembolism	静脉血栓栓塞
WBC	white blood cell	白细胞
WCC	white cell count	白细胞计数
WHO	World Health Organisation	世界卫生组织
XL	extended release	缓释
YMRS	Young Mania Rating Scale	Young 躁狂量表
ZA	zuclopenthixol acetate	醋酸珠氯噻醇

目录

常见精神疾病的药物治疗

精神分裂症及相关精神病性障碍

抗精神病药

引言

抗精神病药分类

20 世纪 90 年代之前,抗精神病药(当时称为强镇静剂)主要根据其化学特性进行分类。第一个抗精神病药氯丙嗪属于吩噻嗪类化合物,由一种三环结构结合一个氮原子和一个硫原子构成。继而陆续开发并上市了其他吩噻嗪类药物,以及化学结构类似的硫杂蒽类药物,如氟哌噻吨。后来,开始根据药理学特征研发出多种不同化学结构的抗精神病药,包括丁酰苯类(氟哌啶醇)、二苯丁基哌啶类(匹莫齐特)和取代的苯甲酰胺类(舒必利和氨磺必利)。

这种根据化学结构分类的方法虽然仍在使用,但已经变得有些多余,因为现有化学单体范围很大,而且新的抗精神病药缺乏清晰的结构-作用相关性。老一代抗精神病药的化学特性与导致运动障碍有关。哌嗪类吩噻嗪(如氟奋乃静、三氟拉嗪)、丁酰苯类和硫杂蒽类最容易引起锥体外系不良反应(extrapyramidal symptoms,EPS),哌啶类吩噻嗪(如哌泊噻嗪)和苯酰胺类导致 EPS 可能性最小,脂肪族吩噻嗪类(如氯丙嗪)和二苯丁基哌啶类(匹莫齐特)则介于两者之间。

药物所致 EPS 相对可能性大小,是最初区分典型/非典型抗精神病药的主要因素。氯氮平早就被视为非典型抗精神病药,因为氯氮平不常导致 EPS,也不能通过动物模型的抗精神病药筛查试验。1990 年氯氮平重新上市,标志着其他不典型抗精神病药开始陆续问世,尽管"不典型"程度各异。其中,可能仅氯氮平和喹硫平最具"非典型"特点,几乎不引起 EPS。其他非典型抗精神病药的作用与剂量相关,但是与不典型抗精神病药不同的是,在产生治疗作用时可能不会出现 EPS。典型与非典型抗精神病药之间真正的区别在于:在批准的剂量范围内容易选择剂量,使其既有效,又不产生 EPS(例如:比较氟哌啶醇与奥氮平)。

在 EPS 易感性中间地带,典型/非典型抗精神病药的二分法不太适用于抗精神病药分类。硫利达嗪在 20 世纪 80 年代被广泛地描述为非典型抗精神病药,但是它属于"传统的"吩噻嗪类化合物。舒必利曾经被当作非典型抗精神病药推销,现在通常被归类为典型抗精神病药。利培酮在最高剂量 16mg/d(美国为 10mg/d)时,几乎就是"典型"抗精神病药。与这些困难相伴的事实是,除对纹状体外 D_2 受体的选择性这个一般而非普遍的发现之外,无论是用药理学还是化学方法,都不能将这些所谓的非典型抗精神病药归纳为一类。与老药相比,非典型抗精神病药的特征,既非提高疗效(氯氮平和一两个其他药物例外),亦非不引起高催乳素血症(利培酮、帕利哌酮和氨磺必利可能比典型抗精神病药更严重)。最后,一些新近推出的药(如匹莫范色林)有抗精神病作用且不易引起 EPS,却与其他抗精神病药在化学、药理学和不良反应方面几乎没有共同点。

为避免上述问题,有研究者将典型与非典型抗精神病药重新分类为第一代抗精神病药(first generation antipsychotics,FGA)和第二代抗精神病药(second generation antipsychotics,SGA)。1990 年之后上市的抗精神病药都归类为 SGA(即所有非典型药物),但这种新的分类命名法免除了与非典型性有关的内涵,不论非典型的含义是什么。然而,FGA/SGA 分类也存在问题,因为它们仅从上市时间来定义两类药物——这几乎是最复杂的药理学分类系统。更为重要的是,上市时间往往与首次合成时间相距甚远。氯氮平是最老的抗精神病药之一(合成于 1959 年),在它还方兴未艾之时,奥氮平就在 1971 年取得了专利。这两种药物当然都是 SGA,而且显然是最现代的抗精神病药。

本版指南保留了 FGA/SGA 分类,但更多的是出于传统,而非特定科学依据。同时,由于大多数人了解哪些药物属于何种类别,故这种分类便于记忆。当然,在选择处方药物或在与患者及照料者讨论时,显然比较合理的方法是考虑具体抗精神病药的特性。考虑到这一点,强烈推荐使用“基于神经科学的命名法(neuroscience-based nomenclature,NbN)”[1],这是一种反映药理学活性的命名系统。

抗精神病药的选择

英国国家卫生与临床优化研究所(National Institute for Health and Clinical Excellence,NICE)用药依从性指南建议[2],患者应该尽可能地参与给其选择处方药物的决策过程,临床医师也应该认识到患者对疾病和药物的观念会影响其治疗依从性。与这种涵盖所有保健服务的一般性建议一致,NICE 精神分裂症指南强调:重要的是患者的选择,而不是推荐一类或一种抗精神病药作为一线治疗[3]。

在精神分裂症和其他精神病性障碍的治疗中,无论急性期还是维持期,抗精神病药都是有效的。不同抗精神病药在药理学、药物代谢、总体疗效/有效性及耐受性方面可能有所不同,但更重要的是在不同的患者之间,其疗效和耐受性会有所不同。这种个体治疗反应的不同,意味着没有任何明确的一线抗精神病药可以适用于所有患者。

相对疗效

继临床抗精神病药治疗干预效果(Clinical Antipsychotic Treatment Intervention Effectiveness,CATIE)[4] 和精神分裂症患者最新抗精神病药使用的成本效用研究(Cost Utility of the Latest Antipsychotic Drugs in Schizophrenia Study,CUtLASS)[5] 的独立发表,世界精神病学协会审查了 51 种 FGA 和 11 种 SGA 相对疗效的证据,得出的结论是:若能(通过仔细调整剂量)使 EPS 最小,并避免使用抗胆碱能药,则没有令人信服的证据支持 SGA 优于 FGA[6]。作为一类药物,SGA 引起 EPS 和迟发性运动障碍(tardive dyskinesia,TD)的可能性较小[7],但是引起代谢方面不良反应的可能性较大,二者在某种程度上相互抵消了。一项荟萃分析发现,对于首次发病的精神病性障碍,FGA 与 SGA 之间的整体疗效差异并不明显,只有奥氮平和氨磺必利显示出少许优势[8]。之后一项针对首次发病的网络荟萃分析发现，奥氮平和氨磺必利具有少许疗效优势，氟哌啶醇的整体表现则较差[9]。

将氯氮平之外的其他第二代抗精神病药进行互相比较时，奥氮平的疗效似乎略优于阿立哌唑、利培酮、喹硫平和齐拉西酮，而利培酮疗效略优于喹硫平和齐拉西酮[10]。以 FGA 为对照的药物试验提示，奥氮平、利培酮和氨磺必利的疗效优于老一代药物[11,12]。一项网络荟萃分析明显证实了这些结果，排序依次为氯氮平、氨磺必利和奥氮平[11]。仅仅这三种药物相对于氟哌啶醇具有明确的疗效优势。这些差异的幅度均很小（但是可能具有实质性差异，因而足以具有临床意义），必须将其与具体抗精神病药之间差异很大的不良反应加以权衡。一项 2019 年发表的网络荟萃分析纳入了 32 种抗精神病药，其中氨磺必利是对阳性症状最有效的药物，而氯氮平对阴性症状和总体症状改善最佳[14]。奥氮平和利培酮对阳性症状的疗效排名也很高。舒必利、氯氮平、氨磺必利、奥氮平和多巴胺受体部分激动剂对抑郁症状的（有利）作用最大，可能反映出这些药物相对缺乏抗精神病药所致的烦躁不安（neuroleptic-induced dysphoria），而大多数 FGA 常常引起这种烦躁不安[15]。较晚上市的药物，其预期疗效往往较差，导致该现象的原因是 1970 年以来安慰剂效应大幅增加[16]。

氯氮平显然是难治性精神分裂症的首选药物[17]，但奇怪的是，这并不是一项普遍的研究发现[18]，可能与许多阳性对照试验的性质和质量有关[19,20]。

第一代和第二代抗精神病药都存在一些不良反应，包括体重增加、脂质代谢异常、高血糖或糖尿病[21,22]、高催乳素血症、股骨颈骨折[23]、性功能异常、EPS（包括恶性综合征）[24]、抗胆碱能作用、静脉血栓栓塞[25]、过度镇静和直立性低血压等。不良反应的确切特点与具体药物有关（见"不良反应"），但是对照研究认为其差异并不明显[26]（参阅对一些不良反应风险排序的大规模荟萃分析[13,27]）。

不良反应是中断治疗的常见原因[28]，特别是在疗效欠佳时[13]。然而，患者并非总是自发报告不良反应[29]；对于不良反应的发生率和重要性，精神科医师的看法和患者的体验迥然不同[30]。系统的询问、体格检查和必要的生化检查，是准确地评估不良反应是否存在、其严重程度或患者自我感受到的严重程度如何的唯一途径。由患者填写的一些清单，如格拉斯哥抗精神病药不良反应评定量表（Glasgow antipsychotics side-effect scale，GASS）[31]，可能是评估过程中有用的第一步。由临床医师填写的抗精神病药非神经系统不良反应量表（Antipsychotic Non-Neurological Side Effects Rating Scale，ANNSERS）有助于更详细地评估[32]。

临床上患者对抗精神病药治疗不依从现象十分常见，此时采用长效制剂以保证药物进入患者体内是绝对有益的。与口服抗精神病药相比，强有力的证据表明，长效制剂与复发和再住院风险降低有关[33-35]。SGA 长效注射剂的问世，在某种程度上改变了人们对长效制剂的印象，后者曾经有时候被看成是对一些患者的惩罚。这些药物在耐受性方面的优势可能与其治疗剂量范围更清晰有部分关系，这意味处方最佳剂量的可能性增大（阿立哌唑被许可的剂量为每月 300mg 或 400mg，相比之下，氟哌噻吨在英国的许可剂量为每 4 周 50mg 至每周 400mg）。氟哌噻吨的最佳剂量大约为每 2 周 40mg[27]，仅为最大许可剂量的 5%。

如前所述，如果在使用两种或以上抗精神病药进行序贯治疗后，患者的症状仍未得到足够的改善，氯氮平将是最有效的治疗[36-38]，NICE 指南也推荐在这种情况下使用氯氮平[3]。对于氯氮平的这种疗效优势，其生物学基础尚不清楚[39]。奥氮平可能是使用氯氮平之前应该使用的两种抗精神病药之一[10,40]。氨磺必利可能也值得一试：它在荟萃分析中的排名很高，一项试验发现继续使用氨磺必利与换用奥氮平效果相当[41]。这项试验也提示氯氮平可能最好作为第二种药物来使用,因为与继续使用首次处方的药物相比,换用其他药物并没有益处。

　　本章涵盖了精神分裂症的抗精神病药治疗、抗精神病药相关不良反应的特点以及如何应对不良反应。

参考文献

1. Zohar J, et al. A review of the current nomenclature for psychotropic agents and an introduction to the Neuroscience-based Nomenclature. *Eur Neuropsychopharmacol* 2015; 25:2318–2325.

2. National Institute for Clinical Excellence. Medicines adherence: involving patients in decisions about prescribed medicines and supporting adherence. Clinical Guidance [CG76]. 2009 (last checked March 2019); https://www.nice.org.uk/Guidance/CG76.

3. National Institute for Health and Care Excellence. Psychosis and schizophrenia in adults: prevention and management. Clinical Guidance [CG178]. 2014 (last checked March 2019); https://www.nice.org.uk/guidance/cg178.

4. Lieberman JA, et al. Effectiveness of antipsychotic drugs in patients with chronic schizophrenia. *N Engl J Med* 2005; 353:1209–1223.

5. Jones PB, et al. Randomized controlled trial of the effect on Quality of Life of second- vs first-generation antipsychotic drugs in schizophrenia: Cost Utility of the Latest Antipsychotic Drugs in Schizophrenia Study (CUtLASS 1). *Arch Gen Psychiatry* 2006; 63:1079–1087.

6. Tandon R, et al. World Psychiatric Association Pharmacopsychiatry Section statement on comparative effectiveness of antipsychotics in the treatment of schizophrenia. *Schizophr Res* 2008; 100:20–38.

7. Tarsy D, et al. Epidemiology of tardive dyskinesia before and during the era of modern antipsychotic drugs. *Handb Clin Neurol* 2011; 100:601–616.

8. Zhang JP, et al. Efficacy and safety of individual second-generation vs. first-generation antipsychotics in first-episode psychosis: a systematic review and meta-analysis. *Int J Neuro Psychopharmacol* 2013; 16:1205–1218.

9. Zhu Y, et al. Antipsychotic drugs for the acute treatment of patients with a first episode of schizophrenia: a systematic review with pairwise and network meta-analyses. *Lancet Psychiatry* 2017; 4:694–705.

10. Leucht S, et al. A meta-analysis of head-to-head comparisons of second-generation antipsychotics in the treatment of schizophrenia. *Am J Psychiatry* 2009; 166:152–163.

11. Davis JM, et al. A meta-analysis of the efficacy of second-generation antipsychotics. *Arch Gen Psychiatry* 2003; 60:553–564.

12. Leucht S, et al. Second-generation versus first-generation antipsychotic drugs for schizophrenia: a meta-analysis. *Lancet* 2009; 373:31–41.

13. Leucht S, et al. Comparative efficacy and tolerability of 15 antipsychotic drugs in schizophrenia: a multiple-treatments meta-analysis. *Lancet* 2013; 382:951–962.

14. Huhn M, et al. Comparative efficacy and tolerability of 32 oral antipsychotics for the acute treatment of adults with multi-episode schizophrenia: a systematic review and network meta-analysis. *Lancet* 2019; 394:939–951.

15. Voruganti L, et al. Neuroleptic dysphoria: towards a new synthesis. *Psychopharmacology* 2004; 171:121–132.

16. Leucht S, et al. Sixty years of placebo-controlled antipsychotic drug trials in acute schizophrenia: systematic review, Bayesian meta-analysis, and meta-regression of efficacy predictors. *Am J Psychiatry* 2017; 174:927–942.

17. Siskind D, et al. Clozapine v. first- and second-generation antipsychotics in treatment-refractory schizophrenia: systematic review and meta-analysis. *Br J Psychiatry* 2016; 209:385–392.

18. Samara MT, et al. Efficacy, acceptability, and tolerability of antipsychotics in treatment-resistant schizophrenia: a network meta-analysis. *JAMA Psychiatry* 2016; 73:199–210.

19. Taylor DM. Clozapine for treatment-resistant schizophrenia: still the gold standard? *CNS Drugs* 2017; 31:177–180.

20. Kane JM, et al. The role of clozapine in treatment-resistant schizophrenia. *JAMA Psychiatry* 2016; 73:187–188.

21. Manu P, et al. Prediabetes in patients treated with antipsychotic drugs. *J Clin Psychiatry* 2012; 73:460–466.

22. Rummel-Kluge C, et al. Head-to-head comparisons of metabolic side effects of second generation antipsychotics in the treatment of schizophrenia: a systematic review and meta-analysis. *Schizophr Res* 2010; 123:225–233.

23. Sorensen HJ, et al. Schizophrenia, antipsychotics and risk of hip fracture: a population-based analysis. *Eur Neuro Psychopharmacol* 2013; 23:872–878.

24. Trollor JN, et al. Comparison of neuroleptic malignant syndrome induced by first- and second-generation antipsychotics. *Br J Psychiatry* 2012; 201:52–56.

25. Masopust J, et al. Risk of venous thromboembolism during treatment with antipsychotic agents. *Psychiatry Clin Neurosci* 2012; 66:541–552.

26. Pope A, et al. Assessment of adverse effects in clinical studies of antipsychotic medication: survey of methods used. *Br J Psychiatry* 2010; 197:67–72.

27. Bailey L, et al. Estimating the optimal dose of flupentixol decanoate in the maintenance treatment of schizophrenia-a systematic review of the literature. *Psychopharmacology* 2019; 236:3081–3092.

28. Falkai P. Limitations of current therapies: why do patients switch therapies? *Eur Neuropsychopharmacol* 2008; 18 Suppl 3:S135–S139.

29. Yusufi B, et al. Prevalence and nature of side effects during clozapine maintenance treatment and the relationship with clozapine dose and plasma concentration. *Int Clin Psychopharmacol* 2007; 22:238–243.

30. Day JC, et al. A comparison of patients' and prescribers' beliefs about neuroleptic side-effects: prevalence, distress and causation. *Acta Psychiatr Scand* 1998; 97:93–97.

31. Waddell L, et al. A new self-rating scale for detecting atypical or second-generation antipsychotic side effects. *J Psychopharmacology* 2008; 22:238–243.

32. Ohlsen RI, et al. Interrater reliability of the Antipsychotic Non-Neurological Side-Effects Rating Scale measured in patients treated with clozapine. *J Psychopharmacol* 2008; 22:323–329.

33. Tiihonen J, et al. Effectiveness of antipsychotic treatments in a nationwide cohort of patients in community care after first hospitalisation due to schizophrenia and schizoaffective disorder: observational follow-up study. *BMJ* 2006; 333:224.

34. Leucht C, et al. Oral versus depot antipsychotic drugs for schizophrenia–a critical systematic review and meta-analysis of randomised long-term trials. *Schizophr Res* 2011; 127:83–92.

35. Leucht S, et al. Antipsychotic drugs versus placebo for relapse prevention in schizophrenia: a systematic review and meta-analysis. *Lancet* 2012; 379:2063–2071.

36. Kane J, et al. Clozapine for the treatment-resistant schizophrenic. A double-blind comparison with chlorpromazine. *Arch Gen Psychiatry* 1988; 45:789–796.

37. McEvoy JP, et al. Effectiveness of clozapine versus olanzapine, quetiapine, and risperidone in patients with chronic schizophrenia who did not respond to prior atypical antipsychotic treatment. *Am J Psychiatry* 2006; 163:600–610.

38. Lewis SW, et al. Randomized controlled trial of effect of prescription of clozapine versus other second-generation antipsychotic drugs in resistant schizophrenia. *Schizophr Bull* 2006; 32:715–723.

39. Stone JM, et al. Review: the biological basis of antipsychotic response in schizophrenia. *J Psychopharmacology* 2010; 24:953–964.

40. Agid O, et al. An algorithm-based approach to first-episode schizophrenia: response rates over 3 prospective antipsychotic trials with a retrospective data analysis. *J Clin Psychiatry* 2011; 72:1439–1444.

41. Kahn RS, et al. Amisulpride and olanzapine followed by open-label treatment with clozapine in first-episode schizophrenia and schizophreniform disorder (OPTiMiSE): a three-phase switching study. *Lancet Psychiatry* 2018; 5:797–807.

一般处方原则

- 应使用**尽可能低**的剂量。每个患者应逐渐加至已知的最低有效剂量(见本章"最低有效剂量");只有经过 1~2 周评估患者疗效差或无效,才应加大剂量。(越来越多的证据表明,治疗 2 周无效是未来预后不良的有力预测因素,除非改变剂量或药物。)

- 定期使用**长效注射剂**时,即使不改变剂量,血浆药物浓度也至少会在起始治疗后 6~12 周内升高(见本章"长效制剂的药代动力学")。因此,在这段时间内增加剂量难以进行评估。首选的方法是先确定疗效和耐受性良好的口服药物剂量,然后给予该药物长效制剂的等效剂量。如果这种方法无法实现,应当使用临床试验确定的最佳剂量作为个体治疗的目标剂量(虽然这一数据在老一代抗精神病药长效制剂中不一定可得)。

- 建议给绝大多数患者使用**一种**抗精神病药(合用或不合用心境稳定剂或镇静剂)。除了某些特殊情况(如氯氮平增效治疗),应避免多种抗精神病药的合用,因为这可能会增加不良反应发生的负担,提高 Q-T 间期延长和心源性猝死的风险(见本章"合并抗精神病药")。

- 抗精神病药的**合用**,仅在一种抗精神病药(包括氯氮平)治疗后疗效欠佳时,才应该考虑。在这种情况下,应仔细评估、记录联合治疗对靶症状的效果和不良反应。如果没有明确的益处,还应转至单一抗精神病药治疗。

- 一般而言,**抗精神病药不应作为镇静剂临时使用**。建议可短期服用苯二氮䓬类药物或一般镇静剂(如异丙嗪)(见本章"快速镇静")。

- 患者对抗精神病药治疗的反应,应采用**经过验证的量表进行评定**,并记录于病案中。

- 接受抗精神病药治疗者,应**密切监测其躯体情况**(包括血压、脉搏、心电图、血糖和血脂)(见本章相应各节)。

- 若要停用抗精神病药,应以双曲线减量方案缓慢减少剂量,以减少撤药反应及疾病反弹的风险。

注:本节未标注参考文献。详细的参考文献及指南见本章对应小节。

最低有效剂量

　　表 1.1 列出了常用抗精神病药治疗首发或复发精神分裂症时可能有效的最低剂量。所推荐的剂量至少对部分患者有效,但是其他患者可能需要更高的剂量。鉴于疗效存在个体差异,全部剂量均应视为大致数值。本章既提供原始文献,也采纳专家共识。本表只包含常用口服抗精神病药。

表 1.1　抗精神病药的最低有效日剂量

药物	首发	复发
第一代抗精神病药		
氯丙嗪[1]	200mg*	300mg
氟哌啶醇[2–7]	2mg	4mg
舒必利[8]	400mg*	800mg
三氟拉嗪[9,10]	10mg*	15mg
第二代抗精神病药		
氨磺必利[11–16]	300mg*	400mg*
阿立哌唑[7,17–22]	10mg	10mg
阿塞那平[7,22,23]	10mg*	10mg
布南色林[24]	未知	8mg
依匹哌唑[25–27]	2mg*	4mg
卡利拉嗪[28,29]	1.5mg*	1.5mg
伊潘立酮[7,21,22,30]	4mg*	8mg
卢美哌隆[31]	未知	42mg*
鲁拉西酮[7,32]	40mg(盐酸)/37mg(基本分子)*	40mg(盐酸)/37mg(基本分子)*
奥氮平[4,7,33–35]	5mg	7.5mg
帕利哌酮[22]	3mg*	3mg
匹莫范色林[36–38]	未知	34mg**
喹硫平[39–44]	150mg(但常用更高剂量[45])	300mg
利培酮[3,7,46–49]	2mg	4mg
齐拉西酮[7,21,50–52]	40mg*	80mg

* 为估计值,现有数据过少。

** FDA 批准可用于帕金森病所致精神病;用于精神分裂症剂量未知。

参考文献

1. Dudley K, et al. Chlorpromazine dose for people with schizophrenia. *Cochrane Database Syst Rev* 2017; 4:Cd007778.

2. McGorry PD. Recommended haloperidol and risperidone doses in first-episode psychosis. *J Clin Psychiatry* 1999; 60:794–795.

3. Schooler N, et al. Risperidone and haloperidol in first-episode psychosis: a long-term randomized trial. *Am J Psychiatry* 2005; **162**:947–953.

4. Keefe RS, et al. Long-term neurocognitive effects of olanzapine or low-dose haloperidol in first-episode psychosis. *Biol Psychiatry* 2006; 59:97–105.

5. Donnelly L, et al. Haloperidol dose for the acute phase of schizophrenia. *Cochrane Database Syst Rev* 2013; Cd001951.

6. Oosthuizen P, et al. A randomized, controlled comparison of the efficacy and tolerability of low and high doses of haloperidol in the treatment of first-episode psychosis. *Int J Neuropsychopharmacol* 2004; 7:125–131.

7. Leucht S, et al. Dose equivalents for second-generation antipsychotics: the minimum effective dose method. *SchizophrBull* 2014; 40:314–326.

8. Soares BG, et al. Sulpiride for schizophrenia. *Cochrane Database Syst Rev* 2000; CD001162.

9. Armenteros JL, et al. Antipsychotics in early onset schizophrenia: systematic review and meta-analysis. *Eur Child Adolesc Psychiatry* 2006; 15:141–148.

10. Koch K, et al. Trifluoperazine versus placebo for schizophrenia. *Cochrane Database Syst Rev* 2014; Cd010226.

11. Mota NE, et al. Amisulpride for schizophrenia. *Cochrane Database Syst Rev* 2002; CD001357.

12. Puech A, et al. Amisulpride, and atypical antipsychotic, in the treatment of acute episodes of schizophrenia: a dose-ranging study vs. haloperidol. The Amisulpride Study Group. *Acta Psychiatr Scand* 1998; 98:65–72.

13. Moller HJ, et al. Improvement of acute exacerbations of schizophrenia with amisulpride: a comparison with haloperidol. PROD-ASLP Study Group. *Psychopharmacology* 1997; 132:396–401.

14. Sparshatt A, et al. Amisulpride – dose, plasma concentration, occupancy and response: implications for therapeutic drug monitoring. *Acta Psychiatr Scand* 2009; 120:416–428.

15. Buchanan RW, et al. The 2009 schizophrenia PORT psychopharmacological treatment recommendations and summary statements. *SchizophrBull* 2010; 36:71–93.

16. Galletly C, et al. Royal Australian and New Zealand College of Psychiatrists clinical practice guidelines for the management of schizophrenia and related disorders. *Aust N Z J Psychiatry* 2016; 50:410–472.

17. Taylor D. Aripiprazole: a review of its pharmacology and clinical utility. *Int J Clin Pract* 2003; 57:49–54.

18. Cutler AJ, et al. The efficacy and safety of lower doses of aripiprazole for the treatment of patients with acute exacerbation of schizophrenia. *CNS Spectr* 2006; 11:691–702.

19. Mace S, et al. Aripiprazole: dose-response relationship in schizophrenia and schizoaffective disorder. *CNS Drugs* 2008; 23:773–780.

20. Sparshatt A, et al. A systematic review of aripiprazole – dose, plasma concentration, receptor occupancy and response: implications for therapeutic drug monitoring. *J Clin Psychiatry* 2010; 71:1447–1456.

21. Liu CC, et al. Aripiprazole for drug-naive or antipsychotic-short-exposure subjects with ultra-high risk state and first-episode psychosis: an open-label study. *J Clin Psychopharmacol* 2013; 33:18–23.

22. Leucht S, et al. Dose-response meta-analysis of antipsychotic drugs for acute schizophrenia. *Am J Psychiatry* 2020; 177:342–353.

23. Citrome L. Role of sublingual asenapine in treatment of schizophrenia. *Neuropsychiatr Dis Treat* 2011; 7:325–339.

24. Tenjin T, et al. Profile of blonanserin for the treatment of schizophrenia. *Neuropsychiatr Dis Treat* 2013; 9:587–594.

25. Correll CU, et al. Efficacy of brexpiprazole in patients with acute schizophrenia: review of three randomized, double-blind, placebo-controlled studies. *Schizophr Res* 2016; 174:82–92.

26. Malla A, et al. The effect of brexpiprazole in adult outpatients with early-episode schizophrenia: an exploratory study. *Int Clin Psychopharmacol* 2016; 31:307–314.

27. Kane JM, et al. A multicenter, randomized, double-blind, controlled phase 3 trial of fixed-dose brexpiprazole for the treatment of adults with acute schizophrenia. *Schizophr Res* 2015; 164:127–135.

28. Garnock-Jones KP. Cariprazine: a review in schizophrenia. *CNS Drugs* 2017; 31:513–525.

29. Citrome L. Cariprazine for acute and maintenance treatment of adults with schizophrenia: an evidence-based review and place in therapy. *Neuropsychiatr Dis Treat* 2018; 14:2563–2577.

30. Crabtree BL, et al. Iloperidone for the management of adults with schizophrenia. *Clin Ther* 2011; 33:330–345.

31. Correll CU, et al. Efficacy and safety of lumateperone for treatment of schizophrenia: a randomized clinical trial. *JAMA Psychiatry* 2020; 77:349–358.

32. Meltzer HY, et al. Lurasidone in the treatment of schizophrenia: a randomized, double-blind, placebo- and olanzapine-controlled study. *Am J Psychiatry* 2011; 168:957–967.

33. Sanger TM, et al. Olanzapine versus haloperidol treatment in first-episode psychosis. *Am J Psychiatry* 1999; 156:79–87.

34. Kasper S. Risperidone and olanzapine: optimal dosing for efficacy and tolerability in patients with schizophrenia. *Int Clin Psychopharmacol* 1998; 13:253–262.

35. Bishara D, et al. Olanzapine: a systematic review and meta-regression of the relationships between dose, plasma concentration, receptor occupancy, and response. *JClinPsychopharmacol* 2013; 33:329–335.

36. Mathis MV, et al. The US Food and Drug Administration's Perspective on the New Antipsychotic Pimavanserin. *J Clin Psychiatry* 2017; 78:e668–e673.

37. Ballard C, et al. Pimavanserin in Alzheimer's Disease Psychosis: efficacy in patients with more pronounced psychotic symptoms. *J Prev Alzheimers Dis* 2019; 6:27–33.

38. Nasrallah HA, et al. Successful treatment of clozapine-nonresponsive refractory hallucinations and delusions with pimavanserin, a serotonin 5HT-2A receptor inverse agonist. *Schizophr Res* 2019; 208:217–220.

39. Small S, et al. Quetiapine in patients with schizophrenia. A high- and low-dose double-blind comparison with placebo. Seroquel Study Group. *Arch Gen Psychiatry* 1997; 54:549–557.

40. Peuskens J, et al. A comparison of quetiapine and chlorpromazine in the treatment of schizophrenia. *Acta Psychiatr Scand* 1997; 96:265–273.

41. Arvanitis LA, et al. Multiple fixed doses of 'Seroquel' (quetiapine) in patients with acute exacerbation of schizophrenia: a comparison with haloperidol and placebo. *Biol Psychiatry* 1997; 42:233–246.

42. Kopala LC, et al. Treatment of a first episode of psychotic illness with quetiapine: an analysis of 2 year outcomes. *Schizophr Res* 2006; 81:29–39.

43. Sparshatt A, et al. Quetiapine: dose-response relationship in schizophrenia. *CNS Drugs* 2008; 22:49–68.

44. Sparshatt A, et al. Relationship between daily dose, plasma concentrations, dopamine receptor occupancy, and clinical response to quetiapine: a review. *J Clin Psychiatry* 2011; 72:1108–1123.

45. Pagsberg AK, et al. Quetiapine extended release versus aripiprazole in children and adolescents with first-episode psychosis: the multicentre, double-blind, randomised tolerability and efficacy of antipsychotics (TEA) trial. *Lancet Psychiatry* 2017; 4:605–618.

46. Lane HY, et al. Risperidone in acutely exacerbated schizophrenia: dosing strategies and plasma levels. *J Clin Psychiatry* 2000; 61:209–214.

47. Williams R. Optimal dosing with risperidone: updated recommendations. *J Clin Psychiatry* 2001; 62:282–289.

48. Ezewuzie N, et al. Establishing a dose-response relationship for oral risperidone in relapsed schizophrenia. *J Psychopharm* 2006; 20:86–90.

49. Li C, et al. Risperidone dose for schizophrenia. *Cochrane Database Syst Rev* 2009; Cd007474.

50. Bagnall A, et al. Ziprasidone for schizophrenia and severe mental illness. *Cochrane Database Syst Rev* 2000; CD001945.

51. Taylor D. Ziprasidone – an atypical antipsychotic. *Pharm J* 2001; 266:396–401.

52. Joyce AT, et al. Effect of initial ziprasidone dose on length of therapy in schizophrenia. *Schizophr Res* 2006; 83:285–292.

最大批准剂量

下表列出了欧盟批准的抗精神病药最大剂量,其依据是截至 2021 年 2 月的欧洲药品管理局药品说明书。

药物	最大剂量
第一代抗精神病药口服制剂	
氯丙嗪	1 000mg/d
氟哌噻吨	18mg/d
氟哌啶醇	20mg/d
左美丙嗪	1 200mg/d
哌氰嗪	300mg/d
奋乃静	24mg/d(64mg/d 用于住院患者)
匹莫齐特	20mg/d
舒必利	2 400mg/d
三氟拉嗪	20mg/d
珠氯噻醇	150mg/d
第二代抗精神病药口服制剂	
氨磺必利	1 200mg/d
阿立哌唑	30mg/d
阿塞那平	20mg/d(舌下)
卡利拉嗪	6mg/d
氯氮平	900mg/d
鲁拉西酮	160mg/d(盐酸)/148mg/d(基本分子)
奥氮平	20mg/d
帕利哌酮	12mg/d
喹硫平	750mg/d 用于精神分裂症(缓释剂 800mg/d)
	800mg/d 用于双相障碍
利培酮	16mg/d
舍吲哚	24mg/d
长效制剂	
阿立哌唑	400mg/m
氟哌噻吨	400mg/w
氟奋乃静	100mg,每 14~35 天 1 次
氟哌啶醇	300mg/4w
帕利哌酮(1 个月剂型)	150mg/m
帕利哌酮(3 个月剂型)	525mg/3m
哌泊噻嗪	200mg/4w
利培酮(杨森)	50mg/2w
珠氯噻醇	600mg/w

　　下表列出了截至 2021 年 2 月欧盟地区以外批准的抗精神病药最大剂量，其依据是美国 FDA 药品说明书。

药物	最大剂量
第二代抗精神病药口服制剂	
布南色林 *	24mg/d 口服 [1]（80mg/d 贴片）[2]
依匹哌唑	4mg/d
伊潘立酮	24mg/d
卢美哌隆	42mg/d
吗茚酮	225mg/d
匹莫范色林	34mg/d
RBP-7000（利培酮 1 个月剂型）	120mg/m
齐拉西酮	160mg/d

＊本书编写时仅在中国、日本和韩国上市。d, day, 日；m, month, 月。

参考文献

1. Inoue Y, et al. Safety and effectiveness of oral blonanserin for schizophrenia: a review of Japanese post-marketing surveillances. *J Pharmacol Sci* 2021; 145:42–51.

2. Nishibe H, et al. Striatal dopamine D2 receptor occupancy induced by daily application of blonanserin transdermal patches: phase 2 study in Japanese patients with schizophrenia. *Int J Neuropsychopharmacol* 2020; 24:108–117.

等效剂量

在不同的第一代抗精神病药之间转换时,等效剂量的知识是有用的。将不同的药物转化成"神经阻滞剂"或"氯丙嗪"的等效剂量估计值(以 mg/d 为单位),其依据来自临床经验、专家组意见(通过不同的方式)和多巴胺结合力研究。

表 1.2 列出了第一代抗精神病药的大致等效剂量[1-4]。从一种 FGA 换成另一种 FGA 时,这些数值只能提供粗略的指导,不能替代临床上根据不良反应和疗效对新药进行的剂量滴定。

表 1.2 第一代抗精神病药的等效剂量

药物	等效剂量(共识)	研究文献中数值范围
氯丙嗪	100mg/d	参考值
氟哌噻吨	3mg/d	2~3mg/d
氟哌噻吨长效制剂	10mg/w	10~20mg/w
氟奋乃静	2mg/d	1~5mg/d
氟奋乃静长效制剂	5mg/w	1~12.5mg/w
氟哌啶醇	2mg/d	1.5~5mg/d
氟哌啶醇长效制剂	15mg/w	5~25mg/w
哌氰嗪	10mg/d	10mg/d
奋乃静	10mg/d	5~10mg/d
匹莫齐特	2mg/d	1.33~2mg/d
哌泊噻嗪长效制剂	10mg/w	10~12.5mg/w
舒必利	200mg/d	133~300mg/d
三氟拉嗪	5mg/d	2.5~5mg/d
珠氯噻醇	25mg/d	25~60mg/d
珠氯噻醇长效制剂	100mg/w	40~100mg/w

d,day,日;W,Week,周。

SGA 等效剂量的临床意义可能差一些,因为它们往往有更准确的、基于证据的批准剂量范围。有几种不同的计算等效剂量的方法,如基于限定日剂量[5],基于最小有效剂量[6,7],或基于平均剂量[8]。这些方法可计算出不同的等效剂量估计值。表 1.3 列出了 SGA 等效剂量的粗略指导[3,4,7-9]。至于确切的等效剂量,存在相当大的分歧,即使此处所引参考文献也如此。氯氮平未纳入其中,因为它具有独特的起始剂量滴定方法,较高的剂量-血浆浓度变异性,以及可能具有独特的作用机制。

在等效剂量方面,FGA 和 SGA 的效能比较具有更大的不确定性。100mg 氯丙嗪可以非常粗略地等效于 1.5mg 利培酮[3]。

表 1.3　第二代抗精神病药的大致等效剂量[3-10]

药物	大致等效剂量
氨磺必利	400mg
阿立哌唑	15mg
阿塞那平	10mg
布南色林	~
依匹哌唑	2mg
卡利拉嗪	1.5mg
氯噻平	100mg
伊潘立酮	12mg
卢美哌隆	~
鲁拉西酮	80mg（74mg 基本分子）
美哌隆	300mg
吗茚酮	50mg
奥氮平	10mg
帕利哌酮长效制剂	100mg/m
匹莫范色林	~
喹硫平	400mg
利培酮口服制剂	4mg
利培酮长效制剂	50mg/2w
利培酮 RBP-7000	120mg/m
齐拉西酮	80mg

~ 表示本书编写时尚不清楚等效剂量。

W，Week，周；m，month，月。

参考文献

1. Foster P. Neuroleptic equivalence. *Pharm J* 1989; **243**:431–432.
2. Atkins M, et al. Chlorpromazine equivalents: a consensus of opinion for both clinical and research implications. *Psychiatric Bull* 1997; **21**:224–226.
3. Patel MX, et al. How to compare doses of different antipsychotics: a systematic review of methods. *Schizophr Res* 2013; **149**:141–148.
4. Gardner DM, et al. International consensus study of antipsychotic dosing. *Am J Psychiatry* 2010; **167**:686–693.
5. Leucht S, et al. Dose equivalents for antipsychotic drugs: the ddd method. *Schizophr Bull* 2016; **42 Suppl 1**:S90–S94.
6. Rothe PH, et al. Dose equivalents for second generation long-acting injectable antipsychotics: the minimum effective dose method. *Schizophr Res* 2018; **193**:23–28.
7. Leucht S, et al. Dose equivalents for second-generation antipsychotics: the minimum effective dose method. *Schizophr Bull* 2014; **40**:314–326.
8. Leucht S, et al. Dose equivalents for second-generation antipsychotic drugs: the classical mean dose method. *Schizophr Bull* 2015; **41**:1397–1402.
9. Woods SW. Chlorpromazine equivalent doses for the newer atypical antipsychotics. *J Clin Psychiatry* 2003; **64**:663–667.
10. Leucht S, et al. Dose-response meta-analysis of antipsychotic drugs for acute schizophrenia. *Am J Psychiatry* 2020; **177**:342–353.

大剂量抗精神病药：处方与监测

"大剂量"抗精神病药处方存在以下两种情况：①单一抗精神病药的剂量超出推荐的最大剂量；②两种或以上的抗精神病药合用，分别计算每种抗精神病药占最大推荐剂量的百分比，累计值大于100%[1]。在临床实践中，抗精神病药联用及按需(必要时使用)处方与大剂量处方密切相关[2,3]。

疗效

目前，尚无明确的证据表明大剂量的抗精神病药比标准剂量对于精神分裂症更为有效。在使用抗精神病药进行快速镇静、预防复发、控制持续攻击行为和处理急性精神病发作时也是如此[1]。即便如此，在英国也有1/4~1/3的住院患者接受了大剂量抗精神病药治疗。2013年，英国对精神分裂症处方审查时发现，在以社区治疗为主的5 000多例患者中，10%的患者服用了大剂量的抗精神病药[4]。

对各种抗精神病药的剂量-效应进行研究发现，剂量超出产品说明书剂量上限时，并不能增加疗效[5,6]。相对低的剂量反而能带来最佳疗效：利培酮4mg/d[7]，喹硫平300mg/d[8]，奥氮平10mg/d[9,10]，等等。类似地，利培酮长效制剂100mg/2w的疗效并不优于50mg/2w[11]，齐拉西酮320mg/d并不优于160mg/d[12]。目前，所有临床使用的抗精神病药(可能除了氯氮平)，其抗精神病作用主要通过对突触后DA受体的拮抗作用(或部分激动作用)产生。越来越多的证据表明，精神分裂症患者的难治性症状并不能用DA通路机制异常来解释[13-16]。因此，对这些患者，增强对DA的阻断不一定有效。同样重要的，质量作用定律表明，达到药效阈值后再增加剂量，多巴胺受体的结合率上升得很少[17]。

Dold等进行了一项荟萃分析，纳入的RCT研究针对标准剂量抗精神病药治疗无效的精神分裂症患者，比较了继续使用该药物的标准剂量或增加剂量的效果。没有证据表明增加剂量可以带来任何收益[18]。有少数随机对照试验比较了大剂量与标准剂量抗精神病药治疗难治性精神分裂症的疗效[1]。其中有些研究认为大剂量时疗效更好[19]，但是这些研究大多做得较早，随机入组患者数较少，研究设计不符合现行标准。一些研究使用的日剂量相当于氯丙嗪10g/d以上。

一项针对首发精神分裂症患者的研究发现，对标准剂量治疗无反应的患者，药物加量至奥氮平30mg/d或利培酮10mg/d，总有效率仅增加4%。相比之下，换用其他抗精神病药(包括氯氮平)时，治疗要成功得多[20]。在一项小样本($n=12$)开放研究中，将喹硫平加量至1 400mg/d，仅1/3的患者获得有限的改善[21]，但其他更大样本的研究则发现大剂量喹硫平并不能增加疗效[8,22,23]。还有一项小样本($n=40$)的随机对照试验，采用大剂量奥氮平(最高45mg/d)与氯氮平进行比较，发现二者对难治性精神分裂症疗效相近；但由于研究所用的样本量较小，尚不能得出二者等效的结论[24]。一篇纳入相关研究的系统综述比较了对于难治性精神分裂症，氯氮平与高于标准剂量的奥氮平的疗效，发现奥氮平(尤其更高剂量)可能是氯氮平治疗的替代品，但氯氮平在疗效上仍然有最有力的证据[25]。

最近对剂量反应的系统分析在很大程度上证实了，所有药物在达到一定剂量以后，其剂量-反应曲线都会达到一个平台[26](奥氮平和鲁拉西酮可能例外，有证据表明这两种药物在许可剂量范围内,较高剂量的疗效某种程度上要好于较低剂量[10,27])。这篇系统综述同时也提示,超过一定剂量可能无法带来额外收益,而这一剂量比前述的剂量要更高,比如利培酮6.3mg/d,喹硫平482mg/d。但重要的是,没有证据支持超许可剂量使用任何药物。

不良反应

抗精神病药治疗中的不良反应大都是剂量相关的,包括 EPS、镇静、直立性低血压、抗胆碱能作用、Q-T 间期延长和因冠心病死亡[28-31]。高剂量抗精神病药治疗明显增加不良反应负担[12,23,28,32,33]。有一些证据表明,当抗精神病药日剂量从非常高(平均氯丙嗪等效剂量2 253mg/d)降至高剂量(平均氯丙嗪等效剂量 1 315mg/d)时,患者的认知和阴性症状均获得改善[34]。

建议

- 大剂量抗精神病药的使用应作为临床实践中的特殊情况,只有经过抗精神病药(包括氯氮平)标准剂量的充分治疗仍无效时,才予以使用。
- 如果处方了大剂量抗精神病药,最好采用经过验证的量表记录目标症状、疗效和不良反应,将其作为标准化实践,以便不断地考量患者治疗中的风险-获益比。密切的躯体情况监测(包括心电图)十分必要。

大剂量抗精神病药的处方流程

在使用大剂量抗精神病药之前,先确定以下因素:
- 已有足够的时间观察疗效(见"起效时间")。
- 至少先后用过两种不同的抗精神病药(如果条件允许,包含奥氮平)。
- 氯氮平无效,或因粒细胞缺乏症或其他严重不良反应而不能耐受。其他不良反应大多能够处理。小部分患者可能会直接拒绝使用氯氮平。
- 患者的治疗依从性应该不存在疑问(监测血药浓度、口服液或分散片、长效制剂等)。
- 不适合使用其他药物,如抗抑郁药或心境稳定剂。
- 心理治疗无效或不适合应用。

使用大剂量抗精神病药的决定权
- 由资深精神科医师做决定。
- 应包括多学科团队。
- 若可能,获得患者的知情同意。

决策程序

- 首先应排除禁忌证（如心电图异常、肝脏损害等）。
- 应考虑及尽量减少合用药物的风险（如可能引起 Q-T 间期延长、电解质紊乱或与细胞色素酶抑制相关的药代相互作用）。
- 在病案中记录使用大剂量抗精神病药的决定，并描述相关的靶症状。建议使用合适的量表。
- 每次增加剂量之后，应等待充分的时间以观察疗效，然后再考虑是否进一步增加剂量。

治疗中的监测

- 应该按照本章"监测"部分中的内容监测躯体情况。
- 所有接受大剂量抗精神病药治疗的患者，均应定期检查心电图（基线，每次增加剂量后达到稳态血浆水平时，然后每 6~12 个月监测 1 次）。若后来合用的药物已知可能引起电解质紊乱或 Q-T 间期延长，应额外增加生化项目或心电图检查。
- 应在 6 周和 3 个月后评定目标症状。若这些症状未充分改善，药物剂量应减至正常范围。

参考文献

1. Royal College of Psychiatrists. Consensus statement on high-dose antipsychotic medication. College Report CR190 2014.
2. Paton C, et al. High-dose and combination antipsychotic prescribing in acute adult wards in the UK: the challenges posed by p.r.n. prescribing. *Br J Psychiatry* 2008; 192:435–439.
3. Roh D, et al. Antipsychotic polypharmacy and high-dose prescription in schizophrenia: a 5-year comparison. *Aust N Z J Psychiatry* 2014; 48:52–60.
4. Patel MX, et al. Quality of prescribing for schizophrenia: evidence from a national audit in England and Wales. *Eur Neuropsychopharmacol* 2014; 24:499–509.
5. Davis JM, et al. Dose response and dose equivalence of antipsychotics. *J Clin Psychopharmacol* 2004; 24:192–208.
6. Gardner DM, et al. International consensus study of antipsychotic dosing. *Am J Psychiatry* 2010; 167:686–693.
7. Ezewuzie N, et al. Establishing a dose-response relationship for oral risperidone in relapsed schizophrenia. *J Psychopharm* 2006; 20:86–90.
8. Sparshatt A, et al. Quetiapine: dose-response relationship in schizophrenia. *CNS Drugs* 2008; 22:49–68.
9. Kinon BJ, et al. Standard and higher dose of olanzapine in patients with schizophrenia or schizoaffective disorder: a randomized, double-blind, fixed-dose study. *J Clin Psychopharmacol* 2008; 28:392–400.
10. Bishara D, et al. Olanzapine: a systematic review and meta-regression of the relationships between dose, plasma concentration, receptor occupancy, and response. *J Clin Psychopharmacol* 2013; 33:329–335.
11. Meltzer HY, et al. A six month randomized controlled trial of long acting injectable risperidone 50 and 100 mg in treatment resistant schizophrenia. *Schizophr Res* 2014; 154:14–22.
12. Goff DC, et al. High-dose oral ziprasidone versus conventional dosing in schizophrenia patients with residual symptoms: the ZEBRAS study. *J Clin Psychopharmacol* 2013; 33:485–490.
13. Egerton A, et al. Dopamine and glutamate in antipsychotic-responsive compared with antipsychotic-nonresponsive psychosis: a multicenter positron emission tomography and magnetic resonance spectroscopy study (STRATA). *Schizophr Bull* 2020; 47:505–516.
14. Kapur S, et al. Relationship between dopamine D2 occupancy, clinical response, and side effects: a double-blind PET study of first-episode schizophrenia. *Am J Psychiatry* 2000; 157:514–520.
15. Demjaha A, et al. Dopamine synthesis capacity in patients with treatment-resistant schizophrenia. *Am J Psychiatry* 2012; 169:1203–1210.
16. Gillespie AL, et al. Is treatment-resistant schizophrenia categorically distinct from treatment-responsive schizophrenia? A systematic review.

BMC Psychiatry 2017; 17:12.

17. Horowitz MA, et al. Tapering Antipsychotic Treatment. *JAMA Psychiatry* 2020; 78:125–126.

18. Dold M, et al. Dose escalation of antipsychotic drugs in schizophrenia: a meta-analysis of randomized controlled trials. *Schizophr Res* 2015; 166:187–193.

19. Aubree JC, et al. High and very high dosage antipsychotics: a critical review. *J Clin Psychiatry* 1980; 41:341–350.

20. Agid O, et al. An algorithm-based approach to first-episode schizophrenia: response rates over 3 prospective antipsychotic trials with a retrospective data analysis. *J Clin Psychiatry* 2011; 72:1439–1444.

21. Boggs DL, et al. Quetiapine at high doses for the treatment of refractory schizophrenia. *Schizophr Res* 2008; 101:347–348.

22. Lindenmayer JP, et al. A randomized, double-blind, parallel-group, fixed-dose, clinical trial of quetiapine at 600 versus 1200 mg/d for patients with treatment-resistant schizophrenia or schizoaffective disorder. *J Clin Psychopharmacol* 2011; 31:160–168.

23. Honer WG, et al. A randomized, double-blind, placebo-controlled study of the safety and tolerability of high-dose quetiapine in patients with persistent symptoms of schizophrenia or schizoaffective disorder. *J Clin Psychiatry* 2012; 73:13–20.

24. Meltzer HY, et al. A randomized, double-blind comparison of clozapine and high-dose olanzapine in treatment-resistant patients with schizophrenia. *J Clin Psychiatry* 2008; 69:274–285.

25. Souza JS, et al. Efficacy of olanzapine in comparison with clozapine for treatment-resistant schizophrenia: evidence from a systematic review and meta-analyses. *CNS Spectr* 2013; 18:82–89.

26. Leucht S, et al. Dose-response meta-analysis of antipsychotic drugs for acute schizophrenia. *Am J Psychiatry* 2020; 177:342–353.

27. Loebel A, et al. Lurasidone dose escalation in early nonresponding patients with schizophrenia: a randomized, placebo-controlled study. *J Clin Psychiatry* 2016; 77:1672–1680.

28. Osborn DP, et al. Relative risk of cardiovascular and cancer mortality in people with severe mental illness from the United Kingdom's General Practice Rsearch Database. *Arch Gen Psychiatry* 2007; 64:242–249.

29. Ray WA, et al. Atypical antipsychotic drugs and the risk of sudden cardiac death. *N Engl J Med* 2009; 360:225–235.

30. Barbui C, et al. Antipsychotic dose mediates the association between polypharmacy and corrected QT interval. *PLoS One* 2016; 11:e0148212.

31. Weinmann S, et al. Influence of antipsychotics on mortality in schizophrenia: systematic review. *Schizophr Res* 2009; 113:1–11.

32. Bollini P, et al. Antipsychotic drugs: is more worse? A meta-analysis of the published randomized control trials. *Psychol Med* 1994; 24:307–316.

33. Baldessarini RJ, et al. Significance of neuroleptic dose and plasma level in the pharmacological treatment of psychoses. *Arch Gen Psychiatry* 1988; 45:79–90.

34. Kawai N, et al. High-dose of multiple antipsychotics and cognitive function in schizophrenia: the effect of dose-reduction. *Prog Neuropsychopharmacol Biol Psychiatry* 2006; 30:1009–1014.

抗精神病药联用（抗精神病药多药治疗）

在精神科临床实践中，抗精神病药联用十分常见[1-3]，且多为长期使用[4]。联用的药物常包括抗精神病药长效制剂[5,6]、喹硫平[7]以及第一代抗精神病药[8]，其中氟哌啶醇和氯丙嗪常在需要时临时使用。

抗精神病药单一使用疗效差

作为英国精神卫生处方监督处（POMH-UK）质量改善项目的一部分[9]，英国国家临床审计发现，大多数规律联用抗精神病药的理由为单一用药效果差，以及从一种药物换成另一种药物的交叉过渡期。抗精神病药联用常见于年轻、男性、病情加重、病情复杂而迁延、功能较差、住院治疗和诊断为精神分裂症的患者[2,7,10-12]。这也在很大程度上印证了抗精神病药联用常常应用在单药治疗效果差的精神分裂症患者上[10,13-15]。

尽管如此，没有良好的证据证明抗精神病药联用比单一用药的疗效更佳[16]。一篇荟萃分析纳入了16个精神分裂症随机对照试验，比较了加用第二种抗精神病药和继续单一用药治疗的疗效，发现联用抗精神病药的总体疗效缺乏双盲/高质量的证据支持[17]。此外，在精神分裂症患者中，即使小心地从联用药物换回单一用药，其效果仍无法确定。两项随机试验发现，大多数患者可以在症状控制良好的情况下从联用药物换回单一用药[18,19]。另一项研究则发现，换回单一用药6个月后，患者的症状加重幅度较大[20]，但是预期这种病情加重能被成功控制[18]。

抗精神病药长期治疗

匈牙利一项基于人群的非干预研究，比较了治疗时间超过一年时，单药治疗与联合用药的疗效。研究者得出的结论是，在精神分裂症患者中，全部原因导致治疗中断的比例SGA单一用药优于联合用药，但联合用药组死亡率和精神科住院率均低于单一用药组[21]。类似地，芬兰一项长达20年的观察性研究报告了62 250例精神分裂症住院治疗患者队列的再住院风险。为了减少选择偏倚，研究者采用了个体内分析，即每个患者作为其自身的对照。主要的发现是，与单药治疗相比，抗精神病药联合用药（尤其是包括氯氮平和抗精神病药长效制剂）与稍低的精神科住院率有关[22]。对于现实世界的发现如何解释，会受到药物适应证的干扰[23]，但是也有一些可能合理的解释。首先联用具有不同受体特点的抗精神病药，可能疗效更好和/或不良反应负担更小，从而导致更好的临床结局。也有可能联合用药增加了服药依从性，患者服用其中至少一种药物的可能性更大[22]。更复杂的推测是，在临床实践中，氯氮平和抗精神病药长效制剂是预防精神分裂症复发最有效的单药治疗手段[24]。因此，在此基础上加用其他药物来减轻代谢不良反应（如加用阿立哌唑），或处理易激惹、焦虑及睡眠障碍（如加用奥氮平或喹硫平），可能让患者更多地参与到治疗中，增加患者对本就更有效的治疗的依从性。

不良反应

有更充足的证据证明抗精神病药联用可能带来伤害。具有临床意义的不良反应与抗精神病药的联用有关,这部分反映了多数联用处方是"大剂量的"[8,25]。文献报告在联用药物的情况下,EPS[26,27],代谢不良反应和糖尿病[20,28,29]、性功能障碍[30]、髋关节骨折[31]、麻痹性肠梗阻[32]、癫痫大发作[33]、Q-T 间期延长[34]、心律失常[13] 的发生率和严重程度升高。从联合用药转换成单一用药可以显著改善认知功能[19]。

有研究认为持续联用抗精神病药会增加死亡率,但证据不一致。两项大样本病例对照研究和一项数据库研究发现,抗精神病药联合治疗的精神分裂症患者,其死亡率较单药治疗的患者没有升高[35-37]。然而,一项对 88 例精神分裂症患者进行的为期 10 年的前瞻性研究报告称,同时接受一种以上抗精神病药治疗与死亡率的显著上升有关[17,38]。这有可能是因为联用药物治疗的精神疾病更严重和更难治疗,但研究人员对这一可能性进行了探索,却发现死亡率与所测量的疾病严重程度指标无关,尽管这些指标多侧重于阴性症状和认知损害。此外,一项研究对大型心理健康匿名数据库(2007—2014 年)中,使用抗精神病药单一或联合治疗 6 个月以上的 10 945 例成年重性精神疾病患者进行数据分析,发现长期规律使用抗精神病药联合治疗与全因死亡率及自然死亡有弱相关性[39]。但作者认为,即使对药物剂量的影响进行控制,其相关性的证据仍然很局限。另一项研究随访 99 例精神分裂症患者达25 年,发现同时服用三种抗精神病药的患者,死亡率是服用一种药物患者的两倍[40]。这些作者也考虑到适应证可能影响结果,猜测抗精神病药联合用药更可能被用于最严重的精神分裂症患者。

考虑到抗精神病药联用与更大的不良反应相关[15,41],标准的做法是在医疗档案中记录每例联用抗精神病药的理由,并明确说明获益和不良反应。这在法医学上是明智的做法,但临床实践中却鲜有人这么做[42]。

临床实践中联合使用抗精神病药

有无数种可能的抗精神病药组合,但是关于整体治疗反应或目标症状群,它们的相对风险-收益数据非常少。临床上联用抗精神病药的弊端包括不良反应负担增加、总治疗剂量增加、药物相互作用风险升高、复杂治疗方案所致的治疗依从性降低以及对药物反应归因困难,导致难以确定最佳的长期治疗方案。

尽管支持性证据有限,联用抗精神病药在许多国家已经成为习惯并应用于临床实践中[43-45]。此外,各种治疗指南的普遍共识是,只有在其他循证的药物治疗(如氯氮平)用尽后,才应该考虑联合使用抗精神病药治疗难治性精神病,但临床实践中并未一致遵循此共识[6,12,13,46-48]。但是需要注意,联用第二种抗精神病药进行氯氮平增效治疗,也许是可以支持的做法[49-53](见本章"氯氮平增效治疗")。其他可能合理的联合用药策略包括联用阿立哌唑以减轻使用氯氮平者的体重[54,55],以及将使用氟哌啶醇[56]或利培酮长效制剂者[57](但不包括氨磺必利[58])的催乳素下降至正常。在这些情况下,合用阿立哌唑可能是有价值、有循证依据的做法,尽管缺乏标准的临床试验证明其安全性。但是在许多情况下,单用阿立哌唑可能是更合理的治疗选择。

结论

目前的共识认为处方一种以上的抗精神病药不太可能提高疗效,反而可能增加躯体疾病,而上述报告的一些发现可能被认为是对该广泛共识的挑战[59,60]。但基于目前关于疗效和潜在严重不良反应的证据,最好避免常规合用除氯氮平外的抗精神病药。

小结

- 尚无充足证据支持除氯氮平外的抗精神病药联用的疗效。
- 大量证据支持抗精神病药联用可能带来潜在伤害,因此一般应避免合用抗精神病药(常常为大剂量)。
- 抗精神病药联用在临床上较常见,目前这种做法尚难以改变。
- 作为最低要求,对所有接受抗精神病联合治疗的患者,应系统评估不良反应(包括心电图监测),并详细记录药物联用对精神病症状的益处。
- 一些抗精神病药联用(如合并阿立哌唑)可增加耐受性,但是对疗效无益。

参考文献

1. Harrington M, et al. The results of a multi-centre audit of the prescribing of antipsychotic drugs for in-patients in the UK. *Psychiatric Bull* 2002; 26:414–418.
2. Gallego JA, et al. Prevalence and correlates of antipsychotic polypharmacy: a systematic review and meta-regression of global and regional trends from the 1970s to 2009. *Schizophr Res* 2012; 138:18–28.
3. Sneider B, et al. Frequency and correlates of antipsychotic polypharmacy among patients with schizophrenia in Denmark: a nation-wide pharmacoepidemiological study. *Eur Neuropsychopharmacol* 2015; 25:1669–1676.
4. Procyshyn RM, et al. Persistent antipsychotic polypharmacy and excessive dosing in the community psychiatric treatment setting: a review of medication profiles in 435 Canadian outpatients. *J Clin Psychiatry* 2010; 71:566–573.
5. Aggarwal NK, et al. Prevalence of concomitant oral antipsychotic drug use among patients treated with long-acting, intramuscular, antipsychotic medications. *J Clin Psychopharmacol* 2012; 32:323–328.
6. Barnes T, et al. Antipsychotic long acting injections: prescribing practice in the UK. *Br J Psychiatry Suppl* 2009; 52:S37–S42.
7. Novick D, et al. Antipsychotic monotherapy and polypharmacy in the treatment of outpatients with schizophrenia in the European Schizophrenia Outpatient Health Outcomes Study. *J Nerv Ment Dis* 2012; 200:637–643.
8. Paton C, et al. High-dose and combination antipsychotic prescribing in acute adult wards in the UK: the challenges posed by p.r.n. prescribing. *Br J Psychiatry* 2008; 192:435–439.
9. Prescribing Observatory for Mental Health. Topic 1g & 3d. Prescribing high dose and combined antipsychotics on adult psychiatric wards. 2017; Prescribing Observatory for Mental Health CCQI1272.
10. Correll CU, et al. Antipsychotic polypharmacy: a comprehensive evaluation of relevant correlates of a long-standing clinical practice. *Psychiatr Clin North Am* 2012; 35:661–681.
11. Baandrup L, et al. Association of antipsychotic polypharmacy with health service cost: a register-based cost analysis. *Eur J Health Econ* 2012; 13:355–363.
12. Kadra G, et al. Predictors of long-term (≥6 months) antipsychotic polypharmacy prescribing in secondary mental healthcare. *Schizophr Res* 2016; 174:106–112.
13. Grech P, et al. Long-term antipsychotic polypharmacy: how does it start, why does it continue? *Ther Adv Psychopharmacol* 2012; 2:5–11.
14. Malandain L, et al. Correlates and predictors of antipsychotic drug polypharmacy in real-life settings: results from a nationwide cohort study. *Schizophr Res* 2018; 192:213–218.
15. Fleischhacker WW, et al. Critical review of antipsychotic polypharmacy in the treatment of schizophrenia. *Int J Neuropsychopharmacol* 2014; 17:1083–1093.
16. Ortiz-Orendain J, et al. Antipsychotic combinations for schizophrenia. *Schizophr Bull* 2018; 44:15–17.
17. Galling B, et al. Antipsychotic augmentation vs. monotherapy in schizophrenia: systematic review, meta-analysis and meta-regression analysis. *World Psychiatry* 2017; 16:77–89.
18. Essock SM, et al. Effectiveness of switching from antipsychotic polypharmacy to monotherapy. *Am J Psychiatry* 2011; 168:702–708.
19. Hori H, et al. Switching to antipsychotic monotherapy can improve attention and processing speed, and social activity in chronic schizophrenia patients. *J Psychiatr Res* 2013; 47:1843–1848.
20. Constantine RJ, et al. The risks and benefits of switching patients with schizophrenia or schizoaffective disorder from two to one antipsychotic medication: a randomized controlled trial. *Schizophr Res* 2015; 166:194–200.
21. Katona L, et al. Real-world effectiveness of antipsychotic monotherapy vs. polypharmacy in schizophrenia: to switch or to combine? A nationwide study in Hungary. *Schizophr Res* 2014; 152:246–254.
22. Tiihonen J, et al. Association of antipsychotic polypharmacy vs monotherapy with psychiatric rehospitalization among adults with schizophrenia. *JAMA Psychiatry* 2019; 76:499–507.
23. Goff DC. Can adjunctive pharmacotherapy reduce hospitalization in schizophrenia?: insights from administrative databases. *JAMA Psychiatry* 2019; 76:468–470.

24. Tiihonen J, et al. Real-world effectiveness of antipsychotic treatments in a nationwide cohort of 29823 patients with schizophrenia. *JAMA Psychiatry* 2017; **74**:686–693.

25. López de Torre A, et al. Antipsychotic polypharmacy: a needle in a haystack? *Gen Hosp Psychiatry* 2012; **34**:423–432.

26. Carnahan RM, et al. Increased risk of extrapyramidal side-effect treatment associated with atypical antipsychotic polytherapy. *Acta Psychiatr Scand* 2006; **113**:135–141.

27. Gomberg RF. Interaction between olanzapine and haloperidol. *J Clin Psychopharmacol* 1999; **19**:272–273.

28. Suzuki T, et al. Effectiveness of antipsychotic polypharmacy for patients with treatment refractory schizophrenia: an open-label trial of olanzapine plus risperidone for those who failed to respond to a sequential treatment with olanzapine, quetiapine and risperidone. *Human Psychopharmacology* 2008; **23**:455–463.

29. Gallego JA, et al. Safety and tolerability of antipsychotic polypharmacy. *Exp Opin Drug Saf* 2012; **11**:527–542.

30. Hashimoto Y, et al. Effects of antipsychotic polypharmacy on side-effects and concurrent use of medications in schizophrenic outpatients. *Psychiatry Clin Neurosci* 2012; **66**:405–410.

31. Sorensen HJ, et al. Schizophrenia, antipsychotics and risk of hip fracture: a population-based analysis. *Eur Neuro Psychopharmacol* 2013; **23**:872–878.

32. Dome P, et al. Paralytic ileus associated with combined atypical antipsychotic therapy. *Prog Neuropsychopharmacol Biol Psychiatry* 2007; **31**:557–560.

33. Hedges DW, et al. New-onset seizure associated with quetiapine and olanzapine. *Ann Pharmacother* 2002; **36**:437–439.

34. Beelen AP, et al. Asymptomatic QTc prolongation associated with quetiapine fumarate overdose in a patient being treated with risperidone. *Hum Exp Toxicol* 2001; **20**:215–219.

35. Baandrup L, et al. Antipsychotic polypharmacy and risk of death from natural causes in patients with schizophrenia: a population-based nested case-control study. *J Clin Psychiatry* 2010; **71**:103–108.

36. Chen Y, et al. Antipsychotics and risk of natural death in patients with schizophrenia. *Neuropsychiatr Dis Treat* 2019; **15**:1863–1871.

37. Tiihonen J, et al. Polypharmacy with antipsychotics, antidepressants, or benzodiazepines and mortality in schizophrenia. *Arch Gen Psychiatry* 2012; **69**:476–483.

38. Waddington JL, et al. Mortality in schizophrenia. Antipsychotic polypharmacy and absence of adjunctive anticholinergics over the course of a 10-year prospective study. *Br J Psychiatry* 1998; **173**:325–329.

39. Kadra G, et al. Long-term antipsychotic polypharmacy prescribing in secondary mental health care and the risk of mortality. *Acta Psychiatr Scand* 2018; **138**:123–132.

40. Joukamaa M, et al. Schizophrenia, neuroleptic medication and mortality. *Br J Psychiatry* 2006; **188**:122–127.

41. Centorrino F, et al. Multiple versus single antipsychotic agents for hospitalized psychiatric patients: case-control study of risks versus benefits. *Am J Psychiatry* 2004; **161**:700–706.

42. Taylor D, et al. Co-prescribing of atypical and typical antipsychotics – prescribing sequence and documented outcome. *Psychiatric Bull* 2002; **26**:170–172.

43. Kreyenbuhl J, et al. Adding or switching antipsychotic medications in treatment-refractory schizophrenia. *Psychiatr Serv* 2007; **58**:983–990.

44. Nielsen J, et al. Psychiatrists' attitude towards and knowledge of clozapine treatment. *J Psychopharmacology* 2010; **24**:965–971.

45. Ascher-Svanum H, et al. Comparison of patients undergoing switching versus augmentation of antipsychotic medications during treatment for schizophrenia. *Neuro Psychiatr Dis Treat* 2012; **8**:113–118.

46. Goren JL, et al. Antipsychotic prescribing pathways, polypharmacy, and clozapine use in treatment of schizophrenia. *Psychiatr Serv* 2013; **64**:527–533.

47. Howes OD, et al. Adherence to treatment guidelines in clinical practice: study of antipsychotic treatment prior to clozapine initiation. *Br J Psychiatry* 2012; **201**:481–485.

48. Thompson JV, et al. Antipsychotic polypharmacy and augmentation strategies prior to clozapine initiation: a historical cohort study of 310 adults with treatment-resistant schizophrenic disorders. *J Psychopharmacology* 2016; **30**:436–443.

49. Shiloh R, et al. Sulpiride augmentation in people with schizophrenia partially responsive to clozapine. A double-blind, placebo-controlled study. *Br J Psychiatry* 1997; **171**:569–573.

50. Josiassen RC, et al. Clozapine augmented with risperidone in the treatment of schizophrenia: a randomized, double-blind, placebo-controlled trial. *Am J Psychiatry* 2005; **162**:130–136.

51. Paton C, et al. Augmentation with a second antipsychotic in patients with schizophrenia who partially respond to clozapine: a meta-analysis. *J Clin Psychopharmacol* 2007; **27**:198–204.

52. Barbui C, et al. Does the addition of a second antipsychotic drug improve clozapine treatment? *Schizophr Bull* 2009; **35**:458–468.

53. Taylor DM, et al. Augmentation of clozapine with a second antipsychotic – a meta-analysis of randomized, placebo-controlled studies. *Acta Psychiatr Scand* 2009; **119**:419–425.

54. Fleischhacker WW, et al. Effects of adjunctive treatment with aripiprazole on body weight and clinical efficacy in schizophrenia patients treated with clozapine: a randomized, double-blind, placebo-controlled trial. *Int J Neuropsychopharmacol* 2010; **13**:1115–1125.

55. Cooper SJ, et al. BAP guidelines on the management of weight gain, metabolic disturbances and cardiovascular risk associated with psychosis and antipsychotic drug treatment. *J Psychopharmacology* 2016; **30**:717–748.

56. Shim JC, et al. Adjunctive treatment with a dopamine partial agonist, aripiprazole, for antipsychotic-induced hyperprolactinemia: a placebo-controlled trial. *Am J Psychiatry* 2007; **164**:1404–1410.

57. Trives MZ, et al. Effect of the addition of aripiprazole on hyperprolactinemia associated with risperidone long-acting injection. *J Clin Psychopharmacol* 2013; **33**:538–541.

58. Chen CK, et al. Differential add-on effects of aripiprazole in resolving hyperprolactinemia induced by risperidone in comparison to benza-

mide antipsychotics. *Prog Neuropsychopharmacol Biol Psychiatry* 2010; 34:1495–1499.

59. Lin SK. Antipsychotic polypharmacy: a dirty little secret or a fashion? *Int J Neuropsychopharmacol* 2020; 23:125–131.

60. Guinart D, et al. Antipsychotic polypharmacy in schizophrenia: why not? *J Clin Psychiatry* 2020; 81:19ac13118.

用抗精神病药预防复发

首次发作的精神病性障碍

在预防复发方面,抗精神病药至少能在短期至中期为患者提供有效的保护[1],且 20 世纪 50 年代抗精神病药的问世似乎改善了整个结局[2]。一项安慰剂对照试验的荟萃分析发现,抗精神病药维持治疗 6~12 个月后,首发精神病性障碍患者的复发率为 26%,而安慰剂治疗者复发率达 61%[3]。目前的专家共识认为,首发精神分裂症应使用抗精神病药治疗至少 1~2 年[4,5],但一项研究发现[6],按照这个共识停用抗精神病药后,1 年的复发率为 80%,2 年的复发率为 98%。2019 年,瑞典的一项人群研究发现,抗精神病药治疗的时间越长,住院的风险越低(比如接受 5 年治疗的患者,其住院率是治疗不到 6 个月的患者的 50%)[7]。

其他研究发现,仅很少部分患者在停药 1~2 年后仍保持稳定状态[8-11](如一项小规模研究发现,在停用利培酮长效注射剂后,94% 的患者在 2 年内复发,97% 的患者在 3 年内复发[12])。2018 年,一项纳入 8 个随机对照研究的荟萃分析结果则要乐观一些:在 18~24 个月内,接受治疗的患者复发率为 35%,中断治疗的复发率为 61%[13]。

一项研究在为期 2 年的随机对照试验结束之后,继续进行 5 年的随访,患者有的维持治疗,有的减少药量或完全停用,结果发现维持治疗组在短期复发预防方面具有显著优势,但在中期复发预防方面这种优势消失。另外,药物减量或停用组在随访时接受的抗精神病药剂量更低,且患者的功能结局更为良好[14]。对于这些结果有许多解释,但是目前能得出的最主要结论是,对于首发精神分裂症患者,减少抗精神病药剂量是一种可能的选择。这项研究遭到了严厉的批评[15],当然,还有其他研究表明停用抗精神病药会带来严重的后果[16],但是这些研究的随访时间较短、样本量较小。尽管如此,有些首发精神分裂症患者并不需要长期抗精神病药治疗就能保持稳定,有研究者指出该数字高达 18%~30%[17]。

没有可靠的患者因素与首发患者停用抗精神病药的后果相关(大麻使用除外[18]),但有很多证据支持继续使用抗精神病药,而非停用它们[19]。有迹象表明,使用双曲线渐减方案在很长的时间内减停药物(见"停用抗精神病药"),可能创造出停药的最佳机会[20,21]。

值得注意的是,对复发的定义,常集中在阳性症状的严重程度上,而明显忽视了认知症状和阴性症状:阳性症状更可能导致患者住院,而认知症状和阴性症状对患者生活质量的整体影响更大(对于这些症状,抗精神病药治疗效果较差,甚至会使其加重)。

在抗精神病药的选择方面,一项随机对照试验结果认为,在首发精神分裂症(不含难治性病例)的中期治疗中,氯氮平与氯丙嗪比较并无明显优势[22]。但是在一项大样本首次住院精神分裂症患者的长期自然观察中发现,与其他口服抗精神病药相比,氯氮平和奥氮平组的再住院率明显要低[23]。在同一项研究中,尽管存在适应证因素的影响(长效制剂会被处方给依从性差的患者,而口服制剂则用于依从性较好的患者[23]),接受长效抗精神病药治疗的患者,再住院率要低于口服药物治疗的患者。随后的研究发现,相比利培酮口服制剂,利培酮长效制剂治疗首发精神分裂症患者具有明显优势[24];帕利哌酮长效制剂相比口服制剂,在治疗"新近诊断的精神分裂症"时具有较小但显著的优势[25]。最近的研究发现,氨磺必利可以带来良好的临床结局,且在最初没有达到缓解的情况下,继续服用氨磺必利与换用奥氮平一样有效[26]。

在临床实践中,医师很少对首发患者给出明确的精神分裂症诊断,大多数医师或患者至少试图在治疗 1 年内停用抗精神病药[27]。在理想情况下,患者应缓慢减少药物剂量,有关家庭成员和医疗工作者应当知道患者停药(极可能通过使用长效注射剂来做到)。至关重要的是患者、照料者和相关健康工作者如何识别复发的早期迹象并寻求帮助。抗精神病药不应被视为唯一的干预手段,具有循证医学证据的心理社会干预和心理干预显然也非常重要[28]。

反复发作的精神分裂症

精神分裂症首次发病后,大多数患者会病情反复。若患者有残留症状、不良反应负担较大并对治疗态度不够积极,则复发的风险较大[29]。伴随着每次复发,患者的基线功能水平衰退[30],这种衰退大多见于病后 10 年内。自杀风险(约 10%)也集中在首次发作后的 10 年中。如果能规律使用抗精神病药,会在短期、中期乃至长期(较不确定)内防止复发[3,31]。那些有针对性(即仅在症状重新出现时)使用抗精神病药者,其结局比预防性使用抗精神病药者要差[32,33],发生迟发性运动障碍的风险也可能更高。同样,低剂量抗精神病药的疗效不如标准剂量[34]。

下表列出了有关抗精神病药维持治疗的利和弊,来源于 Leucht 等(2012 年)的荟萃分析[3]。

	获益				弊端		
结果	抗精神病药	安慰剂	NNT	不良反应	抗精神病药	安慰剂	NNH*
7~12 个月复发率	27%	64%	3	运动障碍	16%	9%	17
再住院率	10%	26%	5	抗胆碱能作用	24%	16%	11
精神状态改善	30%	12%	4	镇静	13%	9%	20
暴力/攻击行为	2%	12%	11	体重增加	10%	6%	20

NNT,需治疗人数;NNH,致成伤害需治疗人数。

* 可能被明显低估,因为在临床试验中极少系统评定不良反应[35]。

在维持治疗中,长效制剂较口服制剂更具优势,这极有可能是因为能够确保药物进入患者体内(或者至少能确保知道用药)。临床试验的荟萃分析结果显示,长效制剂的相对和绝对复发风险分别比口服制剂低 30% 和 10%[3,36]。因此,长效制剂可能更受临床医师和患者欢迎。

小结

- 精神分裂症患者若停用抗精神病药,其复发率极高。
- 抗精神病药显著降低复发率、再住院率和暴力/攻击行为。
- 抗精神病药长效制剂预防复发的效果最好。

一项大型荟萃分析认为,使用新型抗精神病药的复发风险与老一代药物相近[3]。(注意:没有复发不等于功能良好[37]。)在反复发作的精神分裂症患者中,达到临床缓解的比例很小,且不同的抗精神病药之间不尽相同。CATIE 研究报告,达到临床缓解并保持 6 个月以上的患者比例,奥氮平组为 12%,喹硫平组为 8%,利培酮组为 6%[38]。此处见到的奥氮平的优势,与急性期疗效的网络荟萃分析结果一致[39]。

抗精神病药治疗的依从性

精神分裂症患者对抗精神病药治疗的不依从率很高。在出院 10 天后,就有 25% 的患者部分或完全不按医嘱用药,出院后 1 年增至 50%,出院后 2 年增至 75%[40]。不依从不仅增加了复发风险,而且增加了复发时疾病的严重程度和住院时间[40]。自杀未遂的风险也增加 4 倍[40]。

预防复发的药物剂量

许多患者在急性精神病发作时,会接受过高剂量的药物(特别是老药)[41,42]。急性期以后,就需要在治疗有效性与不良反应之间进行平衡。与较高剂量的老药相比,较低剂量(氟哌啶醇 8mg/d 或等效剂量)治疗的患者不良反应较少[43],主观体验更好,社会适应更佳[44]。很低的剂量会增加精神病复发的风险[41,45,46]。迄今尚无充分证据支持低于标准剂量的新药能有效地预防复发。急性期有效的剂量通常应该继续作为预防复发的剂量[47,48],但是首次发作后的预防例外,有证据支持可以非常慎重地减少剂量用于预防复发。最近有一些证据支持在反复发作的精神分裂症中减少剂量[49],撰写本文时,一些临床试验正在进行中[50-52]。

如何停药? 何时停药[53]?

决定停用抗精神病药前,必须对每一位患者进行全面的风险-获益分析。在长期治疗后停用抗精神病药,应是渐进的过程,同时进行密切的监测。突然停药后 6 个月内的复发率是逐步停药后的 2 倍(逐步停药指口服抗精神病药减停过程至少 3 周,或直接停用长效制剂)[54]。一项对复发率的分析发现,换成安慰剂后,帕利哌酮每 3 个月一次的长效剂组复发时间远远晚于每月一次的长效剂组和口服组[55]。总体复发率降低。突然停药也可能引起一些患者出现撤药症状(如头痛、恶心、失眠)[56]。

应考虑以下因素[53]:

- 患者的临床症状是否完全缓解? 如果是,持续了多长时间? 可排除长期存在、并非令患者痛苦不堪、既往药物治疗无效的症状。
- 不良反应(EPS、迟发性运动障碍、镇静、肥胖等)的严重程度?
- 以往发病的表现形式? 要考虑起病的速度、症状持续的时间和严重程度,以及对自身和他人构成的危险。
- 以往是否尝试过减量? 如果是,结果如何?
- 患者目前的社会环境如何? 是处于相对稳定期,还是预期会遇到应激性生活事件?
- 复发的社会成本如何? (例如,患者是否为家庭中唯一养家糊口者?)
- 患者或照料者能否监测症状? 如果能,他们是否会寻求专业帮助?

与首次发病的患者一样,患者、照料者和相关工作人员应该知道复发的早期征象,以及如何寻求专业帮助。要知道,针对复发症状进行的治疗,其疗效远远不如持续的复发预防[10]。对于病史中有过攻击行为、严重自杀未遂以及残留精神病性症状的患者,应考虑终身治疗。

非主流观点

　　虽然显而易见抗精神病药能有效减轻症状的严重程度,降低复发率,但有少数观点认为,抗精神病药可能让患者对精神病变得更为敏感。这种观点认为,停用抗精神病药后的复发,可以被看成是一种撤药反应,其原因是多巴胺受体超敏,尽管证据还不明确[57]。这种现象可以解释为什么在首次发病的患者中,采用较低剂量的抗精神病药时,结局会更好;但也提示了,抗精神病药最终可能使结局更糟糕。这种现象也可以解释突然停药带来的不良后果[54]。这些观察反过来让人们质疑一些长期研究的有效性,因为在这些研究中,积极和成功的治疗突然停止,所导致的反跳现象和撤药反应,可能至少是观察到复发率高的部分原因[58]。

　　"超敏性精神病"的概念在数十年前曾广为讨论[59,60],最近又出现复苏[57]。引人注目的是,用于治疗非精神科疾病的多巴胺受体拮抗剂,也可能引起与撤药有关的精神病[61-63]。虽然这些理论和观点并不能改变本节的治疗建议,但是它们确实强调对所有患者需要尽可能使用最低的剂量,并平衡观察到的收益和不良反应,包括那些临床上不明显的不良反应(如可能带来的大脑结构改变[64])。临床医师应当对这些可能性保持开放的态度,即抗精神病药长期治疗可能加重、至少不改善精神分裂症患者的结局。

参考文献

1. Karson C, et al. Long-term outcomes of antipsychotic treatment in patients with first-episode schizophrenia: a systematic review. *Neuropsychiatr Dis Treat* 2016; 12:57–67.

2. Taylor M, et al. Are we getting any better at staying better? The long view on relapse and recovery in first episode nonaffective psychosis and schizophrenia. *Ther Adv Psychopharmacol* 2019; 9:2045125319870033.

3. Leucht S, et al. Antipsychotic drugs versus placebo for relapse prevention in schizophrenia: a systematic review and meta-analysis. *Lancet* 2012; 379:2063–2071.

4. American Psychiatric Association. Clinical practice guidelines: treatment of patients with schizophrenia. 2019; https://www.psychiatry.org/psychiatrists/practice/clinical-practice-guidelines.

5. Sheitman BB, et al. The evaluation and treatment of first-episode psychosis. *Schizophr Bull* 1997; 23:653–661.

6. Gitlin M, et al. Clinical outcome following neuroleptic discontinuation in patients with remitted recent-onset schizophrenia. *Am J Psychiatry* 2001; 158:1835–1842.

7. Hayes JF, et al. Psychiatric hospitalization following antipsychotic medication cessation in first episode psychosis. *J Psychopharmacology* 2019; 33:532–534.

8. Wunderink L, et al. Guided discontinuation versus maintenance treatment in remitted first-episode psychosis: relapse rates and functional outcome. *J Clin Psychiatry* 2007; 68:654–661.

9. Chen EY, et al. Maintenance treatment with quetiapine versus discontinuation after one year of treatment in patients with remitted first episode psychosis: randomised controlled trial. *BMJ* 2010; 341:c4024.

10. Gaebel W, et al. Relapse prevention in first-episode schizophrenia–maintenance vs intermittent drug treatment with prodrome-based early intervention: results of a randomized controlled trial within the German Research Network on Schizophrenia. *J Clin Psychiatry* 2011; 72:205–218.

11. Caseiro O, et al. Predicting relapse after a first episode of non-affective psychosis: a three-year follow-up study. *J Psychiatr Res* 2012; 46:1099–1105.

12. Emsley R, et al. Symptom recurrence following intermittent treatment in first-episode schizophrenia successfully treated for 2 years: a 3-year open-label clinical study. *J Clin Psychiatry* 2012; 73:e541–e547.

13. Kishi T, et al. Effect of discontinuation v. maintenance of antipsychotic medication on relapse rates in patients with remitted/stable first-episode psychosis: a meta-analysis. *Psychol Med* 2019; 49:772–779.

14. Wunderink L, et al. Recovery in remitted first-episode psychosis at 7 years of follow-up of an early dose reduction/discontinuation or maintenance treatment strategy: long-term follow-up of a 2-year randomized clinical trial. *JAMA Psychiatry* 2013; 70:913–920.

15. Correll CU, et al. What is the risk-benefit ratio of long-term antipsychotic treatment in people with schizophrenia? *World Psychiatry* 2018; 17:149–160.

16. Boonstra G, et al. Antipsychotic prophylaxis is needed after remission from a first psychotic episode in schizophrenia patients: results from an aborted randomised trial. *Int J Psychiatry Clin Pract* 2011; 15:128–134.

17. Murray RM, et al. Should psychiatrists be more cautious about the long-term prophylactic use of antipsychotics? *Br J Psychiatry* 2016; 209:361–365.

18. Bowtell M, et al. Rates and predictors of relapse following discontinuation of antipsychotic medication after a first episode of psychosis.

Schizophr Res 2018; 195:231–236.

19. Emsley R, et al. How long should antipsychotic treatment be continued after a single episode of schizophrenia? *Curr Opin Psychiatry* 2016; 29:224–229.
20. Horowitz MA, et al. Tapering antipsychotic treatment. *JAMA Psychiatry* 2020; 78:125–126.
21. Liu CC, et al. Achieving the lowest effective antipsychotic dose for patients with remitted psychosis: a proposed guided dose-reduction algorithm. *CNS Drugs* 2020; 34:117–126.
22. Girgis RR, et al. Clozapine v. chlorpromazine in treatment-naive, first-episode schizophrenia: 9-year outcomes of a randomised clinical trial. *Br J Psychiatry* 2011; 199:281–288.
23. Tiihonen J, et al. A nationwide cohort study of oral and depot antipsychotics after first hospitalization for schizophrenia. *Am J Psychiatry* 2011; 168:603–609.
24. Subotnik KL, et al. Long-acting injectable risperidone for relapse prevention and control of breakthrough symptoms after a recent first episode of schizophrenia. A randomized clinical trial. *JAMA Psychiatry* 2015; 72:822–829.
25. Schreiner A, et al. Paliperidone palmitate versus oral antipsychotics in recently diagnosed schizophrenia. *Schizophr Res* 2015; 169:393–399.
26. Kahn RS, et al. Amisulpride and olanzapine followed by open-label treatment with clozapine in first-episode schizophrenia and schizophreniform disorder (OPTiMiSE): a three-phase switching study. *Lancet Psychiatry* 2018; 5:797–807.
27. Johnson DAW, et al. Professional attitudes in the UK towards neuroleptic maintenance therapy in schizophrenia. *Psychiatric Bull* 1997; 21:394–397.
28. National Institute for Health and Care Excellence. Psychosis and schizophrenia in adults: prevention and management. Clinical Guidance [CG178]. 2014 (last checked March 2019); https://www.nice.org.uk/guidance/cg178.
29. Schennach R, et al. Predictors of relapse in the year after hospital discharge among patients with schizophrenia. *Psychiatr Serv* 2012; 63:87–90.
30. Wyatt RJ. Neuroleptics and the natural course of schizophrenia. *Schizophr Bull* 1991; 17:325–351.
31. Almerie MQ, et al. Cessation of medication for people with schizophrenia already stable on chlorpromazine. *Schizophr Bull* 2008; 34:13–14.
32. Jolley AG, et al. Trial of brief intermittent neuroleptic prophylaxis for selected schizophrenic outpatients: clinical and social outcome at two years. *Br Med J* 1990; 301:837–842.
33. Herz MI, et al. Intermittent vs maintenance medication in schizophrenia. Two-year results. *Arch Gen Psychiatry* 1991; 48:333–339.
34. Schooler NR, et al. Relapse and rehospitalization during maintenance treatment of schizophrenia. The effects of dose reduction and family treatment. *Arch Gen Psychiatry* 1997; 54:453–463.
35. Pope A, et al. Assessment of adverse effects in clinical studies of antipsychotic medication: survey of methods used. *Br J Psychiatry* 2010; 197:67–72.
36. Leucht C, et al. Oral versus depot antipsychotic drugs for schizophrenia–a critical systematic review and meta-analysis of randomised long-term trials. *Schizophr Res* 2011; 127:83–92.
37. Schooler NR. Relapse prevention and recovery in the treatment of schizophrenia. *J Clin Psychiatry* 2006; 67 Suppl 5:19–23.
38. Levine SZ, et al. Extent of attaining and maintaining symptom remission by antipsychotic medication in the treatment of chronic schizophrenia: evidence from the CATIE study. *Schizophr Res* 2011; 133:42–46.
39. Leucht S, et al. Comparative efficacy and tolerability of 15 antipsychotic drugs in schizophrenia: a multiple-treatments meta-analysis. *Lancet* 2013; 382:951–962.
40. Leucht S, et al. Epidemiology, clinical consequences, and psychosocial treatment of nonadherence in schizophrenia. *J Clin Psychiatry* 2006; 67 Suppl 5:3–8.
41. Baldessarini RJ, et al. Significance of neuroleptic dose and plasma level in the pharmacological treatment of psychoses. *Arch Gen Psychiatry* 1988; 45:79–90.
42. Harrington M, et al. The results of a multi-centre audit of the prescribing of antipsychotic drugs for in-patients in the UK. *Psychiatric Bull* 2002; 26:414–418.
43. Geddes J, et al. Atypical antipsychotics in the treatment of schizophrenia: systematic overview and meta-regression analysis. *Br Med J* 2000; 321:1371–1376.
44. Hogarty GE, et al. Dose of fluphenazine, familial expressed emotion, and outcome in schizophrenia. Results of a two-year controlled study. *Arch Gen Psychiatry* 1988; 45:797–805.
45. Marder SR, et al. Low- and conventional-dose maintenance therapy with fluphenazine decanoate. Two-year outcome. *Arch Gen Psychiatry* 1987; 44:518–521.
46. Uchida H, et al. Low Dose vs Standard Dose of antipsychotics for relapse prevention in schizophrenia: meta-analysis. *Schizophr Bull* 2011; 37:788–799.
47. Rouillon F, et al. Strategies of treatment with olanzapine in schizophrenic patients during stable phase: results of a pilot study. *Eur Neuropsychopharmacol* 2008; 18:646–652.
48. Wang CY, et al. Risperidone maintenance treatment in schizophrenia: a randomized, controlled trial. *Am J Psychiatry* 2010; 167:676–685.
49. Huhn M, et al. Reducing antipsychotic drugs in stable patients with chronic schizophrenia or schizoaffective disorder: a randomized controlled pilot trial. *Eur Arch Psychiatry Clin Neurosci* 2021; 271:293–302.
50. Stürup AE, et al. TAILOR – tapered discontinuation versus maintenance therapy of antipsychotic medication in patients with newly diagnosed schizophrenia or persistent delusional disorder in remission of psychotic symptoms: study protocol for a randomized clinical trial. *Trials* 2017; 18:445.

51. Begemann MJH, et al. To continue or not to continue? Antipsychotic medication maintenance versus dose-reduction/discontinuation in first episode psychosis: HAMLETT, a pragmatic multicenter single-blind randomized controlled trial. *Trials* 2020; 21:147.
52. Moncrieff J, et al. Randomised controlled trial of gradual antipsychotic reduction and discontinuation in people with schizophrenia and related disorders: the RADAR trial (Research into Antipsychotic Discontinuation and Reduction). *BMJ Open* 2019; 9:e030912.
53. Wyatt RJ. Risks of withdrawing antipsychotic medications. *Arch Gen Psychiatry* 1995; 52:205–208.
54. Viguera AC, et al. Clinical risk following abrupt and gradual withdrawal of maintenance neuroleptic treatment. *Arch Gen Psychiatry* 1997; 54:49–55.
55. Weiden PJ, et al. Does half-life matter after antipsychotic discontinuation? A relapse comparison in schizophrenia with 3 different formulations of paliperidone. *J Clin Psychiatry* 2017; 78:e813–e820.
56. Chouinard G, et al. Withdrawal symptoms after long-term treatment with low-potency neuroleptics. *J Clin Psychiatry* 1984; 45:500–502.
57. Yin J, et al. Antipsychotic induced dopamine supersensitivity psychosis: a comprehensive review. *Curr Neuropharmacol* 2017; 15:174–183.
58. Cohen D, et al. Discontinuing psychotropic drugs from participants in randomized controlled trials: a systematic review. *Psychother Psychosom* 2019; 88:96–104.
59. Chouinard G, et al. Neuroleptic-induced supersensitivity psychosis: clinical and pharmacologic characteristics. *Am J Psychiatry* 1980; 137:16–21.
60. Kirkpatrick B, et al. The concept of supersensitivity psychosis. *J Nerv Ment Dis* 1992; 180:265–270.
61. Chaffin DS. Phenothiazine-induced acute psychotic reaction: the 'psychotoxicity' of a drug. *Am J Psychiatry* 1964; 121:26–32.
62. Lu ML, et al. Metoclopramide-induced supersensitivity psychosis. *Ann Pharmacother* 2002; 36:1387–1390.
63. Roy-Desruisseaux J, et al. Domperidone-induced tardive dyskinesia and withdrawal psychosis in an elderly woman with dementia. *Ann Pharmacother* 2011; 45:e51.
64. Huhtaniska S, et al. Long-term antipsychotic use and brain changes in schizophrenia – a systematic review and meta-analysis. *Human Psychopharmacology* 2017; 32:e2574.

阴性症状

精神分裂症的阴性症状表现为正常功能的降低或缺失,构成了精神病理学的重要维度之一。其中一个子维度是"表达缺陷",表现为言语输出或表达减少,情感平淡或迟钝,可以通过表情减少、缺乏眼神交流、自发活动减少和缺乏自主性进行评估。第二个子维度是"意志/动机缺乏",特点为兴趣、欲望和目标的主观减少,以及有目的的行为减少,包括缺少自发的社交互动[1,2]。

持续的阴性症状被认为是精神分裂症患者长期病态和功能预后差的主要原因[3-6]。但阴性症状的病因非常复杂,在着手制订治疗方案之前,必须确定每个患者最可能的原因。在临床上区分原发性和继发性阴性症状是很重要的。原发性阴性症状由持久的功能缺陷状态组成,预示着不良的预后,且随着时间的推移保持稳定;继发性阴性症状继发于阳性症状、抑郁、颓废或药物不良反应,如药物所致帕金森综合征的运动迟缓[5,7]。继发性阴性症状的其他原因包括慢性物质/酒精使用、大剂量抗精神病药、社交剥夺、缺乏刺激以及住院治疗[8]。继发性阴性症状最好的解决方法是消除相关病因。在明确诊断精神分裂症的患者中,3/4 可见不同程度的阴性症状,20% 存在持续的原发性阴性症状[9,10]。

有关阴性症状药物治疗的文献,大多包括急性期疗效研究的亚项分析、相关分析和路径分析[11]。原发性和继发性阴性症状之间通常没有可靠的区分方法,表达缺陷和意志/动机缺乏这两个子维度之间也是同样的情况。几乎没有研究专门招募持续存在阴性症状的患者。对于持续存在的原发性阴性症状,虽然有证据表明一些干预措施有短期疗效,但是长期效果仍缺乏充足证据。总结如下:

- 在首发精神病性障碍中,阴性症状的存在预示着病情恢复和社会功能的结局不佳[4,9]。有证据表明,精神病性障碍越早得到有效治疗,最后发生阴性症状的可能性就越小[12-14]。不过,在解释这些数据时应该记住,早期临床表现以阴性症状为特征,对社会破坏性小,作为精神病的征兆比阳性症状轻微;这些表现可能导致患者延误就诊,精神疾病的未治疗期更长。换言之,具有持续阴性症状的患者原本预后就较差,接受诊断和治疗的时间可能也更晚。
- 抗精神病药虽然可以改善阴性症状,但是限于急性精神障碍发作时的继发性阴性症状[15]。尚没有一致证据证明第二代抗精神病药对阴性症状的疗效优于第一代抗精神病药[16-20]。类似地,早期研究没有发现一致的证据证明哪个第二代抗精神病药更有效[21]。虽然一项纳入 38 项随机对照研究的荟萃分析发现,第二代抗精神病药减轻阴性症状的程度具有统计学意义,但其效应值太小,未达到"随着时间推移,可检测的最小临床改善"的阈值[22]。
- 尽管如此,一项荟萃分析发现[23],有充足的数据支持,某些抗精神病药治疗方案对阴性症状有效,如氨磺必利[24-27]和卡利拉嗪[28,29],奥氮平和喹硫平可能比利培酮有效。阿立哌唑增效治疗同样可能有效[30,31]。
- 氯氮平作为唯一一个治疗难治性精神分裂症有确切优势的药物,对阴性症状是否(至少在短期内)有效,仍不能确定[32-34]。关于氯氮平对阴性症状疗效的研究有一个潜在混杂因素,它较少引起包括运动迟缓在内的帕金森综合征,而这种不良反应在表现上与阴性症状有所重叠,尤其是表达缺陷这一子维度。

第1章

- 抗精神病药以外的药物干预方面,数种调节谷氨酸通路的药物已被作为辅助药物直接进行测试,但结果不理想。相比安慰剂,代谢型谷氨酸2/3(mGlu2/3)受体激动剂对阴性症状没有明显的疗效[35,36]。以其他方式调节 N-甲基-D-天冬氨酸受体(N-methyl-D-aspartic acid receptor,NMDA)的药物也接受了测试:作为抗精神病药的增效剂,随机对照试验结果为阴性的药物包括甘氨酸[37]、D-丝氨酸[38]、莫达非尼[39,40]、阿莫达非尼[41]以及比托派汀[42,43]。小样本预初试验阳性的药物有孕烯诺龙[44]。

- 关于减少谷氨酸传递的药物,拉莫三嗪作为氯氮平增效剂的荟萃分析结果不一致[45,46],美金刚的随机对照试验结果一项有效[47],一项却无效(还是样本量大得多的那项试验)[48]。有荟萃分析提示,加入抗菌和抗炎药米诺环素可以改善阴性症状,但总体样本量仍然较小[49,50]。BeneMin 研究旨在确定,在精神分裂症病程早期使用米诺环素辅助治疗,能否在一年内防止出现阴性症状,但研究结果没有提供任何临床益处的证据[51]。

- 关于抗抑郁药作为抗精神病药增效剂治疗阴性症状的疗效,Cochrane 综述认为,这可能是减轻情感平淡、失语和意志缺失的有效对策[52],但是随机对照试验发现抗抑郁药增效治疗的疗效有限,且证据不一致[53-56]。一项关于安慰剂对照研究的荟萃分析发现,在确诊精神分裂症的患者中,使用抗抑郁药辅助治疗,能有限地减轻阴性症状,但仅在作为第一代抗精神病药的增效治疗时有效[57]。另一项关于相关研究的系统综述认为,有证据表明一些 SSRI 是有效的,如氟伏沙明、西酞普兰、α_2 受体拮抗剂(米氮平和米安色林)[15]。瑞波西汀可能有效[58]。

- 在谷氨酸拮抗剂作为阴性症状的辅助治疗方面,有限的证据表明,托吡酯(一种去甲肾上腺素再摄取抑制剂)可能对包括阴性症状在内的精神分裂症谱系障碍的症状减轻有一定的疗效[59]。

- 荟萃分析支持银杏叶提取物[60]和 COX-2 抑制剂作为抗精神病药增效治疗的效果(尽管效应值很小)[61]。一些小样本随机对照试验证明下述药物有一些效果:司来吉兰[62,63]、普拉克索[64]、局部睾酮[65]、昂丹司琼[66]和格拉司琼[67]。重复经颅磁刺激(rTMS)的研究结果好坏参半,但很有希望[68-70]。经颅直流电刺激(tDCS)治疗阴性症状的证据有限且不确定[15,71]。一项在成年人中进行的大样本($n=250$)试验[72],以及在老年患者中进行的小样本随机对照试验[73],均发现多奈哌齐无效。还有一项随机对照试验发现加兰他敏无效[74]。

与不滥用精神活性物质的患者相比,滥用者出现的阴性症状要少[75]。与其说是药理作用,不如说是这种联系可能至少部分反映了使用精神活性物质(特别是大麻)情况下发生精神病者较少有神经发育风险因素,因此有更好的认知和社会功能[76,77]。

小结及建议

来自英国精神药理学会(British Association for Psychopharmacology,BAP)的2020年精神分裂症治疗指南[78],Veerman 等 2017[8],Aleman 等 2017[15] 和 Remington 等 2016[79]。

- 尚没有以阴性症状为主要结局指标的被较好重复的大型试验或荟萃分析证明(某种治疗手段)可以带来持久的、具有临床意义的益处。
- 一些临床试验发现阴性症状得到了改善,但可能局限于继发性阴性症状。
- 精神病性障碍应尽早识别和治疗,这样多少可以预防阴性症状的发生。

- 对于任何患者,抗精神病药的使用应基于总体疗效和不良反应之间的最佳平衡,且使用可以控制阳性症状的最小剂量。
- 如果阴性症状在精神病性障碍急性发作之后持续存在:
  - 应确保锥体外系症状(特别是动作迟缓)和抑郁症状得到及时发现和处理,同时还应考虑环境对阴性症状的影响(如长期住院、缺乏刺激)。
  - 目前,尚没有充分的证据推荐任何一种药物用来治疗阴性症状。尽管如此,某些情况下可以考虑加用随机对照试验证明有效的药物,如抗抑郁药。但需要确保选用的增效剂通过药代动力学或药效动力学相互作用产生的潜在不良反应最小。

参考文献

1. Messinger JW, et al. Avolition and expressive deficits capture negative symptom phenomenology: implications for DSM-5 and schizophrenia research. *Clin Psychol Rev* 2011; **31**:161–168.
2. Foussias G, et al. Dissecting negative symptoms in schizophrenia: opportunities for translation into new treatments. *J Psychopharmacology* 2015; **29**:116–126.
3. Carpenter WT. The treatment of negative symptoms: pharmacological and methodological issues. *Br J Psychiatry* 1996; **168**:17–22.
4. Galderisi S, et al. Persistent negative symptoms in first episode patients with schizophrenia: results from the European First Episode Schizophrenia Trial. *Eur Neuro PsychoPharmacol* 2013; **23**:196–204.
5. Buchanan RW. Persistent negative symptoms in schizophrenia: an overview. *Schizophr Bull* 2007; **33**:1013–1022.
6. Rabinowitz J, et al. Negative symptoms have greater impact on functioning than positive symptoms in schizophrenia: analysis of CATIE data. *Schizophr Res* 2012; **137**:147–150.
7. Barnes TRE, et al. How to distinguish between the neuroleptic-induced deficit syndrome, depression and disease-related negative symptoms in schizophrenia. *Int Clin Psychopharmacol* 1995; **10 Suppl** 3:115–121.
8. Veerman SRT, et al. Treatment for negative symptoms in schizophrenia: a comprehensive review. *Drugs* 2017; **77**:1423–1459.
9. Rammou A, et al. Negative symptoms in first-episode psychosis: clinical correlates and 1-year follow-up outcomes in London Early Intervention Services. *Early Interv Psychiatry* 2019; **13**:443–452.
10. Bobes J, et al. Prevalence of negative symptoms in outpatients with schizophrenia spectrum disorders treated with antipsychotics in routine clinical practice: findings from the CLAMORS study. *J Clin Psychiatry* 2010; **71**:280–286.
11. Buckley PF, et al. Pharmacological treatment of negative symptoms of schizophrenia: therapeutic opportunity or cul-de-sac? *Acta Psychiatr Scand* 2007; **115**:93–100.
12. Waddington JL, et al. Sequential cross-sectional and 10-year prospective study of severe negative symptoms in relation to duration of initially untreated psychosis in chronic schizophrenia. *Psychol Med* 1995; **25**:849–857.
13. Melle I, et al. Prevention of negative symptom psychopathologies in first-episode schizophrenia: two-year effects of reducing the duration of untreated psychosis. *Arch Gen Psychiatry* 2008; **65**:634–640.
14. Perkins DO, et al. Relationship between duration of untreated psychosis and outcome in first-episode schizophrenia: a critical review and meta-analysis. *Am J Psychiatry* 2005; **162**:1785–1804.
15. Aleman A, et al. Treatment of negative symptoms: where do we stand, and where do we go? *Schizophr Res* 2017; **186**:55–62.
16. Darba J, et al. Efficacy of second-generation-antipsychotics in the treatment of negative symptoms of schizophrenia: a meta-analysis of randomized clinical trials. *Rev Psiquiatr Salud Ment* 2011; **4**:126–143.
17. Leucht S, et al. Second-generation versus first-generation antipsychotic drugs for schizophrenia: a meta-analysis. *Lancet* 2009; **373**:31–41.
18. Erhart SM, et al. Treatment of schizophrenia negative symptoms: future prospects. *Schizophr Bull* 2006; **32**:234–237.
19. Harvey RC, et al. A systematic review and network meta-analysis to assess the relative efficacy of antipsychotics for the treatment of positive and negative symptoms in early-onset schizophrenia. *CNS Drugs* 2016; **30**:27–39.
20. Zhang JP, et al. Efficacy and safety of individual second-generation vs. first-generation antipsychotics in first-episode psychosis: a systematic review and meta-analysis. *Int J Neuro Psychopharmacol* 2013; **16**:1205–1218.
21. Leucht S, et al. A meta-analysis of head-to-head comparisons of second-generation antipsychotics in the treatment of schizophrenia. *Am J Psychiatry* 2009; **166**:152–163.
22. Fusar-Poli P, et al. Treatments of negative symptoms in schizophrenia: meta-analysis of 168 randomized placebo-controlled trials. *Schizophr Bull* 2015; **41**:892–899.
23. Krause M, et al. Antipsychotic drugs for patients with schizophrenia and predominant or prominent negative symptoms: a systematic review and meta-analysis. *Eur Arch Psychiatry Clin Neurosci* 2018; **268**:625–639.
24. Danion JM, et al. Improvement of schizophrenic patients with primary negative symptoms treated with amisulpride. Amisulpride Study Group. *Am J Psychiatry* 1999; **156**:610–616.
25. Speller JC, et al. One-year, low-dose neuroleptic study of in-patients with chronic schizophrenia characterised by persistent negative symptoms. Amisulpride v. haloperidol. *Br J Psychiatry* 1997; **171**:564–568.

26. Leucht S, et al. Amisulpride, an unusual 'atypical' antipsychotic: a meta-analysis of randomized controlled trials. *Am J Psychiatry* 2002; **159**:180–190.

27. Liang Y, et al. Effectiveness of amisulpride in Chinese patients with predominantly negative symptoms of schizophrenia: a subanalysis of the ESCAPE study. *Neuropsychiatr Dis Treat* 2017; **13**:1703–1712.

28. Németh B, et al. Quality-adjusted life year difference in patients with predominant negative symptoms of schizophrenia treated with cariprazine and risperidone. *J Comp Effect Res* 2017; **6**:639–648.

29. Németh G, et al. Cariprazine versus risperidone monotherapy for treatment of predominant negative symptoms in patients with schizophrenia: a randomised, double-blind, controlled trial. *Lancet* 2017; **389**:1103–1113.

30. Zheng W, et al. Efficacy and safety of adjunctive aripiprazole in schizophrenia: meta-analysis of randomized controlled trials. *J Clin Psychopharmacol* 2016; **36**:628–636.

31. Galling B, et al. Antipsychotic augmentation vs. monotherapy in schizophrenia: systematic review, meta-analysis and meta-regression analysis. *World Psychiatry* 2017; **16**:77–89.

32. Siskind D, et al. Clozapine v. first- and second-generation antipsychotics in treatment-refractory schizophrenia: systematic review and meta-analysis. *Br J Psychiatry* 2016; **209**:385–392.

33. Souza JS, et al. Efficacy of olanzapine in comparison with clozapine for treatment-resistant schizophrenia: evidence from a systematic review and meta-analyses. *CNS Spectr* 2013; **18**:82–89.

34. Asenjo Lobos C, et al. Clozapine versus other atypical antipsychotics for schizophrenia. *Cochrane Database Syst Rev* 2010; Cd006633.

35. Adams DH, et al. Pomaglumetad methionil (LY2140023 Monohydrate) and aripiprazole in patients with schizophrenia: a phase 3, multi-center, double-blind comparison. *Schizophr Res Treat* 2014; **2014**:758212.

36. Stauffer VL, et al. Pomaglumetad methionil: no significant difference as an adjunctive treatment for patients with prominent negative symptoms of schizophrenia compared to placebo. *Schizophr Res* 2013; **150**:434–441.

37. Buchanan RW, et al. The Cognitive and Negative Symptoms in Schizophrenia Trial (CONSIST): the efficacy of glutamatergic agents for negative symptoms and cognitive impairments. *Am J Psychiatry* 2007; **164**:1593–1602.

38. Weiser M, et al. A multicenter, add-on randomized controlled trial of low-dose d-serine for negative and cognitive symptoms of schizophrenia. *J Clin Psychiatry* 2012; **73**:e728–e734.

39. Pierre JM, et al. A randomized, double-blind, placebo-controlled trial of modafinil for negative symptoms in schizophrenia. *J Clin Psychiatry* 2007; **68**:705–710.

40. Sabe M, et al. Prodopaminergic drugs for treating the negative symptoms of schizophrenia: systematic review and meta-analysis of randomized controlled trials. *J Clin Psychopharmacol* 2019; **39**:658–664.

41. Kane JM, et al. Adjunctive armodafinil for negative symptoms in adults with schizophrenia: a double-blind, placebo-controlled study. *Schizophr Res* 2012; **135**:116–122.

42. Bugarski-Kirola D, et al. A phase II/III trial of bitopertin monotherapy compared with placebo in patients with an acute exacerbation of schizophrenia – results from the CandleLyte study. *Eur Neuropsychopharmacol* 2014; **24**:1024–1036.

43. Goff DC. Bitopertin: the good news and bad news. *JAMA Psychiatry* 2014; **71**:621–622.

44. Marx CE, et al. Proof-of-concept trial with the neurosteroid pregnenolone targeting cognitive and negative symptoms in schizophrenia. *Neuro Psycho Pharmacology* 2009; **34**:1885–1903.

45. Tiihonen J, et al. The efficacy of lamotrigine in clozapine-resistant schizophrenia: a systematic review and meta-analysis. *Schizophr Res* 2009; **109**:10–14.

46. Veerman SR, et al. Clozapine augmented with glutamate modulators in refractory schizophrenia: a review and metaanalysis. *Pharmacopsychiatry* 2014; **47**:185–194.

47. Rezaei F, et al. Memantine add-on to risperidone for treatment of negative symptoms in patients with stable schizophrenia: randomized, double-blind, placebo-controlled study. *J Clin Psycho Pharmacol* 2013; **33**:336–342.

48. Lieberman JA, et al. A randomized, placebo-controlled study of memantine as adjunctive treatment in patients with schizophrenia. *Neuro Psycho Pharmacology* 2009; **34**:1322–1329.

49. Oya K, et al. Efficacy and tolerability of minocycline augmentation therapy in schizophrenia: a systematic review and meta-analysis of randomized controlled trials. *Human Psycho Pharmacology* 2014; **29**:483–491.

50. Xiang YQ, et al. Adjunctive minocycline for schizophrenia: a meta-analysis of randomized controlled trials. *Eur Neuropsychopharmacol* 2017; **27**:8–18.

51. Deakin B, et al. The benefit of minocycline on negative symptoms of schizophrenia in patients with recent-onset psychosis (BeneMin): a randomised, double-blind, placebo-controlled trial. *Lancet Psychiatry* 2018; **5**:885–894.

52. Rummel C, et al. Antidepressants for the negative symptoms of schizophrenia. *Cochrane Database Syst Rev* 2006; **3**:CD005581.

53. Kishi T, et al. Meta-analysis of noradrenergic and specific serotonergic antidepressant use in schizophrenia. *Int J Neuropsychopharmacol* 2014; **17**:343–354.

54. Sepehry AA, et al. Selective serotonin reuptake inhibitor (SSRI) add-on therapy for the negative symptoms of schizophrenia: a meta-analysis. *J Clin Psychiatry* 2007; **68**:604–610.

55. Singh SP, et al. Efficacy of antidepressants in treating the negative symptoms of chronic schizophrenia: meta-analysis. *Br J Psychiatry* 2010; **197**:174–179.

56. Barnes TRE, et al. Antidepressant Controlled Trial For Negative Symptoms In Schizophrenia (ACTIONS): a double-blind, placebo-controlled, randomised clinical trial. *Health Technol Assess* 2016; **20**:1–46.

57. Galling B, et al. Efficacy and safety of antidepressant augmentation of continued antipsychotic treatment in patients with schizophrenia. *Acta Psychiatr Scand* 2018; **137**:187–205.

58. Zheng W, et al. Adjunctive reboxetine for schizophrenia: meta-analysis of randomized double-blind, placebo-controlled trials. *Pharmacopsychiatry* 2020; **53**:5–13.

59. Afshar H, et al. Topiramate add-on treatment in schizophrenia: a randomised, double-blind, placebo-controlled clinical trial. *J Psychopharmacology* 2009; 23:157–162.

60. Singh V, et al. Review and meta-analysis of usage of ginkgo as an adjunct therapy in chronic schizophrenia. *Int J Neuropsychopharmacol* 2010; 13:257–271.

61. Sommer IE, et al. Nonsteroidal anti-inflammatory drugs in schizophrenia: ready for practice or a good start? A meta-analysis. *J Clin Psychiatry* 2012; 73:414–419.

62. Amiri A, et al. Efficacy of selegiline add on therapy to risperidone in the treatment of the negative symptoms of schizophrenia: a double-blind randomized placebo-controlled study. *Human Psychopharmacology* 2008; 23:79–86.

63. Bodkin JA, et al. Double-blind, placebo-controlled, multicenter trial of selegiline augmentation of antipsychotic medication to treat negative symptoms in outpatients with schizophrenia. *Am J Psychiatry* 2005; 162:388–390.

64. Kelleher JP, et al. Pilot randomized, controlled trial of pramipexole to augment antipsychotic treatment. *Eur Neuro Psychopharmacol* 2012; 22:415–418.

65. Ko YH, et al. Short-term testosterone augmentation in male schizophrenics: a randomized, double-blind, placebo-controlled trial. *J Clin Psychopharmacol* 2008; 28:375–383.

66. Zhang ZJ, et al. Beneficial effects of ondansetron as an adjunct to haloperidol for chronic, treatment-resistant schizophrenia: a double-blind, randomized, placebo-controlled study. *Schizophr Res* 2006; 88:102–110.

67. Khodaie-Ardakani MR, et al. Granisetron as an add-on to risperidone for treatment of negative symptoms in patients with stable schizophrenia: randomized double-blind placebo-controlled study. *J Psychiatr Res* 2013; 47:472–478.

68. Shi C, et al. Revisiting the therapeutic effect of rTMS on negative symptoms in schizophrenia: a meta-analysis. *Psychiatry Res* 2014; 215:505–513.

69. Wobrock T, et al. Left prefrontal high-frequency repetitive transcranial magnetic stimulation for the treatment of schizophrenia with predominant negative symptoms: a sham-controlled, randomized multicenter trial. *Biol Psychiatry* 2015; 77:979–988.

70. Wang J, et al. Efficacy towards negative symptoms and safety of repetitive transcranial magnetic stimulation treatment for patients with schizophrenia: a systematic review. *Shanghai Arch Psychiatry* 2017; 29:61–76.

71. Mondino M, et al. Transcranial direct current stimulation for the treatment of refractory symptoms of schizophrenia. Current evidence and future directions. *Curr Pharm Des* 2015; 21:3373–3383.

72. Keefe RSE, et al. Efficacy and safety of donepezil in patients with schizophrenia or schizoaffective disorder: significant placebo/practice effects in a 12-week, randomized, double-blind, placebo-controlled trial. *Neuro Psycho Pharmacology* 2007; 33:1217–1228.

73. Mazeh D, et al. Donepezil for negative signs in elderly patients with schizophrenia: an add-on, double-blind, crossover, placebo-controlled study. *Int Psychogeriatr* 2006; 18:429–436.

74. Conley RR, et al. The effects of galantamine on psychopathology in chronic stable schizophrenia. *Clin Neuropharmacol* 2009; 32:69–74.

75. Potvin S, et al. A meta-analysis of negative symptoms in dual diagnosis schizophrenia. *Psychol Med* 2006; 36:431–440.

76. Arndt S, et al. Comorbidity of substance abuse and schizophrenia: the role of pre-morbid adjustment. *Psychol Med* 1992; 22:379–388.

77. Leeson VC, et al. The effect of cannabis use and cognitive reserve on age at onset and psychosis outcomes in first-episode schizophrenia. *Schizophr Bull* 2012; 38:873–880.

78. Barnes TRE, et al. Evidence-based guidelines for the pharmacological treatment of schizophrenia: updated recommendations from the British Association for Psychopharmacology. *J Psychopharmacology* 2020; 34:3–78.

79. Remington G, et al. Treating negative symptoms in schizophrenia: an update. *Curr Treat Options Psychiatry* 2016; 3:133–150.

监测

　　下表总结了建议使用抗精神病药治疗者做的监测[1]。然而,在多数国家中,这种监测进行得很少[2-5]。强烈推荐以下的指南,以确保这些药物的安全使用。更多细节、参考文献、背景资料见本章各节。

指标/检验	推荐频率	异常结果的处理	特别注意的药物	不需监测的药物
尿素和电解质 (包括肌酐和肾小球滤过率估计值)	基线和每年常规体检时	分析所有异常的原因	氨磺必利和舒必利经肾排出,若肾小球滤过率下降,应考虑减少剂量	无
全血计数(FBC)[6-11]	基线和每年常规体检时,目的是检测慢性骨髓抑制(某些抗精神病药有轻度风险)	若中性粒细胞少于 1.5×10^9/L,停用可疑药物。若中性粒细胞少于 0.5×10^9/L,转到专科治疗。注意:某些种族中良性白细胞减少症的发生率较高	氯氮平——18周内每周测查;之后每2周1次,至1年;1年后每月1次(各国不同)	无
血脂[12,13] (胆固醇、甘油三酯)尽可能空腹查	基线,3个月,之后每年1次。检测抗精神病药所致血脂改变,并全面监测身体健康状况	提供生活方式指导。考虑更换抗精神病药,或启用他汀类药物	氯氮平、奥氮平——第1年每3个月1次,之后每年1次	有的抗精神病药(如阿立哌唑、鲁拉西酮)与血脂异常间没有确切关联,但是在此患者群体中血脂异常的发生率高[14-16],因此应该监测所有患者
体重[12,14,16] (可能的话包括腰围和BMI)	基线,前3个月需频繁监测,之后每年1次。检测抗精神病药所致体重改变,并全面监测身体健康状况	提供生活方式指导。考虑更换抗精神病药,或饮食/药物干预	氯氮平、奥氮平——前3个月需频繁监测,之后第1年每3个月1次,之后每年1次	阿立哌唑、齐拉西酮、依匹哌唑、卡利拉嗪和鲁拉西酮与体重增加间无确切关联,但仍建议监测,因此患者群体中肥胖的发生率高
血糖 (尽可能空腹查)	基线,4~6个月,之后每年1次。检测抗精神病药所致血糖改变,并全面监测身体健康状况	提供生活方式指导。查空腹或非空腹血糖,以及HbA_{1C}。转给全科或专科医师	氯氮平、奥氮平、氯丙嗪——基线,1个月,之后4~6个月1次	有些抗精神病药与空腹血糖受损没有确切关联,但是在此患者群体中空腹血糖受损发生率高[17,18],因此所有患者均应监测

续表

指标/检验	推荐频率	异常结果的处理	特别注意的药物	不需监测的药物
心电图 [19,20]	基线和达到目标剂量时(临床中罕见心电图改变 [21]);入院初;若药物治疗方案变动,出院前也查	若有异常,应请教或转给心内科专家	氟哌啶醇、匹莫齐特、舍吲哚——必须检查;齐拉西酮——某些情况下必须检查	大多数抗精神病药导致心源性猝死风险升高 [22]。在理想情况下,所有患者最好每年至少查1次
血压	基线,剂量滴定和改变时需频繁监测,以检测抗精神病药引起的血压变化,并全面监测身体健康状况	若严重低血压或高血压(氯氮平),减缓加药速度。若为症状性直立性低血压,考虑换其他抗精神病药;高血压按 NICE 指南处理	氯氮平、氯丙嗪和喹硫平易致直立性低血压	氨磺必利、阿立哌唑、依匹哌唑、卡利拉嗪、鲁拉西酮、三氟拉嗪、舒必利
催乳素	基线,6个月,之后每年1次,目的是检测抗精神病药引起的改变	若证实高催乳素血症且有症状,换药。对于催乳素长期升高者,考虑检测骨密度(如 DEXA 扫描)	氨磺必利、舒必利、利培酮和帕利哌酮易致高催乳素血症	阿塞那平、阿立哌唑、依匹哌唑、卡利拉嗪、氯氮平、鲁拉西酮、喹硫平、奥氮平(<20mg/d)、齐拉西酮一般不升高催乳素,但若出现症状,应测查
肝功能 [23-25]	基线,之后每年常规体检时。检测长期使用抗精神病药引起的变化(罕见)	若提示有肝炎(转氨酶是正常值3倍)或肝功损害(凝血酶原时间/白蛋白改变),应停用可疑药物	氯氮平和氯丙嗪可导致肝功能衰竭	氨磺必利、舒必利
肌酸磷酸激酶(CPK)	基线,疑有恶性综合征时	见"恶性综合征"	高效价第一代抗精神病药易致恶性综合征	无

其他检查:服用氯氮平时应查脑电图 [26,27],有助于决定是否需用丙戊酸盐(尽管其解释显然比较复杂)。服用喹硫平时,应该每年检查**甲状腺**功能,尽管异常的风险极低 [28,29]。

BMI,体重指数;DEXA,双能 X 线吸收测定法。

注:该表为总结概要,详细内容见本章各节。

参考文献

1. National Institute for Clinical Excellence. Psychosis and schizophrenia: what monitoring is required? Clinical Knowledge Summaries. 2014 (last revised November 2020); https://cks.nice.org.uk/topics/psychosis-schizophrenia/prescribing-information/monitoring/#:~:text=References-,What%20monitoring%20is%20required%3F,stabilized%20(whichever%20is%20longer).

2. Bulteau S, et al. Advocacy for better metabolic monitoring after antipsychotic initiation: based on data from a French health insurance database. *Exp Opin Drug Saf* 2021; 20:225–233.

3. Lydon A, et al. Routine screening and rates of metabolic syndrome in patients treated with clozapine and long-acting injectable antipsychotic

medications: a cross-sectional study. *Ir J Psychol Med* 2021; 38:40–48.

4. Poojari PG, et al. Identification of risk factors and metabolic monitoring practices in patients on antipsychotic drugs in South India. *Asian J Psychiatr* 2020; 53:102186.

5. Perry BI, et al. Prolactin monitoring in the acute psychiatry setting. *Psychiatry Res* 2016; 235:104–109.

6. Burckart GJ, et al. Neutropenia following acute chlorpromazine ingestion. *Clin Toxicol* 1981; 18:797–801.

7. Grohmann R, et al. Agranulocytosis and significant leucopenia with neuroleptic drugs: results from the AMUP program. *Psychopharmacology* 1989; 99 Suppl:S109–S112.

8. Esposito D, et al. Risperidone-induced morning pseudoneutropenia. *Am J Psychiatry* 2005; 162:397.

9. Montgomery J. Ziprasidone-related agranulocytosis following olanzapine-induced neutropenia. *Gen Hosp Psychiatry* 2006; 28:83–85.

10. Cowan C, et al. Leukopenia and neutropenia induced by quetiapine. *Prog Neuropsychopharmacol Biol Psychiatry* 2007; 31:292–294.

11. Buchman N, et al. Olanzapine-induced leukopenia with human leukocyte antigen profiling. *Int Clin Psychopharmacol* 2001; 16:55–57.

12. Marder SR, et al. Physical health monitoring of patients with schizophrenia. *Am J Psychiatry* 2004; 161:1334–1349.

13. Fenton WS, et al. Medication-induced weight gain and dyslipidemia in patients with schizophrenia. *Am J Psychiatry* 2006; 163:1697–1704.

14. Weissman EM, et al. Lipid monitoring in patients with schizophrenia prescribed second-generation antipsychotics. *J Clin Psychiatry* 2006; 67:1323–1326.

15. Cohn TA, et al. Metabolic monitoring for patients treated with antipsychotic medications. *Can J Psychiatry* 2006; 51:492–501.

16. Paton C, et al. Obesity, dyslipidaemias and smoking in an inpatient population treated with antipsychotic drugs. *Acta Psychiatr Scand* 2004; 110:299–305.

17. Taylor D, et al. Undiagnosed impaired fasting glucose and diabetes mellitus amongst inpatients receiving antipsychotic drugs. *J Psychopharmacology* 2005; 19:182–186.

18. Citrome L, et al. Incidence, prevalence, and surveillance for diabetes in New York State psychiatric hospitals, 1997–2004. *Psychiatr Serv* 2006; 57:1132–1139.

19. Barnes T, et al. Evidence-based guidelines for the pharmacological treatment of schizophrenia: updated recommendations from the British Association for Psychopharmacology. *J Psychopharmacology* 2020; 34:3–78.

20. Shah AA, et al. QTc prolongation with antipsychotics: is routine ECG monitoring recommended? *J Psychiatr Pract* 2014; 20:196–206.

21. Novotny T, et al. Monitoring of QT interval in patients treated with psychotropic drugs. *Int J Cardiol* 2007; 117:329–332.

22. Ray WA, et al. Atypical antipsychotic drugs and the risk of sudden cardiac death. *N Engl J Med* 2009; 360:225–235.

23. Hummer M, et al. Hepatotoxicity of clozapine. *J Clin Psychopharmacol* 1997; 17:314–317.

24. Erdogan A, et al. Management of marked liver enzyme increase during clozapine treatment: a case report and review of the literature. *Int J Psychiatry Med* 2004; 34:83–89.

25. Regal RE, et al. Phenothiazine-induced cholestatic jaundice. *Clin Pharm* 1987; 6:787–794.

26. Centorrino F, et al. EEG abnormalities during treatment with typical and atypical antipsychotics. *Am J Psychiatry* 2002; 159:109–115.

27. Gross A, et al. Clozapine-induced QEEG changes correlate with clinical response in schizophrenic patients: a prospective, longitudinal study. *Pharmacopsychiatry* 2004; 37:119–122.

28. Twaites BR, et al. The safety of quetiapine: results of a post-marketing surveillance study on 1728 patients in England. *J Psychopharmacology* 2007; 21:392–399.

29. Kelly DL, et al. Thyroid function in treatment-resistant schizophrenia patients treated with quetiapine, risperidone, or fluphenazine. *J Clin Psychiatry* 2005; 66:80–84.

不良反应比较 ——大致指导

药物	镇静	体重增加	静坐不能	帕金森综合征	抗胆碱能作用	低血压	催乳素升高
氨磺必利 *	–	+	+	+	–	–	+++
阿立哌唑	–	–	+	–	–	–	–
阿塞那平 *	+	+	+	–	–	–	+
苯哌利多 *	+	+	+	+++	+	+	+++
依匹哌唑 *							
卡利拉嗪 *	–	–	+	–	–	–	–
氯丙嗪	+++	++	+	++	++	+++	+++
氯氮平	+++	+++	–	–	+++	+++	–
氟哌噻吨 *	+	++	++	++	++	–	+++
氟奋乃静 *	+	+	++	+++	+	–	+++
氟哌啶醇	+	+	+++	+++	+	+	++
伊潘立酮 *	–	++	+	+	–	+	–
卢美哌隆 *	++	–	–	–	–	–	–
洛沙平 *	++	+	+	+++	+	++	+++
鲁拉西酮	+	–	+	+	–	–	–
奥氮平	++	+++	–	–	+	–	+
帕利哌酮	+	++	+	+	+	++	+++
奋乃静	+	+	++	+++	+	+	+++
匹莫范色林 *	–	–	–	–	–	–	–
匹莫齐特 *	+	+	+	+	+	+	+++
哌泊噻嗪 *	++	++	+	++	++	++	+++
丙嗪 *	+++	++	+	+	++	++	++
喹硫平	++	++	–	–	+	++	–
利培酮	+	++	+	+	+	++	+++
舍吲哚 *	–	+	+	–		+++	
舒必利 *	–	+	+	+	–	–	+++
三氟拉嗪	+	+	+	+++	+	+	+++
齐拉西酮 *	+	–	+	–	–	+	+
珠氯噻醇 *	++	++	++	++	++	+	+++

* 可获得性因国家而异。+++ 高发生率/严重程度,++ 中度,+ 低,– 非常低。

注:此表是基于临床经验、制药企业文件和公开发表的研究文献对发生率和/或严重程度进行的大致估计。这是非常粗糙的指导。更准确的信息见各个章节。

本表未提及的不良反应也可能发生,请详细阅读本书关于其他不良反应的章节。

精神分裂症治疗流程

首发精神分裂症

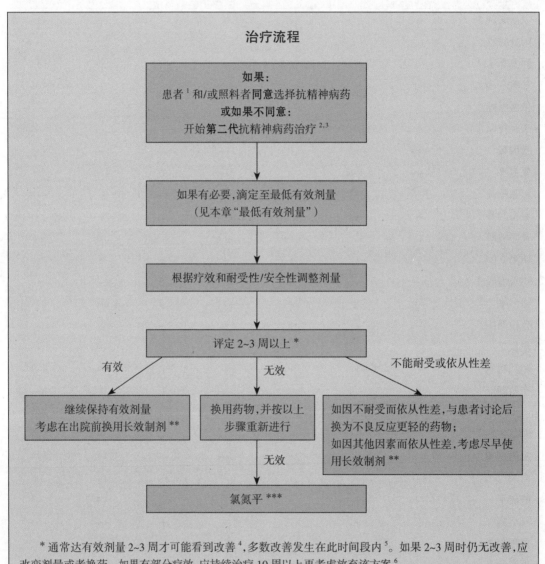

* 通常达有效剂量 2~3 周才可能看到改善[4]，多数改善发生在此时间段内[5]。如果 2~3 周时仍无改善，应改变剂量或者换药。如果有部分疗效，应持续治疗 10 周以上再考虑放弃该方案[6]。

** 在该组患者中早期使用长效制剂可以显著降低复发率和再住院率[7-9]。首发患者可以接受长效制剂[10]。

*** 早期使用氯氮平可能比其他方法更有效[6,11]。不愿使用氯氮平与预后不良相关[12]。

复发或急性加重的精神分裂症（已证实完全依从药物治疗）

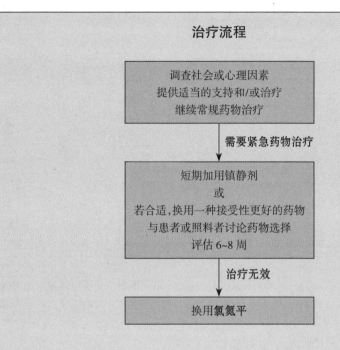

治疗流程

> 调查社会或心理因素
> 提供适当的支持和/或治疗
> 继续常规药物治疗

需要紧急药物治疗

> 短期加用镇静剂
> 或
> 若合适，换用一种接受性更好的药物
> 与患者或照料者讨论药物选择
> 评估 6~8 周

治疗无效

> 换用氯氮平

注：

- 与某些第二代抗精神病药相比，第一代抗精神病药效果稍差[13,14]。第一代抗精神病药也许应作为二线药物使用（或完全不用），因为与第二代抗精神病药相比，其效果可能较差，且引起运动障碍（特别是迟发性运动障碍）的风险高[15,16]。
- 选择治疗时很大程度上要考虑其不良反应和相对毒性。患者似乎有能力基于这些因素做出知情选择[17,18]，但在既往的临床实践中他们很少能参与到药物选择中[19]。让患者做出知情选择似乎可以改善结局[1]。
- 以往治疗不理想的患者（但并未证实为难治性病例），选择奥氮平或利培酮要比喹硫平更好[20]。现有的研究证据表明，奥氮平疗效略优于其他抗精神病药，在决定使用氯氮平之前，应先尝试奥氮平治疗，除非存在禁忌证[21-24]。但需要注意的是，一项随机对照试验发现，继续氨磺必利治疗与换用奥氮平同样有效[6]。
- 在考虑氯氮平治疗前，确定患者对先前治疗的依从性良好，方法是使用长效制剂，或口服治疗时监测血浆药物水平。临床实践中大多数不依从并没有被监测到[23,25]，且表面上对治疗的抵抗可能仅仅因为不充分的治疗[26]。
- 精神分裂症多次发作时，药物起效时间延长，总有效率下降[27]。
- 对于确认的难治性患者（对至少 2 种抗精神病药充分治疗无效），大量证据支持使用氯氮平（且仅能使用氯氮平）[28,29]。

复发或急性加重的精神分裂症（依从性存疑或依从性差）

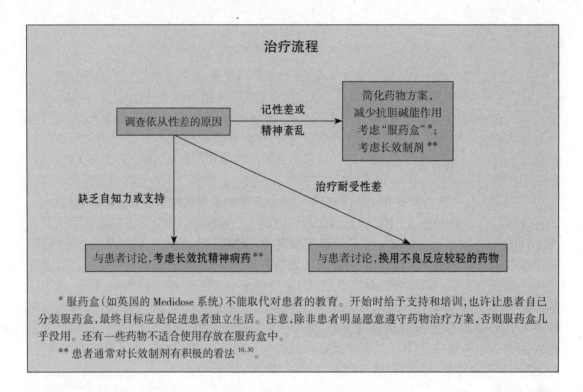

治疗流程

调查依从性差的原因

记性差或
精神紊乱

简化药物方案，
减少抗胆碱能作用
考虑"服药盒"＊；
考虑长效制剂＊＊

缺乏自知力或支持

治疗耐受性差

与患者讨论，考虑长效抗精神病药＊＊

与患者讨论，换用不良反应较轻的药物

　　＊服药盒（如英国的 Medidose 系统）不能取代对患者的教育。开始时给予支持和培训，也许让患者自己分装服药盒，最终目标应是促进患者独立生活。注意，除非患者明显愿意遵守药物治疗方案，否则服药盒几乎没用。还有一些药物不适合使用存放在服药盒中。
　　＊＊患者通常对长效制剂有积极的看法[10,30]。

参考文献

1. Robinson DG, et al. Psychopharmacological treatment in the RAISE-ETP study: outcomes of a manual and computer decision support system based intervention. *Am J Psychiatry* 2018; 175:169–179.

2. Zhu Y, et al. Antipsychotic drugs for the acute treatment of patients with a first episode of schizophrenia: a systematic review with pairwise and network meta-analyses. *Lancet Psychiatry* 2017; 4:694–705.

3. Zhang JP, et al. Efficacy and safety of individual second-generation vs. first-generation antipsychotics in first-episode psychosis: a systematic review and meta-analysis. *Int J Neuropsychopharmacol* 2013; 16:1205–1218.

4. Leucht S, et al. Early-onset hypothesis of antipsychotic drug action: a hypothesis tested, confirmed and extended. *Biol Psychiatry* 2005; 57:1543–1549.

5. Agid O, et al. The 'delayed onset' of antipsychotic action–an idea whose time has come and gone. *J Psychiatry Neurosci* 2006; 31:93–100.

6. Kahn RS, et al. Amisulpride and olanzapine followed by open-label treatment with clozapine in first-episode schizophrenia and schizophreniform disorder (OPTiMiSE): a three-phase switching study. *Lancet Psychiatry* 2018; 5:797–807.

7. Subotnik KL, et al. Long-acting injectable risperidone for relapse prevention and control of breakthrough symptoms after a recent first episode of schizophrenia. a randomized clinical trial. *JAMA Psychiatry* 2015; 72:822–829.

8. Schreiner A, et al. Paliperidone palmitate versus oral antipsychotics in recently diagnosed schizophrenia. *Schizophr Res* 2015; 169:393–399.

9. Alphs L, et al. Treatment effect with paliperidone palmitate compared with oral antipsychotics in patients with recent-onset versus more chronic schizophrenia and a history of criminal justice system involvement. *Early Intervention in Psychiatry* 2018; 12:55–65.

10. Kane JM, et al. Patients with early-phase schizophrenia will accept treatment with sustained-release medication (Long-Acting Injectable Antipsychotics): results from the recruitment phase of the PRELAPSE trial. *J Clin Psychiatry* 2019; 80:18m12546.

11. Agid O, et al. An algorithm-based approach to first-episode schizophrenia: response rates over 3 prospective antipsychotic trials with a retrospective data analysis. *J Clin Psychiatry* 2011; 72:1439–1444.

12. Drosos P, et al. One-year outcome and adherence to pharmacological guidelines in first-episode schizophrenia: results from a consecutive cohort study. *J Clin Psychopharmacol* 2020; 40:534–540.

13. Davis JM, et al. A meta-analysis of the efficacy of second-generation antipsychotics. *Arch Gen Psychiatry* 2003; 60:553–564.

14. Leucht S, et al. Second-generation versus first-generation antipsychotic drugs for schizophrenia: a meta-analysis. *Lancet* 2009; 373:31–41.

15. Schooler N, et al. Risperidone and haloperidol in first-episode psychosis: a long-term randomized trial. *Am J Psychiatry* 2005;

162:947–953.

16. Oosthuizen PP, et al. Incidence of tardive dyskinesia in first-episode psychosis patients treated with low-dose haloperidol. *J Clin Psychiatry* 2003; **64**:1075–1080.

17. Whiskey E, et al. Evaluation of an antipsychotic information sheet for patients. *Int J Psychiatry Clin Pract* 2005; **9**:264–270.

18. Stroup TS, et al. Results of phase 3 of the CATIE schizophrenia trial. *Schizophr Res* 2009; **107**:1–12.

19. Olofinjana B, et al. Antipsychotic drugs – information and choice: a patient survey. *Psychiatric Bulletin* 2005; **29**:369–371.

20. Stroup TS, et al. Effectiveness of olanzapine, quetiapine, risperidone, and ziprasidone in patients with chronic schizophrenia following discontinuation of a previous atypical antipsychotic. *Am J Psychiatry* 2006; **163**:611–622.

21. Haro JM, et al. Remission and relapse in the outpatient care of schizophrenia: three-year results from the Schizophrenia Outpatient Health Outcomes study. *J Clin Psychopharmacol* 2006; **26**:571–578.

22. Novick D, et al. Recovery in the outpatient setting: 36-month results from the Schizophrenia Outpatients Health Outcomes (SOHO) study. *Schizophr Res* 2009; **108**:223–230.

23. Tiihonen J, et al. Effectiveness of antipsychotic treatments in a nationwide cohort of patients in community care after first hospitalisation due to schizophrenia and schizoaffective disorder: observational follow-up study. *BMJ* 2006; **333**:224.

24. Leucht S, et al. A meta-analysis of head-to-head comparisons of second-generation antipsychotics in the treatment of schizophrenia. *Am J Psychiatry* 2009; **166**:152–163.

25. Remington G, et al. The use of electronic monitoring (MEMS) to evaluate antipsychotic compliance in outpatients with schizophrenia. *Schizophr Res* 2007; **90**:229–237.

26. McCutcheon R, et al. Antipsychotic plasma levels in the assessment of poor treatment response in schizophrenia. *Acta Psychiatr Scand* 2018; **137**:39–46.

27. Takeuchi H, et al. Does relapse contribute to treatment resistance? Antipsychotic response in first- vs. second-episode schizophrenia. *Neuropsychopharmacology* 2019; **44**:1036–1042.

28. McEvoy JP, et al. Effectiveness of clozapine versus olanzapine, quetiapine, and risperidone in patients with chronic schizophrenia who did not respond to prior atypical antipsychotic treatment. *Am J Psychiatry* 2006; **163**:600–610.

29. Lewis SW, et al. Randomized controlled trial of effect of prescription of clozapine versus other second-generation antipsychotic drugs in resistant schizophrenia. *Schizophr Bull* 2006; **32**:715–723.

30. Mace S, et al. Positive views on antipsychotic long-acting injections: results of a survey of community patients prescribed antipsychotics. *Ther Adv Psychopharmacol* 2019; **9**:2045125319860977.

第一代抗精神病药的治疗地位

命名

　　所谓第一代（"典型"）和第二代（"非典型"）抗精神病药，并非按药物分类学定义来区分。不管是第一代还是第二代抗精神病药，其包含的药物在药理作用和不良反应方面都有所不同。第一代抗精神病药在 1990 年以前上市，通常易导致急性锥体外系症状、高催乳素血症，长期使用可能导致迟发性运动障碍。人们期望第二代抗精神病药（1990 年以后上市）较少或不导致这些不良反应，但在临床实践中，大多数药物会导致剂量相关的锥体外系症状，有些会引起高催乳素血症（程度通常比第一代抗精神病药更重），都可能导致迟发性运动障碍，但是发生率低于第一代抗精神病药。第二代抗精神病药往往与代谢和心脏并发症有关 [1-3]，尽管并非所有第二代抗精神病药都是如此，但某些第一代抗精神病药却是如此。更为复杂的是，有研究者提出通过仔细的剂量调整，能将第一代抗精神病药的治疗作用和不良反应分开 [4]，从而使得第一代抗精神病药有可能变成第二代抗精神病药（尽管有许多相反的证据 [5-7]）。

　　鉴于这些观察报告，将所谓第一代与第二代抗精神病药分为截然不同的两组并不明智，也没有用处。两者基本区别是急性 EPS 相关的治疗指数宽窄不同。例如，氟哌啶醇发挥效果但又不引起 EPS 时，其剂量范围非常窄（可能 4.0~4.5mg/d）；奥氮平则在较宽的治疗剂量范围（5~40mg/d）内通常不引起 EPS。

　　基于神经科学的命名法（neuroscience-based nomenclature，NbN）（在 iPhone 和其他设备上有免费 APP）可以避免将药物归入第一代或第二代抗精神病药，而是对每个药的药理活性进行描述。毫无疑问，NbN 的广泛应用将提高人们对单个药物作用的理解，并可能防止将来的冗余分类方法。

老一代抗精神病药的作用

　　第一代抗精神病药在精神分裂症治疗中仍在发挥重要的作用。例如，氯丙嗪和氟哌啶醇经常作为 PRN（必要时）处方的选择，氟哌啶醇、珠氯噻醇和氟哌噻吨长效制剂常被使用。若第二代抗精神病药难以耐受（通常是由于代谢改变），或第一代抗精神病药受患者青睐，则第一代抗精神病药可以作为有效的替代品。某些第一代抗精神病药在疗效方面可能逊色于除氯氮平以外的第二代抗精神病药（氨磺必利、奥氮平和利培酮等可能疗效更好 [3,4]），但这种疗效差异非常有限。两项大型实用性临床研究 CATIE[8] 和 CUtLASS[5] 发现，第二代和第一代抗精神病药（分别主要是奋乃静和舒必利）间没有明显的疗效差异。

　　第一代抗精神病药的主要缺点是不可避免地会引起急性锥体外系症状、高催乳素血症和迟发性运动障碍。高催乳素血症在临床上很难避免（药物起效的剂量与引起高催乳素血症的剂量太接近），而且即使未出现临床症状，仍可能明显影响下丘脑功能 [6]。它也与性功能障碍有关 [7]，但需要注意的是，某些第二代抗精神病药导致的自主神经反应也可能引起性功能障碍 [8]。有些第二代抗精神病药（利培酮、帕利哌酮、氨磺必利）引起的催乳素升高比第一代抗精神病药更明显 [9]。

　　所有第一代抗精神病药都是多巴胺的强拮抗剂,容易导致烦躁不安[10]。因此,相比某些第二代抗精神病药,第一代抗精神病药对生活质量的改善可能较小[11]。

　　迟发性运动障碍在第一代抗精神病药中可能要比第二代更常见[12-15](尽管很难定义"非典型"),但是仍然存在一些不确定因素[15-17],而且第一代抗精神病药的剂量是关键性因素。在第二代抗精神病药中,受体的部分激动剂引起迟发性运动障碍的风险可能最低[18]。仔细观察患者并开具最低有效剂量的药物,有助于降低这种严重不良反应的风险[19,20]。即使如此小心,第一代抗精神病药所致迟发性运动障碍的风险仍非常高[21]。

　　关于第二代抗精神病药与仔细调整剂量的第一代抗精神病药的优点,一个很好的例子是一项棕榈酸帕利哌酮和低剂量氟哌啶醇癸酸酯的比较研究[22]。结果发现,帕利哌酮更易导致体重增加和催乳素变化,氟哌啶醇更多引起静坐不能和帕金森综合征,以及更高的迟发性运动障碍发生率。二者的临床疗效相同。

参考文献

1. Blier P, et al. Progress on the neuroscience-based nomenclature (NbN) for psychotropic medications. *Neuropsychopharmacology* 2017; **42**:1927–1928.
2. Caraci F, et al. A new nomenclature for classifying psychotropic drugs. *Br J Clin Pharmacol* 2017; **83**:1614–1616.
3. Davis JM, et al. A meta-analysis of the efficacy of second-generation antipsychotics. *Arch Gen Psychiatry* 2003; **60**:553–564.
4. Leucht S, et al. Second-generation versus first-generation antipsychotic drugs for schizophrenia: a meta-analysis. *Lancet* 2009; **373**:31–41.
5. Jones PB, et al. Randomized controlled trial of the effect on quality of life of second- vs first-generation antipsychotic drugs in schizophrenia: Cost Utility of the Latest Antipsychotic Drugs in Schizophrenia Study (CUtLASS 1). *Arch Gen Psychiatry* 2006; **63**:1079–1087.
6. Smith S, et al. The effects of antipsychotic-induced hyperprolactinaemia on the hypothalamic-pituitary-gonadal axis. *J Clin Psychopharmacol* 2002; **22**:109–114.
7. Smith SM, et al. Sexual dysfunction in patients taking conventional antipsychotic medication. *Br J Psychiatry* 2002; **181**:49–55.
8. Aizenberg D, et al. Comparison of sexual dysfunction in male schizophrenic patients maintained on treatment with classical antipsychotics versus clozapine. *J Clin Psychiatry* 2001; **62**:541–544.
9. Leucht S, et al. Comparative efficacy and tolerability of 15 antipsychotic drugs in schizophrenia: a multiple-treatments meta-analysis. *Lancet* 2013; **382**:951–962.
10. King DJ, et al. Antipsychotic drug-induced dysphoria. *Br J Psychiatry* 1995; **167**:480–482.
11. Grunder G, et al. Effects of first-generation antipsychotics versus second-generation antipsychotics on quality of life in schizophrenia: a double-blind, randomised study. *Lancet Psychiatry* 2016; **3**:717–729.
12. Tollefson GD, et al. Blind, controlled, long-term study of the comparative incidence of treatment-emergent tardive dyskinesia with olanzapine or haloperidol. *Am J Psychiatry* 1997; **154**:1248–1254.
13. Beasley C, et al. Randomised double-blind comparison of the incidence of tardive dyskinesia in patients with schizophrenia during long-term treatment with olanzapine or haloperidol. *Br J Psychiatry* 1999; **174**:23–30.
14. Correll CU, et al. Lower risk for tardive dyskinesia associated with second-generation antipsychotics: a systematic review of 1-year studies. *Am J Psychiatry* 2004; **161**:414–425.
15. Novick D, et al. Tolerability of outpatient antipsychotic treatment: 36-month results from the European Schizophrenia Outpatient Health Outcomes (SOHO) study. *Eur Neuropsychopharmacol* 2009; **19**:542–550.
16. Halliday J, et al. Nithsdale Schizophrenia Surveys 23: movement disorders. 20-year review. *Br J Psychiatry* 2002; **181**:422–427.
17. Miller DD, et al. Extrapyramidal side-effects of antipsychotics in a randomised trial. *Br J Psychiatry* 2008; **193**:279–288.
18. Carbon M, et al. Tardive dyskinesia prevalence in the period of second-generation antipsychotic use: a meta-analysis. *J Clin Psychiatry* 2017; **78**:e264–e278.
19. Jeste DV, et al. Tardive dyskinesia. *Schizophr Bull* 1993; **19**:303–315.
20. Cavallaro R, et al. Recognition, avoidance, and management of antipsychotic-induced tardive dyskinesia. *CNS Drugs* 1995; **4**:278–293.
21. Oosthuizen P, et al. A randomized, controlled comparison of the efficacy and tolerability of low and high doses of haloperidol in the treatment of first-episode psychosis. *Int J Neuropsychopharmacol* 2004; **7**:125–131.
22. McEvoy JP, et al. Effectiveness of paliperidone palmitate vs haloperidol decanoate for maintenance treatment of schizophrenia: a randomized clinical trial. *JAMA* 2014; **311**:1978–1987.

精神分裂症治疗的 NICE 指南 [1]

　　2009 年版的 NICE 指南[1]与以往相比有了一些重要的变化。它不再规定必须以"非典型"抗精神病药作为一线治疗选择。使用两种抗精神病药无效时,只是推荐将氯氮平作为一个选择(而不是直接处方)。这些语义上的差异,分别指出了对第二代抗精神病药不再抱幻想,以及承认在临床实践中应推迟氯氮平的使用。更多地强调患者及其照料者参与处方决策的重要性。一些证据表明这么做的极少[2],但是可以这么做[3]。新版 NICE 指南在 2014 年 2 月面世,并于 2019 年 3 月重审。

NICE 指南相关要点

- 对新近诊断为精神分裂症的患者,应给予口服抗精神病药治疗和心理干预(CBT 或家庭干预)。提供相关的药物信息,与患者及其家属商讨所用药物的治疗获益和不良反应特点。药物的选择应由使用者和保健人员一起决定,并考虑以下内容:
  - 抗精神病药导致下述不良反应的潜在风险:EPS(包括静坐不能)、心血管系统不良反应、代谢相关不良反应(包括体重增加)、内分泌相关不良反应(包括催乳素水平升高)和其他不良反应(包括患者主观不适体验)。
  - 得到患者赞成的照料者的观点。
- 在启用抗精神病药之前,进行以下基线检查并记录:
  - 体重
  - 腰围
  - 脉搏和血压
  - 空腹血糖、HbA_{1C}、血脂、催乳素
  - 评估运动障碍
  - 评估营养状况、饮食和躯体活动水平
- 在启用抗精神病药治疗精神分裂症之前,如果存在以下情况,应对患者进行心电图检查:
  - 在产品特征概要中注明的。
  - 体检发现特定心血管病风险(如有高血压病)。
  - 有心血管病史。
  - 住院治疗的患者。
- 抗精神病药的治疗应明确作为对患者个体的治疗试验,包括以下内容:
  - 记录口服抗精神病药的适应证、预期获益和风险、预计症状发生变化和不良反应出现的时间。
  - 治疗开始阶段,应从药物说明书剂量范围的最低剂量起始,然后,在英国处方集或产品特征概要中标明的剂量范围内缓慢加量。
  - 如果超过英国处方集或产品特征概要中标明的剂量范围,应说明原因并记录备案。
  - 记录继续治疗、换药或停药的原因及效果。
  - 以最佳用药剂量进行 4~6 周的试验(如果完全无效,也许 1/2 的时间就足够了)。
- 在整个治疗过程中,特别是加量阶段,应定期、系统地监测和记录以下内容:

■ 疗效,包括症状和行为的变化。

■ 治疗中的不良反应,包括某些不良反应与精神分裂症临床表现的重叠,如静坐不能与激越或焦虑的重叠。

■ 依从性。

■ 体重,前 6 周每周监测,随后在第 12 周、第 1 年的时候监测,然后每年监测。

■ 每年监测腰围。

■ 脉搏和血压:在第 12 周和第 1 年时监测,然后每年监测。

■ 空腹血糖、HbA_{1C} 和血脂:在第 12 周和第 1 年时监测,然后每年监测。

■ 营养状况、饮食和躯体活动水平。

■ 二级保健人员负责躯体监测 1 年,或者到患者病情稳定为止。

■ 在合适的情况下,与患者及照料者讨论酒精、烟草、处方药、非处方药以及非法药物的使用。讨论它们与所处方药物及心理治疗的潜在相互作用。

■ 不使用抗精神病药的负荷剂量(往往指"快速神经阻滞化")。(注意这一点不适用于奥氮平和帕利哌酮长效制剂的负荷剂量。)

■ 不要常规的一开始就规律合用抗精神病药,除非短期合用(如换药时)。

■ 如果使用氯丙嗪,应告诫可能引起皮肤的光敏性反应。必要时,建议使用防晒霜。

■ 对以下精神分裂症患者,考虑提供抗精神病药长效制剂治疗:

　　■ 在急性期后,喜欢这种治疗方式。

　　■ 已知对口服药物不依从和/或喜欢这种治疗方式。

■ 在进行心理治疗的同时,若先后使用至少两种不同抗精神病药足量治疗疗效仍不充分,才考虑使用氯氮平治疗。需排除非法药物滥用(包括酒精)、其他处方药物的使用及躯体疾病。这两种药物中,至少一种是除氯氮平外的第二代抗精神病药。(见精神分裂症治疗流程——我们建议治疗药物之一应该是奥氮平。)

■ 精神分裂症患者在使用优化剂量的氯氮平治疗后仍无足够疗效时,医疗专家应首先确认患者的治疗依从性(包括血药浓度监测)和心理治疗的参与情况,再加用第二种抗精神病药增强氯氮平疗效。实施这种增效治疗的话,可能需要观察 8~10 周(一些资料认为 6 周可能足够[4])。增效剂应选择与氯氮平常见不良反应不重叠的药物。

参考文献

1. National Institute for Health and Care Excellence. Psychosis and schizophrenia in adults: prevention and management. Clinical Guidance [CG178]. 2014 (last checked March 2019); https://www.nice.org.uk/guidance/cg178.
2. Olofinjana B, et al. Antipsychotic drugs – information and choice: a patient survey. *Psychiatric Bull* 2005;**29**:369–371.
3. Whiskey E, et al. Evaluation of an antipsychotic information sheet for patients. *Int J Psychiatry Clin Pract* 2005;9:264–270.
4. Taylor D, et al. Augmentation of clozapine with a second antipsychotic. A meta analysis. *Acta Psychiatr Scand* 2012;125:15–24.

抗精神病药的治疗反应——加量、换药、联用或等待,哪个正确

对于积极治疗精神分裂症的任何医师而言,临床上最让人进退两难的是,所用抗精神病药治疗不理想时,怎么办? 可能有以下两大原因:首先,是症状控制良好,但不良反应无法耐受;其次,是疗效不理想。幸运的是,对于第一个原因,由于有各种各样的抗精神病药,往往可以找到不良反应能够被患者接受的药物。对于第二个原因疗效不充分,下一步做什么是比较困难的问题。如果患者已经先后接受过两种不同的抗精神病药足量、足疗程治疗,且依从性良好,但是病情仍未充分改善,显然应该考虑选择氯氮平。但是,如果患者不愿意接受氯氮平,临床医师有四种选择:增加所用药物的剂量;换成另一种抗精神病药;加用辅助药物;或只能监测病情,希望外界因素的变化能让病情好转。

何时加量

虽然第一代抗精神病药的最佳剂量始终是一个充满争议的话题,但是第二代抗精神病药的推荐剂量通常基于严格、广泛的临床试验。即便如此,对其最佳剂量的共识也随着时间而变化。例如,利培酮最初上市时,对所有患者推荐的最佳加量方法是从 2mg 至 4mg,再增至 6mg 或更高。但在临床实践中,医师们倾向于使用较低的剂量[1]。相反,喹硫平刚上市时,300mg/d 被认为是最佳剂量。目前的共识倾向于更高的剂量[2],尽管随机对照试验及其他研究证据并不足以支持这种转变[2,3]。尽管如此,大多数临床医师认为在推荐治疗剂量范围内进行增减较为妥当。更重要的问题是,如果达到了推荐剂量的上限且患者能够耐受,但临床疗效仍然有限,这时怎么办?

剂量-疗效观察

Davis 和 Chen[4] 对可找到的 2004 年之前的抗精神病药资料做了系统的荟萃分析,认为能发挥最佳治疗效应的平均剂量是利培酮 4mg、奥氮平 16mg、齐拉西酮 120mg 和阿立哌唑 10~15mg(他们用此分析方法不能确定喹硫平的剂量)[4]。最近有临床试验尝试比较"大剂量"与"标准剂量"抗精神病药的疗效。例如,一个研究组设计了奥氮平的随机、双盲、为期 8 周的固定剂量研究[5],来比较标准剂量与大剂量奥氮平治疗的剂量-疗效关系,奥氮平剂量分别为 10mg、20mg 和 40mg。结果发现,大剂量组没有疗效优势(即 40mg 不优于 10mg),反而有明确证据提示随着剂量增加,不良反应也增加了(体重增加和催乳素升高)。类似地,最初的利培酮注册试验将 2~6mg/d(常用剂量)与 8~16mg/d(大剂量)进行比较,结果发现大剂量组并未进一步增加疗效,反而增加更多的不良反应(EPS 和催乳素升高)。这些研究结果与以往氟哌啶醇固定剂量比较的研究结果是一致的[6],即 8mg/d 以上的剂量不能带来更多获益[7]。

但是,必须明白记住,这些剂量来源于患者被分配到不同剂量的群体研究数据;而不同的是,在临床上只有最初剂量无效时,才考虑增加剂量。Kinon 等[8]针对氟奋乃静标准治疗剂量(当时 20mg/d)无效的患者,采取以下三种方式进行比较:增加氟奋乃静至 80mg/d,换为氟哌啶醇,或保持原治疗剂量观察等待。结果发现三种方法在疗效方面相近。这种结果似乎表明,在群组水平(而非个体水平)没有什么证据支持超出推荐剂量范围的

治疗。这个随机对照试验的证据得到了临床实践规范的印证——Hermes 等分析 CATIE 数据以便找出可以预测医师决定增加剂量的临床因素,发现(在治疗剂量范围内)增加剂量的决定与临床指标相关性很弱[9]。最近一项关于鲁拉西酮治疗成年精神分裂症患者的试验发现,在鲁拉西酮 80mg/d 治疗 2 周疗效不佳时,相比于继续使用 80mg/d 的剂量,增加剂量至 160mg/d 可以显著改善症状[10]。但是这一结果不一定能推广至其他抗精神病药。

2018 年,一项对相关研究的 Cochrane 系统综述总结道,在初始抗精神病药治疗效果不佳时,尚没有高质量证据表明增加药物剂量与继续原来剂量之间存在差异[11]。

血浆药物浓度变异

群组水平的研究证据不能完全左右个体的治疗决定。服用抗精神病药治疗的患者,其血药浓度存在明显的个体间差异。可能会遇到这样的患者,他们在较高剂量(如利培酮 6mg/d 或奥氮平 20mg/d)时的血药浓度,可能分别明显低于利培酮 2mg/d 或奥氮平 10mg/d 的预期血药水平下限,而这一血药浓度可能达不到治疗阈值。对于这样的患者,在告知患者且不良反应可以耐受的前提下,增加该药剂量,使血药浓度上升至特定药物的最佳范围,这种做法是合理的。关于血药浓度及其意义见第 11 章。然而,若患者依从性良好,剂量达到推荐剂量范围的上限,血药浓度也足够,但是缺乏疗效,此时可能的治疗选择有什么?

治疗选择

此时基本上有三种选择:氯氮平,换用另一种抗精神病药,或合用氯氮平以外的另一种抗精神病药。若患者符合使用氯氮平的标准,氯氮平无疑是首选。然而,英国最近对社区居住(不是住院)的患者进行了一项临床审核,涉及 60 个 NHS Trust 医院的 5 000 例患者,发现在符合难治性精神分裂症标准的患者中,40% 并未使用氯氮平。在服用氯氮平者中,绝大多数(85%)是在先后服用两种不同抗精神病药无效之后,等待了比大多数指南建议长得多的时间以后才使用了氯氮平[12]。

总有一些患者不喜欢定期抽血做化验,不喜欢氯氮平的不良反应,也不喜欢服用氯氮平所要求的定期复诊。这些患者只能换用其他抗精神病药,或合并其他抗精神病药。有关换药的数据寥寥无几。虽然在慢性精神分裂症患者的几乎每项临床试验中,都需要把一种抗精神病药换为另一种抗精神病药,但是缺乏严格的研究证据支持哪些换药组合更好(例如,若利培酮无效,换哪种药? 奥氮平、喹硫平、阿立哌唑或齐拉西酮?)如果医师只看由制药企业发起的换药试验,会产生相当混乱的印象,因为此类试验的结果与发起者利益攸关(可见 Heres S 等的"为什么奥氮平优于利培酮,利培酮优于喹硫平,而喹硫平又优于奥氮平:第二代抗精神病药直接对照研究的探索性分析"一文[13])。

CATIE 作为美国公立研究基金资助的对比试验,将服用第一种第二代抗精神病药无效的患者,随机分配到不同的第二种抗精神病药治疗组[14]。换用奥氮平和利培酮的患者,疗效比换用喹硫平和齐拉西酮者好。这种疗效的差别也得到一项荟萃分析的支持:该分析比较第二代与第一代抗精神病药的结论是,除了氯氮平,仅氨磺必利、利培酮和奥氮平在疗效上优于第一代抗精神病药[15]。另一项荟萃分析比较了第二代抗精神病药之间疗效的差异,结果提示奥氮平和利培酮(按顺序)疗效略优于其他第二代抗精神病药[16]。然而,若患者尚未用过奥氮平或者利培酮,且这两个药物在不良反应方面有优势,则合理的决策是换用这两种药物。这两种药物之间的比较资料有限。然而,一些对照、开放研究结果确实显示它们有不对称的优势(即换为奥氮平比转换为利培酮更有效)——这可以提供一些指导,尽管并不完整[17,18]。

奥氮平和利培酮均无效时,目前除了氯氮平,还不清楚应做何种选择。应该换成另一种药物(如阿立哌唑、齐拉西酮或第一代抗精神病药),还是加用另一种抗精神病药? 有趣的是,研究发现,患者因不能耐受(体重增加等)而换用阿立哌唑后,或者疗效没有降低[19,20],或者症状有所改善[21,22]。换药的方法非常重要,加药后换药(阿立哌唑达到治疗剂量后再减停原来的药物)和交叉换药(减停原有药物的同时逐渐增加另一种药物的剂量)效果要好于停用原药后再换用新药物[21]。

在换药之后,最常见的做法是加用其他抗精神病药,因为在日常治疗中,39%~43%的患者使用两种或以上抗精神病药治疗[23]。加用的第二种抗精神病药,通常是为了起到其他作用(如用喹硫平镇静,用阿立哌唑降低催乳素水平等——这些问题在别处讨论)。我们主要关注的是加用另一种抗精神病药能否提高疗效。从理论上讲,因为几乎所有抗精神病药均阻断 D_2 受体(不像降压药,具有不同作用机制),所以合用抗精神病药没有多少道理。抗精神病药联合治疗的研究,常选择临床上方便的合用,或根据临床经验采取的合用,目前最系统的证据是一种抗精神病药联合氯氮平[24,25]——其理论依据是氯氮平对 D_2 受体的占有率低,药物联用增加 D_2 受体占有率可能产生额外的叠加效果[26]。不过,一项荟萃分析纳入的随机对照试验发现,在治疗反应和症状改善方面,与继续单药治疗精神分裂症相比,加用一种第二代抗精神病药(联合用药)的疗效缺乏双盲/高质量证据支持[27]。此外,与抗精神病药单药治疗相比,联合用药似乎与更大的不良反应负担及大剂量处方风险有关[28,29]。

虽然加用第二种抗精神病药进行增效治疗的策略可能需要尽量避免,但在某些情况下,如患者病情急性加重或兴奋激越时,临床医师可能会发现联合治疗是唯一可行的解决方法。也许很常见的情况是,医师接手治疗的患者已经在联用抗精神病药。多数随机对照试验的证据表明,这种情况能被安全地改回抗精神病药单药治疗,至少在大部分情况下不导致症状加重[30-32],尽管这不是一个普遍的发现[33]。Essock 等[32]进行了一项大样本临床试验,共计纳入 127 例服用多种抗精神病药且病情稳定的患者。在 12 个月中,2/3 的患者成功地改成抗精神病药单药治疗。对于改用单药治疗后症状反复的患者,最常用的做法是恢复原先的多药治疗,在此过程中该组患者的病情未出现明显恶化。单一用药的优势是用药较少,对症状控制相当,并能减轻一些体重。

那么,何时应该选择继续当前的治疗方案? 对上述研究证据的回顾提示,不管是增加剂量、换用药物还是合用药物,没有哪种方法会在所有情况下都是明确的赢家。若血药浓度偏低,则增加剂量;若患者未试过奥氮平或利培酮治疗,则考虑换药;若氯氮平治疗无效,则联用药物,这些方法均可能有益。鉴于这些治疗策略的疗效有限,也许同样重要的是来自医师的要求,即应停留在目前的药物治疗方案上,并关注非药物治疗手段:参与个案管理、有针对性的心理治疗以及职业康复,以求增强患者的健康状况。虽然这可能看似被动的选择,但"治疗方案保持不变"产生的伤害往往少于无目的换药。

小结

当治疗不成功时：
■ 如果治疗剂量已经最佳，应考虑继续观察和等待。 ■ 依据耐受性和血药浓度，考虑增加抗精神病药剂量（支持的证据少 [34,35]）。 ■ 如果无效，考虑转换为奥氮平或利培酮治疗（如果尚未使用过）。 ■ 如果无效，应使用氯氮平（支持性证据非常有力）。 ■ 如果氯氮平无效，采用有时限的增效策略（支持性证据并不明确）。

参考文献

1. Ezewuzie N, et al. Establishing a dose-response relationship for oral risperidone in relapsed schizophrenia. *J Psychopharm* 2006;**20**:86–90.

2. Sparshatt A, et al. Quetiapine: dose-response relationship in schizophrenia. *CNS Drugs* 2008;**22**:49–68.

3. Honer WG, et al. A randomized, double-blind, placebo-controlled study of the safety and tolerability of high-dose quetiapine in patients with persistent symptoms of schizophrenia or schizoaffective disorder. *J Clin Psychiatry* 2012;**73**:13–20.

4. Davis JM. Dose response and dose equivalence of antipsychotics. *J Clin Psychopharmacol* 2004;**24**:192–208.

5. Kinon BJ, et al. Standard and higher dose of olanzapine in patients with schizophrenia or schizoaffective disorder: a randomized, double-blind, fixed-dose study. *J Clin Psychopharmacol* 2008;**28**:392–400.

6. Van Putten T, et al. A controlled dose comparison of haloperidol in newly admitted schizophrenic patients. *Arch Gen Psychiatry* 1990;**47**:754–758.

7. Zimbroff DL, et al. Controlled, dose-response study of sertindole and haloperidol in the treatment of schizophrenia. Sertindole Study Group. *Am J Psychiatry* 1997;**154**:782–791.

8. Kinon BJ, et al. Treatment of neuroleptic-resistant schizophrenic relapse. *Psychopharmacol Bull* 1993;**29**:309–314.

9. Hermes E, et al. Predictors of antipsychotic dose changes in the CATIE schizophrenia trial. *Psychiatry Res* 2012;**199**:1–7.

10. Loebel A, et al. Lurasidone dose escalation in early nonresponding patients with schizophrenia: a randomized, placebo-controlled study. *J Clin Psychiatry* 2016;**77**:1672–1680.

11. Samara MT, et al. Increasing antipsychotic dose versus switching antipsychotic for non response in schizophrenia. *Cochrane Database Syst Rev* 2018;**5**:Cd011884.

12. Patel MX, et al. Quality of prescribing for schizophrenia: evidence from a national audit in England and Wales. *Eur Neuropsychopharmacol* 2014;**24**:499–509.

13. Heres S, et al. Why olanzapine beats risperidone, risperidone beats quetiapine, and quetiapine beats olanzapine: an exploratory analysis of head-to-head comparison studies of second-generation antipsychotics. *Am J Psychiatry* 2006;**163**:185–194.

14. Stroup TS, et al. Effectiveness of olanzapine, quetiapine, risperidone, and ziprasidone in patients with chronic schizophrenia following discontinuation of a previous atypical antipsychotic. *Am J Psychiatry* 2006;**163**:611–622.

15. Leucht S, et al. Second-generation versus first-generation antipsychotic drugs for schizophrenia: a meta-analysis. *Lancet* 2009;**373**:31–41.

16. Leucht S, et al. A meta-analysis of head-to-head comparisons of second-generation antipsychotics in the treatment of schizophrenia. *Am J Psychiatry* 2009;**166**:152–163.

17. Hong J, et al. Clinical consequences of switching from olanzapine to risperidone and vice versa in outpatients with schizophrenia: 36-month results from the Worldwide Schizophrenia Outpatients Health Outcomes (W-SOHO) study. *BMC Psychiatry* 2012;**12**:218.

18. Agid O, et al. Antipsychotic response in first-episode schizophrenia: efficacy of high doses and switching. *Eur Neuropsychopharmacol* 2013;**23**:1017–1022.

19. Stroup TS, et al. A randomized trial examining the effectiveness of switching from olanzapine, quetiapine, or risperidone to aripiprazole to reduce metabolic risk: Comparison of Antipsychotics for Metabolic Problems (CAMP). *Am J Psychiatry* 2011;**168**:947–956.

20. Montastruc F, et al. Association of aripiprazole with the risk for psychiatric hospitalization, self-harm, or suicide. *JAMA Psychiatry* 2019;**76**:409–417.

21. Obayashi Y, et al. Switching strategies for antipsychotic monotherapy in schizophrenia: a multi-center cohort study of aripiprazole. *Psychopharmacology* 2020;**237**:167–175.

22. Pae CU, et al. Effectiveness and tolerability of switching to aripiprazole once monthly from antipsychotic polypharmacy and/or other long acting injectable antipsychotics for patients with schizophrenia in routine practice: a retrospective, observation study. *Clin Psychopharmacol Neurosci* 2020;**18**:153–158.

23. Paton C, et al. High-dose and combination antipsychotic prescribing in acute adult wards in the UK: the challenges posed by p.r.n. prescribing. *Br J Psychiatry* 2008;**192**:435–439.

24. Wagner E, et al. Clozapine combination and augmentation strategies in patients with schizophrenia – recommendations from an international expert survey among the Treatment Response and Resistance in Psychosis (TRRIP) Working Group. *Schizophr Bull* 2020; **46**:1459–1470.

25. Taylor DM, et al. Augmentation of clozapine with a second antipsychotic – a meta-analysis of randomized, placebo-controlled studies. *Acta Psychiatr Scand* 2009;119:419–425.

26. Kapur S, et al. Increased dopamine D2 receptor occupancy and elevated prolactin level associated with addition of haloperidol to clozapine. *Am J Psychiatry* 2001;158:311–314.

27. Galling B, et al. Antipsychotic augmentation vs. monotherapy in schizophrenia: systematic review, meta-analysis and meta-regression analysis. *World Psychiatry* 2017;16:77–89.

28. Gallego JA, et al. Safety and tolerability of antipsychotic polypharmacy. *Expert Opinion on Drug Safety* 2012;11:527–542.

29. Barnes TRE, et al. Antipsychotic polypharmacy in schizophrenia: benefits and risks. *CNS Drugs* 2011;25:383–399.

30. Borlido C, et al. Switching from 2 antipsychotics to 1 antipsychotic in schizophrenia: a randomized, double-blind, placebo-controlled study. *J Clin Psychiatry* 2016;77:e14–e20.

31. Hori H, et al. Switching to antipsychotic monotherapy can improve attention and processing speed, and social activity in chronic schizophrenia patients. *J Psychiatr Res* 2013;47:1843–1848.

32. Essock SM, et al. Effectiveness of switching from antipsychotic polypharmacy to monotherapy. *Am J Psychiatry* 2011;168:702–708.

33. Constantine RJ, et al. The risks and benefits of switching patients with schizophrenia or schizoaffective disorder from two to one antipsychotic medication: a randomized controlled trial. *Schizophr Res* 2015;166:194–200.

34. Royal College of Psychiatrists. Consensus statement on high-dose antipsychotic medication. College Report CR190 2014.

35. Barnes TRE, et al. Evidence-based guidelines for the pharmacological treatment of schizophrenia: updated recommendations from the British Association for Psychopharmacology. *J Psychopharmacology* 2020;34:3–78.

急性行为紊乱或暴力行为

急性行为紊乱可以发生在精神疾病、躯体疾病、物质滥用或人格障碍的背景下。患者常有精神病性症状,在被害妄想、幻听、幻视或者幻触的基础上,产生针对他人的攻击行为。本节将讨论如何处理严重精神疾病背景下的行为紊乱。非法物质滥用所致的兴奋/激越将在第 9 章讨论。

若采用适当的心理和行为手段无法减少急性行为紊乱,临床上会采用快速镇静法(RT)。这实际上是最后一步治疗选择。需要快速镇静的患者往往行为过于紊乱,无法做出知情同意并参加 RCT。但是,随着许多创新性方法的应用,近年来关于药物策略的有效性和耐受性的证据越来越多。一份全面的最新共识指南已经发表[1],最近还发表了一篇系统综述和荟萃分析[2]。

口服/吸入治疗

已经发表的一些研究结果提示口服第二代抗精神病药有效[3-6]。在这些研究中,受试者行为紊乱的程度最多是中度,并且所有的受试者均接受了口服药物治疗(这种程度的依从性在临床实践中很少见)。这些研究招募的受试者均接受第二代抗精神病药单药治疗。增加第二种抗精神病药作为"必要时"的治疗,其疗效及安全性尚未在规范的随机对照试验中明确进行研究。

一项单剂量随机对照试验发现,阿那塞平舌下含服治疗急性激越比安慰剂有效[7]。随机对照试验[8-10]和案例研究[11,12]也支持吸入洛沙平治疗中度行为紊乱的有效性。使用这种制剂需要患者合作,且支气管痉挛是已经明确的不良反应,但很少发生。

胃肠外给药治疗

大样本安慰剂随机对照试验支持奥氮平、齐拉西酮和阿立哌唑肌内注射的疗效。综合考虑,这些研究提示,肌内注射抗精神病药的疗效从高到低依次为奥氮平、氟哌啶醇、阿立哌唑、齐拉西酮[2,13]。同样,这些研究中受试者的行为紊乱程度最多达到中度,且药物间的差异很小。

一项大样本观察性研究支持肌内注射奥氮平在临床急症(严重行为紊乱)中的应用是安全有效的[14]。一项研究发现,与单用氟哌啶醇相比,肌内注射咪达唑仑和肌内注射氟哌啶醇联用,对于控制姑息治疗患者的激越效果更好[15]。

几项随机对照试验研究了胃肠外给药在"现实的"急性行为紊乱患者中的疗效。总的来说:

- 与单用咪达唑仑静脉注射相比,咪达唑仑静脉注射合并奥氮平静脉注射,或咪达唑仑静脉注射合并氟哌利多静脉注射,均起效更快,且以后需要用药的次数减少[16]。
- 与氟哌啶醇 5~10mg 合并异丙嗪 50mg 相比,咪达唑仑 7.5~15mg 肌内注射的镇静作用更快(TREC1)[17]。
- 短期使用奥氮平 10mg 时,其疗效与氟哌啶醇 10mg 合并异丙嗪 25~50mg 相同,但疗效持续时间不如后者(TREC4)[18]。

- 氟哌啶醇 5~10mg 合并异丙嗪 50mg，比单用氟哌啶醇 5~10mg 疗效好，耐受性好（6% 的患者出现急性肌张力障碍）（TREC3）[19]。
- 氟哌啶醇 10mg 联合异丙嗪 25~50mg 比劳拉西泮 4mg 疗效好（TREC2）[20]。
- 氯丙嗪 100mg 肌内注射合并氟哌啶醇 5mg 肌内注射及异丙嗪 25mg 肌内注射，疗效并不优于氟哌啶醇 5mg 肌内注射合并异丙嗪 25mg 肌内注射（TREC Lebanon）[21]。
- 咪达唑仑静脉注射合并氟哌利多静脉注射，其镇静作用快于单用氟哌利多静脉注射或单用奥氮平静脉注射。咪达唑仑联合氟哌利多组的患者较少需要额外剂量来达到镇静的效果[22]。
- 在治疗精神分裂症患者的激越时，奥氮平肌内注射的疗效在短期（2h）好于阿立哌唑肌内注射，但在 24h 时二者没有显著差异[23]。
- 一项大样本（n=737）的急诊室研究发现，咪达唑仑 5mg 肌内注射比奥氮平 10mg 肌内注射、齐拉西酮 20mg 肌内注射、氟哌啶醇 5mg 或 10mg 肌内注射均起效更快，疗效更好[24]。
- 一项开放研究发现，氟哌啶醇肌内注射合并劳拉西泮肌内注射疗效与奥氮平肌内注射相似[25]。
- 氟哌利多肌内注射和氟哌啶醇肌内注射疗效相当[26]。

Cochrane 系统评价认为，单用氟哌啶醇能有效地治疗急性行为紊乱，但耐受性差，合并使用异丙嗪（而非劳拉西泮）能够改善耐受性[27,28]。然而，NICE 认为为此使用异丙嗪的证据不能使人信服[29]。对于合并使用氟哌啶醇和异丙嗪，Cochrane 系统评价认为对精神病所致的攻击行为是有效的，且有良好的证据支持。与合并使用氟哌啶醇和异丙嗪相比，使用奥氮平者更可能重新出现攻击行为，并需要进一步接受注射治疗。作者认为"单独使用氟哌啶醇，而不用其他药物减轻其频繁而严重的不良反应，似乎很难说得过去"[30]。Cochrane 系统评价认为阿立哌唑的相关数据较少。证据提示阿立哌唑的疗效优于安慰剂和单用氟哌啶醇，但差于奥氮平。但若要将这些结果推广至现实世界的实践，仍需保持谨慎[31]。

关于奥氮平肌内注射治疗激越的系统综述和荟萃分析发现，奥氮平肌内注射和氟哌啶醇肌内注射疗效相当，但奥氮平肌内注射者较少出现锥体外系不良反应[32]。Cochrane 系统评价提示氟哌利多是有效的，可以用于控制精神病所致的严重行为紊乱和攻击行为[33]。氟哌利多在一些国家被重新开始使用（氟哌利多最初是自己退市的，所以可以重新上市）。

一项荟萃分析考察了肌内注射抗精神病药治疗激越时的安全性，使用氟哌啶醇所致急性肌张力障碍的发生率为 5%，而第二代抗精神病药的结果要好很多[34]。急性锥体外系不良反应往往对于长期依从性不利[35]。此外，大多数国家的氟哌啶醇药品说明书要求使用该药前检查心电图[36,37]，而且不可同时应用其他抗精神病药。肌内注射 10mg 氟哌啶醇后，Q-T 间期延长的平均值达 15ms，但其范围较宽[38]。

需要注意的是，异丙嗪可能会抑制氟哌啶醇的代谢[39]；鉴于氟哌啶醇可能延长 Q-T 间期，药物代谢动力学相互作用可能会有临床意义。虽然单次给药时不太可能成为问题，但是重复给药就可能带来风险。

氟哌利多与 Q-T 间期改变有关（该药既往退市的原因）。在一项背景为医院急症科的观察性研究中，1 009 例使用氟哌利多胃肠外给药的患者中，只有 13 例（1.28%）在用药后出现异常 Q-T 间期，其中 7 例患者存在其他诱因，没有患者出现尖端扭转型室性心动过速[26]。在所有关于氟哌利多的快速镇静研究中，Q-T 间期 >500ms 的总体发生率小于 2%[2]。

目前,很少在快速镇静治疗中使用静脉内给药,但当收益大于风险时,可以考虑将静脉内给药作为最后的手段。一项小样本研究比较了大剂量氟哌啶醇静脉注射和地西泮静脉注射的疗效,发现二者在24h内均有效[40]。两项大型观察性研究调查了在急症科静脉注射奥氮平的安全性。在研究中奥氮平的适应证各种各样,最多的是用于治疗激越。其中一项研究发现[41],使用奥氮平静脉注射治疗激越组(n=265)中,超过1/3的患者在初始奥氮平注射以后需要额外的镇静剂量。17.7%的患者出现缺氧,20.4%的患者使用了辅助供氧。6例患者需要插管(其中2例患者是由于奥氮平治疗)。另一项研究[42]比较了静脉注射奥氮平(n=295)和肌内注射奥氮平(n=489),发现81%的静脉注射患者及84%的肌内注射患者不需要额外的剂量。静脉注射奥氮平的患者出现呼吸抑制的比例较多。5例肌内注射的患者和2例静脉注射的患者需要插管。

在急性精神障碍发作的情况下,大剂量镇静(大于10mg氟哌啶醇、氟哌利多或咪达唑仑)并不比小剂量有效,但会导致更多的不良反应(低血压和血氧饱和度下降)[43]。与此一致的是,一项小样本随机对照试验支持了小剂量氟哌啶醇的疗效,但是氟哌啶醇与咪达唑仑联用时疗效和耐受性更佳[44]。这些数据很大程度上支持在临床紧急情况下使用标准剂量,但需要考虑使用低剂量后进一步物理约束的必要性。

一项小规模观察性研究支持在精神科重症监护室(PICU)应用咪达唑仑含服有效[45]。胃肠外使用咪达唑仑,尤其在大剂量时,容易引起过度镇静伴呼吸抑制[46]。肌内注射劳拉西泮是一种已经确立的治疗,而且TREC2[20]支持其有效性,但是综合所有TREC研究的结果,提示7.5~15mg的咪达唑仑可能疗效更优。一项Cochrane综述分析了苯二氮䓬类药物用于治疗精神病所致攻击和激越的效果,认为大多数临床试验样本量太小,无法突出正面或负面影响的差异;同时,在其他药物的基础上,加用一种苯二氮䓬类药物可能没有明显优势,但可能会导致不必要的不良反应[47]。

对于继发于酒精或毒品急性中毒的行为紊乱,可以指导临床实践的数据较少。一项大样本的给醉酒患者静脉注射镇静剂的观察性研究发现,联合用药(最常见的是氟哌啶醇5mg联合劳拉西泮2mg)的疗效优于两药单用,可以减少后续的镇静需要[48]。一组患者(n=59)接受小剂量氟哌啶醇(口服、肌内注射或静脉给药),以治疗使用苯环利定(PCP)后出现的行为紊乱,结果发现氟哌啶醇治疗有效,而且耐受性良好(轻微低血压和轻微缺氧各1例)[49]。对躁动性谵妄的治疗见第9章。

氯胺酮在医院急诊科被广泛地用于治疗激越。一项系统综述纳入了18项氯胺酮研究[50],发现静脉注射平均315mg氯胺酮,可以在平均7.2min内达到充分镇静。650例患者中超过30%需要插管,超过1%出现喉痉挛。氯胺酮可能不适合在没有插管条件的单位用于快速镇静治疗。

总的来说,目前广泛的共识是咪达唑仑和氟哌利多是见效最快的肌内注射单一药物[51];而氟哌啶醇应避免单独使用,甚至可能也完全放弃联合使用[52]。二线治疗是苯二氮䓬类和抗精神病药联合使用。三线治疗目前可能是静脉注射苯二氮䓬类药物,然后在有插管条件的情况下使用氯胺酮(2~5mg/kg肌内注射)。

实际措施

针对每个患者的治疗计划最好能够提前制订。其目标是预防行为紊乱和减少暴力风险。

护理干预(降低危险行为等级、暂停行为、隔离[53])、增加护理级别、将患者转至 PICU 并给予药物,均是可以采取的选择。需注意避免联合使用抗精神病药,并避免抗精神病药出现累积剂量过高。在快速镇静之后,必须监测常规的躯体指标。需要注意的是,快速镇静往往被患者视作一种惩罚。目前,还鲜有研究关注患者接受快速镇静时的体验。

快速镇静的目标有三部分。

- 减少患者痛苦:心理的或者躯体的(通过自伤或事故)。
- 保持环境安全,减少伤害他人的风险。
- 不对患者造成伤害(使用安全的治疗方案,并监护躯体健康)。

注意:尽管需要快速而有效的治疗,应该避免同时使用两种或以上抗精神病药(抗精神病药联合用药),因为(几乎所有抗精神病药都很常见的)Q-T 间期延长的风险。这在快速镇静中特别重要,因为患者的躯体状态使其容易发生心律失常。

珠氯噻醇醋酸酯

珠氯噻醇醋酸酯(ZA)在英国和欧洲其他国家广泛使用,最广为人知的商品名是Acuphase。珠氯噻醇是硫杂蒽类多巴胺拮抗剂,最早在 20 世纪 60 年代上市。珠氯噻醇醋酸酯不是快速镇静药。其半衰期大约为 20h。肌内注射珠氯噻醇基团成分可以被快速吸收,作用时间 12~24h。通过减慢肌内注射后的吸收速度,其生物半衰期(以及作用的持续时间)取决于从肌内注射部位释放的速率。而这可以通过酯化珠氯噻醇分子来实现,释放速率与酯碳链的长度大致成正比。珠氯噻醇癸酸酯肌内注射以后延迟释放,因此起效慢但作用时间很长。珠氯噻醇醋酸酯(少 8 个碳原子)有望相对迅速地释放,但作用持续时间中等。制药厂的意图是使用珠氯噻醇醋酸酯时,可以避免给行为紊乱的患者重复进行肌内注射。

一项关于珠氯噻醇醋酸酯药物代谢动力学的初步研究,包含 19 例"有必要使用胃肠外神经阻滞剂进行镇静"的患者[54]。结果发现给药 1~2h 后可在血浆中检测到珠氯噻醇,但给药后 36h 左右才达到峰浓度。72h 的血浆药物浓度约为 36h 的 1/3。珠氯噻醇醋酸酯的起效速度不快,17 例患者中有 10 例在 4h 时没有或只出现轻微的精神病性症状改变。镇静效果在 4h 时明显,但在 72h 时效果减弱。

该研究团队又进行了一项随访研究[55],更仔细地调查了珠氯噻醇醋酸酯在 83 例患者中的疗效。作者认为珠氯噻醇醋酸酯使"精神病性症状明显而快速地减轻"。事实上他们在 24h 后才首次评估精神病性症状,因此快速起效的说法没有足够的证据。他们在用药 2h 后评估了镇静作用,观察到统计学上显著的效果:基线时平均镇静分数为 0.0(0= 没有镇静表现),2h 平均镇静分数为 0.6(1= 轻度镇静)。在 8h 时观察到最大的镇静作用(平均分 2.2;2= 中度镇静)。72h 平均分为 1.1。肌张力障碍和肌强直是最常见的不良反应。

两项相互独立的开放性研究发现了相似的结果:缓慢起效并在 24h 达到高峰,72h 仍有明显效果[56,57]。英国的首次研究在 1990 年[58],这项研究发现在给药 8h 后,精神症状评分首次出现显著下降,并继续下降直至 72h 末次评定时。在评估的 25 例患者中,只有 4 例在 1h 内出现镇静的表现(19 例在 2h,22 例在 24h)。

一项研究比较了珠氯噻醇醋酸酯与肌内注射/口服氟哌啶醇及肌内注射/口服珠氯噻醇基本成分的效果(多次给药超过 6 天)[59]。结果发现,两种非酯类的肌内注射/口服制剂在 2h

的镇静效果好于珠氯噻醇醋酸酯,但珠氯噻醇醋酸酯和珠氯噻醇的效果持续时间长于氟哌啶醇,达 144h(但是患者接受珠氯噻醇的剂量更高)。除了珠氯噻醇醋酸酯起效较慢,两种药物没有其他明显区别。三种药物的给药次数差别很大:珠氯噻醇醋酸酯 1~4 次,氟哌啶醇 1~26 次,珠氯噻醇 1~22 次。这是珠氯噻醇醋酸酯的关键(也可能是唯一)的优势:可以减少急性精神病需要重复给药的次数。事实上,这也是首个珠氯噻醇醋酸酯双盲研究的主要发现[60]。在这项研究中,受试者被给予珠氯噻醇醋酸酯或氟哌啶醇肌内注射,并进行超过 3 天的评估。结果发现,在每天的评估中,BPRS 和 CGI 评分的变化几乎相同。不过在 23 例使用珠氯噻醇醋酸酯的患者中,只有 1 例患者需要第二次注射,而使用氟哌啶醇的 21 例患者中,有 7 例需要重复给药。该研究没有比较药物的起效速度。泰国研究者在比较这两种治疗的研究中也发现了类似的结果[61],另外,还有三项中等样本量的研究也有相似发现($n=44$[62], $n=40$[63], $n=50$[64])。在这几项研究中,根据设定的评估时间都无法确定药物何时起效。

一项 Cochrane 综述[65]纳入了上述所有的比较性研究和三项无法获得完整细节的进一步研究[66-68]。作者认为,所有的研究都有方法学缺陷且报道不足,珠氯噻醇醋酸酯并没有表现出"快速起效"。他们指出,珠氯噻醇醋酸酯疗效可能不比其他治疗差,且可能"减少强制注射的次数"。

总的来说,珠氯噻醇醋酸酯在镇静和抗精神病方面存在某种程度的延迟起效,这限制了它在快速镇静上的应用。少数患者在用药 2~4h 后出现明显的镇静,但抗精神病作用需要在 8h 后出现。若对约束患者使用珠氯噻醇醋酸酯,他们在解除约束后的行为可能保持不变,并持续数小时。珠氯噻醇醋酸酯在减少注射所需的约束次数方面有作用,但在快速镇静方面没有作用。

珠氯噻醇醋酸酯使用指南(Acuphase)

珠氯噻醇醋酸酯(ZA)不是快速镇静药物,仅适用于那些已经多次注射短效抗精神病药(如氟哌啶醇、奥氮平)或镇静剂(如劳拉西泮)的急性精神病患者。最好用于过去 Acuphase 治疗效果较好的少数患者。

只有经过足够的时间确认之前所用药物确实已经完全发挥疗效后(静脉注射后 15min;肌内注射后 60min),才应该使用珠氯噻醇醋酸酯。

珠氯噻醇醋酸酯禁用于快速镇静(起效太慢)、有身体抵抗注射行为的患者(有进入血管产生油栓的风险)及未使用过抗精神病药的患者(有持续锥体外系不良反应的风险)。

快速镇静概述

在紧急情况下:评估有无医疗原因[69]。优化常规处方。药物治疗的目的是使患者安静下来,而非过度镇静。

注意:儿童、青少年及老年患者需要使用低剂量药物。胃肠外给药后要监测患者的意识水平和躯体健康情况(见步骤)。

续

干预步骤	
1. 酌情采取降低风险等级、暂停行为、安置等措施	
2. 给予口服药物治疗	
若患者规律服用抗精神病药： **劳拉西泮** 1~2mg **异丙嗪** 25~50mg 单用**咪达唑仑含服**，可以避免肌内注射治疗。剂量：10mg 注意该制剂并未得到许可	若患者未规律服药或注射抗精神病药长效制剂： ■ **奥氮平** 10mg 或 ■ **利培酮** 1~2mg 或 ■ **喹硫平** 50~100mg 或 ■ **氟哌啶醇** 5mg（最好合用异丙嗪 25mg）。注意欧盟产品特征概要对氟哌啶醇的使用建议：治疗前需检查心电图，避免合用抗精神病药 ■ **洛沙平** 10mg **吸入**。注意使用这种制剂需要患者合作，且支气管痉挛是罕见的不良反应（沙丁胺醇吸入器备用）

　　需要时在 45~60min 后重复给药。考虑合用镇静剂和抗精神病药治疗。

　　如果两次用药失败，转到第 3 步；如果患者将自己或其他人置于严重危险中，尽快执行第 3 步。

3. 考虑肌内注射治疗	
劳拉西泮 2mg[ab] **异丙嗪** 50mg[c] **奥氮平** 10mg[d]	若出现苯二氮䓬类药物导致的呼吸抑制，使用氟马西尼治疗 如果患者对苯二氮䓬类耐受，肌内注射异丙嗪是有用的选择 肌内注射奥氮平不可同时肌内注射苯二氮䓬类药物，尤其在喝酒后[70]
阿立哌唑 9.75mg	与奥氮平相比，较少引起低血压，但是疗效较差[5,13,71]
氟哌啶醇 5mg	**氟哌啶醇应放到最后选择** ■ 急性肌张力障碍的发生率较高；可同时肌内注射异丙嗪，保证备有肌内注射的丙环定 ■ 治疗前需检查心电图

　　如果效果不理想，30~60min 后重复给药。如果单药治疗失败，可以考虑联合使用氟哌啶醇和劳拉西泮，或氟哌啶醇和异丙嗪。药物不能混合在同一个注射器内。肌内注射奥氮平禁止与肌内注射苯二氮䓬类药物合用。

4. 考虑静脉注射治疗
■ **地西泮** 10mg 大于 2min 注射完毕[b,e] ■ 如果疗效不充分，5~10min 后重复给药（最多给药 3 次） ■ 需要预备氟马西尼

5. 寻求专家意见[f]
考虑转到内科病房**肌内注射氯胺酮**

注:

a. 仔细阅读药物用法和稀释的指导,各厂家的说明书不同。许多中心使用 4mg。一个备选药物是咪达唑仑 5~15mg,5mg 一般就足够。两种药物抑制呼吸的风险均随剂量增高而增加,但是通常咪达唑仑风险更大。

b. 注意年幼或年老患者,以及那些原有脑损害或者冲动控制问题的患者,因为出现脱抑制反应的情况会更多见[72]。

c. 异丙嗪起效慢,但往往是有效的镇静药物。肌内注射之前不需要稀释。可以重复用药,每天剂量最多 100mg。注射药物后需要等待 1~2h 再评估效果。需要注意的是,曾有报告(尽管罕见)单用异丙嗪也可引起恶性综合征,虽然异丙嗪对多巴胺受体的拮抗作用极弱[73]。另外,要注意异丙嗪和氟哌啶醇的药代动力学相互作用(异丙嗪会减少氟哌啶醇的代谢),如果这两种药物均需重复给药,可能会带来风险。

d. NICE 仅仅推荐用于中度行为紊乱,但是一项大的观察性研究发现,它在临床急症中也有效。

e. 使用地西泮亚微乳注射液(Diazemuls)以避免注射部位反应。劳拉西泮也可以静脉给药。当需要快速起效时,可选择静脉给药,而不是肌内注射。静脉给药也可以保证药物几乎立即输送到其作用部位,有效地避免肌内注射时吸收缓慢造成意外药物蓄积的危险。若用药后未见到效果,可在仅仅 5~10min 后再次静脉给药。咪达唑仑也可以静脉给药,但呼吸抑制常见[1]。

f. 此处的选择有限,尽管肌内注射氯胺酮的广泛使用增加了可选范围。过去会肌内注射异戊巴比妥和副醛,但现在极少使用,药物一般也较难得到。静脉注射奥氮平、氟哌利多和氟哌啶醇是可行的,但不良反应很常见。ECT 也是一种选择。

快速镇静:躯体监测

胃肠外给药后,需监测以下指标:

- **体温**
- **脉搏**
- **血压**
- **呼吸频率**

第 1 个小时内每 15min 监测 1 次,此后每小时监测 1 次,直到患者可以行走。如果患者拒绝生命体征监测,或者由于行为紊乱过于突出而难以接近,应该观察患者有无发热、缺氧、低血压、过度镇静和一般躯体状况等体征或症状。

若患者处于睡眠状态或者**意识丧失**,则需用血氧测定仪来持续监测血氧饱和度。应该有一位护士陪护患者,直到患者可以行走。

若使用胃肠外给药的抗精神病药,尤其剂量较高时,强烈建议监测心电图及血液学指标[74,75]。低钾血症、应激和激越会将患者置于心律失常的风险中[76](见"Q-T 间期延长")。正式建议对所有使用氟哌啶醇的患者进行心电图监测。

右上角：续

快速镇静中的补救措施	
问题	**补救措施**
急性肌张力障碍（包括动眼危象）	给予**丙环定** 5~10mg 肌内注射或静脉注射
呼吸频率降低（<10 次/min）或血氧饱和度下降（<90%）	吸氧，抬高下肢，确保患者不要俯卧 如果怀疑是苯二氮䓬类药物导致的呼吸抑制，给予**氟马西尼**治疗（见使用指导） 如果是其他镇静药物所致：**转移患者到治疗床上并给予机械通气**
脉搏不规律或者缓慢（<50 次/min）	立刻**转移**至专科治疗
血药下降（直立位血压下降 >30mmHg 或舒张压 <50mmHg）	**使患者平躺**，放低床头，密切监测
体温增高	（有恶性综合征风险，且可能发生心律失常） 急查肌酐激酶

氟马西尼使用指导	
适应证	使用劳拉西泮、咪达唑仑或地西泮后，呼吸频率下降至 10 次/min 以下
禁忌证	长期使用苯二氮䓬类药物的癫痫患者
注意	肝功能损害的患者小心增加药物剂量
剂量和给药方式	**起始**：200μg **静脉注射** 15s 以上 ——如果 60s 后未达到所要求的意识清晰程度，则 **追加剂量**：100μg **静脉注射** 15s 以上
重复给药间隔时间	60s
最大剂量	24h 内 1mg（包括 1 次初始剂量和 8 次追加剂量）
不良反应	患者在醒来时可能变得躁动、焦虑或恐惧 规律使用苯二氮䓬类药物的患者可能出现癫痫发作
处理	不良反应通常自行缓解
监测 ■ **监测项目** ■ **监测频率**	 呼吸频率 持续监测直到呼吸频率恢复到基线水平 氟马西尼半衰期很短（明显短于地西泮），呼吸功能可能在恢复后再次恶化

　　注意：如果首次给药后患者的呼吸频率未恢复或患者未清醒，需考虑可能是其他原因导致的镇静。

参考文献

1. Patel MX, et al. Joint BAP NAPICU evidence-based consensus guidelines for the clinical management of acute disturbance: de-escalation and rapid tranquillisation. *J Psychopharmacology* 2018; 32:601–640.

2. Bak M, et al. The pharmacological management of agitated and aggressive behaviour: a systematic review and meta-analysis. *Eur Psychiatry* 2019; 57:78–100.

3. Currier GW, et al. Acute treatment of psychotic agitation: a randomized comparison of oral treatment with risperidone and lorazepam versus intramuscular treatment with haloperidol and lorazepam. *J Clin Psychiatry* 2004; 65:386–394.

4. Ganesan S, et al. Effectiveness of quetiapine for the management of aggressive psychosis in the emergency psychiatric setting: a naturalistic uncontrolled trial. *Int J Psychiatry Clin Pract* 2005; 9:199–203.

5. Simpson JR, Jr., et al. Impact of orally disintegrating olanzapine on use of intramuscular antipsychotics, seclusion, and restraint in an acute inpatient psychiatric setting. *J Clin Psychopharmacol* 2006; 26:333–335.

6. Hsu WY, et al. Comparison of intramuscular olanzapine, orally disintegrating olanzapine tablets, oral risperidone solution, and intramuscular haloperidol in the management of acute agitation in an acute care psychiatric ward in Taiwan. *J Clin Psychopharmacol* 2010; 30:230–234.

7. Pratts M, et al. A single-dose, randomized, double-blind, placebo-controlled trial of sublingual asenapine for acute agitation. *Acta Psychiatr Scand* 2014; 130:61–68.

8. Lesem MD, et al. Rapid acute treatment of agitation in individuals with schizophrenia: multicentre, randomised, placebo-controlled study of inhaled loxapine. *Br J Psychiatry* 2011; 198:51–58.

9. Kwentus J, et al. Rapid acute treatment of agitation in patients with bipolar I disorder: a multicenter, randomized, placebo-controlled clinical trial with inhaled loxapine. *BipolarDisord* 2012; 14:31–40.

10. Allen MH, et al. Efficacy and safety of loxapine for inhalation in the treatment of agitation in patients with schizophrenia: a randomized, double-blind, placebo-controlled trial. *J Clin Psychiatry* 2011; 72:1313–1321.

11. Kahl KG, et al. Inhaled loxapine for acute treatment of agitation in patients with borderline personality disorder: a case series. *J Clin Psychopharmacol* 2015; 35:741–743.

12. Roncero C, et al. Effectiveness of inhaled loxapine in dual-diagnosis patients: a case series. *Clin Neuropharmacol* 2016; 39:206–209.

13. Citrome L. Comparison of intramuscular ziprasidone, olanzapine, or aripiprazole for agitation: a quantitative review of efficacy and safety. *J Clin Psychiatry* 2007; 68:1876–1885.

14. Perrin E, et al. A prospective, observational study of the safety and effectiveness of intramuscular psychotropic treatment in acutely agitated patients with schizophrenia and bipolar mania. *Eur Psychiatry* 2012; 27:234–239.

15. Ferraz Goncalves JA, et al. Comparison of haloperidol alone and in combination with midazolam for the treatment of acute agitation in an inpatient palliative care service. *J Pain Palliat Care Pharmacother* 2016; 30:284–288.

16. Chan EW, et al. Intravenous droperidol or olanzapine as an adjunct to midazolam for the acutely agitated patient: a multicenter, randomized, double-blind, placebo-controlled clinical trial. *Ann Emerg Med* 2013; 61:72–81.

17. TREC Collaborative Group. Rapid tranquillisation for agitated patients in emergency psychiatric rooms: a randomised trial of midazolam versus haloperidol plus promethazine. *BMJ* 2003; 327:708–713.

18. Raveendran NS, et al. Rapid tranquillisation in psychiatric emergency settings in India: pragmatic randomised controlled trial of intramuscular olanzapine versus intramuscular haloperidol plus promethazine. *BMJ* 2007; 335:865.

19. Huf G, et al. Rapid tranquillisation in psychiatric emergency settings in Brazil: pragmatic randomised controlled trial of intramuscular haloperidol versus intramuscular haloperidol plus promethazine. *BMJ* 2007; 335:869.

20. Alexander J, et al. Rapid tranquillisation of violent or agitated patients in a psychiatric emergency setting. Pragmatic randomised trial of intramuscular lorazepam v. haloperidol plus promethazine. *Br J Psychiatry* 2004; 185:63–69.

21. Dib JE, et al. Rapid tranquillisation in a psychiatric emergency hospital in Lebanon: TREC-Lebanon – a pragmatic randomised controlled trial of intramuscular haloperidol and promethazine v. intramuscular haloperidol, promethazine and chlorpromazine. *Psychol Med* 2021: [Epub ahead of print].

22. Taylor DM, et al. Midazolam-droperidol, droperidol, or olanzapine for acute agitation: a randomized clinical trial. *Ann Emerg Med* 2017; 69:318–326.e311.

23. Kittipeerachon M, et al. Intramuscular olanzapine versus intramuscular aripiprazole for the treatment of agitation in patients with schizophrenia: a pragmatic double-blind randomized trial. *Schizophr Res* 2016; 176:231–238.

24. Klein LR, et al. Intramuscular midazolam, olanzapine, ziprasidone, or haloperidol for treating acute agitation in the emergency department. *Ann Emerg Med* 2018; 72:374–385.

25. Huang CL, et al. Intramuscular olanzapine versus intramuscular haloperidol plus lorazepam for the treatment of acute schizophrenia with agitation: an open-label, randomized controlled trial. *J Formos Med Assoc* 2015; 114:438–445.

26. Calver L, et al. The safety and effectiveness of droperidol for sedation of acute behavioral disturbance in the emergency department. *Ann Emerg Med* 2015; 66:230–238.e231.

27. Powney MJ, et al. Haloperidol for psychosis-induced aggression or agitation (rapid tranquillisation). *Cochrane Database Syst Rev* 2012; 11:CD009377.

28. Ostinelli EG, et al. Haloperidol for psychosis-induced aggression or agitation (rapid tranquillisation). *Cochrane Database Syst Rev* 2017; 7:Cd009377.

29. National Institute for Health and Clinical Excellence. Violence and aggression: short-term management in mental health, health and community settings. NICE guideline [NG10]. 2015 (last checked December 2019); https://www.nice.org.uk/guidance/NG10.

30. Huf G, et al. Haloperidol plus promethazine for psychosis-induced aggression. *Cochrane Database Syst Rev* 2016; **11**:Cd005146.

31. Ostinelli EG, et al. Aripiprazole (intramuscular) for psychosis-induced aggression or agitation (rapid tranquillisation). *Cochrane Database Syst Rev* 2018; **1**:Cd008074.

32. Kishi T, et al. Intramuscular olanzapine for agitated patients: a systematic review and meta-analysis of randomized controlled trials. *J Psychiatr Res* 2015; **68**:198–209.

33. Khokhar MA, et al. Droperidol for psychosis-induced aggression or agitation. *Cochrane Database Syst Rev* 2016; **12**:Cd002830.

34. Satterthwaite TD, et al. A meta-analysis of the risk of acute extrapyramidal symptoms with intramuscular antipsychotics for the treatment of agitation. *J Clin Psychiatry* 2008; **69**:1869–1879.

35. Van Harten PN, et al. Acute dystonia induced by drug treatment. *Br Med J* 1999; **319**:623–626.

36. Pharmacovigilance Working Party. Public assessment report on neuroleptics and cardiac safety, in particular QT prolongation, cardiac arrhythmias, ventricular tachycardia and torsades de pointes. 2006.

37. Janssen-Cilag Ltd. Summary of product characteristics. haldol decanoate. 2020; https://www.medicines.org.uk/emc/product/968/smpc.

38. Miceli JJ, et al. Effects of high-dose ziprasidone and haloperidol on the QTc interval after intramuscular administration: a randomized, single-blind, parallel-group study in patients with schizophrenia or schizoaffective disorder. *Clin Ther* 2010; **32**:472–491.

39. Suzuki A, et al. Histamine H1-receptor antagonists, promethazine and homochlorcyclizine, increase the steady-state plasma concentrations of haloperidol and reduced haloperidol. *TherDrug Monit* 2003; **25**:192–196.

40. Lerner Y, et al. Acute high-dose parenteral haloperidol treatment of psychosis. *Am J Psychiatry* 1979; **136**:1061–1064.

41. Martel ML, et al. A large retrospective cohort of patients receiving intravenous olanzapine in the emergency department. *Acad Emerg Med* 2016; **23**:29–35.

42. Cole JB, et al. A prospective observational study of patients receiving intravenous and intramuscular olanzapine in the emergency department. *Ann Emerg Med* 2017; **69**:327–336.e322.

43. Calver L, et al. A prospective study of high dose sedation for rapid tranquilisation of acute behavioural disturbance in an acute mental health unit. *BMC Psychiatry* 2013; **13**:225.

44. Mantovani C, et al. Are low doses of antipsychotics effective in the management of psychomotor agitation? A randomized, rated-blind trial of 4 intramuscular interventions. *J Clin Psychopharmacol* 2013; **33**:306–312.

45. Taylor D, et al. Buccal midazolam for rapid tranquillisation. *Int J Psychiatry Clin Pract* 2008; **12**:309–311.

46. Spain D, et al. Safety and effectiveness of high-dose midazolam for severe behavioural disturbance in an emergency department with suspected psychostimulant-affected patients. *Emerg Med Australas* 2008; **20**:112–120.

47. Zaman H, et al. Benzodiazepines for psychosis-induced aggression or agitation. *Cochrane Database Syst Rev* 2017; **12**:Cd003079.

48. Li SF, et al. Safety and efficacy of intravenous combination sedatives in the ED. *Am J Emerg Med* 2013; **31**:1402–1404.

49. MacNeal JJ, et al. Use of haloperidol in PCP-intoxicated individuals. *Clin Toxicol* 2012; **50**:851–853.

50. Mankowitz SL, et al. Ketamine for rapid sedation of agitated patients in the prehospital and emergency department settings: a systematic review and proportional meta-analysis. *J Emerg Med* 2018; **55**:670–681.

51. Kim HK, et al. Safety and efficacy of pharmacologic agents used for rapid tranquilization of emergency department patients with acute agitation or excited delirium. *Exp Opin Drug Saf* 2021; **20**:123–138.

52. Pierre JM. Time to retire haloperidol? For emergency agitation, evidence suggests newer alternatives may be a better choice. *Curr Psychiatry* 2020; **19**:19+.

53. Huf G, et al. Physical restraints versus seclusion room for management of people with acute aggression or agitation due to psychotic illness (TREC-SAVE): a randomized trial. *Psychol Med* 2012; **42**:2265–2273.

54. Amdisen A, et al. Serum concentrations and clinical effect of zuclopenthixol in acutely disturbed, psychotic patients treated with zuclopenthixol acetate in Viscoleo. *Psychopharmacology* 1986; **90**:412–416.

55. Amdisen A, et al. Zuclopenthixol acetate in viscoleo – a new drug formulation. An open Nordic multicentre study of zuclopenthixol acetate in Viscoleo in patients with acute psychoses including mania and exacerbation of chronic psychoses. *Acta Psychiatr Scand* 1987; **75**:99–107.

56. Lowert AC, et al. Acute psychotic disorders treated with 5% zuclopenthixol acetate in 'Viscoleo' ('Cisordinol-Acutard'), a global assessment of the clinical effect: an open multi-centre study. *Pharmatherapeutica* 1989; **5**:380–386.

57. Balant LP, et al. Clinical and pharmacokinetic evaluation of zuclopenthixol acetate in Viscoleo. *Pharmacopsychiatry* 1989; **22**:250–254.

58. Chakravarti SK, et al. Zuclopenthixol acetate (5% in 'Viscoleo'): single-dose treatment for acutely disturbed psychotic patients. *Curr Med Res Opin* 1990; **12**:58–65.

59. Baastrup PC, et al. A controlled Nordic multicentre study of zuclopenthixol acetate in oil solution, haloperidol and zuclopenthixol in the treatment of acute psychosis. *Acta Psychiatr Scand* 1993; **87**:48–58.

60. Chin CN, et al. A double blind comparison of zuclopenthixol acetate with haloperidol in the management of acutely disturbed schizophrenics. *Med J Malaysia* 1998; **53**:365–371.

61. Taymeeyapradit U, et al. Comparative study of the effectiveness of zuclopenthixol acetate and haloperidol in acutely disturbed psychotic patients. *J Med Assoc Thai* 2002; **85**:1301–1308.

62. Brook S, et al. A randomized controlled double blind study of zuclopenthixol acetate compared to haloperidol in acute psychosis. *Human Psychopharmacol Clin Experimental* 1998; **13**:17–20.

63. Chouinard G, et al. A double-blind controlled study of intramuscular zuclopenthixol acetate and liquid oral haloperidol in the treatment of schizophrenic patients with acute exacerbation. *J Clin Psychopharmacol* 1994; **14**:377–384.

64. Al-Haddad MK, et al. Zuclopenthixol versus haloperidol in the initial treatment of schizophrenic psychoses, affective psychoses and paranoid states: a controlled clinical trial. *Arab J Psychiatry* 1996; **7**:44–54.

65. Jayakody K, et al. Zuclopenthixol acetate for acute schizophrenia and similar serious mental illnesses. *Cochrane Database Syst Rev* 2012; 4:CD000525.

66. Liu P, et al. Observation of clinical effect of clopixol acuphase injection for acute psychosis. *Chin J Pharmacoepidemiology* 1997; 6:202–204.

67. Ropert R, et al. Where zuclopenthixol acetate stands amid the 'modified release' neuroleptics. Congres de Psychiatrie et de Neurolgie de Langue Francaise, LXXXVIth Session, Chambery, France; June 13–17 1988.

68. Berk M. A controlled double blind study of zuclopenthixol acetate compared with clothiapine in acute psychosis including mania and exacerbation of chronic psychosis. Proceedings of XXth Collegium Internationale Neruo-spychopharmacologicum, Melbourne, Australia; June 23–27 1996.

69. Garriga M, et al. Assessment and management of agitation in psychiatry: expert consensus. *World J Biol Psychiatry* 2016; 17:86–128.

70. Wilson MP, et al. Potential complications of combining intramuscular olanzapine with benzodiazepines in emergency department patients. *J Emerg Med* 2012; 43:889–896.

71. Villari V, et al. Oral risperidone, olanzapine and quetiapine versus haloperidol in psychotic agitation. *Prog Neuropsychopharmacol Biol Psychiatry* 2008; 32:405–413.

72. Paton C. Benzodiazepines and disinhibition: a review. *Psychiatric Bulletin* 2002; 26:460–462.

73. Chan-Tack KM. Neuroleptic malignant syndrome due to promethazine. *South Med J* 1999; 92:1017–1018.

74. Appleby L, et al. Sudden unexplained death in psychiatric in-patients. *Br J Psychiatry* 2000; 176:405–406.

75. Yap YG, et al. Risk of torsades de pointes with non-cardiac drugs. Doctors need to be aware that many drugs can cause QT prolongation. *BMJ* 2000; 320:1158–1159.

76. Taylor DM. Antipsychotics and QT prolongation. *Acta Psychiatr Scand* 2003; 107:85–95.

第 1 章

抗精神病药长效制剂

抗精神病药长效制剂(LAI)在临床实践中经常被使用,尤其是在英国、澳大利亚和欧盟。观察性研究发现,相比于口服抗精神病药治疗,抗精神病药 LAI 维持治疗与较少的复发和住院率有关[1-5],尽管研究中有一些混杂因素(如适应证偏倚)。

一项关于随机对照试验的 Cochrane 系统综述,分析了抗精神病药与安慰剂维持治疗精神分裂症的疗效差异,发现抗精神病药 LAI(尤其是氟哌啶醇 LAI 和氟奋乃静 LAI)比口服抗精神病药更有效[6]。不过作者指出,只有对口服和抗精神病药 LAI 的头对头比较才能确定后者是更有效的。而这类随机对照试验多数没有发现抗精神病药 LAI 具有明确的疗效优势[7-9],但可能与研究设计及方法学问题有部分关系[2]。具体来说,双盲随机对照试验多数是短期的,而且研究样本倾向于病情较轻、共病较少且依从性较好的患者[10,11]。以更自然的方式进行随机对照试验,可能会更好地显示长效制剂的优势[12]。不过,以各种方式进行的所有研究都明确表明,使用长效制剂进行维持治疗并不能完全避免复发[13]。

若患者喜欢这种剂型的方便性,或者避免隐蔽的不依从性是临床上的首要问题,建议使用抗精神病药长效制剂[14,15]。虽然 LAI 药物不能保证依从性,但比起口服药物,它至少保证了对依从性的意识。因此,患者对药物的不依从(表现为推迟或拒绝接受注射),作为病情复发的征象或潜在原因,可以被临床医师识别并迅速干预。抗精神病药 LAI 的另一个优势,可能是可以帮助辨别患者疗效不佳的原因,即究竟是因为依从性问题,还是因为疾病难治。许多表现为难治的患者仅仅是因为对口服药物不依从,有时甚至完全如此[16]。此外,抗精神病药 LAI 为执行注射的医护人员提供了仔细观察患者心理状态和不良反应的机会[17]。

不同国家中接受抗精神病药 LAI 治疗的精神分裂症患者比例不同,提示 LAI 的使用受到依从性以外的因素影响。对这些因素的更深入了解,将有助于识别阻碍这种治疗的障碍[18-20]。美国的一项研究发现,美国的首次发病患者很大程度上愿意接受长效制剂治疗[21],提示长效制剂在美国的低使用率可能更多的是由于临床医师不愿意使用,而非患者。

LAI 的处方意见

■ **对于第一代抗精神病药长效制剂,应给予试验剂量**。由于其半衰期长,注射后不良反应可能长时间持续存在。因此,若患者曾有需立即停药的严重不良反应史(如恶性综合征),应避免使用这种治疗。对于第一代抗精神病药,在少量油性溶剂中含少量药物的试验剂量有双重目的:一是了解患者对 EPS 是否易感,二是了解患者对油性溶剂是否敏感。对于第二代抗精神病药长效制剂,并不需要用试验剂量(因为较少引起 EPS,且已知水基不会过敏);但在怀疑患者对口服抗精神病药不依从,且 LAI 制剂的使用将首次确保给药的情况下,使用试验剂量是合适的。对于第一代和第二代抗精神病药 LAI,优先使用口服制剂的等效剂量进行治疗,以评估疗效和耐受性,但这从药代动力学的角度来说并不是必需的。大多数第二代抗精神病药长效制剂可以从一开始就单独使用,但通常需要负荷剂量(如帕利哌酮和阿立哌唑)。

- **从最低治疗剂量起始**。很少有资料证明第一代抗精神病药长效制剂有明确的剂量-疗效关系。有一些资料提示,在药品说明书剂量范围内,低剂量至少与高剂量疗效相同[22-25],但抗精神病药 LAI 的剂量和注射频率是否达到了最佳的获益-风险平衡似乎仍不确定[26-28]。
- **应按产品说明书规定的最长间隔注射药物**。按注册的给药间隔时间,所有 LAI 均可安全使用,记住推荐的最大单次剂量。目前并无证据支持缩短注射间隔时间可以提高疗效。同时,肌内注射部位会产生不适和疼痛,因此减少注射频率是值得的。有报告说一些患者在下次注射的前几天病情会有波动,且每次注射之后,抗精神病药的血药浓度可能会缓慢下降几小时(有些制剂甚至几天)。在这种情况下,患者的病情在注射后不久即明显恢复是没有道理的。更重要的是,在稳定状态下,血浆谷浓度(注射前和刚注射后)通常远高于发挥疗效所需的阈值。
- **只有在足够的评定时间后才能调整用药剂量**。相比于口服制剂,使用 LAI 后,血药达峰时间、治疗作用和稳态血药浓度都会延迟。如果出现不良反应,可能需要减少剂量;增加剂量前,应仔细评定至少一个月,且最好更久。需要注意的是,大多数 LAI 在开始使用且不增加剂量的情况下,血浆药物水平会在数周至数月内逐渐增加。原因与药物的蓄积有关,在注射后至少 6~8 周才可达到稳定血药浓度。因此,在达到稳定的血药浓度之前,增加剂量是不合理的,也不可能进行正确的评估。在治疗过程中,建议监测并记录疗效、不良反应和对躯体健康的影响。
- **长效抗精神病药制剂不推荐用于从未使用过抗精神病药的患者**。在开始使用 LAI 之前,通常使用同一药物的口服剂型 2 周,才能确定是否耐受该药。较为典型的例子是氟哌啶醇、阿立哌唑和帕利哌酮(使用口服利培酮)。

　　加用口服抗精神病药将增加大剂量用药的风险。口服抗精神病药与抗精神病药 LAI 规律联用曾常见于第一代抗精神病药[17,29]。这种策略也许可以用于控制突发症状及更灵活地调整剂量,但其安全性和耐受性并不确定,尤其是在长期使用的情况下[30]。抗精神病药 LAI 和口服制剂的联用很可能会不经意间导致大剂量处方,从而增加不良反应负担,对躯体健康监测造成影响[10,17]。

抗精神病药长效制剂之间的差别

　　第一代抗精神病药长效制剂之间的疗效几乎没有区别,尽管有一些研究提示珠氯噻醇癸酸酯在停药前和住院前时间方面有优势,但这可能是以更大的不良反应负担为代价的[31-33]。Cochrane 数据库完成了对哌泊噻嗪棕榈酸酯[34]、氟哌噻吨癸酸酯[35]、珠氯噻醇癸酸酯[36]、氟哌啶醇癸酸酯[37]和氟奋乃静癸酸酯[38]的综述。

　　第二代抗精神病药长效制剂(阿立哌唑、帕利哌酮、利培酮和奥氮平)之间疗效相当,但导致特定不良反应的可能性不同,如体重增加、代谢不良反应、锥体外系不良反应和血浆催乳素升高[39-42]。例如,帕利哌酮 LAI 与血浆催乳素水平的显著升高有关[41],奥氮平 LAI 可导致体重明显增加,且与注射后谵妄/镇静症状有关,推测为意外局部血管内注射或血管损伤所致[43,44]。由于利培酮 LAI 的药代动力学特性,首次注射后 3 周内需要口服一种抗精神病药(表 1.4)[45,46]。每种第二代抗精神病药的详细剂量将在本章其他部分介绍。

第 1 章

表 1.4 抗精神病药长效制剂:推荐剂量和注射频率 [15]

药物	商品名(英国)	注射部位	试验剂量/mg	剂量范围	注射间隔	评论
阿立哌唑	Abilify Maintena	臀肌	不需要**	300~400mg/m	1 个月	不引起催乳素升高;需要口服负荷剂量
氟哌噻吨癸酸酯	Depixol	臀肌或股肌	20	50mg/4w~400mg/w	2~4w	相比其他 LAI,最大批准剂量很高
氟奋乃静癸酸酯	Modecate	臀肌	12.5	12.5mg/2w~100mg/2w	2~5w	EPS 发生率高
氟哌啶醇癸酸酯	Haldol	臀肌	25*	50~300mg/4w	4w	EPS 发生率高
双羟萘酸奥氮平	ZypAdhera	臀肌	不需要**	150mg/4w~300mg/2w	2~4w	有注射后综合征的风险
棕榈酸帕利哌酮(1 个月剂型)	Xeplion	三角肌或臀肌	不需要**	50~150mg/m	1 个月	治疗起始需负荷剂量
棕榈酸帕利哌酮(3 个月剂型)	Trevicta	三角肌或臀肌	不需要***	175~525mg/3m	3 个月	EPS 发生率较低(相比于其他 FGA)
棕榈酸哌泊噻嗪	Piportil	臀肌	25	50~200mg/4w	4w	? EPS 发生率低(相比于其他 FGA)
利培酮微球	Risperidal Consta	三角肌或臀肌	不需要**	25~50mg/2w	2w	药物释放延迟 2~3 周,需要口服治疗
珠氯噻醇癸酸酯	Clopixol	臀肌或股肌	100	200mg/3w~600mg/w	2~4w	? 疗效略优于第一代长效注射剂

- 以上剂量适用于成人,老年患者的适宜剂量请参阅产品说明书。
- 试验剂量注射后,应等待 4~10 天,再根据治疗反应逐步增加至维持剂量(见各药的产品说明书)。
- 应避免给药间隔时间短于推荐时间,除非特殊情况[例如,注射剂容量高(>3~4mL?)时,可能需要延长间隔时间]。说明书所示最大单次剂量优先于更长的注射间隔时间和较小的注射剂容量。例如,珠氯噻醇 500mg/w 是说明书许可的,但 1 000mg/2w 不是说明书许可的(所用剂量超过最高注册剂量 600mg)。始终要查阅制药企业的官方信息。

* 试验剂量并非制药企业提出。

** LAI 使用前,应确定口服制剂的耐受性和疗效。使用帕利哌酮 LAI 之前,也可以口服利培酮。

*** 在 1 个月剂型治疗满 4 个月以后才应启用。

w,week,周;m,month,月。

参考文献

1. Tiihonen J, et al. Real-world effectiveness of antipsychotic treatments in a nationwide cohort of 29823 patients with schizophrenia. *JAMA Psychiatry* 2017; **74**:686–693.

2. Kirson NY, et al. Efficacy and effectiveness of depot versus oral antipsychotics in schizophrenia: synthesizing results across different research designs. *J Clin Psychiatry* 2013; **74**:568–575.

3. Marcus SC, et al. Antipsychotic adherence and rehospitalization in schizophrenia patients receiving oral versus long-acting injectable antipsychotics following hospital discharge. *J Manag Care Spec Pharm* 2015; **21**:754–768.

4. Nielsen RE, et al. Second-generation LAI are associated to favorable outcome in a cohort of incident patients diagnosed with schizophrenia. *Schizophr Res* 2018; **202**:234–240.

5. Kishimoto T, et al. Effectiveness of long-acting injectable vs oral antipsychotics in patients with schizophrenia: a meta-analysis of prospective and retrospective cohort studies. *Schizophr Bull* 2018; **44**:603–619.

6. Ceraso A, et al. Maintenance treatment with antipsychotic drugs for schizophrenia. *Cochrane Database Syst Rev* 2020; **8**:Cd008016.

7. Ostuzzi G, et al. Does formulation matter? A systematic review and meta-analysis of oral versus long-acting antipsychotic studies. *Schizophr Res* 2017; **183**:10–21.

8. Kishimoto T, et al. Long-acting injectable vs oral antipsychotics for relapse prevention in schizophrenia: a meta-analysis of randomized trials. *Schizophr Bull* 2014; **40**:192–213.

9. Leucht C, et al. Oral versus depot antipsychotic drugs for schizophrenia–a critical systematic review and meta-analysis of randomised long-term trials. *Schizophr Res* 2011; **127**:83–92.

10. Barnes T, et al. Evidence-based guidelines for the pharmacological treatment of schizophrenia: updated recommendations from the British Association for Psychopharmacology. *J Psychopharmacology* 2020; **34**:3–78.

11. Kane JM, et al. Optimizing treatment choices to improve adherence and outcomes in schizophrenia. *J Clin Psychiatry* 2019; **80**:IN18031AH18031C.

12. Kane JM, et al. Effect of long-acting injectable antipsychotics vs usual care on time to first hospitalization in early-phase schizophrenia: a randomized clinical trial. *JAMA Psychiatry* 2020; **77**:1–8.

13. Rubio JM, et al. Psychosis relapse during treatment with long-acting injectable antipsychotics in individuals with schizophrenia-spectrum disorders: an individual participant data meta-analysis. *Lancet Psychiatry* 2020; **7**:749–761.

14. National Institute for Health and Care Excellence. Psychosis and schizophrenia in adults: prevention and management. Clinical Guidance [CG178]. 2014 (last checked March 2019); https://www.nice.org.uk/guidance/cg178.

15. Barnes TR. Evidence-based guidelines for the pharmacological treatment of schizophrenia: recommendations from the British Association for Psychopharmacology. *J Psychopharmacology* 2011; **25**:567–620.

16. McCutcheon R, et al. Antipsychotic plasma levels in the assessment of poor treatment response in schizophrenia. *Acta Psychiatr Scand* 2018; **137**:39–46.

17. Barnes T, et al. Antipsychotic long acting injections: prescribing practice in the UK. *Br J Psychiatry Suppl* 2009; **52**:S37–S42.

18. Brissos S, et al. The role of long-acting injectable antipsychotics in schizophrenia: a critical appraisal. *Ther Adv Psychopharmacol* 2014; **4**:198–219.

19. Haddad P, et al. Prescribing patterns and determinants of use of antipsychotic long-acting injections: an international perspective, in *Antipsychotic Long-acting Injections* (2nd ed.). Oxford University Press; 2016.

20. Patel MX, et al. Attitudes of European physicians towards the use of long-acting injectable antipsychotics. *BMC Psychiatry* 2020; **20**:123.

21. Kane JM, et al. Patients with early-phase schizophrenia will accept treatment with sustained-release medication (Long-Acting Injectable Antipsychotics): results from the recruitment phase of the PRELAPSE trial. *J Clin Psychiatry* 2019; **80**.

22. Kane JM, et al. A multidose study of haloperidol decanoate in the maintenance treatment of schizophrenia. *Am J Psychiatry* 2002; **159**:554–560.

23. Taylor D. Establishing a dose-response relationship for haloperidol decanoate. *Psychiatric Bulletin* 2005; **29**:104–107.

24. McEvoy JP, et al. Effectiveness of paliperidone palmitate vs haloperidol decanoate for maintenance treatment of schizophrenia: a randomized clinical trial. *JAMA* 2014; **311**:1978–1987.

25. Bailey L, et al. Estimating the optimal dose of flupentixol decanoate in the maintenance treatment of schizophrenia—a systematic review of the literature. *Psychopharmacology* 2019; **236**:3081–3092.

26. Uchida H, et al. Monthly administration of long-acting injectable risperidone and striatal dopamine D2 receptor occupancy for the management of schizophrenia. *J Clin Psychiatry* 2008; **69**:1281–1286.

27. Ikai S, et al. Plasma levels and estimated dopamine D(2) receptor occupancy of long-acting injectable risperidone during maintenance treatment of schizophrenia: a 3-year follow-up study. *Psychopharmacology* 2016; **233**:4003–4010.

28. Hill AL, et al. Dose-associated changes in safety and efficacy parameters observed in a 24-week maintenance trial of olanzapine long-acting injection in patients with schizophrenia. *BMC Psychiatry* 2011; **11**:28.

29. Doshi JA, et al. Concurrent oral antipsychotic drug use among schizophrenia patients initiated on long-acting injectable antipsychotics post-hospital discharge. *J Clin Psychopharmacol* 2015; **35**:442–446.

30. Correll CU, et al. Practical considerations for managing breakthrough psychosis and symptomatic worsening in patients with schizophrenia on long-acting injectable antipsychotics. *CNS Spectr* 2018; **24**:354–370.

31. Da Silva Freire Coutinho E, et al. Zuclopenthixol decanoate for schizophrenia and other serious mental illnesses. *Cochrane Database Syst Rev* 2006; CD001164.

32. Shajahan P, et al. Comparison of the effectiveness of depot antipsychotics in routine clinical practice. *Psychiatrist* 2010; **34**:273–279.

33. Adams CE, et al. Systematic meta-review of depot antipsychotic drugs for people with schizophrenia. *Br J Psychiatry* 2001; **179**:290–299.

34. Dinesh M, et al. Depot pipotiazine palmitate and undecylenate for schizophrenia. *Cochrane Database Syst Rev* 2006; CD001720.

35. Mahapatra J, et al. Flupenthixol decanoate (depot) for schizophrenia or other similar psychotic disorders. *Cochrane Database Syst Rev* 2014; 6:CD001470.

36. Coutinho E, et al. Zuclopenthixol decanoate for schizophrenia and other serious mental illnesses. *Cochrane Database Syst Rev* 2000; CD001164.

37. Quraishi S, et al. Depot haloperidol decanoate for schizophrenia. *Cochrane Database Syst Rev* 2000; CD001361.

38. Maayan N, et al. Fluphenazine decanoate (depot) and enanthate for schizophrenia. *Cochrane Database Syst Rev* 2015; Cd000307.

39. Jann MW, et al. Long-acting injectable second-generation antipsychotics: an update and comparison between agents. *CNS Drugs* 2018; **32**:241–257.

40. Correll CU, et al. The use of long-acting injectable antipsychotics in schizophrenia: evaluating the evidence. *J Clin Psychiatry* 2016; **77**:1–24.

41. Nussbaum AM, et al. Paliperidone palmitate for schizophrenia. *Cochrane Database Syst Rev* 2012; Cd008296.

42. Sampson S, et al. Risperidone (depot) for schizophrenia. *Cochrane Database Syst Rev* 2016; 4:Cd004161.

43. Citrome L. Olanzapine pamoate: a stick in time? *Int J Clin Pract* 2009; **63**:140–150.

44. Luedecke D, et al. Post-injection delirium/sedation syndrome in patients treated with olanzapine pamoate: mechanism, incidence, and management. *CNS Drugs* 2015; **29**:41–46.

45. Harrison TS, et al. Long-acting risperidone: a review of its use in schizophrenia. *CNS Drugs* 2004; **18**:113–132.

46. Knox ED, et al. Clinical review of a long-acting, injectable formulation of risperidone. *Clin Ther* 2004; **26**:1994–2002.

抗精神病药长效制剂——药代动力学

药物	商品名(英国)	达峰 时间/天 *	血浆 半衰期/天	达稳态 时间/周 **
阿立哌唑 [1]	Abilify Maintena	7	30~46	~20
月桂酰阿立哌唑 [2-4]	Aristada(美国)	44~50	~54~57	~16
月桂酰阿立哌唑纳米晶 [4-6****]	Aristada Intio(美国)	4	~15~18	
氟哌噻吨癸酸酯 [7,8]	Depixol	4~7	8~17	~8~12
氟奋乃静癸酸酯 [4,9-11]	Modecate	8~12***	7~10	~8
氟哌啶醇癸酸酯 [12,13]	Haldol	7	21	~14
双羟萘酸奥氮平 [4,14,15]	ZypAdhera	2~3	30	~12
棕榈酸帕利哌酮(1 个月剂型) [4,16]	Xeplion	13	25~49	~20
棕榈酸帕利哌酮(3 个月剂型) [17,18]	Trevicta	25	三角肌:84~95 臀肌:118~139	~52
棕榈酸哌泊噻嗪 [19,20]	Piportil	7~14	15	~9
RBP-7000 [4,21](利培酮皮下注射 1 个月剂型)	Perseris(美国)	第一峰 1 天 第二峰 11 天	~8~9	~8
利培酮微球 [22,23]	Risperidal Consta	~30	4	~8
珠氯噻醇癸酸酯 [7,19,24]	Clopixo l	4~7	19	~12

* 达峰时间并不等于达到治疗血药浓度的时间,但是两者都具有剂量依赖性。对于大剂量(负荷剂量),常在达到峰浓度前就可见治疗作用。对于低(试验)剂量,最初的峰浓度可能低于治疗浓度。

** 达到稳态浓度遵循对数原理,而非线性特征:约 90% 的稳态浓度需要 3 个半衰期才能达到。达到稳态浓度所需的时间与剂量和注射频率无关(即,并不会因为单次剂量越大、注射越频繁,就越快达到稳态)。可以给予负荷剂量以快速达到治疗血浆水平,但达到稳态的时间不变。

*** 有研究估计注射后数小时即可达峰浓度 [24,25]。氟奋乃静癸酸酯可能有 2 个峰浓度—— 一个在注射当天,另一个略高的峰浓度出现在约一周以后 [12]。

**** 肌内注射的同时给予 30mg 阿立哌唑单次口服,用于 Aristada 的初始治疗;不用于重复给药。

参考文献

1. Mallikaarjun S, et al. Pharmacokinetics, tolerability and safety of aripiprazole once-monthly in adult schizophrenia: an open-label, parallel-arm, multiple-dose study. *Schizophr Res* 2013; **150**:281–288.

2. Hard ML, et al. Aripiprazole lauroxil: pharmacokinetic profile of this long-acting injectable antipsychotic in persons with schizophrenia. *J Clin Psychopharmacol* 2017; **37**:289–295.

3. Turncliff R, et al. Relative bioavailability and safety of aripiprazole lauroxil, a novel once-monthly, long-acting injectable atypical antipsychotic, following deltoid and gluteal administration in adult subjects with schizophrenia. *Schizophr Res* 2014; **159**:404–410.

4. Correll CU, et al. Pharmacokinetic characteristics of long-acting injectable antipsychotics for schizophrenia: an overview. *CNS Drugs* 2021; **35**:39–59.

5. Alkermes Inc. Highlights of Prescribing Information. ARISTADA INITIO® (aripiprazole lauroxil) extended-release injectable suspension, for intramuscular use. 2020; https://www.aristadahcp.com/downloadables/ARISTADA-INITIO-PI.pdf.

6. Alkermes Inc. ARISTADA INITIO™ (aripiprazole lauroxil) extended-release injectable suspension [product monograph]. 2020; https://www.aristadacaresupport.com/downloadables/ARISTADA-INITIO-ARISTADA-Payer-Hospital-Monograph.pdf.

7. Jann MW, et al. Clinical pharmacokinetics of the depot antipsychotics. *Clin Pharmacokinet* 1985; 10:315–333.

8. Bailey L, et al. Estimating the optimal dose of flupentixol decanoate in the maintenance treatment of schizophrenia—a systematic review of the literature. *Psychopharmacology* 2019; 236:3081–3092.

9. Simpson GM, et al. Single-dose pharmacokinetics of fluphenazine after fluphenazine decanoate administration. *J Clin Psychopharmacol* 1990; 10:417–421.

10. Balant-Gorgia AE, et al. Antipsychotic drugs. Clinical pharmacokinetics of potential candidates for plasma concentration monitoring. *Clin Pharmacokinet* 1987; 13:65–90.

11. Gitlin MJ, et al. Persistence of fluphenazine in plasma after decanoate withdrawal. *J Clin Psychopharmacol* 1988; 8:53–56.

12. Wiles DH, et al. Pharmacokinetics of haloperidol and fluphenazine decanoates in chronic schizophrenia. *Psychopharmacology* 1990; 101:274–281.

13. Nayak RK, et al. The bioavailability and pharmacokinetics of oral and depot intramuscular haloperidol in schizophrenic patients. *J Clin Pharmacol* 1987; 27:144–150.

14. Heres S, et al. Pharmacokinetics of olanzapine long-acting injection: the clinical perspective. *Int Clin Psychopharmacol* 2014; 29:299–312.

15. Mitchell M, et al. Single- and multiple-dose pharmacokinetic, safety, and tolerability profiles of olanzapine long-acting injection: an open-label, multicenter, nonrandomized study in patients with schizophrenia. *ClinTher* 2013; 35:1890–1908.

16. Hoy SM, et al. Intramuscular paliperidone palmitate. *CNS Drugs* 2010; 24:227–244.

17. Ravenstijn P, et al. Pharmacokinetics, safety, and tolerability of paliperidone palmitate 3-month formulation in patients with schizophrenia: a phase-1, single-dose, randomized, open-label study. *J Clin Pharmacol* 2016; 56:330–339.

18. Janssen Pharmaceuticals Inc. Highlights of Prescribing Information. INVEGA TRINZA® (paliperidone palmitate) extended-release injectable suspension for intramuscular use. 2019; https://www.janssenlabels.com/package-insert/product-monograph/prescribing-information/INVEGA+TRINZA-pi.pdf.

19. Barnes TR, et al. Long-term depot antipsychotics. A risk-benefit assessment. *Drug Saf* 1994; 10:464–479.

20. Ogden DA, et al. Determination of pipothiazine in human plasma by reversed-phase high-performance liquid chromatography. *J Pharm Biomed Anal* 1989; 7:1273–1280.

21. US Food and Drug Administration. Clinical pharmacology and biopharmaceutics review(s). perseris. 2018; https://www.accessdata.fda.gov/drugsatfda_docs/nda/2018/210655Orig1s000ClinPharmR.pdf.

22. Ereshefsky L, et al. Pharmacokinetic profile and clinical efficacy of long-acting risperidone: potential benefits of combining an atypical antipsychotic and a new delivery system. *Drugs RD* 2005; 6:129–137.

23. Meyer JM. Understanding depot antipsychotics: an illustrated guide to kinetics. *CNS Spectr* 2013; 18 Suppl 1:58–67.

24. Viala A, et al. Comparative study of the pharmacokinetics of zuclopenthixol decanoate and fluphenazine decanoate. *Psychopharmacology* 1988; 94:293–297.

25. Soni SD, et al. Plasma levels of fluphenazine decanoate. Effects of site of injection, massage and muscle activity. *Br J Psychiatry* 1988; 153:382–384.

使用抗精神病药长效制剂的患者管理

对于所有接受抗精神病药长期治疗的患者,主管精神科医师应该每年至少看一次(最好次数多些),以便评估其进展和治疗情况,并系统全面地评估其耐受性和安全性。对不良反应的评估应包括锥体外系不良反应(主要是帕金森综合征、静坐不能和迟发性运动障碍)。对迟发性运动障碍的评估记录可以使用异常不自主运动量表[1,2]。有些研究发现抗精神病药 LAI 相比口服制剂更容易引起迟发性运动障碍,但仍不明确[3-5];使用同一种抗精神病药时,LAI 和口服制剂导致的迟发性运动障碍风险并没有不同[6,7]。

对于多次发病的大多数精神分裂症患者而言,长期乃至终身治疗是必要的。总的来说,对于病情稳定的患者,有研究者建议维持抗精神病药治疗的剂量应不低于标准每天剂量的50%,因为低于这一水平的治疗与更大的复发风险有关[8]。因此,当抗精神病药剂量减少时,长期随访是非常重要的,尤其是药物剂量减至非常低的时候;因为这种剂量减低与更高的治疗失败风险、住院率和复发率有关[9],而且只在更长的时间内才会变得明显。

但是,对于长期使用长效制剂治疗的患者,若病情稳定,可以考虑减少剂量,因为患者常常接受的是超治疗剂量。在临床试验中,氟哌啶醇癸酸酯的最佳有效剂量是每 4 周 75mg[9,10],棕榈酸帕利哌酮是每月 50mg[11]。如此低的剂量在临床实践中几乎见不到。此外,预防复发所需的纹状体 D_2 受体占有率阈值可能比急性发作期所需的低[12-14]。然而对精神分裂症患者来说,剂量降低至标准剂量以下显然与复发风险更大有关,特别是从长期来看。一项研究比较了低剂量(每 2 周 5mg)和标准剂量(每 2 周 25mg)的氟奋乃静癸酸酯的效果,发现二者的疗效在 1 年时没有差异,但在 2 年时低剂量组明显劣于标准剂量组(复发率分别为 69% 和 36%)[15]。然而,在同一项研究中,当出现症状时增加剂量,高剂量组的优势就没有了。另一项比较低剂量(每 2 周 1.25~5mg)和标准剂量(每 2 周 12.5~50mg)氟奋乃静癸酸酯的研究也发现,低剂量组明显不如标准剂量组,1 年累计复发率分别为 56% 和 7%[16]。类似地,一项随机对照试验比较了 4 组固定月剂量(25mg,50mg,100mg 和 200mg)的氟哌啶醇 LAI 治疗超过 1 年的效果,发现 200mg 标准剂量组的复发率和症状恶化率最低(15%),相比之下 100mg 组为 23%,50mg 组为 25%(但是无统计学意义),且标准剂量组的不良反应发生率只轻微升高[17]。

没有简单的公式可以决定何时或是否减少维持期抗精神病药的剂量。因此,对每一个患者,都应该进行风险与获益分析。应该注意的是,许多患者乐于接受长效制剂[7,18]。

考虑减少剂量时,以下提示可能有所帮助:

- 患者是否没有症状了? 如果是,已经多长时间了? 这里不包括那些长期存在、不导致患者痛苦、既往药物治疗无效的症状。
- 不良反应(包括迟发型运动障碍在内的 EPS,包括肥胖在内的代谢不良反应等)的严重程度、耐受性和致残性如何? 若患者仅报告轻微的或没有报告不良反应,继续治疗通常是合理的,但需要密切监测迟发性运动障碍的表现。
- 以往疾病的表现形式如何? 需要考虑发病的速度、持续时间、发作的严重程度,以及对自身或他人的危险。
- 以前是否尝试过减少药物剂量? 如果是,之前的结果是什么?

■ 患者目前的社会环境如何？是相对平稳期，还是预期会有应激性生活事件发生？

■ 患者复发的社会成本如何？（例如，患者是不是家庭中唯一的经济支柱？）

■ 患者是否有能力监测自己的症状？如果是，患者会寻求帮助吗？

　　如果考虑上述因素之后，决定减少药物剂量，应该让患者的家人参与，并向其清晰说明症状复发或恶化时如何应对。然后合理地采用以下方式：

■ 若尚未停用口服抗精神病药，应首先停用它。

■ 在药品说明书允许的情况下，将注射的时间间隔拉长至 4 周，然后减少每次的注射剂量。

■ 任何时候减量不应超出原治疗剂量的 1/3。注意：利培酮微球注射剂使用时应特殊考虑。

■ 如果可能，减量频率不应超过每 3 个月 1 次，最好每 6 个月 1 次。减药的速度越慢，复发的时间越晚 [19]。

■ 以上过程的最终目标不应该是停用药物，虽然有时会出现这种结果。虽然间歇性、有针对性（有症状时用药）的抗精神病药治疗方法不如连续治疗有效，但可能还是比不治疗好 [20-22]。

　　如果减量过程中患者出现症状，不应将其看作是失败，而是看作确定患者所需最低有效剂量的重要步骤。

　　更多讨论见本章关于长期抗精神病药治疗的部分。

参考文献

1. National Institute of Mental Health. *Abnormal Involuntary Movement Scale (AIMS). (U.S. Public Health Service Publication No. MH-9-17).* Washington, DC: US Government Printing Office; 1974.

2. McEvoy JP. How to assess tardive dyskinesia symptom improvement with measurement-based care. *J Clin Psychiatry* 2020; 81:NU19047BR4C.

3. Novick D, et al. Incidence of extrapyramidal symptoms and tardive dyskinesia in schizophrenia: thirty-six-month results from the European schizophrenia outpatient health outcomes study. *J Clin Psychopharmacol* 2010; 30:531–540.

4. Barnes TR, et al. Long-term depot antipsychotics. A risk-benefit assessment. *Drug Saf* 1994; 10:464–479.

5. Baldessarini RJ, et al. Incidence of extrapyramidal syndromes and tardive dyskinesia. *J Clin Psychopharmacol* 2011; 31:382–384; author reply 384–385.

6. Gopal S, et al. Incidence of tardive dyskinesia: a comparison of long-acting injectable and oral paliperidone clinical trial databases. *Int J Clin Pract* 2014; 68:1514–1522.

7. Patel MX, et al. Why aren't depot antipsychotics prescribed more often and what can be done about it? *Adv Psychiatric Treatment* 2005; 11:203–211.

8. Correll CU, et al. What is the risk-benefit ratio of long-term antipsychotic treatment in people with schizophrenia? *World Psychiatry* 2018; 17:149–160.

9. Taylor D. Establishing a dose-response relationship for haloperidol decanoate. *Psychiatric Bulletin* 2005; 29:104–107.

10. McEvoy JP, et al. Effectiveness of paliperidone palmitate vs haloperidol decanoate for maintenance treatment of schizophrenia: a randomized clinical trial. *JAMA* 2014; 311:1978–1987.

11. Rothe PH, et al. Dose equivalents for second generation long-acting injectable antipsychotics: the minimum effective dose method. *Schizophr Res* 2018; 193:23–28.

12. Takeuchi H, et al. Dose reduction of risperidone and olanzapine and estimated dopamine D_2 receptor occupancy in stable patients with schizophrenia: findings from an open-label, randomized, controlled study. *J Clin Psychiatry* 2014; 75:1209–1214.

13. Mizuno Y, et al. Dopamine D2 receptor occupancy with risperidone or olanzapine during maintenance treatment of schizophrenia: a cross-sectional study. *Prog Neuropsychopharmacol Biol Psychiatry* 2012; 37:182–187.

14. Ikai S, et al. A cross-sectional study of plasma risperidone levels with risperidone long-acting injectable: implications for dopamine D2 receptor occupancy during maintenance treatment in schizophrenia. *J Clin Psychiatry* 2012; 73:1147–1152.

15. Marder SR, et al. Low- and conventional-dose maintenance therapy with fluphenazine decanoate. Two-year outcome. *Arch Gen Psychiatry* 1987; 44:518–521.

16. Kane JM, et al. Low-dose neuroleptic treatment of outpatient schizophrenics: i. preliminary results for relapse rates. *Arch Gen Psychiatry* 1983; 40:893–896.

17. Kane JM, et al. A multidose study of haloperidol decanoate in the maintenance treatment of schizophrenia. *Am J Psychiatry* 2002; 159:554–560.

18. Heres S, et al. The attitude of patients towards antipsychotic depot treatment. *Int Clin Psychopharmacol* 2007; 22:275–282.

19. Weiden PJ, et al. Does half-life matter after antipsychotic discontinuation? A relapse comparison in schizophrenia with 3 different formula-

tions of paliperidone. *J Clin Psychiatry* 2017; 78:e813–e820.

20. National Institute for Health and Care Excellence. Psychosis and schizophrenia in adults: prevention and management. Clinical Guidance [CG178]. 2014 (last checked March 2019); https://www.nice.org.uk/guidance/cg178.

21. Barnes T, et al. Evidence-based guidelines for the pharmacological treatment of schizophrenia: updated recommendations from the British Association for Psychopharmacology. *J Psychopharmacology* 2020; 34:3–78.

22. Sampson S, et al. Intermittent drug techniques for schizophrenia. *Cochrane Database Syst Rev* 2013; Cd006196.

阿立哌唑 LAI

阿立哌唑品牌化

相对于其他第二代抗精神病药 LAI 而言,阿立哌唑不引起催乳素升高和代谢相关不良反应,因而是一种很有用的替代药物。安慰剂对照试验显示,它对急性期及以后的治疗均有效[1]。FDA 已经批准阿立哌唑 LAI 用于成年双相 I 型患者的单药维持治疗[2]。推荐使用阿立哌唑口服 10mg/d,14 天作为初始治疗,以确定耐受性和治疗反应。可采取以下两种方案之一作为阿立哌唑 LAI 起始治疗的剂量[3]。

一处注射起始

在开始那天,注射 400mg 阿立哌唑 LAI,并继续口服阿立哌唑 10~20mg/d,14 天,继而 20mg/d,14 天(一共 28 天),从而在起始阶段维持阿立哌唑的治疗浓度。

或者

两处注射起始

在开始那天,在两个不同的肌肉部位(两个臀肌、两个三角肌或一个臀肌一个三角肌)分别注射 400mg 阿立哌唑 LAI,并口服 20mg 阿立哌唑 1 次。之后不再口服药物。

起始治疗的 1 个月后,开始每个月 400mg 的治疗。

一处注射 + 口服起始方案中,在首次注射后的第 7 天达到血浆峰浓度,在 4 周末达到谷浓度[4]。达到稳态时,血药峰浓度水平将比首次注射后的峰浓度高出 50%,而谷浓度仅比首次注射后的峰浓度略低[4]。剂量调整时应该考虑到这一点。一项人群药代动力学模型研究表明,两处注射起始方案产生的阿立哌唑血药浓度与一处注射起始方法相当[5]。

不能耐受每月 400mg 的患者,可以使用每月 300mg。每月 200mg 则仅用于那些同时服用特异性酶抑制剂的患者。治疗中静坐不能、失眠、恶心和不安的发生率与口服阿立哌唑相近[6,7]。

目前,还没有换用阿立哌唑的正式建议。本章根据现有药代动力学资料的解释,提出以下建议。

换用阿立哌唑 LAI

既往用药	阿立哌唑 LAI 使用建议
口服抗精神病药	交叉换药,先口服阿立哌唑 2 周以上 *
	单处注射起始
	开始阿立哌唑 LAI 治疗,继续口服阿立哌唑 2 周,然后停用口服药
	两处注射起始
	按上述方法在口服阿立哌唑 2 周以后开始阿立哌唑 LAI 治疗,然后停用口服药 **

既往用药	阿立哌唑 LAI 使用建议
抗精神病药长效制剂(除外利培酮 LAI)	在应该注射最后一次长效制剂之日,开始口服阿立哌唑 * **一处注射起始** 2 周后开始阿立哌唑 LAI 治疗,继续口服阿立哌唑 2 周,然后停用口服药 **两处注射起始** 按上述方法在口服阿立哌唑 2 周以后开始阿立哌唑 LAI 治疗,然后停用口服药 **
利培酮 LAI	在最后一次注射利培酮 LAI 4~6 周后,开始口服阿立哌唑 * **一处注射起始** 2 周后开始阿立哌唑 LAI 治疗,继续口服阿立哌唑 2 周,然后停用口服药 **两处注射起始** 按上述方法在口服阿立哌唑 2 周以后开始阿立哌唑 LAI 治疗,然后停用口服药 **

　　* 如果之前已了解患者对阿立哌唑的耐受性和治疗反应,注射之前可能不需要严格执行口服阿立哌唑。但在单处注射起始方案中,阿立哌唑有效血药浓度的到达取决于 4 周的口服治疗。类似地,在两处注射起始方案中,药代动力学模型研究是在起始日血浆水平处于稳态的基础上进行的,而这种稳态是通过口服阿立哌唑达到的。

　　** 如果完全无法口服阿立哌唑(比如患者拒绝),总是使用两处注射起始方案。即使没有事先口服治疗,800mg 的剂量也可以提供治疗血药浓度。

其他阿立哌唑 LAI

　　美国食品药品管理局(FDA)批准了另一种用于治疗精神分裂症的阿立哌唑长效制剂,这种药在美国以外的地方很少使用。月桂酰阿立哌唑是一种前体药物,根据剂量可以按 1 个月、6 周或 2 周的间隔,在三角肌或臀肌进行肌内注射[8,9]。它有四种规格:441mg,662mg,882mg 和 1 064mg;分别含阿立哌唑 300mg,450mg,600mg 和 724mg(见本章长效制剂药代动力学和新型长效制剂部分)。月桂酰阿立哌唑也有特殊的起始治疗方案(Aristada Initio),可以在注射 4 天内提供有效血浆浓度,且不需要口服药物补充[10]。

参考文献

1. Shirley M, et al. Aripiprazole (ABILIFY MAINTENA®): a review of its use as maintenance treatment for adult patients with schizophrenia. *Drugs* 2014; **74**:1097–1110.
2. US Food and Drug Administration. Highlights of Prescribing Information. Abilify Maintena (aripiprazole) for extended-release suspension for intramuscular use. 2020; https://www.accessdata.fda.gov/drugsatfda_docs/label/2020/202971s013lbl.pdf.
3. Otsuka Pharmaceuticals (UK) Ltd. Summary of Product Characteristics. Abilify Maintena 400 mg powder and solvent for prolonged-release suspension for injection. 2020; https://www.medicines.org.uk/emc/product/7965/smpc.
4. Mallikaarjun S, et al. Pharmacokinetics, tolerability and safety of aripiprazole once-monthly in adult schizophrenia: an open-label, parallel-arm, multiple-dose study. *Schizophr Res* 2013; **150**:281–288.
5. Wang Y, et al. The two-injection start of aripiprazole once-monthly provides rapid attainment of therapeutic concentration without the need for 14 day oral Neuropsychopharmacology (ECNP) Congress, 12–15 September 2020, Virtual.
6. Kane JM, et al. Aripiprazole intramuscular depot as maintenance treatment in patients with schizophrenia: a 52-week, multicenter, randomized, double-blind, placebo-controlled study. *J Clin Psychiatry* 2012; **73**:617–624.
7. Potkin SG, et al. Safety and tolerability of once monthly aripiprazole treatment initiation in adults with schizophrenia stabilized on selected atypical oral antipsychotics other than aripiprazole. *Curr Med Res Opin* 2013; **29**:1241–1251.
8. Hard ML, et al. Aripiprazole lauroxil: pharmacokinetic profile of this long-acting injectable antipsychotic in persons with schizophrenia. *J Clin Psychopharmacol* 2017; **37**:289–295.
9. Turncliff R, et al. Relative bioavailability and safety of aripiprazole lauroxil, a novel once-monthly, long-acting injectable atypical antipsychotic, following deltoid and gluteal administration in adult subjects with schizophrenia. *Schizophr Res* 2014; **159**:404–410.
10. Ehret MJ, et al. Aripiprazole Lauroxil NanoCrystal® Dispersion Technology (Aristada Initio®). *Clin Schizophr Relat Psychoses* 2018; **12**:92–96.

奥氮平 LAI

与所有酯类化合物一样,双羟萘酸奥氮平难溶于水。在肌内注射后,双羟萘酸奥氮平的水性悬液即刻并持续释放奥氮平。注射后 1 周内达到血药峰浓度(在大多数人中只需 2~4 天)[1],仅 3 天即可出现疗效[2]。按产品说明书规定仅在臀肌注射;三角肌注射疗效较差[3]。奥氮平 LAI 每 4 周注射 1 次即有效,只有在使用最大剂量时才需 2 周注射 1 次。半衰期大约 30 天[1]。至今尚未与其他抗精神病药长效制剂进行随机对照研究,但自然条件下的数据提示其疗效与帕利哌酮 LAI 相似[4,5]。在一些给药方案中,建议使用负荷剂量(表 1.5)。正式产品说明书/产品特征概要建议,应先口服奥氮平以评定患者的耐受性及疗效。临床上极少这么做,但强烈建议执行。在注射第一次之后,不必同时补充口服药物。

表 1.5 给药方法

口服奥氮平等效剂量	负荷剂量	维持剂量(首剂注射 8 周后)
10mg/d	210mg/2w 或 405mg/4w	300mg/4w(或 150mg/2w)
15mg/d	300mg/2w	405mg/4w(或 210mg/2w)
20mg/d	无至 300mg/2w	300mg/2w

d,day,天;W,Week,周。

换药方法

从口服药物直接换成奥氮平 LAI 通常是可行的,理想的做法是先做口服药物试验。因此,从其他长效制剂(不包括利培酮)换成奥氮平口服或 LAI 时,应在原长效制剂该注射最后一次之日开始。从口服药物换成奥氮平 LAI 也类似——直接换药是可能的,但是在开始奥氮平口服或 LAI 之后,也许最好将前一药物缓慢减量。从利培酮 LAI 换成奥氮平 LAI 时,我们建议从预期的注射日期开始,延后 2 周再开始用奥氮平 LAI(利培酮血药浓度预计在最后一次注射 4~6 周后达峰)。

注射后综合征

注射后综合征(post-injection syndrome)通常发生于双羟萘酸奥氮平注射时不慎进入大量血液中(也许是意外渗入血管[6])。奥氮平血浆浓度可能达到 600μg/L,可导致谵妄和嗜睡[7]。注射后综合征的发生率低于注射例次的 0.1%;几乎所有反应(86%)都在注射后 1h 内出现[8]。我们的研究提示其发生率为注射例次的 0.044%(小于 1/2 000),且 91% 在注射后 1h 内表现明显[9]。注射 3h 后发生的报道非常少,其中一个病例发生在注射 12h 后[10]。

在大多数国家中,奥氮平 LAI 只可以在医疗机构内监督下使用,患者注射后应该观察 3h。基于注射 2h 后发生的病例非常少,有充分的理由把观察时间缩短至 2h(新西兰[11] 和一些其他国家是这样做的)。在 COVID-19 流行期间,已经有研究者建议将观察期缩短[12]。但需要强调的是,注射后综合征可以发生在任何时间,即使在同一个患者多次注射后也可能发生(也就是说,既往奥氮平 LAI 的安全使用不代表注射综合征发生率会降低[13])。

在欧盟,产品特征概述的准确措辞如下[14]:

每次注射后,患者应在医疗机构内由有适当资质的专业人员观察至少 3h,看有无符合奥氮平过量的症状和体征。

患者即将离开医疗机构前,应确认其意识清晰,定向良好,不存在奥氮平过量的症状和体征。如果怀疑药物过量,应继续进行密切的医疗监督和监护,直到检查表明症状和体征已经缓解。对于出现符合奥氮平过量的症状或体征的患者,3h 的观察期应该根据临床情况适当延长。

在注射当日的其他时间内,应告知患者注意继发于注射后不良反应的药物过量的症状和体征、发生问题后应如何获得专业帮助以及避免驾驶或操作机器。

奥氮平 LAI 使用中要求监护,这无疑影响了该药的普及。有趣的是,有些患者在出现了注射后综合征以后仍然选择继续治疗[15]。

出现该综合征的患者除更有可能以前出现过注射部位相关的不良反应以外[16],尚未找到哪些患者因素或医学因素可以预测注射后综合征[7]。有研究认为男性和大剂量药物是注射后综合征的风险因素(该研究调查了 103 505 次注射中发生的 46 次注射后综合征)[9]。

参考文献

1. Heres S, et al. Pharmacokinetics of olanzapine long-acting injection: the clinical perspective. *Int Clin Psychopharmacol* 2014; 29:299–312.

2. Lauriello J, et al. An 8-week, double-blind, randomized, placebo-controlled study of olanzapine long-acting injection in acutely ill patients with schizophrenia. *J Clin Psychiatry* 2008; 69:790–799.

3. Mitchell M, et al. Single- and multiple-dose pharmacokinetic, safety, and tolerability profiles of olanzapine long-acting injection: an open-label, multicenter, nonrandomized study in patients with schizophrenia. *Clin Ther* 2013; 35:1890–1908.

4. Denee TR, et al. Treatment continuation and treatment characteristics of four long acting antipsychotic medications (Paliperidone Palmitate, Risperidone Microspheres, Olanzapine Pamoate and Haloperidol Decanoate) in The Netherlands. *Value Health* 2015; 18:A407.

5. Taipale H, et al. Comparative effectiveness of antipsychotic drugs for rehospitalization in schizophrenia-a nationwide study with 20-year follow-up. *Schizophr Bull* 2017; 44:1381–1387.

6. Luedecke D, et al. Post-injection delirium/sedation syndrome in patients treated with olanzapine pamoate: mechanism, incidence, and management. *CNS Drugs* 2015; 29:41–46.

7. McDonnell DP, et al. Post-injection delirium/sedation syndrome in patients with schizophrenia treated with olanzapine long-acting injection, II: investigations of mechanism. *BMC Psychiatry* 2010; 10:45.

8. Bushes CJ, et al. Olanzapine long-acting injection: review of first experiences of post-injection delirium/sedation syndrome in routine clinical practice. *BMC Psychiatry* 2015; 15:65.

9. Meyers KJ, et al. Postinjection delirium/sedation syndrome in patients with schizophrenia receiving olanzapine long-acting injection: results from a large observational study. *B J Psych Open* 2017; 3:186–192.

10. Garg S, et al. Delayed onset postinjection delirium/sedation syndrome associated with olanzapine pamoate: a case report. *J Clin Psychopharmacol* 2019; 39:523–524.

11. Eli Lilly and Company (NZ) Limited. ZYPREXA RELPREVV® (olanzapine pamoate monohydrate). 2019; https://www.medsafe.govt.nz/Consumers/cmi/z/zyprexarelprevvinj.pdf.

12. Siskind D, et al. Monitoring for post-injection delirium/sedation syndrome with long-acting olanzapine during the COVID-19 pandemic. *Aust N Z J Psychiatry* 2020; 54:759–761.

13. Venkatesan V, et al. Postinjection delirium/sedation syndrome after 31st long-acting olanzapine depot injection. *Clin Neuropharmacol* 2019; 42:64–65.

14. Eli Lilly and Company Limited. Summary of Product Characteristics. ZYPADHERA 210 mg powder and solvent for prolonged release suspension for injection. 2020; https://www.medicines.org.uk/emc/product/6429.

15. Anand E, et al. A 6-year open-label study of the efficacy and safety of olanzapine long-acting injection in patients with schizophrenia: a post hoc analysis based on the European label recommendation. *Neuropsychiatr Dis Treat* 2015; 11:1349–1357.

16. Atkins S, et al. A pooled analysis of injection site-related adverse events in patients with schizophrenia treated with olanzapine long-acting injection. *BMC Psychiatry* 2014; 14:7.

棕榈酸帕利哌酮 LAI

帕利哌酮(9-羟利培酮)是利培酮的主要活性代谢产物。棕榈酸帕利哌酮是帕利哌酮的酯化前体药,有 1 个月和 3 个月两种剂型。在肌肉中,棕榈酸帕利哌酮被酯酶水解为帕利哌酮,随后被吸收入体循环[1]。

帕利哌酮 LAI 1 个月剂型

在使用推荐的起始负荷剂量之后,几天内即可达到其有效血药浓度,因而从药代动力学角度看,在肌内注射开始阶段,不必同时口服帕利哌酮或利培酮[2]。两次起始注射量(三角肌肌内注射)完成后,每月注射一次维持剂量(三角肌或臀部肌内注射)。单次三角肌注射后血药峰浓度比单次臀肌注射高出平均 28%[2]。因此,帕利哌酮 LAI 在第 1 天和第 8 天均采用三角肌注射,有助于药物迅速达到治疗浓度(表 1.6)。最早用药后第 4 天即可观察到精神病性症状改善[2]。

表 1.6　帕利哌酮剂量和用法信息[2]

	剂量	注射途径
起始		
第 1 天	150mg IM	仅三角肌
第 8 天(±4 天)	100mg IM	仅三角肌
维持		
之后每月(±7 天)	50~150mg IM*	三角肌或臀肌 **

* 维持期剂量的判断方法,可能最好是考虑口服利培酮的合适剂量,然后给予等效剂量的帕利哌酮(表 1.7)。治疗前口服帕利哌酮有助于确定给定剂量下的疗效和耐受性。

** 从高剂量口服帕利哌酮或利培酮转换至帕利哌酮 LAI 治疗的患者,可考虑在前 6 个月继续使用三角肌注射[2]。

IM,肌内注射。

表 1.7　近似等效剂量[2,5]

口服利培酮(mg/d) (生物利用度 =70%)[6]	口服帕利哌酮(mg/d) (生物利用度 =28%)[7]	利培酮 LAI(Consta) (mg/2w)	棕榈酸帕利哌酮(mg/m) (生物利用度 =100%)[2]
2	4	25	50
3	6	37.5	75
4	9	50	100
6	12	—	150

W,Week,周;m,month,月。

第二剂起始剂量可以在(在第 1 天注射第一剂之后)第 8 天前后 4 天注射[2]。说明书建议患者可以在每月注射日期的前后 7 天内进行维持剂量注射[2]。这种灵活性可以减少药物遗漏。对药物遗漏的详细建议参照药品说明书[2]。换用棕榈酸帕利哌酮 1 个月剂型的方法见表 1.8。

表 1.8　换用棕榈酸帕利哌酮 1 个月剂型的方法

原用药物	建议换药方法	评论
无	2 个起始剂量：第 1 天 150mg，三角肌注射；第 8 天 100mg，三角肌注射 1 个月后开始维持剂量	生产商建议一般成年人群用 75mg/m[17]。这相当于口服利培酮 3mg/d（表 1.7）。临床实践中 100mg/m 最常见 [18] 维持剂量调整应每月进行。但调整后的全部效应可能在数月内并不明显 [2]
口服帕利哌酮/利培酮	给予 2 个起始剂量后，开始维持剂量治疗（见表 1.7，并给予等效剂量的帕利哌酮 LAI）	在帕利哌酮 LAI 起始期，不必补充口服帕利哌酮或利培酮
口服其他抗精神病药	首次注射帕利哌酮后，在 1~2 周内减少原口服抗精神病药剂量。先给予 2 个起始剂量，然后给予维持剂量	
其他抗精神病长效制剂	该注射下一次原药时，开始帕利哌酮 LAI 治疗（给予维持剂量） 注意：不需要起始剂量	从 FGA 长效制剂转换至帕利哌酮长效剂的剂量难以预测。生产商建议普通成人 75mg/m，但临床实践中更多使用 100mg 和 150mg[18]。若从利培酮 LAI 换药，请见表 1.7，并给予等效剂量 维持剂量调整应每月进行。但调整后的全部效应可能在数月内并不明显 [2]
口服抗精神病药与长效制剂联合治疗	该注射下一次原药时，开始帕利哌酮 LAI（维持剂量） 注意：不需要起始剂量 首次注射帕利哌酮后，在 1~2 周内减少原口服抗精神病药剂量	目标是将帕利哌酮 LAI 作为患者唯一的抗精神病药 应该尽可能按照口服和注射抗精神病药的总剂量控制帕利哌酮的维持剂量（见本章等效剂量表）

m，month，月。

需要注意的点

- 棕榈酸帕利哌酮起始治疗不需要先用试验性剂量（但理想的情况应该是，患者目前口服帕利哌酮或利培酮治疗时病情稳定，或以前口服帕利哌酮或利培酮治疗有效）。
- 注射后血药浓度达峰时间中位数为 13 天 [2]。
- 每年接受注射少于 12 次的患者复发风险升高——正确用药对帕利哌酮每月治疗的疗效至关重要 [3,4]。

在帕利哌酮 LAI 与氟哌啶醇长效制剂的对照研究中，后者采用与帕利哌酮相当的负荷剂量 [8]。在复发预防方面，二者疗效相近，但是帕利哌酮升高催乳素的幅度更大，增加体重更多。氟哌啶醇更易导致静坐不能和急性运动障碍，并且存在迟发性运动障碍发生率升高的趋势。氟哌啶醇平均剂量为每月 75mg，此剂量极少用于临床实践。

有两项研究比较了帕利哌酮 LAI 和阿立哌唑 LAI。第一项随机对照试验发现阿立哌唑每月注射在短期内对生活质量的改善更佳，但阿立哌唑组含有更多年轻患者 [9]。第二项研究比较了两种 LAI 用于精神病及合并物质使用障碍患者的疗效，发现两种药物均能改善生活质量,减少对成瘾物质的渴求,但阿立哌唑更好。在两项研究中,阿立哌唑与帕利哌酮相比都没有明显意义的临床优势 [10]。

帕利哌酮 3 个月剂型

帕利哌酮 3 个月剂型适用于帕利哌酮 1 个月剂型治疗下临床稳定(最好 4 个月以上)的患者,且不需要调整剂量 [1]。建议换用 3 个月剂型之前,1 个月剂型的最后两针剂量保持不变,以便确定所需的维持剂量 [1]。

帕利哌酮 3 个月剂型与 1 个月剂型的耐受性相似,患者通常可以较好地耐受 [12-14],且复发率不高于帕利哌酮 1 个月剂型 [14]。在对缓解因素的预测分析中,从帕利哌酮 1 个月剂型转换成 3 个月剂型后,临床总体印象-疾病严重程度量表(clinical global impression — severity of illness scale,CG I-S)的整体改善提升了缓解的可能性 [15]。

从患者的角度出发,一项定性研究指出,3 个月剂型的优势包括减少了注射的频率和对疾病的关注,没什么劣势。从 1 个月剂型转换至 3 个月剂型不影响患者与医护人员互动的频率和内容 [16]。不应该因为抗精神病药注射频率少了就减少与患者的联系。

在原定下一次帕利哌酮 LAI 1 个月剂型注射时(± 7 天),开始帕利哌酮 LAI 3 个月剂型治疗。帕利哌酮 LAI 3 个月剂型的剂量应基于原帕利哌酮 LAI 1 个月剂型的剂量,见表 1.9。剂量调整不是必要的,以后可以每隔 3 个月进行,但调整后的全部效应可能在数月内并不明显 [11]。

表 1.9 帕利哌酮 LAI 3 个月制剂的剂量

帕利哌酮 LAI 1 个月制剂的剂量	帕利哌酮 LAI 3 个月制剂的剂量
50mg	175mg
75mg	263mg
100mg	350mg
150mg	525mg

用药遗漏时的详细信息见产品说明书。

注射过程对于避免混悬液不完全注射非常重要。需要放松手腕,在垂直方向用力摇匀带帽的预充注射器至少 15s,以确保混悬剂分散均匀。

参考文献

1. Lopez A, et al. Role of paliperidone palmitate 3-monthly in the management of schizophrenia: insights from clinical practice. *Neuropsychiatr Dis Treat* 2019; **15**:449–456.

2. Janssen-Cilag Ltd. Summary of Product Characteristics. Xeplion 25 mg, 50 mg, 75 mg, 100 mg, and 150 mg prolonged-release suspension for injection. 2020; https://www.medicines.org.uk/emc/medicine/31329.

3. Pappa S, et al. Partial compliance with long-acting paliperidone palmitate and impact on hospitalization: a 6-year mirror-image study. *Ther Adv Psychopharmacol* 2020; **10**:2045125320924789.

4. Laing E, et al. Relapse and frequency of injection of monthly paliperidone palmitate-A retrospective case-control study. *Eur Psychiatry* 2021; **64**:e11.

5. Russu A, et al. Maintenance dose conversion between oral risperidone and paliperidone palmitate 1 month: practical guidance based on pharmacokinetic simulations. *Int J Clin Pract* 2018; **72**:e13089.

6. Janssen-Cilag Limited. Summary of product characteristics. risperdal 2mg film-coated tablets. 2020; https://www.medicines.org.uk/emc/product/6858/smpc.

7. Janssen-Cilag Limited. Summary of product characteristics. Invega 3 mg prolonged-release tablets. 2020; https://www.medicines.org.uk/emc/product/6816.

8. McEvoy JP, et al. Effectiveness of paliperidone palmitate vs haloperidol decanoate for maintenance treatment of schizophrenia: a randomized clinical trial. *JAMA* 2014; **311**:1978–1987.

9. Naber D, et al. Qualify: a randomized head-to-head study of aripiprazole once-monthly and paliperidone palmitate in the treatment of schizophrenia. *Schizophr Res* 2015; **168**:498–504.

10. Cuomo I, et al. Head-to-head comparison of 1-year aripiprazole long-acting injectable (LAI) versus paliperidone LAI in comorbid psychosis and substance use disorder: impact on clinical status, substance craving, and quality of life. *Neuropsychiatr Dis Treat* 2018; **14**:1645–1656.

11. Janssen-Cilag Limited. Summary of Product Characteristics. TREVICTA 175mg, 263mg, 350mg, 525mg prolonged release suspension for injection. 2021; https://www.medicines.org.uk/emc/medicine/32050.

12. Lamb YN, et al. Paliperidone palmitate intramuscular 3-monthly formulation: a review in schizophrenia. *Drugs* 2016; **76**:1559–1566.

13. Ravenstijn P, et al. Pharmacokinetics, safety, and tolerability of paliperidone palmitate 3-month formulation in patients with schizophrenia: a phase-1, single-dose, randomized, open-label study. *J Clin Pharmacol* 2016; **56**:330–339.

14. Mathews M, et al. Clinical relevance of paliperidone palmitate 3-monthly in treating schizophrenia. *Neuropsychiatr Dis Treat* 2019; **15**:1365–1379.

15. Nash AI, et al. Predictors of achieving remission in schizophrenia patients treated with paliperidone palmitate 3-month formulation. *Neuropsychiatr Dis Treat* 2019; **15**:731–737.

16. Rise MB, et al. Patients' perspectives on three-monthly administration of antipsychotic treatment with paliperidone palmitate – a qualitative interview study. *Nord J Psychiatry* 2020: [Epub ahead of print].

17. Janssen Pharmaceutical Companies. Highlights of Prescribing Information. INVEGA SUSTENNA (paliperidone palmitate) extended-release injectable suspension, for intramuscular use. 2017; http://www.janssenlabels.com/package-insert/product-monograph/prescribing-information/INVEGA+SUSTENNA-pi.pdf.

18. Taylor DM, et al. Paliperidone palmitate: factors predicting continuation with treatment at 2 years. *Eur Neuropsychopharmacol* 2016; **26**:2011–2017.

利培酮 LAI

利培酮是首个制成长效注射剂的第二代抗精神病药。每 2 周注射 25~50mg 相当于口服利培酮 2~6mg/d[1]。利培酮长效制剂的耐受性也很好，EPS 发生率低于 10%，因不良反应而退出长期试验的比例低于 6%[2]。口服利培酮导致催乳素水平升高[3]，换用利培酮 LAI 也如此[4]，但是从口服剂换成注射剂后，催乳素水平有所下降[5-7]。迟发性运动障碍的发生率较低[8]。与第一代抗精神病药长效制剂尚无直接的随机对照研究；有一些观察性研究进行了比较，但结果不一致。对于原使用第一代抗精神病药长效制剂的稳定期患者，换用利培酮 LAI 的成功率不如继续使用第一代抗精神病药长效制剂[9]，但换用利培酮 LAI 的停药率低于第一代抗精神病药长效制剂[10]。

利培酮 LAI 的剂量-疗效关系存在不确定性。一些临床研究中，将患者随机分组使用不同的固定剂量，结果显示不同剂量组之间的疗效没有差异[11]。有一项随机、固定剂量、为期一年的研究显示，50mg（2 周）组的疗效优于 25mg（2 周）组，但这种差异并未达到统计学显著性[12]。自然观察性研究显示，普遍使用的剂量大于 25mg（2 周）[13,14]。有一项研究认为较高剂量时，患者的治疗结局更优[15,16]。

利培酮 LAI 25mg（2 周）治疗时，血药浓度与口服利培酮 2mg/d 相近或较低[17,18]。有一项纳入治疗药物监测（therapeutic drug monitoring，TDM）患者的研究发现，注射利培酮 LAI 25mg（2 周）的患者中，有 9.5% 的血样中不含利培酮或 9-羟利培酮[19]。在注射 25mg（2 周）者中，纹状体多巴胺 D_2 受体占有率也较低（也许达不到治疗要求）[20,21]。因此，尽管固定剂量研究未发现大于 25mg（2 周）的剂量具有明显的疗效优势，其他参数的结果让人质疑 25mg（2 周）的剂量是否足够治疗全部，甚至大多数患者。虽然这个难题仍未得到解决，但是小心地增加剂量变得非常重要。达到这个目的最有效的方法是，确定所需要的口服利培酮的剂量，然后将其转换成等效的利培酮 LAI 剂量。临床试验已经证明，从口服利培酮 2mg/d 换成利培酮 LAI 25mg（2 周），以及从口服利培酮 4mg/d 换成利培酮 LAI 50mg（2 周）往往是成功的[2,22,23][而从口服利培酮 4mg/d 换成利培酮 LAI 25mg（2 周）则增加了复发风险[24]]。目前，对口服利培酮 6mg/d 转换为利培酮 LAI 的等效剂量仍存问题：理论上应该换成利培酮 LAI 75mg（2 周），但临床试验并未显示出其比低剂量具有优势，而且也超出产品说明书的最高剂量。尽管如此，一项观察性研究报告了使用超过 75mg（2 周）（范围在 75~200mg）治疗患者治疗成功，且 3 年后的继续使用率达 95%[25]。棕榈酸帕利哌酮 150mg（每月）相当于口服利培酮 6mg/d。事实上，有许多理由支持棕榈酸帕利哌酮（9-羟利培酮）可能优于利培酮 LAI（Risperdal Consta）：它在急性期起效，可每月注射 1 次，不需要冷藏，剂量范围更为宽泛（见本章有关棕榈酸帕利哌酮长效注射剂的内容）。

利培酮 LAI 与其他长效制剂有重要区别，应该注意下述几点：

- 利培酮长效制剂并非母药的酯化物。它包含的利培酮被包裹在聚合物中形成微球。这些微球在即将使用前，必须制成水基混悬液。
- 必须储存于冰箱中（要考虑在社区使用的便利性）。
- 规格为 25mg、37.5mg 和 50mg。必须整瓶使用（因为是混悬液）。这意味着在剂量调整方面不太灵活。

- 不需要也没道理使用试验剂量。(需要使用口服利培酮试验耐受性,但不完全符合临床实际。)
- 初次注射后达到治疗血药浓度需要 3~4 周。在初次注射后至少 3 周内,需要继续使用全量的原口服药物。口服抗精神病药有时需要覆盖更长时间(6~8 周)。如果患者注射前未服用口服抗精神病药,应同时给予口服利培酮(关于从其他长效剂换药,见表 1.10。)**因为药物释放延迟很长,对拒绝口服治疗且处于急性发病的患者不应给予利培酮 LAI 治疗。**
- 利培酮 LAI 须每 2 周注射 1 次。产品说明书要求注射时间间隔不得超过 2 周。虽然每月注射一次可能也有效,但临床上注射频率不能随意改变[26]。
- 预测利培酮 LAI 疗效的最有效方式是通过口服利培酮确定治疗剂量和疗效。
- 利培酮 LAI 不适用于难治性精神分裂症患者,尽管有一些研究发现了良好的疗效[27,28]。

　　关于换用利培酮 LAI 治疗的指导,见表 1.10。

表 1.10　如何换用利培酮长效注射剂

原用药物	建议的换药方法	评论
无治疗 (新患者或近期不依从者)	从口服利培酮 2mg/d 起,滴定至有效剂量。若能耐受,使用等效剂量的利培酮 LAI 继续口服利培酮至少 3 周,然后在 1~2 周内逐渐停用。做好继续口服利培酮更长时间的准备	注射前先口服利培酮,确保良好的耐受性 口服 2mg/d 病情稳定者,开始注射 25mg/2w 口服更大剂量者,开始注射 37.5mg/2w,并准备注射 50mg/2w (制药厂的建议可能与此不同——本章指南是建立在许多剂量相关结果和相对血浆水平的研究上的)
口服利培酮	给予等效剂量利培酮 LAI	见上
口服抗精神病药 (非利培酮)	或者: a. 换用口服利培酮,逐渐加至有效剂量。若耐受,给予等效剂量利培酮 LAI 继续口服利培酮至少 3 周,然后在 1~2 周内逐渐停用。做好继续口服利培酮更长时间的准备	从其他药物换成利培酮 LAI 时,剂量评估较困难。一般来说,口服低剂量时,应换成 25mg/2w。此处的"低"指靠近说明书剂量范围下限,或接近最低有效剂量
	或者: b. 给予利培酮 LAI,3~4 周后缓慢停用口服抗精神病药。做好继续口服抗精神病药更长时间的准备	口服较高剂量时,应注射 37.5mg 或 50mg/2w。3~4 周后仍然需要口服抗精神病药时,可能提示需要更高剂量的利培酮 LAI
长效抗精神病药	在最后一次注射原来的长效抗精神病药前一周,给予利培酮 LAI	利培酮 LAI 剂量难以估计。对于原来注射小剂量者(见上),从 25mg/2w 起,然后作必要调整 以往在注册剂量范围中高水平维持者,从 37.5mg/2w 起,做好增加至 50mg/2w 的准备
口服抗精神病药与长效制剂联合治疗	在最后一次注射原来的长效抗精神病药前一周,给予利培酮 LAI 3~4 周后缓慢减少口服抗精神病药。做好继续口服抗精神病药更长时间的准备	目标是将利培酮 LAI 作为患者唯一的抗精神病药。与以前相同,应该尽可能按照口服和注射抗精神病药的总剂量确定利培酮 LAI 的剂量

　　w,week,周。

参考文献

1. Chue P, et al. Comparative efficacy and safety of long-acting risperidone and risperidone oral tablets. *Eur Neuropsychopharmacol* 2005; 15:111–117.

2. Fleischhacker WW, et al. Treatment of schizophrenia with long-acting injectable risperidone: a 12-month open-label trial of the first long-acting second-generation antipsychotic. *J Clin Psychiatry* 2003; 64:1250–1257.

3. Kleinberg DL, et al. Prolactin levels and adverse events in patients treated with risperidone. *J Clin Psychopharmacol* 1999; 19:57–61.

4. Fu DJ, et al. Paliperidone palmitate versus oral risperidone and risperidone long-acting injection in patients with recently diagnosed schizophrenia: a tolerability and efficacy comparison. *Int Clin Psychopharmacol* 2014; 29:45–55.

5. Bai YM, et al. A comparative efficacy and safety study of long-acting risperidone injection and risperidone oral tablets among hospitalized patients: 12-week randomized, single-blind study. *Pharmacopsychiatry* 2006; 39:135–141.

6. Bai YM, et al. Pharmacokinetics study for hyperprolactinemia among schizophrenics switched from risperidone to risperidone long-acting injection. *J Clin Psychopharmacol* 2007; 27:306–308.

7. Peng PW, et al. The disparity of pharmacokinetics and prolactin study for risperidone long-acting injection. *J Clin Psychopharmacol* 2008; 28:726–727.

8. Gharabawi GM, et al. An assessment of emergent tardive dyskinesia and existing dyskinesia in patients receiving long-acting, injectable risperidone: results from a long-term study. *Schizophr Res* 2005; 77:129–139.

9. Covell NH, et al. Effectiveness of switching from long-acting injectable fluphenazine or haloperidol decanoate to long-acting injectable risperidone microspheres: an open-label, randomized controlled trial. *J Clin Psychiatry* 2012; 73:669–675.

10. Suzuki H, et al. Comparison of treatment retention between risperidone long-acting injection and first-generation long-acting injections in patients with schizophrenia for 5 years. *J Clin Psychopharmacol* 2016; 36:405–406.

11. Kane JM, et al. Long-acting injectable risperidone: efficacy and safety of the first long-acting atypical antipsychotic. *Am J Psychiatry* 2003; 160:1125–1132.

12. Simpson GM, et al. A 1-year double-blind study of 2 doses of long-acting risperidone in stable patients with schizophrenia or schizoaffective disorder. *J Clin Psychiatry* 2006; 67:1194–1203.

13. Turner M, et al. Long-acting injectable risperidone: safety and efficacy in stable patients switched from conventional depot antipsychotics. *Int Clin Psychopharmacol* 2004; 19:241–249.

14. Taylor DM, et al. Early clinical experience with risperidone long-acting injection: a prospective, 6-month follow-up of 100 patients. *J Clin Psychiatry* 2004; 65:1076–1083.

15. Taylor DM, et al. Prospective 6-month follow-up of patients prescribed risperidone long-acting injection: factors predicting favourable outcome. *Int J Neuropsychopharmacol* 2006; 9:685–694.

16. Taylor DM, et al. Risperidone long-acting injection: a prospective 3-year analysis of its use in clinical practice. *J Clin Psychiatry* 2009; 70:196–200.

17. Nesvag R, et al. Serum concentrations of risperidone and 9-OH risperidone following intramuscular injection of long-acting risperidone compared with oral risperidone medication. *Acta Psychiatr Scand* 2006; 114:21–26.

18. Castberg I, et al. Serum concentrations of risperidone and 9-hydroxyrisperidone after administration of the long-acting injectable form of risperidone: evidence from a routine therapeutic drug monitoring service. *Ther Drug Monit* 2005; 27:103–106.

19. Bowskill SV, et al. Risperidone and total 9-hydroxyrisperidone in relation to prescribed dose and other factors: data from a therapeutic drug monitoring service, 2002–2010. *Ther Drug Monit* 2012; 34:349–355.

20. Gefvert O, et al. Pharmacokinetics and D2 receptor occupancy of long-acting injectable risperidone (Risperdal Consta™) in patients with schizophrenia. *Int J Neuropsychopharmacol* 2005; 8:27–36.

21. Remington G, et al. A PET study evaluating dopamine D2 receptor occupancy for long-acting injectable risperidone. *Am J Psychiatry* 2006; 163:396–401.

22. Lasser RA, et al. Clinical improvement in 336 stable chronically psychotic patients changed from oral to long-acting risperidone: a 12-month open trial. *Int J Neuropsychopharmacol* 2005; 8:427–438.

23. Lauriello J, et al. Long-acting risperidone vs. placebo in the treatment of hospital inpatients with schizophrenia. *Schizophr Res* 2005; 72:249–258.

24. Bai YM, et al. Equivalent switching dose from oral risperidone to risperidone long-acting injection: a 48-week randomized, prospective, single-blind pharmacokinetic study. *J Clin Psychiatry* 2007; 68:1218–1225.

25. Fernandez-Miranda JJ, et al. Effectiveness, good tolerability, and high compliance of doses of risperidone long-acting injectable higher than 75 mg in people with severe schizophrenia: a 3-year follow-up. *J Clin Psychopharmacol* 2015; 35:630–634.

26. Uchida H, et al. Monthly administration of long-acting injectable risperidone and striatal dopamine D2 receptor occupancy for the management of schizophrenia. *J Clin Psychiatry* 2008; 69:1281–1286.

27. Meltzer HY, et al. A six month randomized controlled trial of long acting injectable risperidone 50 and 100mg in treatment resistant schizophrenia. *Schizophr Res* 2014; 154:14–22.

28. Kimura H, et al. Risperidone long-acting injectable in the treatment of treatment-resistant schizophrenia with dopamine supersensitivity psychosis: results of a 2-year prospective study, including an additional 1-year follow-up. *J Psychopharmacology* 2016; 30:795–802.

利培酮皮下长效注射剂

RBP-7000 或 Perseris 是一种可以一个月皮下注射一次的 LAI，有 90mg 和 120mg 两种规格。90mg 等效于口服利培酮 3mg/d，120mg 等效于口服利培酮 4mg/d[1]。

两种剂型都可以快速起效，且不需要预先口服治疗和口服补充治疗[2,3]。在所有时间点，120mg 剂型均比 90mg 剂型更有效。长期来看，使用每月 120mg 治疗对控制和改善症状量表得分有效[4]。RBP-7000 在理论上明显优于 Risperdal Consta，它起效快，不需要口服补充治疗，且是皮下注射，患者更容易接受[5]，注射时疼痛的风险更低[6]。其缺点在于注射过程需要几个步骤，且对精神科来说，复杂的准备和皮下注射都是相对新鲜的[6]。另一项缺点是无法给予大于 4mg/d 等效剂量的治疗，可能限制了临床应用[7]。（就 C_{max}，C_{min} 和 C_{ave} 来说，3mg/d=90mg/28d；4mg/d=120mg/28d[1,8]）。然而，多巴胺受体结合率与临床疗效大体一致：在稳定状态，90mg 的结合率为 40%~80%；120mg 的结合率为 60%~85%[9]。

大致等效剂量（mg）[10]

口服利培酮（每天）	Risperdal Consta（每 2 周）	棕榈酸帕利哌酮（每月）	RBP-7000（每月）
2	25	50	无数据 *
3	37.5	75	90
4	50	100	120
6	无数据	150	无数据

*Laffont 等[11]认为 90mg 等效于 Risperdal Consta 25mg（每 2 周）。

参考文献

1. US Food and Drug Administration. Cross-discipline team leader review. RBP-7000 (risperidone-ATRIGEL) 2018; https://www.accessdata.fda.gov/drugsatfda_docs/nda/2018/210655Orig1s000SumR.pdf.

2. Nasser AF, et al. Efficacy, safety, and tolerability of RBP-7000 once-monthly risperidone for the treatment of acute schizophrenia: an 8-week, randomized, double-blind, placebo-controlled, multicenter phase 3 study. *J Clin Psychopharmacol* 2016; 36:130–140.

3. Le Moigne A, et al. Reanalysis of a phase 3 trial of a monthly extended-release risperidone injection for the treatment of acute schizophrenia. *J Clin Psychopharmacol* 2021; 41:76–77.

4. Andorn A, et al. Monthly extended-release risperidone (RBP-7000) in the treatment of schizophrenia: results from the phase 3 program. *J Clin Psychopharmacol* 2019; 39:428–433.

5. Tchobaniouk LV, et al. Once-monthly subcutaneously administered risperidone in the treatment of schizophrenia: patient considerations. *Patient Prefer Adherence* 2019; 13:2233–2241.

6. Citrome L. Sustained-release risperidone via subcutaneous injection: a systematic review of RBP-7000 (PERSERIS(™)) for the treatment of schizophrenia. *Clin Schizophr Relat Psychoses* 2018; 12:130–141.

7. Clark I, et al. Newer formulations of risperidone: role in the management of psychotic disorders. *CNS Drugs* 2020; 34:841–852.

8. US Food and Drug Administration. Clinical pharmacology and biopharmaceutics review(s). Perseris 2018; https://www.accessdata.fda.gov/drugsatfda_docs/nda/2018/210655Orig1s000ClinPharmR.pdf.

9. Laffont CM, et al. Population pharmacokinetics and prediction of dopamine D2 receptor occupancy after multiple doses of RBP-7000, a new sustained-release formulation of risperidone, in schizophrenia patients on stable oral risperidone treatment. *Clin Pharmacokinet* 2014; 53:533–543.

10. Karas A, et al. Perseris(TM): a new and long-acting, atypical antipsychotic drug-delivery system. *P & T* 2019; 44:460–466.

11. Laffont CM, et al. Population pharmacokinetic modeling and simulation to guide dose selection for RBP-7000, a new sustained-release formulation of risperidone. *J Clin Pharmacol* 2015; 55:93–103.

新型抗精神病药长效注射制剂

下表提供了部分新型抗精神病药 LAI 制剂的简要信息。

药物	商品名	制剂	给药间隔	注射部位	用药信息	是否需要预混	预先口服治疗是否需要*	预先口服治疗是否可行**	监管状态	其他信息
月桂酰阿立哌唑——缓释注射剂	Aristada Inito	纳米晶分散剂[1]; LinkeRx technology[2]	单次给药	三角肌或臀肌注射	675mg (肌内注射分散剂 =459mg 阿立哌唑)[3]	否	是, 见其他信息	是	2018 年 FDA 批准[4]	Aristada initio 联合口服 30mg 阿立哌唑只能用来作为 Aristada 的起始治疗 (见第 1 章阿立哌唑 LAI),不可用于重复给药[5]
棕榈酸帕利哌酮 6 个月剂型	不适用	微晶混悬液[3]	6 个月	肌内注射	700mg/100mg?[6]	否	否	否——患者在此之前已经接受长效帕利哌酮治疗	正在进行 3 期临床试验[7]	用于帕利哌酮 LAI 1 月剂型或 3 个月剂型治疗稳定的患者[8]
利培酮皮下注射剂 (RBP-7000)	Perseris	混悬液,共聚体; ATRIGEL technology[3]	1 个月	只能用于腹部皮下注射[9]	90mg/120mg	是	否[10]	是	2018 年 FDA 批准[11]	不需要负荷剂量或口服补充治疗。治疗前应对利培酮确定耐受性[9]
利培酮皮下注射缓释剂 (TV-46000)	不适用	混悬液[3]	1 个月或 2 个月[12]	皮下注射	2 次注射方案(TV-46000-A 和 TV-46000-B)处于研究中[13]	否[12]	否[13]	是[13]	正在进行 3 期临床试验[12]	等待 2020 年的 3 期临床试验结果[12]
利培酮	利培酮原位微粒 (Doria)	混悬液[14]	1 个月[14]	三角肌或臀肌注射[15]	75mg/100mg	是	否[16]	是	3 期临床试验完成等待 2020 年欧洲药品监管理局批准[17]	不需要负荷剂量或口服补充治疗。对未使用过利培酮治疗的患者,需进行 3 天口服利培酮试验(2mg/d)确定患者是否过敏[18]

* 只在口服治疗前后检测了 LAI。

** 确定疗效和耐受性的最好方法。

参考文献

1. Krogmann A, et al. Keeping up with the therapeutic advances in schizophrenia: a review of novel and emerging pharmacological entities. *CNS Spectr* 2019; 24:38–69.

2. Alkermes Inc. ARISTADA INITIO™ (aripiprazole lauroxil) extended-release injectable suspension [product monograph]. 2020; https://www.aristadacaresupport.com/downloadables/ARISTADA-INITIO-ARISTADA-Payer-Hospital-Monograph.pdf.

3. Correll CU, et al. Pharmacokinetic characteristics of long-acting injectable antipsychotics for schizophrenia: an overview. *CNS Drugs* 2021; 35:39–59.

4. Pharmaceutical Technology. Alkermes' Aristata Initio approved by FDA for schizophrenia. 2018; https://www.pharmaceutical-technology.com/news/arista-initio-fda-approval-schizophrenia/:~:text=Alkermes'%20Aristada%20Initio%20approved%20by%20FDA%20for%20schizophrenia.,Aristada%20as%20a%20treatment%20for%20adults%20with%20schizophrenia.

5. U.S. Food & Drug Administration. Drug Approval Package: Aripiprazole lauroxil Nanocrystal Dispersion (AL-NCD). 2019; https://www.accessdata.fda.gov/drugsatfda_docs/nda/2018/209830Orig1s000TOC.cfm.

6. Janssen Research & Development LLC. A study of paliperidone palmitate 6-month formulation. 2020; https://www.centerwatch.com/clinical-trials/listings/160465/schizophrenia-study-paliperidone-palmitate-6-month.

7. ClinicalTrial.gov. A study of paliperidone palmitate 6-month formulation. 2020; https://clinicaltrials.gov/ct2/show/NCT04072575.

8. PRNewswire Press release. Janssen submits paliperidone palmitate 6-month (pp6m) supplemental new drug application to U.S. FDA for treatment of schizophrenia in adults. 2020; https://news.yahoo.com/janssen-submits-paliperidone-palmitate-6-120000670.html?guccounter=1&guce_referrer=aHR0cHM6Ly93d3cuYmluZy5jb20vc2VhcmNoNoP3E9UGFsaXBlcmlkb25lK1BhbbG1pdGF0ZSs2LU1vbnRoK0Zvcm11bGF0aW9uJnNyYz1JRS1TZWFyY2hCb3gmRk9STT1JRU5SBRTI&guce_referrer_sig=AQAAAEjhHe6O8HxGLi1o0izgasDe15netPJG3l-MUedGGRDHFMtzWa9biyFopIhgzAbCx2sgWOaiFOxF2PLimzGos4vvuSfNDmbS77QWazTi8BXUH9RqzjgWHJsueeTuPPfHq9OmxpAu-XiwbXTNe1WLVjbFmC7G39qbGtMKyLPH2UDD).

9. Indivior UK Limited. Highlights of prescribing information. Perseris (risperidone) for extended-release injectable suspension for subcutaneous use. 2019; http://www.indivior.com/wp-content/uploads/2018/07/FDA-Label-revised.pdf.

10. Tchobaniouk LV, et al. Once-monthly subcutaneously administered risperidone in the treatment of schizophrenia: patient considerations. *Patient Prefer Adherence* 2019; 13:2233–2241.

11. Indivior. FDA approves PERSERIS (risperidone) for extended-release injectable suspension for the treatment of schizophrenia in adults. 2018; http://indivior.com/wp-content/uploads/2018/07/PERSERIS-Press-Release-FINAL.pdf.

12. Medincell. Building a global pharma leader; through long-acting injectables. January 2019; https://invest.medincell.com/wp-content/uploads/2019/02/19-01-04-JPMprezvdef.pdf.

13. ClinicalTrial.gov. A study to evaluate the safety, tolerability, and effect of risperidone extended-release injectable suspension (TV-46000) for subcutaneous use as maintenance treatment in adult and adolescent patients with schizophrenia. 2020; https://clinicaltrials.gov/ct2/show/NCT03893825.

14. Carabias L, et al. A phase II study to evaluate the pharmacokinetics, safety, and tolerability of risperidone ISM multiple intramuscular injections once every 4 weeks in patients with schizophrenia. *Int Clin Psychopharmacol* 2017; 33:79–87.

15. ClinicalTrial.gov. Study to evaluate the efficacy and safety of risperidone ISM® in patients with acute schizophrenia: open label extension (PRISMA-3_OLE). 2020; https://clinicaltrials.gov/ct2/show/NCT03870880?term=risperidone+ISM&draw=2&rank=1.

16. Llaudo J, et al. Phase I, open-label, randomized, parallel study to evaluate the pharmacokinetics, safety, and tolerability of one intramuscular injection of risperidone ISM at different dose strengths in patients with schizophrenia or schizoaffective disorder (PRISMA-1). *Int Clin Psychopharmacol* 2016; 31:323–331.

17. Rovi. ROVI announces the commencement of the assessment process to obtain marketing authorisation for Doria® in the European Union. 2020; https://www.rovi.es/sites/default/files/Doria%20validation_Press%20release_0.pdf.

18. Correll CU, et al. Efficacy and safety of once-monthly risperidone ISM(®) in schizophrenic patients with an acute exacerbation. *NPJ Schizophr* 2020; 6:37.

扩展阅读

Correll CU, et al. Pharmacokinetic characteristics of long-acting injectable antipsychotics for schizophrenia: an overview. *CNS Drugs* 2021; 35:39–59.

五氟利多每周给药

五氟利多是一种二苯丁哌啶类第一代抗精神病药,在部分国家(如印度)仍有生产,并进口至其他国家。其疗效和耐受性与其他第一代抗精神病药类似[1]。

五氟利多的血浆半衰期异常地长,至少60h[2]。口服之后,12h内达到峰浓度,且单次口服后168h仍能检测到[3]。其长效作用可能是由于可以快速分布到脂肪组织中,而脂肪组织起着药物库的作用[4]。这种特性使得五氟利多可以作为抗精神病药长效注射制剂的替代品,在监督下每周口服一次进行治疗。

一些临床试验研究了每周口服一次五氟利多的效果,其剂量范围通常在每周5~160mg[1]。在这种情况下,其效果至少与第一代抗精神病药长效制剂相当[5,6],且总体耐受性更好[1]。虽然剂量-反应关系仍不清楚,但每周30mg可以取得足够的疗效[7],且至少一项试验使用了每天120mg的剂量(即总共每周840mg)[8]。

正如所料,不良反应包括急性锥体外系不良反应、催乳素升高和迟发性运动障碍。五氟利多通常没有镇静作用。与哌咪清(另一种二苯丁哌啶类药物)类似,五氟利多也会延长Q-T间期[9]。五氟利多具有细胞毒性,可能有抗癌作用[10]。

小结

- 五氟利多可以每周口服1次。
- 监督下每周服用药物的疗效至少与长效注射制剂相当。
- 常用剂量为每周20~40mg。
- 具有第一代抗精神病药的常见不良反应,包括Q-T间期延长。
- 镇静作用小。

在临床实践中,五氟利多通常起始于20mg,在评估后剂量可增加至最多40mg。2~4周后达到稳态血药浓度。需监测的内容包括肝肾功能、心脏代谢变化(如血脂、血糖、超声心动图),以及一般不良反应筛查。

参考文献

1. Soares BG, et al. Penfluridol for schizophrenia. *Cochrane Database Syst Rev* 2006; CD002923.
2. Janssen PA, et al. The pharmacology of penfluridol (R 16341) a new potent and orally long-acting neuroleptic drug. *Eur J Pharmacol* 1970; 11:139–154.
3. Cooper SF, et al. Penfluridol steady-state kinetics in psychiatric patients. *Clin Pharmacol Ther* 1975; 18:325–329.
4. Migdalof BH, et al. Penfluridol: a neuroleptic drug designed for long duration of action. *Drug Metab Rev* 1979; 9:281–299.
5. Iqbal MJ, et al. A long term comparative trial of penfluridol and fluphenazine decanoate in schizophrenic outpatients. *J Clin Psychiatry* 1978; 39:375–379.
6. Quitkin F, et al. Long-acting oral vs injectable antipsychotic drugs in schizophrenics: a one-year double-blind comparison in multiple episode schizophrenics. *Arch Gen Psychiatry* 1978; 35:889–892.
7. Van Praag HM, et al. Controlled trial of penfluridol in acute psychosis. *Br Med J* 1971; 4:710–713.
8. Shopsin B, et al. Penfluridol: an open phase III study in acute newly admitted hospitalized schizophrenic patients. *Psychopharmacology* 1977; 55:157–164.
9. Bhattacharyya R, et al. Resurgence of penfluridol: merits and demerits. *East J Psychiatry* 2015; 18:23–29.
10. Ashraf-Uz-Zaman M, et al. Analogs of penfluridol as chemotherapeutic agents with reduced central nervous system activity. *Bioorg Med Chem Lett* 2018; 28:3652–3657.

电抽搐治疗和精神疾病

来自前瞻性随机对照研究和回顾性研究的证据证明,电抽搐治疗(electric convulsive therapy,ECT)增效抗精神病药治疗对精神分裂症阳性症状有益,包括耐药的精神分裂症[1-7]。然而,关于长期有效性、认知缺陷和生活质量的数据相对缺乏。

一项 Cochrane 系统综述评估了随机对照临床试验,这些试验对比了 ECT 与安慰剂、假 ECT、非药物性干预和抗精神病药对精神分裂症、分裂情感障碍或慢性精神障碍患者的疗效[8]。与安慰剂和假 ECT 组相比,真 ECT 组中更多患者得到了改善,而且有迹象表明,真 ECT 组患者在短期内复发更少,出院可能性更大。该综述的结论是,ECT 联合持续的抗精神病药治疗是治疗精神分裂症的有效选择,特别是当需要全面快速改善和减轻症状,且单用药物治疗仅出现有限的疗效时。

一项自然的镜像研究(2002—2011 年)比较了 2074 例服用抗精神病药并接受 ECT 治疗的精神分裂症住院患者,与继续服用抗精神病药的对照组患者的情况[9]。在治疗后一年内,接受 ECT 治疗的精神病患者住院率下降,但对照组患者没有。在使用氯氮平或中高剂量抗精神病药治疗的患者中,ECT 的效果更明显。

难治性精神分裂症

一项 Cochrane 系统综述研究了将 ECT 添加到难治性精神分裂症(TRS)标准治疗中的利弊[6]。研究人员能够得出有限的结论,即中等质量的 RCT 证据表明 ECT 对中期临床疗效有积极作用。有研究者指出,在得出更有力的结论之前,需要有质量更好的证据。

一些研究集中于 ECT 增效抗精神病药治疗难治性精神分裂症(TRS)的作用[1-3,10,11]。例如,在一个以"阴性症状为主"的难治性精神分裂症患者的相对小样本研究中,多种抗精神病药联合 ECT 增效治疗都可显著降低症状严重程度[12]。一项荟萃分析纳入了针对 TRS 的 RCT,比较了 ECT 和(非氯氮平)抗精神病药联合治疗与同种抗精神病药单药治疗的疗效,发现联合治疗在症状改善、研究定义的反应率和缓解率方面更优[3]。

ECT 增效氯氮平的效果可能至少与其他抗精神病药增效效果相同[4,11,13]。一项回顾性研究评估了氯氮平和 ECT 联合治疗 TRS 患者的有效性和安全性,发现几乎 2/3 的患者有应答(定义为 PANSS 总分降低 30% 或以上)[14]。对这些患者进行二次抽样后随访平均超过 30 个月的数据显示,大多数患者症状改善得以维持或改善得更好。另一个关于 ECT 增效氯氮平的小样本回顾性研究报告称,大约 3/4 的患者出现了急性反应(定义为临床总体印象改善量表的改善[15]),3/4 的应答者这一年随访期内未入院[16]。

在一项随机、单盲的研究中,氯氮平抵抗的难治性精神分裂症患者要么继续单独使用氯氮平治疗,要么联合双侧 ECT 增效治疗[2]。8 周后,半数接受氯氮平加 ECT 治疗的患者达到了预先定义的反应标准(包括简明精神病量表[17]的精神病症状分量表减少 40% 或以上),但单独应用氯氮平组没有一个达到。当单独使用氯氮平组治疗无反应者交叉进入一个为期 8 周的 ECT 开放性试验时,近 1/2 的患者达到了反应标准。

一项针对 ECT 增效氯氮平治疗的系统综述和荟萃分析发现,缺乏对照研究,尽管作者承认此类调查的方法学上存在挑战[18]。他们得出结论,对于单一氯氮平治疗失败的精神分裂症来说，ECT 可能是个有效的增效策略，但需要进一步研究来确定这种策略在 TRS 治疗中的地位。随后的一项关于 ECT 增效治疗氯氮平耐药的精神分裂症的随机对照试验的荟萃分析指出，缺乏假 ECT 作为对照的研究，但得出的结论是这样的治疗策略是有效的且相对安全[19]。

不良反应

尽管 ECT 对维持抗精神病药的增效治疗作用似乎一般有良好的耐受性，少数病例仍报道了不良反应，如暂时的逆行或顺行性遗忘、头痛和恶心[3,11,12,20]；且有报道称，ECT 后有血压升高和持续癫痫发作发生[1]。有证据表明，认知方面的作用通常是轻微且短暂的[19,21]。

小结

总之，有证据支持 ECT 作为药物治疗（特别是氯氮平）的增效方法，对于难治性精神分裂症可能是有效的、相对安全的策略[7,22-24]；但是还需要进一步实施良好的对照试验，以确定这种治疗策略在短期和长期的收益-风险平衡。

参考文献

1. Grover S, et al. Effectiveness of electroconvulsive therapy in patients with treatment resistant schizophrenia: a retrospective study. *Psychiatry Res* 2017; 249:349–353.
2. Petrides G, et al. Electroconvulsive therapy augmentation in clozapine-resistant schizophrenia: a prospective, randomized study. *Focus* 2019; 17:76–82.
3. Zheng W, et al. Electroconvulsive therapy added to non-clozapine antipsychotic medication for treatment resistant schizophrenia: meta-analysis of randomized controlled trials. *PLoS One* 2016; 11:e0156510.
4. Kim HS, et al. Effectiveness of electroconvulsive therapy augmentation on clozapine-resistant schizophrenia. *Psychiatry Investig* 2017; 14:58–62.
5. Vuksan Ćusa B, et al. The effects of electroconvulsive therapy augmentation of antipsychotic treatment on cognitive functions in patients with treatment-resistant schizophrenia. *J Ect* 2018; 34:31–34.
6. Sinclair DJM, et al. Electroconvulsive therapy for treatment-resistant schizophrenia. *Schizophr Bull* 2019; 45:730–732.
7. Grover S, et al. ECT in schizophrenia: a review of the evidence. *Acta Neuropsychiatr* 2019; 31:115–127.
8. Tharyan P, et al. Electroconvulsive therapy for schizophrenia. *Cochrane Database Syst Rev* 2005; Cd000076.
9. Lin HT, et al. Impacts of electroconvulsive therapy on 1-year outcomes in patients with schizophrenia: a controlled, population-based mirror-image study. *Schizophr Bull* 2018; 44:798–806.
10. Masoudzadeh A, et al. Comparative study of clozapine, electroshock and the combination of ECT with clozapine in treatment-resistant schizophrenic patients. *Pak J Biol Sci* 2007; 10:4287–4290.
11. Kaster TS, et al. Clinical effectiveness and cognitive impact of electroconvulsive therapy for schizophrenia: a large retrospective study. *J Clin Psychiatry* 2017; 78:e383–e389.
12. Pawełczyk T, et al. Augmentation of antipsychotics with electroconvulsive therapy in treatment-resistant schizophrenia patients with dominant negative symptoms: a pilot study of effectiveness. *Neuropsychobiology* 2014; 70:158–164.
13. Ahmed S, et al. Combined use of electroconvulsive therapy and antipsychotics (both clozapine and non-clozapine) in treatment resistant schizophrenia: a comparative meta-analysis. *Heliyon* 2017; 3:e00429.
14. Kay SR, et al. The positive and negative syndrome scale (PANSS) for schizophrenia. *Schizophr Bull* 1987; 13:261–276.
15. Guy W. ECDEU Assessment Manual for Psychopharmacology, U.S. Department of Health, Education, and Welfare, Public Health Service, Alcohol, Drug Abuse, and Mental Health Administration, National Institute of Mental Health, Psychopharmacology Research Branch, Division of Extramural Research Programs 1976.
16. Lally J, et al. Augmentation of clozapine with ECT: a retrospective case analysis. *Acta Neuropsychiatr* 2021; 33:31–36.
17. Overall JE, et al. The brief psychiatric rating scale. *Psychol Rep* 1962; 10:812.
18. Lally J, et al. Augmentation of clozapine with electroconvulsive therapy in treatment resistant schizophrenia: a systematic review and meta-analysis. *Schizophr Res* 2016; 171:215–224.
19. Wang G, et al. ECT augmentation of clozapine for clozapine-resistant schizophrenia: a meta-analysis of randomized controlled trials. *J Psychiatr Res* 2018; 105:23–32.
20. Zheng W, et al. Memory impairment following electroconvulsive therapy in Chinese patients with schizophrenia: meta-analysis of randomized controlled trials. *Perspect Psychiatr Care* 2018; 54:107–114.
21. Sanghani SN, et al. Electroconvulsive therapy (ECT) in schizophrenia: a review of recent literature. *Curr Opin Psychiatry* 2018;

31:213–222.

22. Zervas IM, et al. Using ECT in schizophrenia: a review from a clinical perspective. *World J Biol Psychiatry* 2012; 13:96–105.

23. Wagner E, et al. Clozapine combination and augmentation strategies in patients with schizophrenia -recommendations from an international expert survey among the Treatment Response and Resistance in Psychosis (TRRIP) Working Group. *Schizophr Bull* 2020; 46:1459–1470.

24. Arumugham SS, et al. Efficacy and safety of combining clozapine with electrical or magnetic brain stimulation in treatment-refractory schizo-phrenia. *Expert Rev Clin Pharmacol* 2016; 9:1245–1252.

ω-3 脂肪酸(鱼油)在精神分裂症中的应用

鱼油富含 ω-3 脂肪酸,包括二十碳五烯酸(EPA)和二十二碳六烯酸(DHA),也称为多不饱和脂肪酸(PUFA)。这些化合物与神经元膜结构维持、膜蛋白调节以及前列腺素和白细胞三烯的生成有关[1]。大量摄入多不饱和脂肪酸可能具有预防精神病的作用[2],抗精神病药治疗可以纠正 PUFA 的缺陷[3]。动物模型研究提示,PUFA 具有保护作用[4]。它们可用于各种精神疾病的治疗[5,6];病例报告[7-10]、病例系列报告[11]、前瞻性试验都初步提示,它们对精神分裂症具有一定的疗效[12-16]。

治疗

一项有关 EPA 的荟萃分析认为[17],它对确诊的精神分裂症无效,其估计的效应值(0.242)不具有统计学意义。之后,一项随机对照试验纳入了 71 例首发精神分裂症患者,每天给予 2.2g EPA+DHA,持续 6 个月,结果显示干预组患者的症状严重程度有所减轻,PANSS 减分率 50%[18] 的 NNT 为 4。然而,另外一项随机对照试验纳入了 97 例急性精神病性障碍患者,未能证实 EPA 2g/d 疗效优于安慰剂[19];在一项预防复发的研究中,每天服用 EPA 2g+DHA 1g 的价值并不优于安慰剂,甚至复发率更高(分别为 90% 和 75%)[20]。该领域已发表数据的局限性(小样本量、诊断和疾病阶段的异质性、干预组合和剂量的差异)意味着总体结果最多属于不确定[21,22]。对已发表的荟萃分析的系统综述发现,没有证据表明 PUFA 治疗精神分裂症有效[23]。

综合来看,在标准治疗之外加用 EPA 2~3g/d 对精神分裂症治疗可能并无价值。鱼油虽然疗效可疑,但是其价格相对低廉,能较好地耐受[24](可能会有轻微胃肠道症状),并且对躯体健康有益[1,25-29]。

预防

在青少年和青年高危精神病受试者中,采用 EPA 700mg+DHA 480mg/d 进行研究,结果发现[30]与安慰剂相比,该治疗大大地减少了精神病性症状的发生(但是一项评论认为此项研究是"质量非常差的证据"[31])。自从这项单中心研究发表以来,进行了一项大型、多中心的 NEURAPRO 试验[32],给精神病高危成人使用 840mg EPA +560mg DHA 6 个月,结果没有发现任何证据表明其在减少向精神病过渡或改善症状方面的疗效。Cochrane 的结论是,ω-3 脂肪酸"可能会"防止从前驱期转变为精神病,但证据质量很低,这一结论尚未得到证实[33]。

总结

PUFA 不再作为精神分裂症残留症状或预防高危青少年向精神病过渡的治疗推荐[23,34-36]。如果使用,应仔细评定疗效,3 个月以上无效时应该停用,除非因为代谢方面的益处需要继续使用。

建议小结——鱼油（PUFA）

- 对于首次发作精神病性障碍的高危人群
  - 不推荐。如果使用，建议 EPA 700mg/d。
- 对于多次发作的精神分裂症的残留症状（与抗精神病药联用）
  - 不推荐。如果使用，建议剂量为 EPA 2g/d。

参考文献

1. Fenton WS, et al. Essential fatty acids, lipid membrane abnormalities, and the diagnosis and treatment of schizophrenia. *Biol Psychiatry* 2000; **47**:8–21.
2. Hedelin M, et al. Dietary intake of fish, omega-3, omega-6 polyunsaturated fatty acids and vitamin D and the prevalence of psychotic-like symptoms in a cohort of 33,000 women from the general population. *BMC Psychiatry* 2010; **10**:38.
3. Sethom MM, et al. Polyunsaturated fatty acids deficits are associated with psychotic state and negative symptoms in patients with schizophrenia. *Prostaglandins Leukot Essent Fatty Acids* 2010; **83**:131–136.
4. Zugno AI, et al. Omega-3 prevents behavior response and brain oxidative damage in the ketamine model of schizophrenia. *Neuroscience* 2014; **259**:223–231.
5. Freeman MP. Omega-3 fatty acids in psychiatry: a review. *Ann Clin Psychiatry* 2000; **12**:159–165.
6. Ross BM, et al. Omega-3 fatty acids as treatments for mental illness: which disorder and which fatty acid? *Lipids Health Dis* 2007, 6.21.
7. Richardson AJ, et al. Red cell and plasma fatty acid changes accompanying symptom remission in a patient with schizophrenia treated with eicosapentaenoic acid. *Eur Neuropsychopharmacol* 2000; **10**:189–193.
8. Puri BK, et al. Eicosapentaenoic acid treatment in schizophrenia associated with symptom remission, normalisation of blood fatty acids, reduced neuronal membrane phospholipid turnover and structural brain changes. *Int J Clin Pract* 2000; **54**:57–63.
9. Su KP, et al. Omega-3 fatty acids as a psychotherapeutic agent for a pregnant schizophrenic patient. *Eur Neuropsychopharmacol* 2001; **11**:295–299.
10. Cuéllar-Barboza AB, et al. Use of omega-3 polyunsaturated fatty acids as augmentation therapy in treatment-resistant schizophrenia. *Prim Care Companion CNS Disord* 2017; **19**:16l02040.
11. Sivrioglu EY, et al. The impact of omega-3 fatty acids, vitamins E and C supplementation on treatment outcome and side effects in schizophrenia patients treated with haloperidol: an open-label pilot study. *Prog Neuropsychopharmacol Biol Psychiatry* 2007; **31**:1493–1499.
12. Mellor JE, et al. Schizophrenic symptoms and dietary intake of n-3 fatty acids. *Schizophr Res* 1995; **18**:85–86.
13. Peet M, et al. Two double-blind placebo-controlled pilot studies of eicosapentaenoic acid in the treatment of schizophrenia. *Schizophr Res* 2001; **49**:243–251.
14. Fenton WS, et al. A placebo-controlled trial of omega-3 fatty acid (ethyl eicosapentaenoic acid) supplementation for residual symptoms and cognitive impairment in schizophrenia. *Am J Psychiatry* 2001; **158**:2071–2074.
15. Emsley R, et al. Randomized, placebo-controlled study of ethyl-eicosapentaenoic acid as supplemental treatment in schizophrenia. *Am J Psychiatry* 2002; **159**:1596–1598.
16. Berger GE, et al. Ethyl-eicosapentaenoic acid in first-episode psychosis: a randomized, placebo-controlled trial. *J Clin Psychiatry* 2007; **68**:1867–1875.
17. Fusar-Poli P, et al. Eicosapentaenoic acid interventions in schizophrenia: meta-analysis of randomized, placebo-controlled studies. *J Clin Psychopharmacol* 2012; **32**:179–185.
18. Pawelczyk T, et al. A randomized controlled study of the efficacy of six-month supplementation with concentrated fish oil rich in omega-3 polyunsaturated fatty acids in first episode schizophrenia. *J Psychiatr Res* 2016; **73**:34–44.
19. Bentsen H, et al. A randomized placebo-controlled trial of an omega-3 fatty acid and vitamins E+C in schizophrenia. *Transl Psychiatry* 2013; **3**:e335.
20. Emsley R, et al. A randomized, controlled trial of omega-3 fatty acids plus an antioxidant for relapse prevention after antipsychotic discontinuation in first-episode schizophrenia. *Schizophr Res* 2014; **158**:230–235.
21. Bozzatello P, et al. Polyunsaturated fatty acids: what is their role in treatment of psychiatric disorders? *Int J Molecular Sci* 2019; **20**:5257.
22. Hsu MC, et al. Beneficial effects of omega-3 fatty acid supplementation in schizophrenia: possible mechanisms. *Lipids Health Dis* 2020; **19**:159.
23. Firth J, et al. The efficacy and safety of nutrient supplements in the treatment of mental disorders: a meta-review of meta-analyses of randomized controlled trials. *World Psychiatry* 2019; **18**:308–324.
24. Schlögelhofer M, et al. Polyunsaturated fatty acids in emerging psychosis: a safer alternative? *Early Interv Psychiatry* 2014; **8**:199–208.
25. Scorza FA, et al. Omega-3 fatty acids and sudden cardiac death in schizophrenia: if not a friend, at least a great colleague. *Schizophr Res* 2007; **94**:375–376.
26. Caniato RN, et al. Effect of omega-3 fatty acids on the lipid profile of patients taking clozapine. *Aust N Z J Psychiatry* 2006; **40**:691–697.
27. Emsley R, et al. Safety of the omega-3 fatty acid, eicosapentaenoic acid (EPA) in psychiatric patients: results from a randomized, placebo-controlled trial. *Psychiatry Res* 2008; **161**:284–291.
28. Das UN. Essential fatty acids and their metabolites could function as endogenous HMG-CoA reductase and ACE enzyme inhibitors, anti-

arrhythmic, anti-hypertensive, anti-atherosclerotic, anti-inflammatory, cytoprotective, and cardioprotective molecules. *Lipids Health Dis* 2008; 7:37.

29. Xu F, et al. Effects of omega-3 fatty acids on metabolic syndrome in patients with schizophrenia: a 12-week randomized placebo-controlled trial. *Psychopharmacology* 2019; 236:1273–1279.

30. Amminger GP, et al. Long-chain omega-3 fatty acids for indicated prevention of psychotic disorders: a randomized, placebo-controlled trial. *Arch Gen Psychiatry* 2010; 67:146–154.

31. Stafford MR, et al. Early interventions to prevent psychosis: systematic review and meta-analysis. *BMJ* 2013; 346:f185.

32. McGorry PD, et al. Effect of omega-3 polyunsaturated fatty acids in young people at ultrahigh risk for psychotic disorders: the neurapro randomized clinical trial. *JAMA Psychiatry* 2017; 74:19–27.

33. Bosnjak Kuharic D, et al. Interventions for prodromal stage of psychosis. *Cochrane Database Syst Rev* 2019; CD012236.

34. Devoe DJ, et al. Attenuated psychotic symptom interventions in youth at risk of psychosis: a systematic review and meta-analysis. *Early Interv Psychiatry* 2019; 13:3–17.

35. Nasir M, et al. Trim the fat: the role of omega-3 fatty acids in psychopharmacology. *Ther Adv Psychopharmacol* 2019; 9:2045125319869791.

36. Cho M, et al. Adjunctive use of anti-inflammatory drugs for schizophrenia: a meta-analytic investigation of randomized controlled trials. *Aust N Z J Psychiatry* 2019; 53:742–759.

停用抗精神病药

抗精神病药被推荐用于精神分裂症的长期治疗,因为它们可以减轻症状,降低复发风险[1]。然而,抗精神病药有许多不良反应,包括代谢并发症、迟发性运动障碍(TD)、情感迟钝和脑萎缩[2]。有证据表明,减少或停用抗精神病药可以改善患者的社会功能(人际关系、教育或就业、独立生活),在中期不会增加患者的复发率或症状负担[3],但是短期内可能会增加复发的风险[4]。也有证据表明,减少抗精神病药可能会改善认知功能[5]。

此外,抗精神病药预防复发的证据主要为中止试验,其中抗精神病药大多是在一天内停用,所导致的撤药反应可能使停药组表面上复发率升高,夸大了抗精神病药预防复发的作用[6]。患者经常要求减药或停药。鉴于上述情况,这可能是一个合理的选择。谨慎停药应该是高质量用药实践的一个组成部分。

还应该指出的是,虽然 NICE 不推荐给人格障碍患者[8]中长期使用抗精神病药,给痴呆患者也只是谨慎地使用抗精神病药[9],但是英国的抗精神病药处方有 50% 以上给了没有精神病性障碍或躁狂症的患者,用于治疗失眠、焦虑、人格障碍和痴呆症状[7]。以下列出的停药原则也适用于这些患者。

抗精神病药的撤药/停药影响

停止或减少抗精神病药的剂量,会引起各种症状,反映其不同的作用(阻断多巴胺、组胺、乙酰胆碱、5-羟色胺和去甲肾上腺素受体)[10,11]。它们包括自主神经系统症状(腹泻、流涎、出汗)、躯体症状(头痛、恶心、呕吐、厌食)、运动症状(颤抖、不安、运动障碍)和心理症状(焦虑、易怒、烦躁、失眠和精神病性症状)(图 1.1)[10,11]。失眠可能是最常见的撤药症状。

重要的是,抗精神病药的撤药/停药症状可能包括精神病性症状[11,12]。这是由一些案例研究提出的,其中没有精神病性障碍的人因恶心或哺乳困难等原因使用多巴胺拮抗剂治疗,当患者突然停用这些药物时,会出现精神病性症状[13-15]。

在精神病性障碍患者中,当停用抗精神病药时,往往会病情复发。这一现象被广泛地认为揭示了其为潜在的慢性疾病,但停用抗精神病药这一过程本身可能与复发有因果关系[6]。在停药试验中,精神分裂症患者突然停用抗精神病药后复发率显著增高支持了这一点。在一项分析中,4 年内复发者中有 60% 发生在停止用药后的 3 个月内[16],这段时间最有可能显现撤药效应。还有支持的证据是,更缓慢地减药可以降低复发率[16]。

撤药症状的神经生物学

撤药相关的复发归因于长期抗精神病药治疗的神经适应(多巴胺能超敏)在抗精神病药停用后持续存在[17]。事实上,对精神分裂症的分子成像研究发现,服用抗精神病药的受试者 D_2/D_3 受体增加,而未服用抗精神病药的患者则没有[18]。当抗精神病药剂量减少导致 D_2 阻滞减弱时,对多巴胺的超敏反应可能使患者更容易复发精神病[10,17]。

越来越多的证据表明,服用抗精神病药的神经适应作用在停止服用后仍可以持续数月或数年。停止治疗后,动物体内的多巴胺超敏反应持续时间相当于人类一年[19,20]。TD——

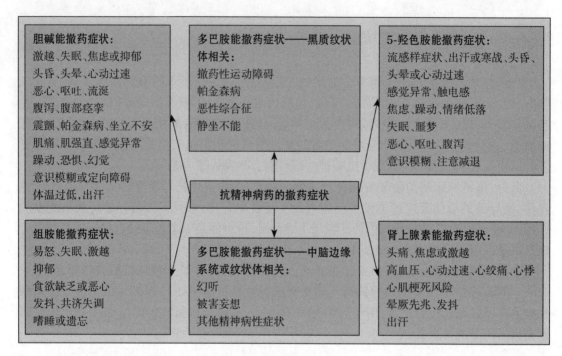

胆碱能撤药症状：
激越、失眠、焦虑或抑郁
头昏、头晕、心动过速
恶心、呕吐、流涎
腹泻、腹部痉挛
震颤、帕金森病、坐立不安
肌痛、肌强直、感觉异常
躁动、恐惧、幻觉
意识模糊或定向障碍
体温过低，出汗

多巴胺能撤药症状——黑质纹状体相关：
撤药性运动障碍
帕金森病
恶性综合征
静坐不能

5-羟色胺能撤药症状：
流感样症状、出汗或寒战、头昏、头晕或心动过速
感觉异常、触电感
焦虑、躁动、情绪低落
失眠、噩梦
恶心、呕吐、腹泻
意识模糊、注意减退

抗精神病药的撤药症状

组胺能撤药症状：
易怒、失眠、激越
抑郁
食欲缺乏或恶心
发抖、共济失调
嗜睡或遗忘

多巴胺能撤药症状——中脑边缘系统或纹状体相关：
幻听
被害妄想
其他精神病性症状

肾上腺素能撤药症状：
头痛、焦虑或激越
高血压、心动过速、心绞痛、心悸
心肌梗死风险
晕厥先兆、发抖
出汗

图 1.1　抗精神病药的撤药症状。改编自 Chouinard et al. (2017)[11]

归因于多巴胺超敏反应——在抗精神病药停用后仍可持续数年[21]。也有证据表明，停用抗精神病药的患者与继续服用抗精神病药的患者相比，三年内的复发率有所增加，之后复发率趋于一致[1]，这表明适应性可能在这一点上消失了。

如果这样的话，抗精神病药停用后复发的风险可以通过逐渐减少剂量来降低，因为这些神经适应在逐渐减少剂量的过程中会慢慢消失，而且阻滞的下降速度也更适度。一项小型分析发现，与突然停药相比，3~9 个月减药的复发率减半[16]，而 4 周减药与突然停药的复发率没有区别[1]。

逐渐减药的模式

PET 成像显示，抗精神病药剂量与 D_2 受体占用率呈双曲线关系[22]。这种双曲线关系也适用于抗精神病药的其他受体靶点（包括组胺能、胆碱能和 5-羟色胺能受体），因为它源于质量作用定律（即当受体靶点饱和时，药物的每一个额外分子的作用就会逐渐减弱）[23]。由于习惯在半对数轴上绘制剂量-效应曲线，这种关系的性质常常被掩盖[23]。抗精神病药的剂量与其治疗效果（以症状量表衡量）之间的双曲线关系也已被证明[24]，这表明临床疗效反映了神经生物学效应模式。

这就对线性减少抗精神病药剂量的基本原理提出了质疑——例如，将奥氮平剂量依次 20mg、15mg、10mg、5mg、0mg 减量。尽管这一方法似乎合理，但剂量与 D_2 阻断效应之间的双曲线关系表明，线性的剂量减少，将导致 D_2 阻滞作用（以及由此产生的临床后果）的下降幅度越来越大（图 1.2A）。事实上，剂量从 5mg 减少到 0mg 时，D_2 阻滞作用下降（52.6%），大于将奥氮平从 40mg 减少到 5mg 所产生的 D_2 阻滞作用下降（37.3%）。D_2 阻滞作用下降的幅度越来越大,更有可能引起复发。

D$_2$ 阻滞作用的线性或"等距"减少,需要抗精神病药按双曲线模式减少剂量(图 1.2B)[25]。这种双曲线性剂量减少模式相当于将剂量连续减半。例如,利培酮剂量依次减至 20mg、10mg、5mg、2.5mg、1.25mg、0.6mg、0.3mg、0mg 时,可使 D$_2$ 阻滞作用降低约 15 个百分点。这种减量模式不太可能引起复发,因为它避免了多巴胺能信号的大幅增加。对这一观点的初步支持来自三个逐步减量抗精神病药的研究:在第一项研究中,实现 6 个月内整体抗精神病药剂量减少 42%,而复发率没有增加[26];在第二项研究中,剂量减少了 25%~62.5%,3/4 的患者没有复发的迹象[27];在第三项研究中,剂量减少了 46.0%~57.6%,减药组与维持剂量组之间 PANSS 总分没有改变[28]。

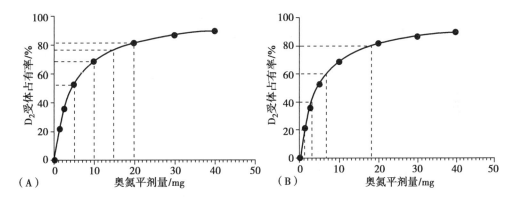

图 1.2　(A) 利培酮线性减量法导致 D$_2$ 受体阻滞作用的下降幅度越来越大。利培酮和 D$_2$ 受体阻滞作用的关系来自 PET 研究荟萃分析的最佳适合线[22]。(B) D$_2$ 受体占用率的线性下降(在本例中,下降率 20%)对应于利培酮的双曲线性减量。在这种情况下,剂量(D$_2$ 受体占有率)分别为 6.9mg(80%)、2.0mg(60%)、0.82mg(40%) 和 0.30mg(20%)。文中给出了与现有药物相对应的这一减药模式的近似值

指数减量模式(即按最近剂量的固定比例减少)将在抗精神病药的所有受体靶点上产生近似线性的下降,从而使其广泛地适用于抗精神病药。值得注意的是,一研究采用了指数减量模式,将部分患者的抗精神病药剂量减少超过 50% 而病情没有复发,具体减量方法是每 6 个月将最近的剂量减少 25%[27]。

在实践中逐渐减量

应告知所有患者,在停止或减少任何抗精神病药剂量时,有出现撤药症状的风险,包括失眠和精神病性症状的增加。氯氮平与最常见且严重的撤药症状有关,可能是因为其有很强的抗胆碱能作用。

应警告患者不要突然停用抗精神病药,因为极有可能导致复发或严重的撤药反应。

何时尝试停药

长期或终身的抗精神病药治疗是现今的现象。20 世纪 60 年代,在急性期治疗有效后,通常会尝试停用抗精神病药,但突然停用往往会导致复发(但有趣的是,并不总是如此[29])。

关于停用抗精神病药,目前尚无循证建议,我们建议仅在缓解6个月(首次发作)或1年(多次发作)的患者中进行尝试。

最初的减量幅度可以根据患者以前的减量经验确定。对于许多患者来说,可以将最近剂量减少约25%(如奥氮平从20mg减到15mg),但是有些患者可能仅需减少10%。减量后,应该监测3个月,观察是否出现撤药症状或精神病性症状恶化。提醒一下:这些症状可能是短暂的撤药效应,不是不可避免的复发迹象,表明有必要恢复常规剂量的药物治疗。如果患者能承受此减量幅度,对其整体精神状态没有显著影响(或者可能只有轻微失眠),那么可以同样的速度进一步减量(如每3个月减量10%~25%)。患者在撤药期间可能需要增加心理社会支持。

如果患者出现明显的撤药症状或精神病性症状加重,则有必要恢复到原来的剂量(或部分剂量)。值得注意的是,这并不排除进一步减量的尝试,但这些尝试应该推迟到病情已经稳定之后,并且减量速度比以前更慢(可能小到目前剂量的5%~10%)。

完全停药前的最后剂量必须非常小,以防止 D_2 阻滞作用大幅度地减少。这可能需要小到原始治疗剂量的1/80(例如0.25mg奥氮平)。服用这些小剂量药物,需要将药片分开,或使用药物的液体制剂。

表1.11和表1.12给出了减药方案的例子,表1.13进行了总结。

表1.11　D_2 受体占有率每减少5个百分点对应的奥氮平剂量

时期	奥氮平剂量/mg	D_2受体占有率/%	时期	奥氮平剂量/mg	D_2受体占有率/%
1	20	81.6	10	2.4	35
2	14	75	11	1.9	30
3	10.5	70	12	1.5	25
4	8.4	65	13	1.1	20
5	6.8	60	14	0.8	15
6	5.5	55	15	0.5	10
7	4.5	50	16	0.24	5
8	3.7	45	17	0	0
9	3	40			

表1.12　D_2受体占有率每减少2.5个百分点对应的奥氮平剂量。按D_2受体占有率"等距"减少原则更大幅度地减量时,可按此方案每隔2~3步进行

时期	奥氮平剂量/mg	D_2受体占有率/%	时期	奥氮平剂量/mg	D_2受体占有率/%
1	20	81.6	5	10.5	70
2	15.5	77.5	6	9.3	67.5
3	13.5	75	7	8.4	65
4	11.9	72.5	8	7.5	62.5

时期	奥氮平剂量/mg	D₂ 受体占有率/%	时期	奥氮平剂量/mg	D₂ 受体占有率/%
9	6.8	60	22	1.7	27.5
10	6.1	57.5	23	1.5	25
11	5.5	55	24	1.3	22.5
12	5	52.5	25	1.1	20
13	4.5	50	26	0.95	17.5
14	4.1	47.5	27	0.8	15
15	3.7	45	28	0.65	12.5
16	3.3	42.5	29	0.5	10
17	3	40	30	0.37	7.5
18	2.7	37.5	31	0.24	5
19	2.4	35	32	0.1	2.5
20	2.2	32.5	33	0	0
21	1.9	30			

表 1.13　奥氮平可能的减量计划摘要

每 2~3 个月减少 5~10mg，直到每天 20mg

每 2~3 个月减少 2.5~5mg，直到每天 10mg

每 2~3 个月减少 1.25~2.5mg，直到每天 5mg

每 2~3 个月减少 0.6~1.25mg，直到每天 2.5mg

每 2~3 个月减少 0.3~0.6mg，直到每天 1.25mg

每 2~3 个月减少 0.15~0.3mg，直到每天 0.6mg

每 2~3 个月减少 0.07~0.15mg，直至**完全停用**

这个过程需要 12~48 个月，取决于患者对减量的耐受程度

参考文献

1. Leucht S, et al. Antipsychotic drugs versus placebo for relapse prevention in schizophrenia: a systematic review and meta-analysis. *Lancet* 2012; 379:2063–2071.
2. Murray RM, et al. Should psychiatrists be more cautious about the long-term prophylactic use of antipsychotics? *Br J Psychiatry* 2016; 209:361–365.
3. Wunderink L, et al. Recovery in remitted first-episode psychosis at 7 years of follow-up of an early dose reduction/discontinuation or maintenance treatment strategy: long-term follow-up of a 2-year randomized clinical trial. *JAMA Psychiatry* 2013; 70:913–920.
4. Wunderink L, et al. Guided discontinuation versus maintenance treatment in remitted first-episode psychosis: relapse rates and functional outcome. *J Clin Psychiatry* 2007; 68:654–661.
5. Omachi Y, et al. Dose reduction/discontinuation of antipsychotic drugs in psychosis; effect on cognition and functional outcomes. *Frontiers in Psychiatry* 2018; 9:447.
6. Moncrieff J. Antipsychotic Maintenance. Treatment: time to rethink? *PLoS Med* 2015; 12:e1001861.
7. Marston L, et al. Prescribing of antipsychotics in UK primary care: a cohort study. *BMJ Open* 2014; 4:e006135.
8. National Institute for Clinical Excellence. Borderline personality disorder: recognition and management. Clinical Guidance 78 [CG78]. 2009

(Last checked July 2018); https://www.nice.org.uk/guidance/CG78.

9. National Institute for Health and Care Excellence. Dementia: assessment, management and support for people living with dementia and their carers [NG97]. 2018; https://www.nice.org.uk/guidance/ng97.

10. Cerovecki A, et al. Withdrawal symptoms and rebound syndromes associated with switching and discontinuing atypical antipsychotics: theoretical background and practical recommendations. *CNS Drugs* 2013; 27:545–572.

11. Chouinard G, et al. Antipsychotic-induced dopamine supersensitivity psychosis: pharmacology, criteria, and therapy. *Psychother Psychosom* 2017; 86:189–219.

12. Moncrieff J. Does antipsychotic withdrawal provoke psychosis? Review of the literature on rapid onset psychosis (supersensitivity psychosis) and withdrawal-related relapse. *Acta Psychiatr Scand* 2006; 114:3–13.

13. Lu ML, et al. Metoclopramide-induced supersensitivity psychosis. *Ann Pharmacother* 2002; 36:1387–1390.

14. Roy-Desruisseaux J, et al. Domperidone-induced tardive dyskinesia and withdrawal psychosis in an elderly woman with dementia. *Ann Pharmacother* 2011; 45:e51.

15. Seeman P Breast is best but taper domperidone when stopping (e-letter). 2014; https://bjgp.org/content/yes-breast-best-taper-domperidone-when-stopping.

16. Viguera AC, et al. Clinical risk following abrupt and gradual withdrawal of maintenance neuroleptic treatment. *Arch Gen Psychiatry* 1997; 54:49–55.

17. Chouinard G, et al. Atypical antipsychotics: CATIE study, drug-induced movement disorder and resulting iatrogenic psychiatric-like symptoms, supersensitivity rebound psychosis and withdrawal discontinuation syndromes. *Psychother Psychosom* 2008; 77:69–77.

18. Howes OD, et al. The nature of dopamine dysfunction in schizophrenia and what this means for treatment. *Arch Gen Psychiatry* 2012; 69:776–786.

19. Joyce JN. D2 but not D3 receptors are elevated after 9 or 11 months chronic haloperidol treatment: influence of withdrawal period. *Synapse* 2001; 40:137–144.

20. Quinn R. Comparing rat's to human's age: how old is my rat in people years? *Nutrition* 2005; 21:775–777.

21. Marsden CD. Is tardive dyskinesia a unique disorder? *Psychopharmacology Suppl* 1985; 2:64–71.

22. Lako IM, et al. Estimating dopamine D_2 receptor occupancy for doses of 8 antipsychotics: a meta-analysis. *J Clin Psychopharmacol* 2013; 33:675–681.

23. Holford N. Pharmacodynamic principles and the time course of delayed and cumulative drug effects. *Translational and Clinical Pharmacology* 2018; 26:56–59.

24. Leucht S, et al. Dose-response meta-analysis of antipsychotic drugs for acute schizophrenia. *Am J Psychiatry* 2020; 177:342–353.

25. Horowitz MA, et al. Tapering antipsychotic treatment. *JAMA Psychiatry* 2021; 78:125–126.

26. Huhn M, et al. Reducing antipsychotic drugs in stable patients with chronic schizophrenia or schizoaffective disorder: a randomized controlled pilot trial. *Eur Arch Psychiatry Clin Neurosci* 2021; 271:293–302.

27. Liu CC, et al. Achieving the lowest effective antipsychotic dose for patients with remitted psychosis: a proposed guided dose-reduction algorithm. *CNS Drugs* 2020; 34:117–126.

28. Ozawa C, et al. Model-guided antipsychotic dose reduction in schizophrenia: a pilot, single-blind randomized controlled trial. *J Clin Psychopharmacol* 2019; 39:329–335.

29. Prien RF, et al. Relapse in chronic schizophrenics following abrupt withdrawal of tranquillizing medication. *Br J Psychiatry* 1969; 115:679–686.

抗精神病药的不良反应

锥体外系不良反应

锥体外系不良反应(EPS)具有以下特点(表 1.14):

- 多与剂量相关。
- 高效价第一代抗精神病药在大剂量使用时最易发生。
- 使用其他抗精神病药,特别是氯氮平、奥氮平、喹硫平和阿立哌唑时,较为少见[1],但一旦发生可能会持续存在[2]。注意:CUtLASS 研究报告,第一代与第二代抗精神病药之间,EPS 发生率没有差异[3](尽管第一代抗精神病药中的舒必利被广泛地使用)。对 EPS 的易感性可能由遗传决定[4]。

　　注意,类似的运动障碍也可能出现在从未服药的精神分裂症患者身上[5-7]。在对首发患者进行的一项研究中,1% 有肌张力障碍,8% 有帕金森综合征,11% 有静坐不能[7]。在这种背景下,帕金森综合征和其他运动异常可能与认知障碍[7,8]和长期社会心理功能不佳有关[9]。在已经明确诊断为精神病性障碍但从未治疗过的患者中,9% 出现自发性运动障碍,17% 出现帕金森综合征[10]。以往有过某种 EPS 的患者,可能更容易出现其他类型的 EPS[11]。物质滥用会增加肌张力障碍、静坐不能和 TD 的风险[12,13]。有证据表明饮酒与静坐不能相关[14,15]。

表 1.14　最常见锥体外系症状

	肌张力障碍 (无法控制的肌肉痉挛)	假性帕金森综合征 (运动迟缓、震颤等)	静坐不能 (坐立不安)[16]	迟发性运动障碍 (异常不自主运动)
症状和体征[17]	身体任何部位肌肉痉挛,如: ■ 眼上翻(动眼危象) ■ 头、颈向一侧扭转(斜颈) 患者可能无法吞咽或清晰讲话。极个别病例出现背部拱起或下颌脱位 急性肌紧张可致痛苦和令人感到恐惧	■ 震颤或强直 ■ 运动迟缓(表情减少,语音单调,躯体运动缓慢,启动困难) ■ 思维迟缓 ■ 流涎 类帕金森病易被误诊为抑郁症或精神分裂症的阴性症状	主观不快、内心不安,有强烈渴望或冲动去活动[1] ■ 坐位时踩脚 ■ 不断交叉/分开双腿 ■ 倒脚摇摆 ■ 不停徘徊 静坐不能易误诊为精神病性激越,并与自杀意念[18]和攻击他人相关[19]	可见各种动作[20],如 ■ 咂嘴或咀嚼 ■ 伸舌(捕蝇动作) ■ 手部舞蹈样运动(弹琴样) ■ 四肢肌张力障碍和舞蹈手足徐动 严重口面运动异常可致难以讲话、进食或呼吸。在压力下运动症状加重
评定量表	无专用量表。一般 EPS 量表有少部分相关内容	Simpson-Angus EPS 评定量表[21]	Barnes 静坐不能量表[22]	异常不自主运动量表(AIMS)[23]

第 1 章

续表

	肌张力障碍 （无法控制的肌肉痉挛）	假性帕金森综合征 （运动迟缓、震颤等）	静坐不能 （坐立不安）[16]	迟发性运动障碍 （异常不自主运动）
患病率（使用第一代抗精神病药）	约 10%，[24] 但多见于[25]： ■ 年轻男性 ■ 从未用过抗精神病药 ■ 使用高效价药物（如氟哌啶醇） 肌张力障碍在老年人中罕见	约 20%[26]，但多见于： ■ 老年女性 ■ 原有神经系统损害（头外伤、卒中等）	差异很大，但使用第一代抗精神病药时急性静坐不能发生率约为 25%[27]，第二代抗精神病药发生率较低 各种抗精神病药导致静坐不能的相对危险性尚不确定[28]，但一致认为奥氮平、喹硫平和氯氮平的发生率最低[29,30]	服用抗精神病药人群中每年为 5%[31]。多见于[32]： ■ 老年 ■ 情感障碍 ■ 精神分裂症 ■ 高剂量 ■ 治疗早期出现急性 EPS 使用第二代抗精神病药者发病率较低[33] 迟发性运动障碍可能与神经认知缺陷有关[34]
发生时间	使用抗精神病药数小时内（若肌内注射或静脉注射，数分钟） 迟发性肌张力障碍发生于抗精神病药治疗后数月至数年	抗精神病药开始使用或增加剂量后数天至数周	急性静坐不能发生于开始服药或增加剂量后数小时至数周；持续数月的静坐不能称为"慢性静坐不能"。迟发性静坐不能往往在治疗后期出现，可能因抗精神病药减量或撤药而加重或引起[16]	数月至数年 停用抗精神病药后逆转的比例不详，可能部分取决于年龄[20]
治疗	根据症状严重程度口服、肌内注射或静脉注射抗胆碱能药[20] ■ 切记患者可能无法吞咽 ■ 静脉注射后 5min 内可见效 ■ 肌内注射后 20min 可见效 ■ 电抽搐治疗可能对迟发性肌张力障碍有效[35,36] ■ 严重症状以简单方法（换用 EPS 风险低的药物）处理无效时，肉毒毒素可能有效[37,38]	据临床情况选择： ■ 减少抗精神病药剂量 ■ 换用类帕金森综合征风险低的抗精神病药（见本章抗精神病药致不良反应的相对可能性） ■ 给予抗胆碱能药。多数患者不需要长期使用抗胆碱能药。应该至少每 3 个月评估一次。不在晚上服用（睡眠时通常无症状）	■ 减少抗精神病药剂量 ■ 换用静坐不能风险低的抗精神病药（见静坐不能与抗精神病药致不良反应的相对可能性） ■ 下述方法可减轻症状[39-41]：低剂量普萘洛尔 30~80mg/d，低剂量氯硝西泮，H_1 受体拮抗剂（如赛庚啶[36]），米氮平[40]，曲唑酮[42,43]，米安色林[44]，苯海拉明可能有效[45] 上述选择均超适应证使用 抗胆碱能药一般无效，除非是整体 EPS 症状中的一部分[46]	■ 停用抗胆碱能药 ■ 减少抗精神病药剂量 ■ 换用迟发性运动障碍风险低的抗精神病药[47-50]；注意研究结果不一[51,52] ■ 氯氮平是最有可能缓解症状的抗精神病药[53,54]，喹硫平也可能有效[55] ■ 缬苯那嗪和氘丁苯那嗪作为附加治疗，均有积极的风险-效益比[53,56-60] ■ 也有一些证据表现丁苯那嗪和银杏叶提取物[61]作为附加治疗可能有效。其他治疗选择[60,62]参考美国神经病学会综述[63]及本章"迟发性运动障碍"

EPS，锥体外系不良反应。

参考文献

1. Leucht S, et al. Comparative efficacy and tolerability of 15 antipsychotic drugs in schizophrenia: a multiple-treatments meta-analysis. *Lancet* 2013; **382**:951–962.

2. Tenback DE, et al. Incidence and persistence of tardive dyskinesia and extrapyramidal symptoms in schizophrenia. *J Psychopharmacol* 2010; **24**:1031–1035.

3. Peluso MJ, et al. Extrapyramidal motor side-effects of first- and second-generation antipsychotic drugs. *Br J Psychiatry* 2012; **200**:387–392.

4. Zivkovic M, et al. The association study of polymorphisms in DAT, DRD2, and COMT genes and acute extrapyramidal adverse effects in male schizophrenic patients treated with haloperidol. *J Clin Psychopharmacol* 2013; **33**:593–599.

5. Cortese L, et al. Relationship of neuromotor disturbances to psychosis symptoms in first-episode neuroleptic-naive schizophrenia patients. *Schizophr Res* 2005; **75**:65–75.

6. Puri BK, et al. Spontaneous dyskinesia in first episode schizophrenia. *J Neurol Neurosurg Psychiatry* 1999; **66**:76–78.

7. Rybakowski JK, et al. Extrapyramidal symptoms during treatment of first schizophrenia episode: Results from EUFEST. Eur Neuropsychopharmacol 2014; **24**:1500–1505.

8. Cuesta MJ, et al. Spontaneous parkinsonism is asociated with cognitive impairment in antipsychotic-naive patients with first-episode psychosis: a 6-month follow-up study. *Schizophr Bull* 2014; **40**:1164–1173.

9. Cuesta MJ, et al. Motor abnormalities in first-episode psychosis patients and long-term psychosocial functioning. *Schizophr Res* 2018; **200**:97–103.

10. Pappa S, et al. Spontaneous Spontaneous Parkinsonism Is Associated With Cognitive Impairment in Antipsychotic-Naive Patients With First-Episode Psychosis: A 6-Month Follow-up Study. Schizophr Bull; 2014; **40**:1164–1173.

11. Kim JH, et al. Prevalence and characteristics of subjective akathisia, objective akathisia, and mixed akathisia in chronic schizophrenic subjects. *Clin Neuropharmacol* 2003; **26**:312–316.

12. Potvin S, et al. Increased extrapyramidal symptoms in patients with schizophrenia and a comorbid substance use disorder. *J Neurol Neurosurg Psychiatry* 2006; **77**:796–798.

13. Potvin S, et al. Substance abuse is associated with increased extrapyramidal symptoms in schizophrenia: a meta-analysis. *Schizophr Res* 2009; **113**:181–188.

14. Hansen LK, et al. Movement disorders in patients with schizophrenia and a history of substance abuse. *Human Psychopharmacology* 2013; **28**:192–197.

15. Duke PJ, et al. South Westminster schizophrenia survey. Alcohol use and its relationship to symptoms, tardive dyskinesia and illness onset. *Br J Psychiatry* 1994; **164**:630–636.

16. Barnes TR, et al. Akathisia variants and tardive dyskinesia. *Arch Gen Psychiatry* 1985; **42**:874–878.

17. Gervin M, et al. Assessment of drug-related movement disorders in schizophrenia. *Adv Psychiatric Treatment* 2000; **6**:332–341.

18. Seemuller F, et al. Akathisia and suicidal ideation in first-episode schizophrenia. *J Clin Psychopharmacol* 2012; **32**:694–698.

19. Leong GB, et al. Neuroleptic-induced akathisia and violence: a review. *J Forensic Sci* 2003; **48**:187–189.

20. Owens DC. Tardive dyskinesia update: the syndrome. *B J Psych Advances* 2018; **25**:57–69.

21. Simpson GM, et al. A rating scale for extrapyramidal side effects. *Acta Psychiatr Scand* 1970; **212**:11–19.

22. Barnes TRE. A rating scale for drug-induced akathisia. *Br J Psychiatry* 1989; **154**:672–676.

23. Guy W. *ECDEU Assessment Manual for Psychopharmacology*. Washington, DC: US Department of Health, Education, and Welfare; 1976:534–537.

24. American Psychiatric Association. Practice guideline for the treatment of patients with schizophrenia. *Am J Psychiatry* 1997; **154** Suppl 4:1–63.

25. Van Harten PN, et al. Acute dystonia induced by drug treatment. *Br Med J* 1999; **319**:623–626.

26. Bollini P, et al. Antipsychotic drugs: is more worse? A meta-analysis of the published randomized control trials. *Psychol Med* 1994; **24**:307–316.

27. Halstead SM, et al. Akathisia: prevalence and associated dysphoria in an in-patient population with chronic schizophrenia. *Br J Psychiatry* 1994; **164**:177–183.

28. Martino D, et al. Movement disorders associated with antipsychotic medication in people with schizophrenia: an overview of Cochrane reviews and meta-analysis. *Can J Psychiatry* 2018; **63**:706743718777392.

29. Hirose S. The causes of underdiagnosing akathisia. *Schizophr Bull* 2003; **29**:547–558.

30. Juncal-Ruiz M, et al. Incidence and risk factors of acute akathisia in 493 individuals with first episode non-affective psychosis: a 6-week randomised study of antipsychotic treatment. *Psychopharmacology* 2017; **234**:2563–2570.

31. Caligiuri M. Tardive Dyskinesia: a task force report of the American Psychiatric Association. *Hosp Community Psychiatry* 1993; **44**:190.

32. Patterson-Lomba O, et al. Risk assessment and prediction of TD incidence in psychiatric patients taking concomitant antipsychotics: a retrospective data analysis. *BMC Neurol* 2019; **19**:174.

33. Widschwendter CG, et al. Antipsychotic-induced tardive dyskinesia: update on epidemiology and management. *Curr Opin Psychiatry* 2019; **32**:179–184.

34. Caroff SN, et al. Treatment outcomes of patients with tardive dyskinesia and chronic schizophrenia. *J Clin Psychiatry* 2011; **72**:295–303.

35. Yasui-Furukori N, et al. The effects of electroconvulsive therapy on tardive dystonia or dyskinesia induced by psychotropic medication: a retrospective study. *Neuropsychiatr Dis Treat* 2014; **10**:1209–1212.

36. Miller CH, et al. Managing antipsychotic-induced acute and chronic akathisia. *Drug Saf* 2000; **22**:73–81.

37. Havaki-Kontaxaki BJ, et al. Treatment of severe neuroleptic-induced tardive torticollis. *Ann Gen Hosp Psychiatry* 2003; 2:9.

38. Hennings JM, et al. Successful treatment of tardive lingual dystonia with botulinum toxin: case report and review of the literature. *Prog Neuropsychopharmacol Biol Psychiatry* 2008; 32:1167–1171.

39. Pringsheim T, et al. The assessment and treatment of antipsychotic-induced akathisia. *Can J Psychiatry* 2018; 63:719–729.

40. Poyurovsky M, et al. Efficacy of low-dose mirtazapine in neuroleptic-induced akathisia: a double-blind randomized placebo-controlled pilot study. *J Clin Psychopharmacol* 2003; 23:305–308.

41. Salem H, et al. Revisiting antipsychotic-induced akathisia: current Issues and prospective challenges. *Curr Neuropharmacol* 2017; 15:789–798.

42. Stryjer R, et al. Treatment of neuroleptic-induced akathisia with the 5-HT2A antagonist trazodone. *Clin Neuropharmacol* 2003; 26:137–141.

43. Stryjer R, et al. Trazodone for the treatment of neuroleptic-induced acute akathisia: a placebo-controlled, double-blind, crossover study. *Clin Neuropharmacol* 2010; 33:219–222.

44. Stryjer R, et al. Mianserin for the rapid improvement of chronic akathisia in a schizophrenia patient. *Eur Psychiatry* 2004; 19:237–238.

45. Vinson DR. Diphenhydramine in the treatment of akathisia induced by prochlorperazine. *J Emerg Med* 2004; 26:265–270.

46. Rathbone J, et al. Anticholinergics for neuroleptic-induced acute akathisia. *Cochrane Database Syst Rev* 2006; CD003727.

47. Glazer WM. Expected incidence of tardive dyskinesia associated with atypical antipsychotics. *J Clin Psychiatry* 2000; **61 Suppl 4**:21–26.

48. Kinon BJ, et al. Olanzapine treatment for tardive dyskinesia in schizophrenia patients: a prospective clinical trial with patients randomized to blinded dose reduction periods. *Prog Neuropsychopharmacol Biol Psychiatry* 2004; 28:985–996.

49. Bai YM, et al. Risperidone for severe tardive dyskinesia: a 12-week randomized, double-blind, placebo-controlled study. *J Clin Psychiatry* 2003; 64:1342–1348.

50. Tenback DE, et al. Effects of antipsychotic treatment on tardive dyskinesia: a 6-month evaluation of patients from the European Schizophrenia Outpatient Health Outcomes (SOHO) Study. *J Clin Psychiatry* 2005; 66:1130–1133.

51. Woods SW, et al. Incidence of tardive dyskinesia with atypical versus conventional antipsychotic medications: a prospective cohort study. *J Clin Psychiatry* 2010; 71:463–474.

52. Pena MS, et al. Tardive dyskinesia and other movement disorders secondary to aripiprazole. *Mov Disord* 2011; 26:147–152.

53. Stegmayer K, et al. Tardive dyskinesia associated with atypical antipsychotics: prevalence, mechanisms and management strategies. *CNS Drugs* 2018; 32:135–147.

54. Simpson GM. The treatment of tardive dyskinesia and tardive dystonia. *J Clin Psychiatry* 2000; **61 Suppl 4**:39–44.

55. Peritogiannis V, et al. Can atypical antipsychotics improve tardive dyskinesia associated with other atypical antipsychotics? Case report and brief review of the literature. *J Psychopharmacol* 2010; 24:1121–1125.

56. Hauser RA, et al. KINECT 3: a phase 3 randomized, double-blind, placebo-controlled trial of valbenazine for tardive dyskinesia. *Am J Psychiatry* 2017; 174:476–484.

57. Josiassen RC, et al. Long-term safety and tolerability of valbenazine (NBI-98854) in subjects with tardive dyskinesia and a diagnosis of schizophrenia or mood disorder. *Psychopharmacol Bull* 2017; 47:61–68.

58. Fernandez HH, et al. Randomized controlled trial of deutetrabenazine for tardive dyskinesia: the ARM-TD study. *Neurology* 2017; 88:2003–2010.

59. Citrome L. Deutetrabenazine for tardive dyskinesia: a systematic review of the efficacy and safety profile for this newly approved novel medication – what is the number needed to treat, number needed to harm and likelihood to be helped or harmed? *Int J Clin Pract* 2017; 71.

60. Ricciardi L, et al. Treatment recommendations for tardive dyskinesia. *Can J Psychiatry* 2019; 64:388–399.

61. Zhang WF, et al. Extract of ginkgo biloba treatment for tardive dyskinesia in schizophrenia: a randomized, double-blind, placebo-controlled trial. *J Clin Psychiatry* 2010.

62. Bergman H, et al. Systematic review of interventions for treating or preventing antipsychotic-induced tardive dyskinesia. *Health Technol Assess* 2017; 21:1–218.

63. Bhidayasiri R, et al. Evidence-based guideline: treatment of tardive syndromes: report of the Guideline Development Subcommittee of the American Academy of Neurology. *Neurology* 2013; 81:463–469.

静坐不能

　　静坐不能是大多数抗精神病药的常见不良反应,但是某些第二代抗精神病药,包括一些最近批准的抗精神病药,似乎发生率较低 [1,2]。在对三项随机、开放试验的汇总分析中 [3],首发精神病患者静坐不能的发生率如下:氟哌啶醇 57%,利培酮 20%,阿立哌唑 18%,齐拉西酮 17%,奥氮平 4%,喹硫平 3.5%。卢美哌隆和匹莫范色林仅在一些国家可用:初步数据表明,卢美哌隆导致静坐不能的风险较低 [4],而匹莫范色林可能改善氟哌啶醇引起的静坐不能 [5]。

　　静坐不能的核心特征是精神不安和烦躁,其特征是不安感 [6,7]。它通常伴有明显的运动不安,严重时可导致患者来回踱步,不能长时间坐着。令人不安的静坐不能的主观体验和自杀意念之间可能相关 [8,9],但仍不确定。

　　有证据表明,避免大剂量抗精神病药、多种抗精神病药联用和快速增加剂量,可预防静坐不能 [6,10-12]。对于任何改善静坐不能的药物治疗方案,甚至那些最常用的方案,如改用引起静坐不能风险较低的抗精神病药,或添加 β-肾上腺素能阻滞剂、5-HT$_{2A}$ 拮抗剂或抗胆碱能药物 [13,14],其获益-风险平衡的证据均有限。下图为药物诱导的持续性静坐不能的治疗方案。

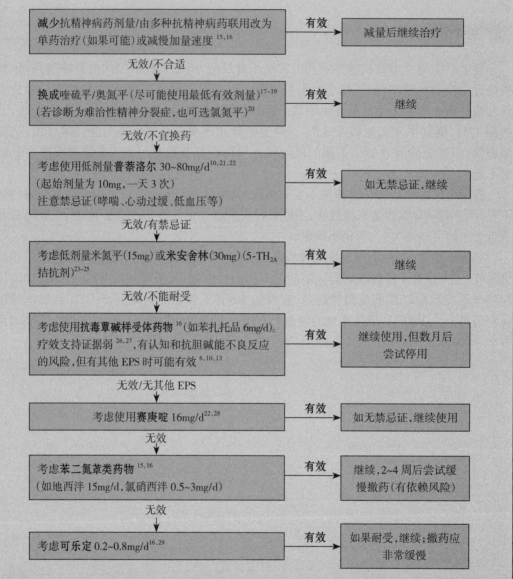

注：

- 静坐不能有时难以明确诊断。目前 EPS 的临床体检表已被提出。对于每个患者，必须仔细了解既往症状、药物疗效和不良反应、合用精神活性物质情况。
- 每一种治疗选择的疗效评估至少需要 1 个月。有些效果可能在几天后出现，但是在慢性静坐不能患者中，疗效观察需要的时间可能要长得多。
- 停止以前对静坐不能无效的治疗后，再开始此流程中的下一个治疗选择。
- 在保证认真监测的情况下，对难治性病例，可以联用不同的治疗手段。
- 对于急性静坐不能，已经研究过其他可能的治疗，包括维生素 B_6 [32,33]、普瑞巴林[34]、苯海拉明[35]、曲唑酮[23,36] 和佐米曲普坦[37,38]。在考虑这些治疗选择之前，应该阅读原始文献。
- 肠道外使用咪达唑仑（1.5mg）成功地预防了静脉注射甲氧氯普胺引起的静坐不能[39]，提示咪达唑仑和苯二氮䓬类药物可能普遍具有特定的治疗效果。
- 在一些病例中，已知躁动/静坐不能是开始使用抗精神病药（如阿立哌唑、卡利拉嗪）时引起的短期效应，可在有限的时间内预防性或治疗性使用苯二氮䓬类药物。临床经验表明，这种做法是有效的。

参考文献

1. Demyttenaere K, et al. Medication-induced akathisia with newly approved antipsychotics in patients with a severe mental illness: a systematic review and meta-analysis. *CNS Drugs* 2019; **33**:549–566.
2. Chow CL, et al. Akathisia and newer second-generation antipsychotic drugs: a review of current evidence. *Pharmacotherapy* 2020; **40**:565–574.
3. Juncal-Ruiz M, et al. Incidence and risk factors of acute akathisia in 493 individuals with first episode non-affective psychosis: a 6-week randomised study of antipsychotic treatment. *Psychopharmacology* 2017; **234**:2563–2570.
4. Correll CU, et al. Efficacy and safety of lumateperone for treatment of schizophrenia: a randomized clinical trial. *JAMA Psychiatry* 2020; **77**:349–358.
5. Abbas A, et al. Pimavanserin tartrate: a 5-HT2A inverse agonist with potential for treating various neuropsychiatric disorders. *Exp Opin Pharmacother* 2008; **9**:3251–3259.
6. Braude WM, et al. Clinical characteristics of akathisia. A systematic investigation of acute psychiatric inpatient admissions. *Br J Psychiatry* 1983; **143**:139–150.
7. Barnes TRE. A rating scale for drug-induced akathisia. *Br J Psychiatry* 1989; **154**:672–676.
8. Seemuller F, et al. Akathisia and suicidal ideation in first-episode schizophrenia. *J Clin Psychopharmacol* 2012; **32**:694–698.
9. Seemuller F, et al. The relationship of akathisia with treatment emergent suicidality among patients with first-episode schizophrenia treated with haloperidol or risperidone. *Pharmacopsychiatry* 2012; **45**:292–296.
10. Miller CH, et al. Managing antipsychotic-induced acute and chronic akathisia. *Drug Saf* 2000; **22**:73–81.
11. Berardi D, et al. Clinical correlates of akathisia in acute psychiatric inpatients. *Int Clin Psychopharmacol* 2000; **15**:215–219.
12. Yoshimura B, et al. Incidence and predictors of acute akathisia in severely ill patients with first-episode schizophrenia treated with aripiprazole or risperidone: secondary analysis of an observational study. *Psychopharmacology* 2019; **236**:723–730.
13. Pringsheim T, et al. The assessment and treatment of antipsychotic-induced akathisia. *Can J Psychiatry* 2018; **63**:719–729.
14. Stroup TS, et al. Management of common adverse effects of antipsychotic medications. *World Psychiatry* 2018; **17**:341–356.
15. Fleischhacker WW, et al. The pharmacologic treatment of neuroleptic-induced akathisia. *J Clin Psychopharmacol* 1990; **10**:12–21.
16. Sachdev P. The identification and management of drug-induced akathisia. *CNS Drugs* 1995; **4**:28–46.
17. Kumar R, et al. Akathisia and second-generation antipsychotic drugs. *Curr Opin Psychiatry* 2009; **22**:293–299.
18. Miller DD, et al. Extrapyramidal side-effects of antipsychotics in a randomised trial. *Br J Psychiatry* 2008; **193**:279–288.
19. Rummel-Kluge C, et al. Second-generation antipsychotic drugs and extrapyramidal side effects: a systematic review and meta-analysis of head-to-head comparisons. *Schizophr Bull* 2012; **38**:167–177.
20. Kane JM, et al. Akathisia: an updated review focusing on second-generation antipsychotics. *J Clin Psychiatry* 2009; **70**:627–643.
21. Adler L, et al. A controlled assessment of propranolol in the treatment of neuroleptic-induced akathisia. *Br J Psychiatry* 1986; **149**:42–45.
22. Fischel T, et al. Cyproheptadine versus propranolol for the treatment of acute neuroleptic-induced akathisia: a comparative double-blind study. *J Clin Psychopharmacol* 2001; **21**:612–615.
23. Laoutidis ZG, et al. 5-HT2A receptor antagonists for the treatment of neuroleptic-induced akathisia: a systematic review and meta-analysis. *Int J Neuropsychopharmacol* 2014; **17**:823–832.
24. Poyurovsky M, et al. Mirtazapine – a multifunctional drug: low dose for akathisia. *CNS Spectr* 2011; **16**:63.
25. Poyurovsky M. Acute antipsychotic-induced akathisia revisited. *Br J Psychiatry* 2010; **196**:89–91.
26. Rathbone J, et al. Anticholinergics for neuroleptic-induced acute akathisia. *Cochrane Database Syst Rev* 2006; CD003727.
27. Baskak B, et al. The effectiveness of intramuscular biperiden in acute akathisia: a double-blind, randomized, placebo-controlled study. *J Clin Psychopharmacol* 2007; **27**:289–294.
28. Weiss D, et al. Cyproheptadine treatment in neuroleptic-induced akathisia. *Br J Psychiatry* 1995; **167**:483–486.
29. Zubenko GS, et al. Use of clonidine in treating neuroleptic-induced akathisia. *Psychiatry Res* 1984; **13**:253–259.
30. Gervin M, et al. Assessment of drug-related movement disorders in schizophrenia. *Adv Psychiatr Treatment* 2000; **6**:332–341.
31. Cunningham Owens DA. *Guide to the extrapyramidal side effects of antipsychotic drugs*. Cambridge University Press; 1999.
32. Miodownik C, et al. Vitamin B6 versus mianserin and placebo in acute neuroleptic-induced akathisia: a randomized, double-blind, controlled study. *Clin Neuropharmacol* 2006; **29**:68–72.
33. Lerner V, et al. Vitamin B6 treatment in acute neuroleptic-induced akathisia: a randomized, double-blind, placebo-controlled study. *J Clin Psychiatry* 2004; **65**:1550–1554.
34. De Berardis D, et al. Reversal of aripiprazole-induced tardive akathisia by addition of pregabalin. *J Neuropsychiatry Clin Neurosci* 2013; **25**:E9–E10.
35. Friedman BW, et al. A randomized trial of diphenhydramine as prophylaxis against metoclopramide-induced akathisia in nauseated emergency department patients. *Ann Emerg Med* 2009; **53**:379–385.
36. Stryjer R, et al. Trazodone for the treatment of neuroleptic-induced acute akathisia: a placebo-controlled, double-blind, crossover study. *Clin Neuropharmacol* 2010; **33**:219–222.
37. Gross-Isseroff R, et al. The 5-HT1D receptor agonist zolmitriptan for neuroleptic-induced akathisia: an open label preliminary study. *Int Clin Psychopharmacol* 2005; **20**:23–25.
38. Avital A, et al. Zolmitriptan compared to propranolol in the treatment of acute neuroleptic-induced akathisia: a comparative double-blind study. *Eur Neuropsychopharmacol* 2009; **19**:476–482.
39. Erdur B, et al. A trial of midazolam vs diphenhydramine in prophylaxis of metoclopramide-induced akathisia. *Am J Emerg Med* 2012; **30**:84–91.

迟发性运动障碍的治疗

与几十年前相比,迟发性运动障碍(TD)现在已是不太常见的问题了 [1,2],这可能是因为第二代抗精神病药的问世和广泛应用,其发生 TD 的风险低于第一代抗精神病药 [3-6]。对已经发生的 TD,治疗常常难以成功,因此必须进行预防、早期发现、早期治疗 [7,8]。有证据表明,TD 与认知损害较重 [7,9]、精神病理学表现更重 [10,11]、死亡率升高有关 [12,13]。

尽管第二代抗精神病药导致 TD 的可能性较小 [14-19],但是它们确实也会导致 TD,总体发生率大约 4% [18],只不过各种药物所致 TD 发生率不同 [20-23]。一项荟萃分析估计,第一代抗精神病药使用者中发生 TD 的年风险为 3.7%~12.5%(取决于药物),第二代抗精神病药使用者中发生 TD 的年风险为 1.7%~4.8% [24]。发生 TD 的风险可能与所用药物的 D_2 受体占有率有关(占有率越大,风险越高) [25]。然而,对相关随机对照试验进行充分的荟萃分析,结果并不支持 SGA 比 FGA 发生 TD 的风险低与后者剂量大有关的观点 [24]。多巴胺部分激动剂(或至少阿立哌唑)可能 TD 发生率最低 [26]。尚不清楚 FGA 和 SGA 长效制剂的 TD 风险是否不同,但可以假设 SGA 长效制剂的 TD 风险可能更低。

TD 可发生在低剂量氟哌啶醇(且既往无急性肌张力障碍 [27])和使用其他多巴胺拮抗剂(如甲氧氯普胺)后 [28]。

TD 也在从未服药的首发 [29,30] 确诊 [31] 精神分裂症患者中见到。

治疗——第一步

大多数权威建议,当发现 TD 早期征象时,最初步骤是停止合用的抗胆碱能药,减少抗精神病药的剂量 [32,33](尽管减少剂量在开始阶段可能会加重 TD 症状)。然而,Cochrane 数据库未发现什么证据能支持减少剂量 [34] 或停用抗胆碱能药 [35] 这种方法,美国神经病学学会也不建议减量 [36]。目前的常用做法是一旦发现 TD,即停止所用的抗精神病药,换成其他引起 TD 可能性小的药物。然而换成特定 SGA 后有益的证据很少 [36]。这方面支持证据最充分的也许是氯氮平 [32,37],但是喹硫平作为另一种对纹状体 DA 拮抗作用较弱的药物也可能有效 [38-44],奥氮平 [39-42,45,46] 和阿立哌唑 [47] 也是可以考虑选择的方法。有些证据支持使用利培酮 [48],但是对于已经发生 TD 的患者,利培酮是不符合逻辑的选择,因为它比氯氮平、喹硫平和奥氮平更易导致急性运动障碍。

治疗——加用其他药物

考虑到没有足够的证据推荐将减少剂量作为 TD 的治疗方法,且换用或停用抗精神病药并非总是有效或适当,因此常需加用其他药物。2020 年的一项荟萃分析发现 [49],只有三种已获许可的 VMAT-2 抑制剂、维生素 E、金刚烷胺和维生素 B_6 有明显的益处。表 1.15 列出了治疗 TD 最常用的辅助药物。

表 1.15　首选用于治疗迟发性运动障碍的其他药物(按字母排序,不分主次)

药物	评论
金刚烷胺 [49-52]	极少使用,但明显有效。剂量为 100~300mg/d

续表

药物	评论
苯二氮䓬类药物 [32,33]	广泛地用于 TD,但 Cochrane 综述认为有限的证据提示其疗效不确定 [53]。必须间歇使用,以避免耐受。最常用的是氯硝西泮 1~4mg/d 和地西泮 6~25mg/d。有更好的证据支持前者 [36,54]
氘丁苯那嗪 [8,52,55-57]	氘丁苯那嗪(VMAT-2 抑制剂)也可以有效治疗 TD。在美国获得 TD 适应证批准 [58]。其支持证据优于丁苯那嗪。半衰期比丁苯那嗪长,但仍需每天服用两次。精神和神经系统不良反应发生率低。剂量是 12~48mg /d
银杏叶提取物 [52,59]	耐受性良好。Cochrane 综述的结论是,尽管银杏叶可以减少 TD 症状,但现有证据不足以支持其作为常规治疗 [50]。中国 3 项随机对照试验的荟萃分析显示,240mg/d 治疗效果良好 [61]
维生素 B$_6$ [62]	得到 Cochrane[63] 和一项荟萃分析 [49] 支持。剂量可达 400mg/d
丁苯那嗪 [64,65]	在英国唯一获批用于中、重度 TD 的治疗药物。可能导致抑郁、嗜睡、帕金森综合征和静坐不能 [54,66]。剂量为 25~200mg/d。利血平(作用机制相似)也有效,但极少使用
缬苯那嗪 [8,56,60,67-70]	有证据支持缬苯那嗪(VMAT-2 抑制剂)作为 TD 治疗有好的获益-风险比。在美国被批准用于 TD 的治疗 [71]。每天一次 80mg 的剂量有效,且对心血管影响温和。抑郁和静坐不能的发生率低
维生素 E [49,72]	虽然有大量的研究,但疗效仍有待确定。Cochrane 认为只有延缓 TD 恶化的证据 [8,73]。剂量为 400~1 600IU/d

治疗——其他可能的选择

　　关于 TD 治疗有大量的建议,这无疑说明标准治疗方法的疗效有限,至少在缬苯那嗪和氘丁苯那嗪问世之前是这样。表 1.16 按字母顺序列出了一些有争议的治疗手段。

表 1.16　TD 治疗的其他选择

药物	评论
氨基酸 [74]	一项小样本随机对照试验支持其使用。毒性低
肉毒毒素 [75-78]	有病例报告能有效地治疗局部运动障碍。目前,可选择用于治疗致残或令人痛苦的局部症状
钙离子拮抗剂 [79]	有几项研究发表,但未被广泛使用。Cochrane 不支持 [80]。一项荟萃分析发现无效 [49]
多奈哌齐 [81-83]	支持证据来自一项开放研究和病例系列研究。一项随机对照试验结果为阴性($n=12$)。剂量为 10mg/d。没有明确的证据表明卡巴拉汀或加兰他敏有效 [84]
鱼油 [85,86]	对使用 EPA 的支持证据非常有限,剂量为 2g/d
氟伏沙明 [87]	有 3 例个案报告。剂量为 100mg/d。注意药物相互作用
加巴喷丁 [88]	支持 GABA 能作用机制改善 TD 的理论。剂量为 900~1 200mg/d。其他 GABA 激动剂的数据不确定 [89]

第1章

续表

药物	评论
左乙拉西坦[90-93]	3篇个案研究。1项随机对照试验。剂量最高 3 000mg/d
褪黑素[94]	一篇纳入 4 项试验的荟萃分析支持使用[95]。通常耐受性好。剂量为 10mg/d。有一些证据认为褪黑素受体基因型决定 TD 风险[96]
纳曲酮[97]	与苯二氮䓬类合用时可能有效。耐受性良好。剂量为 200mg/d
昂丹司琼[98,99]	证据有限，但毒性较低。剂量最高 12mg/d
普萘洛尔[100-102]	以前是一种相对广泛使用的治疗方法。目前只有开放研究，可能值得进行前瞻性随机试验。剂量为 40~120mg/d。注意禁忌证(哮喘、心动过缓、低血压)
槲皮素[103]	具有抗氧化作用的植物提取物。一些病例报告提示其有研究价值[103-105]
羟丁酸钠[106]	有 1 例个案报告。剂量为 8g/d
重复经颅磁刺激(rTMS)[107,108]	关于 TD 患者的 RCT 数据表明，在"一线"药物治疗无效的情况下，双侧半球高频 rTMS 可能是一种可行的治疗方法
唑吡坦[109]	有 3 例报告。剂量为 10~30mg/d

参考文献

1. Merrill RM, et al. Tardive and spontaneous dyskinesia incidence in the general population. *BMC Psychiatry* 2013; **13**:152.

2. Kane JM, et al. Tardive dyskinesia: prevalence, incidence, and risk factors. *J Clin Psychopharmacol* 1988; **8**:52s–56s.

3. De Leon J. The effect of atypical versus typical antipsychotics on tardive dyskinesia: a naturalistic study. *Eur Arch Psychiatry Clin Neurosci* 2007; **257**:169–172.

4. Halliday J, et al. Nithsdale Schizophrenia Surveys 23: movement disorders. 20-year review. *Br J Psychiatry* 2002; **181**:422–427.

5. Kane JM. Tardive dyskinesia circa 2006. *Am J Psychiatry* 2006; **163**:1316–1318.

6. Eberhard J, et al. Tardive dyskinesia and antipsychotics: a 5-year longitudinal study of frequency, correlates and course. *Int Clin Psychopharmacol* 2006; **21**:35–42.

7. Wu JQ, et al. Tardive dyskinesia is associated with greater cognitive impairment in schizophrenia. *Prog Neuropsychopharmacol Biol Psychiatry* 2013; **46**:71–77.

8. Ricciardi L, et al. Treatment recommendations for tardive dyskinesia. *Can J Psychiatry* 2019; **64**:388–399.

9. Strassnig M, et al. Tardive dyskinesia: motor system impairments, cognition and everyday functioning. *CNS Spectr* 2018; **23**:370–377.

10. Yuen O, et al. Tardive dyskinesia and positive and negative symptoms of schizophrenia. A study using instrumental measures. *Br J Psychiatry* 1996; **168**:702–708.

11. Ascher-Svanum H, et al. Tardive dyskinesia and the 3-year course of schizophrenia: results from a large, prospective, naturalistic study. *J Clin Psychiatry* 2008; **69**:1580–1588.

12. Dean CE, et al. Mortality and tardive dyskinesia: long-term study using the US National Death Index. *Br J Psychiatry* 2009; **194**:360–364.

13. Chong SA, et al. Mortality rates among patients with schizophrenia and tardive dyskinesia. *J Clin Psychopharmacol* 2009; **29**:5–8.

14. Beasley C, et al. Randomised double-blind comparison of the incidence of tardive dyskinesia in patients with schizophrenia during long-term treatment with olanzapine or haloperidol. *Br J Psychiatry* 1999; **174**:23–30.

15. Glazer WM. Expected incidence of tardive dyskinesia associated with atypical antipsychotics. *J Clin Psychiatry* 2000; **61 Suppl** 4:21–26.

16. Correll CU, et al. Lower risk for tardive dyskinesia associated with second-generation antipsychotics: a systematic review of 1-year studies. *Am J Psychiatry* 2004; **161**:414–425.

17. Dolder CR, et al. Incidence of tardive dyskinesia with typical versus atypical antipsychotics in very high risk patients. *Biol Psychiatry* 2003; **53**:1142–1145.

18. Correll CU, et al. Tardive dyskinesia and new antipsychotics. *Curr Opin Psychiatry* 2008; **21**:151–156.

19. Carbon M, et al. Tardive dyskinesia prevalence in the period of second-generation antipsychotic use: a meta-analysis. *J Clin Psychiatry* 2017; **78**:e264–e278.

20. Keck ME, et al. Ziprasidone-related tardive dyskinesia (Letter). *Am J Psychiatry* 2004; **161**:175–176.

21. Maytal G, et al. Aripiprazole-related tardive dyskinesia. *CNS Spectr* 2006; **11**:435–439.

22. Fountoulakis KN, et al. Amisulpride-induced tardive dyskinesia. *Schizophr Res* 2006; **88**:232–234.

23. Sachdev P. Early extrapyramidal side-effects as risk factors for later tardive dyskinesia: a prospective study. *Aust N Z J Psychiatry* 2004;

38:445–449.

24. Carbon M, et al. Tardive dyskinesia risk with first- and second-generation antipsychotics in comparative randomized controlled trials: a meta-analysis. *World Psychiatry* 2018; **17**:330–340.

25. Yoshida K, et al. Tardive dyskinesia in relation to estimated dopamine D2 receptor occupancy in patients with schizophrenia: analysis of the CATIE data. *Schizophr Res* 2014; **153**:184–188.

26. Saucedo Uribe E, et al. Preliminary efficacy and tolerability profiles of first versus second-generation long-acting injectable antipsychotics in schizophrenia: a systematic review and meta-analysis. *J Psychiatr Res* 2020; **129**:222–233.

27. Oosthuizen PP, et al. Incidence of tardive dyskinesia in first-episode psychosis patients treated with low-dose haloperidol. *J Clin Psychiatry* 2003; **64**:1075–1080.

28. Kenney C, et al. Metoclopramide, an increasingly recognized cause of tardive dyskinesia. *J Clin Pharmacol* 2008; **48**:379–384.

29. Pappa S, et al. Spontaneous movement disorders in antipsychotic-naive patients with first-episode psychoses: a systematic review. *Psychol Med* 2009; **39**:1065–1076.

30. Puri BK, et al. Spontaneous dyskinesia in first episode schizophrenia. *J Neurol Neurosurg Psychiatry* 1999; **66**:76–78.

31. McCreadie RG, et al. Spontaneous dyskinesia and parkinsonism in never-medicated, chronically ill patients with schizophrenia: 18-month follow-up. *Br J Psychiatry* 2002; **181**:135–137.

32. Duncan D, et al. Tardive dyskinesia: how is it prevented and treated? *Psychiatric Bull* 1997; **21**:422–425.

33. Simpson GM. The treatment of tardive dyskinesia and tardive dystonia. *J Clin Psychiatry* 2000; **61 Suppl 4**:39–44.

34. Bergman H, et al. Antipsychotic reduction and/or cessation and antipsychotics as specific treatments for tardive dyskinesia. *Cochrane Database Syst Rev* 2018; **2**:Cd000459.

35. Bergman H, et al. Anticholinergic medication for antipsychotic-induced tardive dyskinesia. *Cochrane Database Syst Rev* 2018; **1**:Cd000204.

36. Bhidayasiri R, et al. Evidence-based guideline: treatment of tardive syndromes: report of the Guideline Development Subcommittee of the American Academy of Neurology. *Neurology* 2013; **81**:463–469.

37. Pardis P, et al. Clozapine and tardive dyskinesia in patients with schizophrenia: a systematic review. *J Psychopharmacology* 2019; **33**:1187–1198.

38. Vesely C, et al. Remission of severe tardive dyskinesia in a schizophrenic patient treated with the atypical antipsychotic substance quetiapine. *Int Clin Psychopharmacol* 2000; **15**:57–60.

39. Alptekin K, et al. Quetiapine-induced improvement of tardive dyskinesia in three patients with schizophrenia. *Int Clin Psychopharmacol* 2002; **17**:263–264.

40. Nelson MW, et al. Adjunctive quetiapine decreases symptoms of tardive dyskinesia in a patient taking risperidone. *Clin Neuropharmacol* 2003; **26**:297–298.

41. Emsley R, et al. A single-blind, randomized trial comparing quetiapine and haloperidol in the treatment of tardive dyskinesia. *J Clin Psychiatry* 2004; **65**:696–701.

42. Bressan RA, et al. Atypical antipsychotic drugs and tardive dyskinesia: relevance of D2 receptor affinity. *J Psychopharmacology* 2004; **18**:124–127.

43. Sacchetti E, et al. Quetiapine, clozapine, and olanzapine in the treatment of tardive dyskinesia induced by first-generation antipsychotics: a 124-week case report. *Int Clin Psychopharmacol* 2003; **18**:357–359.

44. Gourzis P, et al. Quetiapine in the treatment of focal tardive dystonia induced by other atypical antipsychotics: a report of 2 cases. *Clin Neuropharmacol* 2005; **28**:195–196.

45. Soutullo CA, et al. Olanzapine in the treatment of tardive dyskinesia: a report of two cases. *J Clin Psychopharmacol* 1999; **19**:100–101.

46. Kinon BJ, et al. Olanzapine treatment for tardive dyskinesia in schizophrenia patients: a prospective clinical trial with patients randomized to blinded dose reduction periods. *Prog Neuropsychopharmacol Biol Psychiatry* 2004; **28**:985–996.

47. Chan CH, et al. Switching antipsychotic treatment to aripiprazole in psychotic patients with neuroleptic-induced tardive dyskinesia: a 24-week follow-up study. *Int Clin Psychopharmacol* 2018; **33**:155–162.

48. Bai YM, et al. Risperidone for severe tardive dyskinesia: a 12-week randomized, double-blind, placebo-controlled study. *J Clin Psychiatry* 2003; **64**:1342–1348.

49. Artukoglu BB, et al. Pharmacologic treatment of tardive dyskinesia: a meta-analysis and systematic review. *J Clin Psychiatry* 2020; **81**:19r12798.

50. Angus S, et al. A controlled trial of amantadine hydrochloride and neuroleptics in the treatment of tardive dyskinesia. *J Clin Psychopharmacol* 1997; **17**:88–91.

51. Pappa S, et al. Effects of amantadine on tardive dyskinesia: a randomized, double-blind, placebo-controlled study. *Clin Neuropharmacol* 2010; **33**:271–275.

52. Bhidayasiri R, et al. Updating the recommendations for treatment of tardive syndromes: a systematic review of new evidence and practical treatment algorithm. *J Neurol Sci* 2018; **389**:67–75.

53. Bergman H, et al. Benzodiazepines for antipsychotic-induced tardive dyskinesia. *Cochrane Database Syst Rev* 2018; **1**:Cd000205.

54. Rana AQ, et al. New and emerging treatments for symptomatic tardive dyskinesia. *Drug Des Devel Ther* 2013; **7**:1329–1340.

55. Cummings MA, et al. Deuterium tetrabenazine for tardive dyskinesia. *Clin Schizophr Relat Psychoses* 2018; **11**:214–220.

56. Solmi M, et al. Treatment of tardive dyskinesia with VMAT-2 inhibitors: a systematic review and meta-analysis of randomized controlled trials. *Drug Des Devel Ther* 2018; **12**:1215–1238.

57. Claassen DO, et al. Deutetrabenazine for tardive dyskinesia and chorea associated with Huntington's disease: a review of clinical trial data. *Exp Opin Pharmacother* 2019; **20**:2209–2221.

58. Citrome L. Deutetrabenazine for tardive dyskinesia: a systematic review of the efficacy and safety profile for this newly approved novel medication – what is the number needed to treat, number needed to harm and likelihood to be helped or harmed? *Int J Clin Pract* 2017;

71:e13030.

59. Zhang WF, et al. Extract of Ginkgo biloba treatment for tardive dyskinesia in schizophrenia: a randomized, double-blind, placebo-controlled trial. *J Clin Psychiatry* 2011; **72:**615–621.

60. Soares-Weiser K, et al. Miscellaneous treatments for antipsychotic-induced tardive dyskinesia. *Cochrane Database Syst Rev* 2018; 3:Cd000208.

61. Zheng W, et al. Extract of Ginkgo biloba for tardive dyskinesia: meta-analysis of randomized controlled trials. *Pharmacopsychiatry* 2016; **49:**107–111.

62. Lerner V, et al. Vitamin B(6) in the treatment of tardive dyskinesia: a double-blind, placebo-controlled, crossover study. *Am J Psychiatry* 2001; **158:**1511–1514.

63. Adelufosi AO, et al. Pyridoxal 5 phosphate for neuroleptic-induced tardive dyskinesia. *Cochrane Database Syst Rev* 2015.

64. Jankovic J, et al. Long-term effects of tetrabenazine in hyperkinetic movement disorders. *Neurology* 1997; **48:**358–362.

65. Leung JG, et al. Tetrabenazine for the treatment of tardive dyskinesia. *Ann Pharmacother* 2011; **45:**525–531.

66. Kenney C, et al. Long-term tolerability of tetrabenazine in the treatment of hyperkinetic movement disorders. *Mov Disord* 2007; **22:**193–197.

67. Hauser RA, et al. KINECT 3: a phase 3 randomized, double-blind, placebo-controlled trial of valbenazine for tardive dyskinesia. *Am J Psychiatry* 2017; **174:**476–484.

68. Kane JM, et al. Efficacy of valbenazine (NBI-98854) in treating subjects with tardive dyskinesia and schizophrenia or schizoaffective disorder. *Psychopharmacol Bull* 2017; **47:**69–76.

69. Josiassen RC, et al. Long-term safety and tolerability of valbenazine (NBI-98854) in subjects with tardive dyskinesia and a diagnosis of schizophrenia or mood disorder. *Psychopharmacol Bull* 2017; **47:**61–68.

70. Lindenmayer JP, et al. A long-term, open-label study of valbenazine for tardive dyskinesia. *CNS Spectr* 2020: [Epub ahead of print].

71. Citrome LL. Medication Options and Clinical Strategies for Treating Tardive Dyskinesia. *J Clin Psychiatry* 2020; **81:**TV18059BR18052C.

72. Zhang XY, et al. The effect of vitamin E treatment on tardive dyskinesia and blood superoxide dismutase: a double-blind placebo-controlled trial. *J Clin Psychopharmacol* 2004; **24:**83–86.

73. Soares-Weiser K, et al. Vitamin E for antipsychotic-induced tardive dyskinesia. *Cochrane Database Syst Rev* 2018; 1:Cd000209.

74. Richardson MA, et al. Efficacy of the branched-chain amino acids in the treatment of tardive dyskinesia in men. *Am J Psychiatry* 2003; **160:**1117–1124.

75. Tarsy D, et al. An open-label study of botulinum toxin A for treatment of tardive dystonia. *Clin Neuropharmacol* 1997; **20:**90–93.

76. Brashear A, et al. Comparison of treatment of tardive dystonia and idiopathic cervical dystonia with botulinum toxin type A. *Mov Disord* 1998; **13:**158–161.

77. Hennings JM, et al. Successful treatment of tardive lingual dystonia with botulinum toxin: case report and review of the literature. *Prog Neuropsychopharmacol Biol Psychiatry* 2008; **32:**1167–1171.

78. Beckmann YY, et al. Treatment of intractable tardive lingual dyskinesia with botulinum toxin. *J Clin Psychopharmacol* 2011; **31:**250–251.

79. Essali A, et al. Calcium channel blockers for neuroleptic-induced tardive dyskinesia. *Cochrane Database Syst Rev* 2011; Cd000206.

80. Essali A, et al. Calcium channel blockers for antipsychotic-induced tardive dyskinesia. *Cochrane Database Syst Rev* 2018; 3:Cd000206.

81. Caroff SN, et al. Treatment of tardive dyskinesia with donepezil. *J Clin Psychiatry* 2001; **62:**128–129.

82. Bergman J, et al. Beneficial effect of donepezil in the treatment of elderly patients with tardive movement disorders. *J Clin Psychiatry* 2005; **66:**107–110.

83. Ogunmefun A, et al. Effect of donepezil on tardive dyskinesia. *J Clin Psychopharmacol* 2009; **29:**102–104.

84. Tammenmaa-Aho I, et al. Cholinergic medication for antipsychotic-induced tardive dyskinesia. *Cochrane Database Syst Rev* 2018; 3:Cd000207.

85. Emsley R, et al. The effects of eicosapentaenoic acid in tardive dyskinesia: a randomized, placebo-controlled trial. *Schizophr Res* 2006; **84:**112–120.

86. Vaddadi K, et al. Tardive dyskinesia and essential fatty acids. *Int Rev Psychiatry* 2006; **18:**133–143.

87. Albayrak Y, et al. Beneficial effects of sigma-1 agonist fluvoxamine for tardive dyskinesia and tardive akathisia in patients with schizophrenia: report of three cases. *Psychiatry Investig* 2013; **10:**417–420.

88. Hardoy MC, et al. Gabapentin in antipsychotic-induced tardive dyskinesia: results of 1-year follow-up. *J Affect Disord* 2003; **75:**125–130.

89. Alabed S, et al. Gamma-aminobutyric acid agonists for antipsychotic-induced tardive dyskinesia. *Cochrane Database Syst Rev* 2018; 4:Cd000203.

90. McGavin CL, et al. Levetiracetam as a treatment for tardive dyskinesia: a case report. *Neurology* 2003; **61:**419.

91. Meco G, et al. Levetiracetam in tardive dyskinesia. *Clin Neuropharmacol* 2006; **29:**265–268.

92. Woods SW, et al. Effects of levetiracetam on tardive dyskinesia: a randomized, double-blind, placebo-controlled study. *J Clin Psychiatry* 2008; **69:**546–554.

93. Chen PH, et al. Rapid improvement of neuroleptic-induced tardive dyskinesia with levetiracetam in an interictal psychotic patient. *J Clin Psychopharmacol* 2010; **30:**205–207.

94. Shamir E, et al. Melatonin treatment for tardive dyskinesia: a double-blind, placebo-controlled, crossover study. *Arch Gen Psychiatry* 2001; **58:**1049–1052.

95. Sun CH, et al. Adjunctive melatonin for tardive dyskinesia in patients with schizophrenia: a meta-analysis. *Shanghai Arch Psychiatry* 2017; **29:**129–136.

96. Lai IC, et al. Analysis of genetic variations in the human melatonin receptor (MTNR1A, MTNR1B) genes and antipsychotics-induced tardive dyskinesia in schizophrenia. *World J Biol Psychiatry* 2011; **12:**143–148.

97. Wonodi I, et al. Naltrexone treatment of tardive dyskinesia in patients with schizophrenia. *J Clin Psychopharmacol* 2004; **24**:441–445.

98. Sirota P, et al. Use of the selective serotonin 3 receptor antagonist ondansetron in the treatment of neuroleptic-induced tardive dyskinesia. *Am J Psychiatry* 2000; **157**:287–289.

99. Naidu PS, et al. Reversal of neuroleptic-induced orofacial dyskinesia by 5-HT3 receptor antagonists. *Eur J Pharmacol* 2001; **420**:113–117.

100. Perenyi A, et al. Propranolol in the treatment of tardive dyskinesia. *Biol Psychiatry* 1983; **18**:391–394.

101. Pitts FN, Jr. Treatment of tardive dyskinesia with propranolol. *J Clin Psychiatry* 1982; **43**:304.

102. Hatcher-Martin JM, et al. Propranolol therapy for Tardive dyskinesia: a retrospective examination. *Parkinsonism Relat Disord* 2016; **32**:124–126.

103. Naidu PS, et al. Reversal of haloperidol-induced orofacial dyskinesia by quercetin, a bioflavonoid. *Psychopharmacology* 2003; **167**:418–423.

104. Naidu PS, et al. Quercetin, a bioflavonoid, attenuates haloperidol-induced orofacial dyskinesia. *Neuropharmacology* 2003; **44**:1100–1106.

105. Naidu PS, et al. Reversal of reserpine-induced orofacial dyskinesia and cognitive dysfunction by quercetin. *Pharmacology* 2004; **70**:59–67.

106. Berner JE. A case of sodium oxybate treatment of tardive dyskinesia and bipolar disorder. *J Clin Psychiatry* 2008; **69**:862.

107. Khedr EM, et al. Repetitive transcranial magnetic stimulation for treatment of tardive syndromes: double randomized clinical trial. *J Neur Trans* 2019; **126**:183–191.

108. Brambilla P, et al. Transient improvement of tardive dyskinesia induced with rTMS. *Neurology* 2003; **61**:1155.

109. Waln O, et al. Zolpidem improves tardive dyskinesia and akathisia. *Mov Disord* 2013; **28**:1748–1749.

抗精神病药所致体重增加

体重增加是抗精神病药常见的不良反应,也是心肌代谢性疾病的危险因素[1]。其发生机制尚不清楚[2],一般认为相关病理机制包括 5-HT_{2C} 受体拮抗、H_1 受体拮抗、D_2 受体拮抗和血清瘦素增高(导致瘦素脱敏化)[3-5]。尚无证据表明抗精神病药直接影响代谢功能:体重增加似乎与食物摄入增多,以及一些情况下能量消耗减少有关[6,7]。体重增加的风险与临床疗效相关[8,9](虽然这种相关性可能太小而难以显示临床意义[10]),这可能存在遗传学基础[11]。体重增加在未曾用药患者和治疗的早期阶段更为明显[12-14],女性的风险大于男性[15,16]。

几乎所有临床上使用的抗精神病药都与体重增加有关[12],但不同抗精神病药之间体重增加程度存在很大的差异。用药的患者间也存在明显的个体差异,一部分体重下降,一部分体重不变,一部分体重明显增加。因此,群体研究所得体重增加的平均值可能并非预测患者个体体重增加情况的有用指标。对不同抗精神病药所致体重增加的相对风险的评估大多来自短期临床试验。尽管有以上不足,直接和间接荟萃分析结果表明,根据体重增加的相对风险,这些药物可以被分为三类[17](表 1.17)。

表 1.17 抗精神病药所致体重增加[18-25]

药物	体重增加风险/程度	药物	体重增加风险/程度
氯氮平	高	氨磺必利	低
奥氮平		阿塞那平	
氯丙嗪	中等	布瑞哌唑	
伊潘立酮		阿立哌唑	
舍吲哚		卡利拉嗪	
喹硫平		氟哌啶醇	
利培酮		卢美哌隆	
帕利哌酮		鲁拉西酮	
		舒必利	
		三氟拉嗪	
		齐拉西酮	

如何治疗抗精神病药所致体重增加,参见下一节。

参考文献

1. Barton BB, et al. Update on weight-gain caused by antipsychotics: a systematic review and meta-analysis. *Exp Opin Drug Saf* 2020; **19**:295–314.

2. Correll CU, et al. Antipsychotic drugs and obesity. *Trends Mol Med* 2011; 17:97–107.

3. Nielsen MO, et al. Striatal reward activity and antipsychotic-associated weight change in patients with schizophrenia undergoing initial treatment. *JAMA Psychiatry* 2016; 73:121–128.

4. Ragguett RM, et al. Association between antipsychotic treatment and leptin levels across multiple psychiatric populations: an updated meta-analysis. *Human Psychopharmacology* 2017; 32:e2631.

5. Reynolds GP, et al. Mechanisms underlying metabolic disturbances associated with psychosis and antipsychotic drug treatment. *J*

Psychopharmacology 2017; 269881117722987.

6. Benarroch L, et al. Atypical antipsychotics and effects on feeding: from mice to men. *Psychopharmacology* 2016; 233:2629–2653.

7. Cuerda C, et al. The effects of second-generation antipsychotics on food intake, resting energy expenditure and physical activity. *Eur J Clin Nutr* 2014; 68:146–152.

8. Sharma E, et al. Association between antipsychotic-induced metabolic side-effects and clinical improvement: a review on the Evidence for 'metabolic threshold'. *Asian J Psychiatr* 2014; 8:12–21.

9. Garcia-Rizo C. Antipsychotic-induced weight gain and clinical improvement: a psychiatric paradox. *Frontiers in Psychiatry* 2020; 11:560006.

10. Hermes E, et al. The association between weight change and symptom reduction in the CATIE schizophrenia trial. *Schizophr Res* 2011; 128:166–170.

11. Zhang JP, et al. Pharmacogenetic associations of antipsychotic drug-related weight gain: a systematic review and meta-analysis. *Schizophr Bull* 2016; 42:1418–1437.

12. Bak M, et al. Almost all antipsychotics result in weight gain: a meta-analysis. *PLoS One* 2014; 9:e94112.

13. McEvoy JP, et al. Efficacy and tolerability of olanzapine, quetiapine, and risperidone in the treatment of early psychosis: a randomized, double-blind 52-week comparison. *Am J Psychiatry* 2007; 164:1050–1060.

14. Foley DL, et al. Cardiometabolic risk indicators that distinguish adults with psychosis from the general population, by age and gender. *PLoS One* 2013; 8:e82606.

15. Seeman MV. Secondary effects of antipsychotics: women at greater risk than men. *Schizophr Bull* 2009; 35:937–948.

16. Santini I, et al. The metabolic syndrome in an Italian psychiatric sample: a retrospective chart review of inpatients treated with antipsychotics. *Riv Psichiatr* 2016; 51:37–42.

17. Cooper SJ, et al. BAP guidelines on the management of weight gain, metabolic disturbances and cardiovascular risk associated with psychosis and antipsychotic drug treatment. *J Psychopharmacology* 2016; 30:717–748.

18. Rummel-Kluge C, et al. Head-to-head comparisons of metabolic side effects of second generation antipsychotics in the treatment of schizophrenia: a systematic review and meta-analysis. *Schizophr Res* 2010; 123:225–233.

19. Leucht S, et al. Comparative efficacy and tolerability of 15 antipsychotic drugs in schizophrenia: a multiple-treatments meta-analysis. *Lancet* 2013; 382:951–962.

20. Cutler AJ, et al. Long-term safety and tolerability of iloperidone: results from a 25-week, open-label extension trial. *CNSSpectr* 2013; 18:43–54.

21. McEvoy JP, et al. Effectiveness of paliperidone palmitate vs haloperidol decanoate for maintenance treatment of schizophrenia: a randomized clinical trial. *JAMA* 2014; 311:1978–1987.

22. Lao KS, et al. Tolerability and safety profile of cariprazine in treating psychotic disorders, bipolar disorder and major depressive disorder: a systematic review with meta-analysis of randomized controlled trials. *CNS Drugs* 2016; 30:1043–1054.

23. Leucht S, et al. Sixty years of placebo-controlled antipsychotic drug trials in acute schizophrenia: systematic review, Bayesian meta-analysis, and meta-regression of efficacy predictors. *Am J Psychiatry* 2017; 174:927–942.

24. Garay RP, et al. Therapeutic improvements expected in the near future for schizophrenia and schizoaffective disorder: an appraisal of phase III clinical trials of schizophrenia-targeted therapies as found in US and EU clinical trial registries. *Exp Opin Pharmacother* 2016; 17:921–936.

25. Musil R, et al. Weight gain and antipsychotics: a drug safety review. *Exp Opin Drug Saf* 2015; 14:73–96.

抗精神病药所致体重增加的治疗

体重增加是几乎所有抗精神病药的重要不良反应,其突出后果包括患者形象受损、共病躯体疾病和病死率升高。因此,其预防和治疗成为临床实践中的迫切问题。

监测

患者在开始接受抗精神病药治疗或换药时,至少应该称量和记录体重,理想情况下应记录体重指数(BMI)和腰围[1,2]。在接受治疗后至少前 6 个月内,推荐每 1~2 周监测一次体重[2,3]。治疗早期体重显著增加(如治疗 1 个月后比基线增加 5%)强烈预示体重增加会长期持续,应当考虑相应的预防和治疗措施[4-6]。持续使用抗精神病药者,建议至少每年监测体重[2,3,7]。

临床实践中,对持续用药患者的体重和其他代谢不良反应,其监测往往是不一致且有限的,达不到推荐的最佳方案[8-13]。

治疗和预防

大多数相关资料都集中在如何逆转抗精神病药相关的体重增加问题,但目前可为临床所用的资料则提示,早期干预可能阻止或减少体重增加[14-15]。

患者体重增加时,医师的选择包括换药或制定行为训练项目(或两者同时选择)。换药总是会带来复发或治疗中断的风险[16],但目前已有充分证据支持将原用药物换为阿立哌唑[17,18]、齐拉西酮[19-21]或鲁拉西酮[22,23]时,对逆转体重增加具有明确的疗效。将原用药物换为其他对体重影响较小的抗精神病药也是有益的[2,24,25]。还有一种选择是在原有抗精神病药的基础上加用阿立哌唑,已经发现这种联合治疗在氯氮平和奥氮平治疗患者中减轻了体重[15,26]。

完全停用抗精神病药会逆转体重增加[27,28],但对于大多数多次发作的精神分裂症患者,这种做法并不明智。应该注意到,一些换药和增效治疗策略可减少体重的进一步增加,或者促进体重减轻,但总体的作用有限,许多患者仍会继续超重。如果体重指数要保持或接近正常范围,往往需要增加生活方式干预。

许多生活方式干预措施已经被提出,对其评估都得到了较好的效果[2,14,29-32]。干预措施各不相同,但大多是旨在改善饮食和增加体力活动的"行为生活方式方案"。随机对照试验的荟萃分析显示,这些非药物手段对抗精神病药所致体重增加的预防和干预都有很好的效果。

只有当行为训练或换用对体重增加影响较小的药物失败,或肥胖已经对患者构成明显且迫切的躯体风险时,才考虑药物干预。表 1.18 列出了治疗抗精神病药所致体重增加的可选药物(按英文字母顺序排列)。先前版本中推荐的一些治疗方法(如 H_2 拮抗剂)已从该表中删除,因为临床证据不再支持其使用。

在预防和治疗抗精神病药所致的体重增加方面,二甲双胍是目前可以考虑选用的药物,尽管 GLP-1 激动剂可能最终被证明更有效且具有更好的耐受性。减重手术可能在少数其他干预措施无效的罕见、严重病例中发挥作用[33],然而,其疗效尚不清楚[2]。

表 1.18 抗精神病药所致体重增加的药物治疗(按英文字母顺序排列)

药物	评论
金刚烷胺 [34,35]（100~300mg/d）	可减轻奥氮平相关的体重增加。除失眠和腹部不适外,耐受性良好。可能(至少理论上)会加重精神病性症状。疗效证据弱,不推荐 [2]
α-硫辛酸 [36-38]（1 200mg/d）	可能会导致小幅度的、短期的体重下降。治疗抗精神病药所致体重增加的数据有限。不推荐
加用阿立哌唑 [15,13,39]（5~15mg/d）	随机对照试验结果显示,在使用氯氮平或奥氮平的基础上加用阿立哌唑,对减重和其他代谢指标有正面作用。辅助性治疗似乎是安全的且不会加重精神病。推荐氯氮平或奥氮平导致体重增加时合用,其他抗精神病药导致体重增加时不推荐
倍他司汀 [40,41]（48mg/d）	可能减轻奥氮平所致体重增加。研究数据有限。不推荐
安非他酮 [42,43]	当与控制饮食热量相结合时,似乎对肥胖有效。似乎不会加重精神病性症状,至少用于戒烟时如此 [44]。但对药物所致体重增加的疗效研究少。不推荐
安非他酮+纳曲酮合剂 [45]	已被 FDA 批准作为饮食和锻炼控制体重的补充。没有药物所致体重增加的研究数据。不推荐,但不应被排除
氟伏沙明 [46-48]（50mg/d）	早期的研究数据相互矛盾,但一项短期随机对照试验显示氟伏沙明减少了氯氮平所致体重增加(可能与氯氮平/去甲氯氮平比值升高有关)。联合用药显著增加氯氮平血药浓度,需要极其谨慎。证据基础太有限,不推荐
利拉鲁肽 [49,50]（3mg/d 皮下注射）	GLP-1 激动剂,早前被批准用于治疗 2 型糖尿病,近期被批准作为非糖尿病患者的抗肥胖剂。减重所用剂量(3mg/d)高于治疗糖尿病的剂量(<1.8mg)。药物所致体重增加的研究数据有限。一项随机对照试验显示,应用利拉鲁肽后,长期服用奥氮平或氯氮平导致超重的糖尿病前期患者体重明显减轻 [49]。对其他代谢指标有益处。耐受性良好,但会导致胃肠道功能紊乱。糖尿病前期/糖尿病患者和氯氮平所致体重增加推荐使用。其他 GLP-1 激动剂目前只被批准用于糖尿病,且剂量范围较小。艾塞那肽长效剂(每周 1 次的 GLP-1 激动剂)可能对氯氮平所致体重增加有效 [51],对其他抗精神病药所致体重增加无效 [52]
二甲双胍 [2,32,53,54]（500~2 000mg/d）	对非糖尿病患者的大量研究数据支持其减轻和逆转抗精神病药所致体重增加(主要是奥氮平)。对其他代谢指标也有益。有一些阴性结果,但几项荟萃分析均显示有明确而显著的效果。之后发表了在孤独症谱系障碍儿童青少年中进行的一项结果为阳性的随机对照试验 [55] 和扩展研究 [56]。最适合体重增加和糖尿病的患者,或者有多囊卵巢综合征的患者。注意:二甲双胍会增加维生素 B_{12} 缺乏的风险 [57]
褪黑素 [58-60]（不超过 5mg QN）	一项小型随机对照试验发现可以减少奥氮平引起的体重增加,其他研究为阴性结果。即使有作用也非常有限
甲基纤维素（1 500mg,饭前）	老药,相当难吃。在药物所致体重增加方面无任何资料,其使用曾经相当广泛。可作为容积性缓泻剂,因此可能适用于氯氮平所致体重增加
莫达非尼 [61,62]（不超过 300mg/d）	关于氯氮平所致体重增加,仅有少数阳性数据和一项阴性随机对照试验。不推荐
纳曲酮 [63-64]（25~50mg/d）	有一些阳性结果,但限于两个小型探索性随机对照试验。不推荐

第 1 章

续表

药物	评论
奥利司他 [65-70]（120mg，每天三次，饭前/饭后）	对肥胖有效，特别是与控制食物热量结合时。在药物所致体重增加方面几无研究资料，但却广泛地用于临床，且有部分获得成功。在治疗氯氮平或奥氮平所致体重增加的试验中，仅在男性受试者中有效 [69,70]。如果不限制食物热量，对精神疾病患者的作用非常有限。如果不执行低脂饮食，会引起脂肪泻，并可能导致口服药物吸收不良。总体而言，对氯氮平所致体重增加可能是好的选择，可同时减轻体重和便秘 [71]
瑞波西汀 [15]（4~8mg/d）	可减轻奥氮平所致体重增加。可逆转一些代谢指标的改变 [72]。与倍他司汀合用有效
托吡酯 [32,54,73,74]（不超过 300mg/d）	可减轻体重，即便是药物所致体重增加也有效。随机对照试验的荟萃分析表明，预防效果优于治疗效果。主要问题是托吡酯可引起镇静、意识模糊和认知损害。可能具有抗精神病作用
唑尼沙胺 [75]（100~600mg/d）	具有减轻体重作用的抗癫痫药。一项随机对照试验显示，150mg/d 可明显减轻服用第二代抗精神病药患者的体重。另一项随机对照试验（高达 600mg/d）显示，减少了奥氮平所致体重增加。镇静、腹泻和认知损害是最常见的问题。不推荐

参考文献

1. Marder SR, et al. Physical health monitoring of patients with schizophrenia. *Am J Psychiatry* 2004; 161:1334–1349.

2. Cooper SJ, et al. BAP guidelines on the management of weight gain, metabolic disturbances and cardiovascular risk associated with psychosis and antipsychotic drug treatment. *J Psychopharmacology* 2016; 30:717–748.

3. Galletly C, et al. Royal Australian and New Zealand College of Psychiatrists clinical practice guidelines for the management of schizophrenia and related disorders. *Aust N Z J Psychiatry* 2016; 50:410–472.

4. American Diabetes Association, et al. Consensus Development Conference on antipsychotic drugs and obesity and diabetes. *Diabetes Care* 2004; 27:596–601.

5. Vandenberghe F, et al. Importance of early weight changes to predict long-term weight gain during psychotropic drug treatment. *J Clin Psychiatry* 2015; 76:e1417–e1423.

6. Lipkovich I, et al. Early evaluation of patient risk for substantial weight gain during olanzapine treatment for schizophrenia, schizophreniform, or schizoaffective disorder. *BMC Psychiatry* 2008; 8:78.

7. National Institute for Clinical Excellence. Psychosis and schizophrenia in adults. Quality standard [QS80]. 2015; https://www.nice.org.uk/guidance/qs80.

8. Barnes TR, et al. Screening for the metabolic syndrome in community psychiatric patients prescribed antipsychotics: a quality improvement programme. *Acta Psychiatr Scand* 2008; 118:26–33.

9. Mitchell AJ, et al. Guideline concordant monitoring of metabolic risk in people treated with antipsychotic medication: systematic review and meta-analysis of screening practices. *Psychol Med* 2012; 42:125–147.

10. Barnes TR, et al. Screening for the metabolic side effects of antipsychotic medication: findings of a 6-year quality improvement programme in the UK. *BMJ Open* 2015; 5:e007633.

11. Crawford MJ, et al. Assessment and treatment of physical health problems among people with schizophrenia: national cross-sectional study. *Br J Psychiatry* 2014; 205:473–477.

12. Hammoudeh S, et al. Risk factors of metabolic syndrome among patients receiving antipsychotics: a retrospective study. *Community Ment Health J* 2020; 56:760–770.

13. Ward T, et al. Who is responsible for metabolic screening for mental health clients taking antipsychotic medications? *Int J Ment Health Nurs* 2018; 27:196–203.

14. Bruins J, et al. The effects of lifestyle interventions on (long-term) weight management, cardiometabolic risk and depressive symptoms in people with psychotic disorders: a meta-analysis. *PLoS One* 2014; 9:e112276.

15. Mizuno Y, et al. Pharmacological strategies to counteract antipsychotic-induced weight gain and metabolic adverse effects in schizophrenia: a systematic review and meta-analysis. *Schizophr Bull* 2014; 40:1385–1403.

16. Stroup TS, et al. A randomized trial examining the effectiveness of switching from olanzapine, quetiapine, or risperidone to aripiprazole to reduce metabolic risk: comparison of antipsychotics for metabolic problems (CAMP). *Am J Psychiatry* 2011; 168:947–956.

17. Mukundan A, et al. Antipsychotic switching for people with schizophrenia who have neuroleptic-induced weight or metabolic problems. *Cochrane Database Systematic Rev* 2010; CD006629.

18. Barak Y, et al. Switching to aripiprazole as a strategy for weight reduction: a meta-analysis in patients suffering from schizophrenia. *J Obes*

2011; **2011**:898013.

19. Weiden PJ, et al. Improvement in indices of health status in outpatients with schizophrenia switched to ziprasidone. *J Clin Psychopharmacol* 2003; **23**:595–600.

20. Montes JM, et al. Improvement in antipsychotic-related metabolic disturbances in patients with schizophrenia switched to ziprasidone. *Prog Neuropsychopharmacol Biol Psychiatry* 2007; **31**:383–388.

21. Karayal ON, et al. Switching from quetiapine to ziprasidone: a sixteen-week, open-label, multicenter study evaluating the effectiveness and safety of ziprasidone in outpatient subjects with schizophrenia or schizoaffective disorder. *J Psychiatr Pract* 2011; **17**:100–109.

22. McEvoy JP, et al. Effectiveness of lurasidone in patients with schizophrenia or schizoaffective disorder switched from other antipsychotics: a randomized, 6-week, open-label study. *J Clin Psychiatry* 2013; **74**:170–179.

23. Stahl SM, et al. Effectiveness of lurasidone for patients with schizophrenia following 6 weeks of acute treatment with lurasidone, olanzapine, or placebo: a 6-month, open-label, extension study. *J Clin Psychiatry* 2013; **74**:507–515.

24. Gupta S, et al. Weight decline in patients switching from olanzapine to quetiapine. *Schizophr Res* 2004; **70**:57–62.

25. Ried LD, et al. Weight change after an atypical antipsychotic switch. *Ann Pharmacother* 2003; **37**:1381–1386.

26. Galling B, et al. Antipsychotic augmentation vs. monotherapy in schizophrenia: systematic review, meta-analysis and meta-regression analysis. *World Psychiatry* 2017; **16**:77–89.

27. De Kuijper G, et al. Effects of controlled discontinuation of long-term used antipsychotics on weight and metabolic parameters in individuals with intellectual disability. *J Clin Psychopharmacol* 2013; **33**:520–524.

28. Chen EY, et al. Maintenance treatment with quetiapine versus discontinuation after one year of treatment in patients with remitted first episode psychosis: randomised controlled trial. *BMJ* 2010; **341**:c4024.

29. Werneke U, et al. Behavioural management of antipsychotic-induced weight gain: a review. *Acta Psychiatr Scand* 2003; **108**:252–259.

30. Caemmerer J, et al. Acute and maintenance effects of non-pharmacologic interventions for antipsychotic associated weight gain and metabolic abnormalities: a meta-analytic comparison of randomized controlled trials. *Schizophr Res* 2012; **140**:159–168.

31. Rice J, et al. Integrative management of metabolic syndrome in youth prescribed second-generation antipsychotics. *Med Sci* 2020; **8**:34.

32. Vancampfort D, et al. The impact of pharmacological and non-pharmacological interventions to improve physical health outcomes in people with schizophrenia: a meta-review of meta-analyses of randomized controlled trials. *World Psychiatry* 2019; **18**:53–66.

33. Manu P, et al. Weight gain and obesity in schizophrenia: epidemiology, pathobiology, and management. *Acta Psychiatr Scand* 2015; **132**:97–108.

34. Praharaj SK, et al. Amantadine for olanzapine-induced weight gain: a systematic review and meta-analysis of randomized placebo-controlled trials. *Ther Adv Psychopharmacol* 2012; **2**:151–156.

35. Zheng W, et al. Amantadine for antipsychotic-related weight gain: meta-analysis of randomized placebo-controlled trials. *J Clin Psychopharmacol* 2017; **37**:341–346.

36. Kucukgoncu S, et al. Alpha-lipoic acid (ALA) as a supplementation for weight loss: results from a meta-analysis of randomized controlled trials. *Obes Rev* 2017; **18**:594–601.

37. Kim E, et al. A preliminary investigation of alpha-lipoic acid treatment of antipsychotic drug-induced weight gain in patients with schizophrenia. *J Clin Psychopharmacol* 2008; **28**:138–146.

38. Ratliff JC, et al. An open-label pilot trial of alpha-lipoic acid for weight loss in patients with schizophrenia without diabetes. *Clin Schizophr Relat Psychoses* 2015; **8**:196–200.

39. Zheng W, et al. Efficacy and safety of adjunctive aripiprazole in schizophrenia: meta-analysis of randomized controlled trials. *J Clin Psychopharmacol* 2016; **36**:628–636.

40. Barak N, et al. A randomized, double-blind, placebo-controlled pilot study of betahistine to counteract olanzapine-associated weight gain. *J Clin Psychopharmacol* 2016; **36**:253–256.

41. Lian J, et al. Ameliorating antipsychotic-induced weight gain by betahistine: mechanisms and clinical implications. *Pharmacol Res* 2016; **106**:51–63.

42. Gadde KM, et al. Bupropion for weight loss: an investigation of efficacy and tolerability in overweight and obese women. *Obes Res* 2001; **9**:544–551.

43. Jain AK, et al. Bupropion SR vs. placebo for weight loss in obese patients with depressive symptoms. *Obes Res* 2002; **10**:1049–1056.

44. Tsoi DT, et al. Interventions for smoking cessation and reduction in individuals with schizophrenia. *Cochrane Database Syst Rev* 2013; **2**:CD007253.

45. Greig SL, et al. Naltrexone ER/Bupropion ER: a review in obesity management. *Drugs* 2015; **75**:1269–1280.

46. Hinze-Selch D, et al. Effect of coadministration of clozapine and fluvoxamine versus clozapine monotherapy on blood cell counts, plasma levels of cytokines and body weight. *Psychopharmacology* 2000; **149**:163–169.

47. Lu ML, et al. Effects of adjunctive fluvoxamine on metabolic parameters and psychopathology in clozapine-treated patients with schizophrenia: a 12-week, randomized, double-blind, placebo-controlled study. *Schizophr Res* 2018; **193**:126–133.

48. Lu ML, et al. Adjunctive fluvoxamine inhibits clozapine-related weight gain and metabolic disturbances. *J Clin Psychiatry* 2004; **65**:766–771.

49. Larsen JR, et al. Effect of liraglutide treatment on prediabetes and overweight or obesity in clozapine- or olanzapine-treated patients with schizophrenia spectrum disorder: a randomized clinical trial. *JAMA Psychiatry* 2017; **74**:719–728.

50. Mayfield K, et al. Glucagon-like peptide-1 agonists combating clozapine-associated obesity and diabetes. *J Psychopharmacology* 2016; **30**:227–236.

51. Siskind D, et al. Treatment of clozapine-associated obesity and diabetes with exenatide (CODEX) in adults with schizophrenia: a randomised controlled trial. *Diabetes, Obesity & Metabolism* 2017; **20**:1050–1055.

52. Ishoy PL, et al. Effect of GLP-1 receptor agonist treatment on body weight in obese antipsychotic-treated patients with schizophrenia: a

randomized, placebo-controlled trial. *Diabetes, Obesity & Metabolism* 2017; 19:162–171.

53. Zheng W, et al. Metformin for weight gain and metabolic abnormalities associated with antipsychotic treatment: meta-analysis of randomized placebo-controlled trials. *J Clin Psychopharmacol* 2015; 35:x499–x509.

54. Wang C, et al. Outcomes and safety of concomitant topiramate or metformin for antipsychotics-induced obesity: a randomized-controlled trial. *Ann General Psychiatry* 2020; 19:68.

55. Anagnostou E, et al. Metformin for treatment of overweight induced by atypical antipsychotic medication in young people with autism spectrum disorder: a randomized clinical trial. *JAMA Psychiatry* 2016; 73:928–937.

56. Handen BL, et al. A randomized, placebo-controlled trial of metformin for the treatment of overweight induced by antipsychotic medication in young people with autism spectrum disorder: open-label extension. *J Am Acad Child Adolesc Psychiatry* 2017; 56:849–856.e846.

57. Chapman LE, et al. Association between metformin and vitamin B12 deficiency in patients with type 2 diabetes: a systematic review and meta-analysis. *Diabetes Metab* 2016; 42:316–327.

58. Agahi M, et al. Effect of melatonin in reducing second-generation antipsychotic metabolic effects: a double blind controlled clinical trial. *Diabetes Metab Syndr* 2017; 12:9–15.

59. Wang HR, et al. The role of melatonin and melatonin agonists in counteracting antipsychotic-induced metabolic side effects: a systematic review. *Int Clin Psychopharmacol* 2016; 31:301–306.

60. Porfirio MC, et al. Can melatonin prevent or improve metabolic side effects during antipsychotic treatments? *Neuropsychiatr Dis Treat* 2017; 13:2167–2174.

61. Henderson DC, et al. Effects of modafinil on weight, glucose and lipid metabolism in clozapine-treated patients with schizophrenia. *Schizophr Res* 2011; 130:53–56.

62. Roerig JL, et al. An exploration of the effect of modafinil on olanzapine associated weight gain in normal human subjects. *Biol Psychiatry* 2009; 65:607–613.

63. Taveira TH, et al. The effect of naltrexone on body fat mass in olanzapine-treated schizophrenic or schizoaffective patients: a randomized double-blind placebo-controlled pilot study. *J Psychopharmacology* 2014; 28:395–400.

64. Tek C, et al. A randomized, double-blind, placebo-controlled pilot study of naltrexone to counteract antipsychotic-associated weight gain: proof of concept. *J Clin Psychopharmacol* 2014; 34:608–612.

65. Sjostrom L, et al. Randomised placebo-controlled trial of orlistat for weight loss and prevention of weight regain in obese patients. European Multicentre Orlistat Study Group. *Lancet* 1998; 352:167–172.

66. Hilger E, et al. The effect of orlistat on plasma levels of psychotropic drugs in patients with long-term psychopharmacotherapy. *J Clin Psychopharmacol* 2002; 22:68–70.

67. Pavlovic ZM. Orlistat in the treatment of clozapine-induced hyperglycemia and weight gain. *Eur Psychiatry* 2005; 20:520.

68. Carpenter LL, et al. A case series describing orlistat use in patients on psychotropic medications. *Med Health R I* 2004; 87:375–377.

69. Joffe G, et al. Orlistat in clozapine- or olanzapine-treated patients with overweight or obesity: a 16-week randomized, double-blind, placebo-controlled trial. *J Clin Psychiatry* 2008; 69:706–711.

70. Tchoukhine E, et al. Orlistat in clozapine- or olanzapine-treated patients with overweight or obesity: a 16-week open-label extension phase and both phases of a randomized controlled trial. *J Clin Psychiatry* 2011; 72:326–330.

71. Chukhin E, et al. In a randomized placebo-controlled add-on study orlistat significantly reduced clozapine-induced constipation. *IntClinPsychopharmacol* 2013; 28:67–70.

72. Amrami-Weizman A, et al. The effect of reboxetine co-administration with olanzapine on metabolic and endocrine profile in schizophrenia patients. *Psychopharmacology* 2013; 230:23–27.

73. Correll CU, et al. Efficacy for psychopathology and body weight and safety of topiramate-antipsychotic cotreatment in patients with schizophrenia spectrum disorders: results from a meta-analysis of randomized controlled trials. *J Clin Psychiatry* 2016; 77:e746–e756.

74. Zheng W, et al. Efficacy and safety of adjunctive topiramate for schizophrenia: a meta-analysis of randomized controlled trials. *Acta Psychiatr Scand* 2016; 134:385–398.

75. Buoli M, et al. The use of zonisamide for the treatment of psychiatric disorders: a systematic review. *Clin Neuropharmacol* 2017; 40:85–92.

恶性综合征

　　恶性综合征(NMS)是一种急性体温调节和神经运动控制障碍。特点是在应用抗精神病药后出现肌肉强直、高热、意识改变和自主神经功能障碍,然而在临床表现上有相当大的异质性[1-4]。尽管普遍认为 NMS 是一种急性的、严重的综合征,但在许多病例里,NMS 很少表现出明显的症状和体征。因此,那些"症状丰富"的 NMS 被认为是非恶性症状的极端形式[5]。当然,血清肌酸激酶(CK)升高在无症状 NMS 患者中较为普遍[6]。

　　NMS 是一种罕见但潜在严重甚至致命的抗精神病药不良反应,由多巴胺能拮抗作用介导[1]。危险因素包括男性、脱水、疲惫和意识模糊/激越状态[4,7]。年轻成年男性似乎是高危人群,而对老年人群最有可能是致命的[4,8]。

　　NMS 的发生率和死亡率难以确定,随所用药物的不同和对 NMS 认识的加深而变化。一项药物安全性研究计划的数据显示,1993—2015 年,NMS 的总体发病率为 0.16%[9]。2004—2007 年相似研究报告的发生率为 0.11%[10]。使用高效价第一代抗精神病药的发生率最高,而第二代抗精神病药和低效价第一代抗精神病药发生率较低[3,9,11]。然而,大多数现有抗精神病药均被报道与该综合征有关[12-19],包括最近引入临床的第二代抗精神病药,如齐拉西酮[20,21]、伊潘立酮[22]、阿立哌唑[23-26]、帕利哌酮[27](包括棕榈酸帕利哌酮[28])、阿塞那平[29]和利培酮针剂[30]。使用第二代抗精神病药者中,NMS 死亡率可能较低[3,31-33],除了肌强直和发热较少见[3,32],其他临床表现与第一代抗精神病药相似[32]。在撰写本节时,尚未有资料显示 NMS 与匹莫范色林、卡利拉嗪、布瑞哌唑或卢美哌隆相关[34]。

　　NMS 有时也见于其他药物,如抗抑郁药[35-38]、丙戊酸盐[39,40]、苯妥英[41]和锂盐[42]。SSRI[43]或胆碱能抑制剂[44,45]联合抗精神病药可能会增加发生 NMS 的风险。由第二代抗精神病药和 SSRI 联用所致的 NMS,其症状和发病机制可能和 5-HT 综合征相似[46]。苯二氮䓬类药物是治疗 NMS 的推荐用药,但也有苯二氮䓬类药物和 NMS 相关的报道,可能是由于诊断而混淆,或可用苯二氮䓬类药物戒断的 NMS 样症状解释。[11,48,49]NMS 有时也见于使用非精神药物类多巴胺受体拮抗剂的患者,如甲氧氯普胺(表 1.19)[50]。

表 1.19　恶性综合征

症状和体征[9,51-53] (表现变异很大)[54]	发热、大汗、僵硬、意识模糊、意识波动 血压波动、心动过速 肌酸激酶升高、白细胞升高、肝功能改变
危险因素[8,11,48,52,53,55-57]	高效价第一代抗精神病药、最近加量或快速加量、快速减药、骤停抗胆碱能药、抗精神病药合用 精神病、脑器质性疾病、酒依赖、帕金森病、甲状腺功能亢进、精神运动兴奋、精神发育迟滞 男性、年轻 激越、脱水

续表

治疗 [9,52,58-60] （关于 NMS 的治疗各指南建议不同，且基于有限的证据 [47]）	**在精神科病房：** 停用抗精神病药，监测体温、脉搏、血压。 若还未用苯二氮䓬类药物，考虑使用——文献曾报告用过劳拉西泮肌内注射 [61] **在内科病房或急诊病房：** 输液，溴隐亭 + 丹曲林，苯二氮䓬类药物镇静，必要时人工通气 在众多药物中，左旋多巴、阿扑吗啡和卡马西平都曾用过。ECT 可能对 NMS 有效，即使药物治疗失败后 [62,63]
重新使用抗精神病药 [41,52,58,64]	在大多数情况下，需要重新使用抗精神病药，再次用药的风险是可接受的 停用抗精神病药至少 5 天，最好更久，使 NMS 的症状和体征完全缓解 从非常小的剂量开始，很缓慢地加量，严密监测体温、脉搏和血压。可以监测血清肌酸激酶，但对此存在争议 [53,65]。密切监测生理及生化指标，能有效地减少进展为典型 NMS 的风险 [66,67] 考虑使用的抗精神病药在结构上应该与以前导致 NMS 的药物不同，或使用多巴胺亲和力低的药物（喹硫平或氯氮平）。阿立哌唑也可考虑使用 [68]，但其血浆半衰期较长，可能增加患 NMS 的风险 [11] 避免使用（任何类型的）长效剂及高效价第一代抗精神病药

参考文献

1. Caroff SN, et al. Neuroleptic malignant syndrome. *Med Clin North Am* 1993; **77**:185–202.
2. Gurrera RJ, et al. Thermoregulatory dysfunction in neuroleptic malignant syndrome. *Biol Psychiatry* 1996; **39**:207–212.
3. Belvederi Murri M, et al. Second-generation antipsychotics and neuroleptic malignant syndrome: systematic review and case report analysis. *Drugs in R&D* 2015; **15**:45–62.
4. Ware MR, et al. Neuroleptic malignant syndrome: diagnosis and management. *Prim Care Companion CNS Disord* 2018; **20**.
5. Bristow MF, et al. How 'malignant' is the neuroleptic malignant syndrome? *BMJ* 1993; **307**:1223–1224.
6. Meltzer HY, et al. Marked elevations of serum creatine kinase activity associated with antipsychotic drug treatment. *Neuropsychopharmacology* 1996; **15**:395–405.
7. Keck PE, Jr., et al. Risk factors for neuroleptic malignant syndrome. A case-control study. *Arch Gen Psychiatry* 1989; **46**:914–918.
8. Gurrera RJ. A systematic review of sex and age factors in neuroleptic malignant syndrome diagnosis frequency. *Acta Psychiatr Scand* 2017; **135**:398–408.
9. Schneider M, et al. Neuroleptic malignant syndrome: evaluation of drug safety data from the AMSP program during 1993–2015. *Eur Arch Psychiatry Clin Neurosci* 2020; **270**:23–33.
10. Lao KSJ, et al. Antipsychotics and risk of neuroleptic malignant syndrome: a population-based cohort and case-crossover study. *CNS Drugs* 2020; **34**:1165–1175.
11. Su YP, et al. Retrospective chart review on exposure to psychotropic medications associated with neuroleptic malignant syndrome. *Acta Psychiatr Scand* 2014; **130**:52–60.
12. Sing KJ, et al. Neuroleptic malignant syndrome and quetiapine (Letter). *Am J Psychiatry* 2002; **159**:149–150.
13. Suh H, et al. Neuroleptic malignant syndrome and low-dose olanzapine (Letter). *Am J Psychiatry* 2003; **160**:796.
14. Gallarda T, et al. Neuroleptic malignant syndrome in an 72-year-old-man with Alzheimer's disease: a case report and review of the literature. *Eur Neuropsychopharmacol* 2000; **10 Suppl 3**:357.
15. Stanley AK, et al. Possible neuroleptic malignant syndrome with quetiapine. *Br J Psychiatry* 2000; **176**:497.
16. Sierra-Biddle D, et al. Neuropletic malignant syndrome and olanzapine. *J Clin Psychopharmacol* 2000; **20**:704–705.
17. Hasan S, et al. Novel antipsychotics and the neuroleptic malignant syndrome: a review and critique. *Am J Psychiatry* 1998; **155**:1113–1116.
18. Tsai JH, et al. Zotepine-induced catatonia as a precursor in the progression to neuroleptic malignant syndrome. *Pharmacotherapy* 2005; **25**:1156–1159.
19. Gortney JS, et al. Neuroleptic malignant syndrome secondary to quetiapine. *Ann Pharmacother* 2009; **43**:785–791.
20. Leibold J, et al. Neuroleptic malignant syndrome associated with ziprasidone in an adolescent. *Clin Ther* 2004; **26**:1105–1108.
21. Borovicka MC, et al. Ziprasidone- and lithium-induced neuroleptic malignant syndrome. *Ann Pharmacother* 2006; **40**:139–142.
22. Guanci N, et al. Atypical neuroleptic malignant syndrome associated with iloperidone administration. *Psychosomatics* 2012; **53**:603–605.

23. Spalding S, et al. Aripiprazole and atypical neuroleptic malignant syndrome. *J Am Acad Child Adolesc Psychiatry* 2004; **43**:1457–1458.

24. Chakraborty N, et al. Aripiprazole and neuroleptic malignant syndrome. *Int Clin Psychopharmacol* 2004; **19**:351–353.

25. Rodriguez OP, et al. A case report of neuroleptic malignant syndrome without fever in a patient given aripiprazole. *J Okla State Med Assoc* 2006; **99**:435–438.

26. Srephichit S, et al. Neuroleptic malignant syndrome and aripiprazole in an antipsychotic-naive patient. *J Clin Psychopharmacol* 2006; **26**:94–95.

27. Duggal HS. Possible neuroleptic malignant syndrome associated with paliperidone. *J Neuropsychiatry Clin Neurosci* 2007; **19**:477–478.

28. Langley-degroot M, et al. Atypical neuroleptic malignant syndrome associated with paliperidone long-acting injection: a case report. *J Clin Psychopharmacol* 2016; **36**:277–279.

29. Singh N, et al. Neuroleptic malignant syndrome after exposure to asenapine: a case report. *Prim Care Companion J Clin Psychiatry* 2010; **12**:e1.

30. Mall GD, et al. Catatonia and mild neuroleptic malignant syndrome after initiation of long-acting injectable risperidone: case report. *J Clin Psychopharmacol* 2008; **28**:572–573.

31. Ananth J, et al. Neuroleptic malignant syndrome and atypical antipsychotic drugs. *J Clin Psychiatry* 2004; **65**:464–470.

32. Trollor JN, et al. Comparison of neuroleptic malignant syndrome induced by first- and second-generation antipsychotics. *Br J Psychiatry* 2012; **201**:52–56.

33. Nakamura M, et al. Mortality of neuroleptic malignant syndrome induced by typical and atypical antipsychotic drugs: a propensity-matched analysis from the Japanese Diagnosis Procedure Combination database. *J Clin Psychiatry* 2012; **73**:427–430.

34. Orsolini L, et al. Up-to-date expert opinion on the safety of recently developed antipsychotics. *Exp Opin Drug Saf* 2020; **19**:981–998.

35. Kontaxakis VP, et al. Neuroleptic malignant syndrome after addition of paroxetine to olanzapine. *J Clin Psychopharmacol* 2003; **23**:671–672.

36. Young C. A case of neuroleptic malignant syndrome and serotonin disturbance. *J Clin Psychopharmacol* 1997; **17**:65–66.

37. June R, et al. Neuroleptic malignant syndrome associated with nortriptyline. *Am J Emerg Med* 1999; **17**:736–737.

38. Lu TC, et al. Neuroleptic malignant syndrome after the use of venlafaxine in a patient with generalized anxiety disorder. *J Formos Med Assoc* 2006; **105**:90–93.

39. Verma R, et al. An atypical case of neuroleptic malignant syndrome precipitated by valproate. *BMJ Case Rep* 2014; **2014**:bcr2013202578.

40. Menon V, et al. Atypical neuroleptic malignant syndrome in a young male precipitated by oral sodium valproate. *Aust N Z J Psychiatry* 2016; **50**:1208–1209.

41. Shin HW, et al. Neuroleptic malignant syndrome induced by phenytoin in a patient with drug-induced Parkinsonism. *Neurol Sci* 2014; **35**:1641–1643.

42. Gill J, et al. Acute lithium intoxication and neuroleptic malignant syndrome. *Pharmacotherapy* 2003; **23**:811–815.

43. Stevens DL. Association between selective serotonin-reuptake inhibitors, second-generation antipsychotics, and neuroleptic malignant syndrome. *Ann Pharmacother* 2008; **42**:1290–1297.

44. Stevens DL, et al. Olanzapine-associated neuroleptic malignant syndrome in a patient receiving concomitant rivastigmine therapy. *Pharmacotherapy* 2008; **28**:403–405.

45. Warwick TC, et al. Neuroleptic malignant syndrome variant in a patient receiving donepezil and olanzapine. *Nat Clin Pract Neurol* 2008; **4**:170–174.

46. Odagaki Y. Atypical neuroleptic malignant syndrome or serotonin toxicity associated with atypical antipsychotics? *Curr Drug Saf* 2009; **4**:84–93.

47. Schönfeldt-Lecuona C, et al. Treatment of the neuroleptic malignant syndrome in international therapy guidelines: a comparative analysis. *Pharmacopsychiatry* 2020; **53**:51–59.

48. Nielsen RE, et al. Neuroleptic malignant syndrome-an 11-year longitudinal case-control study. *Can J Psychiatry* 2012; **57**:512–518.

49. Kishimoto S, et al. Postoperative neuroleptic malignant syndrome-like symptoms improved with intravenous diazepam: a case report. *J Anesth* 2013; **27**:768–770.

50. Wittmann O, et al. Neuroleptic malignant syndrome associated with metoclopramide use in a boy: case report and review of the literature. *Am J Ther* 2016; **23**:e1246–e1249.

51. Gurrera RJ. Sympathoadrenal hyperactivity and the etiology of neuroleptic malignant syndrome. *Am J Psychiatry* 1999; **156**:169–180.

52. Levenson JL. Neuroleptic malignant syndrome. *Am J Psychiatry* 1985; **142**:1137–1145.

53. Hermesh H, et al. High serum creatinine kinase level: possible risk factor for neuroleptic malignant syndrome. *J Clin Psychopharmacol* 2002; **22**:252–256.

54. Picard LS, et al. Atypical neuroleptic malignant syndrome: diagnostic controversies and considerations. *Pharmacotherapy* 2008; **28**:530–535.

55. Viejo LF, et al. Risk factors in neuroleptic malignant syndrome. A case-control study. *Acta Psychiatr Scand* 2003; **107**:45–49.

56. Spivak B, et al. Neuroleptic malignant syndrome during abrupt reduction of neuroleptic treatment. *Acta Psychiatr Scand* 1990; **81**:168–169.

57. Spivak B, et al. Neuroleptic malignant syndrome associated with abrupt withdrawal of anticholinergic agents. *Int Clin Psychopharmacol* 1996; **11**:207–209.

58. Olmsted TR. Neuroleptic malignant syndrome: guidelines for treatment and reinstitution of neuroleptics. *South Med J* 1988; **81**:888–891.

59. Lattanzi L, et al. Subcutaneous apomorphine for neuroleptic malignant syndrome. *Am J Psychiatry* 2006; **163**:1450–1451.

60. Kuhlwilm L, et al. The neuroleptic malignant syndrome – a systematic case series analysis focusing on therapy regimes and outcome. *Acta Psychiatr Scand* 2020; **142**:233–241.

61. Francis A, et al. Is lorazepam a treatment for neuroleptic malignant syndrome? *CNS Spectr* 2000; **5**:54–57.

62. BMJ Best Practice. Neuroleptic malignant syndrome. 2020; https://bestpractice.bmj.com/topics/engb/990/pdf/990/Neuroleptic%20malignant%20syndrome.pdf.

63. Morcos N, et al. Electroconvulsive therapy for neuroleptic malignant syndrome: a case series. *J Ect* 2019; 35:225–230.

64. Wells AJ, et al. Neuroleptic rechallenge after neuroleptic malignant syndrome: case report and literature review. *Drug Intell Clin Pharm* 1988; 22:475–480.

65. Klein JP, et al. Massive creatine kinase elevations with quetiapine: report of two cases. *Pharmacopsychiatry* 2006; 39:39–40.

66. Shiloh R, et al. Precautionary measures reduce risk of definite neuroleptic malignant syndrome in newly typical neuroleptic-treated schizophrenia inpatients. *Int Clin Psychopharmacol* 2003; 18:147–149.

67. Hatch CD, et al. Failed challenge with quetiapine after neuroleptic malignant syndrome with conventional antipsychotics. *Pharmacotherapy* 2001; 21:1003–1006.

68. Trutia A, et al. Neuroleptic rechallenge with aripiprazole in a patient with previously documented neuroleptic malignant syndrome. *J Psychiatr Pract* 2008; 14:398–402.

紧张症

紧张症有两种亚型,一种是迟缓或木僵型,表现为精神运动行为减少;另一种是兴奋型,特征是激越、好斗、冲动和明显无目的的过度活动[1,2]。前者往往表现为木僵,主要特征包括缄默、肌强直、明显的精神运动性迟滞、违拗、奇特的姿势、蜡样屈曲和僵住症。木僵虽然在历史上与精神分裂症相关,但也可见于其他精神疾病,如抑郁症、躁狂(较少见)[3-8]、酒精[9]或苯二氮䓬类药物戒断[10]以及转换障碍[3,4,11-17]。如果精神病性木僵不予治疗,将会不可避免地发生躯体并发症,且病情迅速进展。立刻治疗是防止并发症的关键,并发症包括脱水、静脉血栓、肺栓塞、肺炎及最终导致死亡[18]。

紧张症可能由各种全身性、神经性和中毒性疾病引起,包括发育性疾病(如孤独症)、神经变性疾病[19,20]和以下疾病:

- 蛛网膜下腔出血
- 基底核功能紊乱
- 无抽搐的癫痫持续状态
- 闭锁综合征及无动性缄默
- 内分泌代谢疾病,如肝豆状核变性(又称威尔逊病)[21]
- Prader-Willi 综合征
- 抗磷脂综合征[22]
- 自身免疫性脑炎[23]
- 系统性红斑狼疮[24]
- 感染(特别是中枢神经系统感染)
- 痴呆
- 药物戒断状态和药物中毒,如突然停用氯氮平、唑吡坦、苯二氮䓬类药物[25]以及许多非抗精神药物(抗肿瘤药)。

对紧张症的木僵,其治疗取决于病因,但一般会包括苯二氮䓬类药物。苯二氮䓬类药物本身是情感障碍或转换障碍背景下木僵的首选药物[5,6,26]。有人提出苯二氮䓬类药物的作用机制是增强 γ-氨基丁酸(GBA)能递质,或降低脑源性神经营养因子的水平[27]。临床使用经验最多的是劳拉西泮。标准剂量(最多 4mg/d)对许多患者有效,但是可能需要重复使用及使用更高的剂量(8~12mg/d)[28]。一项小型的观察性研究发现[5],对心境障碍(抑郁障碍或双相障碍)所致紧张性木僵采用劳拉西泮-地西泮治疗,肌内注射 2~4mg 劳拉西泮的 12 例患者中 10 例有效。在另一项采用非常相似的治疗方案的研究中,21 名全身性疾病或物质滥用所致紧张症患者中,18 例症状得到缓解[29]。若苯二氮䓬类药物有效,起效会很快。试验剂量的唑吡坦(10mg)可预测对苯二氮䓬类药物的反应[30],而频繁使用唑吡坦可提供有效的治疗[31,32]。静脉注射劳拉西泮也可用于预测疗效[33]。

苯二氮䓬类药物单用对于精神分裂症所致紧张症可能疗效欠佳,有效率为 40%~50%[34]。一项双盲、安慰剂对照、交叉试验显示,劳拉西泮最高 6mg/d 的剂量对于慢性精神分裂症[35]的紧张症无效。同样,在非随机试验中劳拉西泮也效果甚微[36]。一项 Cochrane 综述[37] 搜索了精神分裂症或其他类似重性精神病的紧张症患者用过苯二氮䓬类药物或其他相关治疗方法的随机对照试验。只有一项研究符合要求,其中 17 例患者接受劳拉西泮或奥沙西泮治疗,结果显示效果没有明显差异。作者指出,没有苯二氮䓬类药物与安慰剂或标准治疗相比较的数据。

使精神分裂症更加复杂的是鉴别诊断,包括锥体外系反应和 NMS。关于精神病的紧张性木僵和 NMS 的异同一直存在争议[38-41]。有人创造了两个词,致死性紧张症和恶性紧张症[42],用于描述伴有自主神经功能紊乱或高热的木僵。这种可能致死的疾病难以通过临床表现和实验室检查与 NMS 鉴别,所以有人建议把 NMS 看作是恶性紧张症的一个变异[43]。然而,以前或最近未服用过多巴胺拮抗剂有助于排除 NMS。

近年和以往数十年已出版的大多数资料表明,立刻进行电抽搐治疗对于紧张症仍是最有效的[33,36,44-60]。人们认识到,在 NMS、谵妄性躁狂、有自伤行为的孤独症和边缘性脑炎的背景下发生的紧张症使用电抽搐治疗有效[41]。有人提出对于精神分裂症患者(或接受过抗精神病药治疗的患者),电抽搐治疗的效果可能不如心境障碍患者[61],但是对于苯二氮䓬类药物充分试验无效的紧张型精神分裂症,电抽搐仍被认为是首选的治疗方法[62]。对于恶性紧张症患者,应尽可能地使用充分的电刺激诱发完全的全身发作,使 ECT 的疗效达到最佳[63]。应该优先关注躯体健康,必要时住院治疗,尤其是自主神经功能紊乱,以及在精神科难以处理饮食问题的患者。

应慎重考虑使用抗精神病药。一些作者建议应该完全避免给紧张症患者使用抗精神病药,尽管有阿立哌唑、利培酮、奥氮平、齐拉西酮和氯氮平治疗成功的病例报道[64-69]。支持证据最多的是氯氮平和奥氮平。当每种药物单独使用无效时,与苯二氮䓬类药物合用可能有效[70,71]。

在应用抗精神病药前,应了解病史、既往诊断、既往抗精神病药的疗效以及用药不依从引起木僵的可能性。应该注意,有些躯体疾病的临床表现像木僵(如前所述的例子),必须治疗基础躯体疾病(如狼疮[72])。当抗精神病药治疗期间出现木僵时,若有明确的 NMS 体征,且肌强直伴有自主神经功能紊乱时,应避免使用抗精神病药。若可以排除 NMS,且木僵是对抗精神病药治疗的不依从所致,建议及早重新使用抗精神病药,并考虑苯二氮䓬类药物辅助治疗。当紧张症症状发生于停用氯氮平之后时,这一点可能特别重要[25,73]。也有长期使用苯二氮䓬类药物治疗,撤药后出现紧张症的报道[25]。

紧张性木僵的治疗流程 [74]

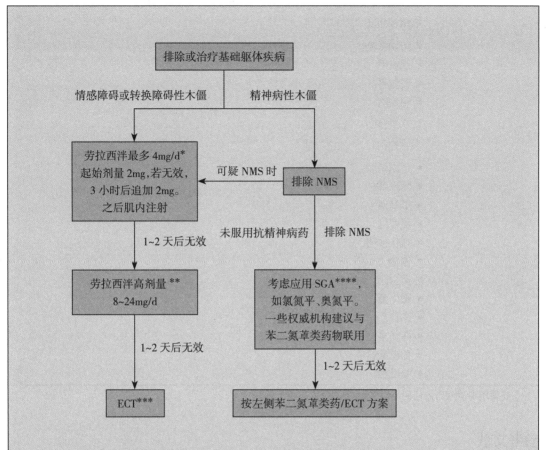

* 劳拉西泮经舌下吸收,无味。这个途径更适用于不合作或不能吞咽的患者。

** 此时可考虑静脉注射地西泮或劳拉西泮。

*** 若有明显的生命危险,马上考虑应用 ECT。

**** 使用抗精神病药治疗紧张性木僵存在相当大的不确定性。抗精神病药可诱发紧张症 [75](紧张型精神分裂症患者发生 NMS 的风险远远高于非紧张型精神分裂症患者 [76]。已有报告除苯二氮䓬类药物之外其他治疗紧张症/木僵的药物,见表 1.20)。当紧张症已经缓解,或苯二氮䓬类药物/电抽搐治疗无效,且有明确的精神病时,选择使用抗精神病药 [74]。

表 1.20 除苯二氮䓬类药物外,已经报告的治疗紧张症/木僵的其他药物

按照英文字母排序——排序与等级或倾向性无关

抗精神病药 [64-69,77-80]

- 阿立哌唑
- 氯氮平
- 奥氮平
- 利培酮
- 齐拉西酮

实验性治疗 [*6,7,31,32,53,81-86]

- 金刚烷胺
- 阿米替林
- 卡马西平
- 氟西汀
- 氟伏沙明
- 锂盐
- 美金刚
- 哌甲酯
- 米氮平
- 曲马多
- 丙戊酸盐
- 唑吡坦

* 在使用本节列出的任何药物之前,务必阅读原始文献。

参考文献

1. Morrison JR. Catatonia. Retarded and excited types. *Arch Gen Psychiatry* 1973; 28:39–41.
2. Walther S, et al. Structure and neural mechanisms of catatonia. *Lancet Psychiatry* 2019; 6:610–619.
3. Takacs R, et al. Catatonia in affective disorders. *Curr Psychiatry Rev* 2013; 9:101–105.
4. Mangas MCC, et al. P-167 – catatonia in bipolar disorder. *Eur Psychiatry* 2012; 27 Suppl 1:1.
5. Huang YC, et al. Rapid relief of catatonia in mood disorder by lorazepam and diazepam. *Biomed J* 2013; 36:35–39.
6. Vasudev K, et al. What works for delirious catatonic mania? *BMJ Case Rep* 2010; 2010.
7. Neuhut R, et al. Resolution of catatonia after treatment with stimulant medication in a patient with bipolar disorder. *Psychosomatics* 2012; 53:482–484.
8. Ghaffarinejad AR, et al. Periodic catatonia. Challenging diagnosis for psychiatrists. *Neurosciences* 2012; 17:156–158.
9. Oldham MA, et al. Alcohol and sedative-hypnotic withdrawal catatonia: two case reports, systematic literature review, and suggestion of a potential relationship with alcohol withdrawal delirium. *Psychosomatics* 2016; 57:246–255.
10. Banerjee D. Etizolam withdrawal catatonia: the first case report. *Asian J Psychiatr* 2018; 37:32–33.
11. Fink M. Rediscovering catatonia: the biography of a treatable syndrome. *Acta Psychiatr Scand Suppl* 2013; 1–47.
12. Bartolommei N, et al. Catatonia: a critical review and therapeutic recommendation. *J Psychopathology* 2012; 18:234–246.
13. Lee J. Dissociative catatonia: dissociative-catatonic reactions, clinical presentations and responses to benzodiazepines. *Aust N Z J Psychiatry* 2011; 45:A42.
14. Suzuki K, et al. Hysteria presenting as a prodrome to catatonic stupor in a depressive patient resolved with electroconvulsive therapy. *J ECT* 2006; 22:276.
15. Alwaki A, et al. Catatonia: an elusive diagnosis. *Neurology* 2013; 80 Suppl 1:P05.127.
16. Dhadphale M. Eye gaze diagnostic sign in hysterical stupor. *Lancet* 1980; 2:374–375.
17. Gomez J. Hysterical stupor and death. *Br J Psychiatry* 1980; 136:105–106.
18. Petrides G, et al. Synergism of lorazepam and electroconvulsive therapy in the treatment of catatonia. *Biol Psychiatry* 1997; 42:375–381.
19. Mazzone L, et al. Catatonia in patients with autism: prevalence and management. *CNS Drugs* 2014; 28:205–215.

20. Dhossche DM, et al. Catatonia in psychiatric illnesses, in SH Fatemi, PJ Clayton, eds. *The medical basis of psychiatry*. Totowa, NJ: Humana Press; 2008:471–486.

21. Shetageri VN, et al. Case report: catatonia as a presenting symptom of Wilsons disease. *Indian J Psychiatry* 2011; 53 Suppl 5:S93–S94.

22. Cardinal RN, et al. Psychosis and catatonia as a first presentation of antiphospholipid syndrome. *Br J Psychiatry* 2009; 195:272.

23. Rogers JP, et al. Catatonia and the immune system: a review. *Lancet Psychiatry* 2019; 6:620–630.

24. Pustilnik S, et al. Catatonia as the presenting symptom in systemic lupus erythematosus. *J Psychiatr Pract* 2011; 17:217–221.

25. Lander M, et al. Review of withdrawal catatonia: what does this reveal about clozapine? *Trans Psychiatry* 2018; 8:139.

26. Sienaert P, et al. Adult catatonia: etiopathogenesis, diagnosis and treatment. *Neuropsychiatry* 2013; 3:391–399.

27. Huang TL, et al. Lorazepam reduces the serum brain-derived neurotrophic factor level in schizophrenia patients with catatonia. *Prog Neuropsychopharmacol Biol Psychiatry* 2009; 33:158–159.

28. Fink M, et al. Neuroleptic malignant syndrome is malignant catatonia, warranting treatments efficacious for catatonia. *Prog Neuropsychopharmacol Biol Psychiatry* 2006; 30:1182–1183.

29. Lin CC, et al. The lorazepam and diazepam protocol for catatonia due to general medical condition and substance in liaison psychiatry. *PLoS One* 2017; 12:e0170452.

30. Javelot H, et al. Zolpidem test and catatonia. *J Clin Pharm Ther* 2015; 40:699–701.

31. Bastiampillai T, et al. Treatment refractory chronic catatonia responsive to zolpidem challenge. *Aust N Z J Psychiatry* 2016; 50:98.

32. Peglow S, et al. Treatment of catatonia with zolpidem. *J Neuropsychiatry Clin Neurosci* 2013; 25:E13.

33. Bush G, et al. Catatonia. II: Treatment with lorazepam and electroconvulsive therapy. *Acta Psychiatr Scand* 1996; 93:137–143.

34. Rosebush PI, et al. Catatonia: re-awakening to a forgotten disorder. *Mov Disord* 1999; 14:395–397.

35. Ungvari GS, et al. Lorazepam for chronic catatonia: a randomized, double-blind, placebo-controlled cross-over study. *Psychopharmacology* 1999; 142:393–398.

36. Dutt A, et al. Phenomenology and treatment of Catatonia: a descriptive study from north India. *Indian J Psychiatry* 2011; 53:36–40.

37. Gibson RC, et al. Benzodiazepines for catatonia in people with schizophrenia and other serious mental illnesses. *Cochrane Database Syst Rev* 2008; CD006570.

38. Luchini F, et al. Catatonia and neuroleptic malignant syndrome: two disorders on a same spectrum? Four case reports. *J Nerv Ment Dis* 2013; 201:36–42.

39. Mishima T, et al. [Diazepam-responsive malignant catatonia in a patient with an initial clinical diagnosis of neuroleptic malignant syndrome: a case report]. *Brain Nerve* 2011; 63:503–507.

40. Rodriguez S, et al. Neuroleptic malignant syndrome or catatonia? A case report. *J Crit Care Med* 2020; 6:190–193.

41. Fink M. Expanding the catatonia tent: recognizing electroconvulsive therapy responsive syndromes. *J Ect* 2020: [Epub ahead of print].

42. Mann SC, et al. Catatonia, malignant catatonia, and neuroleptic malignant syndrome. *Curr Psychiatry Rev* 2013; 9:111–119.

43. Taylor MA, et al. Catatonia in psychiatric classification: a home of its own. *Am J Psychiatry* 2003; 160:1233–1241.

44. Cristancho P, et al. Successful use of right unilateral ECT for catatonia: a case series. *J Ect* 2014; 30:69–72.

45. Philbin D, et al. Catatonic schizophrenia: therapeutic challenges and potentially a new role for electroconvulsive therapy? *BMJ Case Rep* 2013; 2013.

46. Takebayashi M. [Electroconvulsive therapy in schizophrenia]. *Nihon Rinsho* 2013; 71:694–700.

47. Oviedo G, et al. Trends in the administration of electroconvulsive therapy for schizophrenia in Colombia: Descriptive study and literature review. *Eur Arch Psychiatry Clin Neurosci* 2013; 263 Suppl 1:S98.

48. Pompili M, et al. Indications for electroconvulsive treatment in schizophrenia: a systematic review. *SchizophrRes* 2013; 146:1–9.

49. Ogando Portilla N, et al. Electroconvulsive therapy as an effective treatment in neuroleptic malignant syndrome: purposely a case. *Eur Psychiatry* 2013; 28 Suppl 1:1.

50. Unal A, et al. Effective treatment of catatonia by combination of benzodiazepine and electroconvulsive therapy. *J Ect* 2013; 29:206–209.

51. Kaliora SC, et al. The practice of electroconvulsive therapy in Greece. *J ECT* 2013; 29:219–224.

52. Girardi P, et al. Life-saving electroconvulsive therapy in a patient with near-lethal catatonia. *Riv Psichiatr* 2012; 47:535–537.

53. Kumar V, et al. Electroconvulsive therapy in pregnancy. *Indian J Psychiatry* 2011; 53 Suppl 5:S100–S101.

54. Weiss M, et al. Treatment of catatonia with electroconvulsive therapy in adolescents. *J Child Adolesc Psychopharmacol* 2012; 22:96–100.

55. Bauer J, et al. Should the term catatonia be explicitly included in the ICD-10 description of acute transient psychotic disorder F23.0? *Nord J Psychiatry* 2012; 66:68–69.

56. Mohammadbeigi H, et al. Electroconvulsive therapy in single manic episodes: a case series. *Afr J Psychiatry* 2011; 14:56–59.

57. Dragasek J. [Utilisation of electroconvulsive therapy in treatment of depression disorders]. *Psychiatrie* 2011; 15:1211–1219.

58. Sienaert P, et al. A clinical review of the treatment of catatonia. *Front Psychiatry* 2014; 5:181.

59. Luchini F, et al. Electroconvulsive therapy in catatonic patients: efficacy and predictors of response. *World J Psychiatry* 2015; 5:182–192.

60. Lloyd JR, et al. Electroconvulsive therapy for patients with catatonia: current perspectives. *Neuropsychiatr Dis Treat* 2020; 16:2191–2208.

61. Van Waarde JA, et al. Electroconvulsive therapy for catatonia: treatment characteristics and outcomes in 27 patients. *J Ect* 2010; 26:248–252.

62. Jain A, et al. Catatonic Schizophrenia. StatPearls. Treasure Island (FL): statPearls Publishing Copyright © 2020, StatPearls Publishing LLC. 2020.

63. Kellner CH, et al. Electroconvulsive therapy for catatonia. *Am J Psychiatry* 2010; 167:1127–1128.

64. Van Den EF, et al. The use of atypical antipsychotics in the treatment of catatonia. *Eur Psychiatry* 2005; 20:422–429.

65. Caroff SN, et al. Movement disorders associated with atypical antipsychotic drugs. *J Clin Psychiatry* 2002; 63 Suppl 4:12–19.

66. Guzman CS, et al. Treatment of periodic catatonia with atypical antipsychotic, olanzapine. *Psychiatry Clin Neurosci* 2008; 62:482.

67. Babington PW, et al. Treatment of catatonia with olanzapine and amantadine. *Psychosomatics* 2007; 48:534–536.

68. Bastiampillai T, et al. Catatonia resolution and aripiprazole. *Aust N Z J Psychiatry* 2008; 42:907.

69. Strawn JR, et al. Successful treatment of catatonia with aripiprazole in an adolescent with psychosis. *J Child Adolesc Psychopharmacol* 2007; 17:733–735.

70. Spiegel DR, et al. A case of schizophrenia with catatonia resistant to lorazepam and olanzapine monotherapy but responsive to combination treatment: is it time to consider using select second-generation antipsychotics earlier in the treatment algorithm for this patient type? *Clin Neuropharmacol* 2019; 42:57–59.

71. Cevher Binici N, et al. Response of catatonia to amisulpride and lorazepam in an adolescent with schizophrenia. *J Child Adolesc Psychopharmacol* 2018; 28:151–152.

72. Grover S, et al. Catatonia in systemic lupus erythematosus: a case report and review of literature. *Lupus* 2013; 22:634–638.

73. Bilbily J, et al. Catatonia secondary to sudden clozapine withdrawal: a case with three repeated episodes and a literature review. *Case Rep Psychiatry* 2017; 2017:2402731.

74. Rosebush PI, et al. Catatonia and its treatment. *Schizophr Bull* 2010; 36:239–242.

75. Caroff SN, et al. Movement disorders induced by antipsychotic drugs: implications of the CATIE schizophrenia trial. *Neurol Clin* 2011; 29:127–148, viii.

76. Funayama M, et al. Catatonic stupor in schizophrenic disorders and subsequent medical complications and mortality. *Psychosom Med* 2018; 80:370–376.

77. Voros V, et al. [Use of aripiprazole in the treatment of catatonia]. *NeuropsychopharmacolHung* 2010; 12:373–376.

78. Yoshimura B, et al. Is quetiapine suitable for treatment of acute schizophrenia with catatonic stupor? A case series of 39 patients. *Neuropsychiatr Dis Treat* 2013; 9:1565–1571.

79. Todorova K. Olanzapine in the treatment of catatonic stupor – two case reports and discussion. *Eur Neuropsychopharmacol* 2012; 22 Suppl 2:S326.

80. Prakash O, et al. Catatonia and mania in patient with AIDS: treatment with lorazepam and risperidone. *Gen Hosp Psychiatry* 2012; 34:321–326.

81. Daniels J. Catatonia: clinical aspects and neurobiological correlates. *J Neuropsychiatry Clin Neurosci* 2009; 21:371–380.

82. Obregon DF, et al. Memantine and catatonia: a case report and literature review. *J Psychiatr Pract* 2011; 17:292–299.

83. Hervey WM, et al. Treatment of catatonia with amantadine. *Clin Neuropharmacol* 2012; 35:86–87.

84. Consoli A, et al. Lorazepam, fluoxetine and packing therapy in an adolescent with pervasive developmental disorder and catatonia. *J Physiol Paris* 2010; 104:309–314.

85. Lewis AL, et al. Malignant catatonia in a patient with bipolar disorder, B12 deficiency, and neuroleptic malignant syndrome: one cause or three? *J Psychiatr Pract* 2009; 15:415–422.

86. Padhy SK, et al. The catatonia conundrum: controversies and contradictions. *Asian J Psychiatr* 2014; 7:6–9.

心电图改变——Q-T 间期延长

简介

许多抗精神病药与心电图的改变相关,其中一些与严重的室性心律失常及心源性猝死有因果关系。尤其需要指出的是,一些抗精神病药会阻滞心脏的钾离子通道,这与 Q-T 间期延长相关,后者是有时致命的尖端扭转型室性心律失常的危险因素[1]。

病例对照研究发现,大部分抗精神病药会增加心源性猝死的发生率[2-8]。尽管精神分裂症本身可能与 Q-T 间期延长相关[11],但这种风险的增高很可能是抗精神病药引起潜在的心律失常的结果[9,10]。一项针对首发患者的研究表明,使用抗精神病药 2~4 周后会出现明确的 Q-T 间期延长[12]。精神分裂症患者的 Q-T 间期比对照组长(例如,在一项研究[13]中,患者/对照 Q-T 间期为418ms/393ms)。在最近的一项研究中,做过心电图的精神科住院患者中7.6%[14]出现 Q-T 间期延长。

总的来说,Q-T 间期延长的风险与药物剂量相关,但其绝对风险较低,其发生概率明显高于氯氮平所致的致死性粒细胞减少症[8]。一项国家数据库所收集病例的报告表明,根据具体抗精神病药种类和患者年龄不同,尖端扭转型室性心动过速(TdP)的风险在 0~19.2/10 万患者-年[15]。抗精神病药联合用药对 Q-T 间期的影响不确定,[16]但 Q-T 间期延长的程度与总剂量间可能存在函数关系[17]。

在精神卫生机构,受很多因素的影响,监测药物引起的心电图改变是复杂的。首先,精神科医师解释心电图的专业知识可能有限,手动测量 Q-T 间期的专业知识更有限。即使是心血管专科医师测量 Q-T 间期,差距最大也有 20ms[18]。电脑自读式心电监测设备能在某种程度上弥补了专业上的不足,但不同的设备使用了不同的算法和各异的校正公式[19]。另外,与一般内科不同,心电图机并不是在所有的精神科临床区域都随手可得。同时,心电图检查在有些地方也没有时间做(如门诊部)。最后,对急性躁动期、体格检查不合作的患者,可能难以进行心电图检查。

对所有使用抗精神病药的患者,必须进行心电图检查。Q-T 间期的评估应在患者入院时完成(请注意:这是 NICE 精神分裂症指南的建议[20]),此后至少每年复查一次。

Q-T 间期延长

- 心脏 Q-T 间期(Q-T 间期心率校正值通常被称为 Q-T 间期)在判断尖端扭转型心律失常及心源性死亡的风险上,是一项有效却不够精确的预测因子[21]。不同的校正因子和方法会产生显著不同的数值[22]。

- Q-T 间期粗略地反映了心脏复极化的时程。复极化时程延长可导致心室不同结构的电活动位相不一致(离散),从而致使心脏后早期去极化(EAD)的发生,由此可能引发室性期前收缩和尖端扭转型室性心动过速。已经开发出可以更好地预测心律失常的测量指标(Q-T 间期离散度、跨室壁复极离散时间)[13]。

- 关于 Q-T 间期与心律失常之间的确切关系存在着一些争议。非常有限的证据显示,Q-T 间期超过正常上限(男性:440ms;女性:470ms)时,其延长的程度与心律失常风险成指数相关;然而,存在很多众所周知的例外,似乎并不支持该理论 [23](一些药物能够延长 Q-T 间期,但并不增加离散度)。更有力的证据表明,Q-T 间期值大于 500ms 与心律失常风险增加显著相关 [24]。Q-T 间期大于 650ms 更有可能引起尖端扭转型心律失常 [25]。排除一些不确定因素,Q-T 间期测定仍是预估心律失常及猝死风险的重要指标。

- Q-T 间期各个成分可能具有特别重要的意义。T 波从开始到达峰的时间已被证明是心源性猝死相关 Q-T 间期延长的重要方面 [26];T 波从达峰到结束的时间也可以预测心律失常 [13]。
- Q-T 间期的测量和评定受到以下因素的影响:
  - 难以判定 T 波的终点,尤其是存在 U 波时(手动及机器自读式心电图机均如此)[24]。
  - Q-T 间期的正常生理变异:Q-T 间期受到性别、时点、进食、饮酒、月经周期及心电图导联等因素影响 [22,23]。
  - 药源性 Q-T 间期延长的程度与血药浓度相关,在峰浓度时影响最为显著,在谷浓度时影响最小 [22,23]。

其他心电改变

抗精神病药引起的其他心电图改变包括心房颤动、巨大 P 波、T 波改变及传导阻滞 [23]。

量化风险

根据药物对心脏 Q-T 间期影响的现有数据,可将其进行分类(按照报告结果,绝大部分使用 Bazett 公式进行校正):"无影响"药物是指在治疗剂量或超量使用时均未见 Q-T 间期延长报道的药物;"低度影响"药物是指仅在超量使用时发生严重 Q-T 间期延长,或临床正常剂量时平均仅有轻度延长(小于 10ms)的药物;"中度影响"药物是指在正常临床剂量时平均能使 Q-T 间期延长大于 10ms,或在某些情况下正式建议进行心电图监测的药物;"高度影响"药物是指能使 Q-T 间期明显延长的药物(通常是指在正常临床剂量时致使 Q-T 间期延长大于 20ms)。

请注意,如上文所述,对 Q-T 间期的影响未必直接等于尖端扭转型心律失常或猝死 [27],尽管它们常被混为一谈(一个不错的例子便是齐拉西酮——它对 Q-T 间期存在中度影响,却没有心脏毒性的证据 [28])。同时,由于存在 Q-T 间期测量的相关问题,表格中药物的分类难免是大概的。最后,请谨记,即使是在荟萃分析中,不同抗精神病药对 Q-T 间期影响的差异也极少具有统计学意义(表 1.21)[29]。

此外,读者可以参考 RISQ-PATH 研究 [30],该研究为预测患者的 Q-T 间期延长(高于正常范围)提供了一个评分系统。RISQ-PATH 的阴性预测值为 98%,因此可以减少低风险患者的监测。RISQ-PATH 使用 CredibleMeds 对药物造成的 Q-T 间期影响进行分类,这也是推荐的做法 [31]。

阿立哌唑归为低度影响组,此前一直被坚定地归为无影响组。研究数据相当矛盾,大多数研究表明,即使在儿童和青少年中,使用阿立哌唑也会缩短 Q-T 间期 [72]。然而,随后的研究 [62,63,65,66,73] 对阿立哌唑心脏安全性的假设提出了质疑。有意思的是,2020 年的一篇论文分析了 20 年间超过 40 万名住院患者的事件报告,发现在所有抗精神病药中,阿立哌唑的心脏事件发生率最低(0.06%)[74]。

表 1.21 抗精神病药对 Q-T 间期的影响 [13,22,23,32-61]

无影响	中度影响
布瑞哌唑 *	氨磺必利 ****
卡利拉嗪 *	氯丙嗪
鲁拉西酮	氟哌啶醇
卢美哌隆 *	伊潘立酮
	左美丙嗪
低度影响	美哌隆
阿立哌唑 **	匹莫范色林
阿塞那平	喹硫平
氯氮平	齐拉西酮
氟哌噻吨	
氟奋乃静	**高度影响**
奋乃静	任何静脉给药的抗精神病药
丙氯拉嗪	匹莫齐特
奥氮平 ***	舍吲哚
帕利哌酮	任何超过推荐最大剂量的单药或合并用药
利培酮	
舒必利	**未知影响**
	洛沙平
	哌泊噻嗪
	三氟拉嗪
	珠氯噻醇

* 临床经验有限(可能与 Q-T 间期延长有关)。

** 1 例尖端扭转型室性心动过速报道 [62],数据库研究报告 2 例 Q-T 间期延长 [63,64] 并与尖端扭转型室性心动过速相关 [65]。健康志愿者数据显示,阿立哌唑导致 Q-T 间期延长约 8ms [66]。阿立哌唑可能增加 Q-T 间期离散度 [67]。

*** 个别案例 Q-T 间期延长 [37,68],对心脏离子通道 I_{Kr} 有影响 [69],其他数据提示该药对 Q-T 间期没有影响 [23,35,36,70]。

**** 在超量使用时常引发尖端扭转型室性心动过速 [25,71],在临床剂量范围内与尖端扭转型室性心动过速强相关 [65]。

鲁拉西酮归为无影响组 [52],但美国的一项药物说明书研究表明,每天服用 120mg(111mg)的人 Q-T 间期延长 7.5ms [75],每天服用 600mg(555mg)的人 Q-T 间期变化较小(+4.6ms)。而基于患者的研究一致地提示鲁拉西酮对 Q-T 间期没有影响或影响很小 [76-78]。这种出入可能是由于使用不同的校正系数或数据随机变异所致,因为常见于接受安慰剂治疗的患者 [78],并且明显缺少剂量相关的效应提示了这一点。据我们所知,尚未有使用鲁拉西酮出现过 Q-T>500ms 或尖端扭转型室性心动过速的报道。

布瑞哌唑归为无影响组,但要注意的是,一项包含 16 例患者的研究发现,Q-T 间期(霍奇斯公式计算)延长了 10.1ms,并且跨室壁复极离散时间延长 [13]。其他全部数据均提示布瑞哌唑对 Q-T 间期无影响。

其他危险因素

许多生理或病理因素均与 Q-T 间期改变及心律失常相关(表 1.22),并且许多非精神药物也与 Q-T 间期延长密不可分(表 1.23) [24]。在抗精神病药引起的尖端扭转型心律失常中,这些额外的危险因素似乎总是存在[79]。

表 1.22 Q-T 间期延长及心律失常的生理性危险因素

心脏	其他
长 Q-T 间期综合征	高强度体力活动
心动过缓	应激或休克
缺血性心肌病	神经性厌食
心肌炎	年龄的两端——儿童和老年人可能更易产生 Q-T
心肌梗死	间期改变
左心室肥大	女性
代谢	
低钾血症	
低镁血症	
低钙血症	

注:低钾血症相关的 Q-T 间期延长更多见于急性精神病住院患者[80]。另外,请注意,还有许多常规检查发现不了的躯体因素和遗传因素可能会导致患者更易患心律失常[81,82]。

表 1.23 与 Q-T 间期延长有关的非精神药物(最新信息请查阅相关网站)

抗生素	抗心律失常药
红霉素	奎尼丁
克拉霉素	丙吡胺
氨苄西林	普鲁卡因胺
复方新诺明	索他洛尔
喷他脒	胺碘酮
(4 种喹诺酮类药可影响 Q-T 间期——详见药厂文献)	溴苄铵
抗疟药	**其他**
氯喹	金刚烷胺
甲氟喹	环孢素
奎宁	苯海拉明
	羟嗪
	美沙酮
	尼卡地平
	他莫昔芬

注:$β_2$ 受体激动剂和拟交感神经药可能会使 Q-T 间期延长的患者出现尖端扭转型心律失常。

心电图监测

所有被处方抗精神病药的患者均需进行 Q-T 间期检测:

- 入院时
- 若之前存在异常或已知存在其他危险因素,每年体检时

新近使用有中度或高度 Q-T 间期延长风险的抗精神病药达到治疗剂量,或新近合用抗精神病药,均应在一周内检测 Q-T 间期。表 1.24 介绍了抗精神病药所致 Q-T 间期延长的处理方法(表 1.24)。

表 1.24　接受抗精神病药治疗的患者出现 Q-T 间期延长的处理方法

Q-T 间期	处理方法	转诊给心血管医师
<440ms（男）或 <470ms（女）	除非 T 波形态异常，否则无须处理	若有疑问，考虑转诊
>440ms（男）或 470~500ms（女）	考虑将治疗药物减量，或换用对 Q-T 间期影响较小的药物；复查 ECG	考虑转诊
>500ms	复查 ECG；停用可疑药物，换用对 Q-T 间期影响较小的药物	即刻转诊
T 波形态异常	审核治疗方案。考虑将治疗药物减量，或换用对 Q-T 间期影响较小的药物	即刻转诊

代谢抑制

药物引起的 Q-T 间期延长通常取决于血药浓度。因此，药物相互作用非常重要，尤其是药物代谢受抑制使得对 Q-T 间期有影响的药物浓度升高时。常见的抑制药物代谢的药物有氟伏沙明、氟西汀、帕罗西汀及丙戊酸盐。

其他心血管风险因素

抗精神病药所致的心律失常及心源性猝死是非常值得思考的问题。至于心血管病，请注意，与不确定的 Q-T 间期改变相比，吸烟、肥胖或糖耐量异常使患者患病和死亡的风险更大。详见相关章节的讨论内容。

小结

- 在缺乏确凿证据的前提下，假设所有的抗精神病药均与心源性猝死相关。
- 尽可能地处方最低剂量，并且避免药物合用/药物代谢方面的相互作用。
- 入院时即完善心电图检查；若之前存在心电图异常或其他危险因素，每年复查。
- 使用中度或高度风险的抗精神病药时，在达到治疗剂量后的一周内应检测 Q-T 间期。

参考文献

1. Sicouri S, et al. Mechanisms underlying the actions of antidepressant and antipsychotic drugs that cause sudden cardiac arrest. *Arrhythm Electrophysiol Rev* 2018; 7:199–209.
2. Reilly JG, et al. Thioridazine and sudden unexplained death in psychiatric in-patients. *Br J Psychiatry* 2002; 180:515–522.
3. Murray-Thomas T, et al. Risk of mortality (including sudden cardiac death) and major cardiovascular events in atypical and typical antipsychotic users: a study with the general practice research database. *Cardiovasc Psychiatry Neurol* 2013; 2013:247486.
4. Ray WA, et al. Antipsychotics and the risk of sudden cardiac death. *Arch Gen Psychiatry* 2001; 58:1161–1167.
5. Hennessy S, et al. Cardiac arrest and ventricular arrhythmia in patients taking antipsychotic drugs: cohort study using administrative data. *BMJ* 2002; 325:1070.
6. Straus SM, et al. Antipsychotics and the risk of sudden cardiac death. *Arch Intern Med* 2004; 164:1293–1297.
7. Liperoti R, et al. Conventional and atypical antipsychotics and the risk of hospitalization for ventricular arrhythmias or cardiac arrest. *Arch Intern Med* 2005; 165:696–701.
8. Ray WA, et al. Atypical antipsychotic drugs and the risk of sudden cardiac death. *N Engl J Med* 2009; 360:225–235.
9. Schneeweiss S, et al. Antipsychotic agents and sudden cardiac death–how should we manage the risk? *N Engl J Med* 2009; 360:294–296.

10. Nakagawa S, et al. Antipsychotics and risk of first-time hospitalization for myocardial infarction: a population-based case-control study. *J Intern Med* 2006; **260**:451–458.

11. Fujii K, et al. QT is longer in drug-free patients with schizophrenia compared with age-matched healthy subjects. *PLoSOne* 2014; **9**:e98555.

12. Zhai D, et al. QTc interval lengthening in first-episode schizophrenia (FES) patients in the earliest stages of antipsychotic treatment. *Schizophr Res* 2017; **179**:70–74.

13. Okayasu H, et al. Effects of antipsychotics on arrhythmogenic parameters in schizophrenia patients: beyond corrected QT interval. *Neuropsychiatr Dis Treat* 2021; **17**:239–249.

14. Ansermot N, et al. Prevalence of ECG abnormalities and risk factors for QTc interval prolongation in hospitalized psychiatric patients. *Ther Adv Psychopharmacol* 2019; **9**:2045125319891386.

15. Danielsson B, et al. Drug use and torsades de pointes cardiac arrhythmias in Sweden: a nationwide register-based cohort study. *BMJ Open* 2020; **10**:e034560.

16. Takeuchi H, et al. Antipsychotic polypharmacy and corrected QT interval: a systematic review. *Can J Psychiatry* 2015; **60**:215–222.

17. Barbui C, et al. Antipsychotic dose mediates the association between polypharmacy and corrected QT interval. *PLoS One* 2016; **11**:e0148212.

18. Goldenberg I, et al. QT interval: how to measure it and what is 'normal'. *J Cardiovasc Electrophysiol* 2006; **17**:333–336.

19. Nielsen J, et al. Assessing QT interval prolongation and its associated risks with antipsychotics. *CNS Drugs* 2011; **25**:473–490.

20. National Institute for Health and Care Excellence. Psychosis and schizophrenia in adults: prevention and management. Clinical Guidance [CG178]. 2014 (last checked March 2019); https://www.nice.org.uk/guidance/cg178.

21. Malik M, et al. Evaluation of drug-induced QT interval prolongation: implications for drug approval and labelling. *Drug Saf* 2001; **24**:323–351.

22. Haddad PM, et al. Antipsychotic-related QTc prolongation, torsade de pointes and sudden death. *Drugs* 2002; **62**:1649–1671.

23. Taylor DM. Antipsychotics and QT prolongation. *Acta Psychiatr Scand* 2003; **107**:85–95.

24. Botstein P. Is QT interval prolongation harmful? A regulatory perspective. *Am J Cardiol* 1993; **72**:50B-52B.

25. Joy JP, et al. Prediction of torsade de pointes from the QT interval: analysis of a case series of amisulpride overdoses. *Clin Pharmacol Ther* 2011; **90**:243–245.

26. O'Neal WT, et al. Association between QT-interval components and sudden cardiac death: the ARIC Study (Atherosclerosis Risk in Communities). *Circ Arrhythmia Electrophysiol* 2017; **10**:e005485

27. Witchel HJ, et al. Psychotropic drugs, cardiac arrhythmia, and sudden death. *J Clin Psychopharmacol* 2003; **23**:58–77.

28. Strom BL, et al. Comparative mortality associated with ziprasidone and olanzapine in real-world use among 18,154 patients with schizophrenia: the Ziprasidone Observational Study of Cardiac Outcomes (ZODIAC). *Am J Psychiatry* 2011; **168**:193–201.

29. Chung AK, et al. Effects on prolongation of Bazett's corrected QT interval of seven second-generation antipsychotics in the treatment of schizophrenia: a meta-analysis. *J Psychopharmacology* 2011; **25**:646–666.

30. Vandael E, et al. Development of a risk score for QTc-prolongation: the RISQ-PATH study. *Int J Clin Pharm* 2017; **39**:424–432.

31. CredibleMeds®. CredibleMeds. 2021; https://www.crediblemeds.org.

32. Hui WK, et al. Melperone: electrophysiologic and antiarrhythmic activity in humans. *J Cardiovasc Pharmacol* 1990; **15**:144–149.

33. Glassman AH, et al. Antipsychotic drugs: prolonged QTc interval, torsade de pointes, and sudden death. *Am J Psychiatry* 2001; **158**:1774–1782.

34. Warner B, et al. Investigation of the potential of clozapine to cause torsade de pointes. *Adverse Drug React Toxicol Rev* 2002; **21**:189–203.

35. Harrigan EP, et al. A randomized evaluation of the effects of six antipsychotic agents on QTc, in the absence and presence of metabolic inhibition. *J Clin Psychopharmacol* 2004; **24**:62–69.

36. Lindborg SR, et al. Effects of intramuscular olanzapine vs. haloperidol and placebo on QTc intervals in acutely agitated patients. *Psychiatry Res* 2003; **119**:113–123.

37. Dineen S, et al. QTc prolongation and high-dose olanzapine (Letter). *Psychosomatics* 2003; **44**:174–175.

38. Gupta S, et al. Quetiapine and QTc issues: a case report (Letter). *J Clin Psychiatry* 2003; **64**:612–613.

39. Su KP, et al. A pilot cross-over design study on QTc interval prolongation associated with sulpiride and haloperidol. *Schizophr Res* 2003; **59**:93–94.

40. Chong SA, et al. Prolonged QTc intervals in medicated patients with schizophrenia. *Human Psychopharmacology* 2003; **18**:647–649.

41. Stollberger C, et al. Antipsychotic drugs and QT prolongation. *Int Clin Psychopharmacol* 2005; **20**:243–251.

42. Isbister GK, et al. Amisulpride deliberate self-poisoning causing severe cardiac toxicity including QT prolongation and torsades de pointes. *Med J Aust* 2006; **184**:354–356.

43. Ward DI. Two cases of amisulpride overdose: a cause for prolonged QT syndrome. *Emerg Med Australas* 2005; **17**:274–276.

44. Vieweg WV, et al. Torsade de pointes in a patient with complex medical and psychiatric conditions receiving low-dose quetiapine. *Acta Psychiatr Scand* 2005; **112**:318–322.

45. Huang BH, et al. Sulpiride induced torsade de pointes. *Int J Cardiol* 2007; **118**:e100–e102.

46. Kane JM, et al. Long-term efficacy and safety of iloperidone: results from 3 clinical trials for the treatment of schizophrenia. *J Clin Psychopharmacol* 2008; **28**:S29–S35.

47. Kim MD, et al. Blockade of HERG human K+ channel and IKr of guinea pig cardiomyocytes by prochlorperazine. *Eur J Pharmacol* 2006; **544**:82–90.

48. Meltzer H, et al. Efficacy and tolerability of oral paliperidone extended-release tablets in the treatment of acute schizophrenia: pooled data from three 6-week placebo-controlled studies. *J Clin Psychiatry* 2006; **69**:817–829.

49. Chapel S, et al. Exposure-response analysis in patients with schizophrenia to assess the effect of asenapine on QTc prolongation. *J Clin Pharmacol* 2009; **49**:1297–1308.

50. Ozeki Y, et al. QTc prolongation and antipsychotic medications in a sample of 1017 patients with schizophrenia. *Prog Neuropsychopharmacol*

Biol Psychiatry 2010; **34**:401–405.

51. Girardin FR, et al. Drug-induced long QT in adult psychiatric inpatients: the 5-year cross-sectional ECG Screening Outcome in Psychiatry study. *Am J Psychiatry* 2013; **170**:1468–1476.

52. Leucht S, et al. Comparative efficacy and tolerability of 15 antipsychotic drugs in schizophrenia: a multiple-treatments meta-analysis. *Lancet* 2013; **382**:951–962.

53. Grande I, et al. QTc prolongation: is clozapine safe? Study of 82 cases before and after clozapine treatment. *Human Psychopharmacology* 2011; **26**:397–403.

54. Hong HK, et al. Block of hERG K+ channel and prolongation of action potential duration by fluphenazine at submicromolar concentration. *Eur J Pharmacol* 2013; **702**:165–173.

55. Vieweg WV, et al. Risperidone, QTc interval prolongation, and torsade de pointes: a systematic review of case reports. *Psychopharmacology* 2013; **228**:515–524.

56. Suzuki Y, et al. QT prolongation of the antipsychotic risperidone is predominantly related to its 9-hydroxy metabolite paliperidone. *HumPsychopharmacol* 2012; **27**:39–42.

57. Polcwiartek C, et al. The cardiac safety of aripiprazole treatment in patients at high risk for torsade: a systematic review with a meta-analytic approach. *Psychopharmacology* 2015; **232**:3297–3308.

58. Danielsson B, et al. Antidepressants and antipsychotics classified with torsades de pointes arrhythmia risk and mortality in older adults – a Swedish nationwide study. *Br J Clin Pharmacol* 2016; **81**:773–783.

59. Citrome L. Cariprazine in schizophrenia: clinical efficacy, tolerability, and place in therapy. *Adv Ther* 2013; **30**:114–126.

60. Das S, et al. Brexpiprazole: so far so good. *Ther Adv Psychopharmacol* 2016; **6**:39–54.

61. Meyer JM, et al. Lurasidone: a new drug in development for schizophrenia. *Expert Opinion on Investigational Drugs* 2009; **18**:1715–1726.

62. Nelson S, et al. Torsades de pointes after administration of low-dose aripiprazole. *AnnPharmacother* 2013; **47**:e11.

63. Hategan A, et al. Aripiprazole-associated QTc prolongation in a geriatric patient. *J Clin Psychopharmacol* 2014; **34**:766–768.

64. Suzuki Y, et al. Dose-dependent increase in the QTc interval in aripiprazole treatment after risperidone. *Prog Neuropsychopharmacol Biol Psychiatry* 2011; **35**:643–644.

65. Raschi E, et al. The contribution of national spontaneous reporting systems to detect signals of torsadogenicity: issues emerging from the ARITMO project. *Drug Saf* 2016; **39**:59–68.

66. Belmonte C, et al. Evaluation of the relationship between pharmacokinetics and the safety of aripiprazole and its cardiovascular effects in healthy volunteers. *J Clin Psychopharmacol* 2016; **36**:608–614.

67. Germano E, et al. ECG parameters in children and adolescents treated with aripiprazole and risperidone. *Prog Neuropsychopharmacol Biol Psychiatry* 2014; **51**:23–27.

68. Su KP, et al. Olanzapine-induced QTc prolongation in a patient with Wolff-Parkinson-White syndrome. *Schizophr Res* 2004; **66**:191–192.

69. Morissette P, et al. Olanzapine prolongs cardiac repolarization by blocking the rapid component of the delayed rectifier potassium current. *Journal of Psychopharmacology* 2007; **21**:735–741.

70. Bar KJ, et al. Influence of olanzapine on QT variability and complexity measures of heart rate in patients with schizophrenia. *J Clin Psychopharmacol* 2008; **28**:694–698.

71. Berling I, et al. Prolonged QT risk assessment in antipsychotic overdose using the qt nomogram. *Ann Emerg Med* 2015; **66**:154–164.

72. Jensen KG, et al. Corrected QT changes during antipsychotic treatment of children and adolescents: a systematic review and meta-analysis of clinical trials. *J Am Acad Child Adolesc Psychiatry* 2015; **54**:25–36.

73. Karz AJ, et al. Effects of aripiprazole on the QTc: a case report. *J Clin Psychiatry* 2015; **76**:1648–1649.

74. Friedrich ME, et al. Cardiovascular adverse reactions during antipsychotic treatment: results of AMSP, a drug surveillance program between 1993 and 2013. *Int J Neuropsychopharmacol* 2020; **23**:67–75.

75. Sunovion Pharmaceuticals Inc. Highlights of Prescribing Information: LATUDA (lurasidone hydrochloride) tablets. 2019; http://www.latuda.com/LatudaPrescribingInformation.pdf.

76. Potkin SG, et al. Double-blind comparison of the safety and efficacy of lurasidone and ziprasidone in clinically stable outpatients with schizophrenia or schizoaffective disorder. *Schizophr Res* 2011; **132**:101–107.

77. Nakamura M, et al. Lurasidone in the treatment of acute schizophrenia: a double-blind, placebo-controlled trial. *J Clin Psychiatry* 2009; **70**:829–836.

78. Meltzer HY, et al. Lurasidone in the treatment of schizophrenia: a randomized, double-blind, placebo- and olanzapine-controlled study. *Am J Psychiatry* 2011; **168**:957–967.

79. Hasnain M, et al. Quetiapine, QTc interval prolongation, and torsade de pointes: a review of case reports. *Ther Adv Psychopharmacol* 2014; **4**:130–138.

80. Hatta K, et al. Prolonged QT interval in acute psychotic patients. *Psychiatry Res* 2000; **94**:279–285.

81. Priori SG, et al. Low penetrance in the long-QT syndrome: clinical impact. *Circulation* 1999; **99**:529–533.

82. Frassati D, et al. Hidden cardiac lesions and psychotropic drugs as a possible cause of sudden death in psychiatric patients: a report of 14 cases and review of the literature. *Can J Psychiatry* 2004; **49**:100–105.

抗精神病药对血脂的影响

精神分裂症患者中心血管病的患病率和死亡率高于普通人群[1]。血脂异常与肥胖、高血压、吸烟、糖尿病及久坐不动的生活方式一样,均是明确的心血管病危险因素。高密度脂蛋白(HDL)的降低和甘油三酯的升高均包含在代谢综合征的定义中[2]。大部分精神分裂症患者都具有数种上述危险因素,可被视为心血管病的高危人群。血脂异常是可以治疗的,已知对其进行干预可降低患病率和死亡率[3]。积极治疗对糖尿病患者非常重要,在精神分裂症患者中,糖尿病的发病率比普通人群高 2~3 倍。

抗精神病药对血脂的影响

不同抗精神病药对总胆固醇、低密度脂蛋白(LDL)、HDL 以及甘油三酯的影响不尽相同[4]。在一代抗精神病药当中,吩噻嗪类药物能升高甘油三酯及低密度脂蛋白(LDL),降低高 HDL[5],但是具体的影响却很难被量化[6]。氟哌啶醇似乎对血脂水平影响很小[5]。尽管第二代抗精神病药对血脂影响的数据相对较多,但它们源自不同的出处,报告方式也不尽相同,所以很难直接比较这些药物。这些药物虽然也会升高胆固醇水平,但是对甘油三酯的影响最大。甘油三酯升高通常与肥胖及糖尿病相关。从现有数据可知,氯氮平和奥氮平[4,7]对血脂水平的影响最大,而喹硫平、利培酮次之[8,9]。阿立哌唑、鲁拉西酮和齐拉西酮对血脂的影响最小[4,7,10-15],并且有可能轻度逆转既往使用抗精神病药所致的血脂异常[14,16,17]。卡利拉嗪、依匹哌唑对血脂的影响似乎也相对不大[4,18-21]。伊潘立酮可引起体重增加,但并不导致胆固醇和甘油三酯同等升高[4,22,23]。早期的 RCT 研究提示,与安慰剂相比,短期使用卢美哌隆不会导致胆固醇和甘油三酯升高[24]。

奥氮平

奥氮平在短期(12 周)和中期(16 周)内可使甘油三酯水平升高 40%[25,26]。血脂继续升高长达一年[27]。高达 2/3 使用奥氮平的患者出现甘油三酯升高[28],但仅有 10% 发生严重的高甘油三酯血症[29]。尽管奥氮平所致的体重增加通常都与胆固醇[26,30]及甘油三酯[29]的升高有关,但严重的高甘油三酯血症可独立于体重增加而发生[29]。在一项研究中,使用奥氮平或利培酮治疗的患者体重增加的程度相似,但奥氮平组(105mg/dL)的血清甘油三酯水平是利培酮组(32mg/dL)的 4 倍[31]。喹硫平[32]似乎比奥氮平对血脂的影响较小一些,但是数据存在冲突[33]。

一项英国的病例对照研究显示,用奥氮平治疗的精神分裂症患者出现高脂血症的可能性较不用抗精神病药者高出 5 倍,较使用第一代抗精神病药治疗的患者高 3 倍[34]。与未服药或服用第一代抗精神病药相比,利培酮治疗与高脂血症增加无显著相关性。

氯氮平

经过 5 年的氯氮平治疗后,患者的平均甘油三酯水平将会翻倍,而胆固醇水平也至少升高 10%[35]。使用氯氮平治疗的患者甘油三酯升高的程度几乎是使用第一代抗精神病药患者的两倍[36,37]。胆固醇水平也同样升高[7]。

对于肥胖、糖尿病或已有高脂血症的患者,处方氯氮平或奥氮平前需要特别慎重[38]。

筛查与监测

所有的患者需在基线、换用新抗精神病药治疗 3 个月后化验血脂,此后每年复查一次。使用氯氮平或奥氮平的患者,最好在治疗的第一年每 3 个月化验一次血脂,之后每年复查一次。短期内胆固醇不太可能出现具有临床意义的改变,但是甘油三酯可明显增加[39]。实际上,无论处方的是何种药物或诊断如何,血脂异常在长期使用抗精神病药的患者中十分广泛[40-42]。筛查这些潜在的严重药物不良反应在临床实践中还不是常规的[43],但这是 NICE 强烈推荐的[44]。

严重的甘油三酯血症(空腹水平 >5mmol/L)是胰腺炎的危险因素。请注意,抗精神病药所致的血脂异常可独立于体重增加而发生[45]。

血脂异常的治疗

胆固醇水平升高的患者可从改善饮食结构、改变生活方式或使用他汀类药物治疗中获益[46,47]。在这一患者群体中,他汀类药物治疗是有效的,但也可能存在药物相互作用[48]。对高胆固醇血症进行系统性诊断和治疗的大纲已被制定[49],其依据是 NICE 指南[50]。另外,《英国国家处方手册》中可见相关的风险表格及治疗指南。有证据表明,当高危患者[51]的血清胆固醇水平达到 4mmol/L 时就应开始治疗,该浓度也是 NICE 关于心血管事件二级预防的上限水平[52]。NICE 并未提出明确的一级预防的目标水平,但近期建议对于 10 年内罹患心血管病风险大于 10% 的人群,均应使用他汀类药物治疗[52]。将胆固醇水平降至 3.5mmol/L 以下,能够使得冠心病或卒中的风险减低 1/3。当仅有甘油三酯升高时,减少饱和脂肪的摄入、食用鱼油和贝特类药物都是有效的治疗手段[27,53,54],但是没有证据表明这些能减低死亡率。这些患者同时也需要进行糖耐量的检查及糖尿病的筛查。

若在抗精神病药治疗期间患者出现了中、重度血脂异常,首先应考虑换用对血脂影响较小的药物。尽管不作为难治性患者的推荐策略,但氯氮平所致的高脂血症可在换用利培酮后得到改善[55]。也许换用其他药物也能达到同样的效果,但对此缺乏相关的数据[56]。对于抗精神病药所致的血脂异常,D_2 受体部分激动剂,如阿立哌唑(在英国之外,还可选择卢美哌隆和齐拉西酮)是现有情况下的换药选择[17,57]。有证据提示,在使用氯氮平或奥氮平时,合用阿立哌唑可能降低胆固醇和甘油三酯水平[16,47,58];使用抗精神病药治疗时,合用二甲双胍可改善总胆固醇和甘油三酯水平[47,59]。(见英国精神药理协会治疗指南[47]相关章节关于上述两种方法利弊的讨论)

小结

监测药物	推荐监测方法
氯氮平 奥氮平	基线查空腹血脂,之后每 3 个月复查,1 年后每年复查
其他抗精神病药	在基线和 3 个月时检测血脂,之后每年复查[57]

参考文献

1. Brown S, et al. Causes of the excess mortality of schizophrenia. *Br J Psychiatry* 2000; 177:212–217.
2. Alberti KG, et al. The metabolic syndrome–a new worldwide definition. *Lancet* 2005; 366:1059–1062.
3. Durrington P. Dyslipidaemia. *Lancet* 2003; 362:717–731.
4. Pillinger T, et al. Comparative effects of 18 antipsychotics on metabolic function in patients with schizophrenia, predictors of metabolic dysregulation, and association with psychopathology: a systematic review and network meta-analysis. *Lancet Psychiatry* 2020; 7:64–77.
5. Sasaki J, et al. Lipids and apolipoproteins in patients treated with major tranquilizers. *Clin Pharmacol Ther* 1985; 37:684–687.
6. Henkin Y, et al. Secondary dyslipidemia: inadvertent effects of drugs in clinical practice. *JAMA* 1992; 267:961–968.
7. Chaggar PS, et al. Effect of antipsychotic medications on glucose and lipid levels. *J Clin Pharmacol* 2011; 51:631–638.
8. Smith RC, et al. Effects of olanzapine and risperidone on lipid metabolism in chronic schizophrenic patients with long-term antipsychotic treatment: a randomized five month study. *Schizophr Res* 2010; 120:204–209.
9. Perez-Iglesias R, et al. Glucose and lipid disturbances after 1 year of antipsychotic treatment in a drug-naive population. *Schizophr Res* 2009; 107:115–121.
10. Olfson M, et al. Hyperlipidemia following treatment with antipsychotic medications. *Am J Psychiatry* 2006; 163:1821–1825.
11. L'Italien GJ, et al. Comparison of metabolic syndrome incidence among schizophrenia patients treated with aripiprazole versus olanzapine or placebo. *J Clin Psychiatry* 2007; 68:1510–1516.
12. Fenton WS, et al. Medication-induced weight gain and dyslipidemia in patients with schizophrenia. *Am J Psychiatry* 2006; 163:1697–1704.
13. Meyer JM, et al. Change in metabolic syndrome parameters with antipsychotic treatment in the CATIE Schizophrenia Trial: prospective data from phase 1. *Schizophr Res* 2008; 101:273–286.
14. Potkin SG, et al. Double-blind comparison of the safety and efficacy of lurasidone and ziprasidone in clinically stable outpatients with schizophrenia or schizoaffective disorder. *Schizophr Res* 2011; 132:101–107.
15. Correll CU, et al. Long-term safety and effectiveness of lurasidone in schizophrenia: a 22-month, open-label extension study. *CNS Spectr* 2016; 21:393–402.
16. Fleischhacker WW, et al. Effects of adjunctive treatment with aripiprazole on body weight and clinical efficacy in schizophrenia patients treated with clozapine: a randomized, double-blind, placebo-controlled trial. *Int J Neuropsychopharmacol* 2010; 13:1115–1125.
17. Chen Y, et al. Comparative effectiveness of switching antipsychotic drug treatment to aripiprazole or ziprasidone for improving metabolic profile and atherogenic dyslipidemia: a 12-month, prospective, open-label study. *J Psychopharmacol* 2012; 26:1201–1210.
18. Lao KS, et al. Tolerability and safety profile of cariprazine in treating psychotic disorders, bipolar disorder and major depressive disorder: a systematic review with meta-analysis of randomized controlled trials. *CNS Drugs* 2016; 30:1043–1054.
19. Earley W, et al. Tolerability of cariprazine in the treatment of acute bipolar I mania: a pooled post hoc analysis of 3 phase II/III studies. *J Affect Disord* 2017; 215:205–212.
20. McEvoy J, et al. Brexpiprazole for the treatment of schizophrenia: a review of this novel serotonin-dopamine activity modulator. *Clin Schizophr Relat Psychoses* 2016; 9:177–186.
21. Correll CU, et al. Efficacy and safety of brexpiprazole for the treatment of acute schizophrenia: a 6-week randomized, double-blind, placebo-controlled trial. *Am J Psychiatry* 2015; 172:870–880.
22. Citrome L. Iloperidone: chemistry, pharmacodynamics, pharmacokinetics and metabolism, clinical efficacy, safety and tolerability, regulatory affairs, and an opinion. *Expert Opin Drug Metab Toxicol* 2010; 6:1551–1564.
23. Cutler AJ, et al. Long-term safety and tolerability of iloperidone: results from a 25-week, open-label extension trial. *CNS Spectr* 2013; 18:43–54.
24. Correll CU, et al. Efficacy and safety of lumateperone for treatment of schizophrenia: a randomized clinical trial. *JAMA Psychiatry* 2020; 77:349–358.
25. Sheitman BB, et al. Olanzapine-induced elevation of plasma triglyceride levels. *Am J Psychiatry* 1999; 156:1471–1472.
26. Osser DN, et al. Olanzapine increases weight and serum triglyceride levels. *J Clin Psychiatry* 1999; 60:767–770.
27. Meyer JM. Effects of atypical antipsychotics on weight and serum lipid levels. *J Clin Psychiatry* 2001; 62 Suppl 27:27–34.
28. Melkersson KI, et al. Elevated levels of insulin, leptin, and blood lipids in olanzapine-treated patients with schizophrenia or related psychoses. *J Clin Psychiatry* 2000; 61:742–749.
29. Meyer JM. Novel antipsychotics and severe hyperlipidemia. *J Clin Psychopharmacol* 2001; 21:369–374.
30. Kinon BJ, et al. Long-term olanzapine treatment: weight change and weight-related health factors in schizophrenia. *J Clin Psychiatry* 2001; 62:92–100.
31. Meyer JM. A retrospective comparison of weight, lipid, and glucose changes between risperidone- and olanzapine-treated inpatients: metabolic outcomes after 1 year. *J Clin Psychiatry* 2002; 63:425–433.
32. Atmaca M, et al. Serum leptin and triglyceride levels in patients on treatment with atypical antipsychotics. *J Clin Psychiatry* 2003; 64:598–604.
33. De Leon J, et al. A clinical study of the association of antipsychotics with hyperlipidemia. *Schizophr Res* 2007; 92:95–102.
34. Koro CE, et al. An assessment of the independent effects of olanzapine and risperidone exposure on the risk of hyperlipidemia in schizophrenic patients. *Arch Gen Psychiatry* 2002; 59:1021–1026.
35. Henderson DC, et al. Clozapine, diabetes mellitus, weight gain, and lipid abnormalities: a five-year naturalistic study. *Am J Psychiatry* 2000; 157:975–981.
36. Ghaeli P, et al. Serum triglyceride levels in patients treated with clozapine. *Am J Health Syst Pharm* 1996; 53:2079–2081.

37. Spivak B, et al. Diminished suicidal and aggressive behavior, high plasma norepinephrine levels, and serum triglyceride levels in chronic neuroleptic-resistant schizophrenic patients maintained on clozapine. *Clin Neuropharmacol* 1998; **21**:245–250.

38. Baptista T, et al. Novel antipsychotics and severe hyperlipidemia: comments on the Meyer paper. *J Clin Psychopharmacol* 2002; **22**:536–537.

39. Meyer JM, et al. The effects of antipsychotic therapy on serum lipids: a comprehensive review. *Schizophr Res* 2004; **70**:1–17.

40. Paton C, et al. Obesity, dyslipidaemias and smoking in an inpatient population treated with antipsychotic drugs. *Acta Psychiatr Scand* 2004; **110**:299–305.

41. De Hert M, et al. The METEOR study of diabetes and other metabolic disorders in patients with schizophrenia treated with antipsychotic drugs. I. Methodology. *Int J Methods Psychiatr Res* 2010; **19**:195–210.

42. Jin H, et al. Comparison of longer-term safety and effectiveness of 4 atypical antipsychotics in patients over age 40: a trial using equipoise-stratified randomization. *J Clin Psychiatry* 2013; **74**:10–18.

43. Barnes TR, et al. Screening for the metabolic side effects of antipsychotic medication: findings of a 6-year quality improvement programme in the UK. *BMJ Open* 2015; **5**:e007633.

44. National Institute for Health and Care Excellence. Psychosis and schizophrenia in adults: prevention and management. Clinical Guidance 178 [CG178]. 2014; https://www.nice.org.uk/guidance/cg178.

45. Birkenaes AB, et al. Dyslipidemia independent of body mass in antipsychotic-treated patients under real-life conditions. *J Clin Psychopharmacol* 2008; **28**:132–137.

46. Ojala K, et al. Statins are effective in treating dyslipidemia among psychiatric patients using second-generation antipsychotic agents. *J Psychopharmacol* 2008; **22**:33–38.

47. Cooper SJ, et al. BAP guidelines on the management of weight gain, metabolic disturbances and cardiovascular risk associated with psychosis and antipsychotic drug treatment. *J Psychopharmacol* 2016; **30**:717–748.

48. Tse L, et al. Pharmacological treatment of antipsychotic-induced dyslipidemia and hypertension. *Int Clin Psychopharmacol* 2014; **29**:125–137.

49. Ryan A, et al. Dyslipidaemia and cardiovascular risk. *BMJ* 2018; **360**:k835.

50. Rabar S, et al. Lipid modification and cardiovascular risk assessment for the primary and secondary prevention of cardiovascular disease: summary of updated NICE guidance. *BMJ* 2014; **349**:g4356.

51. Group HPSC. MRC/BHF Heart Protection Study of cholesterol lowering with simvastatin in 20,536 high-risk individuals: a randomised placebo-controlled trial. *Lancet* 2002; **360**:7–22.

52. National Institute for Health and Care Excellence. Cardiovascular disease: risk assessment and reduction, including lipid modification. Clinical guideline [CG181] 2014 (Last updated 2016); https://www.nice.org.uk/Guidance/CG181.

53. Caniato RN, et al. Effect of omega-3 fatty acids on the lipid profile of patients taking clozapine. *Aust N Z J Psychiatry* 2006; **40**:691–697.

54. Freeman MP, et al. Omega-3 fatty acids for atypical antipsychotic-associated hypertriglyceridemia. *Ann Clin Psychiatry* 2015; **27**:197–202.

55. Ghaeli P, et al. Elevated serum triglycerides with clozapine resolved with risperidone in four patients. *Pharmacotherapy* 1999; **19**:1099–1101.

56. Weiden PJ. Switching antipsychotics as a treatment strategy for antipsychotic-induced weight gain and dyslipidemia. *J Clin Psychiatry* 2007; **68 Suppl 4**:34–39.

57. Newcomer JW, et al. A multicenter, randomized, double-blind study of the effects of aripiprazole in overweight subjects with schizophrenia or schizoaffective disorder switched from olanzapine. *J Clin Psychiatry* 2008; **69**:1046–1056.

58. Henderson DC, et al. Aripiprazole added to overweight and obese olanzapine-treated schizophrenia patients. *J Clin Psychopharmacol* 2009; **29**:165–169.

59. Jiang WL, et al. Adjunctive metformin for antipsychotic-induced dyslipidemia: a meta-analysis of randomized, double-blind, placebo-controlled trials. *Trans Psychiatry* 2020; **10**:117.

糖尿病与糖耐量异常

精神分裂症

精神分裂症患者发生胰岛素抵抗和糖尿病的概率相对较高[1-2]，并且这种现象在抗精神病药问世及广泛使用前就存在[3-5]。生活方式干预（减轻体重、增加运动）能有效地预防糖尿病的发生[6,7]，并适合所有精神分裂症患者使用。

抗精神病药

有关糖尿病和抗精神病药的研究资料非常多，但不尽完美[8-12]。主要问题是关于糖尿病的发病率与患病率的研究假定糖尿病筛查是全面的或者统一的，但是在临床实践中不可能做到[7]。许多研究没有说明影响糖尿病的其他危险因素[11]。因此药物之间的微小差异很难证实，但也可能这种差异根本就不重要：接受抗精神病药治疗的所有精神分裂症患者患糖尿病的风险均可能增加。

关于抗精神病药引起糖尿病的机制尚不明确，可能包括 $5HT_{2A}/5HT_{2C}$ 的拮抗、高血脂、体重增加及瘦素抵抗[13]。出现胰岛素抵抗可不伴有体重增加[14]。

第一代抗精神病药

很久以前就发现吩噻嗪类衍生物与糖耐量异常和糖尿病相关[15]。随着第一代抗精神病药的出现和广泛使用，糖尿病的患病率明显增加[16]。脂肪胺类吩噻嗪药物糖耐量异常的发生率要高于氟奋乃静和氟哌啶醇[17]。有研究报道其他第一代抗精神病药（如洛沙平）可引起高血糖[18]，有些资料证实氟哌啶醇与高血糖有关[19]。一些研究甚至表明，第一代和第二代抗精神病药引起糖尿病的倾向性没有差异[20,21]；而其他数据表明，在使用第二代抗精神病药的患者中，糖尿病的发生率轻度升高，且有统计学意义[22]。

第二代抗精神病药

氯氮平

氯氮平与高血糖、糖耐量异常、糖尿病酮症酸中毒明显相关[23]。有研究发现，服用氯氮平的精神分裂症患者，尤其是年轻患者，与服用其他第二代或第一代抗精神病药者相比，患糖尿病的风险性似乎更高[24-27]，但是也有不一致的报道[28,29]。

多达 1/3 的精神分裂症患者在治疗 5 年后可能发展为糖尿病[30]。很多病例在治疗的头 6 个月出现，也有些在治疗一月内发生[31]，有一部分仅在治疗多年后出现[29]。因酮症酸中毒而死亡的病例也有报道[31]。虽然肥胖、糖尿病家族史等因素明显地增加了服用氯氮平的精神分裂症患者患糖尿病的风险[33]，但是氯氮平引起的糖尿病未必与这些因素有关[23,32]。

氯氮平可升高胰岛素水平，其程度取决于氯氮平浓度[34,35]。在葡萄糖耐量试验中，氯氮平升高血糖和胰岛素水平的可能性大于第一代抗精神病药[36]。对于服用氯氮平的精神分裂症患者，因为糖尿病的患病率高，要常规进行糖尿病检测[37]。

奥氮平

与氯氮平类似,奥氮平也可引起糖耐量异常、糖尿病及糖尿病酮症酸中毒[38]。奥氮平与氯氮平可直接引起胰岛素抵抗[39,40]。与服用第一代抗精神病药的精神分裂症患者相比,尤其是年轻患者[25],服用奥氮平患糖尿病的风险性更高[41]。服用奥氮平的精神分裂症患者发展为糖尿病的时间还不明确,但出现糖耐量异常可不伴有肥胖及糖尿病家族史[23,32]。与利培酮相比,奥氮平引起糖尿病的可能性更大[42-46]。在葡萄糖耐量试验中,奥氮平升高血糖和胰岛素水平的幅度高于第一代抗精神病药[36,47]。

利培酮

有研究发现(主要是病例报道),利培酮与糖耐量异常[48]、糖尿病[49]及酮症酸中毒[50]发生有关。利培酮引起上述不良反应的病例报道要明显少于氯氮平或奥氮平[51]。至少有一项研究发现,利培酮引起的空腹血糖改变要明显少于奥氮平,但也有一些研究发现这两种药物间无差异[52]。

虽然 40 岁以下服用利培酮的患者可能患糖尿病的风险升高[25],但利培酮对糖尿病的影响并不大于第一代抗精神病药[25,41,43]。与健康志愿者相比(不是与服用第一代抗精神病药的患者相比),利培酮对空腹血糖及葡萄糖耐量试验后的血糖水平有不良影响[36]。

喹硫平

与利培酮一样,喹硫平与新发糖尿病和酮症酸中毒有关[53-55]。服用喹硫平致上述不良反应的病例报道要明显少于奥氮平或氯氮平。喹硫平与糖尿病的相关性要高于第一代抗精神病药[25,56]。有两项研究表明喹硫平与奥氮平在糖尿病的发生率上无差异[52,57]。喹硫平致糖尿病的风险可能与剂量相关,剂量 400mg/d 以上与糖化血红蛋白(HbA_{1C})的改变明确相关[58]。

其他第二代抗精神病药

氨磺必利不会升高血糖水平[59],且似乎与糖尿病的发生无关[60]。有一例病例报道服用舒必利的患者出现酮症酸中毒[61]。有资料表明阿立哌唑[62-65]与齐拉西酮[66,67]都不会改变体内血糖代谢平衡。阿立哌唑甚至可以改善其他抗精神病药导致的糖尿病[68](但是已有报道阿立哌唑引起酮症酸中毒[69-71])。一项大样本的病例对照研究证实,服用氨磺必利和阿立哌唑都不会增加糖尿病的风险[72]。氨磺必利、阿立哌唑及齐拉西酮三种药物可推荐给有糖尿病病史或糖尿病素质的精神分裂症患者使用,或者替代易致糖尿病的其他抗精神病药。资料表明鲁拉西酮[73,74]与阿塞那平[75,76]都不会影响血糖代谢平衡。同样,依匹哌唑[77]和卡利拉嗪[78,79]的前期数据提示其对糖耐量的影响很小。因此,对于使用氯氮平、奥氮平或喹硫平治疗、伴有前驱期糖尿病或糖尿病的患者,可建议换用其他心血管代谢疾病风险较小的药物,例如阿立哌唑、依匹哌唑、卡利拉嗪、鲁拉西酮或齐拉西酮[80]。

拉西酮似乎对血糖指标没有影响,但这方面临床经验有限[81]。

预测与抗精神病药相关的糖尿病

与老年精神分裂症患者相比(抗精神病药可能不增加老年患者患糖尿病的风险[84]),年轻患者患糖尿病的风险明显升高 [82,83]。当给予各种抗精神病药时,首发精神分裂症患者似乎更易发生糖尿病 [85-87]。在抗精神病药治疗期间,精神分裂症患者体重迅速增加及血浆甘油三酯水平升高似乎能预测糖尿病的发生 [88]。

监测

在西方社会,糖尿病是一个日益严峻的问题,它与肥胖、年龄(老年)、教育水平(低)及某些种族相关性很强 [89,90]。主要因为动脉硬化,糖尿病明显地升高了心血管病的死亡率 [91]。类似地,抗精神病药使用也增加了心血管病的死亡率 [92-94]。因此,降低血糖水平及减少其他危险因素(肥胖、高胆固醇血症)的干预方式是必需的 [95]。

对于服用抗精神病药患者的糖尿病监测方法还未达成共识 [96],而且正式指南中的建议也有很大的变化 [97]。鉴于先前在英国 [8,98-100] 和其他地方 [101] 的糖尿病检测状况比较棘手,关于检测需要做哪些、何时做的争论看来不得要领。现在迫切需要通过各种方法提高监测水平,因此任何糖尿病检测方法都能使用,包括尿糖检测和随机血糖检测(表 1.25)。

在理想的情况下,所有的患者都应该进行口服葡萄糖耐量试验(OGTT),因为它是所有检测方法中最敏感的 [102,103]。空腹血浆葡萄糖(FPG)虽然敏感性差些,但仍然推荐使用 [104]。空腹血糖出现任何异常,均应进行口服葡萄糖耐量试验。

对于急性起病、行为紊乱的患者,空腹化验往往是困难的,因此可进行随机血糖检测或糖化血红蛋白(HbA_{1C})检测(不需要空腹)。糖化血红蛋白检测(HbA_{1C})在诊断和监测糖尿病上被公认为是一种实用的方法 [105]。监测频率取决于患者的身体因素(比如体重增加)及已知的危险因素(比如糖尿病家族史、血脂异常、吸烟)。所有患者至少应每年进行糖尿病检测。另外,应该要求所有患者留意和报告糖尿病的症状和体征(乏力、念珠菌感染、口渴、多尿)。

抗精神病药相关糖尿病的治疗

对糖耐量异常的患者,换用致糖尿病风险低的抗精神病药常常有效。在这方面,最有力的证据是换用阿立哌唑 [106-107],也可以换用齐拉西酮 [107] 或者鲁拉西酮 [74]。此外,建议使用标准的抗糖尿病治疗 [80]。吡格列酮 [108] 在治疗糖尿病方面有特殊优势,但需注意这种药物潜在的肝脏毒性。GLP-1 激动剂,例如利拉鲁肽,也使用得越来越多 [109]。

表 1.25　向服用抗精神病药患者推荐使用的糖尿病监测方法

建议的监测	理想状态	最低要求
基线	OGTT 或 FPG 不能空腹检测时,检测糖化血红蛋白(HbA_{1C})	尿糖 随机血糖
延续	所有药物使用 4~6 个月时,以及之后每 12 个月监测 OGTT 或 FPG+HbA_{1c} 对于氯氮平和奥氮平或者出现任何其他风险:1 个月时监测 OGTT 或 FPG,之后每 4~6 个月监测 为了持续定期筛查,适合做 HbA_{1c} 检测,要注意该检测不适合作为短期变化的检查	每 12 个月监测 UG 或 RPG,并监测症状

FPG,空腹血浆葡萄糖;OGTT,口服葡萄糖耐量试验;RPG,随机血浆葡萄糖。

小结：抗精神病药——糖尿病与糖耐量异常的风险

高风险	氯氮平，奥氮平
中风险	喹硫平，利培酮，吩噻嗪类抗精神病药
低风险	高效价的第一代抗精神病药（比如氟哌啶醇）
极低风险	阿立哌唑，氨磺必利，阿塞那平，依匹哌唑，卡利拉嗪，卢美哌隆，鲁拉西酮，齐拉西酮

参考文献

1. Schimmelbusch WH, et al. The positive correlation between insulin resistance and duration of hospitalization in untreated schizophrenia. *Br J Psychiatry* 1971; **118**:429–436.
2. Waitzkin L. A survey for unknown diabetics in a mental hospital. I. Men under age fifty. *Diabetes* 1966; **15**:97–104.
3. Kasanin J. The blood sugar curve in mental disease. II. The schizophrenia (dementia praecox) groups. *Arch Neurol Psychiatry* 1926; **16**:414–419.
4. Braceland FJ, et al. Delayed action of insulin in schizophrenia. *Am J Psychiatry* 1945; **102**:108–110.
5. Kohen D. Diabetes mellitus and schizophrenia: historical perspective. *Br J Psychiatry Suppl* 2004; **47**:S64–S66.
6. Knowler WC, et al. 10-year follow-up of diabetes incidence and weight loss in the Diabetes Prevention Program Outcomes Study. *Lancet* 2009; **374**:1677–1686.
7. Glechner A, et al. Effects of lifestyle changes on adults with prediabetes: a systematic review and meta-analysis. *Prim Care Diabetes* 2018; **12**:393–408.
8. Taylor D, et al. Testing for diabetes in hospitalised patients prescribed antipsychotic drugs. *Br J Psychiatry* 2004; **185**:152–156.
9. Haddad PM. Antipsychotics and diabetes: review of non-prospective data. *Br J Psychiatry Suppl* 2004; **47**:S80–S86.
10. Bushe C, et al. Association between atypical antipsychotic agents and type 2 diabetes: review of prospective clinical data. *Br J Psychiatry* 2004; **184**:S87–S93.
11. Gianfrancesco F, et al. The influence of study design on the results of pharmacoepidemiologic studies of diabetes risk with antipsychotic therapy. *Ann Clin Psychiatry* 2006; **18**:9–17.
12. Hirigo AT, et al. The magnitude of undiagnosed diabetes and Hypertension among adult psychiatric patients receiving antipsychotic treatment. *Diabetol Metab Syndr* 2020; **12**:79.
13. Buchholz S, et al. Atypical antipsychotic-induced diabetes mellitus: an update on epidemiology and postulated mechanisms. *Intern Med J* 2008; **38**:602–606.
14. Teff KL, et al. Antipsychotic-induced insulin resistance and postprandial hormonal dysregulation independent of weight gain or psychiatric disease. *Diabetes* 2013; **62**:3232–3240.
15. Arneson GA. Phenothiazine derivatives and glucose metabolism. *J Neuropsychiatr* 1964; **5**:181.
16. Lindenmayer JP, et al. Hyperglycemia associated with the use of atypical antipsychotics. *J Clin Psychiatry* 2001; **62 Suppl 23**:30–38.
17. Keskiner A, et al. Psychotropic drugs, diabetes and chronic mental patients. *Psychosomatics* 1973; **14**:176–181.
18. Tollefson G, et al. Nonketotic hyperglycemia associated with loxapine and amoxapine: case report. *J Clin Psychiatry* 1983; **44**:347–348.
19. Lindenmayer JP, et al. Changes in glucose and cholesterol levels in patients with schizophrenia treated with typical or atypical antipsychotics. *Am J Psychiatry* 2003; **160**:290–296.
20. Carlson C, et al. Diabetes mellitus and antipsychotic treatment in the United Kingdom. *Eur Neuropsychopharmacol* 2006; **16**:366–375.
21. Ostbye T, et al. Atypical antipsychotic drugs and diabetes mellitus in a large outpatient population: a retrospective cohort study. *Pharmacoepidemiol Drug Saf* 2005; **14**:407–415.
22. Smith M, et al. First- v. second-generation antipsychotics and risk for diabetes in schizophrenia: systematic review and meta-analysis. *Br J Psychiatry* 2008; **192**:406–411.
23. Mir S, et al. Atypical antipsychotics and hyperglycaemia. *Int Clin Psychopharmacol* 2001; **16**:63–74.
24. Lund BC, et al. Clozapine use in patients with schizophrenia and the risk of diabetes, hyperlipidemia, and hypertension: a claims-based approach. *Arch Gen Psychiatry* 2001; **58**:1172–1176.
25. Sernyak MJ, et al. Association of diabetes mellitus with use of atypical neuroleptics in the treatment of schizophrenia. *Am J Psychiatry* 2002; **159**:561–566.
26. Gianfrancesco FD, et al. Differential effects of risperidone, olanzapine, clozapine, and conventional antipsychotics on type 2 diabetes: findings from a large health plan database. *J Clin Psychiatry* 2002; **63**:920–930.
27. Guo JJ, et al. Risk of diabetes mellitus associated with atypical antipsychotic use among patients with bipolar disorder: a retrospective, population-based, case-control study. *J Clin Psychiatry* 2006; **67**:1055–1061.
28. Wang PS, et al. Clozapine use and risk of diabetes mellitus. *J Clin Psychopharmacol* 2002; **22**:236–243.
29. Sumiyoshi T, et al. A comparison of incidence of diabetes mellitus between atypical antipsychotic drugs: a survey for clozapine, risperidone, olanzapine, and quetiapine (Letter). *J Clin Psychopharmacol* 2004; **24**:345–348.
30. Henderson DC, et al. Clozapine, diabetes mellitus, weight gain, and lipid abnormalities: a five-year naturalistic study. *Am J Psychiatry* 2000;

157:975–981.

31. Koller E, et al. Clozapine-associated diabetes. *Am J Med* 2001; 111:716–723.

32. Sumiyoshi T, et al. The effect of hypertension and obesity on the development of diabetes mellitus in patients treated with atypical antipsychotic drugs (Letter). *J Clin Psychopharmacol* 2004; 24:452–454.

33. Zhang R, et al. The prevalence and clinical-demographic correlates of diabetes mellitus in chronic schizophrenic pauents receiving clozapine. *Human Psychopharmacology* 2011; 26:392–396.

34. Melkersson KI, et al. Different influences of classical antipsychotics and clozapine on glucose-insulin homeostasis in patients with schizophrenia or related psychoses. *J Clin Psychiatry* 1999; 60:783–791.

35. Melkersson K. Clozapine and olanzapine, but not conventional antipsychotics, increase insulin release in vitro. *Eur Neuropsychopharmacol* 2004; 14:115–119.

36. Newcomer JW, et al. Abnormalities in glucose regulation during antipsychotic treatment of schizophrenia. *Arch Gen Psychiatry* 2002; 59:337–345.

37. Lamberti JS, et al. Diabetes mellitus among outpatients receiving clozapine: prevalence and clinical-demographic correlates. *J Clin Psychiatry* 2005; 66:900–906.

38. Wirshing DA, et al. Novel antipsychotics and new onset diabetes. *Biol Psychiatry* 1998; 44:778–783.

39. Engl J, et al. Olanzapine impairs glycogen synthesis and insulin signaling in L6 skeletal muscle cells. *Mol Psychiatry* 2005; 10:1089–1096.

40. Vestri HS, et al. Atypical antipsychotic drugs directly impair insulin action in adipocytes: effects on glucose transport, lipogenesis, and antilipolysis. *Neuropsychopharmacology* 2007; 32:765–772.

41. Koro CE, et al. Assessment of independent effect of olanzapine and risperidone on risk of diabetes among patients with schizophrenia: population based nested case-control study. *BMJ* 2002; 325:243.

42. Meyer JM. A retrospective comparison of weight, lipid, and glucose changes between risperidone- and olanzapine-treated inpatients: metabolic outcomes after 1 year. *J Clin Psychiatry* 2002; 63:425–433.

43. Gianfrancesco F, et al. Antipsychotic-induced type 2 diabetes: evidence from a large health plan database. *J Clin Psychopharmacol* 2003; 23:328–335.

44. Leslie DL, et al. Incidence of newly diagnosed diabetes attributable to atypical antipsychotic medications. *Am J Psychiatry* 2004; 161:1709–1711.

45. Duncan E, et al. Relative risk of glucose elevation during antipsychotic exposure in a Veterans Administration population. *Int Clin Psychopharmacol* 2007; 22:1–11.

46. Meyer JM, et al. Change in metabolic syndrome parameters with antipsychotic treatment in the CATIE Schizophrenia Trial: prospective data from phase 1. *Schizophr Res* 2008; 101:273–286.

47. Ebenbichler CF, et al. Olanzapine induces insulin resistance: results from a prospective study. *J Clin Psychiatry* 2003; 64:1436–1439.

48. Mallya A, et al. Resolution of hyperglycemia on risperidone discontinuation: a case report. *J Clin Psychiatry* 2002; 63:453–454.

49. Wirshing DA, et al. Risperidone-associated new-onset diabetes. *Biol Psychiatry* 2001; 50:148–149.

50. Croarkin PE, et al. Diabetic ketoacidosis associated with risperidone treatment? *Psychosomatics* 2000; 41:369–370.

51. Koller EA, et al. Risperidone-associated diabetes mellitus: a pharmacovigilance study. *Pharmacotherapy* 2003; 23:735–744.

52. Lambert BL, et al. Diabetes risk associated with use of olanzapine, quetiapine, and risperidone in veterans health administration patients with schizophrenia. *Am J Epidemiol* 2006; 164:672–681.

53. Henderson DC. Atypical antipsychotic-induced diabetes mellitus: how strong is the evidence? *CNS Drugs* 2002; 16:77–89.

54. Koller EA, et al. A survey of reports of quetiapine-associated hyperglycemia and diabetes mellitus. *J Clin Psychiatry* 2004; 65:857–863.

55. Nanasawa H, et al. Development of diabetes mellitus associated with quetiapine: a case series. *Medicine* 2017; 96:e5900.

56. Citrome L, et al. Relationship between antipsychotic medication treatment and new cases of diabetes among psychiatric inpatients. *Psychiatr Serv* 2004; 55:1006–1013.

57. Bushe C, et al. Comparison of metabolic and prolactin variables from a six-month randomised trial of olanzapine and quetiapine in schizophrenia. *J Psychopharmacology* 2010; 24:1001–1009.

58. Guo Z, et al. A real-world data analysis of dose effect of second-generation antipsychotic therapy on hemoglobin A1C level. *Prog Neuropsychopharmacol Biol Psychiatry* 2011; 35:1326–1332.

59. Vanelle JM, et al. A double-blind randomised comparative trial of amisulpride versus olanzapine for 2 months in the treatment of subjects with schizophrenia and comorbid depression. *Eur Psychiatry* 2006; 21:523–530.

60. De Hert MA, et al. Prevalence of the metabolic syndrome in patients with schizophrenia treated with antipsychotic medication. *Schizophr Res* 2006; 83:87–93.

61. Toprak O, et al. New-onset type II diabetes mellitus, hyperosmolar non-ketotic coma, rhabdomyolysis and acute renal failure in a patient treated with sulpiride. *Nephrol Dial Transplant* 2005; 20:662–663.

62. Keck PE, Jr., et al. Aripiprazole: a partial dopamine D2 receptor agonist antipsychotic. *Exp Opin Investig Drugs* 2003; 12:655–662.

63. Pigott TA, et al. Aripiprazole for the prevention of relapse in stabilized patients with chronic schizophrenia: a placebo-controlled 26-week study. *J Clin Psychiatry* 2003; 64:1048–1056.

64. Van WR, et al. Major changes in glucose metabolism, including new-onset diabetes, within 3 months after initiation of or switch to atypical antipsychotic medication in patients with schizophrenia and schizoaffective disorder. *J Clin Psychiatry* 2008; 69:472–479.

65. Baker RA, et al. Atypical antipsychotic drugs and diabetes mellitus in the US Food and Drug Administration Adverse Event Database: a Systematic Bayesian Signal Detection Analysis. *Psychopharmacol Bull* 2009; 42:11–31.

66. Simpson GM, et al. Randomized, controlled, double-blind multicenter comparison of the efficacy and tolerability of ziprasidone and olanzapine in acutely ill inpatients with schizophrenia or schizoaffective disorder. *Am J Psychiatry* 2004; 161:1837–1847.

67. Sacher J, et al. Effects of olanzapine and ziprasidone on glucose tolerance in healthy volunteers. *Neuropsychopharmacology* 2008;

33:1633–1641.

68. De Hert M, et al. A case series: evaluation of the metabolic safety of aripiprazole. *Schizophr Bull* 2007; 33:823–830.

69. Church CO, et al. Diabetic ketoacidosis associated with aripiprazole. *Diabet Med* 2005; 22:1440–1443.

70. Reddymasu S, et al. Elevated lipase and diabetic ketoacidosis associated with aripiprazole. *J Pancreas* 2006; 7:303–305.

71. Campanella LM, et al. Severe hyperglycemic hyperosmolar nonketotic coma in a nondiabetic patient receiving aripiprazole. *Ann Emerg Med* 2009; 53:264–266.

72. Kessing LV, et al. Treatment with antipsychotics and the risk of diabetes in clinical practice. *Br J Psychiatry* 2010; 197:266–271.

73. McEvoy JP, et al. Effectiveness of lurasidone in patients with schizophrenia or schizoaffective disorder switched from other antipsychotics: a randomized, 6-week, open-label study. *J Clin Psychiatry* 2013; 74:170–179.

74. Stahl SM, et al. Effectiveness of lurasidone for patients with schizophrenia following 6 weeks of acute treatment with lurasidone, olanzapine, or placebo: a 6-month, open-label, extension study. *J Clin Psychiatry* 2013; 74:507–515.

75. McIntyre RS, et al. Asenapine for long-term treatment of bipolar disorder: a double-blind 40-week extension study. *J Affect Disord* 2010; 126:358–365.

76. McIntyre RS, et al. Asenapine versus olanzapine in acute mania: a double-blind extension study. *Bipolar Disorders* 2009; 11:815–826.

77. Garnock-Jones KP. Brexpiprazole: a review in schizophrenia. *CNS Drugs* 2016; 30:335–342.

78. Lao KS, et al. Tolerability and safety profile of cariprazine in treating psychotic disorders, bipolar disorder and major depressive disorder: a systematic review with meta-analysis of randomized controlled trials. *CNS Drugs* 2016; 30:1043–1054.

79. Earley W, et al. Tolerability of cariprazine in the treatment of acute bipolar I mania: a pooled post hoc analysis of 3 phase II/III studies. *J Affect Disord* 2017; 215:205–212.

80. Cernea S, et al. Pharmacological management of glucose dysregulation in patients treated with second-generation antipsychotics. *Drugs* 2020; 80:1763–1781.

81. Correll CU, et al. Efficacy and safety of lumateperone for treatment of schizophrenia: a randomized clinical trial. *JAMA Psychiatry* 2020; 77:349–358.

82. Hammerman A, et al. Antipsychotics and diabetes: an age-related association. *Ann Pharmacother* 2008; 42:1316–1322.

83. Galling B, et al. Type 2 diabetes mellitus in youth exposed to antipsychotics: a systematic review and meta-analysis. *JAMA Psychiatry* 2016; 73:247–259.

84. Albert SG, et al. Atypical antipsychotics and the risk of diabetes in an elderly population in long-term care: a retrospective nursing home chart review study. *J Am Med Dir Assoc* 2009; 10:115–119.

85. De Hert M, et al. Typical and atypical antipsychotics differentially affect long-term incidence rates of the metabolic syndrome in first-episode patients with schizophrenia: a retrospective chart review. *Schizophr Res* 2008; 101:295–303.

86. Saddichha S, et al. Metabolic syndrome in first episode schizophrenia – a randomized double-blind controlled, short-term prospective study. *Schizophr Res* 2008; 101:266–272.

87. Saddichha S, et al. Diabetes and schizophrenia – effect of disease or drug? Results from a randomized, double-blind, controlled prospective study in first-episode schizophrenia. *Acta Psychiatr Scand* 2008; 117:342–347.

88. Reaven GM, et al. In search of moderators and mediators of hyperglycemia with atypical antipsychotic treatment. *J Psychiatr Res* 2009; 43:997–1002.

89. Mokdad AH, et al. The continuing increase of diabetes in the US. *Diabetes Care* 2001; 24:412.

90. Mokdad AH, et al. Diabetes trends in the U.S.: 1990–1998. *Diabetes Care* 2000; 23:1278–1283.

91. Beckman JA, et al. Diabetes and atherosclerosis: epidemiology, pathophysiology, and management. *JAMA* 2002; 287:2570–2581.

92. Henderson DC, et al. Clozapine, diabetes mellitus, hyperlipidemia, and cardiovascular risks and mortality: results of a 10-year naturalistic study. *J Clin Psychiatry* 2005; 66:1116–1121.

93. Lamberti JS, et al. Prevalence of the metabolic syndrome among patients receiving clozapine. *Am J Psychiatry* 2006; 163:1273–1276.

94. Goff DC, et al. A comparison of ten-year cardiac risk estimates in schizophrenia patients from the CATIE study and matched controls. *Schizophr Res* 2005; 80:45–53.

95. Haupt DW, et al. Hyperglycemia and antipsychotic medications. *J Clin Psychiatry* 2001; 62 Suppl 27:15–26.

96. Cohn TA, et al. Metabolic monitoring for patients treated with antipsychotic medications. *Can J Psychiatry* 2006; 51:492–501.

97. De Hert M, et al. Guidelines for screening and monitoring of cardiometabolic risk in schizophrenia: systematic evaluation. *Br J Psychiatry* 2011; 199:99–105.

98. Barnes TR, et al. Screening for the metabolic syndrome in community psychiatric patients prescribed antipsychotics: a quality improvement programme. *Acta Psychiatr Scand* 2008; 118:26–33.

99. Barnes TR, et al. Screening for the metabolic side effects of antipsychotic medication: findings of a 6-year quality improvement programme in the UK. *BMJ Open* 2015; 5:e007633.

100. Crawford MJ, et al. Assessment and treatment of physical health problems among people with schizophrenia: national cross-sectional study. *Br J Psychiatry* 2014; 205:473–477.

101. Morrato EH, et al. Metabolic screening after the ADA's consensus statement on antipsychotic drugs and diabetes. *Diabetes Care* 2009; 32:1037–1042.

102. De Hert M, et al. Oral glucose tolerance tests in treated patients with schizophrenia: data to support an adaptation of the proposed guidelines for monitoring of patients on second generation antipsychotics? *Eur Psychiatry* 2006; 21:224–226.

103. Pillinger T, et al. Impaired glucose homeostasis in first-episode schizophrenia: a systematic review and meta-analysis. *JAMA Psychiatry* 2017; 74:261–269.

104. Marder SR, et al. Physical health monitoring of patients with schizophrenia. *Am J Psychiatry* 2004; 161:1334–1349.

105. National Institute for Health and Care Excellence. Type 2 diabetes: the management of type 2 diabetes. Clinical guideline [CG87]. 2009

(Last updated: December 2014); https://www.nice.org.uk/guidance/CG87.

106. Stroup TS, et al. Effects of switching from olanzapine, quetiapine, and risperidone to aripiprazole on 10-year coronary heart disease risk and metabolic syndrome status: results from a randomized controlled trial. *Schizophr Res* 2013; **146**:190–195.

107. Chen Y, et al. Comparative effectiveness of switching antipsychotic drug treatment to aripiprazole or ziprasidone for improving metabolic profile and atherogenic dyslipidemia: a 12-month, prospective, open-label study. *J Psychopharmacol* 2012; **26**:1201–1210.

108. Smith RC, et al. Effects of pioglitazone on metabolic abnormalities, psychopathology, and cognitive function in schizophrenic patients treated with antipsychotic medication: a randomized double-blind study. *SchizophrRes* 2013; **143**:18–24.

109. Larsen JR, et al. Effect of liraglutide treatment on prediabetes and overweight or obesity in clozapine- or olanzapine-treated patients with schizophrenia spectrum disorder: a randomized clinical trial. *JAMA Psychiatry* 2017; **74**:719–728.

抗精神病药所致的血压变化

直立性低血压

直立性低血压(姿势性低血压)是抗精神病药以及一些抗抑郁药的常见心血管不良反应之一。直立性低血压通常在开始加药期间急性发作,但也有证据表明其可能会成为慢性问题[1]。症状包括头晕、乏力、头痛以及视觉障碍。患者可能无法准确地表达症状,主观报道的姿势性头晕与测量到的姿势性低血压程度呈弱相关[2]。

对疑似患者建议进行血压监测以确诊直立性低血压(即平卧 5min 后站起的 2~5min 内,患者收缩压降低 >20mmHg,或舒张压降低 >10mmHg[3])。直立性低血压可能会导致晕厥以及与跌倒相关的受伤。直立性低血压同时也与冠心病、心力衰竭以及死亡风险增加相关[4]。

缓慢加量是避免或最小化直立性低血压常用且往往有效的策略。然而,在一些患者中,体位性低血压可能限制药物剂量,难以达到最佳疗效。可能的干预方式见表 1.26 及表 1.27。

表 1.26　体位性低血压的危险因素[2]

治疗因素	■ 肌内注射给药(更快达到药物浓度峰值)
	■ 药物过快加量
	■ 联合使用抗精神病药
	■ 药物相互作用(例如, β 受体阻断剂及其他降压药)
患者因素	■ 高龄(年轻患者常出现窦性心动过速,而体位性血压改变极小)
	■ 与自主神经功能障碍相关的疾病(例如,帕金森病)
	■ 脱水
	■ 心血管病

表 1.27　抗精神病药所致直立性低血压的干预方法[2]

降低治疗风险	■ 限制初始剂量,并根据耐受性缓慢加量(多数患者会逐渐耐受降压效果)
	■ 出现低血压时,考虑暂时降低药物剂量
	■ 避免使用对 α_1 肾上腺素受体拮抗作用强的抗精神病药
	■ 少量多次给药,或者使用缓释剂,以降低血浆药物水平峰值
非药物疗法	■ 患者教育。如:早上先在床沿坐几分钟再站起来,缓慢地从坐位站起来
	■ 体位性低血压建议使用腹带或加压袜
	■ 建议没有液体限制的患者增加液体摄入至 1.25~2.5L/d
药物疗法 有明确的治疗指征,没有替代治疗(如氯氮平),或其他干预方式无效者	■ 补充氯化钠可缓解抗抑郁药所致的直立性低血压
	■ 当其他方法无效时,可使用氟氢可的松治疗氯氮平所致直立性低血压(必须检测电解质与血压)
	■ 一例病例报告使用米多君(一种 α_1 受体激动剂)来处理 TCA 所致的直立性低血压。值得注意的是,米多君在与抗精神病药一起使用时,可导致急性肌张力障碍[5]。其他拟交感神经药也被用于治疗直立性低血压,但是目前还缺少治疗精神药物相关病例的证据

目前,报道最多的是与突触后 α_1 肾上腺素能受体亲和力强的抗精神病药。在第二代抗精神病药中,报道案例最多的是氯氮平(24%)、喹硫平(27%)以及伊潘立酮(19.5%),最少的是鲁拉西酮(<2%)和阿塞那平(<2%)[2]。有关第一代抗精神病药的定量数据有限,但低效价的吩噻嗪类(如氯丙嗪)被认为最容易导致直立性低血压[6]。所有报道的发生率多少与药物滴定的方案有关。

高血压

研究发现以下两种途径与抗精神病药引起或恶化高血压有关。

- **血压长时间平稳上升**。这可能与体重增加有关。超重增加了发生高血压的风险。采用 Framingham 数据建立了影响幅度的模型:每30位体重增加4kg的患者中,就有1位在未来10年内发展为高血压[7]。注意这是很轻的体重增加,绝大多数服用抗精神病药的患者体重增加超过4kg,这进一步增加了发展为高血压的风险。

- **使用新药或者增加剂量时不可预测的血压急速上升**。血压短期上升发生在首次服药后的几个小时至1个月内。下面内容介绍引起血压升高的药理学机制和最易引起高血压的药物。

体位性低血压通常与抗精神病药拮抗突触后 α_1 肾上腺素受体有关。一些抗精神病药也能拮抗突触前 α_2 肾上腺素受体,可能导致去甲肾上腺素释放增加和血管收缩。由于拮抗 α_2 受体的抗精神病药也都拮抗 α_1 受体,故服药后患者会发生怎样的改变很难预测,但有小部分患者发展为高血压。有些抗精神病药更易引起血压升高,毋庸置疑,患者的个体因素也很重要。

受体结合研究表明,氯氮平、奥氮平及利培酮对 α_2 肾上腺素受体[8]亲和力最强,因此也许能够预测这些药物最有可能引起高血压。大多数病例报道,患者在服用氯氮平前血压正常,服用氯氮平后血压会急剧上升,停药后血压又回到正常[9-17]。也有报道,停用氯氮平后再用,血压仍会再上升,同时伴有儿茶酚胺的升高。阿立哌唑[18-21]、舒必利[22,23]、利培酮[24]、喹硫平[13]及齐拉西酮[25]也有引起高血压的病例报告。

英国药品和健康产品管理局(Medical and Healthcare Products Regulatory Agency MHRA)黄卡系统的资料表明,氯氮平在抗精神病药中与高血压关系最大。为数不多的病例报告阿立哌唑、奥氮平、喹硫平和利培酮可引起高血压[26]。在这些报道中,并不清楚抗精神病药使用后多久出现高血压,可能是千变万化的。

在抗精神病药长期治疗中,不管服用何种抗精神病药,有30%~40%的患者患上高血压[27]。一项横断面研究发现,只有奋乃静[28]可增加高血压的风险,但这项发现不能用药理机制解释。

原发性高血压患者使用抗精神病药是没有禁忌的,但使用氯氮平需极其谨慎。合用 SSRI 类药物可能会增加高血压的风险,其机制可能是抑制抗精神病药的代谢[13]。理论上,α_2 受体拮抗作用至少可能是氯氮平引起的心动过速和恶心的部分原因[29]。

与抗精神病药相关的高血压治疗应该参照标准方案。应尽可能地换用心血管代谢风险更小的抗精神病药[30]。有明确的证据表明,缬沙坦与替米沙坦在治疗抗精神病药引起的高血压方面是有效的[31]。

参考文献

1. Silver H, et al. Postural hypotension in chronically medicated schizophrenics. *J Clin Psychiatry* 1990; 51:459–462.
2. Gugger JJ. Antipsychotic pharmacotherapy and orthostatic hypotension: identification and management. *CNS Drugs* 2011; 25:659–671.
3. Freeman R, et al. Consensus statement on the definition of orthostatic hypotension, neurally mediated syncope and the postural tachycardia syndrome. *Clin Auton Res* 2011; 21:69–72.
4. Ricci F, et al. Cardiovascular morbidity and mortality related to orthostatic hypotension: a meta-analysis of prospective observational studies. *Eur Heart J* 2015; 36:1609–1617.
5. Stroup TS, et al. Management of common adverse effects of antipsychotic medications. *World Psychiatry* 2018; 17:341–356.
6. Casey DE. The relationship of pharmacology to side effects. *J Clin Psychiatry* 1997; 58 **Suppl** 10:55–62.
7. Fontaine KR, et al. Estimating the consequences of anti-psychotic induced weight gain on health and mortality rate. *Psychiatry Res* 2001; **101**:277–288.
8. Abi-Dargham A, et al. Mechanisms of action of second generation antipsychotic drugs in schizophrenia: insights from brain imaging studies. *Eur Psychiatry* 2005; 20:15–27.
9. Yuen JWY, et al. Clozapine-induced cardiovascular side effects and autonomic dysfunction: a systematic review. *Front Neurosci* 2018; 12:203.
10. Gupta S, et al. Paradoxical hypertension associated with clozapine. *Am J Psychiatry* 1994; **151**:148.
11. George TP, et al. Hypertension after initiation of clozapine. *Am J Psychiatry* 1996; **153**:1368–1369.
12. Shiwach RS. Treatment of clozapine induced hypertension and possible mechanisms. *Clin Neuropharmacol* 1998; 21:139–140.
13. Coulter D. Atypical antipsychotics may cause hypertension. *Prescriber Update* 2003; 24:4.
14. Li JK, et al. Clozapine: a mimicry of phaeochromocytoma. *Aust N Z J Psychiatry* 1997; 31:889–891.
15. Hoorn EJ, et al. Hypokalemic hypertension related to clozapine: a case report. *J Clin Psychopharmacol* 2014; 34:390–392.
16. Sakalkale A, et al. Pseudophaeochromocytoma: a clinical dilemma in clozapine therapy. *Aust N Z J Psychiatry* 2017; 51 (**Suppl1**).
17. Visscher AJ, et al. Periorbital oedema and treatment-resistant hypertension as rare side effects of clozapine. *Aust N Z J Psychiatry* 2011; 45:1097–1098.
18. Hsiao YL, et al. Aripiprazole augmentation induced hypertension in major depressive disorder: a case report. *Prog Neuropsychopharmacol Biol Psychiatry* 2011; 35:305–306.
19. Yasui-Furukori N, et al. Worsened hypertension control induced by aripiprazole. *Neuropsychiatr Dis Treat* 2013; 9:505–507.
20. Seven H, et al. Aripiprazole-induced asymptomatic hypertension: a case report. *Psychopharmacol Bull* 2017; 47:53–56.
21. Alves BB, et al. Use of atypical antipsychotics and risk of hypertension: a case report and review literature. *SAGE Open Medical Case Reports* 2019; 7:2050313x19841825.
22. Mayer RD, et al. Acute hypertensive episode induced by sulpiride – a case report. *Human Psychopharmacology* 1989; 4:149–150.
23. Corvol P, et al. [Hypertensive episodes initiated by sulpiride (Dogmatil)]. *Ann Med Interne* 1973; **124**:647–649.
24. Thomson SR, et al. Risperidone induced hypertension in a young female: a case report. *Adv Sci Lett* 2017; 23:1980–1982.
25. Villanueva N, et al. Probable association between ziprasidone and worsening hypertension. *Pharmacotherapy* 2006; 26:1352–1357.
26. Medicines and Healthcare Products Regulatory Agency. Drug Analysis Profiles (iDAPs) 2021; https://www.gov.uk/drug-analysis-prints.
27. Kelly AC, et al. A naturalistic comparison of the long-term metabolic adverse effects of clozapine versus other antipsychotics for patients with psychotic illnesses. *J Clin Psychopharmacol* 2014; 34:441–445.
28. Boden R, et al. A comparison of cardiovascular risk factors for ten antipsychotic drugs in clinical practice. *Neuropsychiatr Dis Treat* 2013; 9:371–377.
29. Pandharipande P, et al. Alpha-2 agonists: can they modify the outcomes in the postanesthesia care unit? *Curr Drug Targets* 2005; 6:749–754.
30. Whelton PK, et al. 2017 ACC/AHA/AAPA/ABC/ACPM/AGS/APhA/ASH/ASPC/NMA/PCNA guideline for the prevention, detection, evaluation, and management of high blood pressure in adults: a report of the American College of Cardiology/American Heart Association Task Force on Clinical Practice Guidelines. *J Am Coll Cardiol* 2018; 71:e127–e248.
31. Tse L, et al. Pharmacological treatment of antipsychotic-induced dyslipidemia and hypertension. *Int Clin Psychopharmacol* 2014; 29:125–137.

精神病中的低钠血症

低钠血症可发生于下述情况:

- **水中毒**指饮水超过肾脏的最大清除能力。血清和尿液渗透压较低。横断面研究发现,长期患病、住院的精神疾病患者水中毒的发生率为 6%~17%[1,2]。一项纵向研究发现,约有10% 的严重精神分裂症患者有间歇性、继发于液体过剩的低钠血症[3]。主要的病因几乎是不清楚的。有假设认为这是,至少部分原因是,由抗精神病药的抗胆碱能不良反应的极端代偿所导致[4]。另一种理论认为,突触后的多巴胺受体阻滞导致了受体超敏,增加了突触前多巴胺的释放,提高了下丘脑中的多巴胺含量,促使口渴和多饮。一些观察支持了该理论:许多病例发生在病史较长且接受高 D_2 受体亲和力抗精神病药治疗的患者当中,而氯氮平对多饮的改善与其对精神病性症状的改善无关[5]。

- 药物导致的**抗利尿激素分泌异常综合征(SIADH)**,此时肾脏潴留了大量无溶质的水。这就导致血清渗透压低,尿液渗透压相对高。在急性期精神疾病患者中,估计抗利尿激素分泌异常综合征的患病率高达 11%[6]。抗抑郁药引起 SIADH 的危险因素(年龄增长、女性、躯体共病率及多药合用)似乎与抗精神病药关系不大[7]。抗利尿激素分泌异常综合征通常发生在使用药物后最初几周内。病例报告和病例系列研究显示,奋乃静、氟哌啶醇、匹莫齐特、利培酮、帕利哌酮、喹硫平、奥氮平、阿立哌唑、卡利拉嗪和氯氮平与抗利尿激素分泌失调有关[7-26]。系统综述[27] 和一些病例对照研究[28,29] 发现,抗精神病药使患低钠血症的风险明显增加。另一项综述[30] 证实,药物导致的低钠血症与尿液浓缩有关,抗精神病药致低钠血症的风险比水中毒高 5 倍。总的来说,抗精神病药所致低钠血症的发生率在 0.004%[31]~26.1%[32]。使用去氨升压素(对抗氯氮平导致的遗尿)也能引起低钠血症[33]。其他药物,包括抗抑郁药以及抗癫痫药(尤其是卡马西平[34])也被报道有影响[35],且该风险在联合用药时有累加效应[36,37]。

- 严重**高脂血症**或**高血糖**导致继发性的血浆容积增加和"假性低钠血症"[4]。这两种情况在服用抗精神病药的患者中比一般人群多见,因此要排除这两方面的原因。

轻、中度低钠血症可使患者出现精神错乱、恶心、头痛及昏睡等症状。随着血钠的下降,上述症状会越来越严重,甚至可出现癫痫发作和昏迷。

所有服用抗精神病药的患者均需要监测血钠。出现精神错乱或昏睡的征象时,应该做全面的诊断分析,包括检测血钠和尿液渗透压(表 1.28)。

表 1.28　抗精神病药致低钠血症的治疗方法[4,6]

低钠血症原因	相关抗精神病药	治疗方法
水中毒 (血清和尿液 渗透压降低)	只有纯理论性的证据支持抗精神病药是病因 少数患者(如精神性多饮)的主要病因	■ **限制液体**并密切监测血钠浓度,特别是昼夜变化(白天钠浓度下降)。若血钠浓度 <125mmol/L,需要紧急向专科转诊。注意:有报告显示,纠正低钠血症过快时,可引起渗透性脱髓鞘综合征[38] ■ 考虑使用**氯氮平**治疗:它可使升高血浆渗透压至正常范围,升高尿液渗透压(一般不能达到正常范围)[39,40]。其效果与减少液体摄入一致。该作用显然与精神状态的改善无关[41] ■ 奥氮平[42]和利培酮[43]的研究结果不一[7]。喹硫平[44]有一项阳性病例报告。与氯氮平相比,这些证据太弱 ■ 没有证据表明减少或增加抗精神病药剂量能使水中毒患者的血钠浓度改善[45],但是有人建议减少抗精神病药的种类和剂量可能会减少多巴胺受体超敏以及药物不良反应[5] ■ 一些关于精神性多饮的指南中收录了有关**地美环素**使用[46,47]的报告[48]。然而,地美环素通过对 ADH 影响而发挥作用,增加液体排泄。后者在这些患者中已经超负荷。于是,在没有 SIADH 的情况下,对使用地美环素的依据存在争议(文献中的一些病例,可能因为未确诊 SIADH 而使得判断变得更加复杂[49])。一项小型 RCT 研究显示其效果不佳[50]
抗利尿激素分泌异常综合征 (血清渗透压低,尿液渗透压相对较高)	所有抗精神病药	■ 若程度轻,**限制液体**,并密切监测血钠。若血钠 <125mmol/L,紧急转诊到专科 ■ **换用不同的抗精神病药**。没有充分资料指导选择。注意可能会发生交叉过敏(患者可能先天容易发生该病,选择药物相对不重要) ■ 考虑**地美环素**(详见标准处方指南) ■ 锂盐可能有效的[7],但需注意其潜在毒性——低钠血症易导致锂中毒

ADH,抗利尿激素;SIADH,抗利尿激素分泌异常综合征。

　　最近引入的托伐普坦[51]等所谓伐普坦类药物(即非肽类精氨酸血管升压素拮抗剂,因为其引起低渗利尿,也被称为促排水利尿药[52])可能有望治疗不同病因的低钠血症,包括由药物相关的 SIADH 以及精神性多饮引起的低钠血症[53]。有研究报告使用碳酸酐酶抑制剂乙酰唑胺取得成功[54,55]。也有关于厄贝沙坦[56]、普萘洛尔[57]、可乐定[58]、依那普利[58]、卡托普利[59]治疗精神性多饮不同程度取得成功的案例报告。

参考文献

1. De Leon J, et al. Polydipsia and water intoxication in psychiatric patients: a review of the epidemiological literature. *Biol Psychiatry* 1994; 35:408–419.
2. Patel JK. Polydipsia, hyponatremia, and water intoxication among psychiatric patients. *Hosp Community Psychiatry* 1994; 45:1073–1074.
3. De Leon J. Polydipsia–a study in a long-term psychiatric unit. *Eur Arch Psychiatry Clin Neurosci* 2003; 253:37–39.
4. Siegel AJ, et al. Primary and drug-induced disorders of water homeostasis in psychiatric patients: principles of diagnosis and management. *Harv Rev Psychiatry* 1998; 6:190–200.
5. Kirino S, et al. Relationship between polydipsia and antipsychotics: a systematic review of clinical studies and case reports. *Prog Neuropsychopharmacol Biol Psychiatry* 2020; 96:109756.
6. Siegler EL, et al. Risk factors for the development of hyponatremia in psychiatric inpatients. *Arch Intern Med* 1995; 155:953–957.

7. Madhusoodanan S, et al. Hyponatraemia associated with psychotropic medications. A review of the literature and spontaneous reports. *Adv Drug React Toxicol Rev* 2002; 21:17–29.

8. Bachu K, et al. Aripiprazole-induced syndrome of inappropriate antidiuretic hormone secretion (SIADH). *Am J Ther* 2006; 13:370–372.

9. Dudeja SJ, et al. Olanzapine induced hyponatraemia. *Ulster Med J* 2010; 79:104–105.

10. Yam FK, et al. Syndrome of inappropriate antidiuretic hormone associated with aripiprazole. *AmJHealth SystPharm* 2013; 70:2110–2114.

11. Kaur J, et al. Paliperidone inducing concomitantly syndrome of inappropriate antidiuretic hormone, neuroleptic malignant syndrome, and rhabdomyolysis. *Case Reports in Critical Care* 2016; 2016:2587963.

12. Lin MW, et al. Aripiprazole-related hyponatremia and consequent valproic acid-related hyperammonemia in one patient. *Aust N Z J Psychiatry* 2017; 51:296–297.

13. Koufakis T. Quetiapine-Induced Syndrome of Inappropriate Secretion of Antidiuretic Hormone. *Case reports in psychiatry* 2016; 2016:4803132

14. Chen LC, et al. Polydipsia, hyponatremia and rhabdomyolysis in schizophrenia: a case report. *World J Psychiatry* 2014; 4:150–152.

15. Bakhla AK, et al. A suspected case of olanzapine induced hyponatremia. *Indian J Pharmacol* 2014; 46:441–442.

16. Kane JM, et al. Efficacy and safety of cariprazine in acute exacerbation of schizophrenia: results from an international, phase iii clinical trial. *J Clin Psychopharmacol* 2015; 35:367–373.

17. Tibrewal P, et al. Paliperidone-Induced Hyponatremia. *Prim Care Companion CNS Disord* 2017; 19:16l02088.

18. McNally MA, et al. Olanzapine-induced hyponatremia presenting with seizure requiring intensive care unit admission. *Cureus* 2020; 12:e8212.

19. Sachdeva A, et al. Hyponatremia with olanzapine – a suspected association. *Shanghai Arch Psychiatry* 2017; 29:177–179.

20. Kumar PNS, et al. Hyponatremia secondary to SIADH in a schizophrenic patient treated with Quetiapine. *Asian J Psychiatr* 2018; 35:89–90.

21. Mazhar F, et al. Paliperidone-associated hyponatremia: report of a fatal case with analysis of cases reported in the literature and to the US Food and Drug Administration Adverse Event Reporting System. *J Clin Psychopharmacol* 2020; 40:202–205.

22. Chowdhury W, et al. Management of persistent hyponatremia induced by long-acting injectable risperidone therapy. *Cureus* 2018; 10:e2657.

23. Anil SS, et al. A case report of rapid-onset hyponatremia induced by low-dose olanzapine. *J Family Med Primary Care* 2017; 6:878–880.

24. Kang SG, et al. Addendum: low-dose quetiapine-induced syndrome of inappropriate antidiuretic hormone in a patient with traumatic brain syndrome. *Clin Psychopharmacol Neurosci* 2021; 19:179.

25. Aruachán S, et al. Hyponatraemia associated with the use of quetiapine: case report. *Rev Colomb Psiquiatr* 2020; 49:297–300.

26. Zhu X, et al. Rhabdomyolysis and elevated liver enzymes after rapid correction of hyponatremia due to pneumonia and concurrent use of aripiprazole: a case report. *Aust N Z J Psychiatry* 2018; 52:206.

27. Meulendijks D, et al. Antipsychotic-induced hyponatraemia: a systematic review of the published evidence. *Drug Saf* 2010; 33:101–114.

28. Mannesse CK, et al. Hyponatraemia as an adverse drug reaction of antipsychotic drugs: a case-control study in VigiBase. *Drug Saf* 2010; 33:569–578.

29. Falhammar H, et al. Antipsychotics and severe hyponatremia: a Swedish population-based case-control study. *Eur J Intern Med* 2019; 60:71–77.

30. Atsariyasing W, et al. A systematic review of the ability of urine concentration to distinguish antipsychotic- from psychosis-induced hyponatremia. *Psychiatry Res* 2014; 217:129–133.

31. Letmaier M, et al. Hyponatraemia during psychopharmacological treatment: results of a drug surveillance programme. *IntJNeuropsychopharmacol* 2012; 15:739–748.

32. Serrano A, et al. Safety of long-term clozapine administration. Frequency of cardiomyopathy and hyponatraemia: two cross-sectional, naturalistic studies. *Aust N Z J Psychiatry* 2014; 48:183–192.

33. Sarma S, et al. Severe hyponatraemia associated with desmopressin nasal spray to treat clozapine-induced nocturnal enuresis. *Aust N Z J Psychiatry* 2005; 39:949.

34. Yang HJ, et al. Antipsychotic use is a risk factor for hyponatremia in patients with schizophrenia: a 15-year follow-up study. *Psychopharmacology* 2017; 234:869–876.

35. Shepshelovich D, et al. Medication-induced SIADH: distribution and characterization according to medication class. *Br J Clin Pharmacol* 2017; 83:1801–1807.

36. Yamamoto Y, et al. Prevalence and risk factors for hyponatremia in adult epilepsy patients: large-scale cross-sectional cohort study. *Seizure* 2019; 73:26–30.

37. Fabrazzo M, et al. The unmasking of hidden severe hyponatremia after long-term combination therapy in exacerbated bipolar patients: a case series. *Int Clin Psychopharmacol* 2019; 34:206–210.

38. Zaidi AN. Rhabdomyolysis after correction of hyponatremia in psychogenic polydipsia possibly complicated by ziprasidone. *Ann Pharmacother* 2005; 39:1726–1731.

39. Canuso CM, et al. Clozapine restores water balance in schizophrenic patients with polydipsia-hyponatremia syndrome. *J Neuropsychiatry Clin Neurosci* 1999; 11:86–90.

40. Fujimoto M, et al. Clozapine improved the syndrome of inappropriate antidiuretic hormone secretion in a patient with treatment-resistant schizophrenia. *Psychiatry Clin Neurosci* 2016; 70:469.

41. Spears NM, et al. Clozapine treatment in polydipsia and intermittent hyponatremia. *J Clin Psychiatry* 1996; 57:123–128.

42. Littrell KH, et al. Effects of olanzapine on polydipsia and intermittent hyponatremia. *J Clin Psychiatry* 1997; 58:549.

43. Kawai N, et al. Risperidone failed to improve polydipsia-hyponatremia of the schizophrenic patients. *Psychiatry Clin Neurosci* 2002; 56:107–110.

44. Montgomery JH, et al. Adjunctive quetiapine treatment of the polydipsia, intermittent hyponatremia, and psychosis syndrome: a case report.

J Clin Psychiatry 2003; **64**:339–341.

45. Canuso CM, et al. Does minimizing neuroleptic dosage influence hyponatremia? *Psychiatry Res* 1996; **63**:227–229.

46. Nixon RA, et al. Demeclocycline in the prophylaxis of self-induced water intoxication. *Am J Psychiatry* 1982; **139**:828–830.

47. Vieweg WV, et al. The use of demeclocycline in the treatment of patients with psychosis, intermittent hyponatremia, and polydipsia (PIP syndrome). *Psychiatr Q* 1988; **59**:62–68.

48. Srinivasan S, et al. Psychogenic polydipsia. 2019; https://bestpractice.bmj.com/topics/en-gb/865.

49. Walter-Ryan WG. Water intoxication, demeclocycline, and antidiuretic hormone. *Am J Psychiatry* 1983; **140**:815.

50. Alexander RC, et al. A double blind, placebo-controlled trial of demeclocycline treatment of polydipsia-hyponatremia in chronically psychotic patients. *Biol Psychiatry* 1991; **30**:417–420.

51. Josiassen RC, et al. Tolvaptan: a new tool for the effective treatment of hyponatremia in psychotic disorders. *Expert Opin Pharmacother* 2010; **11**:637–648.

52. Decaux G, et al. Non-peptide arginine-vasopressin antagonists: the vaptans. *Lancet* 2008; **371**:1624–1632.

53. Bhatia MS, et al. Psychogenic polydipsia – management challenges. *Shanghai Arch Psychiatry* 2017; **29**:180–183.

54. Ahmed SE, et al. Acetazolamide: treatment of psychogenic polydipsia. *Cureus* 2017; **9**:e1553.

55. Takagi S, et al. Treatment of psychogenic polydipsia with acetazolamide: a report of 5 cases. *Clin Neuropharmacol* 2011; **34**:5–7.

56. Kruse D, et al. Treatment of psychogenic polydipsia: comparison of risperidone and olanzapine, and the effects of an adjunctive angiotensin-II receptor blocking drug (irbesartan). *Aust N Z J Psychiatry* 2001; **35**:65–68.

57. Shevitz SA, et al. Compulsive water drinking treated with high dose propranolol. *J Nerv Ment Dis* 1980; **168**:246–248.

58. Greendyke RM, et al. Polydipsia in chronic psychiatric patients: therapeutic trials of clonidine and enalapril. *Neuropsychopharmacology* 1998; **18**:272–281.

59. Sebastian CS, et al. Comparison of enalapril and captopril in the management of self-induced water intoxication. *Biol Psychiatry* 1990; **27**:787–790.

拓展阅读

Sailer C, et al. Primary polydipsia in the medical and psychiatric patient: characteristics, complications and therapy. *Swiss Med Wkly* 2017; **147**:w14514

Srinivasan S, et al. Psychogenic polydipsia. *BMJ Best Practice* 2019; https://bestpractice.bmj.com/topics/en-gb/865.

高催乳素血症

多巴胺抑制催乳素的释放,因而预期多巴胺拮抗剂能够提高血浆中催乳素的水平。催乳素升高的程度可能与药物剂量相关[1]。对于大多数抗精神病药而言,使催乳素增高的阈活性(D_2 受体占有率)与治疗活性非常接近[2]。基因差异也可能起部分作用[3]。表 1.29 根据对催乳素的影响将抗精神病药分组。

表 1.29　已明确对催乳素影响不大的抗精神病药[4-11]

催乳素无影响(催乳素升高罕见)	催乳素升高(风险低,影响小)	催乳素升高(风险高,影响大)
阿立哌唑	鲁拉西酮	氨磺必利
阿塞纳平	奥氮平	帕利哌酮
依匹唑哌	齐拉西酮	利培酮
卡利拉嗪		舒必利
氯氮平		第一代抗精神病药
伊潘立酮		
卢美哌隆		
哌马色林		
喹硫平		

通常表面上看来,高催乳素血症是无症状的(即患者不会主动报告问题),并且一些证据表明,高催乳素血症不会影响主观生活质量[12]。但是,血浆催乳素水平持续升高与下丘脑-垂体-性腺轴的抑制有关[13]。其症状包括性功能障碍[14](但需要注意其他药理作用也能导致性功能障碍[15])、月经紊乱[4,16]、乳房发育和溢乳[16]以及妊娠妄想[17]。长期不良后果包括骨密度降低[18,19],以及患乳腺癌的风险可能增加[20]。

应激、妊娠及哺乳、癫痫发作、肾功能损害以及其他躯体疾病[7,21,22](包括催乳素瘤)也可能引起催乳素升高。当检测催乳素水平时,应该在早晨取血,并尽量减少静脉穿刺时的压力[22]。

禁忌证

在下列患者群体中应当避免使用催乳素升高风险高的药物:

- **25 岁以下的患者(即在骨密度达到峰值之前)**
- **骨质疏松患者**
- **激素依赖型乳腺癌病史的患者**
- **青年女性**

治疗

对高催乳素血症的患者的治疗主要基于患者的症状以及长期风险,而不是血浆催乳素水平。

下文中,我们提出抗精神病药所致高催乳素血症的处理流程。在需要治疗高催乳素血症时,首选换用较少升高催乳素水平的药物,但是换药总有导致病情波动,甚至复发的风险[23]。次选在原有治疗上加用阿立哌唑[24]。阿立哌唑降低催乳素的作用是剂量依赖性的:

3mg/d 有效,但 6mg/d 效果更好。不需要用更高的剂量 [25]。减少骨密度长期风险的其他方法也值得关注,例如戒烟、增加负重训练,以及保障充分的钙与维生素 D_3 摄入 [18,26]。

对于那些需要继续使用升高催乳素的抗精神病药,同时不能耐受阿立哌唑的患者,多巴胺激动剂可能有效 [27-29]。金刚烷胺、卡麦角林和溴隐亭都被使用过,但每种药物都有加重精神病的可能性(不过没有在试验中报道过)。研究发现,一种植物制剂芍药甘草汤也是有效的 [30-31],但目前证据有限。一项针对使用抗精神病药的糖尿病女性患者的研究提示,大剂量的二甲双胍(2.5~3g/d)可降低催乳素水平 [32]。

治疗总结

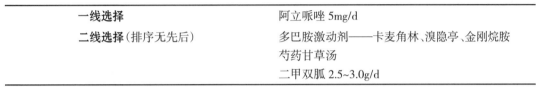

一线选择	阿立哌唑 5mg/d
二线选择(排序无先后)	多巴胺激动剂——卡麦角林、溴隐亭、金刚烷胺
	芍药甘草汤
	二甲双胍 2.5~3.0g/d

抗精神病药所致高催乳素血症的处理见图 1.3。

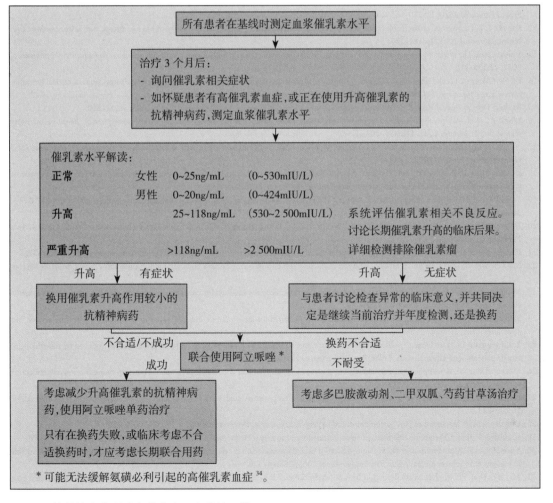

图 1.3　抗精神病药所致高催乳素血症的处理 [33]

参考文献

1. Suzuki Y, et al. Differences in plasma prolactin levels in patients with schizophrenia treated on monotherapy with five second-generation antipsychotics. *Schizophr Res* 2013; 145:116–119.

2. Tsuboi T, et al. Hyperprolactinemia and estimated dopamine D2 receptor occupancy in patients with schizophrenia: analysis of the CATIE data. *Prog Neuropsychopharmacol Biol Psychiatry* 2013; 45:178–182.

3. Young RM, et al. Prolactin levels in antipsychotic treatment of patients with schizophrenia carrying the DRD2*A1 allele. *Br J Psychiatry* 2004; 185:147–151.

4. Haddad PM, et al. Antipsychotic-induced hyperprolactinaemia: mechanisms, clinical features and management. *Drugs* 2004; 64:2291–2314.

5. Holt RI, et al. Antipsychotics and hyperprolactinaemia: mechanisms, consequences and management. *Clin Endocrinol* 2011; 74:141–147.

6. Leucht S, et al. Comparative efficacy and tolerability of 15 antipsychotic drugs in schizophrenia: a multiple-treatments meta-analysis. *Lancet* 2013; 382:951–962.

7. Peuskens J, et al. The effects of novel and newly approved antipsychotics on serum prolactin levels: a comprehensive review. *CNS Drugs* 2014; 28:421–453.

8. Citrome L. Cariprazine: chemistry, pharmacodynamics, pharmacokinetics, and metabolism, clinical efficacy, safety, and tolerability. *Exp Opin Drug Metab Toxicol* 2013; 9:193–206.

9. Marder SR, et al. Brexpiprazole in patients with schizophrenia: overview of short- and long-term phase 3 controlled studies. *Acta Neuropsychiatr* 2017; 29:278–290.

10. Vanover KE, et al. Dopamine D(2) receptor occupancy of lumateperone (ITI-007): a positron emission tomography study in patients with schizophrenia. *Neuropsychopharmacology* 2019; 44:598–605.

11. Yunusa I, et al. Pimavanserin: a novel antipsychotic with potentials to address an unmet need of older adults with dementia-related psychosis. *Front Pharmacol* 2020; 11:87.

12. Kaneda Y. The impact of prolactin elevation with antipsychotic medications on subjective quality of life in patients with schizophrenia. *Clin Neuropsychopharmacol* 2003; 26:182–184.

13. Smith S, et al. The effects of antipsychotic-induced hyperprolactinaemia on the hypothalamic-pituitary-gonadal axis. *J Clin Psychopharmacol* 2002; 22:109–114.

14. De Hert M, et al. Second-generation and newly approved antipsychotics, serum prolactin levels and sexual dysfunctions: a critical literature review. *Exp Opin Drug Saf* 2014; 13:605–624.

15. Baldwin D, et al. Sexual side-effects of antidepressant and antipsychotic drugs. *Adv Psychiatric Treat* 2003; 9:202–210.

16. Wieck A, et al. Antipsychotic-induced hyperprolactinaemia in women: pathophysiology, severity and consequences. Selective literature review. *Br J Psychiatry* 2003; 182:199–204.

17. Ali JA, et al. Delusions of pregnancy associated with increased prolactin concentrations produced by antipsychotic treatment. *Int J Neuropsychopharmacol* 2003; 6:111–115.

18. De Hert M, et al. Relationship between antipsychotic medication, serum prolactin levels and osteoporosis/osteoporotic fractures in patients with schizophrenia: a critical literature review. *Exp Opin Drug Saf* 2016; 15:809–823.

19. Tseng PT, et al. Bone mineral density in schizophrenia: an update of current meta-analysis and literature review under guideline of PRISMA. *Medicine* 2015; 94:e1967.

20. De Hert M, et al. Relationship between prolactin, breast cancer risk, and antipsychotics in patients with schizophrenia: a critical review. *Acta Psychiatr Scand* 2016; 133:5–22.

21. Holt RI. Medical causes and consequences of hyperprolactinaemia. A context for psychiatrists. *J Psychopharmacology* 2008; 22:28–37.

22. Melmed S, et al. Diagnosis and treatment of hyperprolactinemia: an Endocrine Society clinical practice guideline. *J Clin Endocrinol Metab* 2011; 96:273–288.

23. Montejo AL, et al. Multidisciplinary consensus on the therapeutic recommendations for iatrogenic hyperprolactinemia secondary to antipsy-chotics. *Front Neuroendocrinol* 2017; 45:25–34.

24. Sá Esteves P, et al. Low doses of adjunctive aripiprazole as treatment for antipsychotic-induced hyperprolactinemia: a literature review. *Eur Psychiatry* 2015; 30 Suppl 1:393.

25. Yasui-Furukori N, et al. Dose-dependent effects of adjunctive treatment with aripiprazole on hyperprolactinemia induced by risperidone in female patients with schizophrenia. *J Clin Psychopharmacol* 2010; 30:596–599.

26. Meaney AM, et al. Bone mineral density changes over a year in young females with schizophrenia: relationship to medication and endocrine variables. *Schizophr Res* 2007; 93:136–143.

27. Hamner MB, et al. Hyperprolactinaemia in antipsychotic-treated patients: guidelines for avoidance and management. *CNS Drugs* 1998; 10:209–222.

28. Duncan D, et al. Treatment of psychotropic-induced hyperprolactinaemia. *Psychiatric Bulletin* 1995; 19:755–757.

29. Cavallaro R, et al. Cabergoline treatment of risperidone-induced hyperprolactinemia: a pilot study. *J Clin Psychiatry* 2004; 65:187–190.

30. Yuan HN, et al. A randomized, crossover comparison of herbal medicine and bromocriptine against risperidone-induced hyperprolactinemia in patients with schizophrenia. *J Clin Psychopharmacol* 2008; 28:264–370.

31. Man SC, et al. Peony-glycyrrhiza decoction for antipsychotic-related hyperprolactinemia in women with schizophrenia: a randomized con-trolled trial. *J Clin Psychopharmacol* 2016; 36:572–579.

32. Krysiak R, et al. The effect of metformin on prolactin levels in patients with drug-induced hyperprolactinemia. *Eur J Intern Med* 2016;

30:94–98.

33. Walters J, et al. Clinical questions and uncertainty–prolactin measurement in patients with schizophrenia and bipolar disorder. *J Psychopharmacology* 2008; **22**:82–89.

34. Chen CK, et al. Differential add-on effects of aripiprazole in resolving hyperprolactinemia induced by risperidone in comparison to benzamide antipsychotics. *Prog Neuropsychopharmacol Biol Psychiatry* 2010; **34**:1495–1499.

性功能障碍

尽管缺乏常模数据,原发性性功能障碍是常见的[1]。躯体疾病、精神疾病、药物滥用和处方药物都能引起性功能障碍[2]。据估计,30%~82%[3]的精神分裂症患者存在性功能障碍,而普通人群只有30%[4];但要注意的是,这两组人群的患病率因数据收集方法而异(自发报告的人数少,用保密问卷时人数增多,当直接询问时,人数进一步增多[2])。在一项针对精神病患者的研究中,37%的人主动说存在性功能问题,而当直接询问时,发现46%的人存在性功能障碍[5]。

如果可能(问卷可能有用),应该确定基线性功能,因为性功能可以影响生活质量[6]和药物依从性(性功能障碍是治疗脱落的主要原因之一)[7,8]。如患者抱怨性功能障碍,可能表明潜在的躯体或精神疾病加重或治疗不彻底[9,10]。性功能问题也可能是药物治疗引起的,而干预可大大地提高患者的生活质量[11]。

人类的性反应

人类的性反应分为四期,见表1.30[2,12,13]。

表1.30 人类的性反应

性欲	■ 男性与睾酮水平相关
	■ 多巴胺可使其升高,催乳素可使其降低
	■ 社会心理背景和社会心理适应可显著影响性欲
性兴奋	■ 男性受睾酮影响,女性受雌激素影响
	■ 其他可能的机制包括:中枢多巴胺刺激、胆碱能/肾上腺素能平衡调控、外周 α_1 激动作用和一氧化氮通路
	■ 机体病理变化(如高血压或糖尿病)可有明显影响
性高潮	■ 可能与催产素有关
	■ 5-羟色胺活性升高、催乳素升高和 α_1 受体阻滞可导致性高潮抑制
消退	■ 高潮后被动发生

注:在各期都有很多其他激素和神经递质发生复杂的相互作用。

精神病的影响

性功能障碍在首发精神分裂症患者中是一种公认的现象[14,15]。据报道,在已经确诊的患者中,高达82%的男性和96%的女性患者有性功能障碍,伴有生活质量下降[6]。抗精神病药的不良反应并不是唯一的原因,因为在未用药的患者中性功能障碍发病率也很高(17%~70%)[16]。男性[17]抱怨性欲望下降、无法勃起、出现早泄,女性比较笼统地抱怨性享受降低[17,18]。女性精神病患者的生育能力下降[19]。精神病患者不太能够建立良好的性心理关系,抗精神病药能改善一些患者的性功能[20]。对一些精神病患者进行性功能评估显然是困难的。亚利桑那性体验量表(ASEX)可能在这方面有所帮助[21]。

抗精神病药的影响

据报道,绝大部分抗精神病药均可引起性功能障碍,服用第一代抗精神病药的人,高达45%存在性功能障碍[22]。个体易感性差异大,所有的影响均是可逆的。但需要注意的是,躯体疾病和抗精神病药以外的药物均可引起性功能障碍,很多研究没有控制这两个因素,因而难以比较不同抗精神病药所致性功能障碍的发生率[23]。

抗精神病药可降低多巴胺能传递,这本身就能降低性欲,但也可能通过负反馈升高催乳素水平。一些研究表明,高催乳素血症与性功能障碍有关[24],据估计,抗精神病药引起的性功能障碍中,40%与催乳素水平升高有关[4]。高催乳素血症也可引起女性闭经、男性和女性乳房增大及溢乳[25]。虽然已有研究认为抗精神病药影响性功能障碍的倾向与其升高催乳素的倾向相关,即利培酮 > 氟哌啶醇 > 奥氮平 > 喹硫平 > 阿立哌唑[9,23,26],但应当注意的是,在CUtLASS-1研究中,第一代抗精神病药(主要是舒必利,也有其他已知与催乳素升高相关的第一代抗精神病药)对性功能障碍的影响并不比第二代抗精神病药严重(70%的患者使用了不升高催乳素的药物)。其实,这两组的性功能障碍在为期一年的研究中都有所改善[20]。阿立哌唑单用[27]或联合其他抗精神病药[28,29]时,相对地没有性功能方面的不良反应。卡利拉嗪在理论上是一种很合适的替代品(目前还没有换药研究)[30]。

抗胆碱能作用可引起性兴奋障碍[31](同时服用抗胆碱药可能导致性功能障碍[32]),阻断外周 α_1 受体的药物引起男性勃起和射精问题[11]。对外周 α_1 受体和胆碱能受体均有拮抗作用的药物能引起阴茎异常勃起[33]。抗精神病药引起的镇静和体重增加可能会降低性欲[33]。这些原则可用于预测不同抗精神病药的性功能不良反应(表 1.31)。需要记住的是,改用能更好地控制精神病性症状的抗精神病药本身可能有助于性功能障碍。

表 1.31　抗精神病药在性功能方面的不良反应

药物	问题种类
阿立哌唑	■ 对催乳素或 α_1 受体均无影响。未见性功能方面不良反应的报道。将其他抗精神病药换成阿立哌唑可改善性功能[27,29,34,35]。阿立哌唑可引起性欲亢进的个案报道已发表[36,37]
阿塞那平	■ 似乎对催乳素水平没有显著影响[38]
	■ 没有性功能障碍个案报道
布瑞哌唑	■ 与阿立哌唑的作用机制相似(5-HT$_{1A}$ 激动剂,5-HT$_{2A}$ 拮抗剂以及 D$_2$ 部分激动剂)
	■ 造成可忽略不计的催乳素升高[39]
	■ 临床试验中未报告性功能障碍问题[40]
卡利拉嗪	■ 与阿立哌唑的作用机制相似(5-HT$_{1A}$ 激动剂,5-HT$_{2A}$ 拮抗剂以及部分的 D$_2$ 激动剂)
	■ 与高催乳素血症无关[41]
	■ 没有性功能障碍的个案报道
氯氮平	■ 显著的 α_1 肾上腺素能受体阻滞和抗胆碱能作用[42]。对催乳素无影响[43]
	■ 问题可能少于第一代抗精神病药[44]
氟哌啶醇	■ 与吩噻嗪类类似[45],但其抗胆碱作用降低[46]
	■ 报道的性功能障碍发生率高达 70%[47]

续表

药物	问题种类
鲁拉西酮	■ 似乎对催乳素水平没有显著影响 [48]
	■ 没有性功能障碍的个案报道 [49]
奥氮平	■ 由于没有催乳素的相关影响,因此相对其他药物(例如氟哌啶醇)较少发生性功能障碍 [45]
	■ 罕见阴茎异常勃起的报道 [50,51]
	■ 报道的性功能障碍发生率大于50% [47]
帕利哌酮	■ 催乳素升高与利培酮相似
	■ 一项小型研究 [52] 和一份病例报告 [53] 显示,从利培酮口服或利培酮长效注射剂换成帕利培酮长效注射剂后,性功能障碍减少
吩噻嗪类 (如氯丙嗪)	■ 高催乳素血症和抗胆碱能作用。有报道显示低剂量时导致性高潮延迟,之后有正常性高潮,但高剂量时不射精 [18]
	■ 有报道显示硫利达嗪、利培酮和氯丙嗪可引起阴茎异常勃起(可能由 α_1 肾上腺素受体阻滞引起) [46,54,55]
喹硫平	■ 对血清催乳素水平无影响 [56]
	■ 发生性功能障碍的风险较低 [57-60],但已有研究的结果相互矛盾 [61,62]
利培酮	■ 强力升高血清催乳素水平
	■ 相对其他抗精神病药(奥氮平和喹硫平)抗胆碱能作用较弱
	■ 特异性外周 α_1 肾上腺素受体阻滞能导致中等发生率的射精问题,如逆行射精 [63,64]
	■ 罕见阴茎异常勃起的报道 [33]
	■ 报道的性功能障碍发生率为60%~70% [47]
舒必利/氨磺必利	■ 强力升高血清催乳素水平 [22],但是注意,在 CUtLASS-1 研究中,与 SGA(升高催乳素的能力各不相同)相比,舒必利(本研究中主要的 FGA)并未导致更多的性功能障碍 [20]
噻吨类(如氟哌噻吨)	■ 性兴奋问题和性快感缺失 [65]
卢美哌隆	■ 似乎不影响催乳素 [66]
	■ 在(短期)临床试验中没有性功能不良反应的报道 [67]
哌马色林	■ 不与多巴胺受体结合 [68],因此对催乳素没有影响
	■ 有可能改善抑郁患者的性功能 [69]
伊洛哌酮	■ 通常不影响催乳素 [70]
	■ 不良事件报告数据库中有一些性功能障碍的报告 [71],有逆行射精的病例报告 [72]

治疗

在治疗性功能障碍之前,必须进行全面评估,以确定最可能的原因。假设躯体疾病已被排除(糖尿病、高血压、心血管病等)或被治疗(例如肥胖 [73]),则以下原则适用。

性功能障碍偶尔自发缓解 [33],但可能需要 6 个月时间才能变得明显(如果有的话) [30],并且这可能与疾病严重程度的减轻有关,而不是与对抗精神病药本身的耐受有关。当症状持续时,最明显的第一步是适当减少剂量或停止服用引起性功能障碍的药物。下一步是换一种不太可能引起性功能障碍的药物(表 1.30)。另一种选择是加入 5~10mg 阿立哌唑,这能使催乳素水平恢复正常,改善性功能[74-77]。如仍无效或不可行,可以试用"解毒剂":例如赛庚啶(5-HT$_2$ 拮抗剂,4~16mg/d)已被用于 SSRI 引起的性功能障碍,但常引起镇静。有证据表明,米氮平(同样是 5-HT$_2$ 拮抗剂以及 α$_2$ 受体阻滞剂)可以缓解第一代抗精神病药治疗患者的性高潮障碍[78]。使用金刚烷胺、安非他酮、丁螺环酮、氯贝胆碱和育亨宾均获得不同程度的成功,但这些药物也有一些不良反应和与其他药物的相互作用。由于高催乳素血症可导致性功能障碍,有一项随机对照试验评估了司来吉兰(增加多巴胺活性)对性功能障碍的作用,但结果为阴性[79]。研究显示睾酮贴片能增加女性性欲,但需要注意可能会显著增加患乳腺癌的风险(表 1.32)[80,81]。

支持"解毒剂"的证据很差[33,101]。需要注意的是,阳性试验由于样本量小、试验持续时间短以及缺乏混杂因素控制(年龄、合并用药、因基线性功能障碍以外的原因更换抗精神病药),其结果的普遍性受到限制[101]。由于使用不同的评估工具来测量结果,研究之间的数据比较变得更加复杂[102]。

西地那非(伟哥)或前列地尔(凯威捷)等药物仅对勃起障碍有效(它们对性欲和中枢性性兴奋没有影响)。性功能障碍门诊使用的心理方法可能不适合有精神健康问题的患者参加[11]。

表 1.32　抗精神病药所致性功能障碍的治疗

药物	药理	潜在治疗对象	不良反应
前列地尔[1,13]	前列腺素	勃起障碍	疼痛、纤维化、低血压、阴茎异常勃起
金刚烷胺[1,82]	多巴胺激动剂	催乳素引起的性欲和性兴奋降低(多巴胺提高性欲并促进射精)	精神病性症状复发、胃肠道反应、紧张、失眠、皮疹
氯贝胆碱[83]	胆碱能,或肾上腺素能神经传递的胆碱能增强	抗胆碱能作用引起的性兴奋问题和性快感缺失(因三环类抗抑郁药、抗精神病药等)	恶心、呕吐、腹绞痛、心动过缓、视物模糊、出汗
溴隐亭[11]	多巴胺激动剂	催乳素引起的性欲和性兴奋降低	精神病性症状复发、胃肠道反应
安非他酮[84,85]	去甲肾上腺素和多巴胺再摄取抑制剂	选择性 5-羟色胺再摄取抑制剂引起的性功能障碍(证据不足)	注意力集中问题、睡眠减少、震颤
丁螺环酮[86]	5HT$_{1a}$ 部分激动剂	选择性 5-羟色胺再摄取抑制剂所致性功能障碍,特别是性欲减退和性快感缺失	恶心、头晕、头痛
赛庚啶[1,86,87]	5HT$_2$ 拮抗剂	5-色胺传递增加(如选择性 5-羟色胺再摄取抑制)引起的性功能障碍,特别是性快感缺失	镇静和疲劳,抵消抗抑郁药的治疗效果
氟班色林(在美国获得许可)[88]	5HT$_{1A}$ 激动剂,5HT$_{2A}$ 拮抗剂,多巴胺拮抗剂	绝经前妇女性欲的缺乏或丧失。对服用抗抑郁药的女性似乎是安全的[89]	低血压、晕厥、镇静、头晕、恶心、口干

续表

药物	药理	潜在治疗对象	不良反应
西地那非[13,90-93]、他达拉非[94]、洛地那非[95]、伐地那非[96]	磷酸二酯酶抑制剂	任何病因引起的勃起功能障碍。女性性快感缺乏。催乳素升高时有效	轻度头痛、头晕、鼻塞
育亨宾[1,13,97-99]	中枢和外周 α_2 肾上腺素受体拮抗剂	选择性五羟色胺再摄取抑制剂引起的性功能障碍,特别是勃起障碍、性欲降低和性快感缺失(证据不足)	焦虑、恶心、细震颤、血压升高、出汗、乏力
哌马色林[69]	$5HT_{2A}$ 和 $5HT_{2C}$ 的反向激动剂	对抗抑郁药物反应不足的抑郁症患者的性功能障碍。性功能改善与抑郁症疗效无关,尚未证实	外周水肿、恶心、意识模糊
布美诺肽[100]	黑皮质素受体激动剂	绝经前女性性欲低下。没有关于精神疾病患者使用药物的公开数据	脸红、恶心、头痛

注:上述药物最好在性功能障碍专家的护理或监督下使用。

参考文献

1. Baldwin DS, et al. Effects of antidepressant drugs on sexual function. *Int J Psychiatry Clin Pract* 1997; 1:47–58.
2. Pollack MH, et al. Genitourinary and sexual adverse effects of psychotropic medication. *Int J Psychiatry Med* 1992; 22:305–327.
3. Dumontaud M, et al. Sexual dysfunctions in schizophrenia: beyond antipsychotics. A systematic review. *Prog Neuropsychopharmacol Biol Psychiatry* 2020; 98:109804.
4. Nunes LV, et al. Strategies for the treatment of antipsychotic-induced sexual dysfunction and/or hyperprolactinemia among patients of the schizophrenia spectrum: a review. *J Sex Marital Ther* 2012; 38:281–301.
5. Montejo AL, et al. Frequency of sexual dysfunction in patients with a psychotic disorder receiving antipsychotics. *J Sex Med* 2010; 7:3404–3413.
6. Olfson M, et al. Male sexual dysfunction and quality of life in schizophrenia. *J Clin Psychiatry* 2005; 66:331–338.
7. Montejo AL, et al. Incidence of sexual dysfunction associated with antidepressant agents: a prospective multicenter study of 1022 outpatients. Spanish Working Group for the Study of Psychotropic-Related Sexual Dysfunction. *J Clin Psychiatry* 2001; 62 Suppl 3:10–21.
8. Souaiby L, et al. Sexual dysfunction in patients with schizophrenia and schizoaffective disorder and its association with adherence to antipsychotic medication. *J Mental Health* 2020; 29:623–630.
9. Baggaley M. Sexual dysfunction in schizophrenia: focus on recent evidence. *Human Psychopharmacology* 2008; 23:201–209.
10. Ucok A, et al. Sexual dysfunction in patients with schizophrenia on antipsychotic medication. *Eur Psychiatry* 2007; 22:328–333.
11. Segraves RT. Effects of psychotropic drugs on human erection and ejaculation. *Arch Gen Psychiatry* 1989; 46:275–284.
12. Stahl SM. The psychopharmacology of sex, Part 1: neurotransmitters and the 3 phases of the human sexual response. *J Clin Psychiatry* 2001; 62:80–81.
13. Garcia-Reboll L, et al. Drugs for the treatment of impotence. *Drugs Aging* 1997; 11:140–151.
14. Bitter I, et al. Antipsychotic treatment and sexual functioning in first-time neuroleptic-treated schizophrenic patients. *Int Clin Psychopharmacol* 2005; 20:19–21.
15. Dembler-Stamm T, et al. Sexual dysfunction in unmedicated patients with schizophrenia and in healthy controls. *Pharmacopsychiatry* 2018; 51:251–256.
16. Vargas-Cáceres S, et al. The impact of psychosis on sexual functioning: a systematic review. *J Sex Med* 2021; S1743-6095(1720) 31126-31127.
17. Macdonald S, et al. Nithsdale schizophrenia surveys 24: sexual dysfunction. Case-control study. *Br J Psychiatry* 2003; 182:50–56.
18. Smith S. Effects of antipsychotics on sexual and endocrine function in women: implications for clinical practice. *J Clin Psychopharmacol* 2003; 23:S27–S32.
19. Howard LM, et al. The general fertility rate in women with psychotic disorders. *Am J Psychiatry* 2002; 159:991–997.
20. Peluso MJ, et al. Non-neurological and metabolic side effects in the Cost Utility of the Latest Antipsychotics in Schizophrenia Randomised Controlled Trial (CUtLASS-1). *SchizophrRes* 2013; 144:80–86.

21. Byerly MJ, et al. An empirical evaluation of the Arizona sexual experience scale and a simple one-item screening test for assessing antipsychotic-related sexual dysfunction in outpatients with schizophrenia and schizoaffective disorder. *Schizophr Res* 2006; 81:311–316.
22. Smith SM, et al. Sexual dysfunction in patients taking conventional antipsychotic medication. *Br J Psychiatry* 2002; 181:49–55.
23. Serretti A, et al. A meta-analysis of sexual dysfunction in psychiatric patients taking antipsychotics. *Int Clin Psychopharmacol* 2011; 26:130–140.
24. Zhang Y, et al. Prolactin and thyroid stimulating hormone (TSH) levels and sexual dysfunction in patients with schizophrenia treated with conventional antipsychotic medication: a cross-sectional study. *Med Sci Monit* 2018; 24:9136–9143.
25. Collaborative Working Group on Clinical Trial Evaluations. Adverse effects of the atypical antipsychotics. *J Clin Psychiatry* 1998; 59 Suppl 12:17–22.
26. Knegtering H, et al. Are sexual side effects of prolactin-raising antipsychotics reducible to serum prolactin? *Psychoneuroendocrinology* 2008; 33:711–717.
27. Hanssens L, et al. The effect of antipsychotic medication on sexual function and serum prolactin levels in community-treated schizophrenic patients: results from the Schizophrenia Trial of Aripiprazole (STAR) study (NCT00237913). *BMC Psychiatry* 2008; 8:95.
28. Mir A, et al. Change in sexual dysfunction with aripiprazole: a switching or add-on study. *J Psychopharm* 2008; 22:244–253.
29. Byerly MJ, et al. Effects of aripiprazole on prolactin levels in subjects with schizophrenia during cross-titration with risperidone or olanzapine: analysis of a randomized, open-label study. *Schizophr Res* 2009; 107:218–222.
30. Montejo AL, et al. Management strategies for antipsychotic-related sexual dysfunction: a clinical approach. *J Clin Med* 2021; 10:308.
31. Aldridge SA. Drug-induced sexual dysfunction. *Clin Pharm* 1982; 1:141–147.
32. Fond G, et al. Sexual dysfunctions are associated with major depression, chronic inflammation and anticholinergic consumption in the real-world schizophrenia FACE-SZ national cohort. *Prog Neuropsychopharmacol Biol Psychiatry* 2019; 94:109654.
33. Baldwin D, et al. Sexual side-effects of antidepressant and antipsychotic drugs. *Adv Psychiatric Treat* 2003; 9:202–210.
34. Rykmans V, et al. A comparison of switching strategies from risperidone to aripiprazole in patients with schizophrenia with insufficient efficacy/tolerability on risperidone (cn138–169). *Eur Psychiatry* 2008; 23:S111–S111.
35. Potkin SG, et al. Reduced sexual dysfunction with aripiprazole once-monthly versus paliperidone palmitate: results from QUALIFY. *Int Clin Psychopharmacol* 2017; 32:147–154.
36. Chen CY, et al. Improvement of serum prolactin and sexual function after switching to aripiprazole from risperidone in schizophrenia: a case series. *Psychiatry ClinNeurosci* 2011; 65:95–97.
37. Vrignaud L, et al. [Hypersexuality associated with aripiprazole: a new case and review of the literature]. *Therapie* 2014; 69:525–527.
38. Ajmal A, et al. Psychotropic-induced hyperprolactinemia: a clinical review. *Psychosomatics* 2014; 55:29–36.
39. Kane JM, et al. A multicenter, randomized, double-blind, controlled phase 3 trial of fixed-dose brexpiprazole for the treatment of adults with acute schizophrenia. *Schizophr Res* 2015; 164:127–135.
40. Citrome L. Brexpiprazole for schizophrenia and as adjunct for major depressive disorder: a systematic review of the efficacy and safety profile for this newly approved antipsychotic – what is the number needed to treat, number needed to harm and likelihood to be helped or harmed? *Int J Clin Pract* 2015; 69:978–997.
41. Nasrallah HA, et al. The safety and tolerability of cariprazine in long-term treatment of schizophrenia: a post hoc pooled analysis. *BMC Psychiatry* 2017; 17:305.
42. Coward DM. General pharmacology of clozapine. *British J Psychiatry Supp* 1992; 160:5–11.
43. Meltzer HY, et al. Effect of clozapine on human serum prolactin levels. *Am J Psychiatry* 1979; 136:1550–1555.
44. Aizenberg D, et al. Comparison of sexual dysfunction in male schizophrenic patients maintained on treatment with classical antipsychotics versus clozapine. *J Clin Psychiatry* 2001; 62:541–544.
45. Crawford AM, et al. The acute and long-term effect of olanzapine compared with placebo and haloperidol on serum prolactin concentrations. *Schizophr Res* 1997; 26:41–54.
46. Mitchell JE, et al. Antipsychotic drug therapy and sexual dysfunction in men. *Am J Psychiatry* 1982; 139:633–637.
47. Serretti A, et al. Sexual side effects of pharmacological treatment of psychiatric diseases. *Clin Pharmacol Ther* 2011; 89:142–147.
48. Citrome L, et al. Long-term safety and tolerability of lurasidone in schizophrenia: a 12-month, double-blind, active-controlled study. *Int Clin Psychopharmacol* 2012; 27:165–176.
49. Clayton AH, et al. Safety of flibanserin in women treated with antidepressants: a randomized, placebo-controlled study. *J Sex Med* 2018; 15:43–51.
50. Dossenbach M, et al. Effects of atypical and typical antipsychotic treatments on sexual function in patients with schizophrenia: 12-month results from the Intercontinental Schizophrenia Outpatient Health Outcomes (IC-SOHO) study. *Eur Psychiatry* 2006; 21:251–258.
51. Aurobindo Pharma – Milpharm Ltd. Summary of product characteristics. Olanzapine 10 mg tablets. 2020; http://www.medicines.org.uk/emc/medicine/27661/SPC/Olanzapine++10+mg+tablets.
52. Montalvo I, et al. Changes in prolactin levels and sexual function in young psychotic patients after switching from long-acting injectable risperidone to paliperidone palmitate. *Int Clin Psychopharmacol* 2013; 28:46–49.
53. Shiloh R, et al. Risperidone-induced retrograde ejaculation. *Am J Psychiatry* 2001; 158:650.
54. Loh C, et al. Risperidone-induced retrograde ejaculation: case report and review of the literature. *Int Clin Psychopharmacol* 2004; 19:111–112.
55. Thompson JW, Jr., et al. Psychotropic medication and priapism: a comprehensive review. *J Clin Psychiatry* 1990; 51:430–433.
56. Peuskens J, et al. A comparison of quetiapine and chlorpromazine in the treatment of schizophrenia. *Acta Psychiatr Scand* 1997; 96:265–273.
57. Bobes J, et al. Frequency of sexual dysfunction and other reproductive side-effects in patients with schizophrenia treated with risperidone, olanzapine, quetiapine, or haloperidol: the results of the EIRE study. *J Sex Marital Ther* 2003; 29:125–147.

58. Byerly MJ, et al. An open-label trial of quetiapine for antipsychotic-induced sexual dysfunction. *J Sex Marital Ther* 2004; 30:325–332.
59. Knegtering R, et al. A randomized open-label study of the impact of quetiapine versus risperidone on sexual functioning. *J Clin Psychopharmacol* 2004; 24:56–61.
60. Montejo Gonzalez AL, et al. A 6-month prospective observational study on the effects of quetiapine on sexual functioning. *J Clin Psychopharmacol* 2005; 25:533–538.
61. Atmaca M, et al. A new atypical antipsychotic: quetiapine-induced sexual dysfunctions. *Int J Impot Res* 2005; 17:201–203.
62. Kelly DL, et al. A randomized double-blind 12-week study of quetiapine, risperidone or fluphenazine on sexual functioning in people with schizophrenia. *Psychoneuroendocrinology* 2006; 31:340–346.
63. Tran PV, et al. Double-blind comparison of olanzapine versus risperidone in the treatment of schizophrenia and other psychotic disorders. *J Clin Psychopharmacol* 1997; 17:407–418.
64. Raja M. Risperidone-induced absence of ejaculation. *Int Clin Psychopharmacol* 1999; 14:317–319.
65. Aizenberg D, et al. Sexual dysfunction in male schizophrenic patients. *J Clin Psychiatry* 1995; 56:137–141.
66. Correll CU, et al. Safety and tolerability of lumateperone 42 mg: an open-label antipsychotic switch study in outpatients with stable schizophrenia. *Schizophr Res* 2021; 228:198–205.
67. Correll CU, et al. Efficacy and safety of lumateperone for treatment of schizophrenia: a randomized clinical trial. *JAMA Psychiatry* 2020; 77:349–358.
68. Cruz MP. Pimavanserin (Nuplazid): a treatment for hallucinations and delusions associated with Parkinson's disease. *P & T* 2017; 42:368–371.
69. Freeman MP, et al. Improvement of sexual functioning during treatment of MDD with adjunctive pimavanserin: a secondary analysis. *Depress Anxiety* 2020; 37:485–495.
70. Peuskens J, et al. The effects of novel and newly approved antipsychotics on serum prolactin levels: a comprehensive review. *CNS Drugs* 2014; 28:421–453.
71. Subeesh V, et al. Novel adverse events of iloperidone: a disproportionality analysis in US Food and Drug Administration Adverse Event Reporting System (FAERS) Database. *Current Drug Safety* 2019; 14:21–26.
72. Freeman SA. Iloperidone-induced retrograde ejaculation. *Int Clin Psychopharmacol* 2013; 28:156.
73. Theleritis C, et al. Sexual dysfunction and central obesity in patients with first episode psychosis. *Eur Psychiatry* 2017; 42:1–7.
74. Shim JC, et al. Adjunctive treatment with a dopamine partial agonist, aripiprazole, for antipsychotic-induced hyperprolactinemia: a placebo-controlled trial. *Am J Psychiatry* 2007; 164:1404–1410.
75. Yasui-Furukori N, et al. Dose-dependent effects of adjunctive treatment with aripiprazole on hyperprolactinemia induced by risperidone in female patients with schizophrenia. *J Clin Psychopharmacol* 2010; 30:596–599.
76. Trives MZ, et al. Effect of the addition of aripiprazole on hyperprolactinemia associated with risperidone long-acting injection. *J Clin Psychopharmacol* 2013; 33:538–541.
77. Kelly DL, et al. Adjunct aripiprazole reduces prolactin and prolactin-related adverse effects in premenopausal women with psychosis: results from the DAAMSEL clinical trial. *J Clin Psychopharmacol* 2018; 38:317–326.
78. Terevnikov V, et al. Add-on mirtazapine improves orgasmic functioning in patients with schizophrenia treated with first-generation antipsychotics. *Nord J Psychiatry* 2017; 71:77–80.
79. Kodesh A, et al. Selegiline in the treatment of sexual dysfunction in schizophrenic patients maintained on neuroleptics: a pilot study. *Clin Neuropharmacol* 2003; 26:193–195.
80. Davis SR, et al. Testosterone for low libido in postmenopausal women not taking estrogen. *N Eng J Med* 2008; 359:2005–2017.
81. Schover LR. Androgen therapy for loss of desire in women: is the benefit worth the breast cancer risk? *FertilSteril* 2008; 90:129–140.
82. Valevski A, et al. Effect of amantadine on sexual dysfunction in neuroleptic-treated male schizophrenic patients. *Clin Neuropharmacol* 1998; 21:355–357.
83. Gross MD. Reversal by bethanechol of sexual dysfunction caused by anticholinergic antidepressants. *Am J Psychiatry* 1982; 139:1193–1194.
84. Masand PS, et al. Sustained-release bupropion for selective serotonin reuptake inhibitor-induced sexual dysfunction: a randomized, double-blind, placebo-controlled, parallel-group study. *Am J Psychiatry* 2001; 158:805–807.
85. Rezaei O, et al. The effect of bupropion on sexual function in patients with Schizophrenia: a randomized clinical trial. *Eur J Psychiatry* 2017; 32.
86. Rothschild AJ. Sexual side effects of antidepressants. *J Clin Psychiatry* 2000; 61 Suppl 11:28–36.
87. Lauerma H. Successful treatment of citalopram-induced anorgasmia by cyproheptadine. *Acta Psychiatr Scand* 1996; 93:69–70.
88. IBM Watson Health. IBM Micromedex Solutions. 2020; https://www.ibm.com/watson-health/about/micromedex.
89. Clayton AH, et al. Effect of lurasidone on sexual function in major depressive disorder patients with subthreshold hypomanic symptoms (mixed features): results from a placebo-controlled trial. *J Clin Psychiatry* 2018; 79:18m12132.
90. Nurnberg HG, et al. Sildenafil for women patients with antidepressant-induced sexual dysfunction. *Psychiatr Serv* 1999; 50:1076–1078.
91. Salerian AJ, et al. Sildenafil for psychotropic-induced sexual dysfunction in 31 women and 61 men. *J Sex Marital Ther* 2000; 26:133–140.
92. Gopalakrishnan R, et al. Sildenafil in the treatment of antipsychotic-induced erectile dysfunction: a randomized, double-blind, placebo-controlled, flexible-dose, two-way crossover trial. *Am J Psychiatry* 2006; 163:494–499.
93. Mazzilli R, et al. Erectile dysfunction in patients taking psychotropic drugs and treated with phosphodiesterase-5 inhibitors. *Arch Ital Urol Androl* 2018; 90:44–48.
94. De Boer MK, et al. Efficacy of tadalafil on erectile dysfunction in male patients using antipsychotics: a double-blind, placebo-controlled, crossover pilot study. *J Clin Psychopharmacol* 2014; 34:380–382.
95. Nunes LV, et al. Adjunctive treatment with lodenafil carbonate for erectile dysfunction in outpatients with schizophrenia and spectrum: a

randomized, double-blind, crossover, placebo-controlled trial. *J Sex Med* 2013; **10**:1136–1145.

96. Mitsonis CI, et al. Vardenafil in the treatment of erectile dysfunction in outpatients with chronic schizophrenia: a flexible-dose, open-label study. *J Clin Psychiatry* 2008; **69**:206–212.

97. Jacobsen FM. Fluoxetine-induced sexual dysfunction and an open trial of yohimbine. *J Clin Psychiatry* 1992; **53**:119–122.

98. Michelson D, et al. Mirtazapine, yohimbine or olanzapine augmentation therapy for serotonin reuptake-associated female sexual dysfunction: a randomized, placebo controlled trial. *J Psychiatr Res* 2002; **36**:147–152.

99. Woodrum ST, et al. Management of SSRI-induced sexual dysfunction. *Ann Pharmacother* 1998; **32**:1209–1215.

100. Kingsberg SA, et al. Bremelanotide for the treatment of hypoactive sexual desire disorder: two randomized phase 3 trials. *Obstet Gynecol* 2019; **134**:899–908.

101. Allen K, et al. Management of antipsychotic-related sexual dysfunction: systematic review. *J Sex Med* 2019; **16**:1978–1987.

102. Basson R, et al. Women's sexual dysfunction associated with psychiatric disorders and their treatment. *Womens Health* 2018; **14**:1745506518762664.

扩展阅读

Clayton AH, et al. Sexual dysfunction due to psychotropic medications. *Psychiatr Clin North Am* 2016; **39**:427–463.

肺炎

2018 年对 14 项研究进行的荟萃分析表明,与未使用抗精神病药相比,使用抗精神病药与肺炎发病率增加近一倍有关[1]。同样的分析发现使用第一代抗精神病药和第二代抗精神病药的肺炎发病率没有差异,病死率也没有增加。对向美国食品药品管理局自发报告的后续分析发现,服用氯氮平、奥氮平和多种抗精神病药(与氟哌啶醇相比)的患者报告的肺炎发病率较高[2]。据报道,氯氮平[3-5]、其他抗精神病药[6]以及涉及第一代抗精神病药和第二代抗精神病药的多药合用[4,5,7]的剂量增大时,肺炎的风险升高;心境稳定剂[5]联合用药时,肺炎风险也升高。在双相障碍患者中,三类药物合用的风险高于任何两类药物合用[5]。

一项针对双相障碍患者的研究发现,氯氮平、奥氮平和氟哌啶醇与肺炎的发生率增高有关,而锂盐具有保护作用[5]。另一项研究表明,氨磺必利与肺炎发生无关[4]。在一项研究中,再次使用氯氮平者(复发性)肺炎的风险高于首次使用氯氮平者[3]。在被诊断为肺炎的病人中,精神分裂症本身似乎增加了并发症的风险(例如进入重症监护室)[8],但是无论是诊断还是年龄,似乎都不能改变抗精神病药对肺炎的影响[9]。同样,无论是否是阿尔茨海默病患者,抗精神病药相关肺炎的风险均增加[10]。

最近出现的一些数据在某种程度上质疑了抗精神病药使用与肺炎风险之间明显的因果关联。有一项研究观察了 8 000 例患者在服用各种抗精神病药之前与之后的肺炎患病率,发现总体上(或者对于任意一种抗精神病药)并没有任何变化。一个病例对照研究发现,抗精神病药使用的持续时间只是增加肺炎风险的三个因素之一(另外两个是疾病的严重程度和共病指数)[11]。

在此研究中,抗精神病药治疗的持续时间可以被视为疾病持续时间的指标。还需要注意的是,在新型冠状病毒感染期间,有一些抗精神病药显示出抗病毒活性[12,13]。

抗精神病药增加患肺炎风险的机制尚不清楚。可能包括镇静(H_1 拮抗作用最强的药物风险可能最高)[4,7]、肌张力障碍或运动障碍、口干导致食团运送障碍从而增加吸入的风险(氯氮平则为多涎)、一般身体健康状况较差[4]或者对免疫反应的不明影响[7,14]。然而,抗精神病药会增加吸入性肺炎而不是其他类型肺炎的风险,这一事实支持这是可能的(也许是唯一的)机制[15]。使用氯氮平时,肺炎也可能继发于便秘[16]。氯氮平也与抗体缺乏和抗生素的大量使用密切相关[17]。

在任何时期服用任何抗精神病药(尤其是氯氮平[18])的所有患者可能都会增加患肺炎的风险。所有患者均应仔细监测胸部感染迹象,并及时开始有效的治疗。可以考虑使用肺炎球菌疫苗,尽管没有证据支持其在这组患者中的益处。以前使用氯氮平引起肺炎的患者,再次使用氯氮平时需要格外警惕。若对胸部感染的严重程度或类型有任何疑问,应该考虑及早转诊至普通内科治疗。

小结

- 所有抗精神病药的使用均可增加患肺炎的风险。
- 监测所有患者胸部感染的体征并及时治疗。

参考文献

1. Dzahini O, et al. Antipsychotic drug use and pneumonia: systematic review and meta-analysis. *J Psychopharmacology* 2018; **32**:1167–1181.

2. Cepaityte D, et al. Exploring a safety signal of antipsychotic-associated pneumonia: a pharmacovigilance-pharmacodynamic study. *Schizophr Bull* 2020: [Epub ahead of print].

3. Hung GC, et al. Antipsychotic reexposure and recurrent pneumonia in schizophrenia: a nested case-control study. *J Clin Psychiatry* 2016; **77**:60–66.

4. Kuo CJ, et al. Second-generation antipsychotic medications and risk of pneumonia in schizophrenia. *Schizophr Bull* 2013; **39**:648–657.

5. Yang SY, et al. Antipsychotic drugs, mood stabilizers, and risk of pneumonia in bipolar disorder: a nationwide case-control study. *J Clin Psychiatry* 2013; **74**:e79–e86.

6. Huybrechts KF, et al. Comparative safety of antipsychotic medications in nursing home residents. *J Am Geriatr Soc* 2012; **60**:420–429.

7. Trifiro G, et al. Association of community-acquired pneumonia with antipsychotic drug use in elderly patients: a nested case-control study. *Ann Intern Med* 2010; **152**:418–440.

8. Chen YH, et al. Poor clinical outcomes among pneumonia patients with schizophrenia. *Schizophr Bull* 2011; **37**:1088–1094.

9. Nose M, et al. Antipsychotic drug exposure and risk of pneumonia: a systematic review and meta-analysis of observational studies. *Pharmacoepidemiol Drug Saf* 2015; **24**:812–820.

10. Tolppanen AM, et al. Antipsychotic use and risk of hospitalization or death due to pneumonia in persons with and those without Alzheimer disease. *Chest* 2016; **150**:1233–1241.

11. Chan HY, et al. Is antipsychotic treatment associated with risk of pneumonia in people with serious mental illness?: the roles of severity of psychiatric symptoms and global functioning. *J Clin Psychopharmacol* 2019; **39**:434–440.

12. Plaze M, et al. Repurposing chlorpromazine to treat COVID-19: the reCoVery study. *Encephale* 2020; **46**:169–172.

13. Otręba M, et al. Antiviral activity of chlorpromazine, fluphenazine, perphenazine, prochlorperazine, and thioridazine towards RNA-viruses. A review. *Eur J Pharmacol* 2020; **887**:173553.

14. Knol W, et al. Antipsychotic drug use and risk of pneumonia in elderly people. *J Am Geriatr Soc* 2008; **56**:661–666.

15. Herzig SJ, et al. Antipsychotics and the risk of aspiration pneumonia in individuals hospitalized for nonpsychiatric conditions: a cohort study. *J Am Geriatr Soc* 2017; **65**:2580–2586.

16. Galappathie N, et al. Clozapine-associated pneumonia and respiratory arrest secondary to severe constipation. *Med Sci Law* 2014; **54**:105–109.

17. Ponsford M, et al. Clozapine is associated with secondary antibody deficiency. *Br J Psychiatry* 2018; **214**:1–7.

18. De Leon J, et al. Pneumonia may be more frequent and have more fatal outcomes with clozapine than with other second-generation antipsychotics. *World Psychiatry* 2020; **19**:120–121.

扩展阅读

Schoretsanitis G, et al. An update on the complex relationship between clozapine and pneumonia. *Expert Rev Clin Pharmacol* 2021; **14**:145–149.

换用抗精神病药

由于耐受性差而换用抗精神病药的建议总结。

不良反应	建议用药		备选用药
急性锥体外系反应 [1-8] 肌张力障碍、帕金森症、运动迟缓	阿立哌唑 布瑞哌唑 卡利拉嗪 奥氮平 喹硫平	氯氮平 鲁拉西酮 齐拉西酮	
静坐不能 [2,9,10]	奥氮平 喹硫平	氯氮平 布瑞哌唑	
血脂异常 [7,8,11-16]	氨磺必利 阿立哌唑 * 鲁拉西酮 齐拉西酮	阿塞那平 布瑞哌唑 卡利拉嗪	
糖耐量受损 [7,8,15,17-21]	氨磺必利 阿立哌唑 * 鲁拉西酮 齐拉西酮	布瑞哌唑 卡利拉嗪 氟哌啶醇	
高催乳素血症 [7,8,15,22-28]	阿立哌唑 * 布瑞哌唑 卡利拉嗪 鲁拉西酮 喹硫平	氯氮平 奥氮平 齐拉西酮	
体位性低血压 [8,15,29]	氨磺必利 阿立哌唑 布瑞哌唑 卡利拉嗪 鲁拉西酮	氟哌啶醇 舒必利 三氟拉嗪	
Q-T 间期延长 [27,30-37]	布瑞哌唑 卡利拉嗪 鲁拉西酮 帕立哌酮	任何药物小剂量单药治疗均非 Q-T 间期延长的 正式禁忌证(监测心电图)	
镇静 [7,8,27]	氨磺必利 阿立哌唑 布瑞哌唑 卡利拉嗪 利培酮 舒必利	氟哌啶醇 三氟拉嗪 齐拉西酮	

续表

不良反应	建议用药	备选用药
性功能障碍 [8,38-44]	阿立哌唑 布瑞哌唑 卡利拉嗪 鲁拉西酮 喹硫平	氯氮平
迟发性运动障碍 [45-49]	氯氮平	阿立哌唑 奥氮平 喹硫平
体重增加 [16,35,37,50-57]	氨磺必利 阿立哌唑 * 布瑞哌唑 卡利拉嗪 氟哌啶醇 鲁拉西酮 齐拉西酮	阿塞那平 氟哌啶醇 三氟拉嗪

　* 有证据显示，无论是换用还是合用阿立哌唑，都可以有效地降低体重、催乳素水平，改善血脂和降低血糖水平 [58-61]。

　　由于卢美哌隆和哌马色林的可用性有限，所以并未在表中列出。这两种药物都很少或不引起锥体外系反应或静坐不能，对催乳素或血压没有影响，极少导致体重增加和代谢紊乱 [62,63]。哌马色林延长 Q-T 间期 [64]，然而卢美哌隆似乎对心电图没有影响 [65]。

参考文献

1. Stanniland C, et al. Tolerability of atypical antipsychotics. *Drug Saf* 2000; **22**:195–214.
2. Tarsy D, et al. Effects of newer antipsychotics on extrapyramidal function. *CNS Drugs* 2002; **16**:23–45.
3. Caroff SN, et al. Movement disorders associated with atypical antipsychotic drugs. *J Clin Psychiatry* 2002; **63 Suppl 4**:12–19.
4. Lemmens P, et al. A combined analysis of double-blind studies with risperidone vs. placebo and other antipsychotic agents: factors associated with extrapyramidal symptoms. *Acta Psychiatr Scand* 1999; **99**:160–170.
5. Taylor DM. Aripiprazole: a review of its pharmacology and clinical use. *Int J Clin Pract* 2003; **57**:49–54.
6. Meltzer HY, et al. Lurasidone in the treatment of schizophrenia: a randomized, double-blind, placebo- and olanzapine-controlled study. *Am J Psychiatry* 2011; **168**:957–967.
7. Garnock-Jones KP. Cariprazine: a review in schizophrenia. *CNS Drugs* 2017; **31**:513–525.
8. Garnock-Jones KP. Brexpiprazole: a review in schizophrenia. *CNS Drugs* 2016; **30**:335–342.
9. Buckley PF. Efficacy of quetiapine for the treatment of schizophrenia: a combined analysis of three placebo-controlled trials. *Curr Med Res Opin* 2004; **20**:1357–1363.
10. Pringsheim T, et al. The assessment and treatment of antipsychotic-induced akathisia. *Can J Psychiatry* 2018; **63**:719–729.
11. Rettenbacher MA, et al. Early changes of plasma lipids during treatment with atypical antipsychotics. *Int Clin Psychopharmacol* 2006; **21**:369–372.
12. Ball MP, et al. Clozapine-induced hyperlipidemia resolved after switch to aripiprazole therapy. *Ann Pharmacother* 2005; **39**:1570–1572.
13. Chrzanowski WK, et al. Effectiveness of long-term aripiprazole therapy in patients with acutely relapsing or chronic, stable schizophrenia: a 52-week, open-label comparison with olanzapine. *Psychopharmacology* 2006; **189**:259–266.
14. De Hert M, et al. A case series: evaluation of the metabolic safety of aripiprazole. *Schizophr Bull* 2007; **33**:823–830.
15. Citrome L, et al. Long-term safety and tolerability of lurasidone in schizophrenia: a 12-month, double-blind, active-controlled study. *Int Clin Psychopharmacol* 2012; **27**:165–176.
16. Kemp DE, et al. Weight change and metabolic effects of asenapine in patients with schizophrenia and bipolar disorder. *J Clin Psychiatry* 2014; **75**:238–245.

17. Haddad PM. Antipsychotics and diabetes: review of non-prospective data. *Br J Psychiatry Suppl* 2004; 47:S80–S86.

18. Berry S, et al. Improvement of insulin indices after switch from olanzapine to risperidone. *Eur Neuropsychopharmacol* 2002; 12:316.

19. Gianfrancesco FD, et al. Differential effects of risperidone, olanzapine, clozapine, and conventional antipsychotics on type 2 diabetes: findings from a large health plan database. *J Clin Psychiatry* 2002; 63:920–930.

20. Mir S, et al. Atypical antipsychotics and hyperglycaemia. *Int Clin Psychopharmacol* 2001; 16:63–74.

21. Cernea S, et al. Pharmacological management of glucose dysregulation in patients treated with second-generation antipsychotics. *Drugs* 2020; 80:1763–1781.

22. Turrone P, et al. Elevation of prolactin levels by atypical antipsychotics. *Am J Psychiatry* 2002; 159:133–135.

23. David SR, et al. The effects of olanzapine, risperidone, and haloperidol on plasma prolactin levels in patients with schizophrenia. *Clin Ther* 2000; 22:1085–1096.

24. Hamner MB, et al. Hyperprolactinaemia in antipsychotic-treated patients: guidelines for avoidance and management. *CNS Drugs* 1998; 10:209–222.

25. Trives MZ, et al. Effect of the addition of aripiprazole on hyperprolactinemia associated with risperidone long-acting injection. *J Clin Psychopharmacol* 2013; 33:538–541.

26. Suzuki Y, et al. Differences in plasma prolactin levels in patients with schizophrenia treated on monotherapy with five second-generation antipsychotics. *Schizophr Res* 2013; 145:116–119.

27. Leucht S, et al. Comparative efficacy and tolerability of 15 antipsychotic drugs in schizophrenia: a multiple-treatments meta-analysis. *Lancet* 2013; 382:951–962.

28. Keks N, et al. Comparative tolerability of dopamine D2/3 receptor partial agonists for schizophrenia. *CNS Drugs* 2020; 34:473–507.

29. Citrome L. Cariprazine: chemistry, pharmacodynamics, pharmacokinetics, and metabolism, clinical efficacy, safety, and tolerability. *Exp Opin Drug Metab Toxicol* 2013; 9:193–206.

30. Glassman AH, et al. Antipsychotic drugs: prolonged QTc interval, torsade de pointes, and sudden death. *Am J Psychiatry* 2001; 158:1774–1782.

31. Antipsychotics TD. QT prolongation. *Acta Psychiatr Scand* 2003; 107:85–95.

32. Titier K, et al. Atypical antipsychotics: from potassium channels to torsade de pointes and sudden death. *Drug Saf* 2005; 28:35–51.

33. Ray WA, et al. Atypical antipsychotic drugs and the risk of sudden cardiac death. *N Engl J Med* 2009; 360:225–235.

34. Loebel A, et al. Efficacy and safety of lurasidone 80 mg/day and 160 mg/day in the treatment of schizophrenia: a randomized, double-blind, placebo- and active-controlled trial. *Schizophr Res* 2013; 145:101–109.

35. Das S, et al. Brexpiprazole: so far so good. *Ther Adv Psychopharmacol* 2016; 6:39–54.

36. Citrome L. Cariprazine for the treatment of schizophrenia: a review of this dopamine D3-preferring D3/D2 receptor partial agonist. *Clin Schizophr Relat Psychoses* 2016; 10:109–119.

37. Huhn M, et al. Comparative efficacy and tolerability of 32 oral antipsychotics for the acute treatment of adults with multi-episode schizophrenia: a systematic review and network meta-analysis. *Lancet* 2019; 394:939–951.

38. Byerly MJ, et al. An open-label trial of quetiapine for antipsychotic-induced sexual dysfunction. *J Sex Marital Ther* 2004; 30:325–332.

39. Byerly MJ, et al. Sexual dysfunction associated with second-generation antipsychotics in outpatients with schizophrenia or schizoaffective disorder: an empirical evaluation of olanzapine, risperidone, and quetiapine. *Schizophr Res* 2006; 86:244–250.

40. Montejo Gonzalez AL, et al. A 6-month prospective observational study on the effects of quetiapine on sexual functioning. *J Clin Psychopharmacol* 2005; 25:533–538.

41. Dossenbach M, et al. Effects of atypical and typical antipsychotic treatments on sexual function in patients with schizophrenia: 12-month results from the Intercontinental Schizophrenia Outpatient Health Outcomes (IC-SOHO) study. *Eur Psychiatry* 2006; 21:251–258.

42. Kerwin R, et al. A multicentre, randomized, naturalistic, open-label study between aripiprazole and standard of care in the management of community-treated schizophrenic patients Schizophrenia Trial of Aripiprazole: (STAR) study. *Eur Psychiatry* 2007; 22:433–443.

43. Hanssens L, et al. The effect of antipsychotic medication on sexual function and serum prolactin levels in community-treated schizophrenic patients: results from the Schizophrenia Trial of Aripiprazole (STAR) study (NCT00237913). *BMC Psychiatry* 2008; 8:95.

44. Loebel A, et al. Effectiveness of lurasidone vs. quetiapine XR for relapse prevention in schizophrenia: a 12-month, double-blind, noninferiority study. *Schizophr Res* 2013; 147:95–102.

45. Lieberman J, et al. Clozapine pharmacology and tardive dyskinesia. *Psychopharmacology* 1989; 99 Suppl 1:S54–S59.

46. O'Brien J, et al. Marked improvement in tardive dyskinesia following treatment with olanzapine in an elderly subject. *Br J Psychiatry* 1998; 172:186.

47. Sacchetti E, et al. Quetiapine, clozapine, and olanzapine in the treatment of tardive dyskinesia induced by first-generation antipsychotics: a 124-week case report. *Int Clin Psychopharmacol* 2003; 18:357–359.

48. Witschy JK, et al. Improvement in tardive dyskinesia with aripiprazole use. *Can J Psychiatry* 2005; 50:188.

49. Ricciardi L, et al. Treatment recommendations for tardive dyskinesia. *Can J Psychiatry* 2019; 64:388–399.

50. Taylor DM, et al. Atypical antipsychotics and weight gain – a systematic review. *Acta Psychiatr Scand* 2000; 101:416–432.

51. Allison D, et al. Antipsychotic-induced weight gain: a comprehensive research synthesis. *Am J Psychiatry* 1999; 156:1686–1696.

52. Brecher M, et al. The long term effect of quetiapine (Seroquel™) monotherapy on weight in patients with schizophrenia. *Int J Psychiatry Clin Pract* 2000; 4:287–291.

53. Casey DE, et al. Switching patients to aripiprazole from other antipsychotic agents: a multicenter randomized study. *Psychopharmacology* 2003; 166:391–399.

54. Newcomer JW, et al. A multicenter, randomized, double-blind study of the effects of aripiprazole in overweight subjects with schizophrenia or schizoaffective disorder switched from olanzapine. *J Clin Psychiatry* 2008; 69:1046–1056.

55. McEvoy JP, et al. Effectiveness of lurasidone in patients with schizophrenia or schizoaffective disorder switched from other antipsychotics: a randomized, 6-week, open-label study. *J Clin Psychiatry* 2013; **74**:170–179.

56. McEvoy JP, et al. Effectiveness of paliperidone palmitate vs haloperidol decanoate for maintenance treatment of schizophrenia: a randomized clinical trial. *JAMA* 2014; **311**:1978–1987.

57. Nasrallah HA, et al. The safety and tolerability of cariprazine in long-term treatment of schizophrenia: a post hoc pooled analysis. *BMC Psychiatry* 2017; **17**:305.

58. Shim JC, et al. Adjunctive treatment with a dopamine partial agonist, aripiprazole, for antipsychotic-induced hyperprolactinemia: a placebo-controlled trial. *Am J Psychiatry* 2007; **164**:1404–1410.

59. Fleischhacker WW, et al. Weight change on aripiprazole-clozapine combination in schizophrenic patients with weight gain and suboptimal response on clozapine: 16-week double-blind study. *Eur Psychiatry* 2008; **23 Suppl 2**:S114–S115.

60. Henderson DC, et al. Aripiprazole added to overweight and obese olanzapine-treated schizophrenia patients. *J Clin Psychopharmacol* 2009; **29**:165–169.

61. Preda A, et al. A safety evaluation of aripiprazole in the treatment of schizophrenia. *Exp Opin Drug Saf* 2020; **19**:1529–1538.

62. Correll CU, et al. Safety and tolerability of lumateperone 42 mg: an open-label antipsychotic switch study in outpatients with stable schizophrenia. *Schizophr Res* 2021; **228**:198–205.

63. Mathis MV, et al. The US Food and Drug Administration's perspective on the new antipsychotic pimavanserin. *J Clin Psychiatry* 2017; **78**:e668–e673.

64. Cruz MP. Pimavanserin (nuplazid): a treatment for hallucinations and delusions associated with parkinson's disease. *P & T* 2017; **42**:368–371.

65. Greenwood J, et al. Lumateperone: a novel antipsychotic for schizophrenia. *Ann Pharmacother* 2021; **55**:98–104.

静脉血栓栓塞

关联证据

在 1965 年,抗精神病药治疗首次和血栓风险升高相联系 [1]——经过超过十年的观察期,1 590 例患者中 3.1% 发生血栓,其中 9 例(0.6%)患者死亡。然而,持续使用抗精神病药代表着严重而持续的精神疾病,所以观察到的与抗精神病药之间的相关性可能反映了所用药物治疗的疾病的内在病理过程。在某种程度上,抗精神病药治疗与其治疗的疾病对血栓栓塞风险的相对贡献仍有待明确界定。

在一项对近 3 万例患者进行的里程碑式的病例对照研究中 [2],尝试控制年龄和性别的影响(但不控制所诊断的精神疾病)。与对照组相比,服用抗精神病药的患者血栓栓塞的风险总体上显著增加[优势比(OR)7.1]。风险的增加是由低效价吩噻嗪类药物[硫利达嗪、氯丙嗪(OR 24.1)]的作用引起的,主要出现在治疗的前几周。静脉血栓栓塞的绝对风险非常小——只有 0.14% 的患者出现这种情况。二次分析表明与诊断无关(并非所有的处方都是针对精神分裂症)。

随后一项对 7 项病例对照研究进行的荟萃分析 [3] 证实,低效价药物会增加血栓栓塞风险(OR 2.91),并表明使用所有类型抗精神病药的血栓栓塞风险虽相对低但显著增加。此后一项对 17 项研究进行的荟萃分析 [4] 发现,抗精神病药无论是总体上(OR 1.54),还是第一代抗精神病药(OR 1.74)和第二代抗精神病药(OR 1.74)分别计算,患血栓栓塞的风险均略有所增加。血栓栓塞的风险明显随着年龄的增长而降低。研究者认为最好的说法是抗精神病药可能会增加大约 50% 的风险,但剩余的混杂因素不能被忽略(即其他因素可能已经解释了所见的影响)。

从那时起,又有几项病例对照研究证实血栓栓塞风险轻微增加,总体风险很小 [5-7],其中一项研究报告,老年人服用抗精神病药时,发生血栓栓塞的风险为每万名患者年中有 43 例 [7]。其他值得注意的发现包括,丙氯拉嗪(并非总是,甚至经常用于治疗精神病性障碍的药物)与血栓的相关性显著增加 [5],以及与抗精神病药剂量相关的风险增加(高剂量患者的风险增加了 4 倍)[6]。与丙氯拉嗪的相关性在之前一项英国的研究中得到过证实 [8]。这些发现进一步支持了假说:抗精神病药(不仅仅是它们治疗的疾病)会造成血栓栓塞风险增加。病理性凝血的最高风险可能发生在治疗的前 3 个月左右 [9,10]。

最新数据

在 2021 年初,发表了两篇荟萃分析。他们的发现如下。

参考文献	包含的研究数量	相对风险(与没用药比较)第一代抗精神病药	相对风险(与没用药比较)第二代抗精神病药	相对风险(与没用药比较)所有抗精神病药	解释
Di et al., 2021[9]	22	1.83 静脉血栓/肺栓塞	1.75 静脉血栓 3.79 肺栓塞 2.60 静脉血栓/肺栓塞	1.53 静脉血栓 3.69 肺栓塞 1.60 静脉血栓/肺栓塞	年轻患者(年龄 <60 岁)的风险最高。低效价第一代抗精神病药风险最高

续

参考文献	包含的研究数量	相对风险(与没用药比较)第一代抗精神病药	相对风险(与没用药比较)第二代抗精神病药	相对风险(与没用药比较)所有抗精神病药	解释
Liu et al., 2021[10]	28	1.47 静脉血栓/肺栓塞	1.62 静脉血栓/肺栓塞	1.55 静脉血栓 3.68 肺栓塞 2.01 静脉血栓/肺栓塞	与持续性用药患者相比,首次服用抗精神病药的患者有更高的风险。与低剂量相比,高剂量有更高的风险

机制

已经提出了一些机制来解释抗精神病药和血栓之间的相关性。表 1.33 概述了所提出的机制。

表 1.33　关于抗精神病药相关静脉血栓栓塞提出的机制 [11-13]

镇静 *	磷脂抗体升高
肥胖 *	血小板聚集增强 **
高催乳素血症 *	血浆同型半胱氨酸升高

* 一些证据表明,这些因素不是抗精神病药诱导血栓栓塞的机制 [14]。

* * 体外数据表明,不同的抗精神病药对血小板聚集的影响截然不同 [12]。

结果

血栓栓塞风险的增加反映在许多已发表的肺栓塞 [15]、卒中 [16] 和心肌梗死 [17,18] 发病率升高的报告中。

总结

几乎可以肯定,抗精神病药与静脉血栓的风险(虽然小但是重要)增加以及肺栓塞、卒中和心肌梗死的危险相关。风险在治疗早期和年轻人中似乎最大,并且可能与剂量有关。

临床实践要点

- 密切监测所有开始抗精神病药治疗的患者(特别是年轻的患者)的静脉血栓栓塞症状。
  - 小腿疼痛或肿胀
  - 突发呼吸困难
  - 心肌梗死征兆(胸痛、恶心等)
  - 卒中征兆(突发单侧无力等)
- 使用最小治疗剂量。
- 鼓励良好的饮水习惯和身体活动。

参考文献

1. Häfner H, et al. Thromboembolic complications in neuroleptic treatment. *Compr Psychiatry* 1965; 6:25–34.

2. Zornberg GL, et al. Antipsychotic drug use and risk of first-time idiopathic venous thromboembolism: a case-control study. *Lancet* 2000; 356:1219–1223.

3. Zhang R, et al. Antipsychotics and venous thromboembolism risk: a meta-analysis. *Pharmacopsychiatry* 2011; 44:183–188.

4. Barbui C, et al. Antipsychotic drug exposure and risk of venous thromboembolism: a systematic review and meta-analysis of observational studies. *Drug Saf* 2014; 37:79–90.

5. Ishiguro C, et al. Antipsychotic drugs and risk of idiopathic venous thromboembolism: a nested case-control study using the CPRD. *Pharmacoepidemiol Drug Saf* 2014; 23:1168–1175.

6. Wang MT, et al. Use of antipsychotics and risk of venous thromboembolism in postmenopausal women. A population-based nested case-control study. *Thromb Haemost* 2016; 115:1209–1219.

7. Letmaier M, et al. Venous thromboembolism during treatment with antipsychotics: results of a drug surveillance programme. *World J Biol Psychiatry* 2018; 19: 175–186.

8. Parker C, et al. Antipsychotic drugs and risk of venous thromboembolism: nested case-control study. *BMJ* 2010; 341:c4245.

9. Di X, et al. Antipsychotic use and risk of venous thromboembolism: a meta-analysis. *Psychiatry Res* 2021; 296:113691.

10. Liu Y, et al. Current antipsychotic agent use and risk of venous thromboembolism and pulmonary embolism: a systematic review and meta-analysis of observational studies. *Ther Adv Psychopharmacol* 2021; 11:2045125320982720.

11. Hagg S, et al. Risk of venous thromboembolism due to antipsychotic drug therapy. *Exp Opin Drug Saf* 2009; 8:537–547.

12. Dietrich-Muszalska A, et al. The first- and second-generation antipsychotic drugs affect ADP-induced platelet aggregation. *World J Biol Psychiatry* 2010; 11:268–275.

13. Tromeur C, et al. Antipsychotic drugs and venous thromboembolism. *Thromb Res* 2012; 130:S29–S31.

14. Ferraris A, et al. Antipsychotic use among adult outpatients and venous thromboembolic disease: a retrospective cohort study. *J Clin Psychopharmacol* 2017; 37:405–411.

15. Borras L, et al. Pulmonary thromboembolism associated with olanzapine and risperidone. *J Emerg Med* 2008; 35:159–161.

16. Douglas IJ, et al. Exposure to antipsychotics and risk of stroke: self controlled case series study. *BMJ* 2008; 337:a1227.

17. Brauer R, et al. Antipsychotic drugs and risks of myocardial infarction: a self-controlled case series study. *Eur Heart J* 2015; 36:984–992.

18. Huang KL, et al. Myocardial infarction risk and antipsychotics use revisited: a meta-analysis of 10 observational studies. *J Psychopharmacology* 2017; 31:1544–1555.

难治性精神分裂症和氯氮平

氯氮平开始用药方案

氯氮平给药方案

氯氮平的许多不良反应都有剂量依赖性,且与加药速度有关。不良反应往往在治疗开始时容易出现且较严重。标准维持量对从未使用过氯氮平的患者甚至可能致命[1]。为了尽量减少这些问题,在开始治疗时从低剂量开始、缓慢加量是非常重要的。

氯氮平通常从 12.5mg 每晚 1 次开始。氯氮平具有降压作用,因此在用药后 6h 内应每小时监测一次血压。氯氮平首次使用如果是在夜间,那么通常不用监测血压。第 2 天,氯氮平的剂量可以增加到 12.5mg,每天两次。如果患者耐受,氯氮平的剂量可每天增加 25~50mg,直到 300mg/d。加量过程在 2~3 周内完成。如需要继续加量,应缓慢进行,每周增加 50~100mg。为了保证充分地治疗,目标血药浓度应达到 350μg/L,但是在较低血药浓度时即可出现疗效。由于性别和吸烟情况不同,患者达到该血药浓度的平均(存在显著差异)用药剂量差别很大,剂量范围为 250mg/d(女性非吸烟者)至 550mg/d(男性吸烟者)[2]。氯氮平的每天总剂量应分开使用(通常是每天 2 次),但如果镇静是个问题,则较大剂量应放在夜间服用。

表 1.34 是氯氮平的初始治疗建议。该方案较为保守,有人用过更快的加药策略。在下述情况下,加药速度应该更慢:严重镇静或其他剂量相关不良反应、老年人、年幼患者、身体虚弱、对其他抗精神病药耐受差的患者。如果患者不能耐受某一剂量,则需减小到之前能耐受的剂量。如果不良反应缓解,可以更慢的速度再次增加剂量。

如患者因某种原因停止服用氯氮平小于 2 天,则重新使用时的剂量应和停药前的剂量一样,不要补足漏服的剂量。但若超过 2 天,则需重新开始缓慢加药(但可快于从未用过氯氮平的患者)。见本章"在治疗中停药后重新使用氯氮平"相关内容。

表 1.34　氯氮平的初始应用建议(住院患者)

天	早晨剂量/mg	晚上剂量/mg	天	早晨剂量/mg	晚上剂量/mg
1	—	12.5	10	75	100
2	12.5	12.5	11	100	100
3	25	25	12	100	125
4	25	25	13	125	125[a]
5	25	50	14	125	150
6	25	50	15	150	150
7	50	50	18	150	200[b]
8	50	75	21	200	200
9	75	75	28	200	250[c]

[a] 女性非吸烟患者的目标剂量(250mg/d)。

[b] 男性非吸烟患者的目标剂量(350mg/d)。

[c] 女性吸烟患者的目标剂量(450mg/d)。

参考文献

1. Stanworth D, Hunt NC, Flanagan RJ. Clozapine – a dangerous drug in a clozapine-naive subject. *Forensic Sci Int* 2011; 214:e23–e5.
2. Rostami-Hodjegan A, Amin AM, Spencer EP, et al. Influence of dose, cigarette smoking, age, sex, and metabolic activity on plasma clozapine concentrations: a predictive model and nomograms to aid clozapine dose adjustment and to assess compliance in individual patients. *J Clin Psychopharmacol* 2004; 24:70–78.

肌内注射氯氮平

　　肌内注射氯氮平是对拒绝口服药物的难治性精神病患者的一种短期干预,目的是在治疗完成后转为口服氯氮平[1]。尽管证据相对有限,但最近的观察数据表明,开始使用肌内注射氯氮平治疗不会对长期坚持口服治疗产生不利影响[1,2]。肌内注射氯氮平在短期安全性和耐受性方面与口服氯氮平相似[3]。**重要的是,肌内注射氯氮平应该根据个人情况决定是否使用,并且限于所有其他方法都失败且预计对氯氮平治疗有反应的患者将其视为最后手段[1]**。这种制剂在英国等许多国家都未经许可,因此应采取足够的预防措施,并获得患者或护理者的同意。

　　成年人肌内注射氯氮平的一般建议总结在表 1.35 中。

表 1.35　对肌内注射氯氮平的一般建议

规格	25mg/mL
最大剂量 *	每个部位 100mg(4mL)
口服等效剂量	氯氮平的口服生物利用度约为肌内注射液的 50%,例如,每天 50mg 肌内注射液 = 每天 100mg 片剂/口服溶液
给药部位 †	制造商说明臀肌深部注射
最长疗程 ‡	每次注射前,患者应口服氯氮平。氯氮平注射的时间应尽可能短(最多连续 2 周)
给药频率	为了尽量减少注射次数,最好每日 1 次
监测	每次给药后,应在前 2h 内每 15min 观察一次患者,以检查有无过量镇静 常规氯氮平监测也适用

* 对于超过 100mg 的剂量,可以分开注射到两个部位。
† 系列病例报告数据显示,经大腿外侧或三角肌注射——注意注射时疼[2]。
‡ 系列病例报告数据显示肌内注射氯氮平最长达 96 天[2,3]。
注:如果需要肌内注射苯二氮䓬类药物,在肌内注射氯氮平和苯二氮䓬类药物之间至少间隔 1h。

参考文献

1. Casetta C, et al. A retrospective study of intramuscular clozapine prescription for treatment initiation and maintenance in treatment-resistant psychosis. *Br J Psychiatry* 2020; 217:506–513.
2. Henry R, et al. Evaluation of the effectiveness and acceptability of intramuscular clozapine injection: illustrative case series. *B J Psych Bulletin* 2020; 44:239–243.
3. Schulte PF, et al. Compulsory treatment with clozapine: a retrospective long-term cohort study. *Int J Law Psychiatry* 2007; 30:539–545.

优化氯氮平治疗

氯氮平单用

目标剂量 （注意，最好根据患者耐受程度和血药浓度调整剂量）	• 在英国平均剂量约 450mg/d[1] • 疗效通常出现于剂量为 150~900mg/d[2] • 老年人、女性、不吸烟者、使用某些酶抑制剂的患者需要更低的剂量[3,4]（见氯氮平加量方法）
血药浓度	• 大多数研究指出出现疗效的阈值范围为 350~420μg/L[5,6]，最高可达 500μg/L[7] • 在无法达到治疗浓度的男性吸烟患者中，代谢抑制剂（如氟伏沙明[8] 或西咪替丁[9]）可同时使用，但需十分谨慎[10] • 血浆去甲氯氮平浓度的重要性尚不明确，但氯氮平/去甲氯氮平的比例可辅助评估近期用药的依从性

氯氮平的增效剂

临床上常见单用氯氮平时效果不佳，因此使用氯氮平"增效剂"成为普遍的做法。虽然使用增效剂的证据越来越多，但仍不足以制订治疗选择的流程或方案。在临床上，氯氮平增效治疗的效果往往令人失望，症状的严重程度极少出现明显变化。支持这种临床印象的是，很多研究结果模棱两可，最多是略有疗效。荟萃分析显示抗精神病药增效治疗无效[11]，长期研究[12] 认为其作用小，总体上疗效很小[13]，或者对特定症状群有轻微疗效[14]。需要注意的是，该领域的高质量研究很少——当只包括大型高质量研究时，大多数荟萃分析报告药理学增效无益[15]。一项关于难治性精神分裂症多巴胺活性的研究表明，多巴胺并没有过量产生[16,17]。因此多巴胺拮抗剂可能无效。

建议对所有增效剂的使用都要仔细监测，若无明显效果，则在 3~6 个月后停用。在氯氮平治疗中加用其他药物时，应该预计到会加重整体的不良反应负担，因此不宜继续使用无效的治疗。有些病例加用增效剂可减轻一些不良反应的严重程度（如体重增加、血脂异常——见下），或减少氯氮平的剂量。在氯氮平治疗时加入阿立哌唑，可能在逆转代谢影响方面特别有效[18,19]。最近发布的国际共识指南建议：（在优化血药浓度后）根据残留症状选择合适的增强剂；针对阳性症状添加氨磺必利或阿立哌唑，针对阴性症状添加抗抑郁药，针对自杀观念或攻击行为添加心境稳定剂[15]。

表 1.36 显示了单用最佳剂量氯氮平治疗 3~6 个月无满意效果时的治疗选择（原著按字母排序）。

表 1.36 建议选择的氯氮平增效剂

选择	注解
加氨磺必利[20-25] （400~800mg/d）	• 一些证据和临床经验提示，加用氨磺必利可能是值得的。有 3 项小样本的随机对照研究（其中最大的一项研究提示无效），其中两项研究发现不良反应加重（包括对心脏的不良反应）[26,27] • 可减少氯氮平剂量[28]

续表

选择	注解
加阿立哌唑[18,29-31] (15~30mg/d)	■ 虽然一项荟萃分析提示有些作用,但治疗有利的证据非常有限[32]。降低体重和低密度脂蛋白胆固醇[32]。长效注射已被使用[33,34]
加氟哌啶醇[31,35,36] (2~3mg/d)	■ 治疗有益的证据很弱
加拉莫三嗪[37-39] (25~300mg/d)	■ 对部分有效或无效者可能有用。可减少饮酒量[40]。有一些模棱两可的报告[41-43],一些荟萃分析提示有中等效应值[44],但这一结果在很大程度上受到两项外围研究的影响[45]
加 ω-3 甘油三酯[46,47] (2~3g/d EPA)	■ 对抗精神病药(包括氯氮平)无效或部分有效的患者中有效,但支持证据较弱且存争议
加利培酮[48,49] (2~6mg/d)	■ 一项随机对照研究支持,但也有两项随机对照研究却是阴性结果,有效率极低[50,51]。少量研究报道可增加氯氮平的血药浓度。也可选择长期注射剂[34,52];帕利哌酮长效注射已被使用[34,53]。
加舒必利[54] (400mg/d)	■ 可能对部分有效或无效患者有效。得到 4 个随机试验的支持(1 个英语,3 个中文)[55]。总体疗效较弱
加托吡酯[56-60] (50~300mg/d)	■ 随机对照试验结果 2 项阳性,2 项阴性。可加重一些患者的精神病症状[38,61]。两项荟萃分析(包括迄今为止我们还未看到的中国数据)[45,62]表明,对阳性和阴性症状有很强的疗效,还显著减轻体重(但通常伴有精神运动迟缓和注意力困难)
加丙戊酸钠[45-63] (400~800mg/d)	■ 来自 5 项中国的随机对照试验[45]的综合效应表明可缓解阳性症状,但大多数研究质量不高。Cochrane 建议在抗精神病药中添加丙戊酸钠总的来说是有益的,特别是针对兴奋和攻击性[64]
加齐拉西酮[65-68] (80~160mg/d)	■ 3 项随机对照研究支持[68,69]。与 Q-T 间期延长相关。很少应用

注:
■ 始终考虑使用心境稳定剂和/或抗抑郁药,特别是认为情绪紊乱是症状的部分原因时[70-72]。
■ 其他选项包括添加**匹莫齐特**、**奥氮平**或**舍吲哚**。均不建议使用:匹莫齐特和舍吲哚具有严重的心脏毒性,加用奥氮平的支持性证据差[73]且可加剧代谢不良反应。关于匹莫齐特[74,75]和舍吲哚[76]的若干研究显示无效。一个小样本随机对照试验支持使用**银杏提取物**[77],另外两项试验支持使用**美金刚**[78,79]。另一项研究表明增加**乙酰左旋肉碱**可能有益[80],一项病例研究报告**甲状腺素**治疗效果良好[81]。一项随机对照试验描述了**苯甲酸钠**的成功使用[82]。**米诺环素**可能无效[63,83]。**甘氨酸**可能对阳性症状有效,但研究的质量较差[84]。一个小样本系列病例报告(n=6)发现添加**哌马色林**有益[85]。

参考文献

1. Taylor D, et al. A prescription survey of the use of atypical antipsychotics for hospital inpatients in the United Kingdom. *Int J Psychiatry Clin Pract* 2000; 4:41–46.
2. Murphy B, et al. Maintenance doses for clozapine. *Psychiatric Bull* 1998; 22:12–14.
3. Taylor D. Pharmacokinetic interactions involving clozapine. *Br J Psychiatry* 1997; 171:109–112.
4. Lane HY, et al. Effects of gender and age on plasma levels of clozapine and its metabolites: analyzed by critical statistics. *J Clin Psychiatry* 1999; 60:36–40.
5. Taylor D, et al. The use of clozapine plasma levels in optimising therapy. *Psychiatric Bull* 1995; 19:753–755.
6. Spina E, et al. Relationship between plasma concentrations of clozapine and norclozapine and therapeutic response in patients with schizophrenia resistant to conventional neuroleptics. *Psychopharmacology* 2000; 148:83–89.

7. Perry PJ. Therapeutic drug monitoring of antipsychotics. *Psychopharmacol Bull* 2001; 35:19–29.

8. Polcwiartek C, et al. The clinical potentials of adjunctive fluvoxamine to clozapine treatment: a systematic review. *Psychopharmacology* 2016; 233:741–750.

9. Watras M, et al. A therapeutic interaction between cimetidine and clozapine: case study and review of the literature. *Ther Adv Psychopharmacol* 2013; 3:294–297.

10. Gee S, et al. Optimising treatment of schizophrenia: the role of adjunctive fluvoxamine. *Psychopharmacology* 2016; 233:739–740.

11. Barbui C, et al. Does the addition of a second antipsychotic drug improve clozapine treatment? *Schizophr Bull* 2009; 35:458–468.

12. Paton C, et al. Augmentation with a second antipsychotic in patients with schizophrenia who partially respond to clozapine: a meta-analysis. *J Clin Psychopharmacol* 2007; 27:198–204.

13. Taylor D, et al. Augmentation of clozapine with a second antipsychotic. A meta analysis. *Acta Psychiatr Scand* 2012; 125:15–24.

14. Bartoli F, et al. Adjunctive second-generation antipsychotics for specific symptom domains of schizophrenia resistant to clozapine: a meta-analysis. *J Psychiatr Res* 2019; 108:24–33.

15. Wagner E, et al. Clozapine combination and augmentation strategies in patients with schizophrenia –recommendations from an international expert survey among the Treatment Response and Resistance in Psychosis (TRRIP) working group. *Schizophr Bull* 2020; 46:1459–1470.

16. Demjaha A, et al. Dopamine synthesis capacity in patients with treatment-resistant schizophrenia. *Am J Psychiatry* 2012; 169:1203–1210.

17. Demjaha A, et al. Antipsychotic treatment resistance in schizophrenia associated with elevated glutamate levels but normal dopamine function. *Biol Psychiatry* 2014; 75:e11–e13.

18. Fleischhacker WW, et al. Effects of adjunctive treatment with aripiprazole on body weight and clinical efficacy in schizophrenia patients treated with clozapine: a randomized, double-blind, placebo-controlled trial. *Int J Neuropsychopharmacol* 2010; 13:1115–1125.

19. Correll CU, et al. Selective effects of individual antipsychotic cotreatments on cardiometabolic and hormonal risk status: results from a systematic review and meta-analysis. *Schizophr Bull* 2013; 39 (Suppl 1):S29–S30.

20. Matthiasson P, et al. Relationship between dopamine D2 receptor occupancy and clinical response in amisulpride augmentation of clozapine non-response. *J Psychopharm* 2001; 15:S41.

21. Munro J, et al. Amisulpride augmentation of clozapine: an open non-randomized study in patients with schizophrenia partially responsive to clozapine. *Acta Psychiatr Scand* 2004; 110:292–298.

22. Zink M, et al. Combination of clozapine and amisulpride in treatment-resistant schizophrenia–case reports and review of the literature. *Pharmacopsychiatry* 2004; 37:26–31.

23. Ziegenbein M, et al. Augmentation of clozapine with amisulpride in patients with treatment-resistant schizophrenia: an open clinical study. *German J Psychiatry* 2006; 9:17–21.

24. Kampf P, et al. Augmentation of clozapine with amisulpride: a promising therapeutic approach to refractory schizophrenic symptoms. *Pharmacopsychiatry* 2005; 38:39–40.

25. Assion HJ, et al. Amisulpride augmentation in patients with schizophrenia partially responsive or unresponsive to clozapine. A randomized, double-blind, placebo-controlled trial. *Pharmacopsychiatry* 2008; 41:24–28.

26. Barnes TR, et al. Amisulpride augmentation in clozapine-unresponsive schizophrenia (AMICUS): a double-blind, placebo-controlled, randomised trial of clinical effectiveness and cost-effectiveness. *Health Technol Assess* 2017; 21:1–56.

27. Barnes TRE, et al. Amisulpride augmentation of clozapine for treatment-refractory schizophrenia: a double-blind, placebo-controlled trial. *Ther Adv Psychopharmacol* 2018; 8:185–197.

28. Croissant B, et al. Reduction of side effects by combining clozapine with amisulpride: case report and short review of clozapine-induced hypersalivation-a case report. *Pharmacopsychiatry* 2005; 38:38–39.

29. Chang JS, et al. Aripiprazole augmentation in clozapine-treated patients with refractory schizophrenia: an 8-week, randomized, double-blind, placebo-controlled trial. *J Clin Psychiatry* 2008; 69:720–731.

30. Muscatello MR, et al. Effect of aripiprazole augmentation of clozapine in schizophrenia: a double-blind, placebo-controlled study. *Schizophr Res* 2011; 127:93–99.

31. Cipriani A, et al. Aripiprazole versus haloperidol in combination with clozapine for treatment-resistant schizophrenia: a 12-month, randomized, naturalistic trial. *J Clin Psychopharmacol* 2013; 33:533–537.

32. Srisurapanont M, et al. Efficacy and safety of aripiprazole augmentation of clozapine in schizophrenia: a systematic review and meta-analysis of randomized-controlled trials. *J Psychiatr Res* 2015; 62:38–47.

33. Balcioglu YH, et al. One plus one sometimes equals more than two: long-acting injectable aripiprazole adjunction in clozapine-resistant schizophrenia. *Clin Neuropharmacol* 2020; 43:166–168.

34. Grimminck R, et al. Combination of clozapine with long-acting injectable antipsychotics in treatment-resistant schizophrenia: preliminary evidence from health care utilization indices. *Prim Care Companion CNS Disord* 2020; 22:19m02560.

35. Rajarethinam R, et al. Augmentation of clozapine partial responders with conventional antipsychotics. *Schizophr Res* 2003; 60:97–98.

36. Barbui C, et al. Aripiprazole versus haloperidol in combination with clozapine for treatment-resistant schizophrenia in routine clinical care: a randomized, controlled trial. *J Clin Psychopharmacol* 2011; 31:266–273.

37. Dursun SM, et al. Clozapine plus lamotrigine in treatment-resistant schizophrenia. *Arch Gen Psychiatry* 1999; 56:950.

38. Dursun SM, et al. Augmenting antipsychotic treatment with lamotrigine or topiramate in patients with treatment-resistant schizophrenia: a naturalistic case-series outcome study. *J Psychopharm* 2001; 15:297–301.

39. Tiihonen J, et al. Lamotrigine in treatment-resistant schizophrenia: a randomized placebo-controlled crossover trial. *Biol Psychiatry* 2003; 54:1241–1248.

40. Kalyoncu A, et al. Use of lamotrigine to augment clozapine in patients with resistant schizophrenia and comorbid alcohol dependence: a potent anti-craving effect? *J Psychopharmacology* 2005; 19:301–305.

41. Goff DC, et al. Lamotrigine as add-on therapy in schizophrenia: results of 2 placebo-controlled trials. *J Clin Psychopharmacol* 2007;

27:582–589.

42. Heck AH, et al. Addition of lamotrigine to clozapine in inpatients with chronic psychosis. *J Clin Psychiatry* 2005; **66**:1333.

43. Vayisoglu S, et al. Lamotrigine augmentation in patients with schizophrenia who show partial response to clozapine treatment. *Schizophr Res* 2013; **143**:207–214.

44. Tiihonen J, et al. The efficacy of lamotrigine in clozapine-resistant schizophrenia: a systematic review and meta-analysis. *Schizophr Res* 2009; **109**:10–14.

45. Zheng W, et al. Clozapine augmentation with antiepileptic drugs for treatment-resistant schizophrenia: a meta-analysis of randomized controlled trials. *J Clin Psychiatry* 2017; **78**:e498–e505.

46. Peet M, et al. Double-blind placebo controlled trial of N-3 polyunsaturated fatty acids as an adjunct to neuroleptics. *Schizophr Res* 1998; **29**:160–161.

47. Puri BK, et al. Sustained remission of positive and negative symptoms of schizophrenia following treatment with eicosapentaenoic acid. *Arch Gen Psychiatry* 1998; **55**:188–189.

48. Josiassen RC, et al. Clozapine augmented with risperidone in the treatment of schizophrenia: a randomized, double-blind, placebo-controlled trial. *Am J Psychiatry* 2005; **162**:130–136.

49. Raskin S, et al. Clozapine and risperidone: combination/augmentation treatment of refractory schizophrenia: a preliminary observation. *Acta Psychiatr Scand* 2000; **101**:334–336.

50. Anil Yagcioglu AE, et al. A double-blind controlled study of adjunctive treatment with risperidone in schizophrenic patients partially responsive to clozapine: efficacy and safety. *J Clin Psychiatry* 2005; **66**:63–72.

51. Honer WG, et al. Clozapine alone versus clozapine and risperidone with refractory schizophrenia. *N Engl J Med* 2006; **354**:472–482.

52. Se HK, et al. The combined use of risperidone long-acting injection and clozapine in patients with schizophrenia non-adherent to clozapine: a case series. *J Psychopharmacology* 2010; **24**:981–986.

53. Bioque M, et al. Clozapine and paliperidone palmitate antipsychotic combination in treatment-resistant schizophrenia and other psychotic disorders: a retrospective 6-month mirror-image study. *Eur Psychiatry* 2020; **63**:e71

54. Shiloh R, et al. Sulpiride augmentation in people with schizophrenia partially responsive to clozapine. A double-blind, placebo-controlled study. *Br J Psychiatry* 1997; **171**:569–573.

55. Wang J, et al. Sulpiride augmentation for schizophrenia. *Schizophr Bull* 2010; **36**:229–230.

56. Tiihonen J, et al. Topiramate add-on in treatment-resistant schizophrenia: a randomized, double-blind, placebo-controlled, crossover trial. *J Clin Psychiatry* 2005; **66**:1012–1015.

57. Afshar H, et al. Topiramate add-on treatment in schizophrenia: a randomised, double-blind, placebo-controlled clinical trial. *J Psychopharmacology* 2009; **23**:157–162.

58. Muscatello MR, et al. Topiramate augmentation of clozapine in schizophrenia: a double-blind, placebo-controlled study. *J Psychopharmacology* 2011; **25**:667–674.

59. Hahn MK, et al. Topiramate augmentation in clozapine-treated patients with schizophrenia: clinical and metabolic effects. *J Clin Psychopharmacol* 2010; **30**:706–710.

60. Behdani F, et al. Effect of topiramate augmentation in chronic schizophrenia: a placebo-controlled trial. *Arch Iran Med* 2011; **14**:270–275.

61. Millson RC, et al. Topiramate for refractory schizophrenia. *Am J Psychiatry* 2002; **159**:675.

62. Zheng W, et al. Efficacy and safety of adjunctive topiramate for schizophrenia: a meta-analysis of randomized controlled trials. *Acta Psychiatr Scand* 2016; **134**:385–398.

63. Siskind DJ, et al. Augmentation strategies for clozapine refractory schizophrenia: a systematic review and meta-analysis. *Aust N Z J Psychiatry* 2018; **52**:751–767.

64. Wang Y, et al. Valproate for schizophrenia. *Cochrane Database Syst Rev* 2016; **11**:Cd004028.

65. Zink M, et al. Combination of ziprasidone and clozapine in treatment-resistant schizophrenia. *Human Psychopharmacology* 2004; **19**:271–273.

66. Ziegenbein M, et al. Clozapine and ziprasidone: a useful combination in patients with treatment-resistant schizophrenia. *J Neuropsychiatry Clin Neurosci* 2006; **18**:246–247.

67. Ziegenbein M, et al. Combination of clozapine and ziprasidone in treatment-resistant schizophrenia: an open clinical study. *Clin Neuropharmacol* 2005; **28**:220–224.

68. Zink M, et al. Efficacy and tolerability of ziprasidone versus risperidone as augmentation in patients partially responsive to clozapine: a randomised controlled clinical trial. *J Psychopharm* 2009; **23**:305–314.

69. Muscatello MR, et al. Augmentation of clozapine with ziprasidone in refractory schizophrenia: a double-blind, placebo-controlled study. *J Clin Psychopharmacol* 2014; **34**:129–133.

70. Citrome L. Schizophrenia and valproate. *Psychopharmacol Bull* 2003; **37 Suppl 2**:74–88.

71. Tranulis C, et al. Somatic augmentation strategies in clozapine resistance–what facts? *Clin Neuropharmacol* 2006; **29**:34–44.

72. Suzuki T, et al. Augmentation of atypical antipsychotics with valproic acid. An open-label study for most difficult patients with schizophrenia. *Human Psychopharmacology* 2009; **24**:628–638.

73. Gupta S, et al. Olanzapine augmentation of clozapine. *Ann Clin Psychiatry* 1998; **10**:113–115.

74. Friedman JI, et al. Pimozide augmentation of clozapine inpatients with schizophrenia and schizoaffective disorder unresponsive to clozapine monotherapy. *Neuropsychopharmacology* 2011; **36**:1289–1295.

75. Gunduz-Bruce H, et al. Efficacy of pimozide augmentation for clozapine partial responders with schizophrenia. *Schizophr Res* 2013; **143**:344–347.

76. Nielsen J, et al. Augmenting clozapine with sertindole: a double-blind, randomized, placebo-controlled study. *J Clin Psychopharmacol* 2012; **32**:173–178.

77. Doruk A, et al. A placebo-controlled study of extract of ginkgo biloba added to clozapine in patients with treatment-resistant schizophrenia. *Int Clin Psychopharmacol* 2008; 23:223–227.

78. De Lucena D, et al. Improvement of negative and positive symptoms in treatment-refractory schizophrenia: a double-blind, randomized, placebo-controlled trial with memantine as add-on therapy to clozapine. *J Clin Psychiatry* 2009; 70:1416–1423.

79. Veerman SR, et al. Adjunctive memantine in clozapine-treated refractory schizophrenia: an open-label 1-year extension study. *Psychol Med* 2017; 47:363–375.

80. Bruno A, et al. Acetyl-L-carnitine augmentation of clozapine in partial-responder schizophrenia: a 12-week, open-label uncontrolled preliminary study. *Clin Neuropharmacol* 2016; 39:277–280.

81. Seddigh R, et al. Levothyroxine augmentation in clozapine resistant schizophrenia: a case report and review. *Case Rep Psychiatry* 2015; 2015:678040.

82. Lin CH, et al. Sodium benzoate, a D-Amino acid oxidase inhibitor, added to clozapine for the treatment of schizophrenia: a randomized, double-blind, placebo-controlled trial. *Biol Psychiatry* 2018; 84:422–432.

83. Kelly DL, et al. Adjunctive minocycline in clozapine-treated schizophrenia patients with persistent symptoms. *J Clin Psychopharmacol* 2015; 35:374–381.

84. Correll CU, et al. Efficacy of 42 pharmacologic cotreatment strategies added to antipsychotic monotherapy in schizophrenia: systematic overview and quality appraisal of the meta-analytic evidence. *JAMA Psychiatry* 2017; 74:675–684.

85. Nasrallah HA, et al. Successful treatment of clozapine-nonresponsive refractory hallucinations and delusions with pimavanserin, a serotonin 5HT-2A receptor inverse agonist. *Schizophr Res* 2019; 208:217–220.

氯氮平的替代治疗

对于经过充分的标准抗精神病药治疗证明无效的精神分裂症,强有力的证据证明氯氮平有效。在已确定治疗无效的情况下,氯氮平治疗不应延迟或停止[1,2]。虽然临床上普遍使用新型(或最新)抗精神病药而不是用氯氮平,但缺乏令人信服的研究支持。当不能使用氯氮平(由于毒性或患者拒服或拒绝遵守强制性监测)时,可以尝试使用其他药物或联合用药(表 1.37),但临床上的治疗效果常不理想。通常缺乏疗效、安全性/耐受性的长期数据。

虽然根据现有数据无法区分不同治疗方案的优劣,特别是选择抗精神病药[3,4],但是联合用药之前,采用单一用药的方案似乎更为明智。奥氮平可能是最常单用的抗精神病药,而且通常是超剂量使用。如果奥氮平治疗无效,那么下一步可能会添加第二种抗精神病药(例如氨磺必利),尽管联合抗精神病药治疗方案的风险-效益平衡尚不清楚[5]。一项关于氯氮平无效后抗精神病药治疗的研究大体上证实了这些发现,支持对于不明原因停用氯氮平的患者,重新服用氯氮平和奥氮平是最有效和最安全的治疗选择[6]。在不常规使用的药物中,米诺环素和昂丹司琼具有低毒性和良好耐受性的优势。在临床上需要优先考虑避免隐性的不依从时,可以选择抗精神病药长效针剂。

以下列举的治疗药物大多还在试验期,一些药物还难以获得(如甘氨酸、丝氨酸、肌氨酸等)。在使用下述任何治疗方案之前,读者应当参考所引用的原始文献。要特别注意,当超说明书用药时,需告知患者,确保他们理解试验性治疗的潜在不良反应。

难治性精神分裂症的非氯氮平治疗是一个热门的研究领域。谷氨酸能药物(尽管 Bitopetin 是无效的[7])可能和 $5HT_{2A}$ 反向激动剂一样有希望[8]。

表 1.37　氯氮平的替代治疗

治疗方案	注释
别嘌醇 300~600mg/d (**+ 抗精神病药**)[9-12]	增加腺苷能神经传递,可减少多巴胺的效应。三项 RCT[9,10,12] 支持
氨磺必利[13] (最大量 1 200mg/d)	只有一项小样本的开放性实验
抗精神病药复合用药	多种抗精神病药合用过。数据有限,大多是个案报告、开放和自然观察
阿立哌唑[14,15] (15~30mg/d)	一项 RCT 显示,对使用利培酮或奥氮平(+ 其他药物)无效的患者有中度疗效。更高剂量(60mg/d)也有人使用[16]
阿塞那平(+ 抗精神病药)[17]	两项病例报告
贝沙罗汀 75mg/d[18] (**+ 抗精神病药**)	维 A 酸受体激动剂。对非难治性但治疗欠佳的患者进行的一项 RCT 表明,对阳性症状有重要的作用
布南色林 (**+ 抗精神病药**)[19]	在日本和韩国获得许可的非典型抗精神病药。一项系列病例报告发现它是有效的,并有良好的耐受性
认知行为疗法[20]	始终应该考虑非药物治疗
塞来昔布 + 利培酮[21] (400mg+6mg/d)	COX-2 抑制剂调节免疫反应,并可阻止谷氨酸相关的细胞死亡。一项 RCT 显示对所有主要症状群有效。与心血管病的死亡率增加相关

续表

治疗方案	注释
深部脑刺激（DBS）	以伏隔核和次级前扣带回皮质为靶向进行深部脑刺激，7 例抗药性患者中 4 例有效 [22]
多奈哌齐 5~10mg/d（+ 抗精神病药）[23-25]	三项 RCT，一项不支持 [24]，两项支持 [23,25]，提示对认知功能和阴性症状有轻微疗效
D-丙氨酸 100mg/（kg·d）（+ 抗精神病药）[26]	甘氨酸（NMDA）激动剂。一项 RCT 有效
D-丝氨酸 30mg/（kg·d）（+ 奥氮平）[27]	甘氨酸（NMDA）激动剂。一项 RCT 有效
D-丝氨酸，单一用药，最大量 3g[28]	在一项 RCT 中改善阴性症状，对阳性症状的疗效不如高剂量的奥氮平
电痉挛治疗 [29]	开放性研究认为有中等效果，回顾性研究也是如此 [30]。在实际治疗中常常作为最后的治疗方法，短期 [31] 和长期 [32] 治疗都可能有效
雌二醇 100~200μg 经皮贴剂/d（+ 抗精神病药）[33]	雌激素可能具有精神保护和/或抗精神病作用。对育龄妇女进行的 RCT（$n=183$）表明，对阳性症状有益，尤其是高剂量时。注意禁忌证包括绝经后、静脉血栓史、卒中、乳腺癌、偏头痛先兆。长期服用雌二醇（未控制）会增加子宫内膜增生和恶性肿瘤的风险——考虑咨询内分泌学家。缺乏在男性中证据
法莫替丁 100mg bid+ 抗精神病药 [34]	H_2 受体拮抗剂。一项短期（4 周）的 RCT 研究提示可降低 PANSS 和 CGI 评分
银杏制剂（+ 抗精神病药）[6,7]	与氟哌啶醇合用可能有效。不太可能增加不良反应，但临床经验有限
鲁拉西酮最多 240mg/d[35]（+ 伏硫西汀）	一项比较标准剂量和高剂量鲁拉西酮的 RCT 在给药 24 周后，两者抗药性的改善程度相当 [36]。似乎耐受性良好，可能有效，但不包括氯氮平对照组。在一个小样本系列病例报告中，鲁拉西酮合用伏硫西汀有效 [37]
美金刚 20mg/d（+ 抗精神病药）[38-40]	美金刚是一种 NMDA 拮抗剂。两项随机 RCT 对照试验研究，样本较大（$n=138$）的研究提示无效；样本较小（$n=21$）的研究显示，与氯氮平合用时能改善阴性和阳性症状。另一项针对非难治性精神分裂症的研究显示，当与利培酮合用时，美金刚能改善阴性症状
米安色林 +FGA 30mg/d[32]	$5HT_2$ 受体拮抗剂。一项小样本 RCT 提示有效
米诺环素 200mg/d（+ 抗精神病药）[41,42]	可能有抗炎和神经保护作用。一项开放性试验（$n=22$）和一项 RCT（$n=54$）研究提示对阴性症状和认知功能效果良好。另外还有一项是氯氮平增效剂的 RCT[43]。对早期精神病的神经保护作用有 RCT 证据支持 [44]
米氮平 30mg/d（+ 抗精神病药）[45-47]	$5HT_2$ 受体拮抗剂。两项 RCT，一项无效 [46]，一项有效 [45]。效果主要体现在阳性症状
N-乙酰半胱氨酸 2g/d（+ 抗精神病药）[40]	一项 RCT 提示对改善阴性症状和静坐不能有些疗效。另一项 RCT 显示对慢性精神分裂症有效 [48]。有用到 600mg/d 的成功案例 [49]。大型 RCT 正在进行中 [50]
奥氮平 [51-56] 5~25mg/d	有一些实施良好的试验支持，但临床实践效果不佳。一些患者显示中度疗效

续表

治疗方案	注释
奥氮平 [57-63] 30~60mg/d	文献发现有矛盾，但可能有效。高剂量奥氮平不是非典型抗精神病药 [64]，并且耐受性较差 [65]（存在严重代谢改变 [63]）
奥氮平 + 氨磺必利 [66]（最大量 800mg/d）	小型开放性试验显示有效
奥氮平 + 阿立哌唑 [67]	单个病例报告显示有效。可能减少代谢毒性
奥氮平 + 甘氨酸 [68]［0.8g/（kg·d）］	小型双盲交叉试验提示临床上可改善阴性症状
奥氮平 + 拉莫三嗪 [65,69]（最大量 400mg/d）	矛盾的研究结果，相当牵强。拉莫三嗪的耐受性好，有一定的理论基础
奥氮平 + 利培酮 [70]（不同剂量）	小型研究表明，一些患者先后使用单个药物失败后，联合用药可能有效
奥氮平 + 舒必利 [71]（600mg/d）	一些证据表明这种联用可以改善情绪症状
ω-3-甘油酸三酯 [72,73]	提示有效，但数据有限
昂丹司琼 8mg/d（+ 抗精神病药）	一项对 RCT 的系统综述显示可改善阴性症状和一般精神病理。对认知功能的作用尚无定论 [74]
帕利哌酮长效注射剂	少数患者从氯氮平转为帕利培酮 3 个月一次，内分泌和肝功能参数改善，抗精神病药接触量降低。无关于临床结果的数据 [75]
哌马色林（+ 抗精神病药）	在 10 例患者中，哌马色林单独或作为氯氮平或其他抗精神病药的辅助治疗有临床改善，其中有 6 例患者用氯氮平无效 [76]
丙戊茶碱 + 利培酮 [77]（900mg+6mg/d）	一项 RCT 提示对阳性症状有些疗效
喹硫平 [78-81]	证据非常有限，临床经验也不支持。也有使用高剂量（>1 200mg/d）的案例，但不会更有效 [82]
喹硫平 + 氨磺必利 [83]	一项对 19 例患者的自然观察提示有效。平均剂量为喹硫平 700mg，氨磺必利 950mg
喹硫平 + 氟哌啶醇 [84]	两项病例报告
雷洛昔芬 60~120mg/d（+ 抗精神病药）[85]	选择性雌激素受体调节剂，可以提供雌二醇的益处而无长期风险。一例关于绝经后难治性精神分裂症病例的报告 [85]。在非难治性病例中的数据相当矛盾，有两个部分重叠的阳性结果试验 [86,87] 和一个阴性结果试验 [88]。一项针对难治性女性的阳性结果 RCT[89]。缺乏男性试验证据
利鲁唑 100mg/d + 利培酮最多 6mg/d[90]	谷氨酸调节剂。一项 RCT 显示能改善阴性症状
利培酮 [91-93] 4~8mg/d	在真正难治性精神分裂症中疗效存疑，但有一些证据支持。还可尝试联合甘氨酸 [68]、拉莫三嗪 [60] 或其他非典型药物 [94]
利培酮长效注射剂 50/100mg 2/52[95]	一项 RCT 显示两种剂量对难治性精神分裂症都有良好的效果。100mg 剂量的血浆药物水平接近 6~8mg/d 口服利培酮
利坦色林 + 利培酮（12mg+6mg/d）[96]	$5HT_{2A/2C}$ 受体拮抗剂。一项 RCT 提示对阴性症状有点疗效

续表

治疗方案	注释
肌氨酸(2g/d)[97,98] (+抗精神病药)	增加甘氨酸活性。两项 RCT 支持
舍吲哚[99] (12~24mg/d)	一项大型的 RCT(1996—1998 年实施,2011 年发表)提示效果良好,等同利培酮。大约一半受试者有效。另一项 RCT[100] 显示,与氯氮平合用时无效。几乎无临床实践经验
托吡酯(300mg/d) (+抗精神病药)[101]	一项 RCT 显示少许效果。导致体重减轻。可能有认知方面的不良反应
经颅磁刺激[102-104]	相互矛盾的结果
熊去氧胆酸[105]	一个案例报告
丙戊酸盐[106]	疗效存疑,但有明显情绪症状时可能有用
抑肝散 (+抗精神病药)[107]	日本草药,D_2 和 $5HT_{1A}$ 部分激动剂,$5HT_{2A}$ 和谷氨酸受体拮抗剂。对兴奋/敌对症状存在一些潜在益处
佐替平 300mg/d[108]	一项研究显示,一些患者从氯氮平换为佐替平并未出现病情恶化
齐拉西酮 80~160mg/d[109-111]	两项良好的 RCT。一项 [111] 显示在难治性精神分裂症中效果优于氯丙嗪,另一项 [109] 提示在治疗不耐受或难治的受试者中疗效与氯氮平相当。然而,在实践中疗效欠佳。超剂量使用并无优势 [112]

CGI,临床总体印象量表;COX,环氧化酶;FGA,第一代抗精神病药;NMDA,N-甲基-D-天冬氨酸;PANSS,阳性症状和阴性症状量表;RCT,随机对照试验。

所有治疗方案按字母顺序排列,排名不分先后

难治性精神分裂症——氯氮平的替代治疗:总结

治疗	示例	注释	证据强弱
单用氯氮平以外的抗精神病药(标准或高剂量)	阿立哌唑 15~30mg/d 奥氮平 25~40mg/d	除氯氮平外,任何抗精神病药对难治性精神分裂症的疗效证据都很少。一些数据提示奥氮平高于许可剂量时有效,但存在代谢不良反应的风险	非常弱 ±
氯氮平以外的抗精神病药合用	氨磺必利 + 奥氮平 喹硫平 + 氨磺必利 阿立哌唑 + 奥氮平	合用在临床实践中常见。对照试验提供的证据非常有限,但是开放性研究和实际数据证明有些疗效。不良反应负担增加	弱 +
抗炎药作为抗精神病药的辅助药物	N-乙酰半胱氨酸、非甾体抗炎药米诺环素、雌激素、阿司匹林、ω-3 脂肪酸	一组具有炎症特性的药物曾被尝试用作辅助药物。可能对阴性和认知症状有好处,但样本量较小	非常弱 ±
NMDA 受体调节剂作为辅助用药	美金刚、甘氨酸、D-丝氨酸和肌氨酸	很少用在临床实践中。有可能对阴性症状起作用	非常弱 ±

续表

治疗	示例	注释	证据强弱
物理治疗	电痉挛治疗,重复经颅磁刺激,经颅直流电刺激,深部脑刺激	作为氯氮平的辅助治疗,电痉挛治疗的证据最好。其他的仍然主要是实验性的	中等 ++
辅助抗抑郁药	米氮平、伏硫西汀、5-羟色胺再摄取抑制剂	有限的数据证实了对阴性症状和认知症状略有疗效	弱 +
辅助抗癫痫药	拉莫三嗪、托吡酯、丙戊酸钠、卡马西平	数据难以解释,包括氯氮平和氯氮平以外的抗精神病药。充其量略有疗效	弱 +
心理治疗	认知行为疗法	相互矛盾的发现,作用小	非常弱 ±

参考文献

1. Yoshimura B, et al. The critical treatment window of clozapine in treatment-resistant schizophrenia: secondary analysis of an observational study. *Psychiatry Res* 2017; 250:65–70.
2. Howes OD, et al. Adherence to treatment guidelines in clinical practice: study of antipsychotic treatment prior to clozapine initiation. *BrJPsychiatry* 2012; 201:481–485.
3. Molins C, et al. Response to antipsychotic drugs in treatment-resistant schizophrenia: conclusions based on systematic review. *Schizophr Res* 2016; 178:64–67.
4. Samara MT, et al. Efficacy, acceptability, and tolerability of antipsychotics in treatment-resistant schizophrenia: a network meta-analysis. *JAMA Psychiatry* 2016; 73:199–210.
5. Galling B, et al. Antipsychotic augmentation vs. monotherapy in schizophrenia: systematic review, meta-analysis and meta-regression analysis. *World Psychiatry* 2017; 16:77–89.
6. Luykx JJ, et al. In the aftermath of clozapine discontinuation: comparative effectiveness and safety of antipsychotics in patients with schizophrenia who discontinue clozapine. *Br J Psychiatry* 2020; 217:498–505.
7. Bugarski-Kirola D, et al. Efficacy and safety of adjunctive bitopertin versus placebo in patients with suboptimally controlled symptoms of schizophrenia treated with antipsychotics: results from three phase 3, randomised, double-blind, parallel-group, placebo-controlled, multicentre studies in the SearchLyte clinical trial programme. *Lancet Psychiatry* 2016; 3:1115–1128.
8. Garay RP, et al. Potential serotonergic agents for the treatment of schizophrenia. *Exp Opin Invest Drugs* 2016; 25:159–170.
9. Akhondzadeh S, et al. Beneficial antipsychotic effects of allopurinol as add-on therapy for schizophrenia: a double blind, randomized and placebo controlled trial. *Prog Neuropsychopharmacol Biol Psychiatry* 2005; 29:253–259.
10. Brunstein MG, et al. A clinical trial of adjuvant allopurinol therapy for moderately refractory schizophrenia. *J Clin Psychiatry* 2005; 66:213–219.
11. Buie LW, et al. Allopurinol as adjuvant therapy in poorly responsive or treatment refractory schizophrenia. *Ann Pharmacother* 2006; 40:2200–2204.
12. Dickerson FB, et al. A double-blind trial of adjunctive allopurinol for schizophrenia. *Schizophr Res* 2009; 109:66–69.
13. Kontaxakis VP, et al. Switching to amisulpride monotherapy for treatment-resistant schizophrenia. *Eur Psychiatry* 2006; 21:214–217.
14. Kane JM, et al. Aripiprazole for treatment-resistant schizophrenia: results of a multicenter, randomized, double-blind, comparison study versus perphenazine. *J Clin Psychiatry* 2007; 68:213–223.
15. Hsu WY, et al. Aripiprazole in treatment-refractory schizophrenia. *J Psychiatr Pract* 2009; 15:221–226.
16. Crossman AM, et al. Tolerability of high-dose aripiprazole in treatment-refractory schizophrenic patients. *J Clin Psychiatry* 2006; 67:1158–1159.
17. Smith EN, et al. Asenapine augmentation and treatment-resistant schizophrenia in the high-secure hospital setting. *Ther Adv Psychopharmacol* 2014; 4:193–197.
18. Lerner V, et al. The retinoid X receptor agonist bexarotene relieves positive symptoms of schizophrenia: a 6-week, randomized, double-blind, placebo-controlled multicenter trial. *J Clin Psychiatry* 2013; 74:1224–1232.
19. Tachibana M, et al. Effectiveness of blonanserin for patients with drug treatment-resistant schizophrenia and dopamine supersensitivity: a retrospective analysis. *Asian J Psychiatr* 2016; 24:28–32.
20. Valmaggia LR, et al. Cognitive-behavioural therapy for refractory psychotic symptoms of schizophrenia resistant to atypical antipsychotic medication. Randomised controlled trial. *Br J Psychiatry* 2005; 186:324–330.
21. Akhondzadeh S, et al. Celecoxib as adjunctive therapy in schizophrenia: a double-blind, randomized and placebo-controlled trial. *Schizophr Res* 2007; 90:179–185.
22. Corripio I, et al. Deep brain stimulation in treatment resistant schizophrenia: a pilot randomized cross-over clinical trial. *EBioMedicine* 2020;

51:102568.

23. Lee BJ, et al. A 12-week, double-blind, placebo-controlled trial of donepezil as an adjunct to haloperidol for treating cognitive impairments in patients with chronic schizophrenia. *J Psychopharmacology* 2007; **21:**421–427.

24. Keefe RSE, et al. Efficacy and safety of donepezil in patients with schizophrenia or schizoaffective disorder: significant placebo/practice effects in a 12-week, randomized, double-blind, placebo-controlled trial. *Neuropsychopharmacology* 2007; **33:**1217–1228.

25. Akhondzadeh S, et al. A 12-week, double-blind, placebo-controlled trial of donepezil adjunctive treatment to risperidone in chronic and stable schizophrenia. *Prog Neuropsychopharmacol Biol Psychiatry* 2008; **32:**1810–1815.

26. Tsai GE, et al. D-alanine added to antipsychotics for the treatment of schizophrenia. *Biol Psychiatry* 2006; **59:**230–234.

27. Heresco-Levy U, et al. D-serine efficacy as add-on pharmacotherapy to risperidone and olanzapine for treatment-refractory schizophrenia. *Biol Psychiatry* 2005; **57:**577–585.

28. Ermilov M, et al. A pilot double-blind comparison of d-serine and high-dose olanzapine in treatment-resistant patients with schizophrenia. *Schizophr Res* 2013; **150:**604–605.

29. Zheng W, et al. Electroconvulsive therapy added to non-clozapine antipsychotic medication for treatment resistant schizophrenia: meta-analysis of randomized controlled trials. *PLoS One* 2016; **11:**e0156510.

30. Grover S, et al. Effectiveness of electroconvulsive therapy in patients with treatment resistant schizophrenia: a retrospective study. *Psychiatry Res* 2017; **249:**349–353.

31. Chanpattana W, et al. Electroconvulsive therapy in treatment-resistant schizophrenia: prediction of response and the nature of symptomatic improvement. *J Ect* 2010; **26:**289–298.

32. Ravanic DB, et al. Long-term efficacy of electroconvulsive therapy combined with different antipsychotic drugs in previously resistant schizophrenia. *Psychiatr Danub* 2009; **21:**179–186.

33. Kulkarni J, et al. Estradiol for treatment-resistant schizophrenia: a large-scale randomized-controlled trial in women of child-bearing age. *Mol Psychiatry* 2015; **20:**695–702.

34. Meskanen K, et al. A randomized clinical trial of histamine 2 receptor antagonism in treatment-resistant schizophrenia. *J Clin Psychopharmacol* 2013; **33:**472–478.

35. Meltzer H, et al. W162 – lurasidone is an effective treatment for treatment resistant schizophrenia. *Neuropsychopharmacology* 2015; **40 (Suppl 1):**S546.

36. Meltzer HY, et al. Lurasidone improves psychopathology and cognition in treatment-resistant schizophrenia. *J Clin Psychopharmacol* 2020; **40:**240–249.

37. Lowe P, et al. When the drugs don't work: treatment-resistant schizophrenia, serotonin and serendipity. *Ther Adv Psychopharmacol* 2018; **8:**63–70.

38. Lieberman JA, et al. A randomized, placebo-controlled study of memantine as adjunctive treatment in patients with schizophrenia. *Neuropsychopharmacology* 2009; **34:**1322–1329.

39. De Lucena D, et al. Improvement of negative and positive symptoms in treatment-refractory schizophrenia: a double-blind, randomized, placebo-controlled trial with memantine as add-on therapy to clozapine. *J Clin Psychiatry* 2009; **70:**1416–1423.

40. Rezaei F, et al. Memantine add-on to risperidone for treatment of negative symptoms in patients with stable schizophrenia: randomized, double-blind, placebo-controlled study. *J Clin Psychopharmacol* 2013; **33:**336–342.

41. Levkovitz Y, et al. A double-blind, randomized study of minocycline for the treatment of negative and cognitive symptoms in early-phase schizophrenia. *J Clin Psychiatry* 2010; **71:**138–149.

42. Miyaoka T, et al. Minocycline as adjunctive therapy for schizophrenia: an open-label study. *Clin Neuropharmacol* 2008; **31:**287–292.

43. Kelly DL, et al. Adjunctive minocycline in clozapine-treated schizophrenia patients with persistent symptoms. *J Clin Psychopharmacol* 2015; **35:**374–381.

44. Chaudhry IB, et al. Minocycline benefits negative symptoms in early schizophrenia: a randomised double-blind placebo-controlled clinical trial in patients on standard treatment. *J Psychopharmacol* 2012; **26:**1185–1193.

45. Joffe G, et al. Add-on mirtazapine enhances antipsychotic effect of first generation antipsychotics in schizophrenia: a double-blind, randomized, placebo-controlled trial. *Schizophr Res* 2009; **108:**245–251.

46. Berk M, et al. Mirtazapine add-on therapy in the treatment of schizophrenia with atypical antipsychotics: a double-blind, randomised, placebo-controlled clinical trial. *Human Psychopharmacology* 2009; **24:**233–238.

47. Delle CR, et al. Add-on mirtazapine enhances effects on cognition in schizophrenic patients under stabilized treatment with clozapine. *Exp Clin Psychopharmacol* 2007; **15:**563–568.

48. Sepehrmanesh Z, et al. Therapeutic effect of adjunctive N-acetyl cysteine (NAC) on symptoms of chronic schizophrenia: a double-blind, randomized clinical trial. *Prog Neuropsychopharmacol Biol Psychiatry* 2018; **82:**289–296.

49. Bulut M, et al. Beneficial effects of N-acetylcysteine in treatment resistant schizophrenia. *World J Biol Psychiatry* 2009; **10:**626–628.

50. Rossell SL, et al. N-acetylcysteine (NAC) in schizophrenia resistant to clozapine: a double blind randomised placebo controlled trial targeting negative symptoms. *BMC Psychiatry* 2016; **16:**320.

51. Breier A, et al. Comparative efficacy of olanzapine and haloperidol for patients with treatment-resistant schizophrenia. *Biol Psychiatry* 1999; **45:**403–411.

52. Conley RR, et al. Olanzapine compared with chlorpromazine in treatment-resistant schizophrenia. *Am J Psychiatry* 1998; **155:**914–920.

53. Sanders RD, et al. An open trial of olanzapine in patients with treatment-refractory psychoses. *J Clin Psychopharmacol* 1999; **19:**62–66.

54. Taylor D, et al. Olanzapine in practice: a prospective naturalistic study. *Psychiatric Bull* 1999; **23:**178–180.

55. Bitter I, et al. Olanzapine versus clozapine in treatment-resistant or treatment-intolerant schizophrenia. *Prog Neuropsychopharmacol Biol Psychiatry* 2004; **28:**173–180.

56. Tollefson GD, et al. Double-blind comparison of olanzapine versus clozapine in schizophrenic patients clinically eligible for treatment with

第
1
章

clozapine. *Biol Psychiatry* 2001; **49**:52–63.

57. Sheitman BB, et al. High-dose olanzapine for treatment-refractory schizophrenia. *Am J Psychiatry* 1997; **154**:1626.

58. Fanous A, et al. Schizophrenia and schizoaffective disorder treated with high doses of olanzapine. *J Clin Psychopharmacol* 1999; **19**:275–276.

59. Dursun SM, et al. Olanzapine for patients with treatment-resistant schizophrenia: a naturalistic case-series outcome study. *Can J Psychiatry* 1999; **44**:701–704.

60. Conley RR, et al. The efficacy of high-dose olanzapine versus clozapine in treatment-resistant schizophrenia: a double-blind crossover study. *J Clin Psychopharmacol* 2003; **23**:668–671.

61. Kumra S, et al. Clozapine and 'high-dose' olanzapine in refractory early-onset schizophrenia: a 12-week randomized and double-blind comparison. *Biol Psychiatry* 2008; **63**:524–529.

62. Kumra S, et al. Clozapine versus 'high-dose' olanzapine in refractory early-onset schizophrenia: an open-label extension study. *J Child Adolesc Psychopharmacol* 2008; **18**:307–316.

63. Meltzer HY, et al. A randomized, double-blind comparison of clozapine and high-dose olanzapine in treatment-resistant patients with schizophrenia. *J Clin Psychiatry* 2008; **69**:274–285.

64. Bronson BD, et al. Adverse effects of high-dose olanzapine in treatment-refractory schizophrenia. *J Clin Psychopharmacol* 2000; **20**:382–384.

65. Kelly DL, et al. Adverse effects and laboratory parameters of high-dose olanzapine vs. clozapine in treatment-resistant schizophrenia. *Ann Clin Psychiatry* 2003; **15**:181–186.

66. Zink M, et al. Combination of amisulpride and olanzapine in treatment-resistant schizophrenic psychoses. *Eur Psychiatry* 2004; **19**:56–58.

67. Duggal HS. Aripirazole-olanzapine combination for treatment of schizophrenia. *Can J Psychiatry* 2004; **49**:151.

68. Heresco-Levy U, et al. High-dose glycine added to olanzapine and risperidone for the treatment of schizophrenia. *Biol Psychiatry* 2004; **55**:165–171.

69. Dursun SM, et al. Augmenting antipsychotic treatment with lamotrigine or topiramate in patients with treatment-resistant schizophrenia: a naturalistic case-series outcome study. *J Psychopharm* 2001; **15**:297–301.

70. Suzuki T, et al. Effectiveness of antipsychotic polypharmacy for patients with treatment refractory schizophrenia: an open-label trial of olanzapine plus risperidone for those who failed to respond to a sequential treatment with olanzapine, quetiapine and risperidone. *Human Psychopharmacology* 2008; **23**:455–463.

71. Kotler M, et al. Sulpiride augmentation of olanzapine in the management of treatment-resistant chronic schizophrenia: evidence for improvement of mood symptomatology. *Int Clin Psychopharmacol* 2004; **19**:23–26.

72. Mellor JE, et al. Omega-3 fatty acid supplementation in schizophrenic patients. *Human Psychopharmacology* 1996; **11**:39–46.

73. Puri BK, et al. Sustained remission of positive and negative symptoms of schizophrenia following treatment with eicosapentaenoic acid. *Arch Gen Psychiatry* 1998; **55**:188–189.

74. Zheng W, et al. Adjunctive ondansetron for schizophrenia: a systematic review and meta-analysis of randomized controlled trials. *J Psychiatr Res* 2019; **113**:27–33.

75. Martínez-Andrés JA, et al. Switching from clozapine to paliperidone palmitate-3-monthly improved obesity, hyperglycemia and dyslipidemia lowering antipsychotic dose equivalents in a treatment-resistant schizophrenia cohort. *Int Clin Psychopharmacol* 2020; **35**:163–169.

76. Nasrallah HA, et al. Successful treatment of clozapine-nonresponsive refractory hallucinations and delusions with pimavanserin, a serotonin 5HT-2A receptor inverse agonist. *Schizophr Res* 2019; **208**:217–220.

77. Salimi S, et al. A placebo controlled study of the propentofylline added to risperidone in chronic schizophrenia. *Prog Neuropsychopharmacol Biol Psychiatry* 2008; **32**:726–732.

78. Reznik I, et al. Long-term efficacy and safety of quetiapine in treatment-refractory schizophrenia: a case report. *Int J Psychiatry Clin Pract* 2000; **4**:77–80.

79. De Nayer A, et al. Efficacy and tolerability of quetiapine in patients with schizophrenia switched from other antipsychotics. *Int J Psychiatry Clin Pract* 2003; **7**:59–66.

80. Larmo I, et al. Efficacy and tolerability of quetiapine in patients with schizophrenia who switched from haloperidol, olanzapine or risperidone. *Human Psychopharmacology* 2005; **20**:573–581.

81. Boggs DL, et al. Quetiapine at high doses for the treatment of refractory schizophrenia. *Schizophr Res* 2008; **101**:347–348.

82. Lindenmayer JP, et al. A randomized, double-blind, parallel-group, fixed-dose, clinical trial of quetiapine at 600 versus 1200 mg/d for patients with treatment-resistant schizophrenia or schizoaffective disorder. *J Clin Psychopharmacol* 2011; **31**:160–168.

83. Quintero J, et al. The effectiveness of the combination therapy of amisulpride and quetiapine for managing treatment-resistant schizophrenia: a naturalistic study. *J Clin Psychopharmacol* 2011; **31**:240–242.

84. Aziz MA, et al. Remission of positive and negative symptoms in refractory schizophrenia with a combination of haloperidol and quetiapine: two case studies. *J Psychiatr Pract* 2006; **12**:332–336.

85. Tharoor H, et al. Raloxifene trial in postmenopausal woman with treatment-resistant schizophrenia. *Arch Women's Mental Health* 2015; **18**:741–742.

86. Usall J, et al. Raloxifene as an adjunctive treatment for postmenopausal women with schizophrenia: a 24-week double-blind, randomized, parallel, placebo-controlled trial. *Schizophr Bull* 2016; **42**:309–317.

87. Usall J, et al. Raloxifene as an adjunctive treatment for postmenopausal women with schizophrenia: a double-blind, randomized, placebo-controlled trial. *J Clin Psychiatry* 2011; **72**:1552–1557.

88. Weiser M, et al. Raloxifene plus antipsychotics versus placebo plus antipsychotics in severely ill decompensated postmenopausal women with schizophrenia or schizoaffective disorder: a randomized controlled trial. *J Clin Psychiatry* 2017; **78**:e758–e765.

89. Kulkarni J, et al. Effect of adjunctive raloxifene therapy on severity of refractory schizophrenia in women: a randomized clinical trial. *JAMA*

Psychiatry 2016; 73:947–954.

90. Farokhnia M, et al. A double-blind, placebo controlled, randomized trial of riluzole as an adjunct to risperidone for treatment of negative symptoms in patients with chronic schizophrenia. *Psychopharmacology* 2014; 231:533–542.

91. Breier AF, et al. Clozapine and risperidone in chronic schizophrenia: effects on symptoms, parkinsonian side effects, and neuroendocrine response. *Am J Psychiatry* 1999; 156:294–298.

92. Bondolfi G, et al. Risperidone versus clozapine in treatment-resistant chronic schizophrenia: a randomized double-blind study. The Risperidone Study Group. *Am J Psychiatry* 1998; 155:499–504.

93. Conley RR, et al. Risperidone, quetiapine, and fluphenazine in the treatment of patients with therapy-refractory schizophrenia. *Clin Neuropharmacol* 2005; 28:163–168.

94. Lerner V, et al. Combination of 'atypical' antipsychotic medication in the management of treatment-resistant schizophrenia and schizoaffective disorder. *Prog Neuropsychopharmacol Biol Psychiatry* 2004; 28:89–98.

95. Meltzer HY, et al. A six month randomized controlled trial of long acting injectable risperidone 50 and 100mg in treatment resistant schizophrenia. *Schizophr Res* 2014; 154:14–22.

96. Akhondzadeh S, et al. Effect of ritanserin, a 5HT2A/2C antagonist, on negative symptoms of schizophrenia: a double-blind randomized placebo-controlled study. *Prog Neuropsychopharmacol Biol Psychiatry* 2008; 32:1879–1883.

97. Lane HY, et al. Sarcosine or D-serine add-on treatment for acute exacerbation of schizophrenia: a randomized, double-blind, placebo-controlled study. *Arch Gen Psychiatry* 2005; 62:1196–1204.

98. Tsai G, et al. Glycine transporter I inhibitor, N-methylglycine (sarcosine), added to antipsychotics for the treatment of schizophrenia. *Biol Psychiatry* 2004; 55:452–456.

99. Kane JM, et al. A double-blind, randomized study comparing the efficacy and safety of sertindole and risperidone in patients with treatment-resistant schizophrenia. *J Clin Psychiatry* 2011; 72:194–204.

100. Nielsen J, et al. Augmenting clozapine with sertindole: a double-blind, randomized, placebo-controlled study. *J Clin Psychopharmacol* 2012; 32:173–178.

101. Tiihonen J, et al. Topiramate add-on in treatment-resistant schizophrenia: a randomized, double-blind, placebo-controlled, crossover trial. *J Clin Psychiatry* 2005; 66:1012–1015.

102. Franck N, et al. Left temporoparietal transcranial magnetic stimulation in treatment-resistant schizophrenia with verbal hallucinations. *Psychiatry Res* 2003; 120:107–109.

103. Fitzgerald PB, et al. A double-blind sham-controlled trial of repetitive transcranial magnetic stimulation in the treatment of refractory auditory hallucinations. *J Clin Psychopharmacol* 2005; 25:358–362.

104. Tuppurainen H, et al. Repetitive navigated αTMS in treatment-resistant schizophrenia. *Brain Stimulation* 2017; 10:397–398.

105. Khosravi M. Ursodeoxycholic acid augmentation in treatment-refractory schizophrenia: a case report. *J Med Case Rep* 2020; 14:137.

106. Basan A, et al. Valproate as an adjunct to antipsychotics for schizophrenia: a systematic review of randomized trials. *Schizophr Res* 2004; 70:33–37.

107. Miyaoka T, et al. Efficacy and safety of yokukansan in treatment-resistant schizophrenia: a randomized, multicenter, double-blind, placebo-controlled trial. *Evid Based Complement Alternat Med* 2015; 2015:201592.

108. Lin CC, et al. Switching from clozapine to zotepine in patients with schizophrenia: a 12-week prospective, randomized, rater blind, and parallel study. *J Clin Psychopharmacol* 2013; 33:211–214.

109. Sacchetti E, et al. Ziprasidone vs clozapine in schizophrenia patients refractory to multiple antipsychotic treatments: the MOZART study. *Schizophr Res* 2009; 110:80–89.

110. Loebel AD, et al. Ziprasidone in treatment-resistant schizophrenia: a 52-week, open-label continuation study. *J Clin Psychiatry* 2007; 68:1333–1338.

111. Kane JM, et al. Efficacy and tolerability of ziprasidone in patients with treatment-resistant schizophrenia. *Int Clin Psychopharmacol* 2006; 21:21–28.

112. Goff DC, et al. High-dose oral ziprasidone versus conventional dosing in schizophrenia patients with residual symptoms: the ZEBRAS study. *J Clin Psychopharmacol* 2013; 33:485–490.

氯氮平中断治疗后重新使用

如果患者需要停止服用氯氮平,应建议他们联系其处方医师。部分原因是如果突然停止氯氮平治疗,需要监测胆碱能反弹的症状,如恶心、呕吐、腹泻、出汗和头痛[1,2],以及可能出现的肌张力障碍、运动障碍和紧张症状[3-6]。另外,如果氯氮平治疗停止 48h 以上,则剂量需要从 12.5mg 开始重新加量[7,8]。

根据耐受情况,将剂量重新加到治疗水平时,速度可能比初始治疗更快一些。虽然有证据表明,对于未用过氯氮平和重新服用氯氮平的患者,加量更快可能是安全的[3],但由于不良反应,加量过快可能会导致不必要的停药。某些患者需要采取更谨慎的加量方法,如老年人、帕金森病患者以及不清楚药物的潜在益处即开始服用氯氮平的门诊患者[9,10]。

氯氮平在停用一段时间后再次使用时,既要考虑重新产生抗精神病作用,又要确保加量过程中的安全。关键是灵活运用:根据患者以前耐受的剂量调整剂量。虽然存在慢、快、超快加量的例子[8],但是最好根据患者耐受性进行个性化加量。概括地说,从 12.5mg 开始。如果初始剂量没有引起镇静、心率或血压等问题,则下一剂量增加至 25mg。如果 25mg 剂量的耐受性良好,那么下一次可以服用 50mg,依此类推。每天两次用药可使加量速度达到最佳,但一些中心每天三次给药。后一种计划更有可能产生累积效应。如果不能耐受加量计划中的某一剂量,则下一剂量通常应延迟,不得增加(可能减少)。

通常最好一次用一个剂量,连成系列,而不是写一个完整的给药方案,然后可能不得不更改。

参考文献

1. Shiovitz TM, et al. Cholinergic rebound and rapid onset psychosis following abrupt clozapine withdrawal. *Schizophr Bull* 1996; **22**:591–595.
2. Galova A, et al. A case report of cholinergic rebound syndrome following abrupt low-dose clozapine discontinuation in a patient with type I bipolar affective disorder. *BMC Psychiatry* 2019; **19**:73.
3. Ahmed S, et al. Clozapine withdrawal-emergent dystonias and dyskinesias: a case series. *J Clin Psychiatry* 1998; **59**:472–477.
4. Shrivastava M, et al. Relapse of tardive dyskinesia due to reduction in clozapine dose. *Indian J Pharmacol* 2009; **41**:201–202.
5. Boazak M, et al. Catatonia due to clozapine withdrawal: a case report and literature review. *Psychosomatics* 2019; **60**:421–427.
6. Lander M, et al. Review of withdrawal catatonia: what does this reveal about clozapine? *Trans Psychiatry* 2018; **8**:139.
7. Mylan Products Ltd. Clozaril 25mg and 100mg tablets. 2020; https://www.medicines.org.uk/emc/medicine/32564.
8. Rubio JM, et al. How and when to use clozapine. *Acta Psychiatr Scand* 2020; **141**:178–189.
9. Gee SH, et al. Patient attitudes to clozapine initiation. *Int Clin Psychopharmacol* 2017; **32**:337–342.
10. Schulte PF, et al. Comment on 'effectiveness and safety of rapid clozapine titration in schizophrenia'. *Acta Psychiatr Scand* 2014; **130**:69–70.

社区患者如何开始氯氮平治疗

开始社区治疗的禁忌

- 病史中有癫痫发作、严重心脏病、不稳定型糖尿病、麻痹性肠梗阻、恶血质、抗精神病药恶性综合征或其他可增加严重不良反应风险的疾病(在医院严密监测下开始用药时也是可能的)。
- 既往增加氯氮平或其他抗精神病药剂量时产生严重不良反应。
- 不可靠或无序的生活习惯,可能会影响药物治疗依从性或监测方案。
- 严重的酒精或其他物质(如可卡因)滥用,可能增加不良反应的风险。

适合开始社区治疗的情况(下述所有问题的答案都应该是肯定的)

- 患者是否依从口服用药和监测要求?
- 患者是否已经理解定期身体监测和血液检查的必要性?
- 患者是否已经理解可能出现的不良反应,并且知道如何处理(尤其是罕见但严重的不良反应)?
- 患者是否随时能联系到(如当需要追踪结果时)?
- 患者是否可以在加量初期每天复诊?
- 患者是否每周都能取药,或药物是否能送到患者家里?
- 在工作时间之外,患者若出现可能严重的不良反应,是否可能寻求帮助(例如:出现心肌炎或感染的征兆时,如发热、全身乏力、胸痛)?

初始准备工作

　　筛查风险因素,提供基线评估:

- 体格检查、全血细胞计数(见下)、肝功、尿素和电解质、血脂、血糖/HbA_{1c}。考虑检查肌钙蛋白、C 反应蛋白(CRP)、β 利钠肽、红细胞沉降率(ESR)(作为后期检查的基线)。
- ECG——尤其是用于筛查既往有无心肌梗死或心室异常。
- 如果有临床指征,做超声心动图检查。

必须进行血液监测并登记

- 在相关监测单位登记。
- 使用氯氮平之前进行基线血液检查(白细胞计数和分类)。
- 在开始 18 周内每周 1 次验血,当年其他时间每两周 1 次。此后一般每个月检测 1 次。
- 告知患者的全科医师。

剂量调整

　　在社区使用氯氮平,需要缓慢而灵活地加量。在加量期,原来的抗精神病药应缓慢停用(长效注射剂通常在开始加药时停用)。氯氮平能导致显著的体位性低血压。最初的监测有部分原因是为了及时发现并处理这种不良反应。

　　在社区开始使用氯氮平有两种基本方法。一种是早晨在诊所里首次给药,监测患者至少 3h。如果这个剂量可以耐受,患者就可以带药回家睡前服用。这一给药计划在表 1.38 中

表 1.38　建议在社区开始用氯氮平的加药方案(注意:在患者耐受的情况下,许多患者的加量速度要快得多)

天数	星期几	早晨剂量/mg	晚上剂量/mg	监测	原抗精神病药剂量百分比
1	一	6.25	6.25	A	100
2	二	6.25	6.25	A	
3	三	6.25	6.25	A	
4	四	6.25	12.5	A,B,FBC	
5	五	12.5	12.5	A 检查第 4 天以来的结果,提醒患者周末非工作时间安排	
6	六	12.5	12.5	不需常规监测,除非临床需要	
7	日	12.5	12.5	不需常规监测,除非临床需要	
8	一	12.5	25	A	75*
9	二	12.5	25	A	
10	三	25	25	A	
11	四	25	37.5	A,B,FBC	
12	五	25	37.5	A 检查第 1 天以来的结果,提醒患者周末非工作时间安排	
13	六	25	37.5	不需常规监测,除非临床需要	
14	日	25	37.5	不需常规监测,除非临床需要	
15	一	37.5	37.5	A	50*
16	二	37.5	37.5	若无问题不需看	
17	三	37.5	50	A	
18	四	37.5	50	若无问题不需看	
19	五	50	50	A,B,FBC	
20	六	50	50	不需常规监测,除非临床需要	
21	日	50	50	不需常规监测,除非临床需要	
22	一	50	75	A	25*
23	二	50	75	若无问题不需看	
24	三	75	75	A	
25	四	75	75	若无问题不需看	
26	五	75	100	A,B,FBC	
27	六	75	100	不需常规监测,除非临床需要	
28	日	75	100	不需常规监测,除非临床需要	

此后的增量应维持在 25~50mg/d(通常是 25mg/d),直至达到治疗剂量(以血药浓度为准)。注意首过代谢饱和导致的血药浓度突然增加(注意镇静或其他不良反应的增加)。

注:

A,应在给药前测量脉搏、不同体位的血压和体温,理想情况下,应在给药后 30min~6h 测量上述指标。询问不良反应。

B,精神状况,体重,检查并积极处理不良反应(如,行为建议,缓慢增加氯氮平剂量或减少其他抗精神病药剂量,开始辅助治疗——见本章"氯氮平不良反应")。考虑检查肌钙蛋白、CRP、β 利钠肽。

* 可能需要根据不良反应和精神状况做出调整。

FBC,全血细胞计数。

有描述。这是一个非常谨慎的计划,大部分患者可以耐受更快的加量。第二种给药方法是患者在睡前首次服药,因此可以避免服药后密切观察躯体状况。随后的剂量和监测同方法一。最初给药都应该在一周的前几天(如周一),这样能保证足够的工作人员和监测。

不良反应

镇静、流涎和低血压在治疗早期十分常见。这些不良反应常常容易处理(见本章“常见不良反应”),但在社区加药时需要格外注意。考虑使用公认量表对不良反应进行定期、系统的评估,如格拉斯哥抗精神病药不良量表——氯氮平(GASS-C)。

若出现以下情况,正式照料者(通常是社区精神科护士)应当告知开处方者:

- **体温高于 38℃**(十分常见,并且本身不能作为停用氯氮平的充分理由)
- **脉搏 >100 次/min**(同样常见,本身不能作为停用的理由,但有时可能与心肌炎有关)
- **体位性的血压下降 >30mmHg**
- **患者明显过度镇静**
- **任何便秘迹象**
- **流感样症状(不适、疲劳等)**
- **胸痛、呼吸困难、气促**
- **任何其他不可耐受的不良反应。**
- **吸烟习惯改变**

第一个月,医师至少要每周看 1 次患者,对身体和精神状况进行评估。

推荐的额外监测指标

基线	1 个月	3 个月	4~6 个月	12 个月
体重/BMI/腰围	体重/BMI/腰围	体重/BMI/腰围	体重/BMI/腰围	体重/BMI/腰围
血糖/血脂	血糖/血脂		血糖/血脂	血糖/血脂
肝功能化验			肝功能化验	

BMI,体重指数。

在治疗的前 6 周,尤其当怀疑心肌炎时,考虑每周监测血浆肌钙蛋白、β 利钠肽、C 反应蛋白(见本章“心肌炎”)。

从其他抗精神病药换用氯氮平

- 换用方案很大程度上取决于患者的精神状况。
- 考虑相加的抗精神病药不良反应(如低血压、镇静、对 Q-T 间期的影响)。
- 考虑药物相互作用(例如,一些 SSRI 类药物会增加氯氮平水平)。
- 开始使用氯氮平前,应该停用所有长效注射剂、舍吲哚、匹莫齐特、齐拉西酮。
- 其他抗精神病药与氯氮平可以在不同程度上谨慎地交叉换药。当氯氮平与其他已知能影响 Q-T 间期的药物合用时,须谨慎监测 ECG。

严重的心脏不良反应

　　密切关注患者心肌炎的症状和体征,尤其在前两个月。医师应当建议患者,如出现心肌炎的相关症状和体征时,要随时告知医务人员,必要时在非工作时间要求检查。这些症状或体征包括持久的心动过速(尽管一般是良性的)、心悸、气短、发热、心律失常、类似心肌梗死的症状、胸痛和其他难以解释的心力衰竭症状。(见本章"氯氮平:严重血液系统和心血管不良反应")。

氯氮平的不良反应

常见的不良反应

不良反应	出现时间	处理
镇静	发生在用药头几个月,可持续存在,但通常在一定程度上逐渐减弱	可早晨给予小剂量。如果早晨苏醒困难,则晚上早些给药。尽可能减少剂量 有报道使用兴奋剂(哌甲酯[1])和倍他司汀[2]的成功案例,但缺乏长期数据。莫达非尼无效[3]
流涎	发生在用药头几个月,可持续存在,但通常逐渐减弱。发生在夜间的流涎往往非常令人苦恼	0.3mg 东莨菪碱,吮吸、吞咽,最多一天 3 次。其他处理方法见本章"流涎"。注意:抗胆碱能药会加重便秘和认知损害
便秘	前 4 个月风险最高[4]通常会持续存在,因此需要持续监测和治疗	用药之前告知患者可能存在的风险,定期筛查,确保摄入足够的纤维素、液体和保持运动。刺激性缓泻剂(番泻叶)是一线用药,必要时加上润滑性泻药(多库酯钠)和/或渗透性泻药(聚乙二醇)[5]。避免使用膨胀性泻药,因为便秘的根本原因是胃动力下降。停用其他可能导致便秘的药物,并尽可能减少氯氮平的用量。有效治疗和预防便秘十分必要,因为可能导致死亡[4,6-9]。见本章"氯氮平所致便秘"
低血压	前 4 周	建议患者缓慢站起。减少剂量,或减慢加药速度。增加液体摄入量至每天 2 L。[10] 严重时考虑使用吗氯贝胺和牛肉汁[11]、氟氢可的松、去氨升压素或腹带[10]。长期下去,体重增加可能导致高血压
高血压[12]	前 4 周,有时更久	密切监测,必要时尽可能缓慢加量。有时需要降压治疗[13]
心动过速	前 4 周,但有时持续存在	在治疗早期十分常见,通常是良性的。可能与剂量相关[14]。若休息时持续心动过速,并伴有发热、低血压、胸痛,常提示心肌炎[15,16](见本章"心血管不良反应")。建议心内科就诊。若心动过速发生在胸痛或心力衰竭的情况下,应停用氯氮平。良性的窦性心动过速可用比索洛尔[17]或阿替洛尔治疗[18],但是证据不足[19,20]。当有低血压或禁忌证不能使用 β 受体阻滞剂时,可用伊伐布雷定治疗[21]。注意,长期心动过速本身也可引起心肌病[22]或者其他心血管疾病[10]
体重增加	通常在治疗的第一年出现,但有可能持续存在	饮食咨询十分必要。若能在体重增加前给予饮食建议,则效果更好。体重增加常见,且往往显著(头 10 周 >4.5kg[23])。有许多治疗方法(见本章"体重增加的治疗"部分)
发热[24]	前 4 周	氯氮平可引起炎症反应(如升高 C 反应蛋白、白介素-6[25]和嗜酸性粒细胞)[25-27]。可给予对乙酰氨基酚治疗,但要检查全血细胞计数,防止中性粒细胞缺乏。减慢加药速度[28]。这种发热通常与血液病无关[29],但要注意心肌炎、恶性综合征、肺炎和其他罕见炎症性器官损害(见本章"罕见不良反应"部分)

续表

不良反应	出现时间	处理
癫痫发作[30]	任何时候都可能出现[31]	与剂量、血浆药物浓度、快速加量有关[32]。若氯氮平剂量大（≥500mg/d）或血药浓度高（≥500μg/L），可考虑预防性使用托吡酯、拉莫三嗪、加巴喷丁或丙戊酸盐*。有人认为，氯氮平血药浓度低于 1 300μg/L 时，癫痫发作的风险为 1/20，不足以支持一级预防[33]。癫痫发作后，停氯氮平一天，再次使用时从以前剂量的 50% 开始；给予抗癫痫药**。EEG 异常在氯氮平使用者中常见[34,35]
恶心	前 6 周	可给予止吐药。若之前有 EPS，避免使用普鲁氯嗪和甲氧氯普胺。若存在潜在的心脏病风险或 Q-T 间期延长，应避免使用多潘立酮。昂丹司琼是不错的选择，但是可能会加重便秘。有 1 例心肌炎患者仅有的症状是恶心、呕吐[36]
夜尿症	任何时候都可能出现	减量或调整用药，避免深度镇静。睡前避免饮水。考虑晚上按时如厕。可自发缓解，[37]但也可能持续数月或数年[38]。约 1/5 服氯氮平的人会出现夜尿症[39]。严重病例用去氨升压素鼻喷雾剂（10~20μg 每晚）通常有效[40]，但并非没有风险：可能导致低钠血症[41]。抗胆碱能药可能有效[42]，但文献资料较少支持，且可能加重便秘和镇静。麻黄碱[43]、伪麻黄碱[44]和阿立哌唑[45,46]也可使用
胃-食管反流性疾病[47,48]	任何时候	通常给予质子泵抑制剂，但有些是 CYP1A2 诱导剂，可能增加中性粒细胞减少和粒细胞缺乏的风险[49,50]。作为 H_2 受体拮抗剂[51]，氯氮平导致胃-食管反流性疾病（GORD）的原因尚不清楚
肌阵挛[32,52-54]	在剂量或血浆药物浓度增加期间	可能出现在完全强直阵挛发作之前。减少剂量。抗癫痫药可能会有所帮助，并会降低病情发展为癫痫发作的可能。丙戊酸盐是首选，拉莫三嗪可能加重某些类型的肌阵挛
肺炎[55-62]	通常在治疗早期出现，但也可能出现在任何时候	可能是唾液误吸所致（这可能是肺炎有时候表现为剂量相关的原因[63,64]），很少由便秘引起[65]。肺炎是使用氯氮平患者的常见死因[56]。在使用氯氮平的患者中，感染可能更普遍[66]，并且抗生素的使用也随之增加[67]。注意：呼吸道感染可能引起氯氮平水平的升高[68-71]。（可能是人为因素：感染期间吸烟通常停止，但可能是由于炎症导致 CYP1A2 活性下降[72,73]）。氯氮平通常在肺炎消退后继续有效，但是复发的可能性更大[74-76]

　* 丙戊酸钠常规剂量为 1 000~2 000mg/d。血药浓度可作为调整剂量的大致依据，目标浓度为 50~100mg/L。使用缓释剂（如丙戊酸钠缓释剂）可增加服药依从性，可每天 1 次，耐受性更好。

　** 分裂情感障碍使用丙戊酸盐；育龄妇女、氯氮平无效或阴性症状持续存在，可加用拉莫三嗪；如需减轻体重，可使用托吡酯（但要注意认知损害）；若其他抗惊厥药难以耐受，可用加巴喷丁。

参考文献

1. Sarfati D, et al. Methylphenidate as treatment for clozapine-induced sedation in patients with treatment-resistant schizophrenia. *Clin Schizophr Relat Psychoses* 2018: [Epub ahead of print].

2. Poyurovsky M, et al. Beneficial effect of betahistine, a structural analog of histamine, in clozapine-related sedation. *Clin Neuropharmacol* 2019; 42:145.

3. Freudenreich O, et al. Modafinil for clozapine-treated schizophrenia patients: a double-blind, placebo-controlled pilot trial. *J Clin Psychiatry*

2009; 70:1674–1680.

4. Palmer SE, et al. Life-threatening clozapine-induced gastrointestinal hypomotility: an analysis of 102 cases. *J Clin Psychiatry* 2008; 69:759–768.

5. Taylor D, et al. *The Maudsley Practice Guidelines for Physical Health Conditions in Psychiatry.* United Kingdom Wiley – Blackwell; 2020.

6. Townsend G, et al. Case report: rapidly fatal bowel ischaemia on clozapine treatment. *BMC Psychiatry* 2006; 6:43.

7. Rege S, et al. Life-threatening constipation associated with clozapine. *Aust Psychiatry* 2008; 16:216–219.

8. Leung JS, et al. Rapidly fatal clozapine-induced intestinal obstruction without prior warning signs. *Aust N Z J Psychiatry* 2008; 42:1073–1074.

9. Flanagan RJ, et al. Gastrointestinal hypomotility: an under-recognised life-threatening adverse effect of clozapine. *Forensic Sci Int* 2011; 206:e31–e36.

10. Ronaldson KJ. Cardiovascular disease in clozapine-treated patients: evidence, mechanisms and management. *CNS Drugs* 2017; 31:777–795.

11. Taylor D, et al. Clozapine-induced hypotension treated with moclobemide and Bovril. *Br J Psychiatry* 1995; 167:409–410.

12. Gonsai NH, et al. Effects of dopamine receptor antagonist antipsychotic therapy on blood pressure. *J Clin Pharm Ther* 2017; 43:1–7.

13. Henderson DC, et al. Clozapine and hypertension: a chart review of 82 patients. *J Clin Psychiatry* 2004; 65:686–689.

14. Nilsson BM, et al. Tachycardia in patients treated with clozapine versus antipsychotic long-acting injections. *Int Clin Psychopharmacol* 2017; 32:219–224.

15. Medicines CoSo. Clozapine and cardiac safety: updated advice for prescribers. *Curr Prob Pharmacovigilance* 2002; 28:8.

16. Hagg S, et al. Myocarditis related to clozapine treatment. *J Clin Psychopharmacol* 2001; 21:382–388.

17. Nilsson BM, et al. Persistent tachycardia in clozapine treated patients: a 24-hour ambulatory electrocardiogram study. *Schizophr Res* 2018; 199:403–406.

18. Stryjer R, et al. Beta-adrenergic antagonists for the treatment of clozapine-induced sinus tachycardia: a retrospective study. *Clin Neuropharmacol* 2009; 32:290–292.

19. Lally J, et al. Pharmacological interventions for clozapine-induced sinus tachycardia. *Cochrane Database Syst Rev* 2016; Cd011566.

20. Yuen JWY, et al. Clozapine-induced cardiovascular side effects and autonomic dysfunction: a systematic review. *Front Neurosci* 2018; 12:203.

21. Lally J, et al. Ivabradine, a novel treatment for clozapine-induced sinus tachycardia: a case series. *Ther Adv Psychopharmacol* 2014; 4:117–122.

22. Shinbane JS, et al. Tachycardia-induced cardiomyopathy: a review of animal models and clinical studies. *J Am Coll Cardiol* 1997; 29:709–715.

23. Allison D, et al. Antipsychotic-induced weight gain: a comprehensive research synthesis. *Am J Psychiatry* 1999; 156:1686–1696.

24. Verdoux H, et al. Clinical determinants of fever in clozapine users and implications for treatment management: a narrative review. *Schizophr Res* 2019; 211:1–9.

25. Hung YP, et al. Role of cytokine changes in clozapine-induced fever: a cohort prospective study. *Psychiatry Clin Neurosci* 2017; 71:395–402.

26. Kohen I, et al. Increases in C-reactive protein may predict recurrence of clozapine-induced fever. *Ann Pharmacother* 2009; 43:143–146.

27. Kluge M, et al. Effects of clozapine and olanzapine on cytokine systems are closely linked to weight gain and drug-induced fever. *Psychoneuroendocrinology* 2009; 34:118–128.

28. Chung JP, et al. The incidence and characteristics of clozapine – induced fever in a local psychiatric unit in Hong Kong. *Can J Psychiatry* 2008; 53:857–862.

29. Tham JC, et al. Clozapine-induced fevers and 1-year clozapine discontinuation rate. *J Clin Psychiatry* 2002; 63:880–884.

30. Grover S, et al. Association of clozapine with seizures: a brief report involving 222 patients prescribed clozapine. *East Asian Arch Psychiatry* 2015; 25:73–78.

31. Pacia SV, et al. Clozapine-related seizures: experience with 5,629 patients. *Neurology* 1994; 44:2247–2249.

32. Varma S, et al. Clozapine-related EEG changes and seizures: dose and plasma-level relationships. *Ther Adv Psychopharmacol* 2011; 1:47–66.

33. Caetano D. Use of anticonvulsants as prophylaxis for seizures in patients on clozapine. *Australas Psychiatry* 2014; 22:78–83.

34. Centorrino F, et al. EEG abnormalities during treatment with typical and atypical antipsychotics. *Am J Psychiatry* 2002; 159:109–115.

35. Jackson A, et al. EEG changes in patients on antipsychotic therapy: a systematic review. *Epilepsy Behav* 2019; 95:1–9.

36. Van Der Horst MZ, et al. Isolated nausea and vomiting as the cardinal presenting symptoms of clozapine-induced myocarditis: a case report. *BMC Psychiatry* 2020; 20:568.

37. Warner JP, et al. Clozapine and urinary incontinence. *Int Clin Psychopharmacol* 1994; 9:207–209.

38. Jeong SH, et al. A 2-year prospective follow-up study of lower urinary tract symptoms in patients treated with clozapine. *J Clin Psychopharmacol* 2008; 28:618–624.

39. Harrison-Woolrych M, et al. Nocturnal enuresis in patients taking clozapine, risperidone, olanzapine and quetiapine: comparative cohort study. *Br J Psychiatry* 2011; 199:140–144.

40. Steingard S. Use of desmopressin to treat clozapine-induced nocturnal enuresis. *J Clin Psychiatry* 1994; 55:315–316.

41. Sarma S, et al. Severe hyponatraemia associated with desmopressin nasal spray to treat clozapine-induced nocturnal enuresis. *Aust N Z J Psychiatry* 2005; 39:949.

42. Praharaj SK, et al. Amitriptyline for clozapine-induced nocturnal enuresis and sialorrhoea. *Br J Clin Pharmacol* 2007; 63:128–129.

43. Fuller MA, et al. Clozapine-induced urinary incontinence: incidence and treatment with ephedrine. *J Clin Psychiatry* 1996; 57:514–518.

44. Hanes A, et al. Pseudoephedrine for the treatment of clozapine-induced incontinence. *Innov Clin Neurosci* 2013; 10:33–35.

45. Palaniappan P. Aripiprazole as a treatment option for clozapine-induced enuresis. *Indian J Pharmacol* 2015; 47:574–575.

46. Lee MJ, et al. Use of aripiprazole in clozapine induced enuresis: report of two cases. *J Korean Med Sci* 2010; 25:333–335.

47. Taylor D, et al. Use of antacid medication in patients receiving clozapine: a comparison with other second-generation antipsychotics. *J Clin Psychopharmacol* 2010; 30:460–461.

48. Van Veggel M, et al. Clozapine and gastro-oesophageal reflux disease (GORD) – an investigation of temporal association. *Acta Psychiatr Scand* 2013; 127:69–77.

49. Wicinski M, et al. Potential mechanisms of hematological adverse drug reactions in patients receiving clozapine in combination with proton pump inhibitors. *J Psychiatr Pract* 2017; 23:114–120.

50. Shuman MD, et al. Exploring the potential effect of polypharmacy on the hematologic profiles of clozapine patients. *J Psychiatr Pract* 2014; 20:50–58.

51. Humbert-Claude M, et al. Involvement of histamine receptors in the atypical antipsychotic profile of clozapine: a reassessment in vitro and in vivo. *Psychopharmacology* 2011; 220:225–241.

52. Osborne IJ, et al. Clozapine-induced myoclonus: a case report and review of the literature. *Ther Adv Psychopharmacol* 2015; 5:351–356.

53. Praharaj SK, et al. Clozapine-induced myoclonus: a case study and brief review. *Prog Neuropsychopharmacol Biol Psychiatry* 2010; 34:242–243.

54. Sajatovic M, et al. Clozapine-induced myoclonus and generalized seizures. *Biol Psychiatry* 1996; 39:367–370.

55. Hinkes R, et al. Aspiration pneumonia possibly secondary to clozapine-induced sialorrhea. *J Clin Psychopharmacol* 1996; 16:462–463.

56. Taylor DM, et al. Reasons for discontinuing clozapine: matched, case-control comparison with risperidone long-acting injection. *Br J Psychiatry* 2009; 194:165–167.

57. Stoecker ZR, et al. Clozapine usage increases the incidence of pneumonia compared with risperidone and the general population: a retrospective comparison of clozapine, risperidone, and the general population in a single hospital over 25 months. *Int Clin Psychopharmacol* 2017; 32:155–160.

58. Kaplan J, et al. Clozapine-associated aspiration pneumonia: case series and review of the literature. *Psychosomatics* 2017; 58:199–203.

59. Gurrera RJ, et al. Aspiration pneumonia: an underappreciated risk of clozapine treatment. *J Clin Psychopharmacol* 2016; 36:174–176.

60. Aldridge G, et al. Clozapine-induced pneumonitis. *Aust N Z J Psychiatry* 2013; 47:1215–1216.

61. Saenger RC, et al. Aspiration pneumonia due to clozapine-induced sialorrhea. *Clin Schizophr Relat Psychoses* 2016; 9:170–172.

62. Patel SS, et al. Physical complications in early clozapine treatment: a case report and implications for safe monitoring. *Ther Adv Psychopharmacol* 2011; 1:25–29.

63. Trigoboff E, et al. Sialorrhea and aspiration pneumonia: a case study. *Innov Clin Neurosci* 2013; 10:20–27.

64. Kuo CJ, et al. Second-generation antipsychotic medications and risk of pneumonia in schizophrenia. *Schizophr Bull* 2013; 39:648–657.

65. Galappathie N, et al. Clozapine-associated pneumonia and respiratory arrest secondary to severe constipation. *Med Sci Law* 2014; 54:105–109.

66. Landry P, et al. Increased use of antibiotics in clozapine-treated patients. *Int Clin Psychopharmacol* 2003; 18:297–298.

67. Nielsen J, et al. Increased use of antibiotics in patients treated with clozapine. *Eur Neuropsychopharmacol* 2009; 19:483–486.

68. Raaska K, et al. Bacterial pneumonia can increase serum concentration of clozapine. *Eur J Clin Pharmacol* 2002; 58:321–322.

69. De Leon J, et al. Serious respiratory infections can increase clozapine levels and contribute to side effects: a case report. *Prog Neuropsychopharmacol Biol Psychiatry* 2003; 27:1059–1063.

70. Ruan CJ, et al. Pneumonia can cause clozapine intoxication: a case report. *Psychosomatics* 2017; 58:652–656.

71. Leung JG, et al. Necrotizing pneumonia in the setting of elevated clozapine levels. *J Clin Psychopharmacol* 2016; 36:176–178.

72. De Leon J, et al. A rational use of clozapine based on adverse drug reactions, pharmacokinetics, and clinical pharmacopsychology. *Psychother Psychosom* 2020; 89:200–214.

73. Clark SR, et al. Elevated clozapine levels associated with infection: a systematic review. *Schizophr Res* 2018; 192:50–56.

74. Hung GC, et al. Antipsychotic reexposure and recurrent pneumonia in schizophrenia: a nested case-control study. *J Clin Psychiatry* 2016; 77:60–66.

75. Galappathie N, et al. Clozapine re-trial in a patient with repeated life threatening pneumonias. *Acta Biomed* 2014; 85:175–179.

76. Schmidinger S, et al. Pulmonary embolism and aspiration pneumonia after reexposure to clozapine: pulmonary adverse effects of clozapine. *J Clin Psychopharmacol* 2014; 34:385–387.

少见或罕见的不良反应

不良反应	出现时间	评论
粒细胞缺乏症/嗜中性粒细胞减少症(延迟性)[1-4]	通常在治疗的前3个月出现,但也可能在任意时间出现	甚至治疗1年后,也偶有氯氮平明确引起血液病的报道。风险可能升高9年[5]。在一些病例中,氯氮平可能并不是病因[6,7]。见本章"血液系统不良反应"
结肠炎/胃肠坏死[8-15]	通常在治疗1个月内出现,但也可能在任意时间出现[16]	案例报道越来越多。因有潜在的死亡风险,任何严重或慢性的腹泻都应立即转诊至专科医师。使用抗胆碱能药可增加结肠炎和肠坏死的风险[17]
谵妄[18-20]	任何时候	报道非常普遍(8%~10%[18,21]),但如果缓慢加药并监测血药浓度,临床上很少出现。老年和躯体共病增加了谵妄的风险。确保处理谵妄常见因素(见本章"谵妄")
嗜酸性粒细胞增多症[22-24]	头几周[25,26]	较常见,但意义不明。有人认为嗜酸性粒细胞增多预示中性粒缺细胞减少,但存在争议。通常是良性,但需检查炎性器官损害的征象[27](心肌炎[28]、间质性肾炎[26,29]、间质性肺病、肝炎、胰腺[30])。可能与结肠炎和相关症状有关[15,31]。6例药物超敏综合征报道[32]。在器官无炎症的情况下,重新用药有可能成功[33]。同时服用抗抑郁药可能会增加风险[34,35]
心搏骤停[36,37]	任何时候	有2例报道都发生在酷暑时。可能被误诊为恶性综合征(2例肌酸激酶均增高)
肝衰竭或肝酶异常[38-44]	用药头几个月	肝功能良性改变常见(最多50%的患者),但仍然值得监测,因为有非常小的暴发性肝衰竭的风险[45]。皮疹可能与氯氮平相关的肝炎有关[46]。见本章"肝损害"部分
低体温[47]	任何时候	在药物警戒数据库中有少许案例报道。可能是致命的
间质性肾炎[29,48-56]	通常发生在服药前3周,也可能长达3个月[26,57]	为数不多的报道与氯氮平有关。免疫介导。只用药几次就可能发生。症状包括发热、心动过速、恶心、呕吐、腹泻、肌酐升高、排尿困难和嗜酸性粒细胞增多。可能不会出现与肾炎相关的典型皮疹[26]。没有再次用药获得成功的案例报道
间质性肺病	通常发生在服药后的前几个月,也可能在治疗后期出现	6例报道[58]。可能由误吸或者免疫反应引起。症状无特异性:气短、发热、咳嗽、乏力。也有过肺炎的报道[59]
眼部影响	任何时候	有1例眼部色素沉着报道[60],5例眼眶周围水肿[61]。氯氮平可能导致干眼症[62]

续表

不良反应	出现时间	评论
胰腺炎[63-70]	通常发生在用药头6周,也可能在治疗后期出现[71]	几例无症状或有症状胰腺炎的报道。症状包括发热、腹痛腹胀、恶心、呕吐、C反应蛋白增加、脂肪酶和/或淀粉酶升高。丙戊酸钠可能增加风险[26]。大多数再次用药均失败[66,72-74],但有1例获得成功[75]
腮腺肿大[76-82]	通常发生在最初几周,但也可能更晚[83]	几例报道。机制不明,可能与免疫相关,或与唾液黏稠导致钙沉积有关。可能复发。可自发缓解[84]。以特拉唑嗪联合苯扎托品治疗唾液过多可能有效
心包炎和心包渗出[85-93]	任何时候	文献中有数例报道。症状包括乏力、胸痛、呼吸困难和心动过速,也可能无症状[94]。征象包括炎症标志物(尤其是超敏肌钙蛋白I)和B型利钠肽原水平升高[95]。超声心动图可明确/排除渗出。再次用药有可能成功[96,97]
口吃[98-106]	任何时候	个案报告。可能是锥体外系不良反应或癫痫样活动的结果。查血药浓度,考虑减量或使用抗癫痫药,这可能是即将发生全身性癫痫发作的警示信号[107]
血小板减少症[108-111]	头3个月	数据极少,但临床相当常见(1年以上发生率3%[112]~8%[113])。可能是短暂的,没有临床意义,但在一些病例中持续存在[114,115],其他病例再次用药导致复发[116]。血小板增多症也有过报道[117]
皮肤反应[118]	任何时候	精神分裂症患者中皮肤病的发生率普遍较高[119]。4例血管炎报道中[120-123],患者出现下肢融合性红斑。史蒂文斯-约翰逊综合征1例[124],玫瑰糠疹两例[125,126],丘疹1例[127],发疹性脓疱病1例[128],Sweet综合征死亡1例[129]。超敏反应综合征中皮疹常有报道[32]
血栓栓塞[130-134]	任何时候[135]	体重增加和镇静可能导致该风险。机制可能是通过$5HT_{2A}$受体活化增加血小板聚集[136]。氯氮平增加肺血栓栓塞的风险比一般人群高28倍[137]。风险可能与剂量相关[138]。存在其他危险因素(手术、制动)时,预防性抗血栓治疗阈值应该更低。栓塞后持续治疗是可能的[139],但应咨询血液科医师,因为如果没有预防性抗血栓治疗,可能会复发[140,141]

参考文献

1. Thompson A, et al. Late onset neutropenia with clozapine. *Can J Psychiatry* 2004; 49:647–648.

2. Bhanji NH, et al. Late-onset agranulocytosis in a patient with schizophrenia after 17 months of clozapine treatment. *J Clin Psychopharmacol* 2003; 23:522–523.

3. Sedky K, et al. Clozapine-induced agranulocytosis after 11 years of treatment (Letter). *Am J Psychiatry* 2005; 162:814.

4. De Araujo CF, et al. Delayed-onset severe neutropenia associated with clozapine with successful rechallenge at lower dose. *J Clin Psychopharmacol* 2021; 41:77–79.

5. Kang BJ, et al. Long-term patient monitoring for clozapine-induced agranulocytosis and neutropenia in Korea: when is it safe to discontinue CPMS? *Human Psychopharmacology* 2006; 21:387–391.

6. Panesar N, et al. Late onset neutropenia with clozapine. *Aust N Z J Psychiatry* 2011; 45:684.

7. Tourian L, et al. Late-onset agranulocytosis in a patient treated with clozapine and lamotrigine. *J Clin Psychopharmacol* 2011; 31:665–667.

8. Hawe R, et al. Response to clozapine-induced microscopic colitis: a case report and review of the literature. *J Clin Psychopharmacol* 2008; 28:454–455.

9. Shah V, et al. Clozapine-induced ischaemic colitis. *BMJ Case Rep* 2013; 2013:bcr2012007933.

10. Linsley KR, et al. Clozapine-associated colitis: case report and review of the literature. *J Clin Psychopharmacol* 2012; 32:564–566.

11. Baptista T. A fatal case of ischemic colitis during clozapine administration. *Rev Bras Psiquiatr* 2014; 36:358.

12. Rodriguez-Sosa JT, et al. Apropos of a case: relationship of ischemic colitis with clozapine. *Actas Esp Psiquiatr* 2014; 42:325–326.

13. Osterman MT, et al. Clozapine-induced acute gastrointestinal necrosis: a case report. *J Med Case Rep* 2017; 11:270.

14. Holz K, et al. Clozapine associated with microscopic colitis in the setting of biopsy-proven celiac disease. *J Clin Psychopharmacol* 2018; 38:150–152.

15. Rask SM, et al. Clozapine-related diarrhea and colitis: report of 4 cases. *J Clin Psychopharmacol* 2020; 40:293–296.

16. Verdoux H, et al. Clinical determinants of fever in clozapine users and implications for treatment management: a narrative review. *Schizophr Res* 2019; 211:1–9.

17. Peyriere H, et al. Antipsychotics-induced ischaemic colitis and gastrointestinal necrosis: a review of the French pharmacovigilance database. *Pharmacoepidemiol Drug Saf* 2009; 18:948–955.

18. Centorrino F, et al. Delirium during clozapine treatment: incidence and associated risk factors. *Pharmacopsychiatry* 2003; 36:156–160.

19. Shankar BR. Clozapine-induced delirium. *J Neuropsychiatry Clin Neurosci* 2008; 20:239–240.

20. Khanra S, et al. An unusual case of delirium after restarting clozapine. *Clin Psychopharmacol Neurosci* 2016; 14:107–108.

21. Gaertner HJ, et al. Side effects of clozapine. *Psychopharmacology* 1989; 99 Suppl:S97–S100.

22. Hummer M, et al. Does eosinophilia predict clozapine induced neutropenia? *Psychopharmacology* 1996; 124:201–204.

23. Ames D, et al. Predictive value of eosinophilia for neutropenia during clozapine treatment. *J Clin Psychiatry* 1996; 57:579–581.

24. Wysokinski A, et al. Rapidly developing and self-limiting eosinophilia associated with clozapine. *Psychiatry Clin Neurosci* 2015; 69:122.

25. Aneja J, et al. Eosinophilia induced by clozapine: a report of two cases and review of the literature. *J Family Med Primary Care* 2015; 4:127–129.

26. Lally J, et al. Hepatitis, interstitial nephritis, and pancreatitis in association with clozapine treatment: a systematic review of case series and reports. *J Clin Psychopharmacol* 2018; 38:520–527.

27. Marchel D, et al. Multiorgan eosinophilic infiltration after initiation of clozapine therapy: a case report. *BMC Res Notes* 2017; 10:316.

28. Chatterton R. Eosinophilia after commencement of clozapine treatment. *AustNZJPsychiatry* 1997; 31:874–876.

29. Chan SY, et al. Clozapine-induced acute interstitial nephritis. *Hong Kong Med J* 2015; 21:372–374.

30. Lally J, et al. Rechallenge following clozapine-associated eosinophilia: a case report and literature review. *J Clin Psychopharmacol* 2019; 39:504–506.

31. Linsley KR, et al. Clozapine-induced eosinophilic colitis (letter). *Am J Psychiatry* 2005; 162:1386–1387.

32. De Filippis R, et al. Clozapine-related drug reaction with eosinophilia and systemic symptoms (DRESS) syndrome: a systematic review. *Expert Rev Clin Pharmacol* 2020; 13:875–883.

33. McArdle PA, et al. Successful rechallenge with clozapine after treatment associated eosinophilia. *Aust Psychiatry* 2016; 24:365–367.

34. Fabrazzo M, et al. Clozapine versus other antipsychotics during the first 18 weeks of treatment: a retrospective study on risk factor increase of blood dyscrasias. *Psychiatry Res* 2017; 256:275–282.

35. Sanader B, et al. Clozapine-induced DRESS syndrome: a case series from the AMSP multicenter drug safety surveillance project. *Pharmacopsychiatry* 2019; 52:156–159.

36. Kerwin RW, et al. Heat stroke in schizophrenia during clozapine treatment: rapid recognition and management. *J Psychopharmacology* 2004; 18:121–123.

37. Hoffmann MS, et al. Heat stroke during long-term clozapine treatment: should we be concerned about hot weather? *Trends in Psychiatry and Psychotherapy* 2016; 38:56–59.

38. Erdogan A, et al. Management of marked liver enzyme increase during clozapine treatment: a case report and review of the literature. *Int J Psychiatry Med* 2004; 34:83–89.

39. Macfarlane B, et al. Fatal acute fulminant liver failure due to clozapine: a case report and review of clozapine-induced hepatotoxicity. *Gastroenterology* 1997; 112:1707–1709.

40. Chang A, et al. Clozapine-induced fatal fulminant hepatic failure: a case report. *Can J Gastroenterol* 2009; 23:376–378.

41. Chaplin AC, et al. Re: recent case report of clozapine-induced acute hepatic failure. *Can J Gastroenterol* 2010; 24:739–740.

42. Wu Chou AI, et al. Hepatotoxicity induced by clozapine: a case report and review of literature. *Neuropsychiatr Dis Treat* 2014; 10:1585–1587.

43. Kane JP, et al. Clozapine-induced liver injury and pleural effusion. *Mental Illness* 2014; 6:5403.

44. Douros A, et al. Drug-induced liver injury: results from the hospital-based Berlin Case-Control Surveillance Study. *Br J Clin Pharmacol* 2015; 79:988–999.

45. Tucker P. Liver toxicity with clozapine. *Aust N Z J Psychiatry* 2013; 47:975–976.

46. Fong SY, et al. Clozapine-induced toxic hepatitis with skin rash. *J Psychopharmacol* 2005; 19:107.

47. Burk BG, et al. A case report of acute hypothermia during initial inpatient clozapine titration with review of current literature on clozapine-induced temperature dysregulations. *BMC Psychiatry* 2020; 20:290.

48. Hunter R, et al. Clozapine-induced interstitial nephritis – a rare but important complication: a case report. *J Med Case Rep* 2009; 3:8574.

49. Elias TJ, et al. Clozapine-induced acute interstitial nephritis. *Lancet* 1999; 354:1180–1181.

50. Parekh R, et al. Clozapine induced tubulointerstitial nephritis in a patient with paranoid schizophrenia. *BMJ Case Rep* 2014; bcr2013203502.

51. An NY, et al. A case of clozapine induced acute renal failure. *Psychiatry Investig* 2013; **10**:92–94.
52. Kanofsky JD, et al. A case of acute renal failure in a patient recently treated with clozapine and a review of previously reported cases. *Prim Care Companion CNS Disord* 2011; **13**:PCC.10br01091.
53. Au AF, et al. Clozapine-induced acute interstitial nephritis. *Am J Psychiatry* 2004; **161**:1501.
54. Southall KE. A case of interstitial nephritis on clozapine. *Aust N Z J Psychiatry* 2000; **34**:697–698.
55. Fraser D, et al. An unexpected and serious complication of treatment with the atypical antipsychotic drug clozapine. *Clin Nephrol* 2000; **54**:78–80.
56. McLoughlin C, et al. Clozapine-induced interstitial nephritis in a patient with schizoaffective disorder in the forensic setting: a case report and review of the literature. *Ir J Psychol Med* 2019: [Epub ahead of print].
57. Mohan T, et al. Clozapine-induced nephritis and monitoring implications. *Aust N Z J Psychiatry* 2013; **47**:586–587.
58. Can KC, et al. A very rare adverse effect of clozapine, clozapine-induced interstitial lung disease: case report and literature review. *Noro Psikiyatri Arsivi* 2019; **56**:313–315.
59. Torrico T, et al. Clozapine-induced pneumonitis: a case report. *Frontiers in Psychiatry* 2020; **11**:572102.
60. Borovik AM, et al. Ocular pigmentation associated with clozapine. *Med J Aust* 2009; **190**:210–211.
61. Huttlin EA, et al. Periorbital edema associated with clozapine and gabapentins: a case report. *J Clin Psychopharmacol* 2020; **40**:198–199.
62. Ceylan E, et al. The ocular surface side effects of an anti-psychotic drug, clozapine. *Cutan Ocul Toxicol* 2016; **35**:62–66.
63. Bergemann N, et al. Asymptomatic pancreatitis associated with clozapine. *Pharmacopsychiatry* 1999; **32**:78–80.
64. Raja M, et al. A case of clozapine-associated pancreatitis. *Open Neuropsychopharmacol J* 2011; **4**:5–7.
65. Bayard JM, et al. Case report: acute pancreatitis induced by Clozapine. *Acta Gastroenterol Belg* 2005; **68**:92–94.
66. Sani G, et al. Development of asymptomatic pancreatitis with paradoxically high serum clozapine levels in a patient with schizophrenia and the CYP1A2*1F/1F genotype. *J Clin Psychopharmacol* 2010; **30**:737–739.
67. Wehmeier PM, et al. Pancreatitis followed by pericardial effusion in an adolescent treated with clozapine. *J Clin Psychopharmacol* 2003; **23**:102–103.
68. Garlipp P, et al. The development of a clinical syndrome of asymptomatic pancreatitis and eosinophilia after treatment with clozapine in schizophrenia: implications for clinical care, recognition and management. *J Psychopharmacology* 2002; **16**:399–400.
69. Gatto EM, et al. Clozapine and pancreatitis. *Clin Neuropharmacol* 1998; **21**:203.
70. Martin A. Acute pancreatitis associated with clozapine use. *Am J Psychiatry* 1992; **149**:714.
71. Cerulli TR. Clozapine-associated pancreatitis. *Harv Rev Psychiatry* 1999; **7**:61–63.
72. Huang YJ, et al. Recurrent pancreatitis without eosinophilia on clozapine rechallenge. *Prog Neuropsychopharmacol Biol Psychiatry* 2009; **33**:1561–1562.
73. Chengappa KN, et al. Recurrent pancreatitis on clozapine re-challenge. *J Psychopharmacology* 1995; **9**:381–382.
74. Frankenburg FR, et al. Eosinophilia, clozapine, and pancreatitis. *Lancet* 1992; **340**:251.
75. DeRemer CE, et al. Clozapine drug-induced pancreatitis of intermediate latency of onset confirmed by de-challenge and re-challenge. *Int J Clin Pharmacol Ther* 2019; **57**:37–40.
76. Immadisetty V, et al. A successful treatment strategy for clozapine-induced parotid swelling: a clinical case and systematic review. *TherAdvPsychopharmacol* 2012; **2**:235–239.
77. Gouzien C, et al. [Clozapine-induced parotitis: a case study]. *Encephale* 2014; **40**:81–85.
78. Saguem BN, et al. Eosinophilia and parotitis occurring early in clozapine treatment. *Int J Clin Pharm* 2015; **37**:992–995.
79. Vohra A. Clozapine- induced recurrent and transient parotid gland swelling. *African Journal of Psychiatry* 2013; **16**:236, 238.
80. Acosta-Armas AJ. Two cases of parotid gland swelling in patients taking clozapine. *Hosp Med* 2001; **62**:704–705.
81. Patkar AA, et al. Parotid gland swelling with clozapine. *J Clin Psychiatry* 1996; **57**:488.
82. Kathirvel N, et al. Recurrent transient parotid gland swelling with clozapine therapy. *Ir J Psychol Med* 2014; **25**:69–70.
83. Brodkin ES, et al. Treatment of clozapine-induced parotid gland swelling. *Am J Psychiatry* 1996; **153**:445.
84. Vasile JS, et al. Clozapine and the development of salivary gland swelling: a case study. *J Clin Psychiatry* 1995; **56**:511–513.
85. Raju P, et al. Pericardial effusion in patients with schizophrenia: are they on clozapine? *Emerg Med J* 2008; **25**:383–384.
86. Dauner DG, et al. Clozapine-induced pericardial effusion. *J Clin Psychopharmacol* 2008; **28**:455–456.
87. Markovic J, et al. Clozapine-induced pericarditis. *Afr J Psychiatry* 2011; **14**:236–238.
88. Bhatti MA, et al. Clozapine-induced pericarditis, pericardial tamponade, polyserositis, and rash. *J Clin Psychiatry* 2005; **66**:1490–1491.
89. Boot E, et al. Pericardial and bilateral pleural effusion associated with clozapine treatment. *Eur Psychiatry* 2004; **19**:65.
90. Murko A, et al. Clozapine and pericarditis with pericardial effusion. *Am J Psychiatry* 2002; **159**:494.
91. Imon Paul MD, et al. Clozapine induced pericarditis. *Clin Schizophr Relat Psychoses* 2014: **4**;1–6
92. Bath AS, et al. Pericardial effusion: rare adverse effect of clozapine. *Cureus* 2019; **11**:e4890.
93. Johal HK, et al. Clozapine-induced pericarditis: an ethical dilemma. *BMJ Case Rep* 2019; **12**:e229872.
94. Prisco V, et al. Brain natriuretic peptide as a biomarker of asymptomatic clozapine-related heart dysfunction: a criterion for a more cautious administration. *Clin Schizophr Relat Psychoses* 2016; **12**:185–188.
95. Prisco V, et al. Brain natriuretic peptide as a biomarker of asymptomatic clozapine-related heart dysfunction: a criterion for a more cautious administration. *Clin Schizophr Relat Psychoses* 2019; **12**:185–188.
96. Crews MP, et al. Clozapine rechallenge following clozapine-induced pericarditis. *J Clin Psychiatry* 2010; **71**:959–961.
97. Sarathy K, et al. A successful re-trial after clozapine myopericarditis. *J R Coll Physicians Edinb* 2017; **47**:146–147.
98. Kumar T, et al. Dose dependent stuttering with clozapine: a case report. *Asian J Psychiatr* 2013; **6**:178–179.
99. Grover S, et al. Clozapine-induced stuttering: a case report and analysis of similar case reports in the literature. *Gen Hosp Psychiatry* 2012; **34**:703–703.

100. Murphy R, et al. Clozapine-induced stuttering: an estimate of prevalence in the west of Ireland. *Ther Adv Psychopharmacol* 2015; 5:232–236.

101. Rachamallu V, et al. Clozapine-induced microseizures, orofacial dyskinesia, and speech dysfluency in an adolescent with treatment resistant early onset schizophrenia on concurrent lithium therapy. *Case Rep Psychiatry* 2017: 7359095

102. Bar KJ, et al. Olanzapine- and clozapine-induced stuttering. A case series. *Pharmacopsychiatry* 2004; 37:131–134.

103. Chochol MD, et al. Clozapine-associated myoclonus and stuttering secondary to smoking cessation and drug interaction: a case report. *J Clin Psychopharmacol* 2019; 39:275–277.

104. Gica S, et al. Clozapine-associated stuttering: a case report. *Am J Ther* 2020; 27:e624–e627.

105. Das S, et al. Clozapine-induced weight loss and stuttering in a patient with schizophrenia. *Indian J Psychol Med* 2018; 40:385–387.

106. Nagendrappa S, et al. 'I stopped hearing voices, started to stutter' – a case of clozapine-induced stuttering. *Indian J Psychol Med* 2019; 41:97–98.

107. Duggal HS, et al. Clozapine-induced stuttering and seizures. *Am J Psychiatry* 2002; 159:315.

108. Jagadheesan K, et al. Clozapine-induced thrombocytopenia: a pilot study. *Hong Kong J Psychiatry* 2003; 13:12–15.

109. Mihaljevic-Peles A, et al. Thrombocytopenia associated with clozapine and fluphenazine. *Nord J Psychiatry* 2001; 55:449–450.

110. Rudolf J, et al. Clozapine-induced agranulocytosis and thrombopenia in a patient with dopaminergic psychosis. *J Neur Trans* 1997; 104:1305–1311.

111. Assion HJ, et al. Lymphocytopenia and thrombocytopenia during treatment with risperidone or clozapine. *Pharmacopsychiatry* 1996; 29:227–228.

112. Lee J, et al. The effect of clozapine on hematological indices: a 1-year follow-up study. *J Clin Psychopharmacol* 2015; 35:510–516.

113. Grover S, et al. Haematological side effects associated with clozapine: a retrospective study from India. *Asian J Psychiatr* 2020; 48:101906.

114. Kate N, et al. Clozapine associated thrombocytopenia. *J Pharmacol Pharmacother* 2013; 4:149–151.

115. Gonzales MF, et al. Evidence for immune etiology in clozapine-induced thrombocytopenia of 40 months' duration: a case report. *CNS Spectr* 2000; 5:17–18.

116. Hauseux PA, et al. Clozapine rechallenge after thrombocytopenia: a case report. *Schizophr Res* 2020; 222:477–479.

117. Hampson ME. Clozapine-induced thrombocytosis. *Br J Psychiatry* 2000; 176:400.

118. Warnock JK, et al. Adverse cutaneous reactions to antipsychotics. *Am J Clin Dermatol* 2002; 3:629–636.

119. Wu BY, et al. Prevalence and associated factors of comorbid skin diseases in patients with schizophrenia: a clinical survey and national health database study. *Gen Hosp Psychiatry* 2014; 36:415–421.

120. Voulgari C, et al. Clozapine-induced late agranulocytosis and severe neutropenia complicated with streptococcus pneumonia, venous thromboembolism, and allergic vasculitis in treatment-resistant female psychosis. *Case Rep Med* 2015. http://dx.doi.org/10.1155/2015/703218.

121. Penaskovic K, et al. Clozapine-induced allergic vasculitis (letter). *Am J Psychiatry* 2005; 162:1543–1542.

122. Mukherjee S, et al. Leukocytoclastic vasculitis secondary to clozapine. *Indian J Psychiatry* 2019; 61:94–96.

123. Fujimoto S, et al. Clozapine-induced antineutrophil cytoplasmic antibody-associated vasculitis: a case report. *Mod Rheumatol Case Rep* 2020; 4:70–73.

124. Wu MK, et al. The severe complication of Stevens-Johnson syndrome induced by long-term clozapine treatment in a male schizophrenia patient: a case report. *Neuropsychiatr Dis Treat* 2015; 11:1039–1041.

125. Lai YW, et al. Pityriasis rosea-like eruption associated with clozapine: a case report. *Gen Hosp Psychiatry* 2012; 34:703.e705–707.

126. Bhatia MS, et al. Clozapine induced pityriasiform eruption. *Indian J Dermatol* 1997; 42:245–246.

127. Stanislav SW, et al. Papular rash and bilateral pleural effusion associated with clozapine. *Ann Pharmacother* 1999; 33:1008–1009.

128. Bosonnet S, et al. [Acute generalized exanthematic pustulosis after intake of clozapine (leponex) First case]. *Ann Dermatol Venereol* 1997; 124:547–548.

129. Kleinen JM, et al. [Clozapine-induced agranulocytosis and Sweet's syndrome in a 74-year-old female patient A Case Study]. *Tijdschrift Voor Psychiatrie* 2008; 50:119–123.

130. Chate S, et al. Pulmonary thromboembolism associated with clozapine. *J Neuropsychiatry Clin Neurosci* 2013; 25:E3–6.

131. Srinivasaraju R, et al. Clozapine-associated cerebral venous thrombosis. *J Clin Psychopharmacol* 2010; 30:335–336.

132. Werring D, et al. Cerebral venous sinus thrombosis may be associated with clozapine. *J Neuropsychiatry Clin Neurosci* 2009; 21:343–345.

133. Paciullo CA. Evaluating the association between clozapine and venous thromboembolism. *Am J Health Syst Pharm* 2008; 65:1825–1829.

134. Yang TY, et al. Massive pulmonary embolism in a young patient on clozapine therapy. *J Emerg Med* 2004; 27:27–29.

135. Gami RK, et al. Pulmonary embolism and clozapine use: a case report and literature review. *Psychosomatics* 2017; 58:203–208.

136. Hagg S, et al. Risk of venous thromboembolism due to antipsychotic drug therapy. *Exp Opin Drug Saf* 2009; 8:537–547.

137. De Fazio P, et al. Rare and very rare adverse effects of clozapine. *Neuropsychiatr Dis Treat* 2015; 11:1995–2003.

138. Sarvaiya N, et al. Clozapine-associated pulmonary embolism: a high-mortality, dose-independent and early-onset adverse effect. *Am J Ther* 2018; 25:e434–e438.

139. Goh JG, et al. A case report of clozapine continuation after pulmonary embolism in the context of other risk factors for thromboembolism. *Aust N Z J Psychiatry* 2016; 50:1205–1206.

140. Munoli RN, et al. Clozapine-induced recurrent pulmonary thromboembolism. *J Neuropsychiatry Clin Neurosci* 2013; 25:E50–E51.

141. Selten JP, et al. Clozapine and venous thromboembolism: further evidence. *J Clin Psychiatry* 2003; 64:609.

氯氮平:严重的血液系统及心血管不良反应

粒细胞缺乏

氯氮平是有些毒性的,但是可以降低精神分裂症患者的总死亡率,主要是因为降低了自杀率[1-4]。氯氮平可引起严重的、危及生命的不良反应,其中以粒细胞缺乏最为人知,0.4% 的服用者可以出现[5]。遵医嘱服用氯氮平的患者中,粒细胞缺乏相关的死亡率为 0.013%,病死率为 2.1%[6]。已核准的氯氮平监测系统使这一风险明显得到控制,在氯氮平治疗 1 年后出现严重中性粒细胞减少的发生率几乎可以忽略不计[6]。氯氮平导致中性粒细胞减少之后,再次使用有可能成功[7],但是粒细胞缺乏之后不行[8]。氯氮平治疗过程中发生的中性粒细胞减少与使用氯氮平是巧合[9]。

血栓栓塞

有人提出氯氮平与血栓栓塞可能相关[10]。Walker 等[2] 最初发现,致命性肺栓塞的风险约为 1/4 500,是普通人群的 20 倍。在一例非致命性肺栓塞可能与使用氯氮平有关的病例被报告之后[11],瑞典官方发表了相关数据[12]。有 12 例静脉栓塞的报道,其中 5 例是致命的。使用氯氮平的患者发生血栓栓塞的风险为 1/2 000~1/6 000。血栓栓塞可能与氯氮平对磷脂抗体[13] 和血小板聚集[14] 的作用有关。血栓栓塞似乎最可能发生在治疗的头 6 个月[15],但也可能发生在任何时候。其风险可能与剂量无关[15],但一些研究表明与大剂量相关[16]。虽然其他抗精神病药也与血栓栓塞密切相关,但是氯氮平的风险最高[16,17]。

所有药源性血栓栓塞都可能是多因素的[18]。镇静可能导致活动减少,从而发生静脉瘀滞。肥胖、高催乳素血症和吸烟是血栓栓塞的独立风险因素[19,20]。鼓励锻炼和保证饮水充足是基本的预防措施[21]。

心肌炎和心肌病

氯氮平和心肌炎、心肌病相关。氯氮平诱发超敏反应所致心肌炎症,从而导致心肌炎。目前对心肌炎的发生率仍存在争议。澳大利亚的几项研究发现 3% 的使用者出现心肌炎[22-24]。其他地方的研究[25-27] 认为发生率较低,不到 1%。出现这种差异的原因不清楚;有人认为在一些所报告的发生率低的国家,可能由于缺乏强有力的监测而导致漏诊[28]。荟萃分析显示,每 1 000 个患者中发生率低于 1%~7%[29]。心肌炎是潜在的死因(病死率 12.7%[29]),在氯氮平治疗头 6~8 周(中位数 3 周)最有可能发生[30],但也可能发生在任何时候。

心肌病通常以超声心动图确定左心室扩大(射血分数下降)或肥大而做出诊断。它可能发生在心肌炎之后(如果不停用氯氮平),但是还有其他的可能原因,包括持续心动过速、肥胖、糖尿病、个人或家族有心脏病史[28]。发生率数据多来源于澳大利亚,为 0.02%~5%[24,31]。荟萃分析显示,发生率为 6‰,病死率为 7.8%[29]。在治疗中,心肌病可能比心肌炎发生更晚(中位数 9 个月)[30],但与心肌炎一样,也可能发生在任何时候。

尽管发生率报道不一,仍要密切监测患者有无心肌炎迹象,尤其是在治疗的头几个月[32]。心肌炎的症状包括低血压、心动过速、发热、流感样症状、乏力、呼吸困难(伴有呼吸频率增加)

和胸痛[33]。征象包括心电图改变(ST 段压低),影像学和超声示心脏扩大,以及嗜酸性粒细胞增多。服用氯氮平的患者出现很多上述症状,但并不一定会发展为心肌炎[34],相反,没出现这些症状并不能排除心肌炎[35]。但凡出现心力衰竭,应立即停用氯氮平,并转至心内科。重新使用氯氮平有成功的案例[8,36-41](β 受体阻滞剂、ACEI 和盐皮质激素受体拮抗剂可能有用[42-44]),但是也可能再次发生心肌炎[45-48]。重新用药的患者有必要进行超声心动图、C 反应蛋白和肌钙蛋白的检查[49-51]。有效地治疗代谢综合征和糖尿病可能也有帮助[29]。

尸检发现致命性心肌炎可以在没有明确症状的情况下发生,尽管心动过速和发热常出现[52]。澳大利亚墨尔本的团队推出一种监测程序,据说可以通过测量肌钙蛋白 I、肌钙蛋白 T 和 C 反应蛋白而发现全部有症状的心肌炎[53](表 1.39)。在澳大利亚,基线期、6 个月和此后每年常规进行超声心动图检查,但是在缺乏其他症状的情况下进行监测的益处受到了质疑[54]。如果担心可能发生心肌炎,那么在基线期检查超声心动图有利于用药前后的对比,尤其是对那些已有心脏疾病、结构性异常或其他心脏危险因素的患者[55]。除了常规血检(包括 C 反应蛋白和肌钙蛋白)和心电图以外,缺乏监测的资源不应该成为多数患者使用氯氮平的障碍[27]。

表 1.39 心肌炎监测建议 [52,53,66,67]

基线	脉搏、血压、体温、呼吸频率
	全血细胞计数(FBC)
	C 反应蛋白(CRP)
	肌钙蛋白
	超声心动图(若有)
	心电图(ECG)
每天,如果可能	脉搏、血压、体温、呼吸频率
	询问:胸痛、发热、咳嗽、气短、运动能力
第 7、14、21、28 天	C 反应蛋白
	肌钙蛋白
	全血细胞计数
	心电图(如果可能)
如果 C 反应蛋白 >100mg/L,或肌钙蛋白大于正常上限的两倍	停用氯氮平,复查超声
如果发热 + 心动过速 +C 反应蛋白或肌钙蛋白升高(但与上面不同)	每天查 C 反应蛋白和肌钙蛋白

可能增加心肌炎风险的因素包括快速加量、联用丙戊酸钠、老年(每长 10 岁风险增加 31%)[56]。其他精神药物,包括锂盐、利培酮、氟哌啶醇、氯丙嗪、氟奋乃静也与心肌炎有关[57]。最好避免使用其他增加心肌炎风险的药物,但临床上往往很困难。对有心脏病病史、心血管意外事件、吸毒[23]、心脏病家族史的患者,用药时应格外谨慎。

只要超声心动图提示有心力衰竭征兆,都应怀疑心肌病,立即停用氯氮平并转诊。心肌病的表现形式多种多样[58,59],但在早期常无症状[24],所以当出现心悸、胸痛、晕厥、出汗、运动能力下降或呼吸困难时,应当严密排查。严密的心脏监测(包括超声心动图),并使用改善病情的心脏药物,可能会有助于成功地再次使用氯氮平[44,60,61]。

尽管总体死亡率在下降,但是青年人猝死的风险却在上升[62],可能与氯氮平导致的心电图改变有关[63]。虽然总体情况仍不明确,但是需要警惕。当然,其他抗精神病药物也有类似的问题[57,64,65]。

小结

- 使用氯氮平的总死亡率比精神分裂症的总死亡率低。
- 标准监测期间,致死性粒性细胞缺乏症的风险低于 1/8 000。
- 在治疗的患者中致死性肺栓塞的风险大约是 1/4 500。
- 致死性心肌炎或心肌病的风险高达 1/1 000。
- 在氯氮平治疗期间必须谨慎监测,尤其是前 3 个月(见表 1.39)。

参考文献

1. Vermeulen JM, et al. Clozapine and long-term mortality risk in patients with schizophrenia: a systematic review and meta-analysis of studies lasting 1.1–12.5 years. *Schizophr Bull* 2019; **45**:315–329.
2. Walker AM, et al. Mortality in current and former users of clozapine. *Epidemiology* 1997; **8**:671–677.
3. Van Der Zalm Y, et al. Clozapine and mortality: a comparison with other antipsychotics in a nationwide Danish cohort study. *Acta Psychiatr Scand* 2020: [Epub ahead of print].
4. Munro J, et al. Active monitoring of 12760 clozapine recipients in the UK and Ireland. *Br J Psychiatry* 1999; **175**:576–580.
5. Li XH, et al. The prevalence of agranulocytosis and related death in clozapine-treated patients: a comprehensive meta-analysis of observational studies. *Psychol Med* 2020; **50**:583–594.
6. Myles N, et al. Meta-analysis examining the epidemiology of clozapine-associated neutropenia. *Acta Psychiatr Scand* 2018; **138**:101–109.
7. Prokopez CR, et al. Clozapine rechallenge after neutropenia or leucopenia. *J Clin Psychopharmacol* 2016; **36**:377–380.
8. Manu P, et al. Clozapine rechallenge after major adverse effects: clinical guidelines based on 259 cases. *Am J Ther* 2018; **25**:e218–e223.
9. Oloyede E, et al. There is life after the UK clozapine central non-rechallenge database. *Schizophr Bull* 2021: sbab006 [Epub ahead of print].
10. Paciullo CA. Evaluating the association between clozapine and venous thromboembolism. *Am J Health Syst Pharm* 2008; **65**:1825–1829.
11. Lacika S, et al. Pulmonary embolus possibly associated with clozapine treatment (Letter). *Can J Psychiatry* 1999; **44**:396–397.
12. Hagg S, et al. Association of venous thromboembolism and clozapine. *Lancet* 2000; **355**:1155–1156.
13. Davis S, et al. Antiphospholipid antibodies associated with clozapine treatment. *Am J Hematol* 1994; **46**:166–167.
14. Axelsson S, et al. In vitro effects of antipsychotics on human platelet adhesion and aggregation and plasma coagulation. *Clin Exp Pharmacol Physiol* 2007; **34**:775–780.
15. Sarvaiya N, et al. Clozapine-associated pulmonary embolism: a high-mortality, dose-independent and early-onset adverse effect. *Am J Ther* 2018; **25**:e434–e438.
16. Allenet B, et al. Antipsychotic drugs and risk of pulmonary embolism. *PharmacoepidemiolDrug Saf* 2012; **21**:42–48.
17. Dai L, et al. The association and influencing factors between antipsychotics exposure and the risk of VTE and PE: a systematic review and meta-analysis. *Curr Drug Targets* 2020; **21**:930–942.
18. Lacut K. Association between antipsychotic drugs, antidepressant drugs, and venous thromboembolism. *Clin Adv Hematol Oncol* 2008; **6**:887–890.
19. Masopust J, et al. Risk of venous thromboembolism during treatment with antipsychotic agents. *Psychiatry Clin Neurosci* 2012; **66**:541–552.
20. Jonsson AK, et al. Venous thromboembolism in recipients of antipsychotics: incidence, mechanisms and management. *CNS Drugs* 2012; **26**:649–662.
21. Maly R, et al. Assessment of risk of venous thromboembolism and its possible prevention in psychiatric patients. *Psychiatry Clin Neurosci* 2008; **62**:3–8.
22. Ronaldson KJ. Cardiovascular disease in clozapine-treated patients: evidence, mechanisms and management. *CNS Drugs* 2017; **31**:777–795.
23. Khan AA, et al. Clozapine and incidence of myocarditis and sudden death – long term Australian experience. *Int J Cardiol* 2017; **238**:136–139.
24. Youssef DL, et al. Incidence and risk factors for clozapine-induced myocarditis and cardiomyopathy at a regional mental health service in Australia. *Austr Psychiatry* 2016; **24**:176–180.
25. Cohen D, et al. Beyond white blood cell monitoring: screening in the initial phase of clozapine therapy. *J Clin Psychiatry* 2012; **73**:1307–1312.
26. Kilian JG, et al. Myocarditis and cardiomyopathy associated with clozapine. *Lancet* 1999; **354**:1841–1845.
27. Freudenreich O. Clozapine-induced myocarditis: prescribe safely but do prescribe. *Acta Psychiatr Scand* 2015; **132**:240–241.
28. Ronaldson KJ, et al. Clozapine-induced myocarditis, a widely overlooked adverse reaction. *Acta Psychiatr Scand* 2015; **132**:231–240.
29. Siskind D, et al. Systematic review and meta-analysis of rates of clozapine-associated myocarditis and cardiomyopathy. *Aust N Z J Psychiatry*

2020; 54:467–481.

30. La Grenade L, et al. Myocarditis and cardiomyopathy associated with clozapine use in the United States (Letter). N Engl J Med 2001; 345:224–225.

31. Curto M, et al. Systematic review of clozapine cardiotoxicity. Current Psychiatry Reports 2016; 18:68.

32. Marder SR, et al. Physical health monitoring of patients with schizophrenia. Am J Psychiatry 2004; 161:1334–1349.

33. Annamraju S, et al. Early recognition of clozapine-induced myocarditis. J Clin Psychopharmacol 2007; 27:479–483.

34. Wehmeier PM, et al. Chart review for potential features of myocarditis, pericarditis, and cardiomyopathy in children and adolescents treated with clozapine. J Child Adolesc Psychopharmacol 2004; 14:267–271.

35. McNeil JJ, et al. Clozapine-induced myocarditis: characterisation using case-control design. Eur Heart J 2013; 34 (Suppl 1):688.

36. Reinders J, et al. Clozapine-related myocarditis and cardiomyopathy in an Australian metropolitan psychiatric service. Aust N Z J Psychiatry 2004; 38:915–922.

37. Bellissima BL, et al. A systematic review of clozapine-induced myocarditis. Int J Cardiol 2018; 259:122–129.

38. Nguyen B, et al. Successful clozapine re-challenge following myocarditis. Austr Psychiatry 2017; 25:385–386.

39. Otsuka Y, et al. Clozapine-induced myocarditis: follow-up for 3.5 years after successful retrial. J Gen Fam Med 2019; 20:114–117.

40. Noël MC, et al. Clozapine-related myocarditis and rechallenge: a case series and clinical review. J Clin Psychopharmacol 2019; 39:380–385.

41. Hosseini SA, et al. Successful clozapine re-challenge after suspected clozapine-induced myocarditis. Am J Case Rep 2020; 21:e926507.

42. Rostagno C, et al. Beta-blocker and angiotensin-converting enzyme inhibitor may limit certain cardiac adverse effects of clozapine. Gen Hosp Psychiatry 2008; 30:280–283.

43. Floreani J, et al. Successful re-challenge with clozapine following development of clozapine-induced cardiomyopathy. Aust N Z J Psychiatry 2008; 42:747–748.

44. Patel RK, et al. Clozapine and cardiotoxicity – a guide for psychiatrists written by cardiologists. Psychiatry Res 2019; 282:112491.

45. Roh S, et al. Cardiomyopathy associated with clozapine. Exp Clin Psychopharmacol 2006; 14:94–98.

46. Masopust J, et al. Repeated occurrence of clozapine-induced myocarditis in a patient with schizoaffective disorder and comorbid Parkinson's disease. Neuro Endocrinol Lett 2009; 30:19–21.

47. Ronaldson KJ, et al. Observations from 8 cases of clozapine rechallenge after development of myocarditis. JClinPsychiatry 2012; 73:252–254.

48. Nielsen J, et al. Termination of clozapine treatment due to medical reasons: when is it warranted and how can it be avoided? J Clin Psychiatry 2013; 74:603–613; quiz 613.

49. Hassan I, et al. Monitoring in clozapine rechallenge after myocarditis. Austr Psychiatry 2011; 19:370–371.

50. Bray A, et al. Successful clozapine rechallenge after acute myocarditis. Aust N Z J Psychiatry 2011; 45:90.

51. Rosenfeld AJ, et al. Successful clozapine retrial after suspected myocarditis. Am J Psychiatry 2010; 167:350–351.

52. Ronaldson KJ, et al. Clinical course and analysis of ten fatal cases of clozapine-induced myocarditis and comparison with 66 surviving cases. Schizophr Res 2011; 128:161–165.

53. Ronaldson KJ, et al. A new monitoring protocol for clozapine-induced myocarditis based on an analysis of 75 cases and 94 controls. Aust N Z J Psychiatry 2011; 45:458–465.

54. Robinson G, et al. Echocardiography and clozapine: is current clinical practice inhibiting use of a potentially life-transforming therapy? Aust Fam Physician 2017; 46:169–170.

55. Knoph KN, et al. Clozapine-induced cardiomyopathy and myocarditis monitoring: a systematic review. Schizophr Res 2018; 199:17–30.

56. Ronaldson KJ, et al. Rapid clozapine dose titration and concomitant sodium valproate increase the risk of myocarditis with clozapine: a case-control study. Schizophr Res 2012; 141:173–178.

57. Coulter DM, et al. Antipsychotic drugs and heart muscle disorder in international pharmacovigilance: data mining study. BMJ 2001; 322:1207–1209.

58. Pastor CA, et al. Masked clozapine-induced cardiomyopathy. J Am Board Fam Med 2008; 21:70–74.

59. Sagar R, et al. Clozapine-induced cardiomyopathy presenting as panic attacks. J Psychiatr Pract 2008; 14:182–185.

60. Nederlof M, et al. Clozapine re-exposure after dilated cardiomyopathy. BMJ Case Rep 2017; 2017:bcr2017219652.

61. Alawami M, et al. A systematic review of clozapine induced cardiomyopathy. Int J Cardiol 2014; 176:315–320.

62. Modai I, et al. Sudden death in patients receiving clozapine treatment: a preliminary investigation. J Clin Psychopharmacol 2000; 20:325–327.

63. Kang UG, et al. Electrocardiographic abnormalities in patients treated with clozapine. J Clin Psychiatry 2000; 61:441–446.

64. Thomassen R, et al. Antipsychotic drugs and venous thromboembolism (Letter). Lancet 2000; 356:252.

65. Hagg S, et al. Antipsychotic-induced venous thromboembolism: a review of the evidence. CNS Drugs 2002; 16:765–776.

66. Ronaldson KJ, et al. Diagnostic characteristics of clozapine-induced myocarditis identified by an analysis of 38 cases and 47 controls. J Clin Psychiatry 2010; 71:976–981.

67. Yuen JWY, et al. Clozapine-induced cardiovascular side effects and autonomic dysfunction: a systematic review. Front Neurosci 2018; 12:203.

氯氮平引起的多涎

众所周知,氯氮平与明显多涎(流涎)[1]有因果关系。多涎包括嘴中唾液积聚和流口水,晚上尤其明显。它主要发生在服药早期,可能与所用剂量相关。与低剂量相比[2],在标准剂量时,多涎更常见,并与血浆氯氮平浓度升高有关[3]。临床观察发现,多涎随时间推移(通常几个月)严重程度降低,但也可能持续。流涎在社交场合使人感到尴尬,对生活质量[1]有负面影响,并且考虑到它作为吸入性肺炎的促成因素,可能有潜在的生命威胁[4-7]。因此,治疗流涎有一定的紧迫性。

氯氮平导致多涎的药理学机制尚不明确[8]。目前提出的可能机制包括 M_4 毒蕈碱受体激动作用、α_2 肾上腺素能拮抗作用和吞咽反射被抑制[9,10]。虽然至少有一项研究发现氯氮平治疗的前 3 周唾液量就明显增加[13],但是多个试验表明服用氯氮平的患者唾液分泌量并未增加[11,12],因而支持吞咽反射被抑制的假说。

无论哪种机制,能减少唾液分泌的药物都有可能减轻多涎。然而,目前针对流涎还没有药物得到许可,而且鉴于已发表的许多研究存在局限性,暂时无法提出可信的治疗建议[14]。质量一般的证据倾向支持抗毒蕈碱药物,比如丙胺太林和苯海拉明[15,16]。使用抗毒蕈碱药物应考虑到它与氯氮平的作用混淆的风险,因氯氮平有可能导致严重的、可能威胁生命的胃肠动力减退[17,18]。表 1.40 描述了已经验证过的公认的药物治疗方法。可以适当使用非药物方法治疗——包括嚼口香糖,垫高枕头,以及在枕头上铺毛巾以免浸湿卧具[8]。

表 1.40　氯氮平引起的多涎——小结

治疗方法	评论
氨磺必利 100~400mg/d[16,19,20]	支持证据来自 1 项随机安慰剂对照研究、1 项吗氯贝胺对照研究及大量的病例研究[21-25]。氯氮平可减量
阿米替林 25~100mg/d[26-28]	支持的文献有限,不良反应较多,加重便秘
阿托品 舌下给药[29-33] 或以(1mg/10mL)溶液漱口	支持的文献有限,收益风险不确定。很少用。给药问题有过报道[34]
苯海索 5~15mg/d[35]	小型开放性研究显示有效。一些机构使用,但可损害认知功能。小剂量(2mg)可能有效[36]
苯扎托品 2mg/d+ 特拉唑嗪 2mg/d[37]	联合用药优于单一用药。特拉唑嗪为 α_1 受体拮抗剂,故可引起低血压
肉毒毒素[38-41] 两侧腮腺注射(各 150IU)	能有效地治疗神经系统疾病的多涎。文献报道了 6 例成功治疗氯氮平引起多涎的案例
安非他酮 100~150mg/d[42]	个案报道,可降低癫痫阈值
氯苯那敏[16]	抗组胺药和弱抗毒蕈碱药物。1 项高质量研究

续表

治疗方法	评论
可乐定 0.1~0.2mg 贴剂,每周 1 次 或 0.1mg 睡前口服 [43,44]	α_2 受体部分激动剂。支持的文献有限。可加重精神病、抑郁和导致低血压
苯海拉明 [15,16]	抗组胺药和强抗毒蕈碱药物。高质量研究很少
格隆溴铵 0.5~4mg,每天 2 次 [45-49]	一项随机对照试验表明格隆溴铵优于比哌立登,不会恶化认知功能;另一项研究发现,与安慰剂相比,每天 2mg 临床上显著改善"夜间多涎"
胍法辛 1mg,每天 1 次 [50]	α_2 受体激动剂。个案报道。可致低血压
东莨菪碱 0.3mg 吸食或咀嚼,最多每天 3 次或 1.5mg/72h 贴用 [51-54]	外周和中枢抗胆碱能作用。使用非常广泛,但仅有一项双盲对照试验。可引起认知功能损害、嗜睡并加重便秘
异丙托溴铵喷鼻剂 (0.03% 或 0.06%)——0.06% 舌下最多喷 2 下,每天 3 次 或 0.03% 每侧鼻内喷 1 下, 每天 1 次 [55,56]	支持的文献有限。唯一的安慰剂对照试验结果显示阴性 [57]
洛非西定 0.2mg,每天 2 次 [58]	α_2 受体激动剂。数据非常少。可加重精神病、抑郁症并导致低血压
甲氧氯普胺 初始剂量 10mg/d [16,59,60]	双盲、安慰剂对照试验发现显著减少夜间多涎和流涎
吗氯贝胺 150~300mg/d [45]	在一个开放性研究中,14 例患者中 9 例有效。疗效与氨磺必利相同(见上文)
N-乙酰半胱氨酸 [61]	一种能调节谷氨酸能、神经营养和炎症通路的抗氧化剂。一些小样本系列病例报道,流涎明显减少
奥昔布宁 5mg,最多每天 2 次 [62]	个案报道
哌仑西平 50~150mg/d [63-65]	M_1、M_4 选择性受体激动剂。丰富的临床经验证实有效,但有一个随机对照试验显示无效。现仍广泛应用。在英国未批准任何适应证。可致便秘
丙胺太林 7.5mg 睡前服 [15,16]	外周抗胆碱能作用。不作用于中枢。两个随机对照试验(一个结果阳性)。可加重便秘
喹硫平 [51]	可通过减少氯氮平剂量来减轻流涎
舒必利 150~300mg/d [5,16,66,67]	证据来源于一个小的阳性随机对照试验,以及氯氮平与舒必利(高剂量)合用的 Cochrane 综述。可减少氯氮平剂量

参考文献

1. Man WH, et al. Reporting patterns of sialorrhea comparing users of clozapine to users of other antipsychotics: a disproportionality analysis using vigibase. *J Clin Psychopharmacol* 2020; 40:283–286.
2. Subramanian S, et al. Clozapine dose for schizophrenia. *Cochrane Database Syst Rev* 2017; 6:Cd009555.
3. Schoretsanitis G, et al. Elevated clozapine concentrations in clozapine-treated patients with hypersalivation. *Clin Pharmacokinet* 2021; 60:329–335.
4. Hinkes R, et al. Aspiration pneumonia possibly secondary to clozapine-induced sialorrhea. *J Clin Psychopharmacol* 1996; 16:462–463.
5. Saenger RC, et al. Aspiration pneumonia due to clozapine-induced sialorrhea. *Clin Schizophr Relat Psychoses* 2016; 9:170–172.
6. Gurrera RJ, et al. Aspiration pneumonia: an underappreciated risk of clozapine treatment. *J Clin Psychopharmacol* 2016; 36:174–176.
7. Kaplan J, et al. Clozapine-associated aspiration pneumonia: case series and review of the literature. *Psychosomatics* 2017; 58:199–203.
8. Praharaj SK, et al. Clozapine-induced sialorrhea: pathophysiology and management strategies. *Psychopharmacology* 2006; 185:265–273.
9. Davydov L, et al. Clozapine-induced hypersalivation. *Ann Pharmacother* 2000; 34:662–665.
10. Rogers DP, et al. Therapeutic options in the treatment of clozapine-induced sialorrhea. *Pharmacotherapy* 2000; 20:1092–1095.
11. Rabinowitz T, et al. The effect of clozapine on saliva flow rate: a pilot study. *Biol Psychiatry* 1996; 40:1132–1134.
12. Ben Aryeh H, et al. Salivary flow-rate and composition in schizophrenic patients on clozapine: subjective reports and laboratory data. *Biol Psychiatry* 1996; 39:946–949.
13. Praharaj SK, et al. Salivary flow rate in patients with schizrenia on clozapine. *Clin Neuropharmacol* 2010; 33:176–178.
14. Sockalingam S, et al. Review: insufficient evidence to guide use of drugs for clozapine induced hypersalivation. *Evid Based Ment Health* 2009; 12:12.
15. Syed R, et al. Pharmacological interventions for clozapine-induced hypersalivation. *Cochrane Database Syst Rev* 2008; Cd005579.
16. Chen SY, et al. Treatment strategies for clozapine-induced sialorrhea: a systematic review and meta-analysis. *CNS Drugs* 2019; 33:225–238.
17. Palmer SE, et al. Life-threatening clozapine-induced gastrointestinal hypomotility: an analysis of 102 cases. *J Clin Psychiatry* 2008; 69:759–768.
18. West S, et al. Clozapine induced gastrointestinal hypomotility: a potentially life threatening adverse event. A review of the literature. *Gen Hosp Psychiatry* 2017; 46:32–37.
19. Kreinin A, et al. Amisulpride treatment of clozapine-induced hypersalivation in schizophrenia patients: a randomized, double-blind, placebo-controlled cross-over study. *Int Clin Psychopharmacol* 2006; 21:99–103.
20. Kreinin A, et al. Amisulpride versus moclobemide in treatment of clozapine-induced hypersalivation. *World J Biol Psychiatry* 2010; 12:620–626.
21. Praharaj SK, et al. Amisulpride treatment for clozapine-induced sialorrhea. *J Clin Psychopharmacol* 2009; 29:189–190.
22. Aggarwal A, et al. Amisulpride for clozapine induced sialorrhea. *Psychopharmacol Bull* 2009; 42:69–71.
23. Croissant B, et al. Reduction of side effects by combining clozapine with amisulpride: case report and short review of clozapine-induced hypersalivation-a case report. *Pharmacopsychiatry* 2005; 38:38–39.
24. Praharaj SK, et al. Amisulpride improved debilitating clozapine-induced sialorrhea. *Am J Ther* 2011; 18:e84–e85.
25. Kulkarni RR. Low-dose amisulpride for debilitating clozapine-induced sialorrhea: case series and review of literature. *Indian J Psychol Med* 2015; 37:446–448.
26. Copp P, et al. Amitriptyline in clozapine-induced sialorrhoea. *Br J Psychiatry* 1991; 159:166.
27. Praharaj SK, et al. Amitriptyline for clozapine-induced nocturnal enuresis and sialorrhoea. *Br J Clin Pharmacol* 2007; 63:128–129.
28. Sinha S, et al. Very low dose amitriptyline for clozapine-associated sialorrhea. *Curr Drug Saf* 2016; 11:262–263.
29. Antonello C, et al. Clozapine and sialorrhea: a new intervention for this bothersome and potentially dangerous side effect. *J Psychiatry Neurosci* 1999; 24:250.
30. Mustafa FA, et al. Sublingual atropine for the treatment of severe and hyoscine-resistant clozapine-induced sialorrhea. *Afr J Psychiatry* 2013; 16:242.
31. Matos Santana TE, et al. Sublingual atropine in the treatment of clozapine-induced sialorrhea. *Schizophr Res* 2017; 182:144–145.
32. Mubaslat O, et al. The effect of sublingual atropine sulfate on clozapine-induced hypersalivation: a multicentre, randomised placebo-controlled trial. *Psychopharmacology* 2020; 237:2905–2915.
33. Van Der Poorten T, et al. The sublingual use of atropine in the treatment of clozapine-induced sialorrhea: a systematic review. *Clin Case Rep* 2019; 7:2108–2113.
34. Leung JG, et al. Potential problems surrounding the use of sublingually administered ophthalmic atropine for sialorrhea. *Schizophr Res* 2017; 185:202–203.
35. Spivak B, et al. Trihexyphenidyl treatment of clozapine-induced hypersalivation. *Int Clin Psychopharmacol* 1997; 12:213–215.
36. Praharaj SK, et al. Complete resolution of clozapine-induced sialorrhea with low dose trihexyphenidyl. *Psychopharmacol Bull* 2010; 43:73–75.
37. Reinstein M, et al. Comparative efficacy and tolerability of benzatropine and terazosin in the treatment of hypersalivation secondary to clozapine. *Clin Drug Investig* 1999; 17:97–102.
38. Kahl KG, et al. Botulinum toxin as an effective treatment of clozapine-induced hypersalivation. *Psychopharmacology* 2004; 173:229–230.
39. Steinlechner S, et al. Botulinum toxin B as an effective and safe treatment for neuroleptic-induced sialorrhea. *Psychopharmacology* 2010; 207:593–597.

40. Kahl KG, et al. [Pharmacological strategies for clozapine-induced hypersalivation: treatment with botulinum toxin B in one patient and review of the literature]. *Nervenarzt* 2005; 76:205–208.

41. Verma R, et al. Botulinum toxin: a novel therapy for clozapine-induced sialorrhoea. *Psychopharmacology* 2018; 235:369–371.

42. Stern RG, et al. Clozapine-induced sialorrhea alleviated by bupropion–a case report. *Prog Neuropsychopharmacol Biol Psychiatry* 2009; 33:1578–1580.

43. Grabowski J. Clonidine treatment of clozapine-induced hypersalivation. *J Clin Psychopharmacol* 1992; 12:69–70.

44. Praharaj SK, et al. Is clonidine useful for treatment of clozapine-induced sialorrhea? *Journal of Psychopharmacology* 2005; 19:426–428.

45. Duggal HS. Glycopyrrolate for clozapine-induced sialorrhea. *Prog Neuropsychopharmacol Biol Psychiatry* 2007; 31:1546–1547.

46. Robb AS, et al. Glycopyrrolate for treatment of clozapine-induced sialorrhea in three adolescents. *J Child Adolesc Psychopharmacol* 2008; 18:99–107.

47. Liang CS, et al. Comparison of the efficacy and impact on cognition of glycopyrrolate and biperiden for clozapine-induced sialorrhea in schizophrenic patients: a randomized, double-blind, crossover study. *Schizophr Res* 2010; 119:138–144.

48. Man WH, et al. The effect of glycopyrrolate on nocturnal sialorrhea in patients using clozapine: a randomized, crossover, double-blind, placebo-controlled trial. *J Clin Psychopharmacol* 2017; 37:155–161.

49. Praharaj SK, et al. Low-dose glycopyrrolate for clozapine-associated sialorrhea. *J Clin Psychopharmacol* 2014; 34:392.

50. Webber MA, et al. Guanfacine treatment of clozapine-induced sialorrhea. *J Clin Psychopharmacol* 2004; 24:675–676.

51. McKane JP, et al. Hyoscine patches in clozapine-induced hypersalivation. *Psychiatric Bulletin* 2001; 25:277.

52. Gaftanyuk O, et al. Scolpolamine patch for clozapine-induced sialorrhea. *Psychiatr Serv* 2004; 55:318.

53. Segev A, et al. Hyoscine for clozapine-induced hypersalivation: a double-blind, randomized, placebo-controlled cross-over trial. *Int Clin Psychopharmacol* 2019; 34:101–107.

54. Takeuchi I, et al. Effect of scopolamine butylbromide on clozapine-induced hypersalivation in schizophrenic patients: a case series. *Clin Psychopharmacol Neurosci* 2015; 13:109–112.

55. Calderon J, et al. Potential use of ipatropium bromide for the treatment of clozapine-induced hypersalivation: a preliminary report. *Int Clin Psychopharmacol* 2000; 15:49–52.

56. Freudenreich O, et al. Clozapine-induced sialorrhea treated with sublingual ipratropium spray: a case series. *J Clin Psychopharmacol* 2004; 24:98–100.

57. Sockalingam S, et al. Treatment of clozapine-induced hypersalivation with ipratropium bromide: a randomized, double-blind, placebo-controlled crossover study. *J Clin Psychiatry* 2009; 70:1114–1119.

58. Corrigan FM, et al. Clozapine-induced hypersalivation and the alpha 2 adrenoceptor. *Br J Psychiatry* 1995; 167:412.

59. Kreinin A, et al. Double-blind, randomized, placebo-controlled trial of metoclopramide for hypersalivation associated with clozapine. *J Clin Psychopharmacol* 2016; 36:200–205.

60. Hallahan B. Metoclopramide may be effective for clozapine-induced hypersalivation. *Evid Based Ment Health* 2016; 19:124.

61. Uzun Ö, et al. Effect of N-acetylcysteine on clozapine-induced sialorrhea in schizophrenic patients: a case series. *Int Clin Psychopharmacol* 2020; 35:229–231.

62. Leung JG, et al. Immediate-release oxybutynin for the treatment of clozapine-induced sialorrhea. *Ann Pharmacother* 2011; 45:e45.

63. Fritze J, et al. Pirenzepine for clozapine-induced hypersalivation. *Lancet* 1995; 346:1034.

64. Bai YM, et al. Therapeutic effect of pirenzepine for clozapine-induced hypersalivation: a randomized, double-blind, placebo-controlled, crossover study. *J Clin Psychopharmacol* 2001; 21:608–611.

65. Schneider B, et al. Reduction of clozapine-induced hypersalivation by pirenzepine is safe. *Pharmacopsychiatry* 2004; 37:43–45.

66. Kreinin A, et al. Sulpiride addition for the treatment of clozapine-induced hypersalivation: preliminary study. *Isr J Psychiatry Relat Sci* 2005; 42:61–63.

67. Wang J, et al. Sulpiride augmentation for schizophrenia. *Cochrane Database Syst Rev* 2010; CD008125.

氯氮平导致的胃肠动力不足（CIGH）

便秘是氯氮平治疗常见的不良反应，发生率超过 30%，是其他抗精神病药物的 3 倍[1]。其作用机制尚不清楚，但一般认为是药物的抗胆碱[2,3]和抗组胺[4]的联合作用，而氯氮平对 5-HT$_3$ 受体的拮抗作用使得这一发病机制变得更为复杂[2,3,5]。此外，氯氮平的镇静导致久坐的生活方式，它本身也是便秘的危险因素[4]。氯氮平是通过延长肠道通过时间而引发便秘的。80% 的氯氮平服药患者出现肠道通过时间增加，平均通过时间比正常人长 4 倍[6]。

氯氮平引发的便秘远较恶血质常见，且死亡率也较高[4]；便秘严重时，死亡率可达 20%~30%[4,7,8]。最新且规模最大的研究[9]发现，严重动力不足的发生率为 37/10 000，便秘相关死亡的发生率为 7/10 000，死亡率为 18%。显然，要减少由便秘引发的死亡，需要加强对胃肠动力不足的监测。

在使用氯氮平前，应先了解患者消化系统病史，做腹部检查；若患者已有便秘，则在便秘得到解决前，不应使用氯氮平[8]。胃动力不足随时可能发生，但在使用氯氮平的头 4 个月最为严重[8]。在检查全血细胞计数时，采用罗马 III 标准[10]，将有效预防因胃肠动力不足而引发的死亡，但是即使这样也不能保证识别（胃肠）动力不足[11]。

对于氯氮平剂量与便秘的关系，以及血药浓度与便秘的关系，尚无统一意见[8,12,13]。但是胃肠动力不足引发的死亡见于每天使用高剂量的患者（平均 535mg/d）[8,14]。患者死亡时，氯氮平治疗的中位持续时间为 2.5 年[9]。根据病例系列综述，年龄较大、男性、较高的日剂量被认为可能是死亡的危险因素（表 1.41）[14]。

表 1.41　氯氮平所致便秘的危险因素[8,15-18]

年龄增长
女性
抗胆碱能药
高剂量或高血药浓度氯氮平（考虑药物相互作用或戒烟的影响）
高钙血症
胃肠疾病
肥胖
多汗
低纤维饮食
不良的排便习惯
脱水（因多涎而加剧）
糖尿病
甲状腺功能减退
帕金森病
多发性硬化

CIGH 的预防和简单管理

　　缓慢增加氯氮平剂量能有效地减少发生便秘的风险,一般药量增加每天不超过 25mg 或每周不超过 100mg[19]。每天至少食用膳食纤维 20~25g,可增加粪便量,减少胃肠通过时间[18,20](基于初始通过时间,纤维可减少或增加通过时间[21])。如果增加了纤维摄入量,还必须保证摄入足够的液体(1.5~2L/d),以避免肠梗阻[8,18,22]。最好用每天饮食记录监测纤维和液体的摄入量,尤其是在增加氯氮平剂量的时期。此外,规律的锻炼(每周 150min)[23] 亦有助于预防 CIGH[24,25]。

　　主动监测是必不可少的,包括直接询问患者。即使是危及生命的便秘,患者通常也不会自行报告[8]。建议前 4 周每天记录大便情况,之后每周或每月记录。当排便习惯与以往不同时,或每周大便次数少于 3 次时[10],应予以腹部检查[8]。排除肠梗阻后,根据 Porirua 方案建议[26],应同时给予刺激性泻剂和软化性泻剂(如每晚 15mg 番泻叶和每天 3 次多库酯钠,每次 100mg)[8,26,27]。对于慢传输型便秘[2,28],容积性泻剂是无效的,应避免使用。除刺激性泻剂和软化性泻剂组合外,有证据表明乳果糖和聚乙二醇也是有效的[2,29],可考虑使用[26]。大多数 CIGH 患者需要使用刺激性泻剂,如番泻叶或比沙可啶。不应以"长期使用刺激性泻剂通常是被禁止的"为由拒绝使用这些药物。

　　泻药的选择依据还应该有患者既往对药物的反应情况及药物的起效速度[30]。例如,对于需要紧急治疗的患者,不能使用乳果糖,因其需规律服用长达 72h 才起效[31]。刺激性泻剂通常起效最快(6~10h)。泻药剂量应每 48h 增加 1 次,直至症状消失(番泻叶的最大剂量通常为 30mg,多库酯钠为 500mg)。也可以使用甘油栓剂(2×4g),通常在 30min 内起效,但是没有在 CIGH 中使用的数据。事实上,关于抗精神病药相关便秘的泻药选择,已发表的研究很少且质量较差[11]。

可疑急性 CIGH 的处理

　　必须立即就医的症状和体征包括腹痛、腹胀、呕吐、溢出性腹泻、肠鸣音消失、急腹症、恶臭呕吐物和脓毒症症状[7,8,19,32-39]。有从首发症状到死亡仅仅数小时的病例报告[40],所以应当及时评估与处理(包括停用氯氮平)。因此当保守治疗失败或便秘加重而紧急时,应尽早转诊至消化内科或急诊室[8,41]。

严重便秘后再次服用氯氮平

　　一些患者在患严重 CIGH 后成功地再次使用氯氮平,然而这并不是没有风险。因此,对于有 CIGH 既往史或 CIGH 高风险的患者,应采取预防措施。尽量少用导致便秘的药物,并确保先解决其他的危险因素(纤维、液体摄入和运动)。如果未曾正规、足量地试过常规泻药,则应该使用。然而,若这种方法以前失败过,可以使用一些更具实验性的方案。在使用这些治疗方法的任何一种之前,处方医师必须熟悉相关文献(至少需要阅读产品特征概要),并建议邀请胃肠专家参与。

　　英国批准前列腺素 E_1 类似物鲁比前列酮用于治疗成人慢性特发性便秘以及相关症状(因商业原因 2018 年停产),前提是饮食控制或其他非药物治疗(如教育和锻炼)不适合[42]。先前许可适应证的推荐剂量为 24μg、每天 2 次,最长 2 周[42]。据报道,在患严重的 CIGH 后再次服用氯氮平时,鲁比前列酮可有效地避免对其他泻药的需求[43],并在一些中心用于该适应证[43]。

奥利司他是一种减肥药物,众所周知,它具有通便作用,尤其是摄入高脂肪饮食时。据报道,它已成功用于 3 例阿片类药物导致的严重便秘(动力不足引起的便秘)[44]。一项关于奥利司他治疗氯氮平引起的便秘的小样本、随机、安慰剂对照研究发现,在研究终点(第 16 周),奥利司他组便秘、腹泻以及正常大便的发生率优于安慰剂组[45]。但是需要注意:54 例参与者中有 47 例需要传统泻药。还应注意的是,众所周知,奥利司他会减少一些药物的胃肠道吸收。因此,开始使用奥利司他时,需要监测氯氮平的血药浓度。除了临床研究,奥利司他可能特别难以使用,因为不能遵守严格的低脂饮食,胃肠不良反应可能令人感到不快(特别是直肠油性渗漏)。

氯贝胆碱是一种胆碱能激动剂,可以减少 CIGH 患者为保持排便规律所使用的泻药和灌肠剂的量[46]。在这种情况下,氯贝胆碱的使用剂量为 10mg,每天 3 次。只有在其他选择失败并向胃肠专家咨询后才能使用[46]。

普芦卡必利是一种 5-HT_4 受体激动剂,可增加肠道蠕动,批准用于治疗泻药无法足够缓解的慢性便秘。已有普芦卡必利成功用于氯氮平引起的便秘的病例报告[47,48],一项开放性研究表明普芦卡必利的疗效优于乳果糖[49]。

利那洛肽(在英国获得许可用于肠易激综合征的便秘)和普卡那肽(在美国可用于治疗慢性特发性便秘)是口服鸟苷酸环化酶 C 激动剂,迄今为止,没有任何已发表的数据支持它们用于抗精神病药物引起的便秘。

参考文献

1. Shirazi A, et al. Prevalence and predictors of clozapine-associated constipation: a systematic review and meta-analysis. *Int J Molecular Sci* 2016; 17:863.
2. Hibbard KR, et al. Fatalities associated with clozapine-related constipation and bowel obstruction: a literature review and two case reports. *Psychosomatics* 2009; 50:416–419.
3. Rege S, et al. Life-threatening constipation associated with clozapine. *Austr Psychiatry* 2008; 16:216–219.
4. De Hert M, et al. Second-generation antipsychotics and constipation: a review of the literature. *Eur Psychiatry* 2011; 26:34–44.
5. Meltzer HY, et al. Effects of antipsychotic drugs on serotonin receptors. *Pharmacol Rev* 1991; 43:587–604.
6. Every-Palmer S, et al. Clozapine-treated patients have marked gastrointestinal hypomotility, the probable basis of life-threatening gastrointestinal complications: a cross sectional study. *E Bio Med* 2016; 5:125–134.
7. Cohen D, et al. Beyond white blood cell monitoring: screening in the initial phase of clozapine therapy. *J Clin Psychiatry* 2012; 73:1307–1312.
8. Palmer SE, et al. Life-threatening clozapine-induced gastrointestinal hypomotility: an analysis of 102 cases. *J Clin Psychiatry* 2008; 69:759–768.
9. Every-Palmer S, et al. Clozapine-induced gastrointestinal hypomotility: a 22-year bi-national pharmacovigilance study of serious or fatal 'slow gut' reactions, and comparison with international drug safety advice. *CNS Drugs* 2017; 31:699–709.
10. Rome Foundation. Rome IV disorders and criteria. 2020; https://theromefoundation.org.
11. Every-Palmer S, et al. Pharmacological treatment for antipsychotic-related constipation. *Cochrane Database Syst Rev* 2017; 1:Cd011128.
12. Chengappa KN, et al. Anticholinergic differences among patients receiving standard clinical doses of olanzapine or clozapine. *J Clin Psychopharmacol* 2000; 20:311–316.
13. Vella-Brincat J, et al. Clozapine-induced gastrointestinal hypomotility. *Austr Psychiatry* 2011; 19:450–451.
14. West S, et al. Clozapine induced gastrointestinal hypomotility: a potentially life threatening adverse event. A review of the literature. *Gen Hosp Psychiatry* 2017; 46:32–37.
15. Nielsen J, et al. Termination of clozapine treatment due to medical reasons: when is it warranted and how can it be avoided? *J Clin Psychiatry* 2013; 74:603–613; quiz 613.
16. Nielsen J, et al. Risk factors for ileus in patients with schizophrenia. *Schizophr Bull* 2012; 38:592–598.
17. Longmore M, et al. *Oxford handbook of clinical medicine.* Oxford, UK: OUP Oxford; 2010.
18. ZTAS. Zaponex fact sheet – constipation. 2013; https://dokumen.tips/documents/zaponex-fact-sheet-constipation-ztascom-aj-van-beelen-phd-december-2013-m.html.

19. Hayes G, et al. Clozapine-induced constipation. *Am J Psychiatry* 1995; 152:298.

20. Muller-Lissner SA. Effect of wheat bran on weight of stool and gastrointestinal transit time: a meta analysis *Br Med J (Clin Res Ed)* 1988; 296:615–617.

21. Harvey RF, et al. Effects of increased dietary fibre on intestinal transit. *Lancet* 1973; 1:1278–1280.

22. National Prescribing Centre. The management of constipation. *MedRec Bulletin* 2011; 21:1–8.

23. NHS. Exercise: physical activity guidelines for adults aged 19 to 64. 2019; https://www.nhs.uk/live-well/exercise.

24. Fitzsimons J, et al. A review of clozapine safety. *Expert Opinion on Drug Safety* 2005; 4:731–744.

25. Young CR, et al. Management of the adverse effects of clozapine. *Schizophr Bull* 1998; 24:381–390.

26. Every-Palmer S, et al. The porirua protocol in the treatment of clozapine-induced gastrointestinal hypomotility and constipation: a pre- and post-treatment study. *CNS Drugs* 2017; 31:75–85.

27. Swegle JM, et al. Management of common opioid-induced adverse effects. *Am Fam Physician* 2006; 74:1347–1354.

28. Voderholzer WA, et al. Clinical response to dietary fiber treatment of chronic constipation. *Am J Gastroenterol* 1997; 92:95–98.

29. Brandt LJ, et al. Systematic review on the management of chronic constipation in North America. *Am J Gastroenterol* 2005; 100 Suppl 1:S5–S21.

30. Bleakley S, et al. *Clozapine handbook*. Warwickshire, UK: Lloyd-Reinhold Communications LLP; 2013.

31. Intrapharm Laboratories Limited. Summary of Product Characteristics. Lactulose 10 g/15 ml oral solution sachets. 2017; https://www.medicines.org.uk/emc/medicine/25597.

32. Leong QM, et al. Necrotising colitis related to clozapine? A rare but life threatening side effect. *World J Emerg Surg* 2007; 2:21.

33. Shammi CM, et al. Clozapine-induced necrotizing colitis. *J Clin Psychopharmacol* 1997; 17:230–232.

34. Rondla S, et al. A case of clozapine-induced paralytic ileus. *Emerg Med J* 2007; 24:e12.

35. Levin TT, et al. Death from clozapine-induced constipation: case report and literature review. *Psychosomatics* 2002; 43:71–73.

36. Townsend G, et al. Case report: rapidly fatal bowel ischaemia on clozapine treatment. *BMC Psychiatry* 2006; 6:43.

37. Karmacharya R, et al. Clozapine-induced eosinophilic colitis. *Am J Psychiatry* 2005; 162:1386–1387.

38. Erickson B, et al. Clozapine-associated postoperative ileus: case report and review of the literature. *Arch Gen Psychiatry* 1995; 52:508–509.

39. Schwartz BJ, et al. A case report of clozapine-induced gastric outlet obstruction. *Am J Psychiatry* 1993; 150:1563.

40. Drew L, et al. Clozapine and constipation: a serious issue. *Aust N Z J Psychiatry* 1997; 31:149.

41. Ikai S, et al. Reintroduction of clozapine after perforation of the large intestine–a case report and review of the literature. *Ann Pharmacother* 2013; 47:e31.

42. National Institute for Clinical Excellence. Final appraisal determination – lubiprostone for treating chronic idiopathic constipation. 2014; https://www.nice.org.uk/guidance/ta318/documents/constipation-chronic-idiopathic-lubiprostone-final-appraisal-determination-document2.

43. Meyer JM, et al. Lubiprostone for treatment-resistant constipation associated with clozapine use. *Acta Psychiatr Scand* 2014; 130:71–72.

44. Guarino AH. Treatment of intractable constipation with orlistat: a report of three cases *Pain Med* 2005; 6:327–328.

45. Chukhin E, et al. In a randomized placebo-controlled add-on study orlistat significantly reduced clozapine-induced constipation. *Int Clin Psychopharmacol* 2013; 28:67–70.

46. Poetter CE, et al. Treatment of clozapine-induced constipation with bethanechol. *J Clin Psychopharmacol* 2013; 33:713–714.

47. Thomas N, et al. Prucalopride in clozapine-induced constipation. *Aust N Z J Psychiatry* 2018; 52:804.

48. Hui H. Prucalopride for the treatment of clozapine induced constipation: a case report *JOJ Case Studies* 2018; 6:555683.

49. Damodaran I, et al. An open-label, head to head comparison study between prucalopride and lactulose for clozapine induced constipation in patients with treatment resistant schizophrenia. *Healthcare* 2020; 8:533.

氯氮平、中性粒细胞减少症和锂

氯氮平所致中性粒细胞减少症和粒细胞缺乏症的风险

氯氮平所致中性粒细胞减少症的发生率约为 2.7%,其中有 1/2 在治疗的前 18 周内发病,3/4 在治疗 1 年内发病[1]。危险因素包括加勒比黑种人、年轻和基线白细胞计数低[1]。中性粒细胞减少症的发生率与氯氮平剂量无关。大约 0.8% 会发生粒细胞缺乏症。氯氮平导致粒细胞减少或缺乏的机制尚不清楚,可能与免疫介导和细胞毒性作用都有关。此外,发病机制可能存在个体差异性,轻微和重度骨髓抑制的发病机制也可能不同[2]。因中性粒细胞减少症或粒细胞缺乏症而停用氯氮平的患者中,再次服用氯氮平时 1/3 将发生恶血质。若以前发生的是粒细胞缺乏症,则不可避免地会再次发生,且总是较第一次进展迅速、病情严重且持续时间更长[3]。当之前发生的是中性粒细胞减少症时,情况不一定如此[4]。

氯氮平导致中性粒细胞计数低的原因很多,因此容易混淆。单次出现的低计数可能只是偶发现象,不具有临床意义,所有药物都可能出现。多次出现(连续或间断性地),可能见于良性种族性中性粒细胞减少症(BEN,见下文),也可能是由于氯氮平引起的骨髓抑制作用(尤其是连续的进行性下降)。成熟的粒细胞缺乏症可能总是被解释为氯氮平引起的严重骨髓抑制。结果呈现模式很重要:在非 BEN 患者中,粒细胞缺乏症通常先表现为中性粒细胞计数正常,然后中性粒细胞数量急剧下降(通常不超过一周)[5,6],在较长一段时间内接近于零(假设未治疗)。

不遵循这种特征模式的中性粒细胞计数很难解释。冰岛的一项研究发现,氯氮平和其他抗精神病药物引发严重中性粒细胞减少症的风险没有差异,这表明在氯氮平治疗期间发生的中性粒细胞减少可能并非由氯氮平引起[7]。事实上,一项比较氯氮平和其他抗精神病药物引发中性粒细胞减少症风险的荟萃分析发现,与其他抗精神病药物相比,氯氮平与中性粒细胞减少症的相关性并不强[8]。

氯氮平治疗期间粒细胞缺乏症的发病率为 0.4%[9],比先前的认识要低,由此导致死亡的风险为 0.05%,属于罕见事件。超过 80% 的粒细胞缺乏症发生在治疗的前 18 周内[1]。荷兰氯氮平协作组[10]认为,粒细胞缺乏症的风险相当低,精神健全的患者可在治疗 6 个月后停止常规血液学监测。尽管如此,该协作组仍然建议进行低频率的监测,例如在停止常规监测后,仍需每年监测 4 次。

粒细胞缺乏症的危险因素包括年龄增长和亚洲种族[1]。有些患者可能具有遗传倾向[11]。虽然粒细胞缺乏症的发病时间与个体危险因素都不同于中性粒细胞减少症或巧合的中性粒细胞减少,但是在特定患者中,很难确定中性粒细胞减少症不是粒细胞缺乏症的前兆。

为减少血液疾病风险,必须进行血液学监测。然而,在世界范围内,关于监测频率和氯氮平停用阈值的建议存在明显的差异,可能反映了所依据的证据不足[12]。2015 年 10 月,美国食品药品管理局(FDA)对氯氮平监测系统进行了更改,仅强制要求监测绝对中性粒细胞计数,这一举措有效地降低了停用氯氮平的门槛[13]。FDA 建议在中性粒细胞低于 1 000/mm³ 时停用氯氮平(相比之下,英国建议在绝对中性粒细胞计数 <1 500/mm³ 时停用)。FDA 新的法规无疑将改善氯氮平在美国的使用,并可能在国际上产生影响。

有证据表明，氯氮平在世界范围内的使用严重不足，不同国家的处方频率差异很大[14]。这至少部分是由于严格的血液监测要求。2020 年全球爆发的 COVID-19 促使重新评估氯氮平血液学监测，一个团队提议：对于氯氮平治疗一年以上且无中性粒细胞减少病史的患者，监测频率应从每月 1 次减少到 3 个月 1 次[15]。考虑到粒细胞缺乏症在一周以内发生发展，每月进行监测的价值显然是值得怀疑的，特别是对于粒细胞缺乏症总体风险接近于零的患者。

良性种族性中性粒细胞减少症

良性种族性中性粒细胞减少症（BEN）是一种普遍公认的遗传性疾病，其患者中性粒细胞计数相对较低。非洲和中东血统的患病率更高。BEN 的特征是白细胞计数低，可能经常低于正常的下限。这种低白细胞计数模式可以在使用氯氮平之前、期间和之后观察到，并且很可能占观察到的或明显的氯氮平相关中性粒细胞减少症以及停止治疗的一部分。许多国家允许登记 BEN 的情况，为这些患者设定不同的中性粒细胞计数下限。在 BEN 背景下也可能发生真正的氯氮平所致中性粒细胞减少症，但是现有证据表明 BEN 不会增加氯氮平治疗期间发生恶病质的风险[16,17]。

同期使用的药物

氯氮平会合用与血液学不良反应有关的不同类别的药物。这些药物包括：其他抗精神病药、抗癫痫药（如丙戊酸钠和卡马西平）、抗菌剂、胃肠道药物（如质子泵抑制剂）。许多患者在服用氯氮平后会出现中性粒细胞减少症，但并非都与氯氮平有关，甚至并非病理性的。应考虑到上述药物可能的促成作用，如果要再次尝试使用氯氮平，应停用这些药物[18]。

需要管理的事项

在治疗开始前，评估基线血液学指标是很重要的。若怀疑患者患有 BEN，应转诊给血液科进行确认[19]。

鉴别氯氮平毒性反应和与氯氮平无关的中性粒细胞减少症似乎不太可能，但是一些因素很重要。建议联系血液学专家，咨询 BEN 相关问题，排除合用的其他可能导致中性粒细胞减少症的药物。明确诊断为氯氮平所致粒细胞减少症后，不建议使用医源性药物升高白细胞计数。只有在强烈怀疑粒细胞减少症与氯氮平无关时，才可使用锂盐或其他升白细胞药物。既往患过氯氮平所致粒细胞缺乏症的患者，应该禁止再用氯氮平。

锂盐

锂盐可以急性或慢性地升高中性粒细胞计数以及白细胞计数。对锂盐升白细胞的幅度还缺乏量化，但有报道称经锂盐治疗后，中性粒细胞计数均值为 $11.9 \times 10^9/L$，服用氯氮平的患者在加用锂盐后中性粒细胞平均升高 $2 \times 10^9/L$。尽管要求锂的最低血药浓度为 $0.4mmol/L$，但其升白细胞的作用与剂量并没有多大关系。其机制尚不完全明确[20]。

在服用氯氮平时发生中性粒细胞减少症的患者中，锂盐已被用于升高白细胞，从而使氯氮平治疗得以继续。无论是成年人[21-25]还是儿童[26,27]都曾有相关案例报道。几乎所有患者的锂浓度都大于 $0.6mmol/L$。在一个系列病例报告中，因恶血质而停服氯氮平的患者（$n=25$）

在服用锂的情况下再次服用氯氮平时,仅有一例患者再次出现恶血质[28]。若考虑给恶血质患者服用锂盐,应和提供相关监测服务的医学顾问讨论,以确定最佳用药方案。

锂盐似乎并不能预防真正的氯氮平所致粒细胞缺乏症:一例粒细胞缺乏症死亡者正是联合服用锂盐和氯氮平[25],另一例粒细胞缺乏症患者其骨髓对粒细胞集落刺激因子治疗没有反应[29]。

粒细胞集落刺激因子

对于既往有中性粒细胞减少症的患者,使用粒细胞集落刺激因子(G-CSF)以促进持续使用氯氮平治疗,是日益引人注意的策略,但同时也存在一些争议。为了氯氮平治疗而长期规律使用 G-CSF,既有成功的案例[30-32],也有失败的案例[32,33]。不顾中性粒细胞计数偏低或下降而使用 G-CSF,再加上其常见不良反应骨痛[34]和中性粒细胞发育不良[35],会掩盖即将发生的粒细胞减少症或缺乏症,导致严重后果。G-CSF 的长期安全性并未确定——也许应该监测骨密度和脾脏大小。

当中性粒细胞计数低于规定数值,且锂盐不足以防止白细胞计数"跌到"正常范围以下时, "按需要"给予 G-SCF,可以再次试用氯氮平(图 1.4)。同样,这也可能会掩盖严重的粒细胞减少症或缺乏症。在专科病房外,可能实际上也难以这么治疗,因为需要频繁的血液检查(每周 2~3 次),还要直接接触医学评估和 G-SCF。

在考虑使用 G-CSF 前,必须咨询血液学专家,并与提供氯氮平监测服务的医学顾问讨

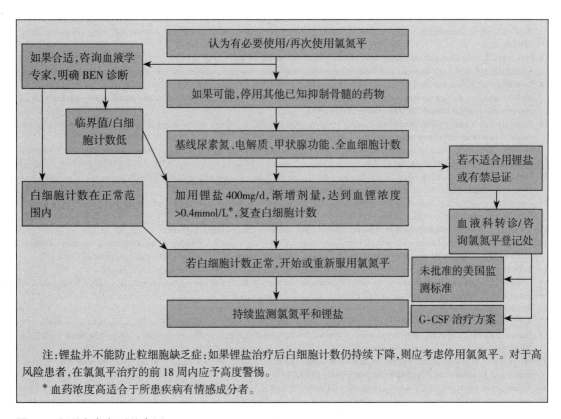

注:锂盐并不能防止粒细胞缺乏症;如果锂盐治疗后白细胞计数仍持续下降,则应考虑停用氯氮平。对于高风险患者,在氯氮平治疗的前 18 周内应予高度警惕。

* 血药浓度高适合于所患疾病有情感成分者。

图 1.4　锂盐与氯氮平的合用

论。应当考虑患者的临床情况。特别是,如果恶病质的第一次发作满足以下任一标准,则认为该患者再次使用氯氮平的风险非常高。这些标准都表明细胞计数低与氯氮平有关:

- 与以往的白细胞计数不一致(即不是重复低白细胞计数模式的一部分);
- 发生于治疗的前18周内;
- 病情严重,中性粒细胞计数 $<0.5 \times 10^9/L$;
- 持续时间长。

以前发生过氯氮平所致中性粒细胞减少症的一些患者,使用G-CSF已经帮助他们成功地再次使用氯氮平[36];但是现有证据表明,对于真正的氯氮平所致粒细胞缺乏症患者,G-CSF并没有这种作用[37]。

G-CSF可用于治疗下述患者:

- 开始时白细胞计数 $<4 \times 10^9/L$,或中性粒细胞计数 $<2.5 \times 10^9/L$;
- 白细胞减少症(白细胞计数 $<3 \times 10^9/L$)或中性粒细胞减少症(中性粒细胞计数 $<1.5 \times 10^9/L$)被认为与良性种族性中性粒细胞减少症有关。这类患者可能是非洲裔或中东裔,没有容易感染的病史,且白细胞形态正常[38];
- 氯氮平治疗时反复出现检测结果呈"琥珀色";
- 检测结果呈"红色"常表明可能与氯氮平无关。

参考文献

1. Munro J, et al. Active monitoring of 12760 clozapine recipients in the UK and Ireland. *Br J Psychiatry* 1999; 175:576–580.
2. Whiskey E, et al. Restarting clozapine after neutropenia: evaluating the possibilities and practicalities. *CNS Drugs* 2007; 21:25–35.
3. Dunk LR, et al. Rechallenge with clozapine following leucopenia or neutropenia during previous therapy. *Br J Psychiatry* 2006; 188:255–263.
4. Prokopez CR, et al. Clozapine rechallenge after neutropenia or leucopenia. *J Clin Psychopharmacol* 2016; 36:377–380.
5. Almaghrebi AH. Safety of a clozapine trial following quetiapine-induced leukopenia: a case report. *Curr Drug Saf* 2019; 14:80–83.
6. Patel NC, et al. Sudden late onset of clozapine-induced agranulocytosis. *Ann Pharmacother* 2002; 36:1012–1015.
7. Ingimarsson O, et al. Neutropenia and agranulocytosis during treatment of schizophrenia with clozapine versus other antipsychotics: an observational study in Iceland. *BMC Psychiatry* 2016; 16:441.
8. Myles N, et al. A meta-analysis of controlled studies comparing the association between clozapine and other antipsychotic medications and the development of neutropenia. *Aust N Z J Psychiatry* 2019; 53:403–412.
9. Li XH, et al. The prevalence of agranulocytosis and related death in clozapine-treated patients: a comprehensive meta-analysis of observational studies. *Psychol Med* 2020; 50:583–594.
10. Netherlands Clozapine Collaboration Group. Guideline for the use of Clozapine version 05-02-2013. 2013; https://www.clozapinepluswerk groep.nl/wp-content/uploads/2013/07/Guideline-for-the-use-of-Clozapine-2013.pdf.
11. Dettling M, et al. Further evidence of human leukocyte antigen-encoded susceptibility to clozapine-induced agranulocytosis independent of ancestry. *Pharmacogenetics* 2001; 11:135–141.
12. Nielsen J, et al. Worldwide differences in regulations of clozapine use. *CNS Drugs* 2016; 30:149–161.
13. FDA. FDA Drug Safety Communication: FDA modifies monitoring for neutropenia associated with schizophrenia medicine clozapine; approves new shared REMS program for all clozapine medicines. 2016; https://www.fda.gov/Drugs/DrugSafety/ucm461853.htm.
14. Bachmann CJ, et al. International trends in clozapine use: a study in 17 countries. *Acta Psychiatr Scand* 2017; 136:37–51.
15. Siskind D, et al. Consensus statement on the use of clozapine during the COVID-19 pandemic. *J Psychiatry Neurosci* 2020; 45:222–223.
16. Manu P, et al. Benign ethnic neutropenia and clozapine use: a systematic review of the evidence and treatment recommendations. *J Clin Psychiatry* 2016; 77:e909–916.
17. Richardson CM, et al. Evaluation of the safety of clozapine use in patients with benign neutropenia. *J Clin Psychiatry* 2016; 77:e1454–e1459.
18. Shuman MD, et al. Exploring the potential effect of polypharmacy on the hematologic profiles of clozapine patients. *J Psychiatr Pract* 2014; 20:50–58.
19. Whiskey E, et al. The importance of the recognition of benign ethnic neutropenia in black patients during treatment with clozapine: case reports and database study. *J Psychopharmacology* 2011; 25:842–845.
20. Paton C, et al. Managing clozapine-induced neutropenia with lithium. *Psychiatric Bull* 2005; 29:186–188.
21. Adityanjee A. Modification of clozapine-induced leukopenia and neutropenia with lithium carbonate. *Am J Psychiatry* 1995; 152:648–649.
22. Silverstone PH. Prevention of clozapine-induced neutropenia by pretreatment with lithium. *J Clin Psychopharmacol* 1998; 18:86–88.

23. Boshes RA, et al. Initiation of clozapine therapy in a patient with preexisting leukopenia: a discussion of the rationale of current treatment options. *Ann Clin Psychiatry* 2001; **13**:233–237.

24. Papetti F, et al. Treatment of clozapine-induced granulocytopenia with lithium (two observations). *Encephale* 2004; **30**:578–582.

25. Kutscher EC, et al. Clozapine-induced leukopenia successfully treated with lithium. *Am J Health Syst Pharm* 2007; **64**:2027–2031.

26. Sporn A, et al. Clozapine-induced neutropenia in children: management with lithium carbonate. *J Child Adolesc Psychopharmacol* 2003; **13**:401–404.

27. Mattai A, et al. Adjunctive use of lithium carbonate for the management of neutropenia in clozapine-treated children. *Human Psychopharmacology* 2009; **24**:584–589.

28. Kanaan RA, et al. Lithium and clozapine rechallenge: a restrospective case analysis. *J Clin Psychiatry* 2006; **67**:756–760.

29. Valevski A, et al. Clozapine-lithium combined treatment and agranulocytosis. *Int Clin Psychopharmacol* 1993; **8**:63–65.

30. Spencer BW, et al. Granulocyte colony stimulating factor (G-CSF) can allow treatment with clozapine in a patient with severe benign ethnic neutropaenia (BEN): a case report. *J Psychopharmacol* 2012; **26**:1280–1282.

31. Hagg S, et al. Long-term combination treatment with clozapine and filgrastim in patients with clozapine-induced agranulocytosis. *Int Clin Psychopharmacol* 2003; **18**:173–174.

32. Joffe G, et al. Add-on filgrastim during clozapine rechallenge in patients with a history of clozapine-related granulocytopenia/agranulocytosis. *Am J Psychiatry* 2009; **166**:236.

33. Mathewson KA, et al. Clozapine and granulocyte colony-stimulating factor: potential for long-term combination treatment for clozapine-induced neutropenia. *J Clin Psychopharmacol* 2007; **27**:714–715.

34. Puhalla S, et al. Hematopoietic growth factors: personalization of risks and benefits. *Mol Oncol* 2012; **6**:237–241.

35. Bain BJ, et al. Neutrophil dysplasia induced by granulocyte colony-stimulating factor. *Am J Hematol* 2010; **85**:354.

36. Myles N, et al. Use of granulocyte-colony stimulating factor to prevent recurrent clozapine-induced neutropenia on drug rechallenge: a systematic review of the literature and clinical recommendations. *Aust N Z J Psychiatry* 2017; 4867417720516.

37. Lally J, et al. The use of granulocyte colony-stimulating factor in clozapine rechallenge: a systematic review. *J Clin Psychopharmacol* 2017; **37**:600–604

38. Hsieh MM, et al. Prevalence of neutropenia in the U.S. population: age, sex, smoking status, and ethnic differences. *Ann Intern Med* 2007; **146**:486–492.

氯氮平与化疗

氯氮平禁止与引起中性粒细胞减少症的药物合用。大多数的化疗会引起明显骨髓抑制。白细胞计数低于 $3 \times 10^9/L$ 时,通常停用氯氮平,这是正式批件或药品说明书中指出的重要安全预防措施。无论是否使用氯氮平,预期许多化疗方案都会使白细胞计数低于该水平。

如果情况允许,在化疗前应停止使用氯氮平。然而,这很可能会使患者病情复发或恶化,从而影响患者做出同意化疗决定的能力。这使得已用氯氮平又需要化疗的患者陷入治疗的困境。许多患者,甚至可能是大多数,在化疗期间继续使用氯氮平。

有很多案例报告支持化疗期间继续使用氯氮平[1-18],但对这些文献的解释可能存在发表偏倚[2]。服用氯氮平的患者在开始化疗之前,有必要制订一个所有参与治疗的医护人员、患者、家属或照料者都同意的治疗计划,这包括肿瘤科医师/内科医师、精神科医师、药剂师以及氯氮平监测机构。当白细胞计数低于正常值下限时应该采取什么措施,应该事先做出计划。治疗计划应当包括血液监测的频率,提高对粒细胞减少症或缺乏症临床后果的警惕,是否及何时应停用氯氮平,以及使用锂盐和 G-SCF 等药物[19,20]以尝试维持正常的中性粒细胞计数。

在英国,氯氮平监测机构通常会要求精神科医师签署"未注册使用"文件,并要求更多的血液监测。并发症似乎罕见,但有一份关于阿霉素、放疗和氯氮平联合治疗后出现持续 6 个月的中性粒细胞减少症的案例报告[8]。G-SCF 已用于治疗与化疗和氯氮平联用相关的粒细胞缺乏症[9,10,21]。使用氯氮平超过一年的患者中,氯氮平所致中性粒细胞减少症极为罕见,患上致命性恶血质的风险可能最低。

小结

- 如果可能,在开始化疗前停止使用氯氮平。但对大多数患者来说停用是不可能的,也是不明智的。
- 在停止氯氮平前,必须考虑精神病复发或恶化的风险。
- 如果患者的精神状态恶化,他们可以撤销对化疗的知情同意。
- 当化疗期间继续使用氯氮平时,强烈建议肿瘤科医师、精神科医师、药剂师、患者和氯氮平监测机构共同协作。

参考文献

1. Wesson ML, et al. Continuing clozapine despite neutropenia. *Br J Psychiatry* 1996; **168**:217–220.
2. Cunningham NT, et al. Continuation of clozapine during chemotherapy: a case report and review of literature. *Psychosomatics* 2014; **55**:673–679.
3. Bareggi C, et al. Clozapine and full-dose concomitant chemoradiation therapy in a schizophrenic patient with nasopharyngeal cancer. *Tumori* 2002; **88**:59–60.
4. Avnon M, et al. Clozapine, cancer, and schizophrenia. *Am J Psychiatry* 1993; **150**:1562–1563.
5. Hundertmark J, et al. Reintroduction of clozapine after diagnosis of lymphoma. *Br J Psychiatry* 2001; **178**:576.
6. McKenna RC, et al. Clozapine and chemotherapy. *Hosp Community Psychiatry* 1994; **45**:831.
7. Haut FA. Clozapine and chemotherapy. *J Drug Devolop Clin Pract* 1995; **7**:237–239.
8. Rosenstock J. Clozapine therapy during cancer treatment. *Am J Psychiatry* 2004; **161**:175.
9. Lee SY, et al. Combined antitumor chemotherapy in a refractory schizophrenic receiving clozapine. *J Korean Neuropsychiatr Assoc* 2000; **39**:234–239.

10. Usta NG, et al. Clozapine treatment of refractory schizophrenia during essential chemotherapy: a case study and mini review of a clinical dilemma. *Ther Adv Psychopharmacol* 2014; **4**:276–281.

11. Rosenberg I, et al. Restarting clozapine treatment during ablation chemotherapy and stem cell transplant for Hodgkin's lymphoma. *Am J Psychiatry* 2007; **164**:1438–1439.

12. Goulet K, et al. Case report: clozapine given in the context of chemotherapy for lung cancer. *Psychooncology* 2008; **17**:512–516.

13. Frieri T, et al. Maintaining clozapine treatment during chemotherapy for non-Hodgkin's lymphoma. *Prog Neuropsychopharmacol Biol Psychiatry* 2008; **32**:1611–1612.

14. Sankaranarayanan A, et al. Clozapine, cancer chemotherapy and neutropenia – dilemmas in management. *PsychiatrDanub* 2013; **25**:419–422.

15. De Berardis D, et al. Safety and efficacy of combined clozapine-azathioprine treatment in a case of resistant schizophrenia associated with Behcet's disease: a 2-year follow-up. *GenHospPsychiatry* 2013; **35**:213–211.

16. Deodhar JK, et al. Clozapine and cancer treatment: adding to the experience and evidence. *Indian J Psychiatry* 2014; **56**:191–193.

17. Monga V, et al. Clozapine and concomitant chemotherapy in a patient with schizophrenia and new onset esophageal cancer. *Psychooncology* 2015; **24**:971–972.

18. Overbeeke MR, et al. Successful clozapine continuation during chemotherapy for the treatment of malignancy: a case report. *Int J Clin Pharm* 2016; **38**:199–202.

19. Whiskey E, et al. Restarting clozapine after neutropenia: evaluating the possibilities and practicalities. *CNS Drugs* 2007; **21**:25–35.

20. Silva E, et al. Clozapine rechallenge and initiation despite neutropenia- a practical, step-by-step guide. *BMC Psychiatry* 2020; **20**:279.

21. Kolli V, et al. Treating chemotherapy induced agranulocytosis with granulocyte colony-stimulating factors in a patient on clozapine. *Psychooncology* 2013; **22**:1674–1675.

第1章

基因检测与氯氮平治疗

　　大量研究试图检测氯氮平疗效和不良反应的遗传预测因子。总体而言,只发现了很小的效应,除非将遗传变异效应以数学方法进行结合,否则临床效用有限。敏感性(准确预测特定结果的可能性)通常很低,但特异性(排除该结果的可能性)通常非常高。这类数值可以与人口发病率数据相结合,以生成阳性预测值(PPV,预测会发生某结果的人群百分比)和阴性预测值(NPV,预测不会发生该结果的人群百分比)。

氯氮平治疗的疗效

　　三个基因变体已被证明确实可以预测氯氮平治疗结果[1]。

HTR2A rs6313c　　CC 基因携带者比 T 基因携带者治疗有效的可能性低
　　　　　　　　CC 146/272 有效,CT/TT 366/596 有效(54% vs 62%)

HTR2A rs6314　　等位基因 C 比 T 更有可能做出应答
　　　　　　　　应答率:C,685/1215;T,55/127(56% vs 43%)

HTR3A rs1062613　等位基因 T 比 C 疗效好
　　　　　　　　等位基因 C 有效 528/841,等位基因 T 有效 134/185(63% vs 72%)

粒细胞缺乏症

　　四种基因变体与粒细胞缺乏症风险的改变具有可信的相关性。某些变体仅在特定族群中发现。

HLA-DQB1　　　序列变异 6672 G > C (REC 21 G)使粒细胞缺乏症的风险比一般人群
　　　　　　　高 1 175%
　　　　　　　敏感度 21.5%,特异度 98.4%[2]
　　　　　　　PPV 5.1%,NPV 99.7%

HLA- DQB1　　5/7 研究认为等位基因 DQB1*0502 与粒细胞缺乏症相关(如 Dettling
　　　　　　　等[3],Yunis 等[4])。效应值可变

HLA-B*59:01　　有该等位基因高度预测粒细胞缺乏症,但在东亚人群中很少见,在白
　　　　　　　种人中几乎不存在
　　　　　　　敏感度 31.8%,特异度 95.3%[5]
　　　　　　　PPV 6.4%,NPV 99.3%

HLA DQB1/HLA-B　单个氨基酸变化 HLA DQB1 126Q 和 HLA-B158T 与粒细胞缺乏症风
　　　　　　　险增加有关。95 个病例中,39 个有一个或者两个等位基因;206 个
　　　　　　　对照中 175 个没有等位基因
　　　　　　　敏感度 41.0%,特异度 85.0%[6,7]。(另有数据为 36% 和 89%[8])
　　　　　　　PPV/NPV 没有给出,但是可以计算

HLA-DQB1 变体和 HLA-B 变体连锁不平衡（LD）[8]，并且可能传达相同的关联信号。LD 中的变体是共同遗传的。

良性种族性中性粒细胞减少症

ACKR1 rs2814778　rs2814778 的 CC 基因型（Duffy Null Status）被认为是导致 BEN 的原因[9]

代谢

氯氮平主要由 CYP1A2 代谢，少部分由 CYP3A4/5 代谢，CYP2D6 几乎没有作用。代谢率通常分为低（PM）、中（IM）或高（EM）三种，每种都与特定的基因变异有关。因此，基因分析可以估计特定个体的氯氮平目标剂量。

细胞色素 p4501A2　PM/IM/EM 状态通常由对 CYP1A2*1 F/1 C/1A/1K 的分析定义[10]

细胞色素 p4503A4　PM/IM/EM 状态

CYP3A4 是氯氮平代谢的次要途径，但代谢状态会影响血药浓度[11]

细胞色素 p4503A5　PM/IM/EM 状态

CYP3A5 PM 状态与氯氮平血药浓度升高相关[12]

其他非 CYP 基因的关联也已得到证实。

NFIB rs28379954 *T > C*　无论是否吸烟，CT 携带者的血药浓度均远低于 TT 携带者[13]

rs2472297 基因型也可以独立预测氯氮平血药浓度[14]。氯氮平血药浓度在 C/C 携带者中最高，在 T/T 携带者中最低（C/T 介于两者之间）。这种单核苷酸多态性位于 15 号染色体上的 CYP1A1 和 CYP1A2 编码基因之间。

其他不良反应

还发现了心肌炎[15]和体重增加[16]的遗传预测因子，但相关性太弱，可能无法临床应用[10]。

（岳伟华　吴仁容　译　田成华　审校）

参考文献

1. Gressier F, et al. Pharmacogenetics of clozapine response and induced weight gain: a comprehensive review and meta-analysis. *Eur Neuropsychopharmacol* 2016; 26:163–185.
2. Athanasiou MC, et al. Candidate gene analysis identifies a polymorphism in HLA-DQB1 associated with clozapine-induced agranulocytosis. *J Clin Psychiatry* 2011; 72:458–463.
3. Dettling M, et al. Genetic determinants of clozapine-induced agranulocytosis: recent results of HLA subtyping in a non-jewish caucasian sample. *Arch Gen Psychiatry* 2001; 58:93–94.
4. Yunis JJ, et al. HLA associations in clozapine-induced agranulocytosis. *Blood* 1995; 86:1177–1183.
5. Saito T, et al. Pharmacogenomic study of clozapine-induced agranulocytosis/granulocytopenia in a Japanese population. *Biol Psychiatry* 2016; 80:636–642.
6. Girardin FR, et al. Cost-effectiveness of HLA-DQB1/HLA-B pharmacogenetic-guided treatment and blood monitoring in US patients taking clozapine. *Pharmacogenomics J* 2019; 19:211–218.
7. Goldstein JI, et al. Clozapine-induced agranulocytosis is associated with rare HLA-DQB1 and HLA-B alleles. *Nat Commun* 2014; 5:4757.
8. Legge SE, et al. Genetics of clozapine-associated neutropenia: recent advances, challenges and future perspective. *Pharmacogenomics* 2019; 20:279–290.
9. Charles BA, et al. Analyses of genome wide association data, cytokines, and gene expression in African-Americans with benign ethnic neutro-

penia. *PLoS One* 2018; **13**:e0194400.

10. Thorn CF, et al. PharmGKB summary: clozapine pathway, pharmacokinetics. *Pharmacogenet Genomics* 2018; **28**:214–222.

11. Tóth K, et al. Potential role of patients' CYP3A-status in clozapine pharmacokinetics. *Int J Neuropsychopharmacol* 2017; **20**:529–537.

12. John AP, et al. Unusually high serum levels of clozapine associated with genetic polymorphism of CYP3A enzymes. *Asian J Psychiatr* 2020; **57**:102126.

13. Smith RL, et al. Identification of a novel polymorphism associated with reduced clozapine concentration in schizophrenia patients-a genome-wide association study adjusting for smoking habits. *Trans Psychiatry* 2020; **10**:198.

14. Pardiñas AF, et al. Pharmacogenomic variants and drug interactions identified through the genetic analysis of clozapine metabolism. *Am J Psychiatry* 2019; **176**:477–486.

15. Lacaze P, et al. Genetic associations with clozapine-induced myocarditis in patients with schizophrenia. *Translational Psychiatry* 2020; **10**:37.

16. Li N, et al. Progress in genetic polymorphisms related to lipid disturbances induced by atypical antipsychotic drugs. *Front Pharmacol* 2020; **10**:1669.

锂盐

作用机制

锂是元素周期表中的第三种元素,与氢和钠属于 ·族。锂盐在人体内广泛参与各种生物活动,有着多种多样的其他生物学效应,使得了解锂在调节情绪和行为中的关键机制极其困难。例如,一些证据表明双相障碍患者较健康人群细胞内钠和钙的浓度升高,而锂则可以降低它们的浓度。基因研究证实双相障碍涉及钙相关基因[1]。糖原合成酶激酶-3(GSK-3)、cAMP 效应元件结合蛋白和 Na^+/K^+ATP 酶相关机制可能在锂的效应中发挥重要的作用。对锂潜在作用机制的回顾,参见 Alda 2015[2]。锂或许可通过保护神经元功能和神经环路[3]而具有神经保护作用。锂还促进海马中新生神经元的产生(神经发生),这对学习、记忆和应激反应[4]具有潜在意义。虽然针对锂对神经可能有保护作用的文献大多基于体外实验或者动物实验,但是一个荟萃分析提示锂可以预防痴呆[5]。然而,值得注意的是,锂的神经毒性,不论是否可逆,均被视为不良反应[6,7]。锂在环境中的含量较低(例如在饮用水中),有报道在群体水平,环境中的锂含量与自杀和痴呆呈负相关[8,9]。

临床适应证

躁狂急性期治疗

锂盐能有效地治疗躁狂发作,其血浆治疗浓度为 0.8~1.0mmol/L。如果需要快速缓解症状,建议使用具有循证基础的一种抗精神病药辅助或单药治疗躁狂发作[10]。快速达到血浆治疗浓度比较困难,并且如果患者不配合,监测也会困难重重。对于不伴有精神病性症状的躁狂发作,或者没有快速循环型证据的患者,锂盐可能有最佳治疗效果[11]。

长期服用锂盐患者急性躁狂发作的治疗

BAP 指南[10]建议在复发的情况下,应迅速检测血锂水平,以了解患者对锂盐治疗的依从性,并可能据此调整剂量。如果血锂水平表明患者对治疗不依从,应查明原因。如果血锂水平正常,但躁狂症状控制不充分,则推荐加用多巴胺受体拮抗剂、多巴胺受体部分受体激动剂或丙戊酸盐[10]。

双相抑郁

锂盐广泛用于双相抑郁,但关于其确切疗效的证据不足 [12,13]。更多证据表明锂盐能预防抑郁发作。

双相障碍的维持治疗

目标是在血锂 0.6~0.8mmol/L [10,14] 达到最高可耐受水平;若反应良好但耐受差,可将其降低至 0.40~0.60mmol/L;若耐受较好但反应差,可将其增加至 0.80~1.00mmol/L。治疗的目的是完全缓解躁狂和抑郁发作 [15]。在临床应用中,锂盐可能是治疗 BD 的最佳药物:Hayes 等 [16] 前瞻性分析了 5 089 例双相障碍患者单药维持治疗的情况:锂(n=1 505),奥氮平(n=1 366),丙戊酸盐(n=1 173)和喹硫平(n=1 075)。发现各个队列中单药治疗失败率达到 75% 的时间为:锂盐单药治疗 2.05 年,奥氮平单药治疗 1.13 年,丙戊酸盐单药治疗 0.98 年,喹硫平单药治疗 0.76 年 [16]。

在单相抑郁中增效抗抑郁药

30%~50% 的患者对一线或二线抗抑郁药无效,而"难治性抑郁症"的结局往往很差 [17]。抗抑郁药治疗抑郁症的循证医学指南,例如 Cleare 等 [18] 建议,作为原有抗抑郁药增效剂,锂盐或喹硫平是最佳选择。锂盐作为选择性 5- 羟色胺再摄取抑制剂(SSRI)或文拉法辛的增效剂,在血锂水平为 0.6~1.0mmol/L 时最有效。为了帮助确定这两种增效剂中哪一种效果更好,正在进行一项比较难治性抑郁中锂盐和喹硫平增效作用的头对头、平行、开放、多中心、随访期为 1 年的随机试验,结果应在 2021 年报告 [19]。对于难治性抑郁,以锂盐作为增效剂时,预示疗效较好的因素包括抑郁症状更重、精神运动迟滞、体重明显减轻、抑郁症家族史和抑郁复发 3 次以上 [20]。当然,对于锂盐使用的依从性也要归入其中。

单相抑郁的预防

在近期的一篇综述中阐述了使用锂对单相抑郁长期治疗的效果 [21]。Cipriani 等(2006)[22] 分析了 8 项随机对照试验(RCT)(n=475),发现锂盐在预防需要住院的复发方面明显优于抗抑郁药,相对危险度为 0.34。Abou-Saleh 等(2017)[23] 建议,如果单相抑郁患者 5 年内有两次复发,或单次重度发作并且存在很强的自杀风险,可以预防性使用锂盐;如果依从性较好,没有不良反应,尤其是怀疑有双相背景时,可长期采用锂盐治疗。

锂盐的其他用途

锂盐还用于治疗攻击和自残行为,近期有研究证实锂有益于 [24] 预防和治疗类固醇所致精神病 [25],升高服用氯氮平者的白细胞计数 [26]。

锂盐和自杀

据估计,15% 的双相障碍患者最终会自杀身亡 [27]。一项临床试验的荟萃分析指出,锂盐能使双相障碍患者自杀未遂和自杀成功的风险降低 80% [28];大型数据库研究显示,与其他心境稳定剂治疗的患者相比,使用锂盐治疗的患者很少自杀成功 [29]。

锂盐也可以防止单相抑郁患者自杀,但是这种保护作用的机制不明[28]。如前文所述,在群体水平,环境中的锂含量与自杀成负相关[8]。

血浆水平

预防性使用锂盐时,其血浆最低有效浓度为 0.4mmol/L,最佳有效浓度范围为 0.6~0.8mmol/L[30]。当血浆水平高于 0.75mmol/L 时,仅增加对躁狂症状的预防作用[31],因此有效预防的目标范围是 0.6~0.8mmol/L[14]。血浆水平的变化似乎会加重复发风险[31]。对于单相抑郁,最佳血浆浓度范围尚不清楚,这方面还有很多研究要做[21]。

与成年人相比,儿童和青少年可能需要更高的血浆药物浓度,以确保中枢神经系统有足够的锂浓度[32]。

锂盐可以被胃肠道迅速吸收,但是分布比较长。若每晚睡前服用一次缓释片,采血测定血锂浓度的时间应该在服药后 10~14h(理想时间为 12h)[10]。

制剂

在英国使用最广泛的两种锂盐商品名为 Priadel 和 Camcolit,它们在药代动力学上的差异没有临床意义。Priadel 的英国制造商试图撤回该产品,目前正在审核中[33]。其他制剂不能被视为具有生物等效性,应该用商品名来开处方。

- 400mg 碳酸锂片剂每片含 10.8mmol 锂。
- 柠檬酸锂液体有两个规格,应该每天给药两次。
  - 5.4mmol/5mL 的液体和 200mg 的碳酸锂等效。
  - 10.8mmol/5mL 的液体和 400mg 的碳酸锂等效。

处方时若不明确拟用哪种规格的液体制剂,可能导致患者所用剂量达不到治疗效果,或者出现中毒。

不良反应

锂盐的大多数不良反应与剂量和血浆浓度相关,包括轻度胃肠道不适、细微震颤、多尿和多饮。每天两次给药时,多尿发生更加频繁[34,35]。普萘洛尔对锂导致的震颤有效。一些皮肤疾病(如银屑病和痤疮)可因锂治疗而加重。锂也可能导致口腔出现金属味、脚踝水肿和体重增加。

锂盐也会导致尿浓缩功能下降——肾源性尿崩症,从而出现口渴和多尿。这种不良反应在中、短期治疗中常常是可逆的,但是在长时间治疗之后或许变成不可逆的(>15 年)[36]。锂盐治疗也会导致肾小球滤过率(GFR)下降,但风险大小尚不确定[36]。当锂浓度 >0.8mmol/L 时,会有肾毒性的较高风险,因此长期锂盐治疗需要定期监测肾功能[37]。

在长期治疗中,锂盐增加了甲状腺功能减退的风险[38];在中年女性中,其风险最高可至20%[39]。在服用锂盐之前(为更好地评估风险)检测甲状腺自身抗体,并且在治疗的第一年更加频繁地监测甲状腺功能(TFT),已经成为临床选择[40]。甲状腺功能减退使用甲状腺素很容易治疗。停用锂盐后,甲状腺功能往往能恢复正常。在罕见情况下,锂盐也会增加甲状腺功能亢进和甲状旁腺功能亢进的风险,有人建议在长期治疗过程中需要监测血钙水平[41,42]。长期血钙水平升高导致的临床后果包括肾结石、骨质疏松、消化不良、高血压和肾损伤。关于锂盐中毒特点的综述,参见 McKnight 等[41]。

锂中毒

一般在锂浓度 >1.5mmol/L 时发生中毒,通常包括胃肠道反应(增加厌食、恶心、腹泻)和中枢神经系统症状(肌无力、嗜睡、意识模糊、共济失调、粗大震颤和肌肉抽搐)[43]。当血锂浓度 >2mmol/L 时,常常发生定向障碍和癫痫发作,可能会进展为昏迷,最终导致死亡。当存在较严重的症状时,要使用渗透性或者强碱性利尿剂(注意不能使用噻嗪类或袢利尿剂)。锂浓度 >3mmol/L 时,需要使用腹膜透析或者血液透析。以上血浆水平仅是指导性的,患者对中毒症状的易感性因人而异。正常血锂浓度下的神经毒性也被描述过,因为血浆锂浓度不能反映脑中锂浓度[44,45]。

中毒的大多数危险因素涉及血钠水平的改变或者人体处理钠的方式。例如低盐饮食、脱水、药物相互作用(见总表)和一些不常见的躯体疾病(如 Addison 病)。

开始使用锂盐治疗时,须告知患者与中毒症状有关的信息和相关的危险因素[46]。这些信息应该每隔一定时期重复告知,以便患者清楚了解。

治疗前检查

在使用锂盐之前,应检查肾功能、甲状腺功能和心脏功能。至少,应该检查估计的肾小球滤过率(eGFR)[47]和甲状腺功能(TFT)。有心血管病风险或者已患心血管病的患者,也建议查心电图。还需要测量基线体重。

锂是一种公认的人类致畸原。应该建议育龄女性使用可靠的避孕方式。见第 7 章。

治疗监测[10]

BAP 指南建议,在处方使用锂盐之前,应检查基线 eGFR、甲状腺功能和血钙。每 6 个月监测一次血锂、eGFR 和 TFT。联用有相互作用的药物、老年或患有慢性肾脏疾病的患者,应更加频繁地监测上述指标。英国患者安全局(NPSA)[48]发布了一项与处方锂盐患者生化监测重要性相关的患者安全性警告。同时也应该监测体重(或体重指数)。已知目前在英国临床实践中,锂盐监测执行欠佳[49],尽管一直以来有一些改善[50]。应用自动提醒系统证明可以提高监测率[51]。锂盐的使用和监测,见表 2.1。

停药

间断性应用锂盐治疗可能会恶化双相障碍患者的自然病程。骤然停用锂盐后的头几个月[52],躁狂复发率也远超预期,即使症状消失长达 5 年的患者也如此[53]。因此,建议如果没有明确的意向持续治疗至少 3 年,最好不要开始锂盐治疗[54]。在急性发病期,违背患者意愿(或者患者明确缺乏药物依从性)开始锂盐治疗时,这个建议具有重要的意义。

用至少 1 个月时间逐步减少锂盐剂量[55],同时避免血浆药物浓度下降超过 0.2mmol/L[31],可以降低复发的风险。与这些建议相反,近期一项自然观察研究发现,那些缓解期达到 2 年以上且缓慢停用锂盐的患者,其复发率比继续用药者至少高 3 倍;复发率的这种明显差异会持续多年。停药前维持高锂浓度的患者尤其容易复发[56]。

美国一项基于处方记录的大型研究发现,1/2 的患者几乎按照处方剂量服用锂盐,1/4

的患者服用处方剂量的 50%~80%,另有 1/4 服用不足 50%。此外,1/3 的患者服用锂盐的总时间少于 6 个月 [57]。一项大型审计发现,在长期服用锂盐的患者中,有 1/10 血浆浓度低于治疗浓度 [58]。显然,在临床实践中依从性不佳限制了锂的作用效果。一项数据库研究显示,服用锂盐直接与自杀风险相关(锂处方越多 = 自杀率更低)[59]。

较少数据支持双相障碍患者停用锂盐后会出现抑郁症状 [52]。几乎没有与单相抑郁患者有关的数据。

表 2.1 锂盐:使用和监测

适应证	躁狂,轻躁狂,预防双相障碍和复发抑郁,减少攻击和自杀行为
用药前检查	估计的肾小球滤过率和甲状腺功能。有心血管病风险或者已患心血管病的患者建议做心电图检查。需要测量基线体重
处方	起初晚上服用 400mg(老年人 200mg)。7 天后监测血浆水平,每次剂量调整 7 天后监测一次,直至达到理想浓度(0.4mmol/L 对单相抑郁有效,0.6~1.0mmol/L 对双相障碍有效,略高浓度治疗难治性躁狂)。最后一次给药 12h 后采集血样。当给予液体制剂时,要清楚说明需用哪种规格
监测	每 6 个月监测血浆锂浓度(联用有相互作用的药物、老年、患有肾损伤或其他相关疾病的患者,需要更加频繁地监测)。估计的肾小球滤过率和甲状腺功能每 6 个月监测一次。体重(或者 BMI)也要监测
停药	缓慢减药至少 1 个月,最好 3 个月。避免血浆水平降低幅度大于 0.2mmol/L

药物相互作用 [60-62]

由于锂盐治疗指数相对较窄,因而与其他药物的药代动力学相互作用可能促进锂中毒。大多数具有临床意义的相互作用是与改变肾脏钠处理的药物发生的。

血管紧张素转换酶抑制剂

血管紧张素转换酶抑制剂(ACEI)可以减轻口渴从而导致轻微脱水;增加肾钠损失,导致肾脏对钠的重吸收增加,从而导致血锂浓度升高。此类影响程度不一,从无影响到锂浓度升高 4 倍。可在数周出现全部作用。心功能不全、脱水和肾功能不全者可能会增加锂中毒风险(可能是因为体液平衡/处理失调)。在老年人,使用 ACEI 类药物导致锂中毒而住院的风险增加 7 倍。ACEI 类药物同样可以促进肾衰竭,因此合并应用锂盐时,应当增加 eGFR 和血锂的监测频率。

以下药物为 ACEI 类药物:卡托普利、昔拉普利、依那普利、福辛普利、咪达普利、赖诺普利、莫西普利、哌林多普利、奎那普利、雷米普利、群多普利。

还需谨慎合用**血管紧张素 II 受体拮抗剂**:坎替沙坦、伊普沙坦、厄贝沙坦、氯沙坦、奥美沙坦、替米沙坦、缬沙坦。

利尿剂

利尿剂可以降低肾脏对锂盐的清除,噻嗪类利尿剂作用比袢利尿剂更明显。应用**噻嗪**

类利尿剂后,血锂浓度常在 10 天内升高,升高幅度不一,25%~400%。

以下药物为噻嗪类(或相关)利尿剂:苄氟噻嗪、氯噻酮、环戊噻嗪、吲达帕胺、美托拉宗、希帕胺。

尽管有病例报告合用袢利尿剂可以引起锂中毒,但很多患者合用袢利尿剂并未出现明显问题。在袢利尿剂使用后第一个月内,药物相互作用的风险最高,因此如果合用这些药物,建议在此期间增加监测血锂浓度。袢利尿剂可以促进钠的流失,进而增加肾脏对钠的重吸收。应用袢利尿剂患者,建议控制钠的摄入;这可能会增加这些患者锂中毒的风险。

以下药物为袢利尿剂:布美他尼、呋喃苯胺酸(呋塞米)和拖拉塞米。

非甾体抗炎药

非甾体抗炎药(NSAID)抑制肾前列腺素的合成,从而减少肾血流量,并可能增加肾脏对钠的重吸收,进而增加锂的重吸收。对于不同患者,上升幅度不一致,无法预测;病例报告的上升幅度为 10%~400%。产生影响的起始时间从几天至几个月。肾功能受损、肾动脉狭窄、心力衰竭、脱水、低盐饮食等因素可能会增加风险。有许多案例报告锂与环氧化酶-2(COX-2)抑制剂之间的相互作用。NSAID 似乎没有像之前报道过那样减弱锂的治疗效果 [63]。

NSAID(或 COX-2 抑制剂)可与锂盐合用,但需要:①定期使用而**不是必要时用**;②必须增加血锂浓度监测频率。

有些 NSAID 无需处方即可购买,因此让患者知道药物之间的潜在相互作用尤为重要(表 2.2)。

以下药物为 NSAID 或 COX-2 抑制剂:醋氯芬酸、阿西美辛、塞来昔布、地昔布洛芬、右酮洛芬、双氯芬酸、二氟尼柳、依托度酸、依托昔布、芬布芬、非诺洛芬、氟比洛芬、布洛芬、吲哚美辛、酮洛芬、罗美昔布、甲芬那酸、美洛昔康、萘丁美酮、萘普生、吡罗昔康、舒林酸、替诺昔康、噻洛芬酸。

卡马西平

卡马西平合并锂盐有神经毒性的报告罕见。大多数报告时代比较久远且包含了高血锂浓度的治疗。但是,需要注意的是,卡马西平能够导致低钠血症,进而引起锂在体内滞留而中毒。类似地,另外一组可导致低钠血症的药物——选择性 5-羟色胺再摄取抑制剂(SSRI),也有导致中枢神经系统中毒的罕见报告。

表 2.2　锂盐:具有临床意义的药物相互作用

药物种类	作用大小	作用时间窗	备注
ACEI 类	■ 不可预知 ■ 血锂浓度升高达 4 倍	数周	■ 老年人因锂中毒住院的风险增加 7 倍 ■ **血管紧张素 II 受体拮抗剂可能有相似风险**
噻嗪类利尿剂	■ 不可预知 ■ 血锂浓度升高达 4 倍	通常前 10 天影响明显	■ 袢利尿剂较安全 ■ 第一个月内影响明显
NSAID	■ 不可预知 ■ 血锂浓度升高,从 10% 至超过 4 倍	不确定;几天至几个月	■ NSAID 必要时使用很普遍 ■ 不用处方即可买到

参考文献

1. Bray NJ, et al. The genetics of neuropsychiatric disorders. *Brain Neurosci Adv* 2019; 2:2398212818799271.

2. Alda M. Lithium in the treatment of bipolar disorder: pharmacology and pharmacogenetics. *Mol Psychiatry* 2015; 20:661–670.

3. Jope RS, et al. Lithium to the rescue. 2016; http://dana.org/Cerebrum/2016/Lithium_to_the_Rescue.

4. Hanson ND, et al. Lithium, but not fluoxetine or the corticotropin-releasing factor receptor 1 receptor antagonist R121919, increases cell proliferation in the adult dentate gyrus. *J Pharmacol Exp Ther* 2011; 337:180–186.

5. Matsunaga S, et al. Lithium as a treatment for Alzheimer's disease: a systematic review and meta-analysis. *J Alzheimer's Dis* 2015; 48:403–410.

6. Netto I, et al. Reversible lithium neurotoxicity: review of the literature. *Prim Care Companion CNS Disord* 2012; 14. PCC.11r01197.

7. Adityanjee, et al. The syndrome of irreversible lithium-effectuated neurotoxicity. *Clin Neuropharmacol* 2005; 28:38–49.

8. Memon A, et al. Association between naturally occurring lithium in drinking water and suicide rates: systematic review and meta-analysis of ecological studies. *Br J Psychiatry* 2020; 1–12. 217:667-678.

9. Kessing LV, et al. Association of lithium in drinking water with the incidence of dementia. *JAMA Psychiatry* 2017; 74:1005–1010.

10. Goodwin GM, et al. Evidence-based guidelines for treating bipolar disorder: revised third edition recommendations from the British Association for Psychopharmacology. *J Psychopharmacol* 2016; 30:495–553.

11. Hui TP, et al. A systematic review and meta-analysis of clinical predictors of lithium response in bipolar disorder. *Acta Psychiatr Scand* 2019; 140:94–115.

12. Bahji A, et al. Comparative efficacy and tolerability of pharmacological treatments for the treatment of acute bipolar depression: a systematic review and network meta-analysis. *J Affect Disord* 2020; 269:154–184.

13. Taylor DM, et al. Comparative efficacy and acceptability of drug treatments for bipolar depression: a multiple-treatments meta-analysis. *Acta Psychiatr Scand* 2014; 130:452–469.

14. Nolen WA, et al. What is the optimal serum level for lithium in the maintenance treatment of bipolar disorder? A systematic review and recommendations from the ISBD/IGSLI Task Force on treatment with lithium. *Bipolar Disord* 2019; 21:394–409.

15. Severus E, et al. Lithium for prevention of mood episodes in bipolar disorders: systematic review and meta-analysis. *Int J Bipolar Disord* 2014; 2:15.

16. Hayes JF, et al. Lithium vs. valproate vs. olanzapine vs. quetiapine as maintenance monotherapy for bipolar disorder: a population-based UK cohort study using electronic health records. *World Psychiatry* 2016; 15:53–58.

17. Dunner DL, et al. Prospective, long-term, multicenter study of the naturalistic outcomes of patients with treatment-resistant depression. *J Clin Psychiatry* 2006; 67:688–695.

18. Cleare A, et al. Evidence-based guidelines for treating depressive disorders with antidepressants: A revision of the 2008 British Association for Psychopharmacology guidelines. *J Psychopharmacol* 2015; 29:459–525.

19. Marwood L, et al. Study protocol for a randomised pragmatic trial comparing the clinical and cost effectiveness of lithium and quetiapine augmentation in treatment resistant depression (the LQD study). *BMC Psychiatry* 2017; 17:231.

20. Bauer M, et al. Role of lithium augmentation in the management of major depressive disorder. *CNS Drugs* 2014; 28:331–342.

21. Young AH. Lithium for long-term treatment of unipolar depression. *Lancet Psychiatry* 2017; 4:511–512.

22. Cipriani A, et al. Lithium versus antidepressants in the long-term treatment of unipolar affective disorder. *Cochrane Database Syst Rev* 2006; CD003492.

23. Abou-Saleh MT, et al. Lithium in the episode and suicide prophylaxis and in augmenting strategies in patients with unipolar depression. *Int J Bipolar Disord* 2017; 5:11.

24. Correll CU, et al. Biological treatment of acute agitation or aggression with schizophrenia or bipolar disorder in the inpatient setting. *Ann Clin Psychiatry* 2017; 29:92–107.

25. Sirois F. Steroid psychosis: a review. *Gen Hosp Psychiatry* 2003; 25:27–33.

26. Aydin M, et al. Continuing clozapine treatment with lithium in schizophrenic patients with neutropenia or leukopenia: brief review of literature with case reports. *Ther Adv Psychopharmacol* 2016; 6:33–38.

27. Harris EC, et al. Excess mortality of mental disorder. *Br J Psychiatry* 1998; 173:11–53.

28. Cipriani A, et al. Lithium in the prevention of suicide in mood disorders: updated systematic review and meta-analysis. *BMJ* 2013; 346:f3646.

29. Hayes JF, et al. Self-harm, unintentional injury, and suicide in bipolar disorder during maintenance mood stabilizer treatment: a UK population-based electronic health records study. *JAMA Psychiatry* 2016; 73:630–637.

30. Nolen WA, et al. The association of the effect of lithium in the maintenance treatment of bipolar disorder with lithium plasma levels: a post hoc analysis of a double-blind study comparing switching to lithium or placebo in patients who responded to quetiapine (Trial 144). *Bipolar Disord* 2013; 15:100–109.

31. Severus WE, et al. What is the optimal serum lithium level in the long-term treatment of bipolar disorder–a review? *Bipolar Disord* 2008; 10:231–237.

32. Moore CM, et al. Brain-to-serum lithium ratio and age: an in vivo magnetic resonance spectroscopy study. *Am J Psychiatry* 2002; 159:1240–1242.

33. Gov.UK Guidance. CMA to investigate the supply of bipolar drug. Press release. 2020; https://www.gov.uk/government/news/cma-to-investigate-the-supply-of-bipolar-drug.

34. Bowen RC, et al. Less frequent lithium administration and lower urine volume. *Am J Psychiatry* 1991; 148:189–192.

35. Ljubicic D, et al. Lithium treatments: single and multiple daily dosing. *Can J Psychiatry* 2008; 53:323–331.

36. Gong R, et al. What we need to know about the effect of lithium on the kidney. *Am J Physiol Renal Physiol* 2016; 311:F1168–F1171.
37. Aiff H, et al. Effects of 10 to 30 years of lithium treatment on kidney function. *J Psychopharmacol* 2015; 29:608–614.
38. Frye MA, et al. Depressive relapse during lithium treatment associated with increased serum thyroid-stimulating hormone: results from two placebo-controlled bipolar I maintenance studies. *Acta Psychiatr Scand* 2009; 120:10–13.
39. Johnston AM, et al. Lithium-associated clinical hypothyroidism. Prevalence and risk factors. *Br J Psychiatry* 1999; 175:336–339.
40. Livingstone C, et al. Lithium: a review of its metabolic adverse effects. *J Psychopharmacol* 2006; 20:347–355.
41. McKnight RF, et al. Lithium toxicity profile: a systematic review and meta-analysis. *Lancet* 2012; 379:721–728.
42. Czarnywojtek A, et al. Effect of lithium carbonate on the function of the thyroid gland: mechanism of action and clinical implications. *J Physiol Pharmacol* 2020; 71: [Epub ahead of print].
43. Ott M, et al. Lithium intoxication: incidence, clinical course and renal function – a population-based retrospective cohort study. *J Psychopharmacol* 2016; 30:1008–1019.
44. Bell AJ, et al. Lithium neurotoxicity at normal therapeutic levels. *Br J Psychiatry* 1993; 162:689–692.
45. Smith FE, et al. 3D (7)Li magnetic resonance imaging of brain lithium distribution in bipolar disorder. *Mol Psychiatry* 2018; 23:2184–2191.
46. Gerrett D, et al. Prescribing and monitoring lithium therapy: summary of a safety report from the National Patient Safety Agency. *BMJ* 2010; 341:c6258.
47. Morriss R, et al. Lithium and eGFR: a new routinely available tool for the prevention of chronic kidney disease. *Br J Psychiatry* 2008; 193:93–95.
48. National Patient Safety Agency. Safer lithium therapy. NPSA/2009/PSA005. 2009 (Last updated August 2018); https://www.sps.nhs.uk/articles/npsa-alert-safer-lithium-therapy-2009.
49. Collins N, et al. Standards of lithium monitoring in mental health trusts in the UK. *BMC Psychiatry* 2010; 10:80.
50. Paton C, et al. Monitoring lithium therapy: the impact of a quality improvement programme in the UK. *Bipolar Disord* 2013; 15:865–875.
51. Kirkham E, et al. Impact of active monitoring on lithium management in Norfolk. *Ther Adv Psychopharmacol* 2013; 3:260–265.
52. Cavanagh J, et al. Relapse into mania or depression following lithium discontinuation: a 7-year follow-up. *Acta Psychiatr Scand* 2004; 109:91–95.
53. Yazici O, et al. Controlled lithium discontinuation in bipolar patients with good response to long-term lithium prophylaxis. *J Affect Disord* 2004; 80:269–271.
54. Goodwin GM. Recurrence of mania after lithium withdrawal. Implications for the use of lithium in the treatment of bipolar affective disorder. *Br J Psychiatry* 1994; 164:149–152.
55. Baldessarini RJ, et al. Effects of the rate of discontinuing lithium maintenance treatment in bipolar disorders. *J Clin Psychiatry* 1996; 57:441–448.
56. Biel MG, et al. Continuation versus discontinuation of lithium in recurrent bipolar illness: a naturalistic study. *Bipolar Disord* 2007; 9:435–442.
57. Sajatovic M, et al. Treatment adherence with lithium and anticonvulsant medications among patients with bipolar disorder. *Psychiatr Serv* 2007; 58:855–863.
58. Paton C, et al. Lithium in bipolar and other affective disorders: prescribing practice in the UK. *J Psychopharmacol* 2010; 24:1739–1746.
59. Kessing LV, et al. Suicide risk in patients treated with lithium. *Arch Gen Psychiatry* 2005; 62:860–866.
60. Medicines Complete. Stockley's drug interactions. 2020; https://www.medicinescomplete.com.
61. Juurlink DN, et al. Drug-induced lithium toxicity in the elderly: a population-based study. *J Am Geriatr Soc* 2004; 52:794–798.
62. Finley PR. Drug interactions with lithium: an update. *Clin Pharmacokinet* 2016; 55:925–941.
63. Kohler-Forsberg O, et al. Nonsteroidal anti-inflammatory drugs (NSAIDs) and paracetamol do not affect 6-month mood-stabilizing treatment outcome among 482 patients with bipolar disorder. *Depress Anxiety* 2017; 34:281–290.

丙戊酸盐

作用机制[1]

丙戊酸盐是一种简单的支链脂肪酸。它的作用机制复杂并且尚未完全弄清。丙戊酸盐抑制 γ-氨基丁酸（GABA）的分解代谢，降低花生四烯酸的更新率，激活细胞外信号调节激酶通路，从而改变突触可塑性，干扰细胞内信号，促进脑源性神经营养因子（BDNF）表达，并且降低蛋白激酶 C 的水平。最近的研究聚焦于丙戊酸盐具有改变与转录调节、细胞骨架修饰和离子平衡有关的多个基因表达的能力。其他被提及的机制包括肌醇的耗竭，以及通过抑制电压门控钠离子通道间接影响非 GABA 通路。

日益增多的文献提及丙戊酸盐作为某些癌症辅助治疗手段的潜力，其相关的机制是抑制组蛋白去乙酰化酶[2-4]，这一特性也可能对神经可塑性产生一些影响[5]。

剂型

丙戊酸盐在英国有三种形式：丙戊酸钠、丙戊酸（获准治疗癫痫）和丙戊酸半钠。丙戊酸半钠和丙戊酸钠均被代谢成丙戊酸，这是所有三种剂型中发挥药理活性的成分[6]。有关情感障碍治疗的临床研究中不定地使用丙戊酸钠、丙戊酸半钠、丙戊酸盐或者丙戊酸。大多数采用丙戊酸半钠。

治疗双相障碍时，美国广泛使用丙戊酸[7]，英国广泛使用丙戊酸钠。需要记住丙戊酸钠和丙戊酸半钠的剂量是不同的，丙戊酸钠含有多余的钠，因此所需剂量要稍高一些（大约 10%）。

尚不清楚丙戊酸、丙戊酸半钠和丙戊酸钠之间是否存在疗效的差异。美国一项大型准实验研究发现，最初接受丙戊酸半钠治疗的住院患者，其住院时间比最初接受丙戊酸治疗的患者长 1/3[8]。注意丙戊酸钠控释片（Epilim Chrono[9]）可以一天一次给药，而丙戊酸钠和丙戊酸半钠需要至少一天两次给药。

适应证

随机对照试验显示丙戊酸盐治疗躁狂有效[10,11]，有效率为 50%，需治疗人数（NNT）为 2~4[12]，但是也存在大样本研究结果为阴性的报道[13]。一项随机对照试验发现，总体上锂盐的疗效优于丙戊酸盐[11]；但一项持续 12 周的大样本（$n=300$）随机开放式研究发现，锂盐和丙戊酸盐治疗急性躁狂是等效的[14]。锂盐治疗无效的患者丙戊酸盐可能有效；在一项小样本安慰剂对照 RCT（$n=36$）中，使用锂盐治疗无效或者不能耐受的患者，换用丙戊酸盐后 YMRS 量表减分率的中位数为 54%，而安慰剂组为 5%[15]。无论是单药治疗[16]，还是作为锂盐的辅助治疗[12]，丙戊酸盐对急性躁狂的疗效不如奥氮平。一项网络荟萃分析报道，丙戊酸盐虽然疗效不如锂盐，但是耐受性优于锂盐[17]。

一篇 4 项小样本 RCT 研究的荟萃分析的结论是：丙戊酸盐对双相抑郁是有效的，具有小到中等的效应值[18]。2020 年一项荟萃分析将双丙戊酸钠在双相抑郁的 21 种治疗方中排在第 5 位[19]。

虽然开放性研究提示丙戊酸盐对于预防双相障碍有效[20]，但是 RCT 研究数据有限[21,22]。

Bowden 等[23]发现,在主要结局指标(出现任何情绪发作的时间)方面,锂盐、丙戊酸盐和安慰剂之间没有明显差异,但是丙戊酸盐在次要结局指标上优于锂盐和安慰剂。这项研究受到质疑,因为纳入了"病得不够重"的患者,以及治疗持续时间不够"长"(1 年)。在另一项为期 47 周的 RCT 研究中[21],丙戊酸盐和奥氮平组之间的复发率没有差异。这项研究未设置安慰剂对照且失访率高,因此难以解释。对这项研究的事后分析发现,丙戊酸盐对快速循环的患者起效比奥氮平快,但该优点未保持住[22]。对于那些非快速循环特征的患者而言,奥氮平治疗 1 年,其躁狂症状的结局优于丙戊酸盐。在另外一项历时 20 个月的锂盐和丙戊酸盐治疗快速循环型患者的 RCT 研究中,复发率和脱落率都高,丙戊酸盐和锂盐的疗效没有差异[24]。最近,BALANCE 研究发现,从数字上看锂盐优于丙戊酸盐,并且锂盐合并丙戊酸盐在统计学上优于丙戊酸盐单一治疗[25]。阿立哌唑合并丙戊酸盐也优于丙戊酸盐单药治疗[26]。

英国国家卫生与临床优化研究所(NICE)推荐丙戊酸盐作为一线选择,用于治疗急性躁狂发作,合并一种抗抑郁药用于治疗急性抑郁发作和预防复发[27],但重要的是不适用于育龄期女性[27,28]。Cochrane 分析认为,丙戊酸盐预防性使用的证据有限[29],但用于该适应证的情况近年大幅增加[30]。在美国,尽管锂盐被推荐为双相障碍患者的一线用药,丙戊酸盐在双相障碍患者中的使用却在不断增加,而锂盐则在减少[31]。

丙戊酸盐有时用于治疗不同病因的攻击行为[32]。一项小样本 RCT(n=16)研究发现,利培酮合并丙戊酸盐增效治疗,与单用利培酮治疗相比,在降低精神分裂症患者的敌意方面没有任何优势[33]。一项镜像研究发现,在安全设置下,丙戊酸盐能够降低精神分裂症或双相障碍患者的激越[34]。

此外,还有一项丙戊酸盐治疗广泛性焦虑障碍的小样本安慰剂对照 RCT 研究显示为阳性结果[35]。

血浆水平

丙戊酸盐的药代动力学是复杂的,遵循一种三腔模型,并且显示具有蛋白结合饱和性。丙戊酸盐血浆浓度监测在应用上被认为比锂盐和卡马西平受到更多限制[36]。尽管数据说服力较弱[36],丙戊酸盐血清浓度和急性躁狂治疗反应之间可能存在线性关系,在血清浓度 <55mg/L 时不会比安慰剂有效,而血清浓度 >94mg/L 时则具有最强的治疗反应[37]。请注意,这是来自实验室的参考范围的上限(对于癫痫)。维持期的最佳血清浓度仍然未知,但是可能至少在 50mg/L[38]。为了快速达到治疗血浆浓度,使用负荷剂量策略通常能较好地耐受。血浆浓度同样也能用来检测不依从性或毒性。

不良反应

丙戊酸盐可产生对胃肠道的刺激和高氨血症[39],两者都能导致恶心。嗜睡和意识模糊偶发于起始剂量大于 750mg/d 的情况。体重增加可能明显[40],特别是与氯氮平合用时。使用丙戊酸盐的患者多达 1/4 会出现剂量相关的震颤[41],其中绝大多数是有问题的意向性或姿势性震颤,但极少发展为与认知下降相关的帕金森病;当丙戊酸盐停用后,这些症状就消失[42]。

脱发伴卷曲样再生以及外周水肿可以出现,还有血小板减少症、白细胞减少症、红细胞发育不全和胰腺炎[43]。丙戊酸盐在女性能够导致雄激素增多症[44],并且与多囊卵巢发病有关。目前,支持这种关联的证据不一。丙戊酸盐是一种主要的人类致畸物(见第 7 章)。丙戊酸盐导致暴发性肝衰竭罕见。接受多种抗癫痫药治疗的婴幼儿发生这种情形的风险最高。任何肝功能指标升高(常见于治疗早期[45])的患者应该接受临床评估,并检查其他的肝功能指标,如白蛋白和凝血时间。

丙戊酸盐的许多不良反应是剂量相关的(血浆峰浓度相关),当血浆浓度 >100mg/L 时,其频率和严重程度都有增加。使用丙戊酸盐缓释制剂每天一次时,血浆峰浓度不像传统剂型那样高,所以能够较好地耐受。

曾有报道丙戊酸盐及其他抗癫痫药与自杀风险增加有关[46],但是不同研究的结果并不一致[47]。抑郁症患者[48]或服用另一种增加抑郁发作风险的抗癫痫药的患者可能是一个高风险的人群[49]。

值得注意的是,丙戊酸盐主要通过肾脏排泄,部分以酮体的形式排泄,因此可能导致尿液检查中尿酮体呈假阳性。

治疗前检查

NICE 推荐基线时检查血常规、肝功能、体重或者 BMI。

治疗中监测

NICE 建议治疗 6 个月后复查血常规和肝功能,并且应该监测 BMI。丙戊酸盐产品特征概要建议,在治疗开始后头 6 个月,肝功能检查应该更频繁;如果转氨酶水平异常,还要测定白蛋白和凝血时间。丙戊酸钠的处方和监测见表 2.3。

停药

尚不清楚骤然停用丙戊酸盐,是否会像停用锂盐一样,恶化双相障碍的自然病程。一项小样本自然回顾性研究提示丙戊酸盐可能会这样[50]。除非有进一步的数据支持,如果要停止丙戊酸盐治疗,应该缓慢减量 1 个月以上。

在育龄期女性中的应用

丙戊酸盐是一种确定的人类致畸原。NICE 建议患有癫痫的女性[51]最好换用其他抗癫痫药,丙戊酸盐不应用于治疗育龄期女性的双相障碍[27]。英国药品和健康产品管理局(MHRA)公布了丙戊酸盐工具包,为患者、全科医师、药剂师和专家提供一套资源[52]。

该工具包以及丙戊酸钠和丙戊酸半钠[9,53]的产品特征概要陈述如下:

- 如果没有专家(神经科医生或者精神科医生)建议,这类药物不作为育龄期女性的首选治疗。
- 备孕并且需要丙戊酸盐的女性,应该预防性使用叶酸。

躁狂期的女性有可能性行为没有节制。非计划妊娠的风险可能高于正常人群(50% 的妊娠是非计划的)。

丙戊酸盐致畸的可能性并没有被广泛认识,许多育龄期女性也不知道需要采取避孕措施或者预防性使用叶酸[54,55]。丙戊酸盐宫内暴露也可能导致儿童的认知功能损害[56],见第 7 章。大多数人现在赞成丙戊酸钠不应用于 50 岁以下的妇女,一些国家正在考虑在这些患者中完全禁止使用。

药物相互作用

丙戊酸盐为高蛋白结合药物，能够被其他蛋白结合药物（如阿司匹林）置换，导致中毒。阿司匹林同样抑制丙戊酸盐代谢：至少需要 300mg 阿司匹林的剂量[57]。其他蛋白结合弱于丙戊酸盐的药物（如华法林），能够被丙戊酸盐置换，导致游离水平升高而中毒。

丙戊酸盐被肝脏代谢。抑制 CYP 酶的药物能够增加丙戊酸盐浓度（如红霉素、氟西汀和西咪替丁）。丙戊酸盐能够抑制葡糖醛酸化，从而升高一些药物的血浆水平，例如抗抑郁药（三环类抗抑郁药，尤其是氯米帕明[58]）、拉莫三嗪[59]、喹硫平[60]、华法林[61] 和苯巴比妥。丙戊酸盐也可显著降低奥氮平的血浆浓度，其机制未知[62]。

药效学的相互作用同样也有。丙戊酸盐的抗惊厥效果能够被降低癫痫发作阈值的药物（如抗精神病药）所拮抗。体重增加能够被其他药物如氯氮平、奥氮平等加重。

表 2.3　丙戊酸钠：处方和监测

适应证	躁狂，轻躁狂，双相抑郁和双相情感障碍的预防；可能降低一些精神障碍的攻击性（数据较弱） 注意：丙戊酸钠仅获准治疗癫痫并且丙戊酸半钠仅获准治疗急性躁狂
用药之前检查	血常规和肝功能检查，需要测量基线体重
用药	根据疗效和不良反应逐渐加量。可用负荷剂量，通常耐受性良好 注意丙戊酸钠控释片可以每天给药一次。其他全部剂型必须每天至少两次 血浆水平可用于保证足够剂量和治疗依从性。应该在即将服药前采血
监测	如果有临床需要，检查血常规和肝功能 体重（或者 BMI）
停用	缓慢减量 1 个月以上

参考文献

1. Rosenberg G. The mechanisms of action of valproate in neuropsychiatric disorders: can we see the forest for the trees? *Cell Mol Life Sci* 2007; 64:2090–2103.
2. Kuendgen A, et al. Valproic acid for the treatment of myeloid malignancies. *Cancer* 2007; 110:943–954.
3. Atmaca A, et al. Valproic acid (VPA) in patients with refractory advanced cancer: a dose escalating phase I clinical trial. *Br J Cancer* 2007; 97:177–182.
4. Hallas J, et al. Cancer risk in long-term users of valproate: a population-based case-control study. *Cancer Epidemiol Biomarkers Prev* 2009; 18:1714–1719.
5. Gervain J, et al. Valproate reopens critical-period learning of absolute pitch. *Front Syst Neurosci* 2013; 7:1–11.
6. Fisher C, et al. Sodium valproate or valproate semisodium: is there a difference in the treatment of bipolar disorder? *Psychiatric Bull* 2003; 27:446–448.
7. Iqbal SU, et al. Divalproex sodium vs. valproic acid: drug utilization patterns, persistence rates and predictors of hospitalization among VA patients diagnosed with bipolar disorder. *J Clin Pharm Ther* 2007; 32:625–632.
8. Wassef AA, et al. Lower effectiveness of divalproex versus valproic acid in a prospective, quasi-experimental clinical trial involving 9,260 psychiatric admissions. *Am J Psychiatry* 2005; 162:330–339.
9. Sanofi. Summary of product characteristics. Epilim Chrono 500mg. 2020; https://www.medicines.org.uk/emc/medicine/6779.
10. Bowden CL, et al. Efficacy of divalproex vs lithium and placebo in the treatment of mania. The Depakote Mania Study Group. *JAMA* 1994; 271:918–924.

11. Freeman TW, et al. A double-blind comparison of valproate and lithium in the treatment of acute mania. *Am J Psychiatry* 1992; 149:108–111.

12. Nasrallah HA, et al. Carbamazepine and valproate for the treatment of bipolar disorder: a review of the literature. *J Affect Disord* 2006; 95:69–78.

13. Hirschfeld RM, et al. A randomized, placebo-controlled, multicenter study of divalproex sodium extended-release in the acute treatment of mania. *J Clin Psychiatry* 2010; 71:426–432.

14. Bowden C, et al. A 12-week, open, randomized trial comparing sodium valproate to lithium in patients with bipolar I disorder suffering from a manic episode. *Int Clin Psychopharmacol* 2008; 23:254–262.

15. Pope HG, Jr., et al. Valproate in the treatment of acute mania. A placebo-controlled study. *Arch Gen Psychiatry* 1991; 48:62–68.

16. Novick D, et al. Translation of randomised controlled trial findings into clinical practice: comparison of olanzapine and valproate in the EMBLEM study. *Pharmacopsychiatry* 2009; 42:145–152.

17. Cipriani A, et al. Comparative efficacy and acceptability of antimanic drugs in acute mania: a multiple-treatments meta-analysis. *Lancet* 2011; 378:1306–1315.

18. Smith LA, et al. Valproate for the treatment of acute bipolar depression: systematic review and meta-analysis. *J Affect Disord* 2010; 122:1–9.

19. Bahji A, et al. Comparative efficacy and tolerability of pharmacological treatments for the treatment of acute bipolar depression: A systematic review and network meta-analysis. *J Affect Disord* 2020; 269:154–184.

20. Calabrese JR, et al. Spectrum of efficacy of valproate in 55 patients with rapid-cycling bipolar disorder. *Am J Psychiatry* 1990; 147:431–434.

21. Tohen M, et al. Olanzapine versus divalproex sodium for the treatment of acute mania and maintenance of remission: a 47-week study. *Am J Psychiatry* 2003; 160:1263–1271.

22. Suppes T, et al. Rapid versus non-rapid cycling as a predictor of response to olanzapine and divalproex sodium for bipolar mania and maintenance of remission: post hoc analyses of 47-week data. *J Affect Disord* 2005; 89:69–77.

23. Bowden CL, et al. A randomized, placebo-controlled 12-month trial of divalproex and lithium in treatment of outpatients with bipolar I disorder. Divalproex Maintenance Study Group. *Arch Gen Psychiatry* 2000; 57:481–489.

24. Calabrese JR, et al. A 20-month, double-blind, maintenance trial of lithium versus divalproex in rapid-cycling bipolar disorder. *Am J Psychiatry* 2005; 162:2152–2161.

25. Geddes JR, et al. Lithium plus valproate combination therapy versus monotherapy for relapse prevention in bipolar I disorder (BALANCE): a randomised open-label trial. *Lancet* 2010; 375:385–395.

26. Marcus R, et al. Efficacy of aripiprazole adjunctive to lithium or valproate in the long-term treatment of patients with bipolar I disorder with an inadequate response to lithium or valproate monotherapy: a multicenter, double-blind, randomized study. *Bipolar Disord* 2011; 13:133–144.

27. National Institute for Health and Care Excellence. Bipolar disorder: assessment and management. Clinical Guidance [CG198]. 2014 (Last updated February 2020); https://www.nice.org.uk/guidance/cg185.

28. National Institute for Health and Care Excellence. Antenatal and postnatal mental health: clinical management and service guidance. Clinical Guidance [CG192]. 2014 (Last updated: February 2020); https://www.nice.org.uk/guidance/cg192.

29. Cipriani A, et al. Valproic acid, valproate and divalproex in the maintenance treatment of bipolar disorder. *Cochrane Database Syst Rev* 2013; 10:CD003196.

30. Hayes J, et al. Prescribing trends in bipolar disorder: cohort study in the United Kingdom THIN primary care database 1995–2009. *PLoSOne* 2011; 6:e28725.

31. Lin Y, et al. Trends in prescriptions of lithium and other medications for patients with bipolar disorder in office-based practices in the United States: 1996–2015. *J Affect Disord* 2020; 276:883–889.

32. Lindenmayer JP, et al. Use of sodium valproate in violent and aggressive behaviors: a critical review. *J Clin Psychiatry* 2000; 61:123–128.

33. Citrome L, et al. Risperidone alone versus risperidone plus valproate in the treatment of patients with schizophrenia and hostility. *Int Clin Psychopharmacol* 2007; 22:356–362.

34. Gobbi G, et al. Efficacy of topiramate, valproate, and their combination on aggression/agitation behavior in patients with psychosis. *J Clin Psychopharmacol* 2006; 26:467–473.

35. Aliyev NA, et al. Valproate (depakine-chrono) in the acute treatment of outpatients with generalized anxiety disorder without psychiatric comorbidity: randomized, double-blind placebo-controlled study. *Eur Psychiatry* 2008; 23:109–114.

36. Haymond J, et al. Does valproic acid warrant therapeutic drug monitoring in bipolar affective disorder? *Ther Drug Monit* 2010; 32:19–29.

37. Allen MH, et al. Linear relationship of valproate serum concentration to response and optimal serum levels for acute mania. *Am J Psychiatry* 2006; 163:272–275.

38. Taylor D, et al. Doses of carbamazepine and valproate in bipolar affective disorder. *Psychiatric Bull* 1997; 21:221–223.

39. Segura-Bruna N, et al. Valproate-induced hyperammonemic encephalopathy. *Acta Neurol Scand* 2006; 114:1–7.

40. El-Khatib F, et al. Valproate, weight gain and carbohydrate craving: a gender study. *Seizure* 2007; 16:226–232.

41. Zadikoff C, et al. Movement disorders in patients taking anticonvulsants. *J Neurol Neurosurg Psychiatry* 2007; 78:147–151.

42. Ristic AJ, et al. The frequency of reversible parkinsonism and cognitive decline associated with valproate treatment: a study of 364 patients with different types of epilepsy. *Epilepsia* 2006; 47:2183–2185.

43. Gerstner T, et al. Valproic acid-induced pancreatitis: 16 new cases and a review of the literature. *J Gastroenterol* 2007; 42:39–48.

44. Joffe H, et al. Valproate is associated with new-onset oligoamenorrhea with hyperandrogenism in women with bipolar disorder. *Biol Psychiatry* 2006; 59:1078–1086.

45. Bjornsson E. Hepatotoxicity associated with antiepileptic drugs. *Acta Neurol Scand* 2008; 118:281–290.

46. Patorno E, et al. Anticonvulsant medications and the risk of suicide, attempted suicide, or violent death. *JAMA* 2010; 303:1401–1409.

47. Gibbons RD, et al. Relationship between antiepileptic drugs and suicide attempts in patients with bipolar disorder. *Arch Gen Psychiatry* 2009; 66:1354–1360.

48. Arana A, et al. Suicide-related events in patients treated with antiepileptic drugs. *N Engl J Med* 2010; 363:542–551.

49. Andersohn F, et al. Use of antiepileptic drugs in epilepsy and the risk of self-harm or suicidal behavior. *Neurology* 2010; 75:335–340.

50. Franks MA, et al. Bouncing back: is the bipolar rebound phenomenon peculiar to lithium? A retrospective naturalistic study. *J Psychopharmacol* 2008; 22:452–456.

51. National Institute for Health and Clinical Excellence. The epilepsies: the diagnosis and management of the epilepsies in adults and children in primary and secondary care. Clinical Guidance 137. 2012 (Last updated February 2016); https://www.nice.org.uk/guidance/cg137.

52. GOV.UK Guidance. Valproate use by women and girls. 2020; https://www.gov.uk/guidance/valproate-use-by-women-and-girls.

53. Sanofi. Summary of product characteristics. Depakote 250mg tablets. 2020; https://www.medicines.org.uk/emc/medicine/25929.

54. James L, et al. Informing patients of the teratogenic potential of mood stabilising drugs; a case notes review of the practice of psychiatrists. *J Psychopharmacol* 2007; 21:815–819.

55. James L, et al. Mood stabilizers and teratogenicity – prescribing practice and awareness amongst practising psychiatrists. *J Mental Health* 2009; 18:137–143.

56. Meador KJ, et al. Cognitive function at 3 years of age after fetal exposure to antiepileptic drugs. *N Engl J Med* 2009; 360:1597–1605.

57. Sandson NB, et al. An interaction between aspirin and valproate: the relevance of plasma protein displacement drug-drug interactions. *Am J Psychiatry* 2006; 163:1891–1896.

58. Fehr C, et al. Increase in serum clomipramine concentrations caused by valproate. *J Clin Psychopharmacol* 2000; 20:493–494.

59. Morris RG, et al. Clinical study of lamotrigine and valproic acid in patients with epilepsy: using a drug interaction to advantage? *Ther Drug Monit* 2000; 22:656–660.

60. Aichhorn W, et al. Influence of age, gender, body weight and valproate comedication on quetiapine plasma concentrations. *Int Clin Psychopharmacol* 2006; 21:81–85.

61. Gunes A, et al. Inhibitory effect of valproic acid on cytochrome P450 2C9 activity in epilepsy patients. *Basic Clin Pharmacol Toxicol* 2007; 100:383–386.

62. Bergemann N, et al. Valproate lowers plasma concentration of olanzapine. *J Clin Psychopharmacol* 2006; 26:432–434.

卡马西平

作用机制[1]

卡马西平是一种电压依赖性钠通道阻滞剂,可以抑制神经元重复放电。它能够减少谷氨酸盐的释放,以及减少多巴胺、去甲肾上腺素的更新。卡马西平与 TCA 的分子结构相似。

奥卡西平(一种卡马西平的结构性衍生物)不仅可以阻断电压依赖性钠通道,而且能够增加钾离子的传导性,并调节高电压激活的钙离子通道。

剂型

卡马西平有液体、咀嚼片、速释和控释制剂。传统剂型一般要每天服用 2~3 次。控释剂可以每天服用 1 或 2 次,并且血药浓度的波动变小可以改善耐受性。这种剂型生物利用度较低,需要增加 10%~15% 的剂量。

适应证

卡马西平主要作为抗癫痫药用于治疗癫痫大发作和局灶性癫痫发作,也可用于治疗三叉神经痛。英国批准卡马西平可以治疗对锂盐无效的双相障碍患者。

两项安慰剂对照随机研究发现,卡马西平缓释剂对躁狂有效,卡马西平组有效率是安慰剂组的 2 倍[2,3]。卡马西平的耐受性很差,眩晕、嗜睡和恶心的发生率较高。另一项研究发现,单用卡马西平与卡马西平联用奥氮平疗效相同[4]。NICE 不推荐将卡马西平作为治疗躁狂的一线药物[5]。Cochrane 的一篇综述得出结论,对于奥卡西平在双相障碍急性期治疗中的疗效和可接受性[6],目前没有足够的方法学质量良好的试验。

开放性研究表明,单用卡马西平对治疗双相抑郁具有一定的疗效[7];注意:支持其他治疗策略的证据更强(见本章"双相抑郁")。对于单相抑郁,卡马西平不管是单用[8],还是联合治疗,均同样有效[9]。

卡马西平通常被认为在预防双相障碍的效果上不如锂盐[10];研究报道卡马西平有效率较低,脱落率较高。一项荟萃分析($n=464$)发现,锂盐和卡马西平的疗效并无显著差异,但接受卡马西平的被试因为不良反应而更易脱落[11]。锂盐被认为在减少自杀行为方面优于卡马西平[12],但是研究数据并不一致[13],而且卡马西平也许也有防自杀的性质[14]。NICE 将卡马西平归类为三线预防用药[5],而这一指导之后出现的数据也支持这一定位[15]。三项小样本研究表明,当与其他心境稳定剂合用时,奥卡西平可能具有预防效果[16-18]。

虽然有数据支持卡马西平在治疗酒精戒断症状方面的应用[19],但起始剂量较高使患者通常难以耐受。Cochrane 分析认为证据不足以支持将卡马西平用于此适应证[20]。卡马西平也被用于治疗精神分裂症患者的攻击行为[21],但研究数据质量较差,且作用模式尚不清楚。另有一些病例报告和开放性病例系列报道了卡马西平在多种精神疾病中的应用,如惊恐障碍、边缘性人格障碍、发作性控制不良综合征等。

血浆浓度

一般认为卡马西平作为抗癫痫药时有效药物浓度范围是 4~12mg/L,但是支持证据并不充分。用于情感障碍患者时,剂量至少为 600mg/d,血浆浓度至少为 7mg/L[22],但是研究结果并不一致[4,8,23]。超过 12mg/L 就有较高的不良反应风险。

卡马西平的血浆浓度在一个剂量区间内变化较大。因此,采血的时间点应该使得某一患者的血药浓度可以重复。最恰当的检测方法是在每天首次服药之前测量低谷期的浓度。

卡马西平为肝酶诱导剂,能够诱导自身及其他药物的代谢,包括一些抗精神病药。开始用药时,其血浆半衰期大约为 30h,长期服用则降为 12h 左右。因此,每次增加剂量 2~4 周后,应检测血药浓度,以保证达到所需浓度。

大多数发表的临床试验表明,卡马西平作为心境稳定剂的有效剂量为 800~1 200mg/d,显著高于英国临床实践中的常用剂量[24]。

不良反应[1]

卡马西平治疗最主要的不良反应为头晕、复视、嗜睡、共济失调、恶心及头痛。通过低剂量起始和缓慢加量,有可能避免这些不良反应。通过每天分次服药或使用控释片,以避免较高的血药浓度,也会有所帮助。口干、水肿和低钠血症也较为常见。性功能障碍也可能发生,这也许是睾酮水平降低所致[25]。大约有 3% 的患者使用卡马西平后出现广泛的红斑疹。严重的剥脱性皮炎极为少见,其易感性是由基因决定的。对于中国汉族或泰裔人群,建议在处方卡马西平前进行基因检测[26]。卡马西平也是一种致畸药物(见第 7 章)。

卡马西平通常会引起慢性的白细胞计数减少[27]。20 000 人中有 1 人会发展为粒细胞缺乏症或再生障碍性贫血。碱性磷酸酶(ALP)和 γ-谷胺转肽酶(GGT)升高比较常见(GGT 升高 2~3 倍并不需要特别关注[28])。多器官的迟发性过敏反应也极为少见,它主要表现为多种皮肤反应、白细胞计数降低和肝功能异常。死亡病例也有报道。这些不良事件并没有明确的时间表[28,29]。

一些抗癫痫药物与自杀行为风险增加有关。卡马西平无此风险,无论是在一般人群中[30,31],还是特定的双相障碍患者中[32]。

治疗前检查

NICE 推荐进行尿素、电解质、血常规和肝功能的基线检查。体重的基线测量也同样需要。

治疗中监测

NICE 推荐 6 个月后复查尿素、电解质、血常规和肝功能,体重(或 BMI)也需要监测。卡马西平的处方和监测见表 2.4。

停药

目前尚不清楚,突然中止卡马西平治疗,是否和突然中止锂盐治疗一样,会加重双相障碍的自然病程。在一个小样本的病例系列中(n=6),一位患者在中止治疗后一个月内出现抑郁[33];另一个小样本病例系列($n=4$)指出,心境障碍患者停药后,有三位在三个月内复发[34]。在没有获得进一步的数据之前,如需终止卡马西平治疗,应该缓慢停药(至少需要一个月)。

表 2.4 卡马西平:处方和监测

适应证	躁狂(非一线用药)、双相抑郁(证据较弱)、单相抑郁(证据较弱)、双相障碍的预防用药(抗精神病药和丙戊酸钠之后的三线用药)、酒精戒断(可能难以耐受)。 卡马西平被批准用于锂盐治疗无效的双相障碍患者
用药前检查	尿素、电解质、血常规和肝功能检查。最好测量体重的基线水平。
处方	根据疗效和不良反应逐渐加量;起始剂量 100~200mg,每天 2 次,目标剂量 400mg,每天 2 次。 注意:缓释剂可以每天服用 1 次或 2 次,其血清水平波动较小,通常耐受性好。 血浆水平可以用来确认足够的剂量和治疗依从性。应在下次服药前立刻采血。 卡马西平诱导自身代谢,每次加量 1 个月后应复查血清浓度
监测	若临床需要,监测尿素、电解质、血常规、肝功能检查 体重(或 BMI)
停用	至少需要 1 个多月的时间来缓慢减药

在育龄期妇女中的应用

卡马西平是一种确定的人类致畸原(见第 7 章)。

躁狂发作的妇女可能表现为性行为不受抑制。意外妊娠的风险可能高于正常人(50% 为意外妊娠)。如果不能避免使用卡马西平,要确保充分避孕(卡马西平和口服避孕药的相互作用在下文中列出),并预防性使用叶酸。

药物相互作用 [35-38]

卡马西平是一种肝细胞色素酶的强诱导剂,通过 CYP3A4 代谢。卡马西平可能会降低某些药物的血浆浓度,导致治疗失败。这些药物包括绝大多数抗抑郁药、大多数抗精神病药、苯二氮䓬类药物、华法林、唑吡坦、一些胆碱酯酶抑制剂、美沙酮、甲状腺素、茶碱、雌激素和其他类固醇。需要避孕的患者应服用至少含有 50μg 雌激素的制剂,或使用非激素避孕方式。抑制 CYP3A4 的药物能够增加卡马西平的血浆浓度,可能会导致中毒,比如氟康唑、西咪替丁、地尔硫䓬、维拉帕米、红霉素和一些选择性 5-羟色胺再摄取抑制剂(SSRI)。

药效学相互作用也会发生。能够降低癫痫发作阈值的药物(如抗精神病药和抗抑郁药)会减弱卡马西平的抗癫痫作用;抑制骨髓的药物(例如氯氮平)会增加卡马西平导致中性粒细胞减少症的风险;增加钠消耗的药物(如利尿剂)可增加低钠血症的风险。有极少的报道指出卡马西平与锂盐合用时有神经毒性,这是罕见的。有关卡马西平相互作用的完整综述,请参阅《精神药物应用临床药代动力学》第 17 章[39]。

由于卡马西平在结构上与 TCA 相似,理论上来说,停用单胺氧化酶抑制剂(MAOI)的 14 天内不能使用卡马西平。

参考文献

1. Novartis Pharmaceuticals UK Limited. Summary of product characteristics. Tegretol tablets 100mg, 200mg, 400mg. 2020; https://www.medi cines.org.uk/emc/medicine/1328.

2. Weisler RH, et al. A multicenter, randomized, double-blind, placebo-controlled trial of extended-release carbamazepine capsules as mono-therapy for bipolar disorder patients with manic or mixed episodes. *J Clin Psychiatry* 2004; 65:478–484.

3. Weisler RH, et al. Extended-release carbamazepine capsules as monotherapy for acute mania in bipolar disorder: a multicenter, randomized, double-blind, placebo-controlled trial. *J Clin Psychiatry* 2005; 66:323–330.

4. Tohen M, et al. Olanzapine plus carbamazepine v. carbamazepine alone in treating manic episodes. *Br J Psychiatry* 2008; 192:135–143.

5. National Institute for Health and Care Excellence. Bipolar disorder: assessment and management. Clinical Guidance 185 [CG185]. 2014 (Last updated February 2020); https://www.nice.org.uk/guidance/cg185.

6. Vasudev A, et al. Oxcarbazepine for acute affective episodes in bipolar disorder. *Cochrane Database Syst Rev* 2011; Cd004857.

7. Dilsaver SC, et al. Treatment of bipolar depression with carbamazepine: results of an open study. *Biol Psychiatry* 1996; 40:935–937.

8. Zhang ZJ, et al. The effectiveness of carbamazepine in unipolar depression: a double-blind, randomized, placebo-controlled study. *J Affect Disord* 2008; 109:91–97.

9. Kramlinger KG, et al. The addition of lithium to carbamazepine. Antidepressant efficacy in treatment-resistant depression. *Arch Gen Psychiatry* 1989; 46:794–800.

10. Nasrallah HA, et al. Carbamazepine and valproate for the treatment of bipolar disorder: a review of the literature. *J Affect Disord* 2006; 95:69–78.

11. Ceron-Litvoc D, et al. Comparison of carbamazepine and lithium in treatment of bipolar disorder: a systematic review of randomized con-trolled trials. *Human Psychopharmacol* 2009; 24:19–28.

12. Kleindienst N, et al. Differential efficacy of lithium and carbamazepine in the prophylaxis of bipolar disorder: results of the MAP study. *Neuropsychobiology* 2000; 42 Suppl 1:2–10.

13. Yerevanian BI, et al. Bipolar pharmacotherapy and suicidal behavior. Part I: lithium, divalproex and carbamazepine. *J Affect Disord* 2007; 103:5–11.

14. Tsai CJ, et al. The rapid suicide protection of mood stabilizers on patients with bipolar disorder: a nationwide observational cohort study in Taiwan. *J Affect Disord* 2016; 196:71–77.

15. Peselow ED, et al. Prophylactic efficacy of lithium, valproic acid, and carbamazepine in the maintenance phase of bipolar disorder: a natural-istic study. *Int Clin Psychopharmacol* 2016; 31:218–223.

16. Vieta E, et al. A double-blind, randomized, placebo-controlled prophylaxis trial of oxcarbazepine as adjunctive treatment to lithium in the long-term treatment of bipolar I and II disorder. *Int J Neuropsychopharmacol* 2008; 11:445–452.

17. Conway CR, et al. An open-label trial of adjunctive oxcarbazepine for bipolar disorder. *J Clin Psychopharmacol* 2006; 26:95–97.

18. Juruena MF, et al. Bipolar I and II disorder residual symptoms: oxcarbazepine and carbamazepine as add-on treatment to lithium in a double-blind, randomized trial. *Prog Neuropsychopharmacol Biol Psychiatry* 2009; 33:94–99.

19. Malcolm R, et al. The effects of carbamazepine and lorazepam on single versus multiple previous alcohol withdrawals in an outpatient ran-domized trial. *J Gen Intern Med* 2002; 17:349–355.

20. Minozzi S, et al. Anticonvulsants for alcohol withdrawal. *Cochrane Database Syst Rev* 2010; CD005064.

21. Brieden T, et al. Psychopharmacological treatment of aggression in schizophrenic patients. *Pharmacopsychiatry* 2002; 35:83–89.

22. Taylor D, et al. Doses of carbamazepine and valproate in bipolar affective disorder. *Psychiatric Bull* 1997; 21:221–223.

23. Simhandl C, et al. The comparative efficacy of carbamazepine low and high serum level and lithium carbonate in the prophylaxis of affective disorders. *J Affect Disord* 1993; 28:221–231.

24. Taylor DM, et al. Prescribing and monitoring of carbamazepine and valproate – a case note review. *Psychiatric Bull* 2000; 24:174–177.

25. Lossius MI, et al. Reversible effects of antiepileptic drugs on reproductive endocrine function in men and women with epilepsy–a prospective randomized double-blind withdrawal study. *Epilepsia* 2007; 48:1875–1882.

26. Hung SI, et al. Genetic susceptibility to carbamazepine-induced cutaneous adverse drug reactions. *Pharmacogenet Genomics* 2006; 16:297–306.

27. Kaufman DW, et al. Drugs in the aetiology of agranulocytosis and aplastic anaemia. *Eur J Haematol Suppl* 1996; 60:23–30.

28. Bjornsson E. Hepatotoxicity associated with antiepileptic drugs. *Acta Neurol Scand* 2008; 118:281–290.

29. Ganeva M, et al. Carbamazepine-induced drug reaction with eosinophilia and systemic symptoms (DRESS) syndrome: report of four cases and brief review. *Int J Dermatol* 2008; 47:853–860.

30. Patorno E, et al. Anticonvulsant medications and the risk of suicide, attempted suicide, or violent death. *JAMA* 2010; 303:1401–1409.

31. Andersohn F, et al. Use of antiepileptic drugs in epilepsy and the risk of self-harm or suicidal behavior. *Neurology* 2010; 75:335–340.

32. Gibbons RD, et al. Relationship between antiepileptic drugs and suicide attempts in patients with bipolar disorder. *Arch Gen Psychiatry* 2009; 66:1354–1360.

33. Macritchie KA, et al. Does 'rebound mania' occur after stopping carbamazepine? A pilot study. *J Psychopharmacol* 2000; 14:266–268.

34. Franks MA, et al. Bouncing back: is the bipolar rebound phenomenon peculiar to lithium? A retrospective naturalistic study. *J Psychopharmacol* 2008; 22:452–456.

35. Spina E, et al. Clinical significance of pharmacokinetic interactions between antiepileptic and psychotropic drugs. *Epilepsia* 2002; 43 Suppl 2:37–44.

36. Patsalos PN, et al. The importance of drug interactions in epilepsy therapy. *Epilepsia* 2002; 43:365–385.

37. Crawford P. Interactions between antiepileptic drugs and hormonal contraception. *CNS Drugs* 2002; **16**:263–272.

38. Citrome L, et al. Pharmacokinetics of aripiprazole and concomitant carbamazepine. *J Clin Psychopharmacol* 2007; **27**:279–283.

39. Taylor D, et al. Clinically significant interactions with mood stabilisers, inM Jann, S Penzak, L Cohen, eds. Applied clinical pharmacokinetics and pharmacodynamics of psychopharmacological agents. Switzerland: ADIS 2016; 423–449.

抗精神病药在双相障碍中的应用

抗精神病药不仅仅有"抗精神病"作用,不同的抗精神病药具有不同特性,如镇静、抗焦虑、抗躁狂、稳定情绪和抗抑郁。一些抗精神病药(喹硫平和奥氮平)具有以上所有药理作用[1]。

有证据支持抗精神病药对双相障碍抑郁相、躁狂相和混合状态都有效,因此从 20 世纪 60 年代开始抗精神病药就被运用于双相障碍急性期和维持期的治疗。

被美国食品药品监督管理局(FDA)批准用于双相障碍的抗精神病药包括阿立哌唑(躁狂、混合发作、维持期),阿塞那平(躁狂,混合状态),卡利拉嗪(抑郁),鲁拉西酮(抑郁),奥氮平(躁狂,混合发作,维持期),奥氮平与氟西汀合剂(抑郁),喹硫平(躁狂,维持期,抑郁),利培酮(躁狂,混合发作),齐拉西酮(躁狂,维持期)。利培酮长效针剂(LAI)被批准用于维持期的单药或辅助治疗,阿立哌唑长效针剂用于维持期的单药治疗。欧盟(EU)的说明书与 FDA 相似,除了奥氮平与氟西汀合剂未被批准用于任何适应证,也没有任何第二代抗精神病药长效针剂被许可用于维持期治疗。

第一代抗精神病药

长期以来,第一代抗精神病药已经被用于治疗躁狂,且一些研究支持它们在急性期的疗效优于安慰剂,与锂盐相当[2,3]。加用锂盐可以增强它们的疗效[4,5]。FGA 被广泛地运用于双相障碍的长期治疗(可能用于预防)[6,7],但是缺乏强有力的数据支持。第一代抗精神病药与双相障碍患者的抑郁和迟发型运动障碍发生有关,这影响了它们的长期使用[7-9]。在实践中 FGA 长效针剂经常使用,但缺少证据支持,并且似乎与抑郁发作的高风险有关[10](见"双相障碍中的抗精神病药长效针剂"章节)。与氟哌啶醇相比,第二代抗精神病药引起抑郁的可能性较小[11]。

第二代抗精神病药

躁狂

网络荟萃分析提示,抗精神病药对躁狂的疗效优于安慰剂,但是与锂盐等其他药物相比没有统计意义上的优势[12]。抗精神病药按有效率依次为:利培酮,氟哌啶醇,卡利拉嗪,奥氮平,阿立哌唑,喹硫平,帕利哌酮,阿塞那平,齐拉西酮。还应注意的是,抗精神病药的有效率与锂盐和抗癫痫药相似[13]。

在 1 周和 3 周时,抗精神病药辅助治疗比心境稳定剂单药治疗有效,在 3 周时心境稳定剂增效治疗比抗精神病药单药治疗有效。联用与更多的不良反应相关,尤其是嗜睡[14]。由于试验中包括了在心境稳定剂治疗失败后躁狂发作的患者,对结局的解读变得困难。

尽管机制很难辨识,但趋同的证据提示抗精神病药的抗躁狂作用与它们对多巴胺系统的作用相关[15,16]。

抑郁

在双相抑郁的急性期治疗中,研究发现有效的抗精神病药有卡利拉嗪、鲁拉西酮、奥氮平（±氟西汀）和喹硫平[13,17]。就机制而言,抗精神病药的抗抑郁作用似乎不是多巴胺介导的作用,因为阿立哌唑以及其他多巴胺阻滞剂类抗精神病药并对双相抑郁的急性期并无疗效[17]。

维持期

值得注意的是,对双相障碍急性期(无论是躁狂相还是抑郁相)有效的药物,对双相障碍的维持期治疗(即预防)也有效[18]。这个观点被一项双相障碍维持期治疗的网络荟萃分析所证实。该分析涵盖的药物包括阿立哌唑、奥氮平、帕利哌酮、喹硫平和利培酮长效针剂。其中除了阿立哌唑和帕利哌酮,都显示了预防复发的作用[19]。应该注意的是,该分析并没有纳入最新的关于阿立哌唑的试验[19](见下文)。

具体的抗精神病药

阿立哌唑

阿立哌唑在躁狂急性期治疗中,无论是单药[20-22]还是作为辅助药物[23]都是有效的,在长程预防中也有效[24,25]。直接将阿立哌唑与锂盐或氟哌啶醇比较并没有发现差异,但是一项小样本 RCT 提示锂盐对躁狂疗效更好[26]。在躁狂的试验中,阿立哌唑与恶心、运动障碍(主要是静坐不能)相关[27]。阿立哌唑长效针剂对双相 I 型也有预防作用,主要是针对躁狂相的预防[28]。

阿塞那平

阿塞那平通过舌下含服给药,对躁狂有治疗效果[29,30]。药效能保持较长时间[31],RCT 证据显示阿塞那平可以预防双相 I 型的抑郁发作和躁狂发作[32]。和其他的抗精神病药相比,阿塞那平不易发生体重增加和代谢紊乱[33]。

卡利拉嗪

在伴有混合特征的躁狂发作中,卡利拉嗪对躁狂和抑郁症状都有疗效[34],并且不易导致体重增加[33]。

氯氮平

最早关于抗精神病药用于双相障碍维持期治疗的观察性研究检查了氯氮平在难治性心境障碍人群中的疗效[35]。15 项研究提供的证据表明,氯氮平对难治性双相障碍中抑郁、躁狂、快速循环状态和精神病性症状有改善作用,但是其中有两项研究使用足量足疗程的药物仍治疗失败[36]。

鲁拉西酮

根据安慰剂对照、鲁拉西酮单药治疗[37],以及作为锂盐、丙戊酸钠辅助治疗[38]的 RCT 证据,鲁拉西酮被 FDA 批准用于双相抑郁急性期治疗,可以单药使用,也可以作为锂盐或双丙戊酸钠的辅助治疗。其主要不良反应包括恶心和静坐不能,对体重和代谢影响甚微[33]。

奥氮平

奥氮平对躁狂有效[39,40]。与其他 FGA 一样，用于躁狂急性期和预防症状(但不是综合征)复发时，奥氮平与心境稳定剂合用效果更好[41,42](但是有一项研究指出，奥氮平与卡马西平合用，疗效并不优于卡马西平单用[43])。有数据表明奥氮平可能有益于长期治疗[44,45]。它可能比锂盐有效[46,47]。当然，奥氮平与明显的代谢不良反应相关，包括体重增加。

喹硫平

有关数据[48-50]表明，喹硫平在治疗双相障碍各方面都非常有效，包括对双相抑郁的预防[51]。喹硫平不易引起锥体外系不良反应，但是对体重和代谢参数会产生明显的影响。

利培酮

利培酮对躁狂有效[52]，特别是与心境稳定剂合用时[53,54]。利培酮的长效针剂同样有效[55](需要注意的是，这种剂型的药代动力学特点使它不适用于躁狂发作的急性期治疗)。长效剂型通常用于预防(在大部分国家中是超适应证使用)。在长程治疗中，它可以有效地预防躁狂发作[18]。帕利哌酮被认为具有类似效果。

其他抗精神病药

使用氨磺必利的研究数据较少[56]；齐拉西酮的数据很多[57]，在美国广泛用于治疗躁狂。伊潘立酮可能对混合发作有效[58]，但是还没有足够的数据去支持它的使用。

参考文献

1. ECNP. Neuroscience based nomenclature, 2nd edition. 2017; http://www.nbn2.com.
2. Cipriani A, et al. Comparative efficacy and acceptability of antimanic drugs in acute mania: a multiple-treatments meta-analysis. *Lancet* 2011; 378:1306–1315.
3. Goodwin GM, et al. Evidence-based guidelines for treating bipolar disorder: revised third edition recommendations from the British Association for Psychopharmacology. *J Psychopharmacol* 2016; 30:495–553.
4. Chou JC, et al. Acute mania: haloperidol dose and augmentation with lithium or lorazepam. *J Clin Psychopharmacol* 1999; 19:500–505.
5. Small JG, et al. A placebo-controlled study of lithium combined with neuroleptics in chronic schizophrenic patients. *Am J Psychiatry* 1975; 132:1315–1317.
6. Soares JC, et al. Adjunctive antipsychotic use in bipolar patients: an open 6-month prospective study following an acute episode. *J Affect Disord* 1999; 56:1–8.
7. Keck PE, Jr., et al. Anticonvulsants and antipsychotics in the treatment of bipolar disorder. *J Clin Psychiatry* 1998; 59 Suppl 6:74–81.
8. Tohen M, et al. Antipsychotic agents and bipolar disorder. *J Clin Psychiatry* 1998; 59 Suppl 1:38–48.
9. Zarate CA, Jr., et al. Double-blind comparison of the continued use of antipsychotic treatment versus its discontinuation in remitted manic patients. *Am J Psychiatry* 2004; 161:169–171.
10. Gigante AD, et al. Long-acting injectable antipsychotics for the maintenance treatment of bipolar disorder. *CNS Drugs* 2012; 26:403–420.
11. Goikolea JM, et al. Lower rate of depressive switch following antimanic treatment with second-generation antipsychotics versus haloperidol. *J Affect Disord* 2013; 144:191–198.
12. Yildiz A, et al. A network meta-analysis on comparative efficacy and all-cause discontinuation of antimanic treatments in acute bipolar mania. *Psychol Med* 2015; 45:299–317.
13. Baldessarini RJ, et al. Pharmacological treatment of adult bipolar disorder. *Mol Psychiatry* 2019; 24:198–217.
14. Ogawa Y, et al. Mood stabilizers and antipsychotics for acute mania: a systematic review and meta-analysis of combination/augmentation therapy versus monotherapy. *CNS Drugs* 2014; 28:989–1003.
15. Ashok AH, et al. The dopamine hypothesis of bipolar affective disorder: the state of the art and implications for treatment. *Mol Psychiatry* 2017; 22:666–679.
16. Jauhar S, et al. A test of the transdiagnostic dopamine hypothesis of psychosis using positron emission tomographic imaging in bipolar affective disorder and schizophrenia. *JAMA Psychiatry* 2017; 74:1206–1213.
17. Taylor DM, et al. Comparative efficacy and acceptability of drug treatments for bipolar depression: a multiple-treatments meta-analysis. *Acta*

Psychiatr Scand 2014; 130:452–469.

18. Taylor MJ. Bipolar treatment efficacy. *Lancet Psychiatry* 2014; 1:418.

19. Miura T, et al. Comparative efficacy and tolerability of pharmacological treatments in the maintenance treatment of bipolar disorder: a systematic review and network meta-analysis. *Lancet Psychiatry* 2014; 1:351–359.

20. Sachs G, et al. Aripiprazole in the treatment of acute manic or mixed episodes in patients with bipolar I disorder: a 3-week placebo-controlled study. *J Psychopharmacol* 2006; 20:536–546.

21. Keck PE, et al. Aripiprazole monotherapy in the treatment of acute bipolar I mania: a randomized, double-blind, placebo- and lithium-controlled study. *J Affect Disord* 2009; 112:36–49.

22. Young AH, et al. Aripiprazole monotherapy in acute mania: 12-week randomised placebo- and haloperidol-controlled study. *Brit J Psychiatry* 2009; 194:40–48.

23. Vieta E, et al. Efficacy of adjunctive aripiprazole to either valproate or lithium in bipolar mania patients partially nonresponsive to valproate/lithium monotherapy: a placebo-controlled study. *Am J Psychiatry* 2008; 165:1316–1325.

24. Keck PE, Jr., et al. Aripiprazole monotherapy for maintenance therapy in bipolar I disorder: a 100-week, double-blind study versus placebo. *J Clin Psychiatry* 2007; 68:1480–1491.

25. Vieta E, et al. Assessment of safety, tolerability and effectiveness of adjunctive aripiprazole to lithium/valproate in bipolar mania: a 46-week, open-label extension following a 6-week double-blind study. *Curr Med Res Opin* 2010; 26:1485–1496.

26. Shafti SS. Aripiprazole versus lithium in management of acute mania: a randomized clinical trial. *East Asian Arch Psychiatry* 2018; 28:80–84.

27. Brown R, et al. Aripiprazole alone or in combination for acute mania. *Cochrane Database Syst Rev* 2013; Cd005000.

28. Calabrese JR, et al. Efficacy and safety of aripiprazole once-monthly in the maintenance treatment of bipolar I disorder: a double-blind, placebo-controlled, 52-week randomized withdrawal study. *J Clin Psychiatry* 2017; 78:324–331.

29. McIntyre RS, et al. Asenapine in the treatment of acute mania in bipolar I disorder: a randomized, double-blind, placebo-controlled trial. *J Affect Disord* 2010; 122:27–38.

30. McIntyre RS, et al. Asenapine versus olanzapine in acute mania: a double-blind extension study. *Bipolar Disord* 2009; 11:815–826.

31. McIntyre RS, et al. Asenapine for long-term treatment of bipolar disorder: a double-blind 40-week extension study. *J Affect Disord* 2010; 126:358–365.

32. Szegedi A, et al. Randomized, double-blind, placebo-controlled trial of asenapine maintenance therapy in adults with an acute manic or mixed episode associated with bipolar I disorder. *Am J Psychiatry* 2018; 175:71–79.

33. Pillinger T, et al. Comparative effects of 18 antipsychotics on metabolic function in patients with schizophrenia, predictors of metabolic dysregulation, and association with psychopathology: a systematic review and network meta-analysis. *Lancet Psychiatry* 2020; 7:64–77.

34. McIntyre RS, et al. Cariprazine for the treatment of bipolar mania with mixed features: a post hoc pooled analysis of 3 trials. *J Affect Disord* 2019; 257:600–606.

35. Zarate CA, Jr., et al. Clozapine in severe mood disorders. *J Clin Psychiatry* 1995; 56:411–417.

36. Li XB, et al. Clozapine for treatment-resistant bipolar disorder: a systematic review. *Bipolar Disord* 2015; 17:235–247.

37. Loebel A, et al. Lurasidone monotherapy in the treatment of bipolar I depression: a randomized, double-blind, placebo-controlled study. *Am J Psychiatry* 2014; 171:160–168.

38. Loebel A, et al. Lurasidone as adjunctive therapy with lithium or valproate for the treatment of bipolar I depression: a randomized, double-blind, placebo-controlled study. *Am J Psychiatry* 2014; 171:169–177.

39. Tohen M, et al. Olanzapine versus placebo in the treatment of acute mania. Olanzapine HGEH Study Group. *Am J Psychiatry* 1999; 156:702–709.

40. Tohen M, et al. Efficacy of olanzapine in acute bipolar mania: a double-blind, placebo-controlled study. The Olanzipine HGGW Study Group. *Arch Gen Psychiatry* 2000; 57:841–849.

41. Tohen M, et al. Efficacy of olanzapine in combination with valproate or lithium in the treatment of mania in patients partially nonresponsive to valproate or lithium monotherapy. *Arch Gen Psychiatry* 2002; 59:62–69.

42. Tohen M, et al. Relapse prevention in bipolar I disorder: 18-month comparison of olanzapine plus mood stabiliser v. mood stabiliser alone. *Br J Psychiatry* 2004; 184:337–345.

43. Tohen M, et al. Olanzapine plus carbamazepine v. carbamazepine alone in treating manic episodes. *Br J Psychiatry* 2008; 192:135–143.

44. Sanger TM, et al. Long-term olanzapine therapy in the treatment of bipolar I disorder: an open-label continuation phase study. *J Clin Psychiatry* 2001; 62:273–281.

45. Vieta E, et al. Olanzapine as long-term adjunctive therapy in treatment-resistant bipolar disorder. *J Clin Psychopharmacol* 2001; 21:469–473.

46. Tohen M, et al. Olanzapine versus lithium in the maintenance treatment of bipolar disorder: a 12-month, randomized, double-blind, controlled clinical trial. *Am J Psychiatry* 2005; 162:1281–1290.

47. McKnight RF, et al. Lithium for acute mania. *Cochrane Database Syst Rev* 2019; 6:Cd004048.

48. Ghaemi SN, et al. The use of quetiapine for treatment-resistant bipolar disorder: a case series. *Ann Clin Psychiatry* 1999; 11:137–140.

49. Sachs G, et al. Quetiapine with lithium or divalproex for the treatment of bipolar mania: a randomized, double-blind, placebo-controlled study. *Bipolar Disorders* 2004; 6:213–223.

50. Altamura AC, et al. Efficacy and tolerability of quetiapine in the treatment of bipolar disorder: preliminary evidence from a 12-month open label study. *J Affect Disord* 2003; 76:267–271.

51. Young AH, et al. A randomised, placebo-controlled 52-week trial of continued quetiapine treatment in recently depressed patients with bipolar I and bipolar II disorder. *World J Biol Psychiatry* 2014; 15:96–112.

52. Segal J, et al. Risperidone compared with both lithium and haloperidol in mania: a double-blind randomized controlled trial. *Clin*

Neuropharmacol 1998; 21:176–180.

53. Sachs GS, et al. Combination of a mood stabilizer with risperidone or haloperidol for treatment of acute mania: a double-blind, placebo-controlled comparison of efficacy and safety. *Am J Psychiatry* 2002; 159:1146–1154.

54. Vieta E, et al. Risperidone in the treatment of mania: efficacy and safety results from a large, multicentre, open study in Spain. *J Affect Disord* 2002; 72:15–19.

55. Quiroz JA, et al. Risperidone long-acting injectable monotherapy in the maintenance treatment of bipolar I disorder. *Biol Psychiatry* 2010; 68:156–162.

56. Vieta E, et al. An open-label study of amisulpride in the treatment of mania. *J Clin Psychiatry* 2005; 66:575–578.

57. Vieta E, et al. Ziprasidone in the treatment of acute mania: a 12-week, placebo-controlled, haloperidol-referenced study. *J Psychopharm* 2010; 24:547–558.

58. Singh V, et al. An open trial of iloperidone for mixed episodes in bipolar disorder. *J Clin Psychopharmacol* 2017; 37:615–619.

抗精神病药长效针剂在双相障碍中的应用

长效针剂在双相障碍中广泛使用,但是在英国并没有任何一种长效针剂被正式批准用于该适应证(阿立哌唑长效针剂 Abilify Maintena 在美国被 FDA 批准[1])。支持它们使用的证据仍非常有限:目前已有几十个开放试验和已发表的病例系列,但是大部分研究包含的样本量都较少[2-4]。尽管如此,回顾性队列研究和人群水平研究也提供了一些证据,支持长效针剂(主要是二代抗精神病药,SGA)在双相障碍维持期的使用[2]。相关的 RCT 有 7 个,但仅 5 个有足够的效力得出可解读的结果(剩余两个总共仅包含 30 例样本[5,6])。这 5 个 RCT 代表了长效针剂治疗双相障碍的最高水平证据。它们的细节罗列在表 2.5。

很难从下表中列出的对照试验中得出确凿的结论。利培酮长效针剂无论是单药治疗还是联合用药都有效,但是只对躁狂、轻躁狂、混合躁狂发作产生保护作用,不减少也不增加抑郁复发的风险。利培酮长效针剂可能效果不如口服奥氮平。目前可以认为帕利哌酮长效针剂可能与利培酮长效针剂有相似的效果。口服帕利哌酮可以预防双相障碍的躁狂复发[7],一些病例报告描述了其长效针剂的良好结局[8]。阿立哌唑长效针剂也能预防躁狂复发,似乎对抑郁的风险没有影响。

表 2.5　双相障碍长效针剂随机对照研究

研究	样本量	长效针剂	对照	疗程	结局
Ahlfors et al. 1981[9]	33(19/14)	氟哌噻吨癸酸酯	锂盐	18 个月	两种治疗都不能改善主要结局(心境发作次数)
MacFadden et al.[10]*	124(65/59)	利培酮(辅助)	安慰剂(辅助)	12 个月	利培酮长效针剂的复发率低于安慰剂(RR=2.3)
Quiroz et al.[11]*	303 (154/149)	利培酮单药治疗	安慰剂单药治疗	24 个月	利培酮总体复发率为 30%,安慰剂为 56%。利培酮不能预防抑郁复发
Vieta et al.[12]*	398(132/135/131)	利培酮单药治疗	安慰剂或口服奥氮平单药	18 个月	任何一种心境发作的复发:口服奥氮平为 23.8%,利培酮长效针剂为 38.9%,安慰剂为 56.4%。奥氮平和利培酮都可以减少心境高涨的风险,但只有奥氮平能减少抑郁的风险
Calabrese et al.[13]*	266 (133/133)	阿立哌唑单药治疗	安慰剂单药治疗	12 个月	任何一种心境发作的复发:阿立哌唑为 26.5%,安慰剂为 51.1%。对预防抑郁复发没有明确的效果。该项 RCT 的后续开放研究(也包括了新使用阿立哌唑的患者)显示了更好的保护效果:87%~98% 的患者在 12 个月内未复发[14]

* 试验由制造商赞助。

双相障碍中 FGA 的数据缺乏,并且总体上质量不高(开放试验,病例系列,回顾性分析)。在这些研究中,与先前的治疗相比,FGA 长效针剂似乎可以减少复发的风险。最大的开放试验[9]（n=85）（参考文献 9 报告了两个研究的结果）提示，氟哌噻吨癸酸酯（20mg，每 2~3 周一次）可以减少心境高涨发作的风险。对于其他 FGA 长效针剂，其他报告描述了相似的作用。一项关于氟哌噻吨长效针剂的 RCT[9] 显示其没有效果，相较于锂盐也没有优势。

综合考虑这项 RCT 以及所有的小样本、非对照观察研究，几乎没有证据支持氟哌噻吨长效针剂增加躁狂复发风险，以及氟哌啶醇长效针剂和氟奋乃静长效针剂增加抑郁复发（或者至少由 FGA 引起抑郁）风险的传说。值得注意的是，系统综述的作者[15,16]重复了这个观点，其根据是在 Ahlfors 等的开放研究[9]中观察到抑郁发作增加了。事实上，这种增加只见于研究对象在试验开始时立即停止锂盐治疗的情况下。尽管如此，口服氟哌啶醇治疗躁狂，比口服 SGA 更可能导致转抑郁相[17]，因此在临床运用时显然需要注意。

目前，没有 FGA 和 SGA 长效针剂之间的对照比较[2-4]。一项我国台湾地区的回顾性队列研究[18]发现，相较于利培酮长效针剂，FGA 长效针剂（50% 氟哌噻吨，25% 氟哌啶醇和 25% 其他）组抑郁复发风险更高，住院可能性更大。再住院的危险比为 1.20（95% CI：1.04~1.38），利培酮再住院率为 0.42，而 FGA 为 0.51。特别注意，治疗中止率很高。在 1 年时，开始时使用利培酮长效针剂者中只有 7.2%、开始时使用 FGA 长效针剂者中只有 2.2% 还在继续原来的治疗。

结论

- 支持 FGA 长效针剂用于双相障碍的证据很弱。
- 非常有限的证据指出，FGA 长效针剂可能在降低躁狂/轻躁狂复发方面有效，但是它们不能预防抑郁的复发，并可能增加其风险。
- 利培酮长效针剂和阿立哌唑长效针剂与安慰剂相比，与减少躁狂/轻躁狂复发风险强烈相关。
- 没有证据表明 SGA 增加抑郁风险。
- 利培酮长效针剂和阿立哌唑长效针剂对抑郁复发的风险没有作用。
- 在双相障碍维持期治疗中，没有证据支持长效针剂相较于口服抗精神病药治疗更有优势。
- 与其他疾病一样，使用长效针剂的优点是依从性明确：长效针剂或者注射了，或者没有注射。

参考文献

1. MDedge Psychiatry. Abilify Maintena OK'd by FDA for adults with bipolar I disorder. 2017; https://www.mdedge.com/psychiatry/article/143846/bipolar-disorder/abilify-maintena-okd-fda-adults-bipolar-i-disorder?sso=true.
2. Keramatian K, et al. Long-acting injectable second-generation/atypical antipsychotics for the management of bipolar disorder: a systematic review. CNS Drugs 2019; 33:431–456.
3. Pacchiarotti I, et al. Long-acting injectable antipsychotics (LAIs) for maintenance treatment of bipolar and schizoaffective disorders: a systematic review. Eur Neuropsychopharmacol 2019; 29:457–470.
4. Prajapati AR, et al. Second-generation antipsychotic long-acting injections in bipolar disorder: systematic review and meta-analysis. Bipolar Disorders 2018; 20:687–696.
5. Esparon J, et al. Comparison of the prophylactic action of flupenthixol with placebo in lithium treated manic-depressive patients. Br J Psychiatry 1986; 148:723–725.
6. Yatham L, et al. Randomised trial of oral vs. injectable antipsychotics in bipolar disorder. Presented at the 6th International Conference on Bipolar Disorder: June 16–18 2005, Pittsburgh, PA; 2005.
7. Berwaerts J, et al. A randomized, placebo- and active-controlled study of paliperidone extended-release as maintenance treatment in patients with bipolar I disorder after an acute manic or mixed episode. J Affect Disord 2012; 138:247–258.
8. Buoli M, et al. Paliperidone palmitate depot in the long-term treatment of psychotic bipolar disorder: a case series. Clin Neuropharmacol

2015; 38:209–211.

9. Ahlfors UG, et al. Flupenthixol decanoate in recurrent manic-depressive illness. A comparison with lithium. *Acta Psychiatr Scand* 1981; **64**:226–237.

10. Macfadden W, et al. A randomized, double-blind, placebo-controlled study of maintenance treatment with adjunctive risperidone long-acting therapy in patients with bipolar I disorder who relapse frequently. *Bipolar Disord* 2009; **11**:827–839.

11. Quiroz JA, et al. Risperidone long-acting injectable monotherapy in the maintenance treatment of bipolar I disorder. *Biol Psychiatry* 2010; **68**:156–162.

12. Vieta E, et al. A randomized, double-blind, placebo-controlled trial to assess prevention of mood episodes with risperidone long-acting injectable in patients with bipolar I disorder. *Eur Neuropsychopharmacol* 2012; **22**:825–835.

13. Calabrese JR, et al. Efficacy and safety of aripiprazole once-monthly in the maintenance treatment of bipolar I disorder: a double-blind, placebo-controlled, 52-week randomized withdrawal study. *J Clin Psychiatry* 2017; **78**:324–331.

14. Calabrese JR, et al. Aripiprazole once-monthly as maintenance treatment for bipolar I disorder: a 52-week, multicenter, open-label study. *Int J Bipolar Disord* 2018; **6**:14.

15. Bond DJ, et al. Depot antipsychotic medications in bipolar disorder: a review of the literature. *Acta Psychiatr Scand Suppl* 2007; **116**: 3–16.

16. Gigante AD, et al. Long-acting injectable antipsychotics for the maintenance treatment of bipolar disorder. *CNS Drugs* 2012; **26**:403–420.

17. Goikolea JM, et al. Lower rate of depressive switch following antimanic treatment with second-generation antipsychotics versus haloperidol. *J Affect Disord* 2013; **144**:191–198.

18. Wu CS, et al. Comparative effectiveness of long-acting injectable risperidone vs. long-acting injectable first-generation antipsychotics in bipolar disorder. *J Affect Disord* 2016; **197**:189–195.

第 2 章

第 2 章

双相障碍患者的躯体指标监测 [1,2]

监测项目	所有患者		根据特定药物额外补充			
	基线	每年复查	抗精神病药	锂盐	丙戊酸盐	卡马西平
甲状腺功能	√	√		在基线和之后每 6 个月；出现异常常需要更加频繁		
肝功能 (LFT)	√	√			第一年每 3 个月复查一次，之后每年	前 3 个月每月复查，之后每年
肾功能 (eGFR)	√	√		在基线和之后每 6 个月；出现恶化迹象或者开始服用相互作用的药物时，需要更加频繁		
电解质、尿素、肌酐 (EUC)	√	√		在基线和之后每 3~6 个月 (包括血清钙)		前 3 个月每月复查，之后每年
血常规 (FBC)	√	√		只在临床需要时	第一年每 3 个月复查一次，之后每年	
血糖	√	√作为例行体检的一部分	在最初服药时和之后每 4~6 个月复查 (奥氮平还需要在 1 个月时复查)；出现血糖升高后需要更加频繁复查			
血脂	√	√作为例行体检的一部分	在最开始和 3 个月时；出现血脂升高需要更加频繁复查			
血压、脉搏	√	√作为例行体检的一部分	右所用抗精神病药与直立性低血压相关，需要在增加剂量期间复查			

续表

监测项目	所有患者		根据特定药物额外补充			
	基线	每年复查	抗精神病药	锂盐	丙戊酸盐	卡马西平
催乳素	只有儿童和青少年需要		在基线和出现催乳素升高的症状时。催乳素升高不太可能出现在喹硫平和阿立哌唑。极偶然出现在奥氮平和阿塞那平。在利培酮和 FGA 中很常见			
心电图	有心血管病或危险因素时		如果有心血管病或危险因素时(或者使用氟哌啶醇)需要在基线监测。如果检测到相关异常,每次增加剂量都应复查心电图	若有心血管病或危险因素,需要在基线监测。如果检测到相关异常,每次增加剂量都应复查心电图		若有心血管病或危险因素,需要在基线监测。若检测到相关异常,每次增加剂量都应复查心电图
腰围或 BMI	√	√ 作为例行体检的一部分	前三个月每个月复查,之后每年	在基线,之后每 6 个月复查,之后每 1 次	第一年每 3 个月复查 1 次,之后每年	在基线,和患者体重快速增加时需要
血药浓度				在初始用药后至少 3~4 天复查,在每次复查,在每次调整剂量后 3~4 天复查,直到血药浓度稳定,之后每一年第一个 3 个月复查 1 次,对大部分患者来说每 6 个月复查一次(见 NICE[2])	根据疗效和耐受性逐步加药。不需要定期检测,除非有效果不佳或中毒的证据	初始用药后两周和每次剂量调整后两周,之后不需要定期检测,除非有疗效不佳、中毒的证据

注:对于使用拉莫三嗪的患者,每年做一次健康检查,不需要其他特殊监测;但是血药浓度可能表明是否可以考虑使用更大剂量。

参考文献

1. Ng F, et al. The International Society for Bipolar Disorders (ISBD) consensus guidelines for the safety monitoring of bipolar disorder treatments. *Bipolar Disord* 2009; 11:559–595.
2. National Institute for Health and Care Excellence. Bipolar disorder: assessment and management. Clinical Guidance [CG185]. 2014 (Last updated February 2020); https://www.nice.org.uk/guidance/cg185.

躁狂或轻躁狂的急性期治疗

药物治疗是躁狂和轻躁狂的主要治疗。抗精神病药和心境稳定剂均有效(尽管这种命名毫无意义,大多数或可能全部抗精神病药具有抗躁狂作用,大多数心境稳定剂能减少躁狂症的精神病性症状)。镇静和抗焦虑药(如苯二氮䓬类药物)可以为这些药物增效。

由于缺乏直接比较研究的证据,难以做出药物选择,从疗效角度不能只推荐一种药物,而不推荐另一种药物。然而,一项多种治疗荟萃分析(允许间接比较)结果显示,奥氮平、利培酮、氟哌啶醇和喹硫平的疗效和可接受性综合优势明显[1]。Cochrane 系统分析提示,单用奥氮平的疗效优于锂盐[2]和丙戊酸盐[3]。奥氮平疗效也可能优于阿塞那平[4]。

抗精神病药与心境稳定剂合用(与心境稳定剂单用相比),对于服用心境稳定剂时复发者明确有益,但是对于未治疗过的患者则疗效不太清楚[5-9]。现有最新国际指南[29]提示,与单药治疗相比,联合治疗"往往起效更快","有效率高 20%"。相反,澳大利亚和新西兰的指南提出,首先试用一种抗精神病药,只有在"单药治疗疗效不足"时,再加用一种心境稳定剂[30]。在实践中,往往有强烈的倾向一开始就采用联合治疗。

该流程图概括了躁狂和轻躁狂的治疗策略(图 2.1)。这些建议基于英国 NICE 指南[6]、英国精神药理学会指南[31]以及引用的个别参考文献。若建议使用抗精神病药,应从批准用于治疗躁狂或双相障碍的药物中选择,即大多数传统药物,包括阿立哌唑、阿塞那平、奥氮平、利培酮和喹硫平。推荐剂量和替代治疗概括在表 2.6 和表 2.7 中。

停止抗抑郁药治疗

患者是否正在使用抗躁狂药*?

否

可以考虑:
一种抗精神病药(如果症状严重或行为紊乱)
或
丙戊酸盐(避免用于育龄妇女)
或
锂盐(如果未来依从性好)
如果疗效不充分:
抗精神药物合并丙戊酸盐或锂盐
所有患者——考虑短期加用苯二氮䓬类药物[21-23]
(劳拉西泮或氯硝西泮)

是

若在用抗精神病药,检查依从性和剂量,必要时增加剂量。可以考虑增加锂盐或丙戊酸盐
若在用锂盐**,测定血浆水平,考虑增加剂量使浓度达到1.0~1.2mmol/L(治疗急性发作),和/或增加一种抗精神病药
若在用丙戊酸盐,检查血浆水平[7,8,24,25],若能耐受,增加剂量,使血药浓度最高达到 125mg/L。考虑加用一种抗精神病药
若在用锂盐或丙戊酸盐,且躁狂严重,检测血药浓度,加用一种抗精神病药[5]
若在用卡马西平,考虑加用抗精神病药(由于抗精神病药浓度下降,可能需要更高的剂量)
所有患者——考虑短期增加苯二氮䓬类药物[21-23]
(劳拉西泮或氯硝西泮)

* 此处抗躁狂药 = 抗精神病药或心境稳定剂。
** 锂盐对于混合状态[26]、物质滥用[27]、快速循环或伴精神病性症状者疗效相对较差[28]。

图 2.1 躁狂或轻躁狂急性期治疗[5-20]

表 2.6　躁狂症的药物治疗:推荐剂量

药物	剂量
锂盐	起始剂量 400mg/d,根据血锂浓度,每隔 3~4 天增加剂量 至少一项研究使用 800mg 作为起始剂量 [32]
丙戊酸盐	**丙戊酸半钠**:250mg,每天 3 次,根据耐受性及血药浓度增加剂量。丙戊酸半钠缓释片 15~30mg/kg 也可能有效 [33],但有一项研究结果为阴性 [34] **丙戊酸钠缓释剂**:500mg/d 起始,按上述方法加量 曾用过更高的所谓负荷剂量,口服 [35-37] 和静脉注射 [38-39] 均有。剂量为 20~30mg/(kg·d) 一项纳入 13 个研究的综述提示,静脉注射丙戊酸盐负荷治疗是有效、安全和耐受性好的治疗方法 [40]
阿立哌唑	15mg/d,根据需要增加到 30mg/d [41],剂量低于 15mg/d 可能无效 [42]
阿塞那平	5mg,每天 2 次,根据需要增加到 10mg,每天 2 次
卡利拉嗪	3mg/d,根据需要增加到 12mg/d [43]
奥氮平	10mg/d,根据需要增加到 15~20mg/d
利培酮	2~3mg/d,根据需要增加到 6mg/d 帕利哌酮治疗躁狂症的证据不足 [44]
喹硫平	**速释剂型**:100mg/d,根据需要增加到 800mg/d。也有更高的起始剂量 [45] **缓释剂型**:300mg/d 开始,第 2 天增加至 600mg/d
氟哌啶醇	5~10mg/d,根据需要增加到 15mg/d
劳拉西泮 [22,23]	最高至 4mg/d(有些中心使用更高的剂量)
氯硝西泮 [21,23]	最高至 8mg/d

表 2.7　躁狂症其他可选治疗
原文以字母顺序排列,不是按照优先推荐排序。选择所列任何治疗前,应咨询专家并阅读原始文献

治疗	说明
别嘌醇 [34] (300~600mg/d)	一项纳入 5 个别嘌醇增效治疗研究的荟萃分析发现效应值小于 0.3 [46]
塞来昔布 (400mg/d) [47]	小样本 RCT(n=46)提示塞来昔布作为丙戊酸盐的增效治疗有益
氯氮平 [48-50]	对于难治性躁狂症或双相障碍是明确的治疗选择。可以快速加量 [51]
依布硒 [52]	抑制肌醇单磷酸酶(类似于锂盐)。有初步证据
加巴喷丁 [53-55] (最多 2.4g/d)	可能仅因抗焦虑作用而有效。很少使用。可能对预防有用 [56]
左乙拉西坦 [57,58] (最高 4 000mg/d)	可能有效,但需对照研究验证。有一例诱发躁狂的报道 [59]
美金刚 [60](10~30mg/d)	证据不一致 [61-63]
褪黑素 6mg/d [64]	初步证据作为增效治疗有益。一个小样本研究得出阴性结果 [65]

续表

治疗	说明
奥卡西平 [66-72]（300~3 000mg/d）	急性期治疗和预防可能有效,但是在年轻患者中进行的一项对照研究结果是阴性的 [73]
苯妥英 [74]（300~400mg/d）	很少使用,数据有限 药代动力学复杂,且治疗窗狭窄
利坦色林 [75]（10mg/d）	一项 RCT 支持。耐受性好。可避免锥体外系反应
他莫昔芬 [76]（20~140mg/d）	可能有效。五项小样本 RCT。量效关系不明确。好的证据支持增效或单药治疗有效,效应值大
托吡酯 [77]（最大剂量 300mg/d）	可能无效,比锂盐效果差 [2]
色氨酸耗竭 [78]	一项小样本 RCT 研究支持
齐拉西酮 [79-81]	三项 RCT 研究支持。在英国以外广泛使用

参考文献

1. Cipriani A, et al. Comparative efficacy and acceptability of antimanic drugs in acute mania: a multiple-treatments meta-analysis. *Lancet* 2011; 378:1306–1315.

2. McKnight RF, et al. Lithium for acute mania. *Cochrane Database Syst Rev* 2019; 6:Cd004048.

3. Jochim J, et al. Valproate for acute mania. *Cochrane Database Syst Rev* 2019; 10:Cd004052.

4. Mahajan V, et al. Efficacy and safety of asenapine versus olanzapine in combination with divalproex for acute mania: a randomized controlled trial. *J Clin Psychopharmacol* 2019; 39:305–311.

5. Smith LA, et al. Acute bipolar mania: a systematic review and meta-analysis of co-therapy vs. monotherapy. *Acta Psychiatr Scand* 2007; 115:12–20.

6. National Institute for Health and Care Excellence. Bipolar disorder: assessment and management. Clinical Guidance [CG185]. 2014 (Last updated February 2020); https://www.nice.org.uk/guidance/cg185.

7. Goodwin GM. Evidence-based guidelines for treating bipolar disorder: revised second edition–recommendations from the British Association for Psychopharmacology. *J Psychopharmacol* 2009; 23:346–388.

8. American Psychiatric Association. Guideline watch: practice guideline for the treatment of patients with bipolar disorder, 2nd edition. Washington, DC: American Psychiatric Association; 2005. doi:10.1176/appi.books.9780890423363.148430.

9. Sachs GS. Decision tree for the treatment of bipolar disorder. *J Clin Psychiatry* 2003; 64 Suppl 8:35–40.

10. Tohen M, et al. A 12-week, double-blind comparison of olanzapine vs haloperidol in the treatment of acute mania. *Arch Gen Psychiatry* 2003; 60:1218–1226.

11. Baldessarini RJ, et al. Olanzapine versus placebo in acute mania treatment responses in subgroups. *J Clin Psychopharmacol* 2003; 23:370–376.

12. Sachs G, et al. Quetiapine with lithium or divalproex for the treatment of bipolar mania: a randomized, double-blind, placebo-controlled study. *Bipolar Disord* 2004; 6:213–223.

13. Yatham LN, et al. Quetiapine versus placebo in combination with lithium or divalproex for the treatment of bipolar mania. *J Clin Psychopharmacol* 2004; 24:599–606.

14. Yatham LN, et al. Risperidone plus lithium versus risperidone plus valproate in acute and continuation treatment of mania. *Int Clin Psychopharmacol* 2004; 19:103–109.

15. Bowden CL, et al. Risperidone in combination with mood stabilizers: a 10-week continuation phase study in bipolar I disorder. *J Clin Psychiatry* 2004; 65:707–714.

16. Hirschfeld RM, et al. Rapid antimanic effect of risperidone monotherapy: a 3-week multicenter, double-blind, placebo-controlled trial. *Am J Psychiatry* 2004; 161:1057–1065.

17. Bowden CL, et al. A randomized, double-blind, placebo-controlled efficacy and safety study of quetiapine or lithium as monotherapy for mania in bipolar disorder. *J Clin Psychiatry* 2005; 66:111–121.

18. Khanna S, et al. Risperidone in the treatment of acute mania: double-blind, placebo-controlled study. *Br J Psychiatry* 2005; 187:229–234.

19. Young RC, et al. GERI-BD: a randomized double-blind controlled trial of lithium and divalproex in the treatment of mania in older patients with bipolar disorder. *Am J Psychiatry* 2017; 174:1086–1093.

20. Conus P, et al. Olanzapine or chlorpromazine plus lithium in first episode psychotic mania: an 8-week randomised controlled trial. *Eur Psychiatry* 2015; 30:975–982.

21. Sachs GS, et al. Adjunctive clonazepam for maintenance treatment of bipolar affective disorder. *J Clin Psychopharmacol* 1990; **10**:42–47.

22. Modell JG, et al. Inpatient clinical trial of lorazepam for the management of manic agitation. *J Clin Psychopharmacol* 1985; **5**:109–113.

23. Curtin F, et al. Clonazepam and lorazepam in acute mania: a Bayesian meta-analysis. *J Affect Disord* 2004; **78**:201–208.

24. Taylor D, et al. Doses of carbamazepine and valproate in bipolar affective disorder. *Psychiatric Bull* 1997; **21**:221–223.

25. Allen MH, et al. Linear relationship of valproate serum concentration to response and optimal serum levels for acute mania. *Am J Psychiatry* 2006; **163**:272–275.

26. Swann AC, et al. Lithium treatment of mania: clinical characteristics, specificity of symptom change, and outcome. *Psychiatry Res* 1986; **18**:127–141.

27. Goldberg JF, et al. A history of substance abuse complicates remission from acute mania in bipolar disorder. *J Clin Psychiatry* 1999; **60**:733–740.

28. Hui TP, et al. A systematic review and meta-analysis of clinical predictors of lithium response in bipolar disorder. *Acta Psychiatr Scand* 2019; **140**:94–115.

29. Yatham LN, et al. Canadian Network for Mood and Anxiety Treatments (CANMAT) and International Society for Bipolar Disorders (ISBD) 2018 guidelines for the management of patients with bipolar disorder. *Bipolar Disord* 2018; **20**:97–170.

30. Malhi GS, et al. The 2020 Royal Australian and New Zealand College of Psychiatrists Clinical Practice Guidelines for mood disorders: bipolar disorder summary. *Bipolar Disord* 2020. **22**:805–821.

31. Goodwin GM, et al. Evidence-based guidelines for treating bipolar disorder: revised third edition recommendations from the British Association for Psychopharmacology. *J Psychopharmacol* 2016; **30**:495–553.

32. Bowden CL, et al. Efficacy of valproate versus lithium in mania or mixed mania: a randomized, open 12-week trial. *Int Clin Psychopharmacol* 2010; **25**:60–67.

33. McElroy SL, et al. Randomized, double-blind, placebo-controlled study of divalproex extended release loading monotherapy in ambulatory bipolar spectrum disorder patients with moderate-to-severe hypomania or mild mania. *J Clin Psychiatry* 2010; **71**:557–565.

34. Hirschfeld RM, et al. A randomized, placebo-controlled, multicenter study of divalproex sodium extended-release in the acute treatment of mania. *J Clin Psychiatry* 2010; **71**:426–432.

35. McElroy SL, et al. A randomized comparison of divalproex oral loading versus haloperidol in the initial treatment of acute psychotic mania. *J Clin Psychiatry* 1996; **57**:142–146.

36. Hirschfeld RM, et al. Safety and tolerability of oral loading divalproex sodium in acutely manic bipolar patients. *J Clin Psychiatry* 1999; **60**:815–818.

37. Hirschfeld RM, et al. The safety and early efficacy of oral-loaded divalproex versus standard-titration divalproex, lithium, olanzapine, and placebo in the treatment of acute mania associated with bipolar disorder. *J Clin Psychiatry* 2003; **64**:841–846.

38. Jagadheesan K, et al. Acute antimanic efficacy and safety of intravenous valproate loading therapy: an open-label study. *Neuropsychobiology* 2003; **47**:90–93.

39. Sekhar S, et al. Efficacy of sodium valproate and haloperidol in the management of acute mania: a randomized open-label comparative study. *J Clin Pharmacol* 2010; **50**:688–692.

40. Fontana E, et al. Intravenous valproate in the treatment of acute manic episode in bipolar disorder: a review. *J Affect Disord* 2020; **260**:738–743.

41. Li DJ, et al. Efficacy, safety and tolerability of aripiprazole in bipolar disorder: an updated systematic review and meta-analysis of randomized controlled trials. *Prog Neuropsychopharmacol Biol Psychiatry* 2017; **79**:289–301.

42. Romeo B, et al. Meta-analysis and review of dopamine agonists in acute episodes of mood disorder: efficacy and safety. *J Psychopharmacol* 2018; **32**:385–396.

43. Vieta E, et al. Effect of cariprazine across the symptoms of mania in bipolar I disorder: analyses of pooled data from phase II/III trials. *Eur Neuropsychopharmacol* 2015; **25**:1882–1891.

44. Chang HY, et al. The efficacy and tolerability of paliperidone in mania of bipolar disorder: a preliminary meta-analysis. *Exp Clin Psychopharmacol* 2017; **25**:422–433.

45. Pajonk FG, et al. Rapid dose titration of quetiapine for the treatment of acute schizophrenia and acute mania: a case series. *J Psychopharmacol* 2006; **20**:119–124.

46. Chen AT, et al. Allopurinol augmentation in acute mania: a meta-analysis of placebo-controlled trials. *J Affect Disord* 2018; **226**:245–250.

47. Arabzadeh S, et al. Celecoxib adjunctive therapy for acute bipolar mania: a randomized, double-blind, placebo-controlled trial. *Bipolar Disord* 2015; **17**:606–614.

48. Mahmood T, et al. Clozapine in the management of bipolar and schizoaffective manic episodes resistant to standard treatment. *Aust N Z J Psychiatry* 1997; **31**:424–426.

49. Green AI, et al. Clozapine in the treatment of refractory psychotic mania. *Am J Psychiatry* 2000; **157**:982–986.

50. Ifteni P, et al. Switching bipolar disorder patients treated with clozapine to another antipsychotic medication: a mirror image study. *Neuropsychiatr Dis Treat* 2017; **13**:201–204.

51. Aksoy Poyraz C, et al. Effectiveness of ultra-rapid dose titration of clozapine for treatment-resistant bipolar mania: case series. *Ther Adv Psychopharmacol* 2015; **5**:237–242.

52. Sharpley AL, et al. A phase 2a randomised, double-blind, placebo-controlled, parallel-group, add-on clinical trial of ebselen (SPI-1005) as a novel treatment for mania or hypomania. *Psychopharmacology (Berl)* 2020; **237**:3773–3782.

53. Macdonald KJ, et al. Newer antiepileptic drugs in bipolar disorder: rationale for use and role in therapy. *CNS Drugs* 2002; **16**:549–562.

54. Cabras PL, et al. Clinical experience with gabapentin in patients with bipolar or schizoaffective disorder: results of an open-label study. *J Clin Psychiatry* 1999; **60**:245–248.

55. Pande AC, et al. Gabapentin in bipolar disorder: a placebo-controlled trial of adjunctive therapy. Gabapentin Bipolar Disorder Study Group.

Bipolar Disord 2000; **2 (3 Pt 2):**249–255.

56. Vieta E, et al. A double-blind, randomized, placebo-controlled, prophylaxis study of adjunctive gabapentin for bipolar disorder. *J Clin Psychiatry* 2006; 67:473–477.

57. Grunze H, et al. Levetiracetam in the treatment of acute mania: an open add-on study with an on-off-on design. *J Clin Psychiatry* 2003; 64:781–784.

58. Goldberg JF, et al. Levetiracetam for acute mania (Letter). *Am J Psychiatry* 2002; **159:**148.

59. Park EM, et al. Acute mania associated with levetiracetam treatment. *Psychosomatics* 2014; **55:**98–100.

60. Koukopoulos A, et al. Antimanic and mood-stabilizing effect of memantine as an augmenting agent in treatment-resistant bipolar disorder. *Bipolar Disord* 2010; 12:348–349.

61. Veronese N, et al. Acetylcholinesterase inhibitors and memantine in bipolar disorder: a systematic review and best evidence synthesis of the efficacy and safety for multiple disease dimensions. *J Affect Disord* 2016; 197:268–280.

62. Serra G, et al. Three-year, naturalistic, mirror-image assessment of adding memantine to the treatment of 30 treatment-resistant patients with bipolar disorder. *J Clin Psychiatry* 2015; 76:e91–e97.

63. Omranifard V, et al. Evaluation of the effect of memantine supplementation in the treatment of acute phase of mania in bipolar disorder of elderly patients: a double-blind randomized controlled trial. *Adv Biomed Res* 2018; 7:148.

64. Moghaddam HS, et al. Efficacy of melatonin as an adjunct in the treatment of acute mania: a double-blind and placebo-controlled trial. *Int Clin Psychopharmacol* 2020; 35:81–88.

65. Quested DJ, et al. Melatonin in acute mania investigation (MIAMI-UK). A randomized controlled trial of add-on melatonin in bipolar disorder. *Bipolar Disord* 2021; 23:176–185

66. Benedetti A, et al. Oxcarbazepine as add-on treatment in patients with bipolar manic, mixed or depressive episode. *J Affect Disord* 2004; 79:273–277.

67. Lande RG. Oxcarbazepine: efficacy, safety, and tolerability in the treatment of mania. *Int J Psychiatry Clin Pract* 2004; 8:37–40.

68. Ghaemi SN, et al. Oxcarbazepine treatment of bipolar disorder. *J Clin Psychiatry* 2003; 64:943–945.

69. Pratoomsri W, et al. Oxcarbazepine in the treatment of bipolar disorder: a review. *Can J Psychiatry* 2006; 51:540–545.

70. Juruena MF, et al. Bipolar I and II disorder residual symptoms: oxcarbazepine and carbamazepine as add-on treatment to lithium in a double-blind, randomized trial. *Prog Neuropsychopharmacol Biol Psychiatry* 2009; 33:94–99.

71. Suppes T, et al. Comparison of two anticonvulsants in a randomized, single-blind treatment of hypomanic symptoms in patients with bipolar disorder. *Aust N Z J Psychiatry* 2007; 41:397–402.

72. Vieta E, et al. A double-blind, randomized, placebo-controlled prophylaxis trial of oxcarbazepine as adjunctive treatment to lithium in the long-term treatment of bipolar I and II disorder. *Int J Neuropsychopharmacol* 2008; 11:445–452.

73. Wagner KD, et al. A double-blind, randomized, placebo-controlled trial of oxcarbazepine in the treatment of bipolar disorder in children and adolescents. *Am J Psychiatry* 2006; 163:1179–1186.

74. Mishory A, et al. Phenytoin as an antimanic anticonvulsant: a controlled study. *Am J Psychiatry* 2000; 157:463–465.

75. Akhondzadeh S, et al. Ritanserin as an adjunct to lithium and haloperidol for the treatment of medication-naive patients with acute mania: a double blind and placebo controlled trial. *BMC Psychiatry* 2003; 3:7.

76. Palacios J, et al. Tamoxifen for bipolar disorder: systematic review and meta-analysis. *J Psychopharmacol* 2019; 33:177–184.

77. Pigott K, et al. Topiramate for acute affective episodes in bipolar disorder in adults. *Cochrane Database Syst Rev* 2016.

78. Applebaum J, et al. Rapid tryptophan depletion as a treatment for acute mania: a double-blind, pilot-controlled study. *Bipolar Disord* 2007; 9:884–887.

79. Keck PE, Jr., et al. Ziprasidone in the treatment of acute bipolar mania: a three-week, placebo-controlled, double-blind, randomized trial. *Am J Psychiatry* 2003; 160:741–748.

80. Potkin SG, et al. Ziprasidone in acute bipolar mania: a 21-day randomized, double-blind, placebo-controlled replication trial. *J Clin Psychopharmacol* 2005; 25:301–310.

81. Vieta E, et al. Ziprasidone in the treatment of acute mania: a 12-week, placebo-controlled, haloperidol-referenced study. *J Psychopharm* 2010; 24:547–558.

快速循环型双相障碍

快速循环型双相障碍通常被定义为,在 12 个月内至少有 4 次(轻)躁狂或抑郁发作(或 4 次清晰的转相)的双相障碍。一般认为,它对药物治疗的反应不如非快速循环型[1,2],且具有更多的抑郁发作和更高的自杀风险[3]。有无快速循环发作双相障碍患者的重要临床区别包括更多的抑郁发作、焦虑障碍发生率高、成瘾、贪食、边缘性人格障碍,非典型特征的抑郁,以及易激惹、危险行为、冲动、激越等症状。与非快速循环型相比,快速循环型患者功能较差,肥胖较多,需要更多的药物治疗[4]。快速循环发作患者往往比其他双相障碍患者需要更高的药物剂量[5]。

表 2.8 列出了快速循环型的药物治疗策略,其依据是非常有限的数据,以及少数药物直接对比研究[6,7]。此治疗策略与已发表的两篇系统综述的结果基本一致[7,8]。2016 年 NICE 指南声称,没有证据支持快速循环型的治疗与比较经典的发作类型不同[9]。目前,没有正式的一线药物或联合治疗——处方部分取决于已经用过什么治疗来预防或治疗心境发作。有证据显示,锂盐治疗快速循环型的疗效不如非快速循环型[44],精神科医师的经验也支持这个观点[45]。

在临床上,治疗效果有时存在个体特异性:患者可能仅对某一种或两种药物有明显反应。约有 1/3 的快速循环型患者可自行缓解或经药物治疗缓解[46],但许多患者可能反复发作[47]。

表 2.8　快速循环型双相障碍的治疗建议

步骤	建议的治疗
步骤 1	所有患者**停用抗抑郁药**[10-14] (一些有争议的证据支持继续使用 SSRI[15,16])
步骤 2	**评估可能的诱因,**如酒精、甲状腺功能紊乱(包括抗甲状腺抗体[17])、外源性应激[2]
步骤 3	**优化心境稳定剂治疗**[18-21](依据血药浓度),和**考虑合用两种心境稳定剂**,如锂盐 + 丙戊酸盐,锂盐 + 拉莫三嗪,丙戊酸盐 + 卡马西平,或转到步骤 4
步骤 4	**考虑其他治疗方案(通常是增效治疗)**(按字母顺序排列,黑体字为优先的治疗选择) 阿立哌唑[22,23](15~30mg/d) 氯氮平[24](常规剂量) 拉莫三嗪[25-27](最大剂量 225mg/d) 左乙拉西坦[28](最大剂量 2 000mg/d) 尼莫地平[29,30](180mg/d) **奥氮平**[18](常规剂量) **喹硫平**[31-34](300~600mg/d) 利培酮[35-37](最大剂量 6mg/d) 甲状腺素[38-40](150~400μg/d) 托吡酯[41](最大剂量 300mg/d)

注:根据患者特点选择药物——目前可以指导药物选择的疗效比较的数据极少。**喹硫平**可能证据最充分[31-33],但没有证据显示其优于阿立哌唑或奥氮平。左乙拉西坦、尼莫地平、甲状腺素和托吡酯的支持数据均很有限。

氯氮平在难治性双相障碍(可能包括快速循环型)中地位明确[42],在急性期和长期治疗均有效[24,43]。

参考文献

1. Calabrese JR, et al. Current research on rapid cycling bipolar disorder and its treatment. *J Affect Disord* 2001; **67**:241–255.
2. Kupka RW, et al. Rapid and non-rapid cycling bipolar disorder: a meta-analysis of clinical studies. *J Clin Psychiatry* 2003; **64**:1483–1494.
3. Coryell W, et al. The long-term course of rapid-cycling bipolar disorder. *Arch Gen Psychiatry* 2003; **60**:914–920.
4. Furio M, et al. Characterization of rapid cycling bipolar patients presenting with major depressive episode within the BRIDGE-II-MIX study. *Bipolar Disord* 2020. [Epub ahead of print].
5. Yasui-Furukori N, et al. Factors Associated with Doses of Mood Stabilizers in Real-world Outpatients with Bipolar Disorder. *Clin Psychopharmacol Neurosci* 2020; **18**:599–606.
6. Tondo L, et al. Rapid-cycling bipolar disorder: effects of long-term treatments. *Acta Psychiatr Scand* 2003; **108**:4–14.
7. Fountoulakis KN, et al. A systematic review of the evidence on the treatment of rapid cycling bipolar disorder. *Bipolar Disord* 2013; **15**:115–137.
8. Fountoulakis KN, et al. The international college of neuro-psychopharmacology (CINP) treatment guidelines for bipolar disorder in adults (CINP-BD-2017), Part 2: review, grading of the evidence, and a Precise Algorithm. *Int J Neuropsychopharmacol* 2017; **20**:121–179.
9. National Institute for Health and Care Excellence. Bipolar disorder: assessment and management. Clinical Guidance [CG185]. 2014 (Last updated February 2020); https://www.nice.org.uk/guidance/cg185.
10. Wehr TA, et al. Can antidepressants cause mania and worsen the course of affective illness? *Am J Psychiatry* 1987; **144**:1403–1411.
11. Altshuler LL, et al. Antidepressant-induced mania and cycle acceleration: a controversy revisited. *Am J Psychiatry* 1995; **152**:1130–1138.
12. Ghaemi SN, et al. Antidepressant discontinuation in bipolar depression: a Systematic Treatment Enhancement Program for Bipolar Disorder (STEP-BD) randomized clinical trial of long-term effectiveness and safety. *J Clin Psychiatry* 2010; **71**:372–380.
13. Ghaemi SN. Treatment of rapid-cycling bipolar disorder: are antidepressants mood destabilizers? *Am J Psychiatry* 2008; **165**:300–302.
14. El-Mallakh RS, et al. Antidepressants worsen rapid-cycling course in bipolar depression: a STEP-BD randomized clinical trial. *J Affect Disord* 2015; **184**:318–321.
15. Amsterdam JD, et al. Efficacy and mood conversion rate during long-term fluoxetine v. lithium monotherapy in rapid- and non-rapid-cycling bipolar II disorder. *Br J Psychiatry* 2013; **202**:301–306.
16. Amsterdam JD, et al. Effectiveness and mood conversion rate of short-term fluoxetine monotherapy in patients with rapid cycling bipolar II depression versus patients with nonrapid cycling bipolar II depression. *J Clin Psychopharmacol* 2013; **33**:420–424.
17. Gan Z, et al. Rapid cycling bipolar disorder is associated with antithyroid antibodies, instead of thyroid dysfunction. *BMC Psychiatry* 2019; **19**:378.
18. Sanger TM, et al. Olanzapine in the acute treatment of bipolar I disorder with a history of rapid cycling. *J Affect Disord* 2003; **73**:155–161.
19. Kemp DE, et al. A 6-month, double-blind, maintenance trial of lithium monotherapy versus the combination of lithium and divalproex for rapid-cycling bipolar disorder and Co-occurring substance abuse or dependence. *J Clin Psychiatry* 2009; **70**:113–121.
20. da Rocha FF, et al. Addition of lamotrigine to valproic acid: a successful outcome in a case of rapid-cycling bipolar affective disorder. *Prog Neuropsychopharmacol Biol Psychiatry* 2007; **31**:1548–1549.
21. Woo YS, et al. Lamotrigine added to valproate successfully treated a case of ultra-rapid cycling bipolar disorder. *Psychiatry Clin Neurosci* 2007; **61**:130–131.
22. Suppes T, et al. Efficacy and safety of aripiprazole in subpopulations with acute manic or mixed episodes of bipolar I disorder. *J Affect Disord* 2008; **107**:145–154.
23. Muzina DJ, et al. Aripiprazole monotherapy in patients with rapid-cycling bipolar I disorder: an analysis from a long-term, double-blind, placebo-controlled study. *Int J Clin Pract* 2008; **62**:679–687.
24. Calabrese JR, et al. Clozapine prophylaxis in rapid cycling bipolar disorder. *J Clin Psychopharmacol* 1991; **11**:396–397.
25. Fatemi SH, et al. Lamotrigine in rapid-cycling bipolar disorder. *J Clin Psychiatry* 1997; **58**:522–527.
26. Calabrese JR, et al. A double-blind, placebo-controlled, prophylaxis study of lamotrigine in rapid-cycling bipolar disorder. Lamictal 614 Study Group. *J Clin Psychiatry* 2000; **61**:841–850.
27. Wang Z, et al. Lamotrigine adjunctive therapy to lithium and divalproex in depressed patients with rapid cycling bipolar disorder and a recent substance use disorder: a 12-week, double-blind, placebo-controlled pilot study. *Psychopharmacol Bull* 2010; **43**:5–21.
28. Braunig P, et al. Levetiracetam in the treatment of rapid cycling bipolar disorder. *J Psychopharmacol* 2003; **17**:239–241.
29. Goodnick PJ. Nimodipine treatment of rapid cycling bipolar disorder. *J Clin Psychiatry* 1995; **56**:330.
30. Pazzaglia PJ, et al. Preliminary controlled trial of nimodipine in ultra-rapid cycling affective dysregulation. *Psychiatry Res* 1993; **49**:257–272.
31. Goldberg JF, et al. Effectiveness of quetiapine in rapid cycling bipolar disorder: a preliminary study. *J Affect Disord* 2008; **105**:305–310.
32. Vieta E, et al. Quetiapine monotherapy in the treatment of patients with bipolar I or II depression and a rapid-cycling disease course: a randomized, double-blind, placebo-controlled study. *Bipolar Disord* 2007; **9**:413–425.
33. Langosch JM, et al. Efficacy of quetiapine monotherapy in rapid-cycling bipolar disorder in comparison with sodium valproate. *J Clin Psychopharmacol* 2008; **28**:555–560.
34. Vieta E, et al. Quetiapine in the treatment of rapid cycling bipolar disorder. *Bipolar Disord* 2002; **4**:335–340.
35. Jacobsen FM. Risperidone in the treatment of affective illness and obsessive-compulsive disorder. *J Clin Psychiatry* 1995; **56**:423–429.
36. Bobo WV, et al. A randomized open comparison of long-acting injectable risperidone and treatment as usual for prevention of relapse, rehospitalization, and urgent care referral in community-treated patients with rapid cycling bipolar disorder. *Clin Neuropharmacol* 2011; **34**:224–233.

37. Vieta E, et al. Treatment of refractory rapid cycling bipolar disorder with risperidone. *J Clin Psychopharmacol* 1998; **18**:172–174.

38. Extein IL. High doses of levothyroxine for refractory rapid cycling. *Am J Psychiatry* 2000; **157**:1704–1705.

39. Walshaw PD, et al. Adjunctive thyroid hormone treatment in rapid cycling bipolar disorder: a double-blind placebo-controlled trial of levo-thyroxine (L-T(4)) and triiodothyronine (T(3)). *Bipolar Disord* 2018; **20**:594–603.

40. Qureshi MM, et al. The chimera of circular insanity and the labours of Thyreoidea. *Bipolar Disord* 2019; **21**:794–796.

41. Chen CK, et al. Combination treatment of clozapine and topiramate in resistant rapid-cycling bipolar disorder. *Clin Neuropharmacol* 2005; **28**:136–138.

42. Delgado A, et al. Clozapine in bipolar disorder: a systematic review and meta-analysis. *J Psychiatr Res* 2020; **125**:21–27.

43. Kılınçel O, et al. The role of clozapine as a mood regulator in the treatment of rapid cycling bipolar affective disorder. *Turk J Psychiatry* 2019; **30**:268–271.

44. Hui TP, et al. A systematic review and meta-analysis of clinical predictors of lithium response in bipolar disorder. *Acta Psychiatr Scand* 2019; **140**:94–115.

45. Montlahuc C, et al. Response to lithium in patients with bipolar disorder: what are psychiatrists' experiences and practices compared to literature review? *Pharmacopsychiatry* 2019; **52**:70–77.

46. Koukopoulos A, et al. Duration and stability of the rapid-cycling course: a long-term personal follow-up of 109 patients. *J Affect Disord* 2003; **73**:75–85.

47. Carvalho AF, et al. Rapid cycling in bipolar disorder: a systematic review. *J Clin Psychiatry* 2014; **75**:e578–e586.

第 2 章

双相抑郁

双相抑郁的抑郁发作与抑郁障碍的抑郁发作诊断标准相同,但在严重程度、病程、复发、药物疗效等方面存在差异。与单相抑郁相比,双相抑郁起病急、发作频繁、病情严重、病程短、容易出现妄想和相反的自主神经症状(如食欲增强、睡眠过多)[1-3]。约有 15% 的双相障碍患者自杀[4],这反映了抑郁发作的严重程度和频率。与躁狂症和单相抑郁相比,双相抑郁产生的社会经济负担更大[5],在时间上占双相障碍有症状时期的大部分[6,7]。

双相抑郁的药物治疗一定程度上存在争议,其原因有两方面。首先,迄今为止专门针对双相抑郁的高质量随机对照试验很少;其次,该疾病需要考虑终身的结局,而不能仅关注不连续抑郁发作的疗效[8]。目前,对于双相抑郁发作中药物的疗效我们知道一些,但是对于长期用药的治疗或有害作用知之甚少。

在英国,NICE 指南建议在起始阶段合用氟西汀与奥氮平,或单用喹硫平(假定尚未使用抗精神病药)[9]。拉莫三嗪被认为是二线治疗。英国精神药理学会指南(BAP)推荐拉莫三嗪作为一线选择,但也警告在长程治疗中需要一种心境稳定剂或抗精神病药以预防躁狂发作[10]。在 BAP 指南中,鲁拉西酮也是一线选择。

更多最新的指南大体上一致,但并非完全一致。加拿大心境与焦虑治疗网络(CANMAT)/国际双相障碍学会(ISBD)指南推荐喹硫平、鲁拉西酮(合用或不合用一种心境稳定剂)、拉莫三嗪和锂盐作为一线治疗[11]。2020 年 RANCP 指南建议锂盐、拉莫三嗪和丙戊酸盐(按照排序)作为一线药物,喹硫平、鲁拉西酮和卡利拉嗪(也是依序)作为二线治疗[12]。

表 2.9 至表 2.11 中列出了双相抑郁治疗选择的一些广义指南。

表 2.9　双相抑郁已证实的治疗(原著按字母顺序排列)

药物/方案	说明
拉莫三嗪[1,13-19]	拉莫三嗪似乎对双相抑郁的治疗和复发预防均有效。不会引起转为躁狂或快速循环发作。拉莫三嗪与西酞普兰疗效相当,与锂盐相比较少引起体重增加。总体来讲,拉莫三嗪的疗效难以明确,因为有许多模棱两可的临床试验[20,21],它们可能没有考虑到药物完全滴定所需的时间。拉莫三嗪可以作为锂盐的增效治疗[22],或者在孕期作为锂盐的替代药[23]。以后一项试验提示拉莫三嗪与喹硫平联合治疗的疗效强[24]。拉莫三嗪抗躁狂效果微弱[25] 小风险的皮疹使治疗变得复杂,它与剂量滴定速度有关。逐渐加量的必要性可能会限制拉莫三嗪的临床应用 另一个复杂的问题是剂量:50mg/d 有效,但 200mg/d 可能更好。在美国剂量最高达 1 200mg/d(平均 250mg/d)。血浆浓度(只有抗癫痫作用的浓度范围是已知的)可以指导更高剂量的需求
锂盐[1,13,26-28]	锂盐治疗双相抑郁可能有效,但支持的数据在方法学上受到质疑[29]。有一些证据显示锂盐可预防抑郁复发,但预防躁狂复发的证据更充分。强有力的证据证明锂盐可有效降低双相障碍患者的自杀率[30,31]

续表

药物/方案	说明
鲁拉西酮	三项随机对照试验研究发现,鲁拉西酮单用[32] 或与心境稳定剂合用[33-34] 均有良好的疗效。另一项随机对照试验研究报道,鲁拉西酮在伴亚综合征轻躁狂症状的双相抑郁中取得良好的效果[35]。汇总分析提示疗效与剂量相关[36]。网络荟萃分析提示,鲁拉西酮疗效优于阿立哌唑、齐拉西酮,但并不优于喹硫平、奥氮平[37]
心境稳定剂 + 抗抑郁药[38-44]	抗抑郁药在双相抑郁中仍广泛应用,尤其是在心境稳定剂治疗基础上出现的严重抑郁发作。尽管抗抑郁药有加速循环或转为躁狂的风险,它仍被认为是有效的。研究发现,心境稳定剂单用与合用抗抑郁药的疗效相当,进一步分析提示较高剂量抗抑郁药可能有效[45-47]。通常最好避免使用三环类抗抑郁药和单胺氧化酶抑制剂。如果要使用抗抑郁药,建议使用选择性 5-羟色胺再摄取抑制剂。文拉法辛和安非他酮也可以使用。文拉法辛可能更容易诱发转躁狂[48,49] 抑郁症状缓解后继续使用抗抑郁药可以预防抑郁复发[50,51],然而只是在没有心境稳定剂的情况下[52]。迄今为止,对于是否继续长期使用抗抑郁药,仍然没有达成共识[53]。最新证据提示,舍曲林单药治疗的转躁率并不高于锂盐 + 舍曲林合并治疗[54] 一些指南推荐双相 II 型抑郁使用抗抑郁药[11],证据显示舍曲林在这些患者中不增加转躁率[54]
奥氮平 ± 氟西汀[13,29,55-58]	奥氮平和氟西汀合剂(symbyax)治疗双相抑郁的疗效优于安慰剂和单用奥氮平,剂量是奥氮平 6mg/d+ 氟西汀 25mg/d,或者奥氮平 12mg/d+ 氟西汀 50mg/d(5/20mg 和 10/40mg 可能也有效)。该合剂可能比拉莫三嗪有效。对预防复发也有效。NICE 建议将其作为一线治疗[9] 与安慰剂对比,单用奥氮平有效[59],但合并氟西汀更好(这可能是双相抑郁使用抗抑郁药的最有力证据)
喹硫平[60-64]	5 项大样本随机对照试验证实,在治疗双相 I 型和双相 II 型抑郁时,喹硫平 300mg/d 和 600mg/d(单药治疗)均有效。后来中国人群一项研究显示,喹硫平 300mg/d 治疗双相 I 型抑郁有效[65]。喹硫平可能优于锂盐和帕罗西汀 喹硫平也预防抑郁和躁狂复发[66,67],因此成为双相抑郁治疗的选择之一。喹硫平与转为躁狂无关
丙戊酸盐[1,13,68-72]	丙戊酸盐单药治疗有效的证据很少,但被一些指南推荐。有几个小样本随机对照试验,许多结果是阴性的,然而荟萃分析结果支持其抗抑郁有效[71]。也许可能预防抑郁复发,但缺乏大量数据支持

表 2.10 双相抑郁的备选治疗- 在使用前参考原始文献

药物/方案	说明
抗抑郁药[73-81]	由于转躁和诱发快速循环的风险,"无对抗的"抗抑郁药(即没有心境稳定剂保护)一般避免用于治疗双相抑郁。也有证据显示,尽管剂量可能是关键,但是与单相抑郁相比,抗抑郁药治疗双相抑郁的疗效很差(可能根本没效)[47]。短期使用氟西汀、文拉法辛和吗氯贝胺似乎有一定的疗效而且安全,甚至单一用药也如此。一项荟萃分析提示,反苯环丙胺效应值大,没有转躁风险[82]。然而,总体上应避免单一使用抗抑郁药,尤其双相障碍 I 型[53]
卡利拉嗪[83]	一项随机对照试验提示,卡利拉嗪 1.5mg/d 治疗双相 I 型抑郁有效。另一项较大样本研究显示,1.5mg/d 和 3mg/d 均有效[84]。最新研究发现 1.5mg/d 患者有效,而 3mg/d 无效[84]

续表

药物/方案	说明
氯胺酮 [85-88]	氯胺酮 0.5mg/kg 静脉注射对难治性双相抑郁有效。有效率很高。分离症状常见但短暂。目前氯胺酮已被接受为难治性双相抑郁的标准治疗 [89,90]。静脉注射其外消旋体可能比鼻内使用艾司氯胺酮有效 [91]。转躁是一个潜在的问题,但可能是远期风险 [92]
普拉克索 [93,94]	两项小样本安慰剂对照试验发现普拉克索治疗双相抑郁有效,平均有效剂量为 1.7mg/d。这两项研究均把普拉克索作为心境稳定剂的增效药物。两项研究均未发现转为躁狂或轻躁狂的风险增加(理论上的考虑),但无足够证据排除这种可能性。一项荟萃分析显示对有效率影响大,但对治愈的影响不强 [95]

表 2.11　双相抑郁的其他可能治疗方案——使用前咨询专家

药物/方案	说明
阿立哌唑 [96-99]	有限的开放研究支持其可用于双相抑郁的增效治疗。RCT 研究是阴性结果。可能无效 [95]
卡马西平 [1,13,100]	偶尔被推荐使用,但数据缺乏且疗效有限。也许和其他心境稳定剂合用时有效
加巴喷丁 [1,101,102]	开放性研究发现,作为心境稳定剂或抗精神病药的增效治疗,疗效一般。平均剂量 1 750mg/d。对双相抑郁的明显疗效可能源于其抗焦虑作用
肌醇 [103]	一项小样本随机探索试验发现,12g/d 的肌醇对双相抑郁有效
米非司酮 [104,105]	一些证据表明其能提高双相抑郁患者的心境,但一项大样本试验没有重复该结论。两项试验都发现米非司酮改善认知功能。所用剂量是 600mg/d
莫达非尼 [106]	对莫达非尼/阿莫达非尼的 5 项研究的荟萃分析提示,其有效和治愈率高,而且耐受性好,不增加转躁风险
ω-3 脂肪酸 [107,108]	一项随机对照试验结果阳性(1g/d 或 2g/d),一项研究结果阴性(6g/d)

双相抑郁的荟萃分析

双相抑郁的荟萃分析因评价疗效的方法不同而受到限制。这就意味着许多有科学价值的研究因参数(结局、病程等)不匹配,不能与其他研究比较,而不能被纳入一些荟萃分析。早期的锂盐研究就是一个重要的例子——用药时间短和交叉设计使其被排除在荟萃分析外。BAP 指南对于网络荟萃分析有点不屑一顾(也许是正确的),因为结果受纳入标准严重影响,而且经常与直接比较的结果相矛盾 [10]。

对 5 项试验(906 名受试者)的荟萃分析发现,尽管结果接近统计学意义,但是抗抑郁药的有效率和治愈率与安慰剂比较没有优势 [98]。另外一项对不涉及抗抑郁药的研究(7 307 名受试者)的分析发现 [109],以下药物在统计上优于安慰剂:奥氮平与氟西汀合剂、丙戊酸盐、喹硫平、鲁拉西酮、奥氮平、阿立哌唑和卡马西平(按照效应值大小由高向低排序)。

2014 年一项网络荟萃分析包括 29 项研究和 8 331 名受试者 [110]。整体上,在效应值和有效率两方面排序最高的药物有奥氮平与氟西汀合剂、鲁拉西酮、奥氮平、丙戊酸盐、SSRI 和喹硫平,其中奥氮平与氟西汀合剂位居第一。最近一项网络荟萃分析包括 50 项研究和 11 448 名受试者 [111],结果发现疗效优于安慰剂的药物有奥氮平与氟西汀合剂、奥氮平、丙戊酸盐、卡利拉嗪、拉莫三嗪、鲁拉西酮和喹硫平。有意思的是,丙米嗪和氟西汀的疗效也优于安慰剂(但具有宽的置信区间)。

药物选择小结

奥氮平 + 氟西汀合剂可能是双相抑郁最有效的治疗选择,但其使用因奥氮平常见的不良反应而受到限制。氟西汀以外的其他 SSRI 可能有效,但除非患者明显获益,否则应该避免使用 [53]。其他一线选择有喹硫平、奥氮平、鲁拉西酮、拉莫三嗪和丙戊酸盐。这些药物在不良反应、耐受性和费用方面有明显差异,给患者处方时这些因素均需要考虑。锂盐同样也有效,但证据相对弱。二线药物包括氯胺酮,莫达非尼也用得越来越多。阿立哌唑、利培酮、齐拉西酮、三环类(丙米嗪除外)和 MAOI 类(反苯环丙胺除外)抗抑郁药可能无效,应避免常规地使用 [110]。

参考文献

1. Malhi GS, et al. Bipolar depression: management options. *CNS Drugs* 2003; **17**:9–25.

2. Perlis RH, et al. Clinical features of bipolar depression versus major depressive disorder in large multicenter trials. *Am J Psychiatry* 2006; **163**:225–231.

3. Mitchell PB, et al. Comparison of depressive episodes in bipolar disorder and in major depressive disorder within bipolar disorder pedigrees. *Br J Psychiatry* 2011; **199**:303–309.

4. Haddad P, et al. Pharmacological management of bipolar depression. *Acta Psychiatr Scand* 2002; **105**:401–403.

5. Hirschfeld RM. Bipolar depression: the real challenge. *Eur Neuropsychopharmacol* 2004; **14 Suppl 2**:S83–S88.

6. Judd LL, et al. The long-term natural history of the weekly symptomatic status of bipolar I disorder. *Arch Gen Psychiatry* 2002; **59**:530–537.

7. Judd LL, et al. A prospective investigation of the natural history of the long-term weekly symptomatic status of bipolar II disorder. *Arch Gen Psychiatry* 2003; **60**:261–269.

8. Baldassano CF, et al. Rethinking the treatment paradigm for bipolar depression: the importance of long-term management. *CNS Spectr* 2004; **9**:11–18.

9. National Institute for Health and Care Excellence. Bipolar disorder: assessment and management. Clinical Guidance [CG185]. 2014 (Last updated February 2020); https://www.nice.org.uk/guidance/cg185.

10. Goodwin GM, et al. Evidence-based guidelines for treating bipolar disorder: revised third edition recommendations from the British Association for Psychopharmacology. *J Psychopharmacol* 2016; **30**:495–553.

11. Yatham LN, et al. Canadian network for mood and anxiety treatments (CANMAT) and International Society for Bipolar Disorders (ISBD) 2018 guidelines for the management of patients with bipolar disorder. *Bipolar Disord* 2018; **20**:97–170.

12. Malhi GS, et al. The 2020 Royal Australian and New Zealand College of Psychiatrists Clinical Practice Guidelines for mood disorders: bipolar disorder summary. *Bipolar Disord* 2020; **22**:805–821.

13. Yatham LN, et al. Bipolar depression: criteria for treatment selection, definition of refractoriness, and treatment options. *Bipolar Disord* 2003; **5**:85–97.

14. Calabrese JR, et al. A double-blind placebo-controlled study of lamotrigine monotherapy in outpatients with bipolar I depression. Lamictal 602 Study Group. *J Clin Psychiatry* 1999; **60**:79–88.

15. Bowden CL, et al. Lamotrigine in the treatment of bipolar depression. *Eur Neuropsychopharmacol* 1999; **9 Suppl 4**:S113–S117.

16. Marangell LB, et al. Lamotrigine treatment of bipolar disorder: data from the first 500 patients in STEP-BD. *Bipolar Disord* 2004; **6**:139–143.

17. Schaffer A, et al. Randomized, double-blind pilot trial comparing lamotrigine versus citalopram for the treatment of bipolar depression. *J Affect Disord* 2006; **96**:95–99.

18. Bowden CL, et al. Impact of lamotrigine and lithium on weight in obese and nonobese patients with bipolar I disorder. *Am J Psychiatry* 2006; **163**:1199–1201.

19. Suppes T, et al. A single blind comparison of lithium and lamotrigine for the treatment of bipolar II depression. *J Affect Disord* 2008; **111**:334–343.

20. Geddes JR, et al. Lamotrigine for treatment of bipolar depression: independent meta-analysis and meta-regression of individual patient data from five randomised trials. *Br J Psychiatry* 2009; **194**:4–9.

21. Calabrese JR, et al. Lamotrigine in the acute treatment of bipolar depression: results of five double-blind, placebo-controlled clinical trials. *Bipolar Disord* 2008; **10**:323–333.

22. van der Loos ML, et al. Efficacy and safety of lamotrigine as add-on treatment to lithium in bipolar depression: a multicenter, double-blind, placebo-controlled trial. *J Clin Psychiatry* 2009; **70**:223–231.

23. Newport DJ, et al. Lamotrigine in bipolar disorder: efficacy during pregnancy. *Bipolar Disord* 2008; **10**:432–436.

24. Geddes JR, et al. Comparative evaluation of quetiapine plus lamotrigine combination versus quetiapine monotherapy (and folic acid versus placebo) in bipolar depression (CEQUEL): a 2 x 2 factorial randomised trial. *Lancet Psychiatry* 2016; 3:31–39.

25. Goodwin GM, et al. A pooled analysis of 2 placebo-controlled 18-month trials of lamotrigine and lithium maintenance in bipolar I disorder. *J Clin Psychiatry* 2004; 65:432–441.

26. Geddes JR, et al. Long-term lithium therapy for bipolar disorder: systematic review and meta-analysis of randomized controlled trials. *Am J Psychiatry* 2004; 161:217–222.

27. Calabrese JR, et al. A placebo-controlled 18-month trial of lamotrigine and lithium maintenance treatment in recently depressed patients with bipolar I disorder. *J Clin Psychiatry* 2003; 64:1013–1024.

28. Prien RF, et al. Lithium carbonate and imipramine in prevention of affective episodes. A comparison in recurrent affective illness. *Arch Gen Psychiatry* 1973; 29:420–425.

29. Grunze H, et al. The world federation of societies of biological psychiatry (WFSBP) guidelines for the biological treatment of bipolar disorders: update 2010 on the treatment of acute bipolar depression. *World J Biol Psychiatry* 2010; 11:81–109.

30. Goodwin FK, et al. Suicide risk in bipolar disorder during treatment with lithium and divalproex. *JAMA* 2003; 290:1467–1473.

31. Kessing LV, et al. Suicide risk in patients treated with lithium. *Arch Gen Psychiatry* 2005; 62:860–866.

32. Loebel A, et al. Lurasidone monotherapy in the treatment of bipolar I depression: a randomized, double-blind, placebo-controlled study. *Am J Psychiatry* 2014; 171:160–168.

33. Loebel A, et al. Lurasidone as adjunctive therapy with lithium or valproate for the treatment of bipolar I depression: a randomized, double-blind, placebo-controlled study. *Am J Psychiatry* 2014; 171:169–177.

34. Suppes T, et al. Lurasidone adjunctive with lithium or valproate for bipolar depression: a placebo-controlled trial utilizing prospective and retrospective enrolment cohorts. *J Psychiatr Res* 2016; 78:86–93.

35. Suppes T, et al. Lurasidone for the treatment of major depressive disorder with mixed features: a randomized, double-blind, placebo-controlled study. *Am J Psychiatry* 2016; 173:400–407.

36. Chapel S, et al. Lurasidone dose response in bipolar depression: a population dose-response analysis. *Clin Ther* 2016; 38:4–15.

37. Ostacher M, et al. Lurasidone compared to other atypical antipsychotic monotherapies for bipolar depression: A systematic review and network meta-analysis. *World J Biol Psychiatry* 2018; 19:586–601.

38. Calabrese JR, et al. International consensus group on bipolar i depression treatment guidelines. *J Clin Psychiatry* 2004; 65:571–579.

39. Nemeroff CB, et al. Double-blind, placebo-controlled comparison of imipramine and paroxetine in the treatment of bipolar depression. *Am J Psychiatry* 2001; 158:906–912.

40. Vieta E, et al. A randomized trial comparing paroxetine and venlafaxine in the treatment of bipolar depressed patients taking mood stabilizers. *J Clin Psychiatry* 2002; 63:508–512.

41. Young LT, et al. Double-blind comparison of addition of a second mood stabilizer versus an antidepressant to an initial mood stabilizer for treatment of patients with bipolar depression. *Am J Psychiatry* 2000; 157:124–126.

42. Fawcett JA. Lithium combinations in acute and maintenance treatment of unipolar and bipolar depression. *J Clin Psychiatry* 2003; **64 Suppl** 5:32–37.

43. Altshuler L, et al. The impact of antidepressant discontinuation versus antidepressant continuation on 1-year risk for relapse of bipolar depression: a retrospective chart review. *J Clin Psychiatry* 2001; 62:612–616.

44. Erfurth A, et al. Bupropion as add-on strategy in difficult-to-treat bipolar depressive patients. *Neuropsychobiology* 2002; **45 Suppl** 1:33–36.

45. Sachs GS, et al. Effectiveness of adjunctive antidepressant treatment for bipolar depression. *N Engl J Med* 2007; 356:1711–1722.

46. Goldberg JF, et al. Adjunctive antidepressant use and symptomatic recovery among bipolar depressed patients with concomitant manic symptoms: findings from the STEP-BD. *Am J Psychiatry* 2007; 164:1348–1355.

47. Tada M, et al. Antidepressant dose and treatment response in bipolar depression: reanalysis of the Systematic Treatment Enhancement Program for Bipolar Disorder (STEP-BD) data. *J Psychiatr Res* 2015; 68:151–156.

48. Post RM, et al. Mood switch in bipolar depression: comparison of adjunctive venlafaxine, bupropion and sertraline. *Br J Psychiatry* 2006; 189:124–131.

49. Leverich GS, et al. Risk of switch in mood polarity to hypomania or mania in patients with bipolar depression during acute and continuation trials of venlafaxine, sertraline, and bupropion as adjuncts to mood stabilizers. *Am J Psychiatry* 2006; 163:232–239.

50. Salvi V, et al. The use of antidepressants in bipolar disorder. *J Clin Psychiatry* 2008; 69:1307–1318.

51. Altshuler LL, et al. Impact of antidepressant continuation after acute positive or partial treatment response for bipolar depression: a blinded, randomized study. *J Clin Psychiatry* 2009; 70:450–457.

52. Ghaemi SN, et al. Long-term antidepressant treatment in bipolar disorder: meta-analyses of benefits and risks. *Acta Psychiatr Scand* 2008; 118:347–356.

53. Pacchiarotti I, et al. The International Society for Bipolar Disorders (ISBD) task force report on antidepressant use in bipolar disorders. *Am J Psychiatry* 2013; 170:1249–1262.

54. Altshuler LL, et al. Switch rates during acute treatment for bipolar II depression with lithium, sertraline, or the two combined: a randomized double-blind comparison. *Am J Psychiatry* 2017; 174:266–276.

55. Tohen M, et al. Efficacy of olanzapine and olanzapine-fluoxetine combination in the treatment of bipolar I depression. *Arch Gen Psychiatry* 2003; 60:1079–1088.

56. Brown EB, et al. A 7-week, randomized, double-blind trial of olanzapine/fluoxetine combination versus lamotrigine in the treatment of bipolar I depression. *J Clin Psychiatry* 2006; 67:1025–1033.

57. Corya SA, et al. A 24-week open-label extension study of olanzapine-fluoxetine combination and olanzapine monotherapy in the treatment of bipolar depression. *J Clin Psychiatry* 2006; 67:798–806.

58. Dube S, et al. Onset of antidepressant effect of olanzapine and olanzapine/fluoxetine combination in bipolar depression. *Bipolar Disord* 2007; **9**:618–627.

59. Tohen M, et al. Randomised, double-blind, placebo-controlled study of olanzapine in patients with bipolar I depression. *Br J Psychiatry* 2012; **201**:376–382.

60. Calabrese JR, et al. A randomized, double-blind, placebo-controlled trial of quetiapine in the treatment of bipolar I or II depression. *Am J Psychiatry* 2005; **162**:1351–1360.

61. Thase ME, et al. Efficacy of quetiapine monotherapy in bipolar I and II depression: a double-blind, placebo-controlled study (the BOLDER II study). *J Clin Psychopharmacol* 2006; **26**:600–609.

62. Suppes T, et al. Effectiveness of the extended release formulation of quetiapine as monotherapy for the treatment of acute bipolar depression. *J Affect Disord* 2010; **121**:106–115.

63. Young AH, et al. A double-blind, placebo-controlled study of quetiapine and lithium monotherapy in adults in the acute phase of bipolar depression (EMBOLDEN I). *J Clin Psychiatry* 2010; **71**:150–162.

64. McElroy SL, et al. A double-blind, placebo-controlled study of quetiapine and paroxetine as monotherapy in adults with bipolar depression (EMBOLDEN II). *J Clin Psychiatry* 2010; **71**:163–174.

65. Li H, et al. Efficacy and safety of quetiapine extended release monotherapy in bipolar depression: a multi-center, randomized, double-blind, placebo-controlled trial. *Psychopharmacology (Berl)* 2016; **233**:1289–1297.

66. Vieta E, et al. Efficacy and safety of quetiapine in combination with lithium or divalproex for maintenance of patients with bipolar I disorder (international trial 126). *J Affect Disord* 2008; **109**:251–263.

67. Suppes T, et al. Maintenance treatment for patients with bipolar I disorder: results from a North American study of quetiapine in combination with lithium or divalproex (trial 127). *Am J Psychiatry* 2009; **166**:476–488.

68. Goodwin GM. Evidence-based guidelines for treating bipolar disorder: revised second edition–recommendations from the British Association for Psychopharmacology. *J Psychopharmacol* 2009; **23**:346–388.

69. Davis LL, et al. Divalproex in the treatment of bipolar depression: a placebo-controlled study. *J Affect Disord* 2005; **85**:259–266.

70. Ghaemi SN, et al. Divalproex in the treatment of acute bipolar depression: a preliminary double-blind, randomized, placebo-controlled pilot study. *J Clin Psychiatry* 2007; **68**:1840–1844.

71. Smith LA, et al. Valproate for the treatment of acute bipolar depression: systematic review and meta-analysis. *J Affect Disord* 2010; **122**:1–9.

72. Muzina DJ, et al. Acute efficacy of divalproex sodium versus placebo in mood stabilizer-naive bipolar I or II depression: a double-blind, randomized, placebo-controlled trial. *J Clin Psychiatry* 2011; **72**:813–819.

73. Amsterdam JD, et al. Short-term fluoxetine monotherapy for bipolar type II or bipolar NOS major depression – low manic switch rate. *Bipolar Disord* 2004; **6**:75–81.

74. Amsterdam JD, et al. Efficacy and safety of fluoxetine in treating bipolar II major depressive episode. *J Clin Psychopharmacol* 1998; **18**:435–440.

75. Amsterdam J. Efficacy and safety of venlafaxine in the treatment of bipolar II major depressive episode. *J Clin Psychopharmacol* 1998; **18**:414–417.

76. Amsterdam JD, et al. Venlafaxine monotherapy in women with bipolar II and unipolar major depression. *J Affect Disord* 2000; **59**:225–229.

77. Silverstone T. Moclobemide vs. imipramine in bipolar depression: a multicentre double-blind clinical trial. *Acta Psychiatr Scand* 2001; **104**:104–109.

78. Ghaemi SN, et al. Antidepressant treatment in bipolar versus unipolar depression. *Am J Psychiatry* 2004; **161**:163–165.

79. Post RM, et al. A re-evaluation of the role of antidepressants in the treatment of bipolar depression: data from the Stanley Foundation Bipolar Network. *Bipolar Disord* 2003; **5**:396–406.

80. Amsterdam JD, et al. Comparison of fluoxetine, olanzapine, and combined fluoxetine plus olanzapine initial therapy of bipolar type I and type II major depression–lack of manic induction. *J Affect Disord* 2005; **87**:121–130.

81. Amsterdam JD, et al. Fluoxetine monotherapy of bipolar type II and bipolar NOS major depression: a double-blind, placebo-substitution, continuation study. *Int Clin Psychopharmacol* 2005; **20**:257–264.

82. Heijnen WT, et al. Efficacy of tranylcypromine in bipolar depression: a systematic review. *J Clin Psychopharmacol* 2015; **35**:700–705.

83. Durgam S, et al. An 8-week randomized, double-blind, placebo-controlled evaluation of the safety and efficacy of cariprazine in patients with bipolar I depression. *Am J Psychiatry* 2016; **173**:271–281.

84. Earley W, et al. Cariprazine treatment of bipolar depression: a randomized double-blind placebo-controlled phase 3 study. *Am J Psychiatry* 2019; **176**:439–448.

85. Diazgranados N, et al. A randomized add-on trial of an N-methyl-D-aspartate antagonist in treatment-resistant bipolar depression. *Arch Gen Psychiatry* 2010; **67**:793–802.

86. Shahani R, et al. Ketamine-associated ulcerative cystitis: a new clinical entity. *Urology* 2007; **69**:810–812.

87. Zarate CA, Jr., et al. Replication of ketamine's antidepressant efficacy in bipolar depression: a randomized controlled add-on trial. *Biol Psychiatry* 2012; **71**:939–946.

88. Permoda-Osip A, et al. Single ketamine infusion and neurocognitive performance in bipolar depression. *Pharmacopsychiatry* 2015; **48**:78–79.

89. Jha MK, et al. Psychopharmacology and experimental therapeutics for bipolar depression. *Focus (American Psychiatric Publishing)* 2019; **17**:232–237.

90. Włodarczyk A, et al. Safety and tolerability of ketamine use in treatment-resistant bipolar depression patients with regard to central nervous system symptomatology: literature review and analysis. *Medicina (Kaunas)* 2020; **56**:67.

91. Bahji A, et al. Comparative efficacy of racemic ketamine and esketamine for depression: a systematic review and meta-analysis. *J Affect Disord* 2021; 278:542–555.

92. Alison McInnes L, et al. Possible affective switch associated with intravenous ketamine treatment in a patient with bipolar I disorder. *Biol Psychiatry* 2016; 79:e71–e72.

93. Goldberg JF, et al. Preliminary randomized, double-blind, placebo-controlled trial of pramipexole added to mood stabilizers for treatment-resistant bipolar depression. *Am J Psychiatry* 2004; 161:564–566.

94. Zarate CA, Jr., et al. Pramipexole for bipolar II depression: a placebo-controlled proof of concept study. *Biol Psychiatry* 2004; 56:54–60.

95. Romeo B, et al. Meta-analysis and review of dopamine agonists in acute episodes of mood disorder: efficacy and safety. *J Psychopharmacol* 2018; 32:385–396.

96. Ketter TA, et al. Adjunctive aripiprazole in treatment-resistant bipolar depression. *Ann Clin Psychiatry* 2006; 18:169–172.

97. Mazza M, et al. Beneficial acute antidepressant effects of aripiprazole as an adjunctive treatment or monotherapy in bipolar patients unresponsive to mood stabilizers: results from a 16-week open-label trial. *Expert Opin Pharmacother* 2008; 9:3145–3149.

98. Sidor MM, et al. Antidepressants for the acute treatment of bipolar depression: a systematic review and meta-analysis. *J Clin Psychiatry* 2011; 72:156–167.

99. Cruz N, et al. Efficacy of modern antipsychotics in placebo-controlled trials in bipolar depression: a meta-analysis. *Int J Neuropsychopharmacol* 2010; 13:5–14.

100. Dilsaver SC, et al. Treatment of bipolar depression with carbamazepine: results of an open study. *Biol Psychiatry* 1996; 40:935–937.

101. Wang PW, et al. Gabapentin augmentation therapy in bipolar depression. *Bipolar Disorders* 2002; 4:296–301.

102. Ashton H, et al. GABA-ergic drugs: exit stage left, enter stage right. *J Psychopharmacol* 2003; 17:174–178.

103. Chengappa KN, et al. Inositol as an add-on treatment for bipolar depression. *Bipolar Disord* 2000; 2:47–55.

104. Young AH, et al. Improvements in neurocognitive function and mood following adjunctive treatment with mifepristone (RU-486) in bipolar disorder. *Neuropsychopharmacology* 2004; 29:1538–1545.

105. Watson S, et al. A randomized trial to examine the effect of mifepristone on neuropsychological performance and mood in patients with bipolar depression. *Biol Psychiatry* 2012; 72:943–949.

106. Nunez NA, et al. Efficacy and tolerability of adjunctive modafinil/armodafinil in bipolar depression: a meta-analysis of randomized controlled trials. *Bipolar Disord* 2020; 22:109–120.

107. Frangou S, et al. Efficacy of ethyl-eicosapentaenoic acid in bipolar depression: randomised double-blind placebo-controlled study. *Br J Psychiatry* 2006; 188:46–50.

108. Keck PE, Jr., et al. Double-blind, randomized, placebo-controlled trials of ethyl-eicosapentanoate in the treatment of bipolar depression and rapid cycling bipolar disorder. *Biol Psychiatry* 2006; 60:1020–1022.

109. Selle V, et al. Treatments for acute bipolar depression: meta-analyses of placebo-controlled, monotherapy trials of anticonvulsants, lithium and antipsychotics. *Pharmacopsychiatry* 2014; 47:43–52.

110. Taylor DM, et al. Comparative efficacy and acceptability of drug treatments for bipolar depression: a multiple-treatments meta-analysis. *Acta Psychiatr Scand* 2014; 130:452–469.

111. Bahji A, et al. Comparative efficacy and tolerability of pharmacological treatments for the treatment of acute bipolar depression: a systematic review and network meta-analysis. *J Affect Disord* 2020; 269:154–184.

第 2 章

双相障碍的预防

普遍一致的观点是在急性发作期有效的药物方案应该继续用于预防。因此,很大程度上每个患者的维持期治疗选择由急性期治疗的疗效与耐受性决定。可能例外的情况包括:躁狂发作缓解后,考虑停止与心境稳定剂合用的抗精神病药(一些权威建议[1]);双相抑郁急性期治疗有效后,停止使用抗抑郁药。这些例外的前提是心境稳定剂继续使用(大多数权威建议,至少含蓄地建议[2])。一些证据显示,从锂盐或丙戊酸盐联合治疗方案中停止抗精神病药,会增加复发风险[3]。

急性发作后残留情绪症状是复发的有力预测因素[4,5]。就单药治疗而言,大多数证据支持锂盐可有效地预防躁狂发作和抑郁发作[6-11]。卡马西平预防效果欠佳[10,12]。尽管丙戊酸盐也可以防范抑郁和躁狂复发[10,16],但它的长期疗效仍不确定[8,9,13-15]。锂盐被证实有预防自杀的优势[17-20],但是和其他心境稳定剂相比,其劣势也许是突然停用后疾病结局可能恶化[21-24](尽管其他药物突然停用的影响可能相似[24])。锂盐早期使用可能发挥增效作用[25]。

独立的 BALANCE 研究发现,丙戊酸钠单用的疗效不如锂盐单用,也不如锂盐与丙戊酸盐合用[14],这使丙戊酸盐作为一线单药治疗受到质疑。一项大样本观察性研究发现,在预防任何心境复发和减少再住院方面,锂盐明显比丙戊酸盐有效[26]。基于此证据以及丙戊酸盐未获批用于预防,丙戊酸盐应该作为二线治疗。

第一代抗精神病药已经在临床上使用且被认为有效,但是客观证据不足[27,28]。第一代抗精神病药长效剂可以预防躁狂复发,但可能加重抑郁发作[29]。有证据支持许多第二代抗精神病药的疗效,尤其是奥氮平[9,30]、喹硫平[31]、阿立哌唑[32]和利培酮[33]。大多数研究探究其与心境稳定剂合用,少有试验支持单药治疗。2017 年一项综述显示,仅奥氮平、喹硫平和利培酮单药治疗可能优于安慰剂[34]。

奥氮平、喹硫平和阿立哌唑有预防复发的适应证,可以预防躁狂发作和抑郁发作[34]。阿塞那平[35]和齐拉西酮[36]可能也有效。不同第二代抗精神病药之间难以选择[34]。

2020 年一篇纳入 41 项研究和 9 821 例受试者的荟萃分析结果显示,所有抗精神病药与心境稳定剂合用时,疗效优于心境稳定剂单药治疗[37]。其中,从统计学结果上看(任何心境发作复发风险),阿立哌唑与丙戊酸盐合用是最佳的维持治疗方案。同时期的另一篇纳入 14 项单药治疗研究的荟萃分析发现,阿立哌唑、奥氮平、鲁拉西酮、利培酮或喹硫平比安慰剂有效,时间持续 6 个月以上[38]。

长效阿立哌唑被证实可以延迟躁狂发作时间,降低躁狂复发率,总体上安全性和耐受性好[39]。利培酮长效注射剂也有随机对照试验[40]和真实世界研究[41]的良好支持。

NICE 指南建议[30]

- 当计划长期用药预防**复发**时,应考虑**那些**在躁狂或双相抑郁发作期间治疗有效的药物。与患者讨论是选择继续使用治疗方案还是换成**锂盐**,并告知患者锂盐是双相障碍长期治疗最有效的药物。

- 推荐**锂盐**作为双相障碍长期治疗的一线用药：如果锂盐疗效欠佳，可考虑加用**丙戊酸盐**；如果对锂盐不耐受，可考虑换用丙戊酸盐或者**奥氮平**；如果**喹硫平**对既往躁狂发作或双相抑郁有效，也可考虑。
- 不要给育龄妇女服用丙戊酸盐。
- 与患者讨论每一种药物可能的获益和风险。
- 后续治疗团队应负责监测**抗精神病药**的有效性和耐受性，直至患者病情稳定。
- 停药之前，与患者讨论如何识别疾病**复发**的早期症状，以及症状出现后该怎么做。
- 如果停药，要逐渐停药，并监测**复发**征兆。
- 停药之后要继续监测患者的症状、情绪及精神状态 2 年。可以在初级保健机构进行。

优化锂盐治疗 [42]

对于双相障碍成年患者，标准的锂盐血清浓度应该是 0.60~0.80mmol/L。如果反应好，但耐受性差，可以降低至 0.40~0.60mmol/L；如果反应不佳，而耐受性好，可以增加至 0.80~1.00mmol/L。对于儿童和青少年患者没有共识，但是国际双相障碍学会（ISBD）/国际锂盐研究工作组建议与成年人一样。对于老年人，建议采取比较保守的方法：一般推荐 0.40~0.60mmol/L，65~79 岁患者最高 0.70 或 0.80mmol/L，80 岁及以上患者最高 0.70mmol/L。

联合治疗

相当大一部分双相障碍患者单用心境稳定剂达不到充分的治疗 [14]，因此常常将两种心境稳定剂合用，或者将一种心境稳定剂与一种抗精神病药合用 [43-46]。另外，有证据表明，若既往合并用药对躁狂发作或者抑郁发作有效，则继续使用此种合用预防复发的效果最好 [31,45]。多药合用时，需要权衡可能增加的药物不良反应。NICE [30] 和 BAP [10] 指南建议，将奥氮平、利培酮、喹硫平或氟哌啶醇与锂盐或丙戊酸钠合用。其他抗精神病药（如阿立哌唑）也可以考虑与锂盐或丙戊酸盐合用，尤其是发现该抗精神病药在躁狂发作或抑郁发作急性期治疗有效时 [31,47]。卡马西平可作为三线用药。拉莫三嗪可能对双相障碍 Ⅱ 型有效 [30]，但似乎仅能明显预防抑郁复发 [48]。鲁拉西酮的长期疗效可能大致相似，包括单药治疗和与一种心境稳定剂合用 [49,50]。

根据目前已有的数据推断，锂盐与一种第二代抗精神病药合用可能是多药治疗的首选。有真实世界研究支持三种药物合用：一项研究发现两种最佳治疗方案，首先是锂盐 + 丙戊酸盐 + 喹硫平，然后是锂盐 + 丙戊酸盐 + 奥氮平 [51]。如果心境稳定剂耐受性差或不能依从，可以考虑抗精神病药单药治疗 [52]。

对抗抑郁药长期治疗的一项荟萃分析发现，抗抑郁药继续治疗更容易诱发躁狂，而不是预防抑郁发作 [53]。双相障碍系统治疗的增强计划（STEP-BD）研究发现，对于快速循环型患者，继续服用抗抑郁药（与停用相比）对患者无明显益处，甚至使结局恶化 [54]。尽管一些双相障碍患者停用抗抑郁药后抑郁可能复发，但是现有证据实际上不支持长期使用抗抑郁药治疗双相障碍 [24]。

精神活性物质滥用增加转躁的风险 [55]。

总结表

双相障碍的预防

一线：锂盐单药治疗

二线：奥氮平、阿立哌唑、利培酮或喹硫平与丙戊酸钠（育龄妇女禁用）或锂盐合用

三线：其他抗精神病药（鲁拉西酮、阿塞那平、齐拉西酮）或其他心境稳定剂（卡马西平、拉莫三嗪）合用

四线：一种抗精神病药与两种心境稳定剂合用

- 始终保持急性期治疗有效的方案预防复发（如心境稳定剂 + 抗精神病药）。
- 尽可能避免长期使用抗抑郁药。

参考文献

1. Malhi GS, et al. The 2020 Royal Australian and New Zealand College of Psychiatrists Clinical Practice Guidelines for mood disorders: bipolar disorder summary. *Bipolar Disord* 2020; 22:805–821.

2. Yatham LN, et al. Canadian network for mood and anxiety treatments (CANMAT) and International Society for Bipolar Disorders (ISBD) 2018 guidelines for the management of patients with bipolar disorder. *Bipolar Disord* 2018; 20:97–170.

3. Kang MG, et al. Lithium vs valproate in the maintenance treatment of bipolar I disorder: a post- hoc analysis of a randomized double-blind placebo-controlled trial. *Aust N Z J Psychiatry* 2020; 54:298–307.

4. Solomon DA, et al. Longitudinal course of bipolar I disorder: duration of mood episodes. *Arch Gen Psychiatry* 2010; 67:339–347.

5. Perlis RH, et al. Predictors of recurrence in bipolar disorder: primary outcomes from the Systematic Treatment Enhancement Program for Bipolar Disorder (STEP-BD). *Am J Psychiatry* 2006; 163:217–224.

6. Young AH, et al. Lithium in mood disorders: increasing evidence base, declining use? *Brit J Psychiatry* 2007; 191:474–476.

7. Biel MG, et al. Continuation versus discontinuation of lithium in recurrent bipolar illness: a naturalistic study. *Bipolar Disord* 2007; 9:435–442.

8. Bowden CL, et al. A randomized, placebo-controlled 12-month trial of divalproex and lithium in treatment of outpatients with bipolar I disorder. Divalproex Maintenance Study Group. *Arch Gen Psychiatry* 2000; 57:481–489.

9. Tohen M, et al. Olanzapine versus divalproex sodium for the treatment of acute mania and maintenance of remission: a 47-week study. *Am J Psychiatry* 2003; 160:1263–1271.

10. Goodwin GM, et al. Evidence-based guidelines for treating bipolar disorder: revised third edition recommendations from the British Association for Psychopharmacology. *J Psychopharmacol* 2016; 30:495–553.

11. Sani G, et al. Treatment of bipolar disorder in a lifetime perspective: is lithium still the best choice? *Clin Drug Investig* 2017; 37:713–727.

12. Hartong EG, et al. Prophylactic efficacy of lithium versus carbamazepine in treatment-naive bipolar patients. *J Clin Psychiatry* 2003; 64:144–151.

13. Cipriani A, et al. Valproic acid, valproate and divalproex in the maintenance treatment of bipolar disorder. *Cochrane Database Syst Rev* 2013; 10:CD003196.

14. Geddes JR, et al. Lithium plus valproate combination therapy versus monotherapy for relapse prevention in bipolar I disorder (BALANCE): a randomised open-label trial. *Lancet* 2010; 375:385–395.

15. Kemp DE, et al. A 6-month, double-blind, maintenance trial of lithium monotherapy versus the combination of lithium and divalproex for rapid-cycling bipolar disorder and Co-occurring substance abuse or dependence. *J Clin Psychiatry* 2009; 70:113–121.

16. Smith LA, et al. Effectiveness of mood stabilizers and antipsychotics in the maintenance phase of bipolar disorder: a systematic review of randomized controlled trials. *Bipolar Disorders* 2007; 9:394–412.

17. Cipriani A, et al. Lithium in the prevention of suicidal behavior and all-cause mortality in patients with mood disorders: a systematic review of randomized trials. *Am J Psychiatry* 2005; 162:1805–1819.

18. Kessing LV, et al. Suicide risk in patients treated with lithium. *Arch Gen Psychiatry* 2005; 62:860–866.

19. Young AH, et al. Lithium in maintenance therapy for bipolar disorder. *J Psychopharmacol* 2006; 20:17–22.

20. Song J, et al. Suicidal behavior during lithium and valproate treatment: a within-individual 8-year prospective study of 50,000 patients with bipolar disorder. *Am J Psychiatry* 2017; 174:795–802.

21. Mander AJ, et al. Rapid recurrence of mania following abrupt discontinuation of lithium. *Lancet* 1988; 2:15–17.

22. Faedda GL, et al. Outcome after rapid vs gradual discontinuation of lithium treatment in bipolar disorders. *Arch Gen Psychiatry* 1993; 50:448–455.

23. Macritchie KA, et al. Does 'rebound mania' occur after stopping carbamazepine? A pilot study. *J Psychopharmacol* 2000; 14:266–268.

24. Franks MA, et al. Bouncing back: is the bipolar rebound phenomenon peculiar to lithium? A retrospective naturalistic study. *J Psychopharmacol*

2008; 22:452–456.

25. Kessing LV, et al. Starting lithium prophylaxis early v. late in bipolar disorder. *Br J Psychiatry* 2014; 205:214–20.

26. Kessing LV, et al. Valproate v. lithium in the treatment of bipolar disorder in clinical practice: observational nationwide register-based cohort study. *Brit J Psychiatry* 2011; 199:57–63.

27. Gao K, et al. Typical and atypical antipsychotics in bipolar depression. *J Clin Psychiatry* 2005; 66:1376–1385.

28. Hellewell JS. A review of the evidence for the use of antipsychotics in the maintenance treatment of bipolar disorders. *J Psychopharmacol* 2006; 20:39–45.

29. Gigante AD, et al. Long-acting injectable antipsychotics for the maintenance treatment of bipolar disorder. *CNS Drugs* 2012; 26:403–420.

30. National Institute for Health and Care Excellence. Bipolar disorder: assessment and management. Clinical Guidance [CG185]. 2014 (Last updated February 2020); https://www.nice.org.uk/guidance/cg185.

31. Vieta E, et al. Efficacy and safety of quetiapine in combination with lithium or divalproex for maintenance of patients with bipolar I disorder (international trial 126). *J Affect Disord* 2008; 109:251–263.

32. McIntyre RS. Aripiprazole for the maintenance treatment of bipolar I disorder: A review. *Clin Ther* 2010; **32 Suppl 1**:S32–S38.

33. Ghaemi SN, et al. Long-term risperidone treatment in bipolar disorder: 6-month follow up. *Int Clin Psychopharmacol* 1997; 12:333–338.

34. Lindstrom L, et al. Maintenance therapy with second generation antipsychotics for bipolar disorder – A systematic review and meta-analysis. *J Affect Disord* 2017; 213:138–150.

35. Szegedi A, et al. Randomized, double-blind, placebo-controlled trial of asenapine maintenance therapy in adults with an acute manic or mixed episode associated with bipolar I disorder. *Am J Psychiatry* 2017; 175:71–79.

36. Bowden CL, et al. Efficacy of valproate versus lithium in mania or mixed mania: a randomized, open 12-week trial. *Int Clin Psychopharmacol* 2010; 25:60–67.

37. Kishi T, et al. Mood stabilizers and/or antipsychotics for bipolar disorder in the maintenance phase: a systematic review and network meta-analysis of randomized controlled trials. *Mol Psychiatry* 2020. [Epub ahead of print].

38. Escudero MAG, et al. Second generation antipsychotics monotherapy as maintenance treatment for bipolar disorder: a systematic review of long-term studies. *Psychiatr Q* 2020; 91:1047–1060.

39. Calabrese JR, et al. Efficacy and safety of aripiprazole once-monthly in the maintenance treatment of bipolar i disorder: a double-blind, placebo-controlled, 52-week randomized withdrawal study. *J Clin Psychiatry* 2017; 78:324–331.

40. Kishi T, et al. Long-acting injectable antipsychotics for prevention of relapse in bipolar disorder: a systematic review and meta-analyses of randomized controlled trials. *Int J Neuropsychopharmacol* 2016; 19.

41. Hsieh MH, et al. Bipolar patients treated with long-acting injectable risperidone in Taiwan: A 1-year mirror-image study using a national claims database. *J Affect Disord* 2017; 218:327–334.

42. Nolen WA, et al. What is the optimal serum level for lithium in the maintenance treatment of bipolar disorder? A systematic review and recommendations from the ISBD/IGSLI Task Force on treatment with lithium. *Bipolar Disord* 2019; 21:394–409.

43. Freeman MP, et al. Mood stabilizer combinations: a review of safety and efficacy. *Am J Psychiatry* 1998; 155:12–21.

44. Muzina DJ, et al. Maintenance therapies in bipolar disorder: focus on randomized controlled trials. *Aust N Z J Psychiatry* 2005; 39:652–661.

45. Tohen M, et al. Relapse prevention in bipolar I disorder: 18-month comparison of olanzapine plus mood stabiliser v. mood stabiliser alone. *Br J Psychiatry* 2004; 184:337–345.

46. Paton C, et al. Lithium in bipolar and other affective disorders: prescribing practice in the UK. *J Psychopharmacol* 2010; 24:1739–1746.

47. Marcus R, et al. Efficacy of aripiprazole adjunctive to lithium or valproate in the long-term treatment of patients with bipolar I disorder with an inadequate response to lithium or valproate monotherapy: a multicenter, double-blind, randomized study. *Bipolar Disord* 2011; 13:133–144.

48. Bowden CL, et al. A placebo-controlled 18-month trial of lamotrigine and lithium maintenance treatment in recently manic or hypomanic patients with bipolar I disorder. *Arch Gen Psychiatry* 2003; 60:392–400.

49. Pikalov A, et al. Long-term use of lurasidone in patients with bipolar disorder: safety and effectiveness over 2 years of treatment. *Int J Bipolar Disord* 2017; 5:9.

50. Calabrese JR, et al. Lurasidone in combination with lithium or valproate for the maintenance treatment of bipolar I disorder. *Eur Neuropsychopharmacol* 2017; 27:865–876.

51. Wingård L, et al. Monotherapy vs. combination therapy for post mania maintenance treatment: a population based cohort study. *Eur Neuropsychopharmacol* 2019; 29:691–700.

52. Jauhar S, et al. Controversies in bipolar disorder; role of second-generation antipsychotic for maintenance therapy. *Int J Bipolar Disord* 2019; 7:10.

53. Ghaemi SN, et al. Long-term antidepressant treatment in bipolar disorder: meta-analyses of benefits and risks. *Acta Psychiatr Scand* 2008; 118:347–356.

54. Ghaemi SN, et al. Antidepressant discontinuation in bipolar depression: a Systematic Treatment Enhancement Program for Bipolar Disorder (STEP-BD) randomized clinical trial of long-term effectiveness and safety. *J Clin Psychiatry* 2010; 71:372–380.

55. Ostacher MJ, et al. Impact of substance use disorders on recovery from episodes of depression in bipolar disorder patients: prospective data from the Systematic Treatment Enhancement Program for Bipolar Disorder (STEP-BD). *Am J Psychiatry* 2010; 167:289–297.

第2章

停用锂盐和心境稳定剂

停药依据

由于承受各种不良反应,患者可能要求停用锂盐或其他心境稳定剂。一项队列研究显示,54% 患者中断锂盐治疗主要由于耐受性问题,包括腹泻(13%)、震颤(11%)、多尿/多饮/尿崩症(9%)、肌酐升高(9%)和体重增加(7%)[1]。另外,尽管锂盐和心境稳定剂能有效地控制急性期症状和预防复发,或许临床医师判定风险与获益的平衡随时间而发生了变化(例如躯体不良反应逐渐增加,其他应对策略形成),因此可以考虑减量或停药。其他病人使用心境稳定剂治疗人格障碍等病,但是缺乏证据。停药应该将撤药反应和复发的风险降至最低(两个关键风险)。

锂盐和其他心境稳定剂的撤药反应

停用锂盐可能引起撤药反应,包括躯体和心理症状(表 2.12)。这些撤药反应包括心境发作(抑郁和躁狂,前者更常见),有时被称为"反弹"效应[2,3]。突然停药后复发的风险远远超过未经治疗者[2]。例如,对双相障碍患者中断锂盐的研究的荟萃分析发现,未治疗患者平均周期(两次发作之间平均时间)是 11.6 个月,而锂盐中断治疗后患者复发时间为 1.7 个月[2]。这意味着复发率增加 7 倍,说明锂盐停用后躁狂和抑郁症状立即发生,主要原因是锂盐的撤药反应。

"反弹"效应的原因一直有不同的解释,包括多巴胺能超敏感性[4],以及锂盐治疗期间神经元细胞膜、细胞转运功能或其他神经递质系统改变[5]。其他心境稳定剂也与"撤药"综合征相关[6]。

表 2.12 锂盐的撤药反应[3,7,8]

躯体	心理
■ 震颤	■ 焦虑
■ 多尿	■ 紧张
■ 肌无力	■ 易激惹
■ 多饮	■ 警觉
■ 口干	■ 睡眠紊乱
	■ 心境高涨/躁狂
	■ 情绪低落

长期治疗的证据

尽管锂盐被认为是预防双相障碍的一线选择[9],但是锂盐和其他心境稳定剂长程治疗的既往证据是基于中断治疗研究,纳入的患者被随机分配组继续或停止治疗[10,11]。这些研究中,锂盐有时被突然停用。如上所述,锂盐突然停用可能产生撤药反应,包括促发心境发作[2]。事实上,在一项突然停用锂盐的研究中,明显的单相抑郁患者出现躁狂发作的比例为 13%[12]。

证据显示其他心境稳定剂突然停用也能促发心境发作[3]。快速停用这些药物的患者复发率明显高于未治疗患者,提示撤药反应可以提高复发的频率和程度[2,13]。维持治疗研究的随访时间很少超过2年,但是自然状态下研究数据(更长随访时间)充分支持锂盐的长期使用[14]。

逐渐停药的时间

突然停药(1~14天)的危害远远大于"逐渐"停药(14~30天)[15-17]。突然停药导致复发时间缩短、研究结束时复发比例明显增加。这些证据充分、可重复的结果支持如下建议:锂盐不应该突然停用(除非发生严重不良反应),撤药一般情况下应该至少持续1个月,如果可行最好时间更长一些。

很少研究观察锂盐逐渐停用的最佳速度和时长。然而,研究发现50%的复发出现在锂盐停用后头3个月,随后逐渐减少[2]。这说明锂盐潜在适应性的消退可能需要这么长时间,用3个月以上时间逐渐减量可能有益。有一项研究发现,中断锂盐治疗2~5个月以上的患者,其复发率高于锂盐维持治疗患者[18]。NICE指南建议逐渐停用的时间应该在4周至3个月,而这项研究结果提示停药速度应该更慢一些[19]。

这样长时间的停药方案在不同医学领域并非罕见:在非精神科疾病中,抗癫痫药逐渐停用需要1个月至4年,停药后头6个月内复发率增加,之后复发率与继续使用抗癫痫药者相同[6]。

逐渐停药实践指南

- 应该告知患者有出现反弹效应的可能,如果锂盐或心境稳定剂停药过快,情感症状复发的风险可能增加。如果这些药物减得更慢一些,那么反弹效应会减少。
- 如何逐渐减量或减量需要多长时间,尚缺乏明确证据。但是,遵循其他精神药物的减药原则,开始时应将当前剂量减少10%~25%,同时监测撤药症状(表2.12)和其他症状2~4周,以确保病情稳定。
- 应该根据对此减量幅度的耐受程度进一步逐渐减量。减量应该使用指数法,将最近的剂量按固定比例(如10%~25%)计算,得出每次减量的幅度。大约每月一次,或直至确定病情稳定(随着总剂量减低,减量幅度也有效地变得越来越小)。
- 偶尔情况下,在完全停药前最后剂量可能非常小,因为小剂量对靶受体的效应相对较大。为达到小剂量,需要使用液体制剂(锂盐)或切片器(丙戊酸盐和卡马西平)。
- 由于锂盐或心境稳定剂减量过程可能导致病情不稳,在逐渐减量期间有必要采取其他策略[20]。为确保病情稳定,在完全停药后必须持续监测几个月。
- 如果撤药或复发的症状出现,暂停减量、剂量小幅增加或恢复之前有效剂量都是可能的对策。减药困难并不妨碍再次尝试减量,但是可能提示需要更缓慢的减量方案。
- 对于双相障碍患者,可以考虑的其他治疗方法包括家庭治疗、人际治疗、认知行为治疗、心理教育和社会节律治疗,以及更具个性化、更特殊的药物治疗方案[21-23]。

(汪作为 方贻儒 译 田成华 审校)

参考文献

1. Öhlund L, et al. Correction to: reasons for lithium discontinuation in men and women with bipolar disorder: a retrospective cohort study. *BMC Psychiatry* 2018; **18**:322.

2. Suppes T, et al. Risk of recurrence following discontinuation of lithium treatment in bipolar disorder. *Arch Gen Psychiatry* 1991; **48**:1082–1088.

3. Franks MA, et al. Bouncing back: is the bipolar rebound phenomenon peculiar to lithium? A retrospective naturalistic study. *J Psychopharmacol* 2008; **22**:452–456.

4. Ferrie L, et al. Effect of chronic lithium and withdrawal from chronic lithium on presynaptic dopamine function in the rat. *J Psychopharmacol* 2005; **19**:229–234.

5. Balon R, et al. Lithium discontinuation: withdrawal or relapse? *Compr Psychiatry* 1988; **29**:330–334.

6. Vernachio K, et al. A review of withdraw strategies for discontinuing antiepileptic therapy in epilepsy and pain management. *Pharm Pharmacol Int J* 2015; **3**:232–235.

7. Baastrup PC, et al. Prophylactic lithium: double blind discontinuation in manic-depressive and recurrent-depressive disorders. *Lancet* 1970; **2**:326–330.

8. Klein E, et al. Discontinuation of lithium treatment in remitted bipolar patients: relationship between clinical outcome and changes in sleep-wake cycles. *J Nerv Ment Dis* 1991; **179**:499–501.

9. Nolen WA, et al. What is the optimal serum level for lithium in the maintenance treatment of bipolar disorder? A systematic review and recommendations from the ISBD/IGSLI Task Force on treatment with lithium. *Bipolar Disord* 2019; **21**:394–409.

10. Geddes JR, et al. Long-term lithium therapy for bipolar disorder: systematic review and meta-analysis of randomized controlled trials. *Am J Psychiatry* 2004; **161**:217–222.

11. Moncrieff J. Lithium: evidence reconsidered. *Br J Psychiatry* 1997; **171**:113–119

12. Faedda GL, et al. Lithium discontinuation: uncovering latent bipolar disorder? *Am J Psychiatry* 2001; **158**:1337–1339.

13. Goodwin GM. Recurrence of mania after lithium withdrawal. Implications for the use of lithium in the treatment of bipolar affective disorder. *Br J Psychiatry* 1994; **164**:149–152.

14. Kessing LV, et al. Effectiveness of maintenance therapy of lithium vs other mood stabilizers in monotherapy and in combinations: a systematic review of evidence from observational studies. *Bipolar Disord* 2018; **20**:419–431

15. Faedda GL, et al. Outcome after rapid vs gradual discontinuation of lithium treatment in bipolar disorders. *Arch Gen Psychiatry* 1993; **50**:448–455.

16. Baldessarini RJ, et al. Illness risk following rapid versus gradual discontinuation of antidepressants. *Am J Psychiatry* 2010; **167**:934–941.

17. Baldessarini RJ, et al. Effects of the rate of discontinuing lithium maintenance treatment in bipolar disorders. *J Clin Psychiatry* 1996; **57**:441–448.

18. Biel MG, et al. Continuation versus discontinuation of lithium in recurrent bipolar illness: a naturalistic study. *Bipolar Disord* 2007; **9**:435–442.

19. National Institute for Health and Care Excellence. Bipolar disorder: assessment and management. Clinical Guidance [CG185]. 2014 (Last updated February 2020); https://www.nice.org.uk/guidance/cg185.

20. Guy A, et al. Guidance for psychological therapists: enabling conversations with clients taking or withdrawing from prescribed psychiatric drugs. London: APPG for Prescribed Drug Dependence; 2019.

21. Reinares M, et al. Psychosocial interventions in bipolar disorder: what, for whom, and when. *J Affect Disord* 2014; **156**:46–55.

22. Cappleman R, et al. Managing bipolar moods without medication: a qualitative investigation. *J Affect Disord* 2015; **174**:241–249.

23. Miklowitz DJ. Adjunctive psychotherapy for bipolar disorder: state of the evidence. *Am J Psychiatry* 2008; **165**:1408–1419.

第 2 章

第 3 章

抑郁和焦虑障碍

针对抑郁障碍的引言

抑郁症在全世界范围内都被认为是主要的公共健康问题。治疗抑郁症的主要手段是处方抗抑郁药;对轻度抑郁症患者,心理治疗也可以替代抗抑郁药作为一线治疗[1]。其他治疗方法[如迷走神经刺激术(vague nerve stimulation,VNS)[2]、重复经颅磁刺激(repetitive transcranial stimulation,rTMS)[3] 等]也已问世,但尚未被广泛应用。

下面介绍处方药物的基本原则,以及英国卫生和保健优化研究院(National Institute ofhealth and Care Excellence,NICE)的抑郁症治疗指南概要。抑郁症用药的基本原则,见表 3.1。

表 3.1 抑郁症用药的基本原则

- 与患者讨论药物的选择,以及其他非药物治疗的可用性和可行性
- 与患者讨论可能的结局,如抑郁症状需要经过几周方能逐步缓解
- 给予可能有效的抗抑郁药剂量(必要时逐渐加量)
- 对于单次发作,症状缓解后,继续治疗至少 6~9 个月(多次发作者可能需要更长时间)
- 抗抑郁药需缓慢停药,常要告知患者停药症状的风险和性质

抑郁症治疗的官方指南

NICE 指南[1]:概述

- 对于最近发病的轻度抑郁症,并不推荐抗抑郁药作为一线治疗。对这类患者,最好选择主动监测、个体化自助、认知行为治疗或者锻炼。
- 抗抑郁药可用于中、重度抑郁症和恶劣心境。
- 若处方抗抑郁药,建议使用非专利的选择性 5-羟色胺再摄取抑制剂。
- 所有患者都应该被告知抗抑郁药的停药反应。
- 对于难治性抑郁症,推荐的策略包括使用锂盐或抗精神病药作为增效剂,或者合用第二种抗抑郁药(见本章"难治性抑郁"部分)。
- 既往已经有 2 次抑郁发作,并存在功能损害的患者,治疗需要至少 2 年。

■ 电痉挛治疗（ECT）已被证明对严重和难治性抑郁症有效。

在撰写本书时，新的 NICE 指南尚处于草稿状态[4]。基本的原则与之前的指南一致，重要的差别点是第一次治疗失败后的药物推荐（见本章"抑郁症的药物治疗"部分）。

本章专注于抗抑郁药的使用，提供有关药物选择、剂量调整、换药策略和治疗顺序的建议。几乎不讨论其他非药物治疗方式，并不意味着它们的疗效不可靠，只是因为（作为一本处方指南）需要把注意力集中在药物相关主题。

参考文献

1. National Institute for Clinical Excellence. Depression: the treatment and management of depression in adults. Clinical Guidance [CG90]. 2009 (last reviewed December 2013); https://www.nice.org.uk/guidance/cg90.

2. George MS, et al. Vagus nerve stimulation for the treatment of depression and other neuropsychiatric disorders. *Expert Rev Neurother* 2007; 7:63–74.

3. Loo CK, et al. A review of the efficacy of transcranial magnetic stimulation (TMS) treatment for depression, and current and future strategies to optimize efficacy. *J Affect Disord* 2005; 88:255–267.

4. National Institute for Health and Care Excellence. Depression in adults: treatment and management – full guideline (Draft for Consultation). 2017; https://www.nice.org.uk/guidance/GID-CGWAVE0725/documents/draft-guideline.

第 3 章

抗抑郁药：概述

疗效

2018 年一项系统综述发现，在患有抑郁症的成年人中，所有抗抑郁药都比安慰剂有效[1]，另一项综述发现，抗抑郁药治疗对轻度、中度或重度抑郁症的益处相同[2]。

对于中度或以上的抑郁症患者，抗抑郁药通常被推荐作为一线治疗，而心理治疗则被用于症状较轻的患者。在中、重度患者中，约 20% 即使不治疗也能缓解，30% 安慰剂治疗有效，50% 抗抑郁药治疗有效[3]。据此计算，相对于真正的无治疗对照组，抗抑郁药的需要治疗人数（number needed to treat，NNT）为 3；相对于安慰剂，抗抑郁药的 NNT 则为 5。需要注意的是，在临床试验中，"有效"被规定为抑郁量表评分降低 50%，这是有些人为的两分法；而且使用连续性量表测量出来的变化值，往往显示出来的活性治疗与安慰剂（其本身对于抑郁症也是有效的治疗）之间的平均差值相对较小。

从历史角度上看，药物与安慰剂的疗效差异可能已经消失，这很大程度上是源于方法学变化[4]。评分量表可能在一定程度上模糊了抗抑郁药的效果。Hieronymus 等[5] 针对 18 个企业资助的、涉及 6 669 名抑郁症患者的帕罗西汀、西酞普兰、舍曲林、氟西汀的安慰剂对照试验进行患者水平的事后分析，探索如果采用"抑郁情绪"（0~4 级）单一条目作为疗效的衡量标准结果会有何影响。采用汉密尔顿抑郁量表（HAMD）-17 项版本的总分作为判断依据，在第 6 周时 32 个对照研究中有 18 个（56%）没有发现活性药物与安慰剂之间的差异；而以抑郁情绪作为唯一的疗效参数时，32 个对照中只有 3 个（9%）是阴性结果。正如前面提到的，即使在使用完整版本抑郁量表的情况下，最近的网络荟萃分析也显示抗抑郁药比安慰剂更有优势，其中阿米替林最有效[1]。

2019 年，PANDA 试验的结果支持将选择性 5-HT 再摄取抑制剂（SSRI）用于较既往更广泛的人群，包括那些不符合抑郁症或广泛性焦虑障碍诊断标准的轻、中度症状的患者[6]。

起效时间

人们普遍认为抗抑郁药起效通常需要 2~4 周。这其实是个误解。所有抗抑郁药的反应都呈现为一种模式，在第 1~2 周症状改善最快，第 4~6 周症状改善最慢。抗抑郁药与安慰剂之间出现具有统计学意义的差异，在单个临床试验中需要 2~4 周（因而有延迟起效的说法）；但是在（统计效力更强的）荟萃分析中，只需要 1~2 周[7,8]。因此，若治疗的患者数量大，并使用详细的量表，在治疗 1 周就能出现具有统计学意义的抗抑郁作用。在仅采用简单观察法的临床实践中，通常需要 2 周才能看到抗抑郁作用[9]。因此，若抗抑郁药治疗 3~4 周后疗效仍不明显，就需要调整抗抑郁药剂量或者换药。然而，重要的是清楚"无效"是由什么构成的。人们发现药物起效有不同的模式[10]，有些患者起效较慢。然而，在那些最终治疗起效的患者中，治疗 4 周时，患者应该已经开始出现至少轻度的症状改善。因此，若患者此时病情没有表现出一点改善，那么该剂量的药物可能永远都不会有效。相反，在治疗 4 周时若病情已有轻度改善（即进步幅度未达"有效"标准），仍会随着治疗进行而出现充分的疗效[11]。一项"巨分析"（mega-analysis）[12] 显示，如果单独考察对抑郁情绪的影响（而非采用汉密尔顿抑郁量表总分),那么抗抑郁药(西酞普兰、帕罗西汀或舍曲林)试验中,快速起效和剂量反应关系都很明显。

抗抑郁药选择和相关不良反应

与老一代的三环类抗抑郁药和单胺氧化酶抑制剂(MAOI)相比,选择性 5-HT 再摄取抑制剂(SSRI)耐受性较好,一般被推荐为抑郁症的一线治疗药物[13]。有一些网络荟萃分析结果[1,14]提示,某些抗抑郁药的疗效可能优于其他抗抑郁药,但是这种差异并非总是能够在头对头研究中得到证实,因此应该谨慎对待这些结果。不同抗抑郁药的不良反应存在差异。例如,帕罗西汀引起的体重增加较多,性功能障碍的发生率较高;舍曲林导致腹泻的发生率高于其他 SSRI[15]。双重再摄取抑制剂,如文拉法辛和度洛西汀,往往耐受性不如 SSRI,但是优于 TCA。所有药物的耐受性均有明显的个体差异,这种差异难以根据某种药物已知的不良反应来预测。往往需要采用灵活的方法,为具体患者选择合适的药物。

除了头痛和胃肠道症状,SSRI 类药物还可引起一些其他不良反应,包括性功能障碍(见本章"抗抑郁药和性功能障碍")、低钠血症(见本章"抗抑郁药和低钠血症")、胃肠道出血(见本章"SSRI 与出血"部分)。TCA 有一些心血管系统不良反应(低血压、心动过速和 QTc 延长),药物过量时毒性特别大[16](见第 13 章"精神药物过量")。目前,极少使用的 MAOI 类药物可能会与含酪胺食物发生相互作用,导致高血压危象,更常见的是导致低血压。所有抗抑郁药均可导致停药症状,短半衰期药物问题最大(见本章"抗抑郁药的停药症状")。有关抗抑郁药临床相关不良反应的摘要,请参阅下文。

药物相互作用

某些 SSRI 是单个或者多个肝脏细胞色素 P450 通路的强抑制剂,且抑制效应的强度与剂量相关。因此,药物共用时,预期会出现一些具有临床意义的相互作用。例如,氟伏沙明是 CYP1A2 的强抑制剂,可导致茶碱血浆浓度升高;氟西汀是 CYP2D6 的强抑制剂,可导致氯氮平使用者癫痫发作的风险升高;帕罗西汀是 CYP2D6 的强抑制剂,可导致他莫昔芬(一种前体药物)治疗失败,增加死亡率[17]。

抗抑郁药也可能导致药效学相互作用。例如,合并使用可能导致电解质紊乱的利尿剂时,可增加 TCA 的心血管毒性。本章后面可以找到临床相关的药物与抗抑郁药相互作用的总结。

从一种抗抑郁药换为另一种抗抑郁药时,需要考察抗抑郁药之间可能的药代动力学和药效动力学相互作用(见本章"换药和停药")。

自杀

抗抑郁药治疗被认为增加了患者(尤其是青少年和青年人)出现自杀观念和自杀行为的风险[18-21],因此,建议警告患者在治疗前几周存在这种不良反应的潜在风险,并使其了解如何在必要时寻求帮助。开始或停止使用抗抑郁药时,自杀率或自伤率往往更高,因此在停止治疗时,应与开始时一样关注风险评估[22]。此外,75 岁及以上开始抗抑郁药治疗的人,更换抗抑郁药可能是自杀风险增加的标志[23]。

所有抗抑郁药均有此风险[24],包括那些适应证并不是抑郁症的药物(如托莫西汀)。应该注意的是：①尽管对一些患者而言,自杀风险相对于安慰剂有所增加,但绝对风险仍然很小。②避免自杀观念和自杀行为最有效的措施是治疗抑郁症[25-27]。③抗抑郁药是目前所有措施中最有效的治疗手段[3,28]。在大多数情况下,自杀风险随着抗抑郁药治疗显著减少[29-31]。需要注意的是,患者如果用一种抗抑郁药在治疗过程中出现或加重了自杀观念,使用其他治疗时也可能有类似的体验[32]。最近的一些数据表明,越来越多完成自杀的年轻女性,在过去几年中自杀前和自杀时都接受过抗抑郁药治疗[33]。在撰写本文时,除了年轻人使用抗抑郁药风险最高,对于抗抑郁药的潜在风险尚无明确共识[34]。

抗抑郁药过量中毒的表现在同一类别内和不同类别之间均存在差异[35]。见第 13 章"精神药物过量"部分。

疗程

抗抑郁药能缓解患者的抑郁症状,但并不能治疗其潜在病因。单次发作临床痊愈之后,还应继续用药 6~9 个月(以覆盖绝大多数单次发作未治疗时的假定病程)。对多次复发患者,现有证据提示患者维持治疗 2 年以上是有益的;目前没有确定疗程的上限是多长时间(见本章"抗抑郁药预防作用"部分)。关于增效治疗的疗程,没有多少研究数据,因此无法提出建议。少数观点认为,从长远看,抗抑郁药会使结局恶化[36]。

下一步治疗

约 1/3 的患者使用第一种抗抑郁药无效。这些患者可选的治疗手段包括增加剂量、换用另一种抗抑郁药或者给予增效治疗。从缓解抑郁的序贯治疗研究(Sequenced Treatment Alternatives to Relieve Depression,STAR*D)中获得的经验是,在治疗无效者中,每次改变治疗,都会对小部分人有效,但该疗效的效应值不大,且不同治疗措施之间的疗效也没有明显差异。见本章"难治性抑郁的治疗"部分。

焦虑谱系障碍中的抗抑郁药使用

抗抑郁药是许多焦虑谱系障碍的一线治疗措施。见本章"焦虑谱系障碍"部分。

参考文献

1. Cipriani A, et al. Comparative efficacy and acceptability of 21 antidepressant drugs for the acute treatment of adults with major depressive disorder: a systematic review and network meta-analysis. *Lancet* 2018; 391:1357–1366.
2. Furukawa TA, et al. Initial severity of major depression and efficacy of new generation antidepressants: individual participant data meta-analysis. *Acta Psychiatr Scand* 2018; 137:450–458.
3. Anderson IM, et al. Evidence-based guidelines for treating depressive disorders with antidepressants: a revision of the 2000 British Association for Psychopharmacology guidelines. *J Psychopharmacology* 2008; 22:343–396.
4. Khan A, et al. Why has the antidepressant-placebo difference in antidepressant clinical trials diminished over the past three decades? *CNS Neurosci Ther* 2010; 16:217–226.
5. Hieronymus F, et al. Consistent superiority of selective serotonin reuptake inhibitors over placebo in reducing depressed mood in patients with major depression. *Mol Psychiatry* 2016; 21:523–530.
6. Lewis G, et al. The clinical effectiveness of sertraline in primary care and the role of depression severity and duration (PANDA): a pragmatic, double-blind, placebo-controlled randomised trial. *Lancet Psychiatry* 2019; 6:903–914.
7. Taylor MJ, et al. Early onset of selective serotonin reuptake inhibitor antidepressant action: systematic review and meta-analysis. *Arch Gen Psychiatry* 2006; 63:1217–1223.
8. Papakostas GI, et al. A meta-analysis of early sustained response rates between antidepressants and placebo for the treatment of major depressive disorder. *J Clin Psychopharmacol* 2006; 26:56–60.
9. Szegedi A, et al. Early improvement in the first 2 weeks as a predictor of treatment outcome in patients with major depressive disorder: a

meta-analysis including 6562 patients. *J Clin Psychiatry* 2009; **70**:344–353.

10. Uher R, et al. Early and delayed onset of response to antidepressants in individual trajectories of change during treatment of major depression: a secondary analysis of data from the Genome-Based Therapeutic Drugs for Depression (GENDEP) study. *J Clin Psychiatry* 2011; **72**:1478–1484.

11. Posternak MA, et al. Response rates to fluoxetine in subjects who initially show no improvement. *J Clin Psychiatry* 2011; **72**:949–954.

12. Hieronymus F, et al. A mega-analysis of fixed-dose trials reveals dose-dependency and a rapid onset of action for the antidepressant effect of three selective serotonin reuptake inhibitors. *Trans Psychiatry* 2016; **6**:e834.

13. National Institute for Health and Care Excellence. Depression in adults: recognition and management. Clinical guideline [CG90]. 2009 (last updated: December 2013); https://www.nice.org.uk/Guidance/cg90.

14. Cipriani A, et al. Comparative efficacy and acceptability of 12 new-generation antidepressants: a multiple-treatments meta-analysis. *Lancet* 2009; **373**:746–758.

15. Gartlehner G, et al. Comparative benefits and harms of second-generation antidepressants: background paper for the American College of Physicians. *Ann Intern Med* 2008; **149**:734–750.

16. Flanagan RJ. Fatal toxicity of drugs used in psychiatry. *Human Psychopharmacology* 2008; **23 Suppl 1**:43–51.

17. Kelly CM, et al. Selective serotonin reuptake inhibitors and breast cancer mortality in women receiving tamoxifen: a population based cohort study. *BMJ* 2010; **340**:c693.

18. Stone M, et al. Risk of suicidality in clinical trials of antidepressants in adults: analysis of proprietary data submitted to US Food and Drug Administration. *BMJ* 2009; **339**:b2880.

19. Carpenter DJ, et al. Meta-analysis of efficacy and treatment-emergent suicidality in adults by psychiatric indication and age subgroup following initiation of paroxetine therapy: a complete set of randomized placebo-controlled trials. *J Clin Psychiatry* 2011; **72**:1503–1514.

20. Barbui C, et al. Selective serotonin reuptake inhibitors and risk of suicide: a systematic review of observational studies. *CMAJ* 2009; **180**:291–297.

21. Umetsu R, et al. Association between selective serotonin reuptake inhibitor therapy and suicidality: analysis of U.S. Food and drug administration adverse event reporting system data. *Biol Pharm Bull* 2015; **38**:1689–1699.

22. Coupland C, et al. Antidepressant use and risk of suicide and attempted suicide or self harm in people aged 20 to 64: cohort study using a primary care database. *BMJ* 2015; **350**:h517.

23. Hedna K, et al. Antidepressants and suicidal behaviour in late life: a prospective population-based study of use patterns in new users aged 75 and above. *Eur J Clin Pharmacol* 2018; **74**:201–208.

24. Schneeweiss S, et al. Variation in the risk of suicide attempts and completed suicides by antidepressant agent in adults: a propensity score-adjusted analysis of 9 years' data. *Arch Gen Psychiatry* 2010; **67**:497–506.

25. Isacsson G, et al. The increased use of antidepressants has contributed to the worldwide reduction in suicide rates. *Br J Psychiatry* 2010; **196**:429–433.

26. Gibbons RD, et al. Suicidal thoughts and behavior with antidepressant treatment: reanalysis of the randomized placebo-controlled studies of fluoxetine and venlafaxine. *Arch Gen Psychiatry* 2012; **69**:580–587.

27. Lu CY, et al. Changes in antidepressant use by young people and suicidal behavior after FDA warnings and media coverage: quasi-experimental study. *BMJ* 2014; **348**:g3596.

28. Isacsson G, et al. Antidepressant medication prevents suicide in depression. *Acta Psychiatr Scand* 2010; **122**:454–460.

29. Simon GE, et al. Suicide risk during antidepressant treatment. *Am J Psychiatry* 2006; **163**:41–47.

30. Mulder RT, et al. Antidepressant treatment is associated with a reduction in suicidal ideation and suicide attempts. *Acta Psychiatr Scand* 2008; **118**:116–122.

31. Tondo L, et al. Suicidal status during antidepressant treatment in 789 Sardinian patients with major affective disorder. *Acta Psychiatr Scand* 2008; **118**:106–115.

32. Perlis RH, et al. Do suicidal thoughts or behaviors recur during a second antidepressant treatment trial? *J Clin Psychiatry* 2012; **73**:1439–1442.

33. Larsson J. Antidepressants and suicide among young women in Sweden 1999–2013. *Int J Risk Saf Med* 2017; **29**:101–106.

34. Spielmans GI, et al. Duty to warn: antidepressant black box suicidality warning is empirically justified. *Front Psychiatry* 2020; **11**:18.

35. Hawton K, et al. Toxicity of antidepressants: rates of suicide relative to prescribing and non-fatal overdose. *Br J Psychiatry* 2010; **196**:354–358.

36. Fava GA. May antidepressant drugs worsen the conditions they are supposed to treat? The clinical foundations of the oppositional model of tolerance. *Ther Adv Psychopharmacol* 2020; [Epub ahead of print].

抗抑郁药公认的最低有效剂量

所建议的抗抑郁药最低有效剂量见表 3.2。

表 3.2   抗抑郁药的最小推荐治疗剂量

抗抑郁药	剂量
三环类	不明确,最少 75~100mg/d[1],可能是 125mg/d[2]
洛非帕明	140mg/d[3]
SSRI	
西酞普兰	20mg/d[4]
艾司西酞普兰	10mg/d[5]
氟西汀	20mg/d[6]
氟伏沙明	50mg/d[7]
帕罗西汀	20mg/d[8]
舍曲林	50mg/d[9]
其他	
阿戈美拉汀	25mg/d[10]
安非他酮	150mg/d[11]
去甲文拉法辛	50mg/d[12]
度洛西汀	60mg/d[13,14]
米那普仑	40mg/d[15]
米氮平	30mg/d[16](15mg?)
吗氯贝胺	300mg/d[17]
瑞波西汀	8mg/d[18]
曲唑酮	150mg/d[19]
文拉法辛	75mg/d[20]
维拉唑酮	20mg/d[15]
伏硫西汀	10mg/d[15]

参考文献

1. Furukawa TA, et al. Meta-analysis of effects and side effects of low dosage tricyclic antidepressants in depression: systematic review. *BMJ* 2002; 325:991.
2. Donoghue J, et al. Suboptimal use of antidepressants in the treatment of depression. *CNS Drugs* 2000; 13:365–368.
3. Lancaster SG, et al. Lofepramine. A review of its pharmacodynamic and pharmacokinetic properties, and therapeutic efficacy in depressive illness. *Drugs* 1989; 37:123–140.
4. Montgomery SA, et al. The optimal dosing regimen for citalopram – a meta-analysis of nine placebo-controlled studies. *Int Clin Psychopharmacol* 1994; 9 Suppl 1:35–40.
5. Burke WJ, et al. Fixed-dose trial of the single isomer SSRI escitalopram in depressed outpatients. *J Clin Psychiatry* 2002; 63:331–336.

6. Altamura AC, et al. The evidence for 20mg a day of fluoxetine as the optimal dose in the treatment of depression. *Br J Psychiatry Suppl* 1988; 109–112.

7. Walczak DD, et al. The oral dose-effect relationship for fluvoxamine: a fixed-dose comparison against placebo in depressed outpatients. *Ann Clin Psychiatry* 1996; 8:139–151.

8. Dunner DL, et al. Optimal dose regimen for paroxetine. *J Clin Psychiatry* 1992; 53 **Suppl**:21–26.

9. Moon CAL, et al. A double-blind comparison of sertraline and clomipramine in the treatment of major depressive disorder and associative anxiety in general practice. *J Psychopharm* 1994; 8:171–176.

10. Loo H, et al. Determination of the dose of agomelatine, a melatoninergic agonist and selective 5-HT(2C) antagonist, in the treatment of major depressive disorder: a placebo-controlled dose range study. *Int Clin Psychopharmacol* 2002; 17:239–247.

11. Hewett K, et al. Eight-week, placebo-controlled, double-blind comparison of the antidepressant efficacy and tolerability of bupropion XR and venlafaxine XR. *J Psychopharmacology* 2009; 23:531–538.

12. Kornstein SG, et al. The effect of desvenlafaxine 50 mg/day on a subpopulation of anxious/depressed patients: a pooled analysis of seven randomized, placebo-controlled studies. *Human Psychopharmacology* 2014; 29:492–501.

13. Goldstein DJ, et al. Duloxetine in the treatment of depression: a double-blind placebo-controlled comparison with paroxetine. *J Clin Psychopharmacol* 2004; 24:389–399.

14. Detke MJ, et al. Duloxetine, 60 mg once daily, for major depressive disorder: a randomized double-blind placebo-controlled trial. *J Clin Psychiatry* 2002; 63:308–315.

15. He H, et al. Efficacy and tolerability of different doses of three new antidepressants for treating major depressive disorder: a PRISMA-compliant meta-analysis. *J Psychiatr Res* 2018; 96:247–259.

16. Furukawa TA, et al. No benefit from flexible titration above minimum licensed dose in prescribing antidepressants for major depression: systematic review. *Acta Psychiatr Scand* 2020; 141:401–409.

17. Priest RG, et al. Moclobemide in the treatment of depression. *Rev Contemporary Pharmacother* 1994; 5:35–43.

18. Schatzberg AF. Clinical efficacy of reboxetine in major depression. *J Clin Psychiatry* 2000; 61 **Suppl** 10:31–38.

19. Brogden RN, et al. Trazodone: a review of its pharmacological properties and therapeutic use in depression and anxiety. *Drugs* 1981; 21:401–429.

20. Feighner JP, et al. Efficacy of once-daily venlafaxine extended release (XR) for symptoms of anxiety in depressed outpatients. *J Affect Disord* 1998; 47:55–62.

第 3 章

抑郁症的药物治疗

图 3.1 概括了抑郁症的药物治疗。

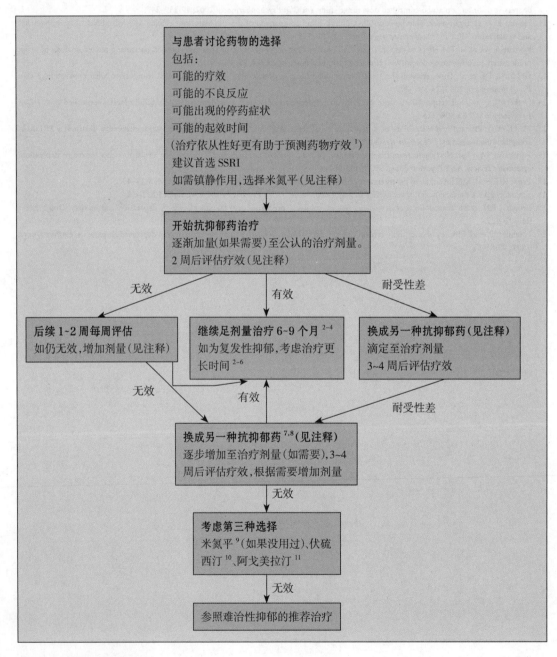

图 3.1 抑郁症的药物治疗

注:

- 蒙哥马利抑郁量表(MADRS)[12]和汉密尔顿抑郁量表(HAMD)[13]是临床试验中常用的疗效评价工具。HAMD 稍显落伍,但熟悉 MADRS 的医生较少(MADRS 可能是评价疾病严重程度及其变化的最好量表)。PHQ-9[14]使用简便,被推荐用于评估抑郁症的症状变化(但它更适合评价症状频率,而非症状的严重程度)。

- 抗抑郁药选择大多受到患者和医师倾向性的影响。但是大多数专家选择 SSRI,或者在需要镇静作用时选择米氮平。最大的网络荟萃分析[15]显示,同时作用于去甲肾上腺素和 5-羟色胺再摄取的药物最有效(排名最靠前的 6 个药中,有 5 个是双通道药物),而阿戈美拉汀和 SSRI 脱落率最低。一项 2018 年发表的有关新一类抗抑郁药的网络荟萃分析[16]显示,左米那普仑、维拉唑酮和伏硫西汀相对老一代抗抑郁药的优势较小。

- 治疗 2 周后的评估有利于预测最终疗效[17]。治疗 2 周后,那些改善幅度没能达到可接受的症状阈值的患者,只有大约 30% 最终有效。如果在治疗 2 周后症状无改善,甚至恶化,最终症状改善的概率更小。

- 如果患者对某个药物耐受性差,已有研究[18]支持可以换成不同类别的药物,这有坚实的理论基础。即便如此,临床上不能耐受某种 SSRI 的患者却可能会耐受另外一种 SSRI。

- 对治疗无效的患者,有证据表明在同一类别的药物中更换是有效的[8,19-22]。但在实践中,最常见的是换成不同类别的药物,这已获得一些分析的支持[23]。美国精神病学会对两种方式均有推荐[2]。2018 版 NICE 指南草案[24]建议,几乎没有令人信服的证据支持不同类别抗抑郁药之间的转换(来自另一项分析的观察[25]),抗抑郁药联合治疗或添加第二代抗精神病药(SGA)是这一阶段更好的选择。在治疗失败时,换药最有力的证据可能是伏硫西汀[10]。

- 在治疗抑郁症时,很少证据支持大多数 SSRI 药物的剂量需要增加[20],至少在采用量表总分作为评价标准时[26]是这样。在采用 HAMD 心境条目作为考察标准时,结果提示 SSRI 药物具有一定的量效关系[27]。也有其他证据提示,增加文拉法辛、艾司西酞普兰和三环类药物的剂量可能有效[3]。一般而言,通过增加药物剂量来获得的疗效较小(SSRI、文拉法辛)或者不存在(如米氮平剂量超过 30mg/d),但剂量增加对耐受性的影响是明确且显著有害的[28]。

- 如果不良反应无法耐受,应尽早换药(如治疗 1~2 周之后);或者治疗 3~4 周时仍毫无改善,也应换药。关于什么时间换药,观点并不一致。但是显然,抗抑郁药起效相当迅速[29-31],2~6 周治疗无效是药物最终无效的良好预测指标[32-34]。若治疗 3~4 周时毫无改善,一般应该更改治疗(英国精神药理学会指南建议为 4 周[3])。若此时已有一定改善,在接下来的 2~3 周内可继续治疗并评估(见本章"抗抑郁药:概述"部分)。

参考文献

1. Leuchter AF, et al. Role of pill-taking, expectation and therapeutic alliance in the placebo response in clinical trials for major depression. *Br J Psychiatry* 2014; 205:443–449.

2. American Psychiatric Association. *Practice guideline for the treatment of patients with major depressive disorder*. Third Edition. Washington, USA: American Psychiatric Association; 2010.

3. Anderson IM, et al. Evidence-based guidelines for treating depressive disorders with antidepressants: a revision of the 2000 British Association for Psychopharmacology guidelines. *J Psychopharmacology* 2008; 22:343–396.

4. Crismon ML, et al. The Texas medication algorithm project: report of the Texas consensus conference panel on medication treatment of major depressive disorder. *J Clin Psychiatry* 1999; 60:142–156.

5. Kocsis JH, et al. Maintenance therapy for chronic depression. A controlled clinical trial of desipramine. *Arch Gen Psychiatry* 1996; 53:769–774.

6. Dekker J, et al. The use of antidepressants after recovery from depression. *Eur J Psychiatry* 2000; 14:207–212.

7. Nelson JC. Treatment of antidepressant nonresponders: augmentation or switch? *J Clin Psychiatry* 1998; 59 Suppl 15:35–41.

8. Joffe RT. Substitution therapy in patients with major depression. *CNS Drugs* 1999; 11:175–180.

9. National Institute for Health and Care Excellence. Depression in adults: recognition and management. Clinical Guidance [CG90]. 2009 (reviewed December 2013); http://www.nice.org.uk/Guidance/cg90.

10. Montgomery SA, et al. A randomised, double-blind study in adults with major depressive disorder with an inadequate response to a single course of selective serotonin reuptake inhibitor or serotonin-noradrenaline reuptake inhibitor treatment switched to vortioxetine or agomelatine. *Human Psychopharmacology* 2014; 29:470–482.

11. Sparshatt A, et al. A naturalistic evaluation and audit database of agomelatine: clinical outcome at 12 weeks. *Acta Psychiatr Scand* 2013;

128:203–211.

12. Montgomery SA, et al. A new depression scale designed to be sensitive to change. *Br J Psychiatry* 1979; **134**:382–389.

13. Hamilton M. Development of a rating scale for primary depressive illness. *Br J Soc Clin Psychol* 1967; **6**:278–296.

14. Kroenke K, et al. The PHQ-9: validity of a brief depression severity measure. *J Gen Intern Med* 2001; **16**:606–613.

15. Cipriani A, et al. Comparative efficacy and acceptability of 21 antidepressant drugs for the acute treatment of adults with major depressive disorder: a systematic review and network meta-analysis. *Lancet* 2018; **391**:1357–1366.

16. Wagner G, et al. Efficacy and safety of levomilnacipran, vilazodone and vortioxetine compared with other second-generation antidepressants for major depressive disorder in adults: a systematic review and network meta-analysis. *J Affect Disord* 2018; **228**:1–12.

17. de Vries YA, et al. Predicting antidepressant response by monitoring early improvement of individual symptoms of depression: individual patient data meta-analysis. *Br J Psychiatry* 2019; **214**:4–10.

18. Köhler-Forsberg O, et al. Efficacy of anti-inflammatory treatment on major depressive disorder or depressive symptoms: meta-analysis of clinical trials. *Acta Psychiatr Scand* 2019; **139**:404–419.

19. Thase ME, et al. Citalopram treatment of fluoxetine nonresponders. *J Clin Psychiatry* 2001; **62**:683–687.

20. Rush AJ, et al. Bupropion-SR, sertraline, or venlafaxine-XR after failure of SSRIs for depression. *N Engl J Med* 2006; **354**:1231–1242.

21. Ruhe HG, et al. Switching antidepressants after a first selective serotonin reuptake inhibitor in major depressive disorder: a systematic review. *J Clin Psychiatry* 2006; **67**:1836–1855.

22. Brent D, et al. Switching to another SSRI or to venlafaxine with or without cognitive behavioral therapy for adolescents with SSRI-resistant depression: the TORDIA randomized controlled trial. *JAMA* 2008; **299**:901–913.

23. Papakostas GI, et al. Treatment of SSRI-resistant depression: a meta-analysis comparing within- versus across-class switches. *Biol Psychiatry* 2008; **63**:699–704.

24. National Institute for Health and Care Excellence. Depression in adults: treatment and management – Full guideline (Draft for Consultation). 2017; https://www.nice.org.uk/guidance/GID-CGWAVE0725/documents/draft-guideline.

25. Bschor T, et al. Switching the antidepressant after nonresponse in adults with major depression: a systematic literature search and meta-analysis. *J Clin Psychiatry* 2018; 79.

26. Adli M, et al. Is dose escalation of antidepressants a rational strategy after a medium-dose treatment has failed? A systematic review. *Eur Arch Psychiatry Clin Neurosci* 2005; **255**:387–400.

27. Hieronymus F, et al. A mega-analysis of fixed-dose trials reveals dose-dependency and a rapid onset of action for the antidepressant effect of three selective serotonin reuptake inhibitors. *Trans Psychiatry* 2016; **6**:e834.

28. Furukawa TA, et al. Optimal dose of selective serotonin reuptake inhibitors, venlafaxine, and mirtazapine in major depression: a systematic review and dose-response meta-analysis. *Lancet Psychiatry* 2019; **6**:601–609.

29. Papakostas GI, et al. A meta-analysis of early sustained response rates between antidepressants and placebo for the treatment of major depressive disorder. *J Clin Psychopharmacol* 2006; **26**:56–60.

30. Taylor MJ, et al. Early onset of selective serotonin reuptake inhibitor antidepressant action: systematic review and meta-analysis. *Arch Gen Psychiatry* 2006; **63**:1217–1223.

31. Posternak MA, et al. Is there a delay in the antidepressant effect? A meta-analysis. *J Clin Psychiatry* 2005; **66**:148–158.

32. Szegedi A, et al. Early improvement in the first 2 weeks as a predictor of treatment outcome in patients with major depressive disorder: a meta-analysis including 6562 patients. *J Clin Psychiatry* 2009; **70**:344–353.

33. Baldwin DS, et al. How long should a trial of escitalopram treatment be in patients with major depressive disorder, generalised anxiety disorder or social anxiety disorder? An exploration of the randomised controlled trial database. *Human Psychopharmacology* 2009; **24**:269–275.

34. Nierenberg AA, et al. Early nonresponse to fluoxetine as a predictor of poor 8-week outcome. *Am J Psychiatry* 1995; **152**:1500–1503.

第 3 章

难治性抑郁的治疗：首选

难治性抑郁的治疗很难成功,结局往往欠佳[1-3],尤其在不遵守循证治疗方案时,更是如此[4]。难治性抑郁并非完全一样,根据其严重程度可分为不同等级[5],形成一个复杂的谱系,其治疗结果与严重程度的等级密切相关[6]。少数症状顽固的单相抑郁患者,实际上有可能是双相抑郁[7,8],标准的抗抑郁药治疗常常无效[9,10](见第 2 章"双相抑郁"部分)。最近有一种将治疗抵抗的(treatment-resistant)抑郁症描述为"治疗困难的"(difficult to treat)抑郁症的趋势,因为前一种描述暗示抑郁症治疗通常是有效的,因此无效在某种程度上是异常的[11]。有人建议放弃治疗抵抗的抑郁症这一诊断(再次提出"治疗困难"的抑郁症这个概念),这会促使临床医师在越来越复杂的治疗方案中尝试越来越多的药物,而不是将康复的期待维持在更现实的水平[12]。

难治性抑郁的治疗在一定程度上受到 STAR*D(Sequenced Treatment Alternatives to Relieve Depression,缓解抑郁的序贯治疗方案)研究结果的启发。STAR*D 是一个实用的有效性研究,它把症状缓解作为主要结局指标。在第一阶段[13],2 786 名被试接受西酞普兰治疗(平均剂量 41.8mg/d),历时 14 周;28% 的被试者症状缓解,47% 的被试者治疗有效(即症状评分降低 50%)。症状未缓解的被试者进入下一步序贯治疗研究(第 2 阶段)[14-18],缓解率见图 3.2。进入第 2 阶段后,很少有差异具有统计学意义。在第 3 阶段[17],发现患者对 T_3 的耐受性显著优于对锂的耐受性。在第 4 阶段[16],反苯环丙胺的疗效和耐受性均不如合用米氮平和文拉法辛。总体上可以看到,缓解率低得令人担忧;但是需要注意的是,该研究的被试者有长期复发性抑郁的病史。

STAR*D 研究表明,难治性抑郁的治疗需要采用灵活的策略(表 3.3),并且某种治疗的疗效难以根据药理学或既往治疗经验进行预测。该项目确定,安非他酮和丁螺环酮增效治疗是值得尝试的选择,也把既往默默无闻的 T_3 增效治疗和去甲替林方案挖掘出来。该研究在一定程度上证实了米氮平和文拉法辛合用的安全性,并在较小程度上证明了这种合用的疗效。

应该指出的是,对 STAR*D 项目有许多有价值的批评,包括没有安慰剂组,治疗和一些评估为开放性的,未能说明患者在第一次就诊后退出的原因,无法解释使用先验次要指标作为主要结果指标的原因,支付给受试者报酬,以及观察到 1 518 名缓解的患者中有 93% 在 12 个月的随访中复发或退出研究[19,20]。这些因素或许不会改变对比较数据的解释,但它进一步强化了使用该研究中的抗抑郁药方案治疗长期、难治性抑郁时,不能期望太高。

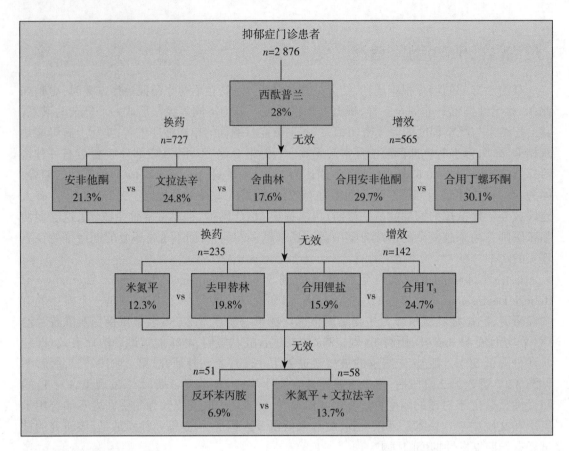

图 3.2　STAR*D 中的缓解率

表 3.3　难治性抑郁——首选:一般已获得发表文献支持的常用治疗方案(排序不分先后)

治疗	优点	缺点
抗抑郁药加**阿立哌唑**[21-27] (2~20mg/d)	▪ 良好的证据基础 ▪ 通常耐受好且安全 ▪ 低剂量(2~10mg/d)可能有效 ▪ 获得最近的荟萃分析支持[28]	▪ 标准剂量(≥10mg/d)常见有静坐不能和躁动不安 ▪ 可能有失眠问题
加用**锂盐**[29] 开始时目标血浆水平为 0.4~0.8mmol/L;若疗效欠佳,最高可增加到 1.0mmol/L	▪ 已经得到确认 ▪ 有充分文献支持 ▪ NICE 推荐[30] ▪ 最近的荟萃分析支持[28]	▪ 血浆水平高时耐受性差 ▪ 可能中毒 ▪ 往往需要向专科医生转诊 ▪ 需要监测血浆水平(以及甲状腺功能、eGFR) ▪ 多种治疗无效者,锂盐增效也可能无效
合用**奥氮平**和**氟西汀**[31] (6.25~12.5mg+25~50mg 经美国批准的日剂量)*	▪ 有充分的研究 ▪ 通常耐受性很好 ▪ 奥氮平 +TCA 也可能有效[32] ▪ 单用奥氮平可能有效[33,34]	▪ 体重增加的风险 ▪ 在美国以外,临床经验有限 ▪ 数据大多与双相抑郁有关

续表

治疗	优点	缺点
加用喹硫平[35-40] （150mg/d 或 300mg/d） 合并 SSRI、SNRI	■ 良好的证据基础 ■ 通常耐受性良好 ■ 对抗抑郁作用似有可信服的解释 ■ 疗效可能优于锂	■ 口干、镇静和便秘可能构成问题 ■ 长期治疗有体重增加的风险
SSRI+ 安非他酮[15,41-45] 最高 400mg/d	■ STAR*D 支持 ■ 耐受性良好 ■ 可改善性功能不良反应	■ 在英国，未被批准用于治疗抑郁症
SSRI 或文拉法辛 + 米安色林[18,45-48]（30mg/d）**或米氮平**（30~45mg/d）	■ NICE 推荐 ■ 通常耐受性良好 ■ 已广泛使用	■ 理论上有 5- 羟色胺综合征的风险（需告知患者） ■ 米安色林有致恶血质风险 ■ 米氮平致体重增加和镇静 ■ 近期一项大型 RCT 研究显示：既往 SSRI/SNRI 治疗无效的患者，加用米氮平无优势[49]

　　* 在没有复合制剂的情况下，将 5mg+20mg 升至 10mg +40mg 似乎是合理的。

　　eGFR，肾小球滤过率估计值；NICE，国家卫生与保健研究所；SNRI，去甲肾上腺素 5- 羟色胺再摄取抑制剂；SSRI，选择性 5- 羟色胺再摄取抑制剂；STAR*D，改善抑郁症的序贯治疗方案；TCA，三环类抗抑郁药；TFT，甲状腺功能试验。

参考文献

1. Dunner DL, et al. Prospective, long-term, multicenter study of the naturalistic outcomes of patients with treatment-resistant depression. *J Clin Psychiatry* 2006; 67:688–695.

2. Wooderson SC, et al. Prospective evaluation of specialist inpatient treatment for refractory affective disorders. *J Affect Disord* 2011; 131:92–103.

3. Fekadu A, et al. What happens to patients with treatment-resistant depression? A systematic review of medium to long term outcome studies. *J Affect Disord* 2009; 116:4–11.

4. Trivedi MH, et al. Clinical results for patients with major depressive disorder in the Texas Medication Algorithm Project. *Arch Gen Psychiatry* 2004; 61:669–680.

5. Fekadu A, et al. A multidimensional tool to quantify treatment resistance in depression: the Maudsley staging method. *J Clin Psychiatry* 2009; 70:177–184.

6. Fekadu A, et al. The Maudsley Staging Method for treatment-resistant depression: prediction of longer-term outcome and persistence of symptoms. *J Clin Psychiatry* 2009; 70:952–957.

7. Angst J, et al. Toward a re-definition of subthreshold bipolarity: epidemiology and proposed criteria for bipolar-II, minor bipolar disorders and hypomania. *J Affect Disord* 2003; 73:133–146.

8. Smith DJ, et al. Unrecognised bipolar disorder in primary care patients with depression. *British J Psychiatry* 2011; 199:49–56.

9. Sidor MM, et al. Antidepressants for the acute treatment of bipolar depression: a systematic review and meta-analysis. *J Clin Psychiatry* 2011; 72:156–167.

10. Taylor DM, et al. Comparative efficacy and acceptability of drug treatments for bipolar depression: a multiple-treatments meta-analysis. *Acta Psychiatr Scand* 2014; 130:452–469.

11. Cosgrove L, et al. Reconceptualising treatment-resistant depression as difficult-to-treat depression. *Lancet Psychiatry* 2021; 8:11–13.

12. Rush AJ, et al. Difficult-to-treat depression: a clinical and research roadmap for when remission is elusive. *Aust N Z J Psychiatry* 2019; 53:109–118.

13. Trivedi MH, et al. Evaluation of outcomes with citalopram for depression using measurement-based care in STAR*D: implications for clinical practice. *Am J Psychiatry* 2006; 163:28–40.

14. Rush AJ, et al. Bupropion-SR, sertraline, or venlafaxine-XR after failure of SSRIs for depression. *N Engl J Med* 2006; 354:1231–1242.

15. Trivedi MH, et al. Medication augmentation after the failure of SSRIs for depression. *N Engl J Med* 2006; 354:1243–1252.

16. Fava M, et al. A comparison of mirtazapine and nortriptyline following two consecutive failed medication treatments for depressed outpatients: a STAR*D report. *Am J Psychiatry* 2006; 163:1161–1172.

17. Nierenberg AA, et al. A comparison of lithium and T(3) augmentation following two failed medication treatments for depression: a STAR*D report. *Am J Psychiatry* 2006; 163:1519–1530.

18. McGrath PJ, et al. Tranylcypromine versus venlafaxine plus mirtazapine following three failed antidepressant medication trials for depression: a STAR*D report. *Am J Psychiatry* 2006; 163:1531–1541.

19. Pigott HE, et al. Efficacy and effectiveness of antidepressants: current status of research. *Psychother Psychosom* 2010; 79:267–279.

20. Pigott HE. The STAR*D trial: it is time to reexamine the clinical beliefs that guide the treatment of major depression. *Can J Psychiatry* 2015; 60:9–13.

21. Marcus RN, et al. The efficacy and safety of aripiprazole as adjunctive therapy in major depressive disorder: a second multicenter, randomized, double-blind, placebo-controlled study. *J Clin Psychopharmacol* 2008; 28:156–165.

22. Hellerstein DJ, et al. Aripiprazole as an adjunctive treatment for refractory unipolar depression. *Prog Neuropsychopharmacol Biol Psychiatry* 2008; 32:744–750.

23. Simon JS, et al. Aripiprazole augmentation of antidepressants for the treatment of partially responding and nonresponding patients with major depressive disorder. *J Clin Psychiatry* 2005; 66:1216–1220.

24. Papakostas GI, et al. Aripiprazole augmentation of selective serotonin reuptake inhibitors for treatment-resistant major depressive disorder. *J Clin Psychiatry* 2005; 66:1326–1330.

25. Berman RM, et al. Aripiprazole augmentation in major depressive disorder: a double-blind, placebo-controlled study in patients with inadequate response to antidepressants. *CNS Spectr* 2009; 14:197–206.

26. Fava M, et al. A double-blind, placebo-controlled study of aripiprazole adjunctive to antidepressant therapy among depressed outpatients with inadequate response to prior antidepressant therapy (ADAPT-A Study). *PsychotherPsychosom* 2012; 81:87–97.

27. Jon DI, et al. Augmentation of aripiprazole for depressed patients with an inadequate response to antidepressant treatment: a 6-week prospective, open-label, multicenter study. *Clin Neuropharmacol* 2013; 36:157–161.

28. Strawbridge R, et al. Augmentation therapies for treatment-resistant depression: systematic review and meta-analysis. *Br J Psychiatry* 2019; 214:42–51.

29. Undurraga J, et al. Lithium treatment for unipolar major depressive disorder: systematic review. *J Psychopharmacology (Oxford, England)* 2019; 33:167–176.

30. National Institute for Clinical Excellence. Depression: the treatment and management of depression in adults. Clinical Guidance [CG90]. 2009 (last reviewed Dec 2013); https://www.nice.org.uk/guidance/cg90.

31. Luan S, et al. Efficacy and safety of olanzapine/fluoxetine combination in the treatment of treatment-resistant depression: a meta-analysis of randomized controlled trials. *Neuropsychiatr Dis Treat* 2017; 13:609–620.

32. Takahashi H, et al. Augmentation with olanzapine in TCA-refractory depression with melancholic features: a consecutive case series. *Human Psychopharmacology* 2008; 23:217–220.

33. Corya SA, et al. A randomized, double-blind comparison of olanzapine/fluoxetine combination, olanzapine, fluoxetine, and venlafaxine in treatment-resistant depression. *Depress Anxiety* 2006; 23:364–372.

34. Thase ME, et al. A randomized, double-blind comparison of olanzapine/fluoxetine combination, olanzapine, and fluoxetine in treatment-resistant major depressive disorder. *J Clin Psychiatry* 2007; 68:224–236.

35. Jensen NH, et al. N-desalkylquetiapine, a potent norepinephrine reuptake inhibitor and partial 5-HT1A agonist, as a putative mediator of quetiapine's antidepressant activity. *Neuropsychopharmacology* 2008; 33:2303–2312.

36. El-Khalili N, et al. Extended-release quetiapine fumarate (quetiapine XR) as adjunctive therapy in major depressive disorder (MDD) in patients with an inadequate response to ongoing antidepressant treatment: a multicentre, randomized, double-blind, placebo-controlled study. *Int J Neuropsychopharmacol* 2010; 13:917–932.

37. Bauer M, et al. Extended-release quetiapine as adjunct to an antidepressant in patients with major depressive disorder: results of a randomized, placebo-controlled, double-blind study. *J Clin Psychiatry* 2009; 70:540–549.

38. Bauer M, et al. A pooled analysis of two randomised, placebo-controlled studies of extended release quetiapine fumarate adjunctive to antidepressant therapy in patients with major depressive disorder. *J Affect Disord* 2010; 127:19–30.

39. Montgomery S, et al. P01-75 – Quetiapine XR or lithium combination with antidepressants in treatment resistant depression. *Eur Psychiatry* 2010; 25:296–296.

40. Doree JP, et al. Quetiapine augmentation of treatment-resistant depression: a comparison with lithium. *Curr Med Res Opin* 2007; 23:333–341.

41. Zisook S, et al. Use of bupropion in combination with serotonin reuptake inhibitors. *Biol Psychiatry* 2006; 59:203–210.

42. Fatemi SH, et al. Venlafaxine and bupropion combination therapy in a case of treatment-resistant depression. *Ann Pharmacother* 1999; 33:701–703.

43. Lam RW, et al. Citalopram and bupropion-SR: combining versus switching in patients with treatment-resistant depression. *J Clin Psychiatry* 2004; 65:337–340.

44. Papakostas GI, et al. The combination of duloxetine and bupropion for treatment-resistant major depressive disorder. *Depress Anxiety* 2006; 23:178–181.

45. Henssler J, et al. Combining antidepressants in acute treatment of depression: a meta-analysis of 38 studies including 4511 patients. *Can J Psychiatry* 2016; 61:29–43.

46. Carpenter LL, et al. A double-blind, placebo-controlled study of antidepressant augmentation with mirtazapine. *Biol Psychiatry* 2002; 51:183–188.

47. Carpenter LL, et al. Mirtazapine augmentation in the treatment of refractory depression. *J Clin Psychiatry* 1999; **60**:45–49.

48. Ferreri M, et al. Benefits from mianserin augmentation of fluoxetine in patients with major depression non-responders to fluoxetine alone. *Acta Psychiatr Scand* 2001; **103**:66–72.

49. Kessler DS, et al. Mirtazapine added to SSRIs or SNRIs for treatment resistant depression in primary care: phase III randomised placebo controlled trial (MIR). *BMJ* 2018; **363**:k4218.

难治性抑郁的治疗：次选（表 3.4）

表 3.4　次选：不太常用，已发表的评价结论支持度不同（排序不分先后）

治疗	优点	缺点
加用**氯胺酮**（0.5mg/kg 静脉注射，时间不少于 40min）[1] **氯胺酮鼻**内滴入（在大多数国家被许可）剂量在 28~84mg[2] 见本章氯胺酮制剂部分	■ 很快起效（数小时内），包括对自杀的疗效 [3,4] ■ 缓解率高 ■ 一些证据表明，若反复给药，可维持疗效 ■ 在这种次麻醉剂量下，通常耐受性好	■ 静脉注射需要在医院使用 ■ 偶见认知影响（意识模糊、解离等）和其他精神症状 [5] ■ 伴有暂时性血压升高、心动过速、心律失常。静脉注射前需做心电图检查 [6] ■ 不良反应可能被低估 [7] ■ 可能需要重复治疗以维持疗效
* 加用**拉莫三嗪**（用过 100mg/d、200mg/d 和 400mg/d）[8]	■ 研究相当充分 ■ 使用非常广泛 ■ 可能是耐受性最佳的增效策略 [9]	■ 缓慢加药 ■ 皮疹风险 ■ 合适的剂量尚不清楚
电抽搐治疗 [10-12]	■ 获得公认 ■ 有效 ■ 有充分的文献支持	■ 在公众当中名声不好 ■ 需要全身麻醉 ■ 需要向专科医师转诊 ■ 通常当作最后的治疗，或需要迅速起效时才使用 ■ 最好与其他治疗联合使用
合用**三碘甲腺原氨酸**（20~50μg/d）[13-19] 使用较高剂量也安全	■ 通常耐受性很好 ■ 充分的文献支持 ■ 可能对双相抑郁有效	■ 需要监测临床和甲功 ■ 通常需要专家指导用药 ■ 一些研究为阴性结果 ■ 在非难治性抑郁中，与单用抗抑郁药比较没有优势 [20]

参考文献

1. Marcantoni WS, et al. A systematic review and meta-analysis of the efficacy of intravenous ketamine infusion for treatment resistant depression: January 2009–January 2019. *J Affect Disord* 2020; 277:831–841.
2. Papakostas GI, et al. Efficacy of esketamine augmentation in major depressive disorder: a meta-analysis. *J Clin Psychiatry* 2020; 81:19r12889.
3. Wilkinson ST, et al. The effect of a single dose of intravenous ketamine on suicidal ideation: a systematic review and individual participant data meta-analysis. *Am J Psychiatry* 2018; 175:150–158.
4. Witt K, et al. Ketamine for suicidal ideation in adults with psychiatric disorders: a systematic review and meta-analysis of treatment trials. *Aust N Z J Psychiatry* 2020; 54:29–45.
5. Beck K, et al. Association of ketamine with psychiatric symptoms and implications for its therapeutic use and for understanding schizophrenia: a systematic review and meta-analysis. *JAMA Network Open* 2020; 3:e204693.
6. Aan Het Rot M, et al. Safety and efficacy of repeated-dose intravenous ketamine for treatment-resistant depression. *Biol Psychiatry* 2010; 67:139–145.
7. Short B, et al. Side-effects associated with ketamine use in depression: a systematic review. *Lancet Psychiatry* 2018; 5:65–78.
8. Goh KK, et al. Lamotrigine augmentation in treatment-resistant unipolar depression: a comprehensive meta-analysis of efficacy and safety. *J Psychopharmacology* 2019; 33:700–713.
9. Papadimitropoulou K, et al. Comparative efficacy and tolerability of pharmacological and somatic interventions in adult patients with treatment-resistant depression: a systematic review and network meta-analysis. *Curr Med Res Opin* 2017; 33:701–711.
10. Folkerts HW, et al. Electroconvulsive therapy vs. paroxetine in treatment-resistant depression – a randomized study. *Acta Psychiatr Scand*

1997; **96**:334–342.

11. Gonzalez-Pinto A, et al. Efficacy and safety of venlafaxine-ECT combination in treatment-resistant depression. *J Neuropsychiatry Clin Neurosci* 2002; **14**:206–209.

12. Eranti S, et al. A randomized, controlled trial with 6-month follow-up of repetitive transcranial magnetic stimulation and electroconvulsive therapy for severe depression. *Am J Psychiatry* 2007; **164**:73–81.

13. Joffe RT, et al. A comparison of triiodothyronine and thyroxine in the potentiation of tricyclic antidepressants. *Psychiatry Res* 1990; **32**:241–251.

14. Anderson IM. Drug treatment of depression: reflections on the evidence. *Adv Psychiatric Treatment* 2003; **9**:11–20.

15. Nierenberg AA, et al. A comparison of lithium and T(3) augmentation following two failed medication treatments for depression: a STAR*D report. *Am J Psychiatry* 2006; **163**:1519–1530.

16. Iosifescu DV, et al. An open study of triiodothyronine augmentation of selective serotonin reuptake inhibitors in treatment-resistant major depressive disorder. *J Clin Psychiatry* 2005; **66**:1038–1042.

17. Abraham G, et al. T3 augmentation of SSRI resistant depression. *J Affect Disord* 2006; **91**:211–215.

18. Kelly TF, et al. Long term augmentation with T3 in refractory major depression. *J Affect Disord* 2009; **115**:230–233.

19. Parmentier T, et al. The use of triiodothyronine (T3) in the treatment of bipolar depression: a review of the literature. *J Affect Disord* 2018; **229**:410–414.

20. Garlow SJ, et al. The combination of triiodothyronine (T3) and sertraline is not superior to sertraline monotherapy in the treatment of major depressive disorder. *J Psychiatr Res* 2012; **46**:1406–1413.

难治性抑郁的治疗:其他报道过的治疗方法

　　作为难治性抑郁症的潜在治疗方案,大量的治疗方式曾被研究。本节中的表 3.5 简要描述了支持证据有限,但在特殊情况下可能值得尝试的策略。医师在使用这些方法之前,必须熟悉原始文献。

表 3.5　其他报道过的治疗方法(排序不分先后)(原文排列基于药物首字母顺序)

治疗	评价
金刚烷胺(最高 300mg/d)[1]	数据有限
死藤水(含致幻剂二甲基色胺)[2,3]	有效,专科医师使用
丁丙诺啡(0.8~2mg/d)[4]	证据合理,但有明显的禁忌证
加用卡麦角林 2mg/d[5]	数据非常有限
D-环丝氨酸(1 000mg/d)[6]	一项小样本的 RCT 研究显示有效
地塞米松 3~4mg/d[7,8]	数据有限
右美沙芬 + 奎尼丁 45/10mg BD[9,10]	有希望的新型治疗。NDMA 拮抗剂。需要奎尼丁作为 CYP2D6 抑制剂来延长右美沙芬的作用
叶酸/甲基叶酸(2mg/d 叶酸?)[12-14]	可能有好处,但试验质量低
东莨菪碱(4μg/kg IV)[15]	越来越多的证据表明其起效快,有一定的疗效
酮康唑 400~800mg/d[16]	很少使用,有肝中毒的风险
联合使用 MAOI 和 TCA,例如三甲丙米嗪和苯乙肼[17-19]	曾广泛使用,但需要特别小心
美卡舍明(最高 10mg/d)[20,21]	一项 21 名患者的探索性研究
米诺环素 200mg/d[22-25]	在动物和人类中进行的几项荟萃分析为阳性结果,最近在双相抑郁的 RCT 研究中失败了
莫达非尼 100~400mg/d[26-30]	见本章"兴奋剂在抑郁症中的应用"的部分
纳曲酮 100mg/d[31,32]	没有对非阿片类滥用者的研究
奈米非肽(40~240mg/d 皮下)[33]	一项 25 名患者的探索性研究
去甲替林 ± 锂盐[34-37]	再度被考察的治疗选择
雌激素(各种方案)[38]	数据有限
ω-3-甘油三酯 EPA[39]	通常与抗抑郁药合用。效果可能是剂量敏感的,总剂量应 <1g/d 且 EPA 含量 >60%
吲哚洛尔(5mg tid 或 7.5mg qd)[30,40-44]	耐受性好,可以在初级保健机构开始治疗。数据主要与加快起效有关。难治性数据互相矛盾

续表

治疗	评价
普拉克索 0.125~5mg/d[38,39]	一项良好的 RCT 研究显示有明确的疗效
赛洛西宾 10/25mg 相隔一周[45]	有效,但仅限专科医师使用
利培酮 0.5~3mg/d+ 抗抑郁药[46-51]	与其他 SGA 相比,RCT 支持力度不那么大
S-腺苷-L-甲硫氨酸 400mg/d IM; 1 600mg/d 口服[52-55]	在难治性抑郁中数据有限 系统综述提示支持力度较弱
SSRI+ 丁螺环酮最高 60mg/d[56,57]	STAR*D 支持 需高剂量但耐受性差(常见头晕)
SSRI+TCA[58]	曾广泛使用
兴奋剂:安非他明,哌甲酯	研究结果不一 见本章"抑郁症中的兴奋剂"部分
TCA——高剂量[59]	曾广泛使用。需进行心脏监测
睾酮凝胶[30,60]	对于睾酮水平低的人有效
噻奈普汀(25~50mg/d)[61,62]	数据极少。很多国家没有噻奈普汀
色氨酸 2~3g tid[63-66]	有长久的成功使用的历史
文拉法辛 >200mg/d[67-70]	可以在初级保健机构开始使用 NICE 推荐 恶心、呕吐;停药反应常见 需进行血压监测
文拉法辛——极高剂量 (高达 600mg/d)[72]	见上文。需进行心脏监测
文拉法辛 +IV氯米帕明[73]	需进行心脏监测
加用锌(25mg Zn+/d)[74]	一项 RCT 研究(n=60)表明其对难治性抑郁效果好
齐拉西酮最高 160mg/d[75-77]	支持证据少,可能没有抗抑郁作用

注:有其他非药物治疗,包括各种心理治疗、重复经颅磁刺激(rTMS)、迷走神经刺激、深部脑刺激和精神外科。但不在本书讨论范围内。

EPA,二十碳五烯酸;IM,肌内注射;IV,静脉注射;MAOI,单胺氧化酶抑制剂;RCT,随机对照试验;SC,皮下注射;SSRI,选择性 5-羟色胺再摄取抑制剂;TCA,三环类抗抑郁药;tid,一天 3 次。

参考文献

1. Stryjer R, et al. Amantadine as augmentation therapy in the management of treatment-resistant depression. *Int Clin Psychopharmacol* 2003; **18**:93–96.
2. Santos RGD, et al. Long-term effects of ayahuasca in patients with recurrent depression: a 5-year qualitative follow-up. *Arch Clin Psychiatry* 2018; **45**:22–24.
3. Palhano-Fontes F, et al. Rapid antidepressant effects of the psychedelic ayahuasca in treatment-resistant depression: a randomized placebo-

controlled trial. *Psychol Med* 2019; 49:655–663.

4. Stanciu CN, et al. Use of buprenorphine in treatment of refractory depression-A review of current literature. *Asian J Psychiatr* 2017; 26:94–98.

5. Takahashi H, et al. Addition of a dopamine agonist, cabergoline, to a serotonin-noradrenalin reuptake inhibitor, milnacipran as a therapeutic option in the treatment of refractory depression: two case reports. *Clin Neuropharmacol* 2003; 26:230–232.

6. Heresco-Levy U, et al. A randomized add-on trial of high-dose D-cycloserine for treatment-resistant depression. *Int J Neuropsychopharmacol* 2013; 16:501–506.

7. Dinan TG, et al. Dexamethasone augmentation in treatment-resistant depression. *Acta Psychiatr Scand* 1997; 95:58–61.

8. Bodani M, et al. The use of dexamethasone in elderly patients with antidepressant-resistant depressive illness. *J Psychopharmacology* 1999; 13:196–197.

9. Murrough JW, et al. Dextromethorphan/quinidine pharmacotherapy in patients with treatment resistant depression: a proof of concept clinical trial. *J Affect Disord* 2017; 218:277–283.

10. Kelly TF, et al. The utility of the combination of dextromethorphan and quinidine in the treatment of bipolar II and bipolar NOS. *J Affect Disord* 2014; 167:333–335.

11. Nofziger JL, et al. Evaluation of dextromethorphan with select antidepressant therapy for the treatment of depression in the acute care psychiatric setting. *Ment Health Clin* 2019; 9:76–81.

12. Firth J, et al. The efficacy and safety of nutrient supplements in the treatment of mental disorders: a meta-review of meta-analyses of randomized controlled trials. *World Psychiatry* 2019; 18:308–324.

13. Roberts E, et al. Caveat emptor: folate in unipolar depressive illness, a systematic review and meta-analysis. *J Psychopharmacology* 2018; 32:377–384.

14. Abou-Saleh MT, et al. Folic acid and the treatment of depression. *J Psychosom Res* 2006; 61:285–287.

15. Drevets WC, et al. Antidepressant effects of the muscarinic cholinergic receptor antagonist scopolamine: a review. *Biol Psychiatry* 2013; 73:1156–1163.

16. Wolkowitz OM, et al. Antiglucocorticoid treatment of depression: double-blind ketoconazole. *Biol Psychiatry* 1999; 45:1070–1074.

17. White K, et al. The combined use of MAOIs and tricyclics. *J Clin Psychiatry* 1984; 45:67–69.

18. Kennedy N, et al. Treatment and response in refractory depression: results from a specialist affective disorders service. *J Affect Disord* 2004; 81:49–53.

19. Connolly KR, et al. If at first you don't succeed: a review of the evidence for antidepressant augmentation, combination and switching strategies. *Drugs* 2011; 71:43–64.

20. George TP, et al. Nicotinic antagonist augmentation of selective serotonin reuptake inhibitor-refractory major depressive disorder: a preliminary study. *J Clin Psychopharmacol* 2008; 28:340–344.

21. Bacher I, et al. Mecamylamine – a nicotinic acetylcholine receptor antagonist with potential for the treatment of neuropsychiatric disorders. *Expert Opin Pharmacother* 2009; 10:2709–2721.

22. Reis DJ, et al. The antidepressant impact of minocycline in rodents: a systematic review and meta-analysis. *Sci Rep* 2019; 9:261.

23. Zazula R, et al. Minocycline as adjunctive treatment for major depressive disorder: pooled data from two randomized controlled trials. *Aust N Z J Psychiatry* 2020; 4867420965697.

24. Strawbridge R, et al. Augmentation therapies for treatment-resistant depression: systematic review and meta-analysis. *Br J Psychiatry* 2019; 214:42–51.

25. Husain MI, et al. Minocycline and celecoxib as adjunctive treatments for bipolar depression: a multicentre, factorial design randomised controlled trial. *Lancet Psychiatry* 2020; 7:515–527.

26. DeBattista C, et al. A prospective trial of modafinil as an adjunctive treatment of major depression. *J Clin Psychopharmacol* 2004; 24:87–90.

27. Ninan PT, et al. Adjunctive modafinil at initiation of treatment with a selective serotonin reuptake inhibitor enhances the degree and onset of therapeutic effects in patients with major depressive disorder and fatigue. *J Clin Psychiatry* 2004; 65:414–420.

28. Menza MA, et al. Modafinil augmentation of antidepressant treatment in depression. *J Clin Psychiatry* 2000; 61:378–381.

29. Taneja I, et al. A randomized, double-blind, crossover trial of modafinil on mood. *J Clin Psychopharmacol* 2007; 27:76–78.

30. Kleeblatt J, et al. Efficacy of off-label augmentation in unipolar depression: a systematic review of the evidence. *Eur Neuropsychopharmacol* 2017; 27:423–441.

31. Pettinati HM, Ph.D., et al. A double-blind, placebo-controlled trial combining sertraline and naltrexone for treating co-occurring depression and alcohol dependence. *Am J Psychiatry* 2010; 167:668–675.

32. Browne CA, et al. Novel targets to treat depression: opioid-based therapeutics. *Harv Rev Psychiatry* 2020; 28:40–59.

33. Feighner JP, et al. Clinical effect of nemifitide, a novel pentapeptide antidepressant, in the treatment of severely depressed refractory patients. *Int Clin Psychopharmacol* 2008; 23:29–35.

34. Nierenberg AA, et al. Nortriptyline for treatment-resistant depression. *J Clin Psychiatry* 2003; 64:35–39.

35. Nierenberg AA, et al. Lithium augmentation of nortriptyline for subjects resistant to multiple antidepressants. *J Clin Psychopharmacol* 2003; 23:92–95.

36. Fava M, et al. A comparison of mirtazapine and nortriptyline following two consecutive failed medication treatments for depressed outpatients: a STAR*D report. *Am J Psychiatry* 2006; 163:1161–1172.

37. Shelton RC, et al. Olanzapine/fluoxetine combination for treatment-resistant depression: a controlled study of SSRI and nortriptyline resistance. *J Clin Psychiatry* 2005; 66:1289–1297.

38. Stahl SM. Basic psychopharmacology of antidepressants, part 2: oestrogen as an adjunct to antidepressant treatment. *J Clin Psychiatry* 1998; 59 Suppl 4:15–24.

第 3 章

39. Liao Y, et al. Efficacy of omega-3 PUFAs in depression: a meta-analysis. *Trans Psychiatry* 2019; **9**:190.

40. McAskill R, et al. Pindolol augmentation of antidepressant therapy. *Br J Psychiatry* 1998; **173**:203–208.

41. Rasanen P, et al. Mitchell B. Balter award–1998. Pindolol and major affective disorders: a three-year follow-up study of 30,485 patients. *J Clin Psychopharmacol* 1999; **19**:297–302.

42. Perry EB, et al. Pindolol augmentation in depressed patients resistant to selective serotonin reuptake inhibitors: a double-blind, randomized, controlled trial. *J Clin Psychiatry* 2004; **65**:238–243.

43. Sokolski KN, et al. Once-daily high-dose pindolol for SSRI-refractory depression. *Psychiatry Res* 2004; **125**:81–86.

44. Whale R, et al. Pindolol augmentation of serotonin reuptake inhibitors for the treatment of depressive disorder: a systematic review. *J Psychopharmacology* 2010; **24**:513–520.

45. Carhart-Harris RL, et al. Psilocybin with psychological support for treatment-resistant depression: an open-label feasibility study. *Lancet Psychiatry* 2016; **3**:619–627.

46. Yoshimura R, et al. Addition of risperidone to sertraline improves sertraline-resistant refractory depression without influencing plasma concentrations of sertraline and desmethylsertraline. *Human Psychopharmacology* 2008; **23**:707–713.

47. Mahmoud RA, et al. Risperidone for treatment-refractory major depressive disorder: a randomized trial. *Ann Intern Med* 2007; **147**:593–602.

48. Ostroff RB, et al. Risperidone augmentation of selective serotonin reuptake inhibitors in major depression. *J Clin Psychiatry* 1999; **60**:256–259.

49. Rapaport MH, et al. Effects of risperidone augmentation in patients with treatment-resistant depression: results of open-label treatment followed by double-blind continuation. *Neuropsychopharmacology* 2006; **31**:2505–2513.

50. Stoll AL, et al. Tranylcypromine plus risperidone for treatment-refractory major depression. *J Clin Psychopharmacol* 2000; **20**:495–496.

51. Keitner GI, et al. A randomized, placebo-controlled trial of risperidone augmentation for patients with difficult-to-treat unipolar, non-psychotic major depression. *J Psychiatr Res* 2009; **43**:205–214.

52. Pancheri P, et al. A double-blind, randomized parallel-group, efficacy and safety study of intramuscular S-adenosyl-L-methionine 1,4-butanedisulphonate (SAMe) versus imipramine in patients with major depressive disorder. *Int J Neuropsychopharmacol* 2002; **5**:287–294.

53. Alpert JE, et al. S-adenosyl-L-methionine (SAMe) as an adjunct for resistant major depressive disorder: an open trial following partial or nonresponse to selective serotonin reuptake inhibitors or venlafaxine. *J Clin Psychopharmacol* 2004; **24**:661–664.

54. Sharma A, et al. S-adenosylmethionine (SAMe) for neuropsychiatric disorders: a clinician-oriented review of research. *J Clin Psychiatry* 2017; **78**:e656–e667.

55. Galizia I, et al. S-adenosyl methionine (SAMe) for depression in adults. *Cochrane Database Syst Rev* 2016; **10**:Cd011286.

56. Trivedi MH, et al. Medication augmentation after the failure of SSRIs for depression. *N Engl J Med* 2006; **354**:1243–1252.

57. Appelberg BG, et al. Patients with severe depression may benefit from buspirone augmentation of selective serotonin reuptake inhibitors: results from a placebo-controlled, randomized, double-blind, placebo wash-in study. *J Clin Psychiatry* 2001; **62**:448–452.

58. Taylor D. Selective serotonin reuptake inhibitors and tricyclic antidepressants in combination – interactions and therapeutic uses. *Br J Psychiatry* 1995; **167**:575–580.

59. Malhi GS, et al. Management of resistant depression. *Int J Psychiatry Clin Pract* 1997; **1**:269–276.

60. Pope HG, Jr., et al. Testosterone gel supplementation for men with refractory depression: a randomized, placebo-controlled trial. *Am J Psychiatry* 2003; **160**:105–111.

61. Tobe EH, et al. Possible usefulness of tianeptine in treatment-resistant depression. *Int J Psychiatry Clin Pract* 2013; **17**:313–316.

62. Woo YS, et al. Tianeptine combination for partial or non-response to selective serotonin re-uptake inhibitor monotherapy. *Psychiatry Clin Neurosci* 2013; **67**:219–227.

63. Angst J, et al. The treatment of depression with L-5-hydroxytryptophan versus imipramine. Results of two open and one double-blind study. *Arch Psychiatr Nervenkr* 1977; **224**:175–186.

64. Alino JJ, et al. 5-Hydroxytryptophan (5-HTP) and a MAOI (nialamide) in the treatment of depressions. A double-blind controlled study. *Int Pharmacopsychiatry* 1976; **11**:8–15.

65. Hale AS, et al. Clomipramine, tryptophan and lithium in combination for resistant endogenous depression: seven case studies. *Br J Psychiatry* 1987; **151**:213–217.

66. Young SN. Use of tryptophan in combination with other antidepressant treatments: a review. *J Psychiatry Neurosci* 1991; **16**:241–246.

67. Poirier MF, et al. Venlafaxine and paroxetine in treatment-resistant depression. Double-blind, randomised comparison. *Br J Psychiatry* 1999; **175**:12–16.

68. Nierenberg AA, et al. Venlafaxine for treatment-resistant unipolar depression. *J Clin Psychopharmacol* 1994; **14**:419–423.

69. Smith D, et al. Efficacy and tolerability of venlafaxine compared with selective serotonin reuptake inhibitors and other antidepressants: a meta-analysis. *Br J Psychiatry* 2002; **180**:396–404.

70. Rush AJ, et al. Bupropion-SR, sertraline, or venlafaxine-XR after failure of SSRIs for depression. *N Engl J Med* 2006; **354**:1231–1242.

71. National Institute for Clinical Excellence. Depression: the treatment and management of depression in adults. Clinical Guidance [CG90]. 2009 (last reviewed Dec 2013); https://www.nice.org.uk/guidance/cg90.

72. Harrison CL, et al. Tolerability of high-dose venlafaxine in depressed patients. *J Psychopharmacology* 2004; **18**:200–204.

73. Fountoulakis KN, et al. Combined oral venlafaxine and intravenous clomipramine-A: successful temporary response in a patient with extremely refractory depression. *Can J Psychiatry* 2004; **49**:73–74.

74. Siwek M, et al. Zinc supplementation augments efficacy of imipramine in treatment resistant patients: a double blind, placebo-controlled study. *J Affect Disord* 2009; **118**:187–195.

75. Papakostas GI, et al. Ziprasidone augmentation of selective serotonin reuptake inhibitors (SSRIs) for SSRI-resistant major depressive disor-

der. *J Clin Psychiatry* 2004; 65:217–221.

76. Dunner DL, et al. Efficacy and tolerability of adjunctive ziprasidone in treatment-resistant depression: a randomized, open-label, pilot study. *J Clin Psychiatry* 2007; 68:1071–1077.

77. Papakostas GI, et al. A 12-week, randomized, double-blind, placebo-controlled, sequential parallel comparison trial of ziprasidone as monotherapy for major depressive disorder. *J Clin Psychiatry* 2012; 73:1541–1547.

氯胺酮

背景

在最近的 20 年里,氯胺酮作为一种非竞争性的 N-甲基-D-天冬氨酸(NMDA)受体拮抗剂和解离麻醉剂,已成为一种新型有效的速效抗抑郁药。2000 年,Berman 及同事报告了一项具有里程碑意义的 RCT 研究,该研究对抑郁症患者给予单次静脉注射亚麻醉剂量的氯胺酮(0.5mg/kg ,静脉滴注时间不少于 40min)[1]。氯胺酮滴注数小时内产生显著的抗抑郁作用,且逐步增强到给药后 3 天。此后,这一发现在涉及单相和双相抑郁(包括难治性个体)的多项试验中获得重复[2-6]。

氯胺酮是一种外消旋混合物,由同样数量的 S-氯胺酮和 R-氯胺酮两种对映体构成,其中 S-氯胺酮与 NMDA 受体的结合力较强。氯胺酮还是难治性抑郁症的超说明书治疗方法,但是 S-氯胺酮鼻喷剂(Spravato™)已被研发出来,在欧美被批准用于难治性抑郁症(与口服抗抑郁药合用)。

机制

目前,氯胺酮和艾司氯胺酮快速抗抑郁作用的确切作用机制尚不清楚,但有人提出这些作用是通过阻断 γ-氨基丁酸(GABA)能中间神经元上的 NMDA 受体介导的,这些中间神经元通常作用于谷氨酸能神经元抑制谷氨酸释放[7]。这种脱抑制作用导致急性皮质谷氨酸激增,激活突触后 α-氨基-3-羧基-5-甲基-4-异噁唑丙酸(AMPA)受体,对下游突触发生和神经可塑性通路产生影响。[7]

给药路径

对于难治性抑郁症,氯胺酮的最佳给药方法尚未完全确定;然而已有获得批准的鼻内艾司氯胺酮给药指南(表 3.6)。静脉注射氯胺酮(不少于 40min 静脉滴注 0.5mg/kg)是其超说明书使用的金标准,具有支持疗效的最佳证据。其他给药途径,包括皮下注射、肌内注射、口服和舌下含服,都需要进一步研究来证明这些途径的相对有效性和安全性,以及每种情况下的最佳给药方案。这些途径在生物利用度、作用持续时间、实用性和患者舒适度方面都有其自身的优势和挑战。虽然在不同给药路径和不同剂量时,尚未确定氯胺酮的固定用药方案,但是在考虑了现有证据和临床经验后,在表 3.6 中提供了用药建议的概要。

不良反应

在抗抑郁药量下使用时,氯胺酮通常会导致明显的分离症状[8]。这些症状包括知觉扭曲,并可能导致严重的焦虑。因此,任何使用氯胺酮的患者都必须在给药期间和给药后 1h 内由受过培训的临床医师进行监测。此外,虽然罕见,但有报道氯胺酮会引发喉痉挛,因此负责监测的临床医师需要接受中级或高级生命支持培训。当通过口服或舌下途径以低剂量给予氯胺酮时,引起严重解离症状的风险较小。因此,在临床监督下给予试验剂量后,就可在非临床环境(家庭)用药,但是应建议患者在给药后至少 1h 不要开车、操作大型机械或参与其他高风险活动。此外,处方医师还必须考虑药物被转移和非法使用的风险。

表 3.6　难治性抑郁症以氯胺酮不同途径给药和艾司氯胺酮鼻内滴注时的用药建议

	剂量	详细	频率	点评
静脉注射 [2-6]	■ 0.5mg/kg,如果无效,增加至 1.0mg/kg ■(老年人从 0.25mg/kg 渐加)	■ 滴注时间不少于 40min	■ 诱导阶段:每周 1 次或 2 次 ■ 维持阶段:根据反应,每周 1 次,然后 2 周 1 次,甚至每月 1 次(考虑在两次静脉滴注期间补充口服/舌下药物)	■ 需要在临床环境下给药 ■ 偶发认知影响(意识错乱、分离等) ■ 可能导致血压一过性增高、心动过速和心律失常。治疗前需检查心电图。在注射前后监测血压 ■ 在滴注期间和静脉滴注后观察 1h
皮下注射 [9,10]	■ 0.5mg/kg,如果无效,增加至 1.0mg/kg ■(老年人从 0.25mg/kg 渐加)	■ 在适当部位进行皮下注射	■ 同上	■ 同上 ■ 比静脉滴注或肌内注射耐受性好
肌内注射 [11,12]	■ 0.5mg/kg,如果无效,增加至 1.0mg/kg ■(老年人从 0.25mg/kg 渐加)	■ 在适当部位进行肌内注射	■ 同上	■ 同上
口服 [13-15]	■ 0.5~5.0mg/kg 取决于给药的策略	■ 口服胶囊	■ 定期小剂量 ■ 0.5~2.0mg /kg,每 1~3 天 1 次 ■ 间断大剂量补充静脉滴注/皮下注射/肌内注射的治疗 ■ 2.0~5.0mg/kg,每周 1~2 次	■ 可在家中服用 ■ 低剂量具有较好的耐受性,然而抗抑郁效果不如静脉注射/皮下注射/肌内注射 ■ 高剂量可能用作具有实践意义的替代方案以维持静脉滴注/皮下注射/肌内注射的疗效。根据疗效/不良反应调整剂量
舌下 [15-17]	■ 0.5~3.0mg/kg,依用药策略而定	■ 氯胺酮溶液(舌下含 5min,后吞咽) ■ 舌下氯胺酮糖	■ 定期小剂量 ■ 0.5~1.5mg/kg,每 1~3 天 1 次 ■ 极低舌下剂量的证据有限(10mg,每 2~3 天 1 次,或每周 1 次) [18] ■ 间断大剂量补充静脉滴注/皮下注射/肌内注射的治疗 ■ 1.5~3.0mg /kg,每周 1~2 次	■ 可在家中服用 ■ 低剂量具有较好的耐受性;然而,推测抗抑郁效果不如静脉注射/皮下注射/肌内注射 ■ 高剂量可能用作具有实践意义的替代方案以维持静脉滴注/皮下注射/肌内注射的疗效。根据疗效/不良反应调整剂量

续表

	剂量	详细	频率	点评
艾司氯胺酮鼻内滴入 [19-22]	■ 56~84mg（老年人使用28mg） ■ *与口服抗抑郁药合用	■ 两喷28mg（每一侧鼻腔一喷） ■ 基于总需要量，可5min后再次使用	■ 先每周2次，再每周1次，然后每两周1次	■ 需在医院内给药 ■ 偶发认知损害（意识错乱，解离等） ■ 与一过性血压升高、心动过速和心律失常有关。治疗前需查心电图。在注射前后监测血压 ■ 在用药后观察2h

　　氯胺酮对血压和心率有显著的影响，建议在给药前对患者进行体格检查，包括基线血压、血细胞计数、肝功能、甲状腺功能和心电图。此外，还建议在氯胺酮给药期间和之后进行生命体征监测（包括血压和心率）。

参考文献

1. Berman RM, et al. Antidepressant effects of ketamine in depressed patients. *Biol Psychiatry* 2000; 47:351–354.
2. Zarate CA, Jr., et al. A randomized trial of an N-methyl-D-aspartate antagonist in treatment-resistant major depression. *Arch Gen Psychiatry* 2006; 63:856–864.
3. Diazgranados N, et al. A randomized add-on trial of an N-methyl-D-aspartate antagonist in treatment-resistant bipolar depression. *Arch Gen Psychiatry* 2010; 67:793–802.
4. Murrough JW, et al. Antidepressant efficacy of ketamine in treatment-resistant major depression: a two-site randomized controlled trial. *Am J Psychiatry* 2013; 170:1134–1142.
5. Singh JB, et al. A double-blind, randomized, placebo-controlled, dose-frequency study of intravenous ketamine in patients with treatment-resistant depression. *Am J Psychiatry* 2016; 173:816–826.
6. Fava M, et al. Double-blind, placebo-controlled, dose-ranging trial of intravenous ketamine as adjunctive therapy in treatment-resistant depression (TRD). *Mol Psychiatry* 2020; 25:1592–1603.
7. Lener MS, et al. Glutamate and gamma-aminobutyric acid systems in the pathophysiology of major depression and antidepressant response to ketamine. *Biol Psychiatry* 2017; 81:886–897.
8. Beck K, et al. Association of ketamine with psychiatric symptoms and implications for its therapeutic use and for understanding schizophrenia: a systematic review and meta-analysis. *JAMA Netw Open* 2020; 3:e204693.
9. Loo CK, et al. Placebo-controlled pilot trial testing dose titration and intravenous, intramuscular and subcutaneous routes for ketamine in depression. *Acta Psychiatr Scand* 2016; 134:48–56.
10. George D, et al. Pilot randomized controlled trial of titrated subcutaneous ketamine in older patients with treatment-resistant depression. *Am J Geriatr Psychiatry* 2017; 25:1199–1209.
11. Glue P, et al. Dose- and exposure-response to ketamine in depression. *Biol Psychiatry* 2011; 70:e9–e10; author reply e11–e12.
12. Cusin C, et al. Long-term maintenance with intramuscular ketamine for treatment-resistant bipolar II depression. *Am J Psychiatry* 2012; 169:868–869.
13. Arabzadeh S, et al. Does oral administration of ketamine accelerate response to treatment in major depressive disorder? Results of a double-blind controlled trial. *J Affect Disord* 2018; 235:236–241.
14. Domany Y, et al. Repeated oral ketamine for out-patient treatment of resistant depression: randomised, double-blind, placebo-controlled, proof-of-concept study. *Br J Psychiatry* 2019; 214:20–26.
15. Rosenblat JD, et al. Oral ketamine for depression: a systematic review. *J Clin Psychiatry* 2019; 80:18r12475.
16. Swainson J, et al. Sublingual ketamine: an option for increasing accessibility of ketamine treatments for depression? *J Clin Psychiatry* 2020; 81:19lr13146.
17. Nguyen L, et al. Off-label use of transmucosal ketamine as a rapid-acting antidepressant: a retrospective chart review. *Neuropsychiatr Dis Treat* 2015; 11:2667–2673.
18. Lara DR, et al. Antidepressant, mood stabilizing and procognitive effects of very low dose sublingual ketamine in refractory unipolar and bipolar depression. *Int J Neuropsychopharmacol* 2013; 16:2111–2117.

19. Canuso CM, et al. Efficacy and safety of intranasal esketamine for the rapid reduction of symptoms of depression and suicidality in patients at imminent risk for suicide: results of a double-blind, randomized, placebo-controlled study. *Am J Psychiatry* 2018; 175:620–630.

20. Daly EJ, et al. Efficacy and safety of intranasal esketamine adjunctive to oral antidepressant therapy in treatment-resistant depression: a randomized clinical trial. *JAMA Psychiatry* 2018; 75:139–148.

21. Popova V, et al. Efficacy and safety of flexibly dosed esketamine nasal spray combined with a newly initiated oral antidepressant in treatment-resistant depression: a randomized double-blind active-controlled study. *Am J Psychiatry* 2019; 176:428–438.

22. Daly EJ, et al. Efficacy of esketamine nasal spray plus oral antidepressant treatment for relapse prevention in patients with treatment-resistant depression: a randomized clinical trial. *JAMA Psychiatry* 2019; 76:893–903.

精神病性抑郁

　　虽然各种严重程度的抑郁症都可能出现精神病性症状[1]，但是有精神病性症状的患者通常比没有精神病性症状的患者病情更重[2]。尽管如此，精神病性抑郁是一种未被充分识别的疾病[3]，其终身患病率高达1%[4]。联合使用抗抑郁药和抗精神病药是通常推荐的一线治疗方案[5]，但是直到目前，支持这一做法的数据相对较少[6,7]。

　　在治疗精神病性抑郁方面，当剂量足够时，TCA可能比新型抗抑郁药疗效更优[6,8,9]。如果以前的充分治疗无效，估计后续治疗有效的可能性也较小[10]。

　　专门探讨新型抗抑郁药和非典型抗精神病药单用或联用治疗精神病性抑郁的研究很少。一项大型RCT研究[11]表明，合用奥氮平和氟西汀的有效率为64%，单用奥氮平的有效率为35%，单用安慰剂的有效率为28%。另一项精神病性抑郁的药物治疗（STOP-PD）研究[12]显示，合用奥氮平和舍曲林的临床缓解率为42%，而单用奥氮平的临床缓解率为24%。这两项研究都没设置单用抗抑郁药组。一些小型的开放试验发现，喹硫平[13]、阿立哌唑[14]、氨磺必利[15]联合　种抗抑郁药治疗有效，并且耐受性相对较好，但是这些研究也没有单用抗抑郁药治疗的数据。一项RCT研究（$n=122$）[9]发现，文拉法辛联合喹硫平的疗效优于单用文拉法辛，但是并不优于单用丙米嗪。对这些结果的可能解释是：支持TCA比文拉法辛疗效好，支持抗抑郁药和抗精神病药联合治疗比单用抗抑郁药效果好。

　　一篇综述对所有联合治疗研究进行总结后指出，抗精神病药和抗抑郁药合用，比单用其中一个效果要好（9项研究中有4项显示联合治疗具有一定的优势[16]）。最近一项荟萃分析认为，一种抗精神病药和一种抗抑郁药合用，疗效优于单用一种抗精神病药（NNT 5）或单用一种抗抑郁药（NNT 7）[17]。NICE建议[18]，在治疗急性期精神病性抑郁时，应当考虑在一种抗抑郁药基础上增加一种抗精神病药。Cochrane同意这一建议，但是鉴于试验的数量和质量有所保留[19]。需要注意的是，这些数据均与急性期治疗相关。

　　事实上，抗抑郁药和抗精神病药联合治疗的最佳疗程尚不明确。NICE建议，对于非精神病性抑郁症，如果单用抗抑郁药没有足够的疗效，可以在抗抑郁药基础上增加抗精神病药作为增效剂；如果在维持期停用一种药物，通常应该停用增效剂。在精神病性抑郁中，STOP-PD研究的继续阶段有证据表明，从舍曲林联合治疗中停用奥氮平后，长期结局会变差[20,21]。这个证据也许足以建议在急性期症状缓解之后继续联合治疗，但在这个问题上尚未达成共识[22]。一个重要的因素是STOP-PD研究中被分配到奥氮平组的年轻人体重显著增加[23]。

　　临床实践中，至少直到近年来，仍然只有小部分精神病性抑郁患者使用了抗精神病药[24]。这不仅反映了临床医师不确定这一治疗策略的风险收益比，也反映出已发表的治疗指南之间缺乏共识[25]。对抑郁症的精神病性症状诊断不足（因此治疗不充分）也是一个明显的问题[3,26]。然而，一些抗精神病药，例如喹硫平和奥氮平，也具有抗抑郁作用（同时有抗精神病作用）。因此，将它们作为抗抑郁治疗的增效剂是有经验基础的（除具有上述试验结果支持外）。

　　与非精神病性抑郁相比，精神病性抑郁的长期预后通常较差[27,28]。药物治疗和心理治疗的联合对精神病性抑郁的疗效不如非精神病性抑郁[29]。精神病性抑郁患者与非精神病性抑郁患者相比更容易尝试和完成自杀[30]。

精神病性抑郁是 ECT 的适应证之一。ECT 不仅对精神病性抑郁有效,而且对精神病性抑郁复发有保护作用,甚至可能优于它对非精神病性抑郁复发的保护作用[31]。一项小型 RCT 研究表明,随访 2 年时,去甲替林联合 ECT 的维持作用优于单用去甲替林[32]。

由于下丘脑-垂体-肾上腺(HPA)轴活动过度在精神病性抑郁中更加常见,新的治疗方法是基于抗糖皮质激素的治疗策略。一项小型、开放研究发现,糖皮质激素受体拮抗剂米非司酮[33]能够快速起效,但是该发现也受到一些批评[34]。疗效可能与米非司酮的血浆水平有关(>1 800ng/mL)[35]。另一项分析表明,米非司酮血浆浓度高于 1 637ng/mL 与疗效密切相关[36],但也有一项试验因米非司酮缺乏疗效而提前停止。

该个案报告称,以充分剂量的抗抑郁药联合抗精神病药治疗无效的患者,用哌甲酯治疗有效[37]。其他案例报告描述了拉莫三嗪[38]以及苯乙肼与阿立哌唑和喹硫平联合用药的成功结果[39]。在一项开放研究中,米诺环素也显示了良好的疗效[40]。

氯胺酮也可能对精神病性抑郁有效。一份报告[41]描述了两名对标准治疗无反应的患者(其中一名患者被诊断为分裂情感性障碍)在静脉使用氯胺酮(0.5mg/kg)后快速起效。另一份报告[42]概述 4 名患者静脉注射或皮下注射艾司氯胺酮(0.5mg/kg)快速起效,其中两人初步诊断是单相抑郁。

其他治疗或增效方案,除了另行介绍的难治性抑郁和精神病,并没有在精神病性抑郁中使用的适应证。

总结

- TCA 可能是精神病性抑郁的首选药物。
- 当 TCA 耐受性差时,SSRI、SNRI 是第二选择。
- 建议在抗抑郁药基础上联合使用奥氮平或喹硫平。
- 合用抗精神病药治疗的最佳剂量和疗程尚不明确。
- 如果在维持期需要停用一种药物,通常应该停用抗精神病药,但有一些证据表明这会使结果恶化。
- 如果需要快速起效,或其他治疗失败,应考虑进行 ECT 治疗。

参考文献

1. Forty L, et al. Is depression severity the sole cause of psychotic symptoms during an episode of unipolar major depression? A study both between and within subjects. *J Affect Disord* 2009; 114:103–109.
2. Gaudiano BA, et al. Depressive symptom profiles and severity patterns in outpatients with psychotic vs nonpsychotic major depression. *Compr Psychiatry* 2008; 49:421–429.
3. Heslin M, et al. Psychotic major depression: challenges in clinical practice and research. *Br J Psychiatry* 2018; 212:131–133.
4. Jääskeläinen E, et al. Epidemiology of psychotic depression – systematic review and meta-analysis. *Psychol Med* 2018; 48:905–918.
5. Cleare A, et al. Evidence-based guidelines for treating depressive disorders with antidepressants: a revision of the 2008 British Association for Psychopharmacology guidelines. *J Psychopharmacology* 2015; 29:459–525.
6. Wijkstra J, et al. Pharmacological treatment for unipolar psychotic depression: systematic review and meta-analysis. *Br J Psychiatry* 2006; 188:410–415.
7. Mulsant BH, et al. A double-blind randomized comparison of nortriptyline plus perphenazine versus nortriptyline plus placebo in the treatment of psychotic depression in late life. *J Clin Psychiatry* 2001; 62:597–604.
8. Birkenhager TK, et al. Efficacy of imipramine in psychotic versus nonpsychotic depression. *J Clin Psychopharmacol* 2008; 28:166–170.
9. Wijkstra J, et al. Treatment of unipolar psychotic depression: a randomized, double-blind study comparing imipramine, venlafaxine, and venlafaxine plus quetiapine. *Acta Psychiatr Scand* 2010; 121:190–200.

10. Blumberger DM, et al. Impact of prior pharmacotherapy on remission of psychotic depression in a randomized controlled trial. *J Psychiatr Res* 2011; **45:**896–901.

11. Rothschild AJ, et al. A double-blind, randomized study of olanzapine and olanzapine/fluoxetine combination for major depression with psychotic features. *J Clin Psychopharmacol* 2004; **24:**365–373.

12. Meyers BS, et al. A double-blind randomized controlled trial of olanzapine plus sertraline vs olanzapine plus placebo for psychotic depression: the study of pharmacotherapy of psychotic depression (STOP-PD). *Arch Gen Psychiatry* 2009; **66:**838–847.

13. Konstantinidis A, et al. Quetiapine in combination with citalopram in patients with unipolar psychotic depression. *Prog Neuropsychopharmacol Biol Psychiatry* 2007; **31:**242–247.

14. Matthews JD, et al. An open study of aripiprazole and escitalopram for psychotic major depressive disorder. *J Clin Psychopharmacol* 2009; **29:**73–76.

15. Politis AM, et al. Combination therapy with amisulpride and antidepressants: clinical observations in case series of elderly patients with psychotic depression. *Prog Neuropsychopharmacol Biol Psychiatry* 2008; **32:**1227–1230.

16. Rothschild AJ. Challenges in the treatment of major depressive disorder with psychotic features. *Schizophr Bull* 2013; **39:**787–796.

17. Farahani A, et al. Are antipsychotics or antidepressants needed for psychotic depression? A systematic review and meta-analysis of trials comparing antidepressant or antipsychotic monotherapy with combination treatment. *J Clin Psychiatry* 2012; **73:**486–496.

18. National Institute for Health and Care Excellence. Depression in adults: recognition and management. Clinical guideline [CG90]. 2009 (Last updated: December 2013); https://www.nice.org.uk/Guidance/cg90.

19. Wijkstra J, et al. Pharmacological treatment for psychotic depression. *Cochrane Database Syst Rev* 2015; Cd004044.

20. Bingham KS, et al. Stabilization treatment of remitted psychotic depression: the STOP-PD study. *Acta Psychiatr Scand* 2018; **138:**267–273.

21. Flint AJ, et al. Effect of continuing olanzapine vs placebo on relapse among patients with psychotic depression in remission: the STOP-PD II randomized clinical trial. *JAMA* 2019; **322:**622–631.

22. Dubovsky SL, et al. Psychotic depression: diagnosis, differential diagnosis, and treatment. *Psychother Psychosom* 2020; 1–18. [Epub ahead print].

23. Flint AJ, et al. Effect of older vs younger age on anthropometric and metabolic variables during treatment of psychotic depression with sertraline plus olanzapine: the STOP-PD II Study. *Am J Geriatr Psychiatry* 2020:S1064-7481(20)30546-7.

24. Andreescu C, et al. Persisting low use of antipsychotics in the treatment of major depressive disorder with psychotic features. *J Clin Psychiatry* 2007; **68:**194–200.

25. Leadholm AK, et al. The treatment of psychotic depression: is there consensus among guidelines and psychiatrists? *J Affect Disord* 2013; **145:**214–220.

26. Rothschild AJ, et al. Missed diagnosis of psychotic depression at 4 academic medical centers. *J Clin Psychiatry* 2008; **69:**1293–1296.

27. Flint AJ, et al. Two-year outcome of psychotic depression in late life. *Am J Psychiatry* 1998; **155:**178–183.

28. Maj M, et al. Phenomenology and prognostic significance of delusions in major depressive disorder: a 10-year prospective follow-up study. *J Clin Psychiatry* 2007; **68:**1411–1417.

29. Gaudiano BA, et al. Differential response to combined treatment in patients with psychotic versus nonpsychotic major depression. *J Nerv Ment Dis* 2005; **193:**625–628.

30. Gournellis R, et al. Psychotic (delusional) depression and suicidal attempts: a systematic review and meta-analysis. *Acta Psychiatr Scand* 2018; **137:**18–29.

31. Birkenhager TK, et al. One-year outcome of psychotic depression after successful electroconvulsive therapy. *J ECT* 2005; **21:**221–226.

32. Navarro V, et al. Continuation/maintenance treatment with nortriptyline versus combined nortriptyline and ECT in late-life psychotic depression: a two-year randomized study. *Am J Geriatr Psychiatry* 2008; **16:**498–505.

33. Belanoff JK, et al. An open label trial of C-1073 (mifepristone) for psychotic major depression. *Biol Psychiatry* 2002; **52:**386–392.

34. Rubin RT. Dr. Rubin replies (Letter). *Am J Psychiatry* 2004; **161:**1722.

35. Blasey CM, et al. A multisite trial of mifepristone for the treatment of psychotic depression: a site-by-treatment interaction. *Contemp Clin Trials* 2009; **30:**284–288.

36. Block T, et al. Mifepristone plasma level and glucocorticoid receptor antagonism associated with response in patients with psychotic depression. *J Clin Psychopharmacol* 2017; **37:**505–511.

37. Huang CC, et al. Adjunctive use of methylphenidate in the treatment of psychotic unipolar depression. *Clin Neuropharmacol* 2008; **31:**245–247.

38. Kajiya T, et al. Effect of lamotrigine in the treatment of bipolar depression with psychotic features: a case report. *Ann General Psychiatry* 2017; **16:**31.

39. Meyer JM, et al. Augmentation of phenelzine with aripiprazole and quetiapine in a treatment-resistant patient with psychotic unipolar depression: case report and literature review. *CNS Spectr* 2017; **22:**391–396.

40. Miyaoka T, et al. Minocycline as adjunctive therapy for patients with unipolar psychotic depression: an open-label study. *Prog Neuropsychopharmacol Biol Psychiatry* 2012; **37:**222–226.

41. Ribeiro CM, et al. The use of ketamine for the treatment of depression in the context of psychotic symptoms: to the editor. *Biol Psychiatry* 2016; **79:**e65–e66.

42. Ajub E, et al. Efficacy of esketamine in the treatment of depression with psychotic features: a case series. *Biol Psychiatry* 2018; **83:**e15–e16.

第3章

更换抗抑郁药

一般指导原则

- 当要换用另一种抗抑郁药时,通常应该避免突然停药,除非出现严重不良事件。建议交叉换药,即逐渐减少无效或不能耐受的药物剂量,同时逐步增加新药的剂量。

举例		第 1 周	第 2 周	第 3 周	第 4 周
停用西酞普兰	40mg od	20mg od	10mg od	5mg od	2.5mg
改用米氮平	—	15mg od	30mg od	30mg od	45mg od(如果需要)

od,每天 1 次。

- 交叉换药的速度最好根据患者的耐受程度确定。这方面研究很少,因此需要慎重。可能需要延长时间以减轻撤药症状。
- 注意,即使是交叉换药,联合使用某些抗抑郁药也属于绝对禁忌。在其他情况下,若药物合用存在理论风险或缺乏经验,也不宜交叉换药。
- 换药的策略不仅取决于换药的原因(疗效不充分、无效、耐受性差或不良反应),而且取决于所涉及抗抑郁药的药代动力学和药效动力学[1-3]。
- 在某些情况下,没必要使用交叉换药。例如,将一种 SSRI 换成另一种 SSRI 时,因为二者作用太相似,后者可以改善前者的停药反应。实际上,对于 SSRI 的停药反应,一直主张突然换用氟西汀治疗[4]。即使两药作用方式相似但不完全相同时,也可以突然停药[5]。因此,在某些情况下,突然停用一种抗抑郁药,换用另一种抗抑郁药并使用常用剂量,不仅耐受良好,还能降低停药反应的风险和程度。
- 同时服用两种抗抑郁药的潜在危险包括药效动力学相互作用(5-羟色胺综合征、低血压、困倦;取决于所涉及的药物)和药代动力学相互作用(如有些 SSRI 类药物增加三环类药物的血浆水平)。
- 阿戈美拉汀似乎不会引起停药反应[6],但仍建议在换药时缓慢停用。从阿戈美拉汀的作用方式来看(褪黑素激动剂,5-HT$_{2C}$ 拮抗剂),预期它不能减轻其他抗抑郁药引起的停药反应。没有理论依据表明阿戈美拉汀与其他抗抑郁药合用可能发生药效学相互作用,但在缺乏有用数据的情况下建议谨慎使用。确实会发生一些药代动力学相互作用,阿戈美拉汀不应与氟伏沙明联用。

■ 5-羟色胺综合征可在使用治疗剂量的单一 5-羟色胺药物时发生,但更多见于 5-羟色胺能药物联合使用或过量使用时。大多数严重的 5-羟色胺综合征病例涉及 MAOI(包括吗氯贝胺)和 SSRI 合用[7,8]。当换药策略需要联合使用 5-羟色胺能药时,建议谨慎使用。

5-羟色胺综合征的症状

	严重程度	症状
严重程度增加 ↓	轻度	失眠、焦虑、恶心、腹泻、高血压、心动过速、反射亢进
	中度	躁动、肌阵挛、震颤、瞳孔散大、面色潮红、出汗、低热(<38.5℃)
	重度	严重高热、意识模糊、强直、呼吸衰竭、昏迷、死亡

应谨慎对待表 3.7 中给出的建议,应该在换药时非常仔细地监测患者。

表 3.7 抗抑郁药:换药和停药 *

更换药物	阿戈美拉汀	安非他酮	氯米帕明	氟西汀	氟伏沙明	MAOI 苯乙肼 环苯丙胺 司来吉兰
阿戈美拉汀[a]		直接换药	直接换药	直接换药	直接换药	直接换药
安非他酮[b]	谨慎交叉换药		谨慎交叉换药,氯米帕明从小剂量开始	谨慎交叉换药	谨慎交叉换药	逐渐减量、停药,2 周后换药
氯米帕明	谨慎交叉换药	谨慎交叉换药		逐渐减量、停药,再换用氟西汀,从 10mg/d 开始	逐渐减量、停药,再从低剂量氟伏沙明开始	逐渐减量、停药,3 周后换药
氟西汀[c]	谨慎交叉换药	停用氟西汀。4~7 天后换安非他酮	停用氟西汀。2 周后换低剂量氯米帕明		停用氟西汀。4~7 天后换低剂量氟伏沙明	停药,5~6 周后换药
氟伏沙明[d]	逐渐减量、停药,4 天后换药	谨慎交叉换药	逐渐减量、停药,后从低剂量起始换用	直接换药		逐渐减量、停药,1 周后换药
MAOI 苯乙肼 环苯丙胺 司来吉兰	谨慎交叉换药	逐渐减量、停药,2 周后换药	逐渐减量、停药,3 周后换药	逐渐减量、停药,2 周后换药	逐渐减量、停药,2 周后换药	逐渐减量、停药,2 周后换药
吗氯贝胺	逐渐减量、停药,24h 后换药	逐渐减量、停药,24h 后换药	逐渐减量、停药,24h 后换药	逐渐减量、停药,24h 后换药	逐渐减量、停药,24h 后换药	逐渐减量、停药,24h 后换药
米氮平	谨慎交叉换药	谨慎交叉换药	谨慎交叉换药	谨慎交叉换药	谨慎交叉换药	逐渐减量、停药,2 周后换药
瑞波西汀[e]	谨慎交叉换药	谨慎交叉换药	谨慎交叉换药	谨慎交叉换药	谨慎交叉换药	逐渐减量、停药,1 周后换药
曲唑酮	谨慎交叉换药	谨慎交叉换药	谨慎交叉换药,氯米帕明从低剂量起始	谨慎交叉换药	谨慎交叉换药	逐渐减量、停药,1 周后换药
其他 SSRI,[f] 伏硫西汀[g]	谨慎交叉换药	谨慎交叉换药	逐渐减量、停药,氯米帕明从低剂量起始	直接换药	直接换药	逐渐减量、停药,1 周后换药[h]

吗氯贝胺	米氮平	瑞波西汀	曲唑酮	其他 SSRI[f] 伏硫西汀	SNRI 度洛西汀 文拉法辛 去甲文拉法辛	TCA(除外 氯米帕明)
直接换药	直接换药	直接换药	直接换药	直接换药	直接换药	直接换药
逐渐减量、停药,然后换药	谨慎交叉换药	谨慎交叉换药	谨慎交叉换药	谨慎交叉换药	谨慎交叉换药	谨慎交叉换药,TCA从低剂量起始
逐渐减量、停药,1周后换药	谨慎交叉换药	谨慎交叉换药	谨慎交叉换药	逐渐减量、停药,然后从低剂量起始	逐渐减量、停药,然后从低剂量起始	谨慎交叉换药
逐渐减量、停药,5~6周后换药	谨慎交叉换药	谨慎交叉换药	谨慎交叉换药	直接停药,4~7天后从低剂量起始	直接停药,4~7天后从低剂量起始	直接停药,4~7天后从低剂量起始
逐渐减量、停药,1周后换药	谨慎交叉换药,米氮平从15mg起始	谨慎交叉换药	谨慎交叉换药	有可能直接换药	有可能直接换药	慎重交叉换药,从低剂量起始
逐渐减量、停药,2周后换药	逐渐减量、停药,2周后换药	逐渐减量、停药,2周后换药	逐渐减量、停药,2周后换药	逐渐减量、停药,2周后换药	逐渐减量、停药,2周后换药	逐渐减量、停药,2周后换药[j]
	逐渐减量、停药,24h后换药	逐渐减量、停药,24h后换药	逐渐减量、停药,24h后换药	逐渐减量、停药,24h后换药	逐渐减量、停药,24h后换药	逐渐减量、停药,24h后换药
逐渐减量、停药,1周后换药		谨慎交叉换药	谨慎交叉换药	谨慎交叉换药	谨慎交叉换药	谨慎交叉换药
逐渐减量、停药,1周后换药	谨慎交叉换药		谨慎交叉换药	谨慎交叉换药	谨慎交叉换药	谨慎交叉换药
逐渐减量、停药,1周后换药	谨慎交叉换药	谨慎交叉换药		谨慎交叉换药	谨慎交叉换药	谨慎交叉换药,TCA从低剂量起始
逐渐减量、停药,1周后换药	谨慎交叉换药	谨慎交叉换药	谨慎交叉换药	有可能直接换药	有可能直接换药	谨慎交叉换药,TCA从低剂量起始

更换药物	阿戈美拉汀	安非他酮	氯米帕明	氟西汀	氟伏沙明	MAOI 苯乙肼 环苯丙胺 司来吉兰
SNRI 度洛西汀[i] 文拉法辛 去甲文拉法辛	谨慎交叉换药	谨慎交叉换药	逐渐减量、停药,氯米帕明从低剂量起始	直接换药	直接换药	逐渐减量、停药,1 周后换药
三环类	谨慎交叉换药	剂量减半时加安非他酮,然后缓慢停用三环类	直接换药	剂量减半时加氟西汀,然后缓慢停用三环类	谨慎交叉换药	逐渐减量、停药,2 周后换用[j]

续表

吗氯贝胺	米氮平	瑞波西汀	曲唑酮	其他 SSRI[f] 伏硫西汀	SNRI 度洛西汀 文拉法辛 去甲文拉法辛	TCA（除外 氯米帕明）
逐渐减量、停药,1 周后换药	谨慎交叉换药	谨慎交叉换药	谨慎交叉换药	直接换药	直接换药	谨慎交叉换药,TCA 从低剂量起始
逐渐减量、停药,1 周后换药	谨慎交叉换药	谨慎交叉换药	剂量减半时加曲唑酮,然后缓慢停用三环类	剂量减半时加SSRI,然后缓慢停用三环类	谨慎交叉换药,SNRI 从低剂量起始	直接换药

注:

* 表中给出的建议部分来自制药商提供的资料和出版数据,部分源于理论。个体用药受多种因素影响,应谨慎处理每种情况。

谨慎交叉换药——通常需要超过 2~4 周。

[a] 阿戈美拉汀不影响单胺类摄取,与 α、β 肾上腺素能受体、组胺受体、胆碱能受体、多巴胺受体和苯二氮䓬类药物受体没有亲和力。该药与其他抗抑郁药相互作用的可能性低,预计不能缓解其他抗抑郁药的停药反应。当从阿戈美拉汀换成其他抗抑郁药时,应谨慎尝试交叉换药。

[b] 安非他酮在英国被许可用于戒烟,但未被许可用于治疗抑郁症。它是 CYP2D6 的抑制剂,交叉换药时需要特别谨慎经该酶代谢的药物。

[c] 注意:由于氟西汀的代谢产物半衰期长,停药后 5 周内仍可能与氟西汀发生药物相互作用。

[d] 氟伏沙明是 CYP1A2 的强抑制剂,对 CYP2C 和 CYP3A4 的抑制作用略弱,发生药物相互作用的可能性高,需特别注意。

[e] 瑞波西汀不建议作为抗抑郁药单独使用。

[f] 西酞普兰、艾司西酞普兰、帕罗西汀和舍曲林。

[g] 伏硫西汀临床经验有限,应格外谨慎。安非他酮和其他 2D6 抑制剂(如氟西汀和帕罗西汀)相互替换时要特别小心[9]。

[h] 若是伏硫西汀应停用 3 周[10]。

[i] 从 SSRI 和文拉法辛突然换为度洛西汀时,可从 60mg/d 开始[5]。

[j] 若是丙米嗪应停用 3 周。

参考文献

1. Cleare A, et al. Evidence-based guidelines for treating depressive disorders with antidepressants: a revision of the 2008 British Association for Psychopharmacology guidelines. *J Psychopharmacology* 2015; **29**:459–525.

2. Harvey BH, et al. New insights on the antidepressant discontinuation syndrome. *Human Psychopharmacology* 2014; **29**:503–516.

3. Malhi GS, et al. Royal Australian and New Zealand College of Psychiatrists clinical practice guidelines for mood disorders. *Aust N Z J Psychiatry* 2015; **49**:1087–1206.

4. Benazzi F. Fluoxetine for the treatment of SSRI discontinuation syndrome. *Int J Neuropsychopharmacol* 2008; **11**:725–726.

5. Perahia DG, et al. Switching to duloxetine from selective serotonin reuptake inhibitor antidepressants: a multicenter trial comparing 2 switching techniques. *J Clin Psychiatry* 2008; **69**:95–105.

6. Goodwin GM, et al. Agomelatine prevents relapse in patients with major depressive disorder without evidence of a discontinuation syndrome: a 24-week randomized, double-blind, placebo-controlled trial. *J Clin Psychiatry* 2009; **70**:1128–1137.

7. Buckley NA, et al. Serotonin syndrome. *BMJ* 2014; **348**:g1626.

8. Abadie D, et al. Serotonin syndrome: analysis of cases registered in the French pharmacovigilance database. *J Clin Psychopharmacol* 2015; **35**:382–388.

9. Chen G, et al. Pharmacokinetic drug interactions involving vortioxetine (Lu AA21004), a multimodal antidepressant. *Clin Drug Investig* 2013; **33**:727–736.

10. Citrome L. Vortioxetine for major depressive disorder: a systematic review of the efficacy and safety profile for this newly approved antidepressant – what is the number needed to treat, number needed to harm and likelihood to be helped or harmed? *Int J Clin Pract* 2014; **68**:60–82.

第 3 章

抗抑郁药停药症状

背景

　　许多药物包括抗抑郁药都有停药症状。"停药症状"(综合征)指患者停用抗抑郁药时出现的症状[1,2]。"停药症状"和"戒断症状"在语义上有重要的差别——后者意味着成瘾,前者则没有。虽然抗抑郁药不是成瘾物质(例如,它们不会引起渴求),但分类和语义差异与患者体验并无关联。停药症状可用"受体反跳(receptor rebound)"[3]加以解释,如有强抗胆碱能不良反应的抗抑郁药停用后出现腹泻。

体征和症状

　　抗抑郁药的停药症状既可能是全新的,也可能类似于疾病的原有症状,后者本来是用药治疗的目标。停药症状可与疾病的复发或者复燃有以下区别:快速发作(数天而不是数周,或药物 3~5 个半衰期内[4]),重新服用抗抑郁药后快速起效(通常在数小时内,数天内必然缓解),出现与原发疾病完全不同的躯体和心理症状(例如大脑过电感、头晕、恶心)。图 3.3 总结了使用 SSRI 和相关药物(例如 SNRI 和其他 5-羟色胺再摄取抑制剂)报告的各种停药症状。使用其他抗抑郁药报道的症状总结在表 3.8 中。

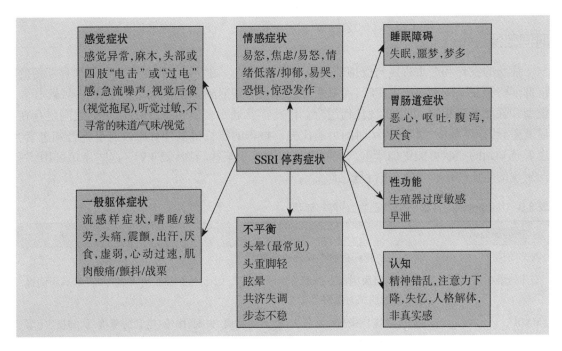

图 3.3　常见停药症状

表 3.8　影响抗抑郁药停药症状发生率和严重程度的因素

药理因素	■ 药物半衰期——与症状的严重程度和发作相关。半衰期较短的药物（例如文拉法辛和度洛西汀）症状通常较严重
- 药代动力学	
- 药物半衰期	■ 其他药代动力学因素——非线性药代动力学
- 药效学	■ 受体亲和力：对 5-羟色胺转运体的亲和力越高，停药症状的风险越高
- 受体亲和力	
治疗因素	
- 治疗持续时间	
- 剂量	
- 减药方法	
患者因素	
- 既往经验和预期效应	

发生率和严重程度

许多患者会出现抗抑郁药停药症状：14 项考察抗抑郁药停药症状发生率的研究报告停药症状发生率为 27%~86%，加权平均值为 56%。尽管报告的发生率在不同药物和研究方法之间差异很大（氟西汀 9%~77%，帕罗西汀 42%~100%[5]），但在某种程度上，停药症状可见于所有抗抑郁药，但阿戈美拉汀可能例外 [4]。

时间范围

症状的发作和严重程度与抗抑郁药的半衰期有关。帕罗西汀和文拉法辛等半衰期短的抗抑郁药会在一两天内产生症状，而氟西汀的症状可延迟到 2~6 周以后 [1]。症状的持续时间、类型和强度各不相同，可以出现任何组合。停药症状通常轻微并有自限性，个体之间也存在显著差异，并且某些症状的持续时间可能比先前报告的要长得多 [6]。如果没有事先告知患者，患者感知到的症状可能更加严重。一些症状较常见于某些药物（表 3.9）。这些症状可用《停药出现的体征和症状量表》进行量化评估 [7]。

表 3.9　其他抗抑郁药（非 SSRI 类药物）的停药症状

抗抑郁药类型	症状
阿戈美拉汀	即使存在，停药症状的风险也非常低 [4]
安非他酮	不常见，但病例报告描述了焦虑、头痛、失眠、易怒和肌肉疼痛 [8,9]，有单一病例报告了急性肌张力障碍 [10]
MAOI*	常见：激越、易激惹、共济失调、运动障碍、失眠、困倦、生动的梦境、认知损害、语速慢、强制言语 偶见：幻觉、妄想 RIMA：吗氯贝胺有流感样症状 [11]
NaSSA（例如米氮平）	惊恐、焦虑、烦躁、易激惹、轻躁狂、失眠、头晕、感觉异常、恶心、呕吐 [10]

续表

抗抑郁药类型	症状
5-羟色胺调节剂(伏硫西汀、维拉唑酮)	尚未报道[10],这些是相对较新的抗抑郁药,临床经验较少。与其他抗抑郁药(如SSRI)药理作用类似,因此不能忽视停药症状的发生[10]。
TCA	一般躯体和胃肠道不适,睡眠障碍表现为起始和中段失眠或过度生动、可怕的梦,静坐不能或帕金森症状,轻躁狂或躁狂,心律失常[10]
曲唑酮	轻躁狂、焦虑、眠浅、噩梦、人格解体、蚁行感、头痛[10]

* 反苯环丙胺在较大剂量时可能具有类似苯丙胺的特征[12],因此可能与真正的"戒断症状"有关。可能会出现谵妄[13]。

临床相关性[14,15]

停药症状可被误认为疾病复燃或者出现新的躯体疾病,导致不必要检查或重新使用抗抑郁药[16]。停药症状可严重到足以影响日常功能,那些出现停药症状的患者可能推断(也许是适当的)抗抑郁药有"成瘾性",继而不希望接受治疗。也有证据表明,停用帕罗西汀会出现急性自杀观念[17]。

谁是风险最高的[10,14-16,18]

尽管所有患者都可能发生停药症状,风险较高的见于短半衰期的药物[7](如帕罗西汀、文拉法辛),尤其是患者服药不规律时。2/3 的患者不时漏服药物[19],许多患者会突然停药[20]。风险较高的还有已经服用抗抑郁药 8 周以上者[21]、服用大剂量抗抑郁药者、抗抑郁药(尤其是 SSRI)治疗早期出现焦虑症状者、服用其他中枢神经系统药物(如降压药、抗组胺药、抗精神病药)者、儿童或青少年[7]、年轻人[22]以及既往出现过停药症状者。

抗抑郁药的停药症状在服用抗抑郁药的母亲所分娩的孩子中较为常见(见第 7 章"妊娠"部分)。

如何避免停药症状[14-16,18]

一般而言,抗抑郁药治疗应逐渐停止[6]。读者可参阅本章"停用抗抑郁药"部分,了解特定抗抑郁药的停药建议。药物半衰期越短,越要遵守这个规则。到减药后期,速度应该更慢,因为只有在抗抑郁药每天总剂量减少幅度较大时(按比例),才会出现停药症状。使用MAOI 治疗的患者,其减药过程需要更长时间。环苯丙胺可能特别难以停药[13]。高危患者(见上)减药需要更加缓慢。阿戈美拉汀突然停用可能不会引起停药反应,但原则上应该缓慢停药——所有抗精神病药都应尽可能缓慢停药。

即使在缓慢停药的情况下,患者已经接受了充分的停药症状教育,仍有可能发生停药症状[7,17]。这可能是因为没有按比例逐渐减量(见本章中关于"停用抗抑郁药"的部分)。

如何治疗停药症状[14-16,23]

这个领域很少有系统性研究。治疗是经验性的。如果症状轻微,应该安慰患者,这些症状在停用抗抑郁药之后是常见的,过几天或几周就会消失。如果症状严重,需要重新使用原来的抗抑郁药（或同一类别中半衰期较长的抗抑郁药），然后在监测这些症状的同时逐步减量[6]。

一些证据支持在三环类药物停药过程中使用抗胆碱能药[24]，在帕罗西汀[25]、舍曲林[25]、氯米帕明[26]、文拉法辛[27]停药过程中使用氟西汀（血浆半衰期较长），使用这些方法似乎都比使用其他类似药物能更少出现停药症状[7]。建议使用替代类药物（例如短期对症使用苯二氮䓬类药物）治疗停药相关的焦虑和失眠[28]。

患者应该知道的要点

- 根据医学定义，抗抑郁药并没有成瘾性（患者对抗抑郁药持负面看法，最常提到的原因是成瘾[29]，1977年英国进行的样本为1 946人的调查中，74%被调查者认为抗抑郁药有成瘾性[30]）。但是需要注意的是，成瘾和停药症状在语义和类属上的差异对患者并不重要。
- 需要告诉患者，在停用抗抑郁药时，可能会出现停药症状（并告知停用所用药物时最可能出现的症状）。
- 抗抑郁药一般不能突然停药：可能出现停药反应，并且更容易疾病复发[31]。
- 若所用抗抑郁药的半衰期短，漏服药或延迟服药也可能出现停药症状。很少有患者体验到给药前的停药症状，否则每天会提前服用抗抑郁药。

参考文献

1. Horowitz MA, et al. Tapering of SSRI treatment to mitigate withdrawal symptoms. *Lancet Psychiatry* 2019; 6:538–546.
2. Massabki I, et al. Selective serotonin reuptake inhibitor 'discontinuation syndrome' or withdrawal. *Br J Psychiatry* 2020; 6:1–4.
3. Zabegalov KN, et al. Understanding antidepressant discontinuation syndrome (ADS) through preclinical experimental models. *Eur J Pharmacol* 2018; 829:129–140.
4. Henssler J, et al. Antidepressant withdrawal and rebound phenomena. *Dtsch Arztebl Int* 2019; 116:355–361.
5. Davies J, et al. A systematic review into the incidence, severity and duration of antidepressant withdrawal effects: are guidelines evidence-based? *Addict Behav* 2019; 97:111–121.
6. National Institute for Health and Care Excellence. Depression in adults: recognition and management. Clinical guideline [CG90]. 2009 (Last updated: December 2013); https://www.nice.org.uk/Guidance/cg90.
7. Fava GA, et al. Withdrawal symptoms after selective serotonin reuptake inhibitor discontinuation: a systematic review. *Psychother Psychosom* 2015; 84:72–81.
8. Berigan TR. Bupropion-associated withdrawal symptoms revisited: a case report. *Prim Care Companion J Clin Psychiatry* 2002; 4:78.
9. Berigan TR, et al. Bupropion-associated withdrawal symptoms: a case report. *Prim Care Companion J Clin Psychiatry* 1999; 1:50–51.
10. Cosci F, et al. Acute and persistent withdrawal syndromes following discontinuation of psychotropic medications. *Psychother Psychosom* 2020; 89:283–306.
11. Curtin F, et al. Moclobemide discontinuation syndrome predominantly presenting with influenza-like symptoms. *J Psychopharmacology* 2002; 16:271–272.
12. Ricken R, et al. Tranylcypromine in mind (Part II): review of clinical pharmacology and meta-analysis of controlled studies in depression. *Eur Neuropsychopharmacol* 2017; 27:714–731.
13. Gahr M, et al. Withdrawal and discontinuation phenomena associated with tranylcypromine: a systematic review. *Pharmacopsychiatry* 2013; 46:123–129.
14. Lejoyeux M, et al. Antidepressant withdrawal syndrome: recognition, prevention and management. *CNS Drugs* 1996; 5:278–292.
15. Haddad PM, et al. Recognising and managing antidepressant discontinuation symptoms. *Adv Psychiatric Treatment* 2007; 13:447–457.
16. Haddad PM. Antidepressant discontinuation syndromes. *Drug Saf* 2001; 24:183–197.
17. Tint A, et al. The effect of rate of antidepressant tapering on the incidence of discontinuation symptoms: a randomised study. *J Psychopharmacology* 2008; 22:330–332.
18. Ogle NR, et al. Guidance for the discontinuation or switching of antidepressant therapies in adults. *J Pharm Pract* 2013; 26:389–396.
19. Meijer WE, et al. Spontaneous lapses in dosing during chronic treatment with selective serotonin reuptake inhibitors. *Br J Psychiatry* 2001; 179:519–522.
20. van Geffen EC, et al. Discontinuation symptoms in users of selective serotonin reuptake inhibitors in clinical practice: tapering versus abrupt discontinuation. *Eur J Clin Pharmacol* 2005; 61:303–307.
21. Kramer JC, et al. Withdrawal symptoms following discontinuation of imipramine therapy. *Am J Psychiatry* 1961; 118:549–550.
22. Read J. How common and severe are six withdrawal effects from, and addiction to, antidepressants? The experiences of a large international

sample of patients. *Addict Behav* 2020; **102**:106–157.

23. Wilson E, et al. A review of the management of antidepressant discontinuation symptoms. *Ther Adv Psychopharmacol* 2015; **5**:357–368.
24. Dilsaver SC, et al. Antidepressant withdrawal symptoms treated with anticholinergic agents. *Am J Psychiatry* 1983; **140**:249–251.
25. Benazzi F. Re: selective serotonin reuptake inhibitor discontinuation syndrome: putative mechanisms and prevention strategies. *Can J Psychiatry* 1999; **44**:95–96.
26. Benazzi F. Fluoxetine for clomipramine withdrawal symptoms. *Am J Psychiatry* 1999; **156**:661–662.
27. Giakas WJ, et al. Intractable withdrawal from venlafaxine treated with fluoxetine. *Psychiatric Annals* 1997; **27**:85–93.
28. Fava GA, et al. Understanding and managing withdrawal syndromes after discontinuation of antidepressant drugs. *J Clin Psychiatry* 2019; **80**.
29. Gibson K, et al. Patient-centered perspectives on antidepressant use. *Int J Mental Health* 2014; **43**:81–99.
30. Paykel ES, et al. Changes in public attitudes to depression during the Defeat Depression Campaign. *Br J Psychiatry* 1998; **173**:519–522.
31. Baldessarini RJ, et al. Illness risk following rapid versus gradual discontinuation of antidepressants. *Am J Psychiatry* 2010; **167**:934–941.

扩展阅读

Fava GA, et al. Withdrawal Symptoms after Selective Serotonin Reuptake Inhibitor Discontinuation: A Systematic Review. *Psychother Psychosom* 2015; **84**:72–81.

Haddad PM, et al. Recognising and managing antidepressant discontinuation symptoms. *Advances in Psychiatric Treatment* 2007; **13**:447–457.

Schatzberg AF, et al. Antidepressant discontinuation syndrome: consensus panel recommendations for clinical management and additional research. *J Clin Psychiatry* 2006; **67 Suppl 4**:27–30.

Shelton RC. The nature of the discontinuation syndrome associated with antidepressant drugs. *J Clin Psychiatry* 2006; **67 Suppl 4**:3–7.

第 3 章

停用抗抑郁药

大约 50% 的患者在减少或停用抗抑郁药后会出现停药反应[1]。对于其中一些(可能多达 50%)患者,症状会很严重并且持续很长时间(数月或数年)[1,2]。对于其他人,症状可能较轻并有自限性。已经确定了一个单独的停药综合征类别,称为急性停药后综合征(post-acute withdrawal syndrome,PAWS),它可以持续数年,并涉及大量的有时使人衰弱的症状,但其病理生理学机制研究较少[3]。

抗抑郁药的许多特征会影响发生停药反应的可能性。患者服用抗抑郁药时间越长、剂量越高,越容易出现停药反应[4,5]。半衰期短和具有胆碱能或肾上腺素能作用的抗抑郁药,往往与更严重的停药反应相关——文拉法辛、度洛西汀和帕罗西汀是最常见的[6,7]。患者突然或快速停药有更多的停药反应[8-10]。可能存在一系列个体生理(和心理)差异,但目前还知之甚少,这也决定了停药反应的严重程度[11]。

减药的理论依据

有一些证据表明,缓慢减量将症状分散到更长时间,可以减少患者出现无法忍受的停药症状的机会[9,10,12]。随机研究表明,与骤然停药相比,减药持续 14 天时,停药症状的程度不是没有减轻,就是减轻甚微[13,14,15]。这些研究的普遍结论是需要更长时间的逐渐减药方案[16,17]。在数月内逐渐减少药物似乎可以降低出现停药症状的风险[9,10,12],但有些患者减药过程需要数年。临床经验表明,长期抗抑郁药治疗的大多数患者需要 3 个月至 2 年才能以可耐受的方式停用。

虽然线性减少药物剂量(例如舍曲林 50mg,37.5mg,25mg,12.5mg,0)似乎是合理的(并且拆分片剂是可行的),但由于抗抑郁药的剂量与其对主要目标 5-羟色胺受体(SERT)的效果之间存在双曲线关系(遵循质量作用定律[18]),这可能会导致更加严重的停药症状(图3.4a)[11]。这与患者报告一致,即在小剂量时减药是该过程中最困难的。

以"平和"的方式减少对目标受体的影响,这样的减药方式更合理:双曲线式减少剂量(图 3.4b)。更容易接近的是以指数(成比例)方式减少剂量——例如每 2~4 周减少最近一次剂量的 10%~20%(表 3.10)。完全停药前最后的剂量必须很小(<1mg),以防止减药到零的

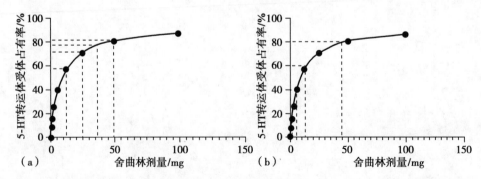

图 3.4　(a)线性减少剂量导致对目标受体作用的下降幅度越来越大,可能与更多的停药反应有关。(b)对目标受体作用的平缓下降需要双曲线剂量降低。停药前的最终剂量需要非常小

时候"下降"大于以前能耐受的下降幅度。这已获得研究证据支持,即逐渐减少到远低于常规治疗剂量(例如舍曲林 0.5mg)的方法,提高了人们停用抗抑郁药的机会[12,19],并最终远离它们[20]。

表 3.10　以舍曲林为例每个时期减少 20%(基于上一次剂量)

时期	剂量/mg	时期	剂量/mg	时期	剂量/mg
1	200	12	17	23	1.5
2	160	13	14	24	1.2
3	128	14	11	25	0.9
4	102	15	9	26	0.75
5	82	16	7	27	0.6
6	66	17	5.5	28	0.5
7	52	18	4.5	29	0.4
8	42	19	3.6	30	0.3
9	34	20	2.9	31	0.25
10	27	21	2.3	32	0
11	21	22	1.8		

　　注:许多患者减量的步骤可能多于这个——每月减少最近一次剂量的 5%~10%。

　　*2~4 周通常是可耐受的;其他可能需要更长时间。从 0.25mg 减少到 0mg 的幅度相当于前一次减量的幅度(剂量减少 20% 大约等于 5-羟色胺转运体抑制降低 3%)。

减药的实践操作

减药前

　　应告知所有患者停用任何抗抑郁药后都可能出现停药症状的风险。一些抗抑郁药,如帕罗西汀和文拉法辛,更为常见严重的停药症状。

　　应警告患者不要突然停用抗抑郁药,因为这种方法被认为最有可能引起严重而持久的停药症状,并增加复发的风险。

　　尽管停用抗抑郁药会引起令人不快的症状,但应该告诉患者,如果逐渐且小心地减量,停药症状可以维持在可耐受的水平。患者在过去可能有过快速减药所带来的负面经历,因此更需要消除其疑虑。

　　很难预测个体逐渐减停抗抑郁药所需的确切时间,但大多数长期用药的患者需要大约 3 个月,有些甚至需要 2 年。这可能有助于设定预期时间。

　　应与患者讨论过去的停药经历,因为这可以作为预测逐渐减量后出现什么停药症状的线索。仔细考察既往尝试停药的过程,可能会发现那些被误诊为复发的停药症状。

　　患者通常需要做一些抗抑郁药逐渐减量的准备,这可能包括减轻工作负荷、家庭责任或增加对非药物处理技能的关注(患者发现了很多有用的方法,包括接纳、呼吸练习、锻炼、业余爱好、记日记以及减少应激)[21,22]。有证据表明正念认知疗法(mindfulness-based cognitive therapy,MB-CT)有助于停用抗抑郁药[23]。

医师和患者都应该意识到,虽然患者在停药期间可能出现负面的心理和身体症状,这并不表明需要足剂量药物(这可能只是表明需要减慢减药的速度)。患者和医师应熟悉各种停药反应(图 3.4),当出现停药症状时,这有助于减轻不必要的焦虑。患者可能在此过程中需要更多专业或其他方面的支持[22]。

减药过程

患者可按停药反应的危险进行大致分层:

对于低风险患者(用药时间 <6 个月,半衰期长的抗抑郁药,过去没有出现显著的停药症状),可以试减 25%。

对于高风险患者(用药时间 >6 个月,半衰期短的抗抑郁药,过去出现过停药症状),建议试减 5%~10%。

所有患者均应监测停药症状 2~4 周,或直到症状完全缓解。监测方法可以每天简单地测评症状(例如十分之几),或使用标准化评估工具,如 DESS[24]。

应根据上述减药测试的可耐受性来确定未来减药的过程。如果开始减药时患者可耐受,观察期结束时无停药症状或症状已经缓解,可继续以相同的比例和相同的速率减少剂量(注意,要以最后使用的剂量计算)。请参阅表 3.10 中的示例方案,舍曲林的简化减药指导方案见框 3.1。如果症状不能耐受,应该放慢减量的速度;如果严重,可能需要重新使用之前的剂量,稳定一段时间后,再采取更谨慎的减药计划。

框 3.1　根据指数模式对舍曲林减药进行的简化指导方案。提供的减少幅度相当于每一步减少 10%~20% 的剂量。一些患者可能需要更小幅度的减药,其他患者则可以耐受更大幅度、更快速度的减药。

- 每 2~4 周减少 12.5~25mg 直到达到 50mg/d
- 每 2~4 周减少 2~5mg 直到达到 15mg/d,然后
- 每 2~4 周减少 1~2mg 直到达到 9mg/d,然后
- 每 2~4 周减少 0.4~1mg 直到达到 4mg/d,然后
- 每 2~4 周减少 0.2~0.4mg 直到达到 2mg/d,然后
- 每 2~4 周减少 0.1~0.25mg 直到完全停药

这个过程通常需要几个月至两年,但有些人需要更长的时间。

处理办法

如果停药症状在某一时间点变得无法忍受,保持当前剂量更长的时间待其缓解;若症状过于严重,需要加回到症状可以耐受时的剂量,并保持该剂量直到症状消失。患者状态稳定后,减药过程需要更加缓慢,减药幅度更小或减药间隔时间更长。一些患者发现自己 1 个月剂量减少的幅度不能超过 5%。

重要的是要记住,即使患者出现严重的停药症状,也不能表示他们不能停用抗抑郁药,而只是表明他们需要缓慢减药,剂量减少的幅度要更小一些。

氟西汀的半衰期长,停药症状的出现可以推迟到数周后,应对此予以注意。由于停药期较长,氟西汀减量幅度较大时,可能相对容易耐受。氟西汀的减量方法也可以是降低给药频率(例如,每周 6 天每天 20mg,每周 5 天每天 20mg,以此类推)。

不幸的是,目前的抗抑郁药片剂无法使用符合药理学知识的减药方案,因此患者需要抗抑郁药液体制剂(或使用荷兰减药带)[19]。对于没有液体剂型的抗抑郁药,必须制作液体剂型,或者改用有液体制剂的药物。许多患者报告,他们自己将药片切碎、称重,或用压碎的药片制作溶液,但是我们并不推荐这种方法。

完全停药之前可能需要非常小的最终剂量,以便避免对递质系统的作用出现较大的下降。对于许多药物,最终剂量可能比 1mg 还要少得多。例如,对于舍曲林剂量每月减少 10% 的患者,最终剂量可能仅仅 0.1mg,对 5-羟色胺转运体作用的减少幅度就与前一次减药时相同[11]。

参考文献

1. Davies J, et al. A systematic review into the incidence, severity and duration of antidepressant withdrawal effects: are guidelines evidence-based? *Addict Behav* 2019; **97**:111–121.
2. Stockmann T, et al. SSRI and SNRI withdrawal symptoms reported on an internet forum. *Int J Risk Saf Med* 2018; **29**:175–180.
3. Cosci F, et al. Acute and persistent withdrawal syndromes following discontinuation of psychotropic medications. *Psychother Psychosom* 2020; **89**:283–306.
4. Weller I, et al. Report of the CSM expert working group on the safety of selective serotonin reuptake inhibitors antidepressants. 2005; https://www.neuroscience.ox.ac.uk/publications/474047.
5. Read J, et al. Adverse effects of antidepressants reported by a large international cohort: emotional blunting, suicidality, and withdrawal effects. *Current Drug Safety* 2018; **13**:176–186.
6. Taylor D, et al. Antidepressant withdrawal symptoms-telephone calls to a national medication helpline. *J Affect Disord* 2006; **95**:129–133.
7. Henssler J, et al. Antidepressant withdrawal and rebound phenomena. *Dtsch Arztebl Int* 2019; **116**:355–361.
8. Himei A, et al. Discontinuation syndrome associated with paroxetine in depressed patients: a retrospective analysis of factors involved in the occurrence of the syndrome. *CNS Drugs* 2006; **20**:665–672.
9. Murata Y, et al. Effects of the serotonin 1A, 2A, 2C, 3A, and 3B and serotonin transporter gene polymorphisms on the occurrence of paroxetine discontinuation syndrome. *J Clin Psychopharmacol* 2010; **30**:11–17.
10. van Geffen EC, et al. Discontinuation symptoms in users of selective serotonin reuptake inhibitors in clinical practice: tapering versus abrupt discontinuation. *Eur J Clin Pharmacol* 2005; **61**:303–307.
11. Horowitz MA, et al. Tapering of SSRI treatment to mitigate withdrawal symptoms. *Lancet Psychiatry* 2019; **6**:538–546.
12. Groot PC, et al. Antidepressant tapering strips to help people come off medication more safely. *Psychosis* 2018; **10**:142–145.
13. Tint A, et al. The effect of rate of antidepressant tapering on the incidence of discontinuation symptoms: a randomised study. *J Psychopharmacology* 2008; **22**:330–332.
14. Baldwin DS, et al. A double-blind, randomized, parallel-group, flexible-dose study to evaluate the tolerability, efficacy and effects of treatment discontinuation with escitalopram and paroxetine in patients with major depressive disorder. *Int Clin Psychopharmacol* 2006; **21**:159–169.
15. Montgomery SA, et al. Absence of discontinuation symptoms with agomelatine and occurrence of discontinuation symptoms with paroxetine: a randomized, double-blind, placebo-controlled discontinuation study. *Int Clin Psychopharmacol* 2004; **19**:271–280.
16. Haddad PM, et al. Recognising and managing antidepressant discontinuation symptoms. *Adv Psychiatric Treatment* 2007; **13**:447–457.
17. Phelps J. Tapering antidepressants: is 3 months slow enough? *Med Hypotheses* 2011; **77**:1006–1008.
18. Holford N. Pharmacodynamic principles and the time course of delayed and cumulative drug effects. *Trans Clin Pharmacology* 2018; **26**:56–59.
19. Groot PC, et al. How user knowledge of psychotropic drug withdrawal resulted in the development of person-specific tapering medication. *Ther Adv Psychopharmacol* 2020; **10**:2045125320932452.
20. Groot PC, et al. Outcome of antidepressant drug discontinuation with taperingstrips after 1–5 years. *Ther Adv Psychopharmacol* 2020; **10**:2045125320954609.
21. Inner Compass Initiative Inc. The withdrawal project. 2019; https://withdrawal.theinnercompass.org.
22. Guy A, et al. *Guidance for psychological therapists: enabling conversations with clients taking or withdrawing from prescribed psychiatric drugs.* London: APPG for Prescribed Drug Dependence; 2019.
23. Maund E, et al. Managing antidepressant discontinuation: a systematic review. *Ann Fam Med* 2019; **17**:52–60.
24. Rosenbaum JF, et al. Selective serotonin reuptake inhibitor discontinuation syndrome: a randomized clinical trial. *Biol Psychiatry* 1998; **44**:77–87.

第 3 章

电抽搐治疗和精神药物

　　在进行 ECT 时,通常会继续使用精神药物。一些药物(特别是抗抑郁药[1,2])能增强 ECT 疗效。

　　表 3.11 总结了 ECT 期间各种精神药物对于发作持续时间的影响。需要注意的是,因为该领域对照良好的研究很少,在考察相关建议时要预先考虑这一点。

　　还要注意的是,麻醉药物的选择对发作持续时间[3-8]、发作后意识模糊程度及 ECT 疗效有很大的影响[9,10]。使用氯胺酮作为麻醉剂最终不会改善 ECT 的结果[11,12],但是在 ECT 早期改善抑郁症状方面可能有短期益处[13]。除了合并的药物,还有许多因素会影响患者 ECT 发作阈值和持续时间[14]。

表 3.11　ECT 中精神药物对癫痫发作持续时间的影响

药物	对 ECT 癫痫发作持续时间的影响	评价[3,15-18]
苯二氮䓬类药物[19]	缩短 证据不一,临床意义不清楚	所有的苯二氮䓬类药物都可能提高发作阈值,因此尽可能不用。许多药物作用时间长,可能需要在开始 ECT 数天前停药。苯二氮䓬类药物还可能使麻醉更加复杂,降低 ECT 的疗效 如果需要镇静,考虑羟嗪。如果必须长期使用苯二氮䓬类药物,继续服药的同时需使用更高的刺激量、双侧刺激
SSRI[2,20-23]	影响极小,可能略微延长	在 ECT 期间使用通常认为是安全的。注意与麻醉剂复杂的药代动力学相互作用。孤立病例报告提示使用氟西汀和帕罗西汀在 ECT 治疗期间发生 5-羟色胺综合征[24,25]
文拉法辛[26]	标准剂量影响极小	有限的数据显示,文拉法辛对发作持续时间没有影响,但剂量超过 300mg/d 时,可能增加心脏停搏的风险[27]。更大剂量时明确会引起癫痫发作。建议监测 ECG
米氮平[2,28]	影响极小——略微延长	在 ECT 中显然是安全的。像其他抗抑郁药一样,可增强 ECT 的疗效。可减轻 ECT 后的恶心和头痛
度洛西汀[29,30]	未知	一个案例报告表明,度洛西汀不会使 ECT 复杂化。另一个个案表明,度洛西汀的使用与室性心动过速有关
TCA[2,21,31]	可能延长	关于 ECT 的数据很少,但是许多 TCA 可以降低发作阈值。TCA 与 ECT 后的心律不齐有关,老年人和心脏病患者应避免使用。对于其他患者,在 ECT 期间最好继续 TCA 治疗。需要进行密切监测。注意低血压和发作时间延长的风险
MAOI[32]	影响极小	与 ECT 相关的数据非常有限,但在 MAOI 治疗期间使用 ECT 具有很长的历史 MAOI 可能并不影响发作持续时间,但是与麻醉中有时会使用的拟交感神经药可能有交互作用,并可能导致高血压危象。司来吉兰经皮吸收剂型似乎是安全的[33] 在 ECT 期间可以继续使用 MAOI,但必须告知麻醉师。注意低血压

续表

药物	对 ECT 癫痫发作持续时间的影响	评价[3,15-18]
锂盐[34-37]	可能延长	关于锂盐和 ECT 的关系,研究结果相互矛盾。联合治疗可能导致谵妄和意识模糊,一些权威建议在 ECT 前48h 停止锂盐治疗。在英国,锂盐治疗期间往往也使用 ECT,但是需从低刺激量开始,并进行密切监测。联合治疗的耐受性通常很好[38]。需要注意的是,锂盐增强了非去极化神经肌肉阻滞剂(如琥珀胆碱)的作用。锂盐治疗同时使用硫喷妥钠或丙泊酚可降低发作阈值
抗精神病药[40-44]	影响不一 吩噻嗪、氯氮平延长 其他未报告有明显影响	发表的研究数据很少,但使用广泛。吩噻嗪类和氯氮平也许最有可能会延长发作,有人建议在 ECT 前停用。然而,也有二者可以安全联用的报告(特别是氯氮平[45,46],现在进行 ECT 时通常会继续氯氮平治疗)。ECT 在氯氮平无效时有作用[47] 一般来说,联合使用 ECT 和抗精神病药是安全的。关于阿立哌唑、喹硫平和齐拉西酮的数据很少,但它们似乎也是安全的。一项病例系列研究显示[48],抗精神病药增加了发作后的认知功能障碍
抗癫痫药[49-52]	缩短	如果作为心境稳定剂,可以继续使用,但需准备使用更大能量的刺激(并不总是需要)。如果用于癫痫,其作用是使发作阈值正常化。可能会有相互作用。丙戊酸盐可能会延长硫喷妥钠的作用;卡马西平可能会抑制神经肌肉阻滞作用。一项小型的 RCT 研究发现卡马西平和丙戊酸盐(全剂量与半剂量)在发作持续时间、发作阈值和认知结果方面没有显著差异[53]。报告显示拉莫三嗪不会引起问题
巴比妥类	缩短	在 ECT 中,所有的巴比妥类都会缩短发作时间,但是仍广泛作为镇静性麻醉剂使用 硫喷妥钠和美索比妥可能与心律失常有关

对于已知会降低发作阈值的药物,最好以低能量(50mC)刺激开始治疗。工作人员应警惕发作延长的可能性,备好静脉注射地西泮。对于已知会升高发作阈值的药物,当然需要更强的刺激。有一些方法能够降低发作阈值或延长发作时间[54],但是对该问题的讨论并不属于本书范围。

电抽搐治疗经常引起意识模糊和定向障碍,引起谵妄较少。同时服用锂盐可能会增加谵妄风险[34]。也有两例 5-羟色胺综合征的案例报告;一例发生在联合使用曲唑酮、安非他酮和喹硫平的患者进行 ECT 治疗后[55],另一例发生在 ECT 治疗期间接受锂盐治疗的患者[56]。密切观察是必不可少的。使用硫胺素(每天 200mg)减少 ECT 后意识模糊[57]的支持性证据很少。去甲替林似乎能增强 ECT 疗效,并减少认知方面的不良反应[1]。认知增强剂(多奈哌齐、美金刚、利斯的明)可能会改善认知功能,并减少 ECT 诱发的认知不良反应(并且似乎是安全的)[58,59]。布洛芬可用于预防头痛[60],鼻内使用舒马曲坦[61]也可以治疗头痛。

参考文献

1. Sackeim HA, et al. Effect of concomitant pharmacotherapy on electroconvulsive therapy outcomes: short-term efficacy and adverse effects. *Arch Gen Psychiatry* 2009; **66**:729–737.

2. Baghai TC, et al. The influence of concomitant antidepressant medication on safety, tolerability and clinical effectiveness of electroconvulsive therapy. *World J Biol Psychiatry* 2006; **7**:82–90.

3. Avramov MN, et al. The comparative effects of methohexital, propofol, and etomidate for electroconvulsive therapy. *Anesth Analg* 1995; **81**:596–602.

4. Stadtland C, et al. A switch from propofol to etomidate during an ECT course increases EEG and motor seizure duration. *J ECT* 2002; **18**:22–25.

5. Gazdag G, et al. Etomidate versus propofol for electroconvulsive therapy in patients with schizophrenia. *J ECT* 2004; **20**:225–229.

6. Conca A, et al. Etomidate vs. thiopentone in electroconvulsive therapy. An interdisciplinary challenge for anesthesiology and psychiatry. *Pharmacopsychiatry* 2003; **36**:94–97.

7. Rasmussen KG, et al. Seizure length with sevoflurane and thiopental for induction of general anesthesia in electroconvulsive therapy: a randomized double-blind trial. *J ECT* 2006; **22**:240–242.

8. Bundy BD, et al. Influence of anesthetic drugs and concurrent psychiatric medication on seizure adequacy during electroconvulsive therapy. *J Clin Psychiatry* 2010; **71**:775–777.

9. Stripp TK, et al. Anaesthesia for electroconvulsive therapy – new tricks for old drugs: a systematic review. *Acta Neuropsychiatr* 2018; **30**:61–69.

10. Eser D, et al. The influence of anaesthetic medication on safety, tolerability and clinical effectiveness of electroconvulsive therapy. *World J Biol Psychiatry* 2010; **11**:447–456.

11. McGirr A, et al. Adjunctive ketamine in electroconvulsive therapy: updated systematic review and meta-analysis. *Br J Psychiatry* 2017; **210**:403–407.

12. Fernie G, et al. Ketamine as the anaesthetic for electroconvulsive therapy: the KANECT randomised controlled trial. *Br J Psychiatry* 2017; **210**:422–428.

13. Zheng W, et al. Adjunctive ketamine and electroconvulsive therapy for major depressive disorder: a meta-analysis of randomized controlled trials. *J Affect Disord* 2019; **250**:123–131.

14. van Waarde JA, et al. Clinical predictors of seizure threshold in electroconvulsive therapy: a prospective study. *Eur Arch Psychiatry Clin Neurosci* 2013; **263**:167–175.

15. Royal College of Psychiatrists. The ECT Handbook (4th Edition) – rCPsych Publications: rCPsych Publications 2019.

16. Kellner CH, et al. ECT–drug interactions: a review. *Psychopharmacol Bull* 1991; **27**:595–609.

17. Naguib M, et al. Interactions between psychotropics, anaesthetics and electroconvulsive therapy: implications for drug choice and patient management. *CNS Drugs* 2002; **16**:229–247.

18. Maidment I. The interaction between psychiatric medicines and ECT. *Hosp Pharm* 1997; **4**:102–105.

19. Tang VM, et al. Should benzodiazepines and anticonvulsants be used during electroconvulsive therapy?: a case study and literature review. *J ECT* 2017; **33**:237–242.

20. Masdrakis VG, et al. The safety of the electroconvulsive therapy-escitalopram combination. *J ECT* 2008; **24**:289–291.

21. Dursun SM, et al. Effects of antidepressant treatments on first-ECT seizure duration in depression. *Prog Neuropsychopharmacol Biol Psychiatry* 2001; **25**:437–443.

22. Jarvis MR, et al. Novel antidepressants and maintenance electroconvulsive therapy: a review. *Ann Clin Psychiatry* 1992; **4**:275–284.

23. Papakostas YG, et al. Administration of citalopram before ECT: seizure duration and hormone responses. *J ECT* 2000; **16**:356–360.

24. Okamoto N, et al. Transient serotonin syndrome by concurrent use of electroconvulsive therapy and selective serotonin reuptake inhibitor: a case report and review of the literature. *Case Reports in Psychiatry* 2012; **2012**:215214.

25. Klysner R, et al. Transient serotonin toxicity evoked by combination of electroconvulsive therapy and fluoxetine. *Case Rep Psychiatry* 2014; **2014**:162502.

26. Gonzalez-Pinto A, et al. Efficacy and safety of venlafaxine-ECT combination in treatment-resistant depression. *J Neuropsychiatry Clin Neurosci* 2002; **14**:206–209.

27. Kranaster L, et al. Venlafaxine-associated post-ictal asystole during electroconvulsive therapy. *Pharmacopsychiatry* 2012; **45**:122–124.

28. Li TC, et al. Mirtazapine relieves post-electroconvulsive therapy headaches and nausea: a case series and review of the literature. *J ECT* 2011; **27**:165–167.

29. Hanretta AT, et al. Combined use of ECT with duloxetine and olanzapine: a case report. *J ECT* 2006; **22**:139–141.

30. Heinz B, et al. Postictal ventricular tachycardia after electroconvulsive therapy treatment associated with a lithium-duloxetine combination. *J ECT* 2013; **29**:e33–e35.

31. Birkenhager TK, et al. Possible synergy between electroconvulsive therapy and imipramine: a case report. *J Psychiatr Pract* 2016; **22**:478–480.

32. Dolenc TJ, et al. Electroconvulsive therapy in patients taking monoamine oxidase inhibitors. *J ECT* 2004; **20**:258–261.

33. Horn PJ, et al. Transdermal selegiline in patients receiving electroconvulsive therapy. *Psychosomatics* 2010; **51**:176–178.

34. Patel RS, et al. Combination of lithium and electroconvulsive therapy (ECT) is associated with higher odds of delirium and cognitive problems in a large national sample across the United States. *Brain Stimul* 2020; **13**:15–19.

35. Jha AK, et al. Negative interaction between lithium and electroconvulsive therapy–a case-control study. *Br J Psychiatry* 1996; **168**:241–243.

36. Rucker J, et al. A case of prolonged seizure after ECT in a patient treated with clomipramine, lithium, L-tryptophan, quetiapine, and thyroxine for major depression. *J ECT* 2008; 24:272–274.

37. Dolenc TJ, et al. The safety of electroconvulsive therapy and lithium in combination: a case series and review of the literature. *J ECT* 2005; 21:165–170.

38. Thirthalli J, et al. A prospective comparative study of interaction between lithium and modified electroconvulsive therapy. *World J Biol Psychiatry* 2011; 12:149–155.

39. Galvez V, et al. Predictors of seizure threshold in right unilateral ultrabrief electroconvulsive therapy: role of concomitant medications and anaesthesia used. *Brain Stimul* 2015; 8:486–492.

40. Havaki-Kontaxaki BJ, et al. Concurrent administration of clozapine and electroconvulsive therapy in clozapine-resistant schizophrenia. *Clin Neuropharmacol* 2006; 29:52–56.

41. Nothdurfter C, et al. The influence of concomitant neuroleptic medication on safety, tolerability and clinical effectiveness of electroconvulsive therapy. *World J Biol Psychiatry* 2006; 7:162–170.

42. Gazdag G, et al. The impact of neuroleptic medication on seizure threshold and duration in electroconvulsive therapy. *Ideggyogy Sz* 2004; 57:385–390.

43. Masdrakis VG, et al. The safety of the electroconvulsive therapy-aripiprazole combination: four case reports. *J ECT* 2008; 24:236–238.

44. Oulis P, et al. Corrected QT interval changes during electroconvulsive therapy-antidepressants-atypical antipsychotics coadministration: safety issues. *J ECT* 2011; 27:e4–e6.

45. Grover S, et al. Combined use of clozapine and ECT: a review. *Acta Neuropsychiatr* 2015; 27:131–142.

46. Flamarique I, et al. Electroconvulsive therapy and clozapine in adolescents with schizophrenia spectrum disorders: is it a safe and effective combination? *J Clin Psychopharmacol* 2012; 32:756–766.

47. Arumugham SS, et al. Efficacy and safety of combining clozapine with electrical or magnetic brain stimulation in treatment-refractory schizophrenia. *Expert Rev Clin Pharmacol* 2016; 9:1245–1252.

48. van Waarde JA, et al. Patient, treatment, and anatomical predictors of outcome in electroconvulsive therapy: a prospective study. *J ECT* 2013; 29:113–121.

49. Penland HR, et al. Combined use of lamotrigine and electroconvulsive therapy in bipolar depression: a case series. *J ECT* 2006; 22:142–147.

50. Zarate CA, Jr., et al. Combined valproate or carbamazepine and electroconvulsive therapy. *Ann Clin Psychiatry* 1997; 9:19–25.

51. Sienaert P, et al. Concurrent use of lamotrigine and electroconvulsive therapy. *J ECT* 2011; 27:148–152.

52. Jahangard L, et al. Comparing efficacy of ECT with and without concurrent sodium valproate therapy in manic patients. *J ECT* 2012; 28:118–123.

53. Rakesh G, et al. Concomitant anticonvulsants with bitemporal electroconvulsive therapy: a randomized controlled trial with clinical and neurobiological application. *J ECT* 2017; 33:16–21.

54. Datto C, et al. Augmentation of seizure induction in electroconvulsive therapy: a clinical reappraisal. *J ECT* 2002; 18:118–125.

55. Cheng YC, et al. Serotonin syndrome after electroconvulsive therapy in a patient on trazodone, bupropion, and quetiapine: a case report. *Clin Neuropharmacol* 2015; 38:112–113.

56. Deuschle M, et al. Electroconvulsive therapy induces transient sensitivity for a serotonin syndrome: a case report. *Pharmacopsychiatry* 2017; 50:41–42.

57. Linton CR, et al. Using thiamine to reduce post-ECT confusion. *Int J Geriatr Psychiatry* 2002; 17:189–192.

58. Prakash J, et al. Therapeutic and prophylactic utility of the memory-enhancing drug donepezil hydrochloride on cognition of patients undergoing electroconvulsive therapy: a randomized controlled trial. *J ECT* 2006; 22:163–168.

59. Niu Y, et al. Prophylactic cognitive enhancers for improvement of cognitive function in patients undergoing electroconvulsive therapy: a systematic review and meta-analysis. *Medicine (Baltimore)* 2020; 99:e19527.

60. Leung M, et al. Pretreatment with ibuprofen to prevent electroconvulsive therapy-induced headache. *J Clin Psychiatry* 2003; 64:551–553.

61. Markowitz JS, et al. Intranasal sumatriptan in post-ECT headache: results of an open-label trial. *J ECT* 2001; 17:280–283.

第 3 章

抑郁症治疗中兴奋剂的使用

兴奋剂能减轻疲劳、促进觉醒、提高心境（与抗抑郁药不同）。自 20 世纪 30 年代以来，安非他明就被用于治疗抑郁症[1]。近来，莫达非尼被作为标准抗抑郁药的辅助治疗手段进行了评估[2]。安非他明具有耐受和依赖倾向，因此现在极少用于抑郁症。该药长期大量使用与偏执性精神病发病有关[3]。哌甲酯现在使用比较广泛，但也可能有类似的缺憾。莫达非尼似乎并不会引起耐受、依赖或精神病，但是它缺少安非他明的欣快作用。阿莫达非尼是莫达非尼的长效异构体，在一些国家已经上市。

兴奋剂与标准抗抑郁药显著的不同是，它通常在几个小时之内就会产生作用，但其抗抑郁作用可能是短暂的。因此，在需要快速起效且依赖性不成问题时（如不治之症伴有的抑郁症），可使用安非他明和哌甲酯，也可以考虑使用氯胺酮（如果能够使用）。对于标准抗抑郁治疗无效的严重、慢性抑郁症（如考虑进行精神外科手术的患者），使用这些药物也可能是合理的。对于更大范围的患者而言，莫达非尼可以合理地作为抗抑郁药的辅助治疗使用，也可以作为嗜睡和疲劳的一种特殊治疗方式使用[4]。

表 3.12 列出了在各种临床情境中，支持（或不支持）使用兴奋剂的情况。一般而言，抑郁症治疗中使用兴奋剂的研究质量较差且无明确结论。考虑到兴奋剂使用的短期和长期安全性均不明确[5,6]，将任何兴奋剂用于抑郁症治疗时都需要慎重考虑。某个药物列入表 3.11 中，不应被视为建议使用。

表 3.12　抑郁症治疗中兴奋剂的使用

临床使用	已评估的方案	评价	建议
单纯性抑郁的单一治疗	莫达非尼 100~200mg/d[8,9]	只有个案报告——疗效未经证实	优先使用标准抗抑郁药。单纯性抑郁避免单用兴奋剂治疗[10]。荟萃分析发现，辅助治疗而非单药治疗与临床显著改善有关[7]
	哌甲酯 20~40mg/d[11,12]	疗效极小	
	右苯丙胺 20mg/d[11]	疗效极小	
加快或增强疗效的辅助治疗	SSRI+ 哌甲酯 10~20mg/d[13,14]	对起效时间没有明确影响	总体来说不推荐使用兴奋剂，但莫达非尼可能有益
	SSRI+ 莫达非尼 400mg/d[15]	疗效优于单用 SSRI	
	三环类 + 哌甲酯 5~15mg/d[16]	单一开放试验表明能加快起效时间	
	SSRI 或 SNRI+ 赖右苯丙胺 20~70mg/d[17]	不优于安慰剂	
辅助治疗有疲乏和嗜睡的抑郁症	SSRI+ 莫达非尼 200mg/d[18,19]	只对嗜睡有效。莫达非尼可诱发自杀观念	可能对疲劳有效，但证据不足。当疲劳突出且其他治疗无效时，可以选择
	SSRI+ 哌甲酯 10~40mg/d[20]	对临终患者的疲劳有明显的效果	

续表

临床使用	已评估的方案	评价	建议
难治性抑郁的辅助治疗	SSRI+ 莫达非尼 100~400mg/d[7,21-26]	主要对疲劳和白天困倦有效10 项研究的荟萃分析显示能显著改善抑郁症状[7]	数据有限。莫达非尼可能对疲劳[27] 和认知改善[28] 有效
	MAOI+ 右苯丙胺 7.5~40mg/d[29] 或赖右苯丙胺 50mg/d[30]	一项系列个案研究和一个病例报告支持	兴奋剂是难治性抑郁的一个治疗选择,但其他治疗选择或有更好的证据支持
	哌甲酯或右苯丙胺 +/ - 抗抑郁药[32]	大的系列个案(n=50)显示对大多数人有效	一项自然主义研究表明哌甲酯可以减少自残或自杀企图[31]
	赖右苯丙胺 20~70mg/d+ 抗抑郁药[7,17,33]	两项荟萃研究发现与安慰剂相比对抑郁有小而无意义的疗效	
双相抑郁的辅助治疗[34,35]	心境稳定剂和/或抗抑郁药 + 莫达非尼 100~200mg/d[36]心境稳定剂 + 阿莫达非尼 150~200mg/d[29]	显著优于安慰剂。没有转躁的证据某些指标优于安慰剂	当其他标准治疗失败时,是一个可能的治疗选择与安慰剂相比,此处引用的荟萃试验分析发现,兴奋剂具有良好的耐受性和总体益处[37]
	心境稳定剂 + 哌甲酯 10~40mg/d[39]	结果不一,阳性结果为主	没有关于治疗出现躁狂症[34,37,38] 的证据
	心境稳定剂和/或抗精神病药 + 赖右苯丙胺 20~70mg/d[40]	与安慰剂相比,患者自评指标改善比率较大	
晚期癌症的单一治疗或附加治疗	哌甲酯 5~30mg/d[41-45]	病例系列和开放性前瞻性研究	对于预期生命只有数周的患者是有效的治疗选择
	右苯丙胺 2.5~20mg/d[46,47]哌甲酯 20mg/d+ 米氮平 30mg/d[48]哌甲酯 20mg/d+SSRI[49]莫达非尼 200mg/d[50]	对心境、疲劳和疼痛有益RCT 表明从联合治疗的第3 天起见效RCT 未显示联合治疗有益仅对那些同时有严重的、与癌症相关疲劳的抑郁症状有效	
老年抑郁症的单一治疗或附加治疗	哌甲酯 1.25~20mg/d[51-53]	三项安慰剂对照研究支持。能快速改善心境和活动	只有标准抗抑郁药无法耐受,或有禁忌证时,才建议使用监测心率加快——一项试验中出现心率显著加快[54]
	哌甲酯 5~40mg+ 西酞普兰 20~60mg/d[54]	一项安慰剂对照研究。与单药治疗相比联合治疗更快起效	
卒中后抑郁的单一治疗	哌甲酯 5~40mg/d[55-58]	受到不同的证据支持,包括两项安慰剂对照试验[55,58]。数天后对情绪起效	优先使用标准抗抑郁药。需要进一步研究,兴奋剂可改善认知和运动功能
	莫达非尼 100mg/d[59]	一个案例报告	

续表

临床使用	已评估的方案	评价	建议
继发于躯体疾病的抑郁症的单一治疗	哌甲酯 5~20mg/d[60] 右苯丙胺 2.5~30mg/d[61,62]	数据有限	兴奋剂不是合适的治疗方法。优先使用标准的抗抑郁药
HIV 相关抑郁症和疲乏的单一治疗	右苯丙胺 2.5~40mg/d[63,64]	受到一项良好的对照研究的支持[64] 对心境和疲劳有益	若疲劳用标准抗抑郁药无效,可选择
脑外伤后抑郁症的单药治疗	哌甲酯 5~20mg/d[65,66]	改善抑郁症状、白天困倦和认知功能	对于此项适应证似乎比抗抑郁药更好,但数据仅限于两项研究

参考文献

1. Satel SL, et al. Stimulants in the treatment of depression: a critical overview. *J Clin Psychiatry* 1989; 50:241–249.
2. Menza MA, et al. Modafinil augmentation of antidepressant treatment in depression. *J Clin Psychiatry* 2000; 61:378–381.
3. Warneke L. Psychostimulants in psychiatry. *Canadian J Psychiatry* 1990; 35:3–10.
4. Goss AJ, et al. Modafinil augmentation therapy in unipolar and bipolar depression: a systematic review and meta-analysis of randomized controlled trials. *J Clin Psychiatry* 2013; 74:1101–1107.
5. Candy M, et al. Psychostimulants for depression. *Cochrane Database Syst Rev* 2008; CD006722.
6. Hardy SE. Methylphenidate for the treatment of depressive symptoms, including fatigue and apathy, in medically ill older adults and terminally ill adults. *Am J Geriatr Pharmacother* 2009; 7:34–59.
7. McIntyre RS, et al. The efficacy of psychostimulants in major depressive episodes: a systematic review and meta-analysis. *J Clin Psychopharmacol* 2017; 37:412–418.
8. Lundt L. Modafinil treatment in patients with seasonal affective disorder/winter depression: an open-label pilot study. *J Affect Disord* 2004; 81:173–178.
9. Kaufman KR, et al. Modafinil monotherapy in depression. *Eur Psychiatry* 2002; 17:167–169.
10. Hegerl U, et al. Why do stimulants not work in typical depression? *Aust N Z J Psychiatry* 2017; 51:20–22.
11. Little KY. d-Amphetamine versus methylphenidate effects in depressed inpatients. *J Clin Psychiatry* 1993; 54:349–355.
12. Robin AA, et al. A controlled trial of methylphenidate (ritalin) in the treatment of depressive states. *J Neurol Neurosurg Psychiatry* 1958; 21:55–57.
13. Lavretsky H, et al. Combined treatment with methylphenidate and citalopram for accelerated response in the elderly: an open trial. *J Clin Psychiatry* 2003; 64:1410–1414.
14. Postolache TT, et al. Early augmentation of sertraline with methylphenidate. *J Clin Psychiatry* 1999; 60:123–124.
15. Abolfazli R, et al. Double-blind randomized parallel-group clinical trial of efficacy of the combination fluoxetine plus modafinil versus fluoxetine plus placebo in the treatment of major depression. *Depress Anxiety* 2011; 28:297–302.
16. Gwirtsman HE, et al. The antidepressant response to tricyclics in major depressives is accelerated with adjunctive use of methylphenidate. *Psychopharmacol Bull* 1994; 30:157–164.
17. Giacobbe P, et al. Efficacy and tolerability of lisdexamfetamine as an antidepressant augmentation strategy: a meta-analysis of randomized controlled trials. *J Affect Disord* 2018; 226:294–300.
18. Dunlop BW, et al. Coadministration of modafinil and a selective serotonin reuptake inhibitor from the initiation of treatment of major depressive disorder with fatigue and sleepiness: a double-blind, placebo-controlled study. *J Clin Psychopharmacol* 2007; 27:614–619.
19. Fava M, et al. Modafinil augmentation of selective serotonin reuptake inhibitor therapy in MDD partial responders with persistent fatigue and sleepiness. *Ann Clin Psychiatry* 2007; 19:153–159.
20. Kerr CW, et al. Effects of methylphenidate on fatigue and depression: a randomized, double-blind, placebo-controlled trial. *J Pain Symptom Manage* 2012; 43:68–77.
21. DeBattista C, et al. Adjunct modafinil for the short-term treatment of fatigue and sleepiness in patients with major depressive disorder: a preliminary double-blind, placebo-controlled study. *J Clin Psychiatry* 2003; 64:1057–1064.
22. Fava M, et al. A multicenter, placebo-controlled study of modafinil augmentation in partial responders to selective serotonin reuptake inhibitors with persistent fatigue and sleepiness. *J Clin Psychiatry* 2005; 66:85–93.
23. Rasmussen NA, et al. Modafinil augmentation in depressed patients with partial response to antidepressants: a pilot study on self-reported symptoms covered by the major depression inventory (MDI) and the symptom checklist (SCL-92). *Nordic J Psychiatry* 2005; 59:173–178.
24. DeBattista C, et al. A prospective trial of modafinil as an adjunctive treatment of major depression. *J Clin Psychopharmacol* 2004; 24:87–90.

25. Markovitz PJ, et al. An open-label trial of modafinil augmentation in patients with partial response to antidepressant therapy. *J Clin Psychopharmacol* 2003; 23:207–209.

26. Ravindran AV, et al. Osmotic-release oral system methylphenidate augmentation of antidepressant monotherapy in major depressive disorder: results of a double-blind, randomized, placebo-controlled trial. *J Clin Psychiatry* 2008; 69:87–94.

27. Ghanean H, et al. Fatigue in patients with major depressive disorder: prevalence, burden and pharmacological approaches to management. *CNS Drugs* 2018; 32:65–74.

28. Vaccarino SR, et al. The potential procognitive effects of modafinil in major depressive disorder: a systematic review. *J Clin Psychiatry* 2019; 80:19r12767.

29. Fawcett J, et al. CNS stimulant potentiation of monoamine oxidase inhibitors in treatment refractory depression. *J Clin Psychopharmacol* 1991; 11:127–132.

30. Israel JA. Combining stimulants and monoamine oxidase inhibitors: a reexamination of the literature and a report of a new treatment combination. *Prim Care Companion CNS Disord* 2015; 17:10.4088/PCC.15br01836.

31. Rohde C, et al. The use of stimulants in depression: results from a self-controlled register study. *Aust N Z J Psychiatry* 2020; 54:808–817.

32. Parker G, et al. Do the old psychostimulant drugs have a role in managing treatment-resistant depression? *Acta Psychiatr Scand* 2010; 121:308–314.

33. Richards C, et al. A randomized, double-blind, placebo-controlled, dose-ranging study of lisdexamfetamine dimesylate augmentation for major depressive disorder in adults with inadequate response to antidepressant therapy. *J Psychopharmacology* 2017; 31:1190–1203.

34. Szmulewicz AG, et al. Dopaminergic agents in the treatment of bipolar depression: a systematic review and meta-analysis. *Acta Psychiatr Scand* 2017; 135:527–538.

35. Perugi G, et al. Use of stimulants in bipolar disorder. *Curr Psychiatry Rep* 2017; 19:7.

36. Frye MA, et al. A placebo-controlled evaluation of adjunctive modafinil in the treatment of bipolar depression. *Am J Psychiatry* 2007; 164:1242–1249.

37. Tsapakis EM, et al. Adjunctive treatment with psychostimulants and stimulant-like drugs for resistant bipolar depression: a systematic review and meta-analysis. *CNS Spectr* 2020: 1–12. [Epub ahead of print].

38. Nunez NA, et al. Efficacy and tolerability of adjunctive modafinil/armodafinil in bipolar depression: a meta-analysis of randomized controlled trials. *Bipolar Disord* 2020; 22:109–120.

39. Dell'Osso B, et al. Assessing the roles of stimulants/stimulant-like drugs and dopamine-agonists in the treatment of bipolar depression. *Curr Psychiatry Rep* 2013; 15:378.

40. McElroy SL, et al. Adjunctive lisdexamfetamine in bipolar depression: a preliminary randomized, placebo-controlled trial. *Int Clin Psychopharmacol* 2015; 30:6–13.

41. Fernandez F, et al. Methylphenidate for depressive disorders in cancer patients. *Psychosomatics* 1987; 28:455–461.

42. Macleod AD. Methylphenidate in terminal depression. *J Pain Symptom Manage* 1998; 16:193–198.

43. Homsi J, et al. Methylphenidate for depression in hospice practice. *Am J Hosp Palliat Care* 2000; 17:393–398.

44. Sarhill N, et al. Methylphenidate for fatigue in advanced cancer: a prospective open-label pilot study. *Am J Hosp Palliat Care* 2001; 18:187–192.

45. Homsi J, et al. A phase II study of methylphenidate for depression in advanced cancer. *Am J Hosp Palliat Care* 2001; 18:403–407.

46. Burns MM, et al. Dextroamphetamine treatment for depression in terminally ill patients. *Psychosomatics* 1994; 35:80–83.

47. Olin J, et al. Psychostimulants for depression in hospitalized cancer patients. *Psychosomatics* 1996; 37:57–62.

48. Ng CG, et al. Rapid response to methylphenidate as an add-on therapy to mirtazapine in the treatment of major depressive disorder in terminally ill cancer patients: a four-week, randomized, double-blinded, placebo-controlled study. *Eur Neuropsychopharmacol* 2014; 24:491–498.

49. Sullivan DR, et al. Randomized, double-blind, placebo-controlled study of methylphenidate for the treatment of depression in SSRI-treated cancer patients receiving palliative care. *Psychooncology* 2017; 26:1763–1769.

50. Conley CC, et al. Modafinil moderates the relationship between cancer-related fatigue and depression in 541 patients receiving chemotherapy. *J Clin Psychopharmacol* 2016; 36:82–85.

51. Padala PR, et al. Methylphenidate for apathy in community-dwelling older veterans with mild Alzheimer's disease: a double-blind, randomized, placebo-controlled trial. *Am J Psychiatry* 2018; 175:159–168.

52. Kaplitz SE. Withdrawn, apathetic geriatric patients responsive to methylphenidate. *J Am Geriatr Soc* 1975; 23:271–276.

53. Wallace AE, et al. Double-blind, placebo-controlled trial of methylphenidate in older, depressed, medically ill patients. *Am J Psychiatry* 1995; 152:929–931.

54. Lavretsky H, et al. Citalopram, methylphenidate, or their combination in geriatric depression: a randomized, double-blind, placebo-controlled trial. *Am J Psychiatry* 2015; 172:561–569.

55. Grade C, et al. Methylphenidate in early poststroke recovery: a double-blind, placebo-controlled study. *Arch Phys Med Rehabil* 1998; 79:1047–1050.

56. Lazarus LW, et al. Efficacy and side effects of methylphenidate for poststroke depression. *J Clin Psychiatry* 1992; 53:447–449.

57. Lingam VR, et al. Methylphenidate in treating poststroke depression. *J Clin Psychiatry* 1988; 49:151–153.

58. Delbari A, et al. Effect of methylphenidate and/or levodopa combined with physiotherapy on mood and cognition after stroke: a randomized, double-blind, placebo-controlled trial. *Eur Neurol* 2011; 66:7–13.

59. Sugden SG, et al. Modafinil monotherapy in poststroke depression. *Psychosomatics* 2004; 45:80–81.

60. Rosenberg PB, et al. Methylphenidate in depressed medically ill patients. *J Clin Psychiatry* 1991; 52:263–267.

61. Woods SW, et al. Psychostimulant treatment of depressive disorders secondary to medical illness. *J Clin Psychiatry* 1986; 47:12–15.

第 3 章

62. Kaufmann MW, et al. The use of d-amphetamine in medically ill depressed patients. *J Clin Psychiatry* 1982; 43:463–464.

63. Wagner GJ, et al. Dexamphetamine as a treatment for depression and low energy in AIDS patients: a pilot study. *J Psychosom Res* 1997; 42:407–411.

64. Wagner GJ, et al. Effects of dextroamphetamine on depression and fatigue in men with HIV: a double-blind, placebo-controlled trial. *J Clin Psychiatry* 2000; 61:436–440.

65. Zhang WT, et al. Efficacy of methylphenidate for the treatment of mental sequelae after traumatic brain injury. *Medicine (Baltimore)* 2017; 96:e6960.

66. Lee H, et al. Comparing effects of methylphenidate, sertraline and placebo on neuropsychiatric sequelae in patients with traumatic brain injury. *Human Psychopharmacology* 2005; 20:97–104.

卒中后抑郁

抑郁本身是卒中的一个明确危险因素[1-4]。此外,卒中的幸存者中至少有 30%~40% 患有抑郁症[5,6],目前已知卒中后抑郁会延缓患者功能康复速度[7]。抗抑郁药可缓解抑郁症状[8],促使患者更快康复[9]。它们还能提高整体认知功能[10,11],促进运动功能恢复[12,13],甚至降低死亡率[14]。尽管益处显著,大多数卒中后抑郁患者并未得到治疗[15]。

预防

卒中后抑郁的高发病率促使我们关注其预防价值。汇总分析数据显示,抗抑郁药具有显著的预防作用[16,17]。去甲替林、氟西汀、艾司西酞普兰、度洛西汀和舍曲林似乎都能够预防卒中后抑郁[18-22]。米氮平可以防止和治疗卒中后抑郁[23]。一项设计良好、多中心、安慰剂对照 RCT 研究发现,艾司西酞普兰可降低轻度抑郁症状的发生率,但不能降低中度或重度抑郁症状的发生率[24]。

一项大型队列研究考察了用过抗抑郁药治疗的老年患者的不良结果,报告称,与 SSRI 或 TCA 相比,米氮平(和文拉法辛)可能增加新发卒中的风险[25]。

米安色林对卒中后抑郁的治疗似乎无效[26]。阿米替林[27]和度洛西汀[28]治疗卒中后中枢性疼痛有效[20]。

不推荐常规使用抗抑郁药预防卒中后抑郁——Cochrane 认为可能有益处,但需注意证据不足[29]。最近的 3 项大型多中心 RCT(未包括在 Cochrane 评价中)显示,使用氟西汀的风险(骨折、跌倒、癫痫发作)超过减少抑郁症发生率的好处[30-32]。

治疗

由于躯体疾病共病以及与其他药物可能发生相互作用(尤其是华法林——框 3.2),卒中后抑郁的治疗十分复杂。在抗抑郁药中,三环类药物被禁用的可能性大于 SSRI[33]。针对氟西汀[12,30,34,35]、西酞普兰[10,36-38]和去甲替林[39,40]的研究或许最充分[41],它们的有效性和安全性良好[42]。SSRI 和去甲替林被广泛推荐用于卒中后抑郁的治疗。瑞波西汀(与去甲替林一样,不影响血小板活性)可能同样有效且耐受性良好[43],但其总体效果尚存疑问[44]。伏硫西汀可能特别令人感兴趣,因为它对认知有额外的益处(独立于对抑郁症的影响)。它似乎也不会对心血管参数产生不利影响,也与华法林或阿司匹林没有相互作用,但目前没有数据支持其治疗卒中后抑郁症的特殊价值。

SSRI 似乎并不会增加(卒中后再次)卒中的风险[45],尽管对此仍有一些担忧和疑问[46-49](卒中可能是栓塞或出血——SSRI 可能会预防栓塞[50,51],但诱发出血[52,53],但是其证据相当薄弱[54]——见本章"SSRI 与出血"部分)。其他不良反应也需注意,特别是跌倒、骨折和癫痫发作[30-32]。

抗抑郁药对卒中后抑郁明确有效[42,55],通常不应拒绝其使用(尽管 Cochrane 对抗抑郁药的疗效态度冷淡[29])。抑郁症的不充分治疗会增加卒中的风险[14,56]。两项多重治疗的荟萃分析表明,考虑到卒中后的疗效和耐受性,帕罗西汀可能是首选药物。但是样本量小且缺乏该领域高质量的研究限制了该建议的强度[57,58](每项分析仅包括一项帕罗西汀试验,而对帕罗西汀的 4 项试验进行的荟萃分析并没有发现获益[59]）。最近对 51 项试验进行的大型多重治疗荟萃分析将米氮平的有效率列为第一，其次是文拉法辛和艾司西酞普兰。但是这些研究仅限于中国患者，因此可能缺乏普遍性[60]。

框 3.2　卒中后抑郁——推荐药物

SSRI*
去甲替林

　*SSRI 会增加新发出血性卒中的风险（绝对风险低），当已知现有卒中为出血性时，SSRI 与华法林或其他抗血小板药物合用时，需要密切关注[61,62]。如果患者在服用华法林，建议使用西酞普兰或艾司西酞普兰（或许相互作用可能性最低[63]），并使用最低有效剂量[49]。与直接作用口服抗凝剂（DOAC）的药代动力学相互作用可能性知之甚少。西酞普兰或艾司西酞普兰可能再次成为首选，因为这两种药物都不影响与 DOAC 代谢相关的酶[64]。

　　进行抗凝治疗或阿司匹林治疗的患者，如果要使用 SSRI，需同时处方质子泵抑制剂护胃。去甲替林似乎不会增加出血风险，是一种替代方法。

参考文献

1. Wium-Andersen MK, et al. An attempt to explain the bidirectional association between ischaemic heart disease, stroke and depression: a cohort and meta-analytic approach. *Br J Psychiatry* 2020; 217:434–441.
2. Pan A, et al. Depression and risk of stroke morbidity and mortality: a meta-analysis and systematic review. *JAMA* 2011; 306:1241–1249.
3. Pequignot R, et al. Depressive symptoms, antidepressants and disability and future coronary heart disease and stroke events in older adults: the Three City Study. *Eur J Epidemiol* 2013; 28:249–256.
4. Li CT, et al. Major depressive disorder and stroke risks: a 9-year follow-up population-based, matched cohort study. *PLoS One* 2012; 7:e46818.
5. Gainotti G, et al. Relation between depression after stroke, antidepressant therapy, and functional recovery. *J Neurol Neurosurg Psychiatry* 2001; 71:258–261.
6. Hayee MA, et al. Depression after stroke-analysis of 297 stroke patients. *Bangladesh Med Res Counc Bull* 2001; 27:96–102.
7. Paolucci S, et al. Post-stroke depression, antidepressant treatment and rehabilitation results. A case-control study. *Cerebrovasc Dis* 2001; 12:264–271.
8. Xu XM, et al. Efficacy and feasibility of antidepressant treatment in patients with post-stroke depression. *Medicine (Baltimore)* 2016; 95:e5349.
9. Gainotti G, et al. Determinants and consequences of post-stroke depression. *Curr Opin Neurol* 2002; 15:85–89.
10. Jorge RE, et al. Escitalopram and enhancement of cognitive recovery following stroke. *Arch Gen Psychiatry* 2010; 67:187–196.
11. Gu SC, et al. Early selective serotonin reuptake inhibitors for recovery after stroke: a meta-analysis and trial sequential analysis. *J Stroke Cerebrovasc Dis* 2018; 27:1178–1189.
12. Chollet F, et al. Fluoxetine for motor recovery after acute ischaemic stroke (FLAME): a randomised placebo-controlled trial. *Lancet Neurol* 2011; 10:123–130.
13. Thilarajah S, et al. Factors associated with post-stroke physical activity: a systematic review and meta-analysis. *Arch Phys Med Rehabil* 2018; 99:1876–1889.
14. Krivoy A, et al. Low adherence to antidepressants is associated with increased mortality following stroke: a large nationally representative cohort study. *Eur Neuropsychopharmacol* 2017; 27:970–976.
15. El Husseini N, et al. Depression and antidepressant use after stroke and transient ischemic attack. *Stroke* 2012; 43:1609–1616.
16. Farooq S, et al. Pharmacological interventions for prevention of depression in high risk conditions: systematic review and meta-analysis. *J Affect Disord* 2020; 269:58–69.
17. Chen Y, et al. Antidepressant prophylaxis for poststroke depression: a meta-analysis. *Int Clin Psychopharmacol* 2007; 22:159–166.
18. Feng R, et al. Effect of sertraline in the treatment and prevention of poststroke depression: a meta-analysis. *Medicine (Baltimore)* 2018; 97:e13453.
19. Narushima K, et al. Preventing poststroke depression: a 12-week double-blind randomized treatment trial and 21-month follow-up. *J Nerv Ment Dis* 2002; 190:296–303.
20. Robinson RG, et al. Escitalopram and problem-solving therapy for prevention of poststroke depression: a randomized controlled trial. *JAMA* 2008; 299:2391–2400.
21. Almeida OP, et al. Preventing depression after stroke: results from a randomized placebo-controlled trial. *J Clin Psychiatry* 2006; 67:1104–1109.
22. Zhang LS, et al. Prophylactic effects of duloxetine on post-stroke depression symptoms: an open single-blind trial. *Eur Neurol* 2013; 69:336–343.

23. Niedermaier N, et al. Prevention and treatment of poststroke depression with mirtazapine in patients with acute stroke. *J Clin Psychiatry* 2004; **65**:1619–1623.

24. Kim JS, et al. Efficacy of early administration of escitalopram on depressive and emotional symptoms and neurological dysfunction after stroke: a multicentre, double-blind, randomised, placebo-controlled study. *Lancet Psychiatry* 2017; **4**:33–41.

25. Coupland C, et al. Antidepressant use and risk of adverse outcomes in older people: population based cohort study. *BMJ* 2011; **343**:d4551.

26. Palomaki H, et al. Prevention of poststroke depression: 1 year randomised placebo controlled double blind trial of mianserin with 6 month follow up after therapy. *J Neurol Neurosurg Psychiatry* 1999; **66**:490–494.

27. Lampl C, et al. Amitriptyline in the prophylaxis of central poststroke pain. Preliminary results of 39 patients in a placebo-controlled, long-term study. *Stroke* 2002; **33**:3030–3032.

28. Kim NY, et al. Effect of duloxetine for the treatment of chronic central poststroke pain. *Clin Neuropharmacol* 2019; **42**:73–76.

29. Allida S, et al. Pharmacological, psychological and non-invasive brain stimulation interventions for preventing depression after stroke. *Cochrane Database Syst Rev* 2020; **5**:Cd003689.

30. EFFECTS Trial Collaboration. Safety and efficacy of fluoxetine on functional recovery after acute stroke (EFFECTS): a randomised, double-blind, placebo-controlled trial. *Lancet Neurol* 2020; **19**:661–669.

31. FOCUS Trial Collaboration. Effects of fluoxetine on functional outcomes after acute stroke (FOCUS): a pragmatic, double-blind, randomised, controlled trial. *Lancet* 2019; **393**:265–274.

32. AFFINITY Trial Collaboration. Safety and efficacy of fluoxetine on functional outcome after acute stroke (AFFINITY): a randomised, double-blind, placebo-controlled trial. *Lancet Neurol* 2020; **19**:651–660.

33. Cole MG, et al. Feasibility and effectiveness of treatments for post-stroke depression in elderly inpatients: systematic review. *J Geriatr Psychiatry Neurol* 2001; **14**:37–41.

34. Wiart L, et al. Fluoxetine in early poststroke depression: a double-blind placebo-controlled study. *Stroke* 2000; **31**:1829–1832.

35. Choi-Kwon S, et al. Fluoxetine improves the quality of life in patients with poststroke emotional disturbances. *Cerebrovasc Dis* 2008; **26**:266–271.

36. Andersen G, et al. Effective treatment of poststroke depression with the selective serotonin reuptake inhibitor citalopram. *Stroke* 1994; **25**:1099–1104.

37. Tan S, et al. Efficacy and safety of citalopram in treating post-stroke depression: a meta-analysis. *Eur Neurol* 2015; **74**:188–201.

38. Cui M, et al. Efficacy and safety of citalopram for the treatment of poststroke depression: a meta-analysis. *J Stroke Cerebrovasc Dis* 2018; **27**:2905–2918.

39. Robinson RG, et al. Nortriptyline versus fluoxetine in the treatment of depression and in short-term recovery after stroke: a placebo-controlled, double-blind study. *Am J Psychiatry* 2000; **157**:351–359.

40. Zhang WH, et al. Nortriptyline protects mitochondria and reduces cerebral ischemia/hypoxia injury. *Stroke* 2008; **39**:455–462.

41. Starkstein SE, et al. Antidepressant therapy in post-stroke depression. *Expert Opin Pharmacother* 2008; **9**:1291–1298.

42. Mead GE, et al. Selective serotonin reuptake inhibitors for stroke recovery. *JAMA* 2013; **310**:1066–1067.

43. Rampello L, et al. An evaluation of efficacy and safety of reboxetine in elderly patients affected by 'retarded' post-stroke depression. A random, placebo-controlled study. *Arch Gerontol Geriatr* 2005; **40**:275–285.

44. Eyding D, et al. Reboxetine for acute treatment of major depression: systematic review and meta-analysis of published and unpublished placebo and selective serotonin reuptake inhibitor controlled trials. *BMJ* 2010; **341**:c4737.

45. Douglas I, et al. The use of antidepressants and the risk of haemorrhagic stroke: a nested case control study. *Br J Clin Pharmacol* 2011; **71**:116–120.

46. Trajkova S, et al. Use of antidepressants and risk of incident stroke: a systematic review and meta-analysis. *Neuroepidemiology* 2019; **53**:142–151.

47. Hoirisch-Clapauch S, et al. Antidepressants: bleeding or thrombosis? *Thromb Res* 2019; **181 Suppl 1**:S23–S28.

48. Hackam DG, et al. Selective serotonin reuptake inhibitors and brain hemorrhage: a meta-analysis. *Neurology* 2012; **79**:1862–1865.

49. Kim JH, et al. Major adverse cardiovascular events in antidepressant users within patients with ischemic heart diseases: a nationwide cohort study. *J Clin Psychopharmacol* 2020; **40**:475–481.

50. He Y, et al. Effect of fluoxetine on three-year recurrence in acute ischemic stroke: a randomized controlled clinical study. *Clin Neurol Neurosurg* 2018; **168**:1–6.

51. Douros A, et al. Degree of serotonin reuptake inhibition of antidepressants and ischemic risk: a cohort study. *Neurology* 2019; **93**:e1010–e1020.

52. Trifiro G, et al. Risk of ischemic stroke associated with antidepressant drug use in elderly persons. *J Clin Psychopharmacol* 2010; **30**:252–258.

53. Wu CS, et al. Association of cerebrovascular events with antidepressant use: a case-crossover study. *Am J Psychiatry* 2011; **168**:511–521.

54. Mortensen JK, et al. Safety of selective serotonin reuptake inhibitor treatment in recovering stroke patients. *Exp Opin Drug Saf* 2015; **14**:911–919.

55. Chen Y, et al. Treatment effects of antidepressants in patients with post-stroke depression: a meta-analysis. *Ann Pharmacother* 2006; **40**:2115–2122.

56. Bangalore S, et al. Cardiovascular hazards of insufficient treatment of depression among patients with known cardiovascular disease: a propensity score adjusted analysis. *Eur Heart J Qual Care Clin Outcomes* 2018; **4**:258–266.

57. Sun Y, et al. Comparative efficacy and acceptability of antidepressant treatment in poststroke depression: a multiple-treatments meta-analysis. *BMJ Open* 2017; **7**:e016499.

58. Deng L, et al. Interventions for management of post-stroke depression: a Bayesian network meta-analysis of 23 randomized controlled trials. *Sci Rep* 2017; **7**:16466.

59. Li L, et al. Effectiveness of paroxetine for poststroke depression: a meta-analysis. *J Stroke Cerebrovasc Dis* 2020; 29:104664.

60. Li X, et al. Comparative efficacy of nine antidepressants in treating Chinese patients with post-stroke depression: a network meta-analysis. *J Affect Disord* 2020; 266:540–548.

61. Jeong HE, et al. Risk of major adverse cardiovascular events associated with concomitant use of antidepressants and non-steroidal anti-inflammatory drugs: a retrospective cohort study. *CNS Drugs* 2020; 34:1063–1074.

62. Quinn GR, et al. Effect of selective serotonin reuptake inhibitors on bleeding risk in patients with atrial fibrillation taking warfarin. *Am J Cardiol* 2014; 114:583–586.

63. Sayal KS, et al. Psychotropic interactions with warfarin. *Acta Psychiatr Scand* 2000; 102:250–255.

64. Fitzgerald JL, et al. Drug interactions of direct-acting oral anticoagulants. *Drug Saf* 2016; 39:841–845.

扩展阅读

Castilla-Guerra. Pharmacological management of post-stroke depression. *Expert Rev Neurother* 2020; 20:157–166.

抗抑郁药：其他用药途径

个别情况下，患者不能或者不愿口服抗抑郁药，或者胃肠道对药物的吸收可能会受到阻碍，而包括心理干预和 ECT 治疗等在内的替代治疗又不可行或者有禁忌证。

一种情况是躯体疾病共病抑郁症[1]，尤其是做过胃肠道切除术的患者。此类患者通常插入胃管。若使用胃内通路，可将抗抑郁药研碎后服用。若使用空肠内导管，需要更加小心，因为吸收的速度和程度发生了变化。在可能的情况下，血浆水平的监测可能有助于区分无效和不吸收。

作为商品的非口服剂型非常少。这类剂型大多在英国没有获得许可，可能难以获取，只能通过药物进口商或从特定制造商获取。另外，使用这些超过适应证或者没有适应证的药物，通常意味着处方医师要对不良反应负责。因此，只有在绝对必要时，才可以使用抗抑郁药的非口服剂型。值得考虑的是，一些通常未标记为"抗抑郁药"的精神药物，在药理上可具有抗抑郁活性，并且更容得到非口服制剂。许多非典型抗精神病药可肌内注射，但是支持用于抑郁症的数据仅限于标准抗抑郁药的口服辅助剂。

抗抑郁药的替代给药方法

舌下

小样本病例报道支持躯体情况不允许口服用药的抑郁症患者舌下服用氟西汀液体剂型的有效性[2]。在这些报道中，使用剂量最高 60mg/d 时，可使血浆氟西汀和去甲氟西汀水平达到推荐治疗浓度下限[2]。氯胺酮注射液也被用于舌下，效果明显[3]。它可能会比其他给药途径（静脉注射或皮下注射）耐受性更好[3]。

口腔

司来吉兰可作为口服冻干剂用于口腔吸收（已获准用于治疗帕金森病），但在 1.25mg 剂量下对 MAO-B 选择性抑制，对中枢神经系统中的 MAO-A 缺乏作用，因此被认为没有抗抑郁活性[4]。一项小型研究发现，10mg/d 口腔分解司来吉兰能显著抑制脑 MAO-A，但尚未研究其临床抗抑郁活性[5]。

多项研究探讨开发了多塞平口腔黏合给药系统[6,7]，但目前还没有商业化产品。一例病例报告描述了口含阿米替林片[8]能达到治疗血药浓度。另一病例使用米氮平分散片，假设它通过口腔吸收[9]，但并没有血浆药物浓度的报告，也没有信息表明米氮平分散片实际上是通过口腔黏膜吸收的（而不是分散在唾液中后再吞服）。

静脉注射和肌内注射

静脉制剂能避免首过效应，导致血药浓度更高[10,11]，也许疗效更好[11,12]，但不一定起效更快[12-14]。众所周知，与静脉给药相关的安慰剂效应很大[15]。请注意，鉴于口服药物通常具有可变的首过效应，计算正确的抗抑郁药肠外剂量是困难的。预计肠胃外剂量远低于口服剂量，并能产生相同的效果。

对严重抑郁的住院患者，静脉用西酞普兰，然后口服西酞普兰维持治疗，是临床上有效的治疗策略[13]。静脉用西酞普兰治疗强迫症症状时,疗效更好,起效更快(与口服相比)[16]。静脉注射剂型的耐受性好,最常见的不良反应是恶心、头痛、震颤、困倦,与口服药物相似[17,18]。在一个病例报告中,一名65岁老年人静脉注射西酞普兰后,出现了急性运动亢进性谵妄[19]。目前已有静脉用艾司西酞普兰剂型,但对它的研究还集中在药代动力学方面[20]。需要注意的是,口服西酞普兰引起的QTc延长发生率高于其他SSRI。如果在躯体状况不好的患者中使用静脉剂型,建议进行心电图监测。

米氮平也有静脉用制剂。有两项研究均采用连续14天、每天缓慢静脉注射米氮平15mg治疗抑郁症,患者耐受性好[21,22]。有报道,米氮平6~30mg/d静脉用药可治疗妊娠呕吐[23,24]。

阿米替林同时有静脉用和肌内注射用制剂(肌内注射剂型也可用于静脉注射),两种用药途径均可用于术后镇痛和抑郁症治疗[25]。肌内注射制剂的浓度(10mg/mL)较低,若要达到抗抑郁药量,药物必须使用较大的容积,这不利于肌内注射[26]。它在世界大部分地区退市。氯米帕明也许是研究最广泛的静脉用抗抑郁药。已有研究显示,静脉用氯米帕明的脉冲负荷剂量(pulse loading doses)使强迫症症状比口服药物减少更多、更快[10,27]。三环类抗抑郁药静脉使用有可能产生严重心脏不良反应,因此必须监测脉搏、血压和心电图。

别孕烯醇酮(商品名为布瑞诺龙,brexanolone)是一种内源性孕酮代谢物,在美国获准用于静脉注射治疗产后抑郁。鉴于其独特的作用机制,不适用于治疗其他类型的抑郁症。

静脉注射伏硫西汀已被用于加快对口服制剂的疗效[28],但这不是市售制剂。

静脉用抗抑郁药的一个理由是其抗抑郁作用起效更快,但这在对照研究中并未得到一致证明[29]。

氯胺酮是一种谷氨酸能N-甲基-D-天冬氨酸(NMDA)受体拮抗剂,对其静脉注射制剂进行的广泛研究结果显示,它的抗抑郁作用起效快,但维持时间短[30]。长期使用的疗效持续时间可能与急性身体不适的患者无关。氯胺酮也可通过鼻内[31]、肌内注射、皮下注射[32,33]、舌下[3,34]以及黏膜途径给药[35]。也曾把静脉用东莨菪碱作为一种抗抑郁药进行研究,对于单相抑郁或者双相抑郁症患者,均能在用药72h内出现抗抑郁疗效[36-38]。

透皮制剂

以凝胶制剂形式出现的阿米替林一般作为各种慢性疼痛治疗的辅助用药用于疼痛门诊[39,40]。其规格通常是50mmol/L或者100mmol/L,有的添加利多卡因。尽管已经证明它具有镇痛作用,但目前尚无此路径用药后血药水平的公开数据发表。盐酸去甲替林已经被制成透皮贴剂用于戒烟[41]。丙米嗪和多塞平的纳米乳剂也被做成了经皮释放剂型,作为镇痛药[42]使用。在本书写作之时,尚无关于去甲替林贴剂、丙米嗪或多塞平纳米乳剂用于抑郁症的研究发表。这些制剂中的任何一种都不太可能达到抗抑郁作用的血药浓度。

口服司来吉兰剂量超过20mg/d时可能是有效的抗抑郁药,但该剂量时酶选择性丧失,需要限制酪氨酸饮食[43,44]。司来吉兰也可以透皮给药,具有较好的疗效和耐受性,在24h内能透入25%~30%的药量,每天给药5天后达到稳态浓度[45]。该途径绕过了首过代谢,能提供一个更高、更持久的司来吉兰血药水平;同时绕开了胃肠道MAO-A系统[46,47]。因此,使用较低剂量贴剂(6mg/24h)时,似乎不需要限制酪氨酸摄入,甚至在使用更高剂量贴剂时,也无高血压反应的报告。使用司来吉兰透皮贴剂高剂量水平(9mg/24h和12mg/24h)的患者应避免使用富含酪氨酸饮食[48],但通常司来吉兰透皮制剂耐受性较好。

经直肠给药

与胃肠道其他部分相比,直肠黏膜缺少丰富的绒毛和微绒毛,从而限制了其表面积。因此,直肠用药制剂需要最大限度地增加活性成分与黏膜的接触。目前,尚无现成的抗抑郁药栓剂,但临时制作是可能的。例如,阿米替林(置于可可脂中)栓剂已经由一家医院药房生产,每次 50mg,每天 2 次,主观上已获得一些成功[49,50]。多塞平胶囊直接通过直肠给药,用于治疗肿瘤相关疼痛(并无特殊剂型),其血浆药物浓度达到了所期待的治疗浓度范围[51]。与之相似,也有报道称,临时制备的丙米嗪或者氯米帕明栓剂产生的血药浓度与口服途径给药相当[52]。在术前口服曲唑酮且病情稳定的患者中,术后成功地使用了曲唑酮栓剂[50,51]。在一个肠道损伤的危重患者中,舍曲林片直肠给药也获得成功[53]。

鼻内

艾司氯胺酮鼻喷剂(Spravato)于 2019 年在英国、2020 年在美国获得许可,用于治疗难治性抑郁症。它需要特定的给药方法(倾斜头部),这对于身体不适的患者可能无法坚持。在撰写本文时,出于对临床和成本效益(长期使用)的担忧,英国国家健康与护理卓越研究所(NICE)尚未推荐鼻内使用氯胺酮用于治疗难治性抑郁症。这可能使得很难在英国医院内获得艾司氯胺酮,但是氯胺酮的其他剂型价格便宜且容易获得(表 3.13)。

表 3.13　抗抑郁药的替代剂型和用药途径

药物名称和途径	用法信息	厂家	注意事项
舌下用氟西汀	剂量最高 60mg/d	使用液体氟西汀剂型	血浆浓度略低于口服
颊侧司来吉兰(口服冻干粉)	10mg(8 × 1.25mg 冻干)/d	Cephalon UK Limited	口腔分解冻干制剂(Zelapar®)获批用于治疗帕金森病。试验数据显示,MAO-A 抑制需要 10mg 冻干制剂——这实际上可能难以给药
颊侧阿米替林	从 25mg 每晚开始,渐加至 125mg/d	仿制产品	将片剂压碎并使其在患者口中溶解以促进口腔吸收。作者报告了一例患者用药后抑郁症状减轻[8]
静脉用阿米替林	25~100mg 溶入 250mL 的 0.9% 氯化钠溶液,缓慢静脉滴注,时间需超过 120min	联系当地进口商	不良反应与剂量相关,基本上与口服药类似。高剂量可出现头晕、困倦。剂量约 100mg 时可发生心动过缓。建议 ECG 监测
静脉用氯米帕明	25mg/2mL 注射剂 起始剂量 25mg,溶入 500mL 的 0.9% 氯化钠溶液,用超过 90min 的时间缓慢静脉滴注 在 10~14 天内,每天增加 25mg,直至 250~300mg[54,55] 另一例报告起始剂量为 50mg/d 静脉注射,5~7 天内,滴定至最大剂量 225mg/d[56]	Novartis Defiante	最常报告的不良反应与口服剂型相似,包括恶心、出汗、坐立不安、脸红、困倦、疲乏、腹部不适和紧张。建议 ECG 监测 第 1 次静脉给药 1 周后发现症状减轻

药物名称和途径	用法信息	厂家	注意事项
静脉用西酞普兰	40mg/mL 注射剂 剂量 20~40mg，溶于 250mL 的 0.9% 氯化钠溶液或 5% 葡萄 糖溶液。治疗强迫症的剂量 最高达 80mg/d。输液速度为 每小时 20mg	Lundbeck（灵北），在 某些国家可用。在 英国尚未获得许可， 可以从德国进口，但 可能需要 3~4 周	最常报告的不良反应是恶心、头 痛、震颤和嗜睡，与口服制剂的不 良反应相似。有 1 例急性运动亢 进性谵妄的病例报告。用于抑郁 症和强迫症。建议 ECG 监测
静脉用艾司西酞普兰	10mg 缓慢滴注，需时超过 60min	Lundbeck（灵北），全 球都未上市	迄今研究只是集中在药代动力学 方面。建议 ECG 监测
静脉用米氮平	6mg/2mL 静脉注射液 15mg/5mL 静脉注射液 15mg 溶于 5% 葡萄糖溶液中， 静脉滴注时间超过 60min。	联系当地进口商	最常报告的不良反应有恶心、镇静 和头晕，与口服药的不良反应相似
静脉用曲唑酮 [57]	25~100mg 溶于 250mL 生理盐 水，滴注时间大约 1.5h，持续 1 周。根据抑郁症状的程度决 定静脉注射剂量。	仅在意大利可用	曲唑酮仅在静脉治疗 1 周后才出 现显著症状改善，耐受性优于氯米 帕明
肌内注射氟哌噻 吨癸酸酯 [58]	每 2 周 5~10mg	Lundbeck Mylan	肌内注射氟哌噻吨具有提升情绪 的作用，并且在这些剂量下耐受性 良好。锥体外系反应罕见。不良 反应有口干、头晕和嗜睡
司来吉兰透皮 贴剂	6mg/24h；9mg/24h；12mg/24h 从 6mg/24h 开始，最短每 2 周 增加 3mg/24h，逐渐增到最大 剂量 12mg/24h [59]	Bristol Myers Squibb， 通过联盟批发商	6mg/24h 的剂量并不需要限制酪氨 酸饮食 在更高的剂量，尽管尚无高血压危 象报道，生产厂家仍然建议避免富 含酪氨酸食物 用药部位反应和失眠是最常见的 不良反应
直肠用阿米替林	剂量最高达 50mg bd	栓剂已经由药店制备	仅有病例报告
直肠用氯米帕明	无详细信息		
直肠用丙米嗪	无详细信息		
直肠用多塞平	无详细信息	胶囊已用于直肠给药	
直肠用舍曲林	起始剂量：每天将 25mg 片剂 置于肠腔。每 3 天加量 1 次， 第 10 天加到最大剂量 100mg	片剂已用于直肠给药	100mg 稳态剂量水平时，可在血清 中检测出舍曲林，但不是代谢物。 血药浓度处于所报告的口服舍曲 林的浓度范围内。没有记录到不 良反应
直肠用曲唑酮	无详细信息	栓剂已经由药店制备	曲唑酮直肠剂型已经用于术后疼 痛或癌性疼痛，而不是用于抗抑郁

第3章

药物名称和途径	用法信息	厂家	注意事项
氯胺酮	静脉注射：0.5mg/kg 滴注时间超过 40min 皮下注射：首剂 0.25mg/kg（范围 12.5~25mg），标准治疗剂量 0.5mg/kg（范围 25~50mg） 舌下：1.5mg/kg	静脉制剂广泛销售	与静脉注射相比，皮下注射氯胺酮较少引起不良反应（解离症状或血压变化）。舌下给药耐受性良好。使用氯胺酮的经验正在增加，但建议在开始前征求专家意见

注：所列全部制剂的可用性因时间和国家而异。

参考文献

1. Cipriani A, et al. Metareview on short-term effectiveness and safety of antidepressants for depression: an evidence-based approach to inform clinical practice. *Can J Psychiatry* 2007; 52:553–562.
2. Pakyurek M, et al. Sublingually administered fluoxetine for major depression in medically compromised patients. *Am J Psychiatry* 1999; 156:1833–1834.
3. Swainson J, et al. Sublingual ketamine: an option for increasing accessibility of ketamine treatments for depression? *J Clin Psychiatry* 2020; 81:19lr13146.
4. Morgan PT. Treatment-resistant depression: response to low-dose transdermal but not oral selegiline. *J Clin Psychopharmacol* 2007; 27:313–314.
5. Fowler JS, et al. Evidence that formulations of the selective MAO-B inhibitor, selegiline, which bypass first-pass metabolism, also inhibit MAO-A in the human brain. *Neuropsychopharmacology* 2015; 40:650–657.
6. Laffleur F, et al. Modified biomolecule as potential vehicle for buccal delivery of doxepin. *Ther Deliv* 2016; 7:683–689.
7. Sanz R, et al. Development of a buccal doxepin platform for pain in oral mucositis derived from head and neck cancer treatment. *Eur J Pharm Biopharm* 2017; 117:203–211.
8. Robbins B, et al. Amitriptyline absorption in a patient with short bowel syndrome. *Am J Gastroenterol* 1999; 94:2302–2304.
9. Das A, et al. Options when anti-depressants cannot be used in conventional ways. Clinical case and review of literature. *Personal Med Psychiatry* 2019; 15–16:22–27.
10. Deisenhammer EA, et al. Intravenous versus oral administration of amitriptyline in patients with major depression. *J Clin Psychopharmacol* 2000; 20:417–422.
11. Koran LM, et al. Rapid benefit of intravenous pulse loading of clomipramine in obsessive-compulsive disorder. *Am J Psychiatry* 1997; 154:396–401.
12. Svestka J, et al. [Citalopram (Seropram) in tablet and infusion forms in the treatment of major depression]. *Cesk Psychiatr* 1993; 89:331–339.
13. Baumann P, et al. A double-blind double-dummy study of citalopram comparing infusion versus oral administration. *J Affect Disord* 1998; 49:203–210.
14. Pollock BG, et al. Acute antidepressant effect following pulse loading with intravenous and oral clomipramine. *Arch Gen Psychiatry* 1989; 46:29–35.
15. Sallee FR, et al. Pulse intravenous clomipramine for depressed adolescents: double-blind, controlled trial. *Am J Psychiatry* 1997; 154:668–673.
16. Bhikram TP, et al. The effect of intravenous citalopram on the neural substrates of obsessive-compulsive disorder. *J Neuropsychiatry Clin Neurosci* 2016; 28:243–247.
17. Guelfi JD, et al. Efficacy of intravenous citalopram compared with oral citalopram for severe depression. Safety and efficacy data from a double-blind, double-dummy trial. *J Affect Disord* 2000; 58:201–209.
18. Kasper S, et al. Intravenous antidepressant treatment: focus on citalopram. *Eur Arch Psychiatry Clin Neurosci* 2002; 252:105–109.
19. Delic M, et al. Delirium during i. v. citalopram treatment: a case report. *Pharmacopsychiatry* 2013; 46:37–38.
20. Sogaard B, et al. The pharmacokinetics of escitalopram after oral and intravenous administration of single and multiple doses to healthy subjects. *J Clin Pharmacol* 2005; 45:1400–1406.
21. Konstantinidis A, et al. Intravenous mirtazapine in the treatment of depressed inpatients. *Eur Neuropsychopharmacol* 2002; 12:57–60.
22. Muhlbacher M, et al. Intravenous mirtazapine is safe and effective in the treatment of depressed inpatients. *Neuropsychobiology* 2006; 53:83–87.
23. Guclu S, et al. Mirtazapine use in resistant hyperemesis gravidarum: report of three cases and review of the literature. *ArchGynecolObstet* 2005; 272:298–300.
24. Schwarzer V, et al. Treatment resistant hyperemesis gravidarum in a patient with type 1 diabetes mellitus: neonatal withdrawal symptoms after successful antiemetic therapy with mirtazapine. *Arch Gynecol Obstet* 2008; 277:67–69.
25. Collins JJ, et al. Intravenous amitriptyline in pediatrics. *J Pain SymptomManage* 1995; 10:471–475.

26. RX List. Elavil. 2021; http://www.rxlist.com.

27. Koran LM, et al. Pulse loading versus gradual dosing of intravenous clomipramine in obsessive-compulsive disorder. *Eur Neuropsychopharmacol* 1998; 8:121–126.

28. Vieta E, et al. Intravenous vortioxetine to accelerate onset of effect in major depressive disorder: a 2-week, randomized, double-blind, placebo-controlled study. *Int Clin Psychopharmacol* 2019; 34:153–160.

29. Moukaddam NJ, et al. Intravenous antidepressants: a review. *Depress Anxiety* 2004; 19:1–9.

30. Murrough JW, et al. Antidepressant efficacy of ketamine in treatment-resistant major depression: a two-site randomized controlled trial. *Am J Psychiatry* 2013; 170:1134–1142.

31. Lapidus KA, et al. A randomized controlled trial of intranasal ketamine in major depressive disorder. *Biol Psychiatry* 2014; 76:970–976.

32. Loo CK, et al. Placebo-controlled pilot trial testing dose titration and intravenous, intramuscular and subcutaneous routes for ketamine in depression. *Acta Psychiatr Scand* 2016; 134:48–56.

33. George D, et al. Pilot randomized controlled trial of titrated subcutaneous ketamine in older patients with treatment-resistant depression. *Am J Geriatr Psychiatry* 2017; 25:1199–1209.

34. Lara DR, et al. Antidepressant, mood stabilizing and procognitive effects of very low dose sublingual ketamine in refractory unipolar and bipolar depression. *Int J Neuropsychopharmacol* 2013; 16:2111–2117.

35. Nguyen L, et al. Off-label use of transmucosal ketamine as a rapid-acting antidepressant: a retrospective chart review. *Neuropsychiatr Dis Treat* 2015; 11:2667–2673.

36. Jaffe RJ, et al. Scopolamine as an antidepressant: a systematic review. *Clin Neuropharmacol* 2013; 36:24–26.

37. Furey ML, et al. Pulsed intravenous administration of scopolamine produces rapid antidepressant effects and modest side effects. *J Clin Psychiatry* 2013; 74:850–851.

38. Drevets WC, et al. Replication of scopolamine's antidepressant efficacy in major depressive disorder: a randomized, placebo-controlled clinical trial. *Biol Psychiatry* 2010; 67:432–438.

39. Gerner P, et al. Topical amitriptyline in healthy volunteers. *Reg Anesth Pain Med* 2003; 28:289–293.

40. Ho KY, et al. Topical amitriptyline versus lidocaine in the treatment of neuropathic pain. *Clin J Pain* 2008; 24:51–55.

41. Melero A, et al. Nortriptyline for smoking cessation: release and human skin diffusion from patches. *Int J Pharm* 2009; 378:101–107.

42. Sandig AG, et al. Transdermal delivery of imipramine and doxepin from newly oil-in-water nanoemulsions for an analgesic and anti-allodynic activity: development, characterization and in vivo evaluation. *Colloids SurfB Biointerfaces* 2013; 103:558–565.

43. Sunderland T, et al. High-dose selegiline in treatment-resistant older depressive patients. *Arch Gen Psychiatry* 1994; 51:607–615.

44. Mann JJ, et al. A controlled study of the antidepressant efficacy and side effects of (-)-deprenyl. A selective monoamine oxidase inhibitor. *Arch Gen Psychiatry* 1989; 46:45–50.

45. Viatris. EMSAM®* (selegiline transdermal system). 2021; https://www.viatris.com/en-us/lm/countryhome/us-products/productcatalog/productdetails?id=bcd487dc-1180-48d3-a0ca-4ac8927c6980.

46. Wecker L, et al. Transdermal selegiline: targeted effects on monoamine oxidases in the brain. *Biol Psychiatry* 2003; 54:1099–1104.

47. Azzaro AJ, et al. Pharmacokinetics and absolute bioavailability of selegiline following treatment of healthy subjects with the selegiline transdermal system (6 mg/24 h): a comparison with oral selegiline capsules. *J Clin Pharmacol* 2007; 47:1256–1267.

48. Amsterdam JD, et al. Selegiline transdermal system in the prevention of relapse of major depressive disorder: a 52-week, double-blind, placebo-substitution, parallel-group clinical trial. *J Clin Psychopharmacol* 2006; 26:579–586.

49. Adams S. Amitriptyline suppositories. *N Engl J Med* 1982; 306:996.

50. Mirassou MM. Rectal antidepressant medication in the treatment of depression. *J Clin Psychiatry* 1998; 59:29.

51. Storey P, et al. Rectal doxepin and carbamazepine therapy in patients with cancer. *N Engl J Med* 1992; 327:1318–1319.

52. Chaumeil JC, et al. Formulation of suppositories containing imipramine and clomipramine chlorhydrates. *Drug Dev Ind Pharm* 1988; 15–17:2225–2239.

53. Leung JG, et al. Rectal bioavailability of sertraline tablets in a critically ill patient with bowel compromise. *J Clin Psychopharmacol* 2017; 37:372–373.

54. Lopes R, et al. The utility of intravenous clomipramine in a case of Cotard's syndrome. *Rev Bras Psiquiatr* 2013; 35:212–213.

55. Fallon BA, et al. Intravenous clomipramine for obsessive-compulsive disorder refractory to oral clomipramine: a placebo-controlled study. *Arch Gen Psychiatry* 1998; 55:918–924.

56. Karameh WK, et al. Intravenous clomipramine for treatment-resistant obsessive-compulsive disorder. *Int J Neuropsychopharmacol* 2015; 19:pyv084.

57. Buoli M, et al. Is trazodone more effective than clomipramine in major depressed outpatients? A single-blind study with intravenous and oral administration. *CNS Spectr* 2019; 24:258–264.

58. Maragakis BP. A double-blind comparison of oral amitriptyline and low-dose intramuscular flupenthixol decanoate in depressive illness. *Curr Med Res Opin* 1990; 12:51–57.

59. Nandagopal JJ, et al. Selegiline transdermal system: a novel treatment option for major depressive disorder. *Exp Opin Pharmacother* 2009; 10:1665–1673.

第 3 章

抗抑郁药的预防作用

首次发作

单次发作的抑郁症在完全缓解后,仍需治疗至少 6~9 个月[1]。如果病情缓解后马上停抗抑郁药,50% 的患者在 3~6 个月内又会出现抑郁症状[1]。一项著名的氟西汀维持治疗的研究[2]表明,在 12 周时停止有效治疗最易复发,其次是在 26 周停药,再次是在 50 周停药(此时安慰剂和活性药物治疗在复发风险方面没有差异)。另一项研究表明,患者只有"在 16~20 周内没有明显症状"时才应尝试停药[3]。即使在治疗的前 6 个月内不持续使用抗抑郁药,也可以预测有较高的复燃率[4]。

复发性抑郁

抑郁症在 15% 的病例中持续存在,在 35% 的病例中复发。首次发作的患者约 50% 能够康复,并且没有再次发作[5]。已知有很多因素增加复发风险,包括抑郁症家族史、复发性心境恶劣、伴发非情感性精神障碍、女性、发作时间长、治疗困难的程度[6]、慢性躯体疾病和社会因素(如缺少可信任关系和心理社会应激源)。一些处方药会促发抑郁[6,7]。

图 3.5 概括了多次发作患者复发的风险:那些被招募入研究的患者至少有过 3 次抑郁发作,2 次发作间隔不到 3 年[8,9]。抑郁症患者心血管病风险增加[10]。与人群常模比较,抑郁症患者自杀死亡率显著增加。

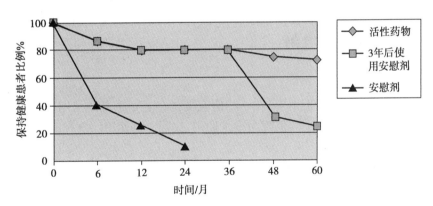

图 3.5 多次抑郁症发作患者的抑郁症复发风险。患者至少有过 3 次抑郁症发作,
2 次发作间隔不到 3 年

对抗抑郁药巩固治疗研究的荟萃分析[11]结论是,继续抗抑郁药治疗使抑郁症复发风险减少了 2/3,约相当于绝对风险的 1/2。此后一项纳入 54 项研究的荟萃分析得出了几乎一致的结论:复发风险减少了 65%[12]。复发风险在停药后前几个月内最大,这个风险与既往治疗时间长短无关[13]。持续服药的获益持续 36 个月以上,不同患者群(首次发作、多次发作、慢性)均类似,尽管这些研究中并没有仅纳入首次发作的患者。需要在首次发作的患者中进行特定研究,以证明治疗超过 6~9 个月会给该患者群带来额外益处。大部分数据都针对成年人。

在老年患者(许多是首次发作)中进行的维持治疗 RCT 研究发现,抗抑郁药巩固治疗的获益超过 2 年,效应值与成年人相仿[14]。一项小样本 RCT 研究($n=22$)也证明了在青少年中预防性使用抗抑郁药的益处[15]。

许多本可从抗抑郁药维持治疗中获益的患者并没有接受维持治疗[16]。确信的是,对长期抑郁症给予最佳治疗,能明显减少抑郁症相关的死亡率[17]。

少数观点认为抗抑郁药的预防作用被高估了,因为维持试验中存在混杂因素——可能会突然停止有效的药物治疗,正是这种停药方式(不一定是停药本身)增加了复发的风险[18,19]。因此,至少部分持续治疗的优势来自改用安慰剂患者的次优治疗。最近的研究采用更长时间(1 个月以上)停止用药[20],但即使这样也可能不足以完全消除停药的负面影响[21]。还有少数派观点认为抗抑郁药最终可能会使所治的疾病恶化[22]。对这一理论的支持来自以下观察:对抗抑郁药的疗效随着既往服用的抗抑郁药数量增加而降低[23]。

长期抗抑郁药治疗的其他可能缺点是,增加了胃肠道出血和脑出血的风险(见本章"SSRI 与出血"部分),另外合用可能增加药物相互作用的风险,从而增加出血和低钠血症的风险。

这些观察结果,再加上已知维持试验主要是在缓解期的患者中进行,强烈建议只有在有明确证据表明获益显著的情况下才能继续抗抑郁治疗。这似乎是一个显而易见的观点,但临床经验表明,长期、无效或部分有效的抗抑郁治疗是常见的。治疗目标是达到或维持缓解。残留症状预示着糟糕的结局和高复发风险[24]。

NICE 建议[25]:

- 近期有 2~3 次抑郁发作的患者、发作期有严重功能损害的患者,均应建议持续服用抗抑郁药至少 2 年。
- 对于维持治疗的患者,应该再次进行评估,考虑其年龄、共病状况和其他危险因素之后,再决定 2 年以后是否需要维持治疗。

预防用药的剂量

成年人剂量与急性治疗期相同[26]。一些研究支持在老年患者中采用较低剂量:度硫平 75mg/d 起到了有效的预防作用[27],但现在很少使用,仅限专科使用。没有证据支持使用低于标准剂量的 SSRI[28]。

停用 ECT 后的复发率与停用抗抑郁药后的情况相似[29]。需要使用抗抑郁药进行预防,最好选择与第一次治疗时失败的药物不同的药物,尽管缺少这方面的数据。

锂盐对单相抑郁症也有一定的预防作用,但与抗抑郁药相比疗效如何,尚不明确[30]。然而,现已证实,锂盐治疗与任何单相抑郁治疗的最佳结果相关[31]。NICE 建议,锂盐不能单独用于单相抑郁的预防[25]。有证据支持锂盐和去甲替林的联合使用[32]。

锂盐维持治疗能预防自杀[26]。

患者应该知道的要点

- 单次抑郁发作应该在临床痊愈后继续治疗至少 6~9 个月。
- 抑郁症的复发风险高,且复发风险随着复发次数增加而增加。
- 有过多次抑郁发作的患者可能需要治疗多年。

- 坚持服用抗抑郁药能大大地增加患者保持健康的机会。
- 抗抑郁药：
  - 有效
  - 不成瘾（但是可以预期停药症状）
  - 已知不会随着时间延长而丧失疗效
  - 已知不会引起新的长期不良反应
- 药物需要以治疗剂量继续服用。若不良反应不能耐受，找到更合适的替代药物是可能的。
- 患者如果决定停药，一定不能突然停药，因为这会导致令人不快的停药反应（见本章"抗抑郁药停药症状"部分），并带来较高的复发风险[33]。药物需要在医生监督下逐渐减少[21]。

参考文献

1. Cleare A, et al. Evidence-based guidelines for treating depressive disorders with antidepressants: a revision of the 2008 British Association for Psychopharmacology guidelines. *J Psychopharmacology* 2015; 29:459–525.

2. Reimherr FW, et al. Optimal length of continuation therapy in depression: a prospective assessment during long-term fluoxetine treatment. *Am J Psychiatry* 1998; 155:1247–1253.

3. Prien RF, et al. Continuation drug therapy for major depressive episodes: how long should it be maintained? *Am J Psychiatry* 1986; 143:18–23.

4. Kim KH, et al. The effects of continuous antidepressant treatment during the first 6months on relapse or recurrence of depression. *J Affect Disord* 2011; 132:121–129.

5. Eaton WW, et al. Population-based study of first onset and chronicity in major depressive disorder. *Arch Gen Psychiatry* 2008; 65:513–520.

6. National Institute for Health and Clinical Excellence. Depression in adults with a chronic physical health problem: recognition and management. Clinical Guidance [CG91]. 2009; http://www.nice.org.uk/CG91.

7. Patten SB, et al. Drug-induced depression. *Psychother Psychosom* 1997; 66:63–73.

8. Frank E, et al. Three-year outcomes for maintenance therapies in recurrent depression. *Arch Gen Psychiatry* 1990; 47:1093–1099.

9. Kupfer DJ, et al. Five-year outcome for maintenance therapies in recurrent depression. *Arch Gen Psychiatry* 1992; 49:769–773.

10. Taylor D. Antidepressant drugs and cardiovascular pathology: a clinical overview of effectiveness and safety. *Acta Psychiatr Scand* 2008; 118:434–442.

11. Geddes JR, et al. Relapse prevention with antidepressant drug treatment in depressive disorders: a systematic review. *Lancet* 2003; 361:653–661.

12. Glue P, et al. Meta-analysis of relapse prevention antidepressant trials in depressive disorders. *Aust N Z J Psychiatry* 2010; 44:697–705.

13. Keller MB, et al. The prevention of recurrent episodes of depression with venlafaxine for two years (PREVENT) study: outcomes from the 2-year and combined maintenance phases. *J Clin Psychiatry* 2007; 68:1246–1256.

14. Reynolds CF, III, et al. Maintenance treatment of major depression in old age. *N Engl J Med* 2006; 354:1130–1138.

15. Cheung A, et al. Maintenance study for adolescent depression. *J Child Adolesc Psychopharmacol* 2008; 18:389–394.

16. Holma IA, et al. Maintenance pharmacotherapy for recurrent major depressive disorder: 5-year follow-up study. *Br J Psychiatry* 2008; 193:163–164.

17. Gallo JJ, et al. Long term effect of depression care management on mortality in older adults: follow-up of cluster randomized clinical trial in primary care. *BMJ* 2013; 346:f2570.

18. Cohen D, et al. Withdrawal effects confounding in clinical trials: another sign of a needed paradigm shift in psychopharmacology research. *Ther Adv Psychopharmacol* 2020; 10:2045125320964097.

19. Hengartner MP. Editorial: antidepressant prescriptions in children and adolescents. *Front Psychiatry* 2020; 11:600283.

20. DeRubeis RJ, et al. Prevention of recurrence after recovery from a major depressive episode with antidepressant medication alone or in combination with cognitive behavioral therapy: phase 2 of a 2-phase randomized clinical trial. *JAMA Psychiatry* 2020; 77:237–245.

21. Horowitz MA, et al. Tapering of SSRI treatment to mitigate withdrawal symptoms. *Lancet Psychiatry* 2019; 6:538–546.

22. Fava GA. May antidepressant drugs worsen the conditions they are supposed to treat? The clinical foundations of the oppositional model of tolerance. *Ther Adv Psychopharmacol* 2020; 10:2045125320970325.

23. Amsterdam JD, et al. Prior antidepressant treatment trials may predict a greater risk of depressive relapse during antidepressant maintenance therapy. *J Clin Psychopharmacol* 2019; 39:344–350.

24. Kennedy N, et al. Residual symptoms at remission from depression: impact on long-term outcome. *J Affect Disord* 2004; 80:135–144.

25. National Institute for Clinical Excellence. Depression: the treatment and management of depression in adults. Clinical Guidance [CG90]; 2009 (last reviewed December 2013); https://www.nice.org.uk/guidance/cg90.

26. Anderson IM, et al. Evidence-based guidelines for treating depressive disorders with antidepressants: a revision of the 2000 British Association for Psychopharmacology guidelines. *J Psychopharmacology* 2008; 22:343–396.

27. Old Age Depression Interest Group. How long should the elderly take antidepressants? A double-blind placebo-controlled study of continu-

ation/prophylaxis therapy with dothiepin. *Br J Psychiatry* 1993; **162**:175–182.

28. Franchini L, et al. Dose-response efficacy of paroxetine in preventing depressive recurrences: a randomized, double-blind study. *J Clin Psychiatry* 1998; **59**:229–232.

29. Nobler MS, et al. *Refractory depression and electroconvulsive therapy*. Chichester: John Wiley & Sons Ltd; 1994.

30. Cipriani A, et al. Lithium versus antidepressants in the long-term treatment of unipolar affective disorder. *Cochrane Database Syst Rev* 2006; CD003492.

31. Young AH. Lithium for long-term treatment of unipolar depression. *Lancet Psychiatry* 2017; **4**:511–512.

32. Sackeim HA, et al. Continuation pharmacotherapy in the prevention of relapse following electroconvulsive therapy: a randomized controlled trial. *JAMA* 2001; **285**:1299–1307.

33. Baldessarini RJ, et al. Illness risk following rapid versus gradual discontinuation of antidepressants. *Am J Psychiatry* 2010; **167**:934–941.

其他药物与抗抑郁药的相互作用

药物可以通过两种不同的方式相互作用。

- **药代动力学相互作用**：指一种药物干扰另一种药物的吸收、分布、代谢或消除。这可能导致药物达不到治疗效果，或者产生中毒。最常见的药代动力学相互作用发生在抑制或诱导肝细胞色素 P450 酶的药物之间（表 3.14 和表 3.15）。其他影响药物代谢的酶系还包括含黄素单氧化酶（FMO）[1] 和葡糖醛酸转移酶（UGT）[2]。尽管后两种酶系均与精神药物的代谢相关，但目前关于药物对其抑制或诱导作用的研究还很少。

表 3.14 抗抑郁药对 CYP 酶活性影响的汇总 [5-7]

抗抑郁药	代谢该药物的酶系统	可抑制的酶系统
SSRI		
西酞普兰	***CYP2C19***, *CYP2D6*, *CYP3A4*	*CYP2D6*（弱）
艾司西酞普兰	***CYP2C19***, *CYP2D6*, *CYP3A4*	*CYP2D6*（弱）
氟西汀	***CYP2D6***, *CYP3A4*	***CYP2D6***（中至强） *CYP2C9*（中）, *CYP3A4*（弱）
氟伏沙明	***CYP2D6***；其他可能参与的酶	***CYP1A2***（强）, ***CYP2C19***（强）, *CYP3A4*（弱）, *CYP2C9*（弱）
帕罗西汀	***CYP2D6***	***CYP2D6***（强）
舍曲林	***CYP3A4***, *CYP2D6*（次要代谢酶）和可能的其他途径	***CYP2D6***（弱）
SNRI		
去甲文拉法辛	***CYP3A4***	*CYP2D6*（弱）
度洛西汀	***CYP1A2***, ***CYP2D6***	*CYP2D6*（中）
左米那普仑	***CYP3A4***, *CYP2C8*, *CYP2C19*, *CYP2D6*	
文拉法辛	***CYP2D6***, *CYP3A4*	*CYP2D6*（弱）
TCA		
阿米替林 氯米帕明	***CYP1A2***, ***CYP2D6***, *CYP3A4*, *CYP2C19*	
去甲丙米嗪	***CYP2D6***	
度硫平	*CYP2D6* 和其他可能途径	
多塞平	*CYP2D6*, *CYP1A2*（次要）, *CYP3A4*（次要）	
丙米嗪	***CYP1A2***, ***CYP2D6***, *CYP3A4*, *CYP2C19*	
去甲替林	***CYP2D6***	
曲米帕明	***CYP2D6***	

续表

抗抑郁药		代谢该药物的酶系统	可抑制的酶系统
其他			
	阿戈美拉汀	*CYP1A2*	
	安非他酮	*CYP2B6*	*CYP2D6*（强）
	艾司氯胺酮	*CYP3A4*,*CYP2B6*	
	米安色林	*CYP2D6*	
	米氮平	*CYP1A2*,*CYP2D6*,*CYP3A4*	*CYP2D6*（弱）
	瑞波西汀	*CYP3A4*	
	曲唑酮	*CYP3A4*	
	伏硫西汀	*CYP2D6*,*CYP2A6*,*CYP2B6*,*CYP2C8*,*CYP2C19*,*CYP3A4*	
	维拉唑酮	*CYP3A4*	*CYP2C8*

黑体字显示的 CYP 是指：
- 主要的代谢酶途径。
- 主要的酶活性。

表 3.15　药代动力学相互作用——重要相互作用概述 [3,15]

CYP1A2	CYP2B6	CYP2C9	CYP 2C19	CYP 2D6	CYP3A4/5/7
遗传多态性超快代谢型可有	占肝脏总 CYP 含量的 2%~10%[16]	5%~10% 高加索人慢代谢型	约 20% 亚洲人和 3%~5% 高加索人慢代谢型	3%~5% 高加索人慢代谢型	占 P450 酶系的 60%
被以下因素诱导：					
卡马西平	卡马西平	苯妥英	阿帕鲁胺	卡马西平	卡马西平
木炭烹饪	依法韦伦	利福平	利福平	苯妥英	苯妥英
吸烟	洛匹那韦		恩扎鲁胺		泼尼松龙
奥美拉唑	利福平		青蒿素		利福平
苯巴比妥	利托那韦		依法韦伦		
苯妥英					
被以下因素抑制：					
西咪替丁	氯吡格雷	西咪替丁	氟康唑	氯丙嗪	红霉素
环丙沙星	噻氯匹定	氟西汀	氟西汀	安非他酮	氟西汀
红霉素	伏立康唑	氟伏沙明	氟伏沙明	度洛西汀	氟伏沙明
氟伏沙明		吗氯贝胺	埃索美拉唑	氟西汀	西柚汁
		舍曲林	吗氯贝胺	氟奋乃静	酮康唑
			奥美拉唑	氟哌啶醇	去甲氟西汀
			伏立康唑	帕罗西汀	帕罗西汀
			阿米达非尼	舍曲林	舍曲林
			依特拉维林	三环类药	三环类药
			异烟肼		
			莫达非尼		
			西咪替丁		

续表

CYP1A2	CYP2B6	CYP2C9	CYP 2C19	CYP 2D6	CYP3A4/5/7
参与代谢：					
阿戈美拉汀	安非他酮	阿戈美拉汀	西酞普兰	氯氮平	钙阻滞剂
苯二氮䓬类	美沙酮	安非他酮	地西泮	可待因	卡马西平
药物	曲马多	西酞普兰	吗氯贝胺	多奈哌齐	氯氮平
咖啡因		地西泮		度洛西汀	多奈哌齐
氯氮平		奥美拉唑		氟哌啶醇	红霉素
度洛西汀		苯妥英		吩噻嗪类	加兰他敏
氟哌啶醇		三环类药		利培酮	美沙酮
米氮平		华法林		他莫昔芬	左米那普仑
奥氮平				三环类	米氮平
雷美替安				曲马多	瑞波西汀
茶碱				曲唑酮	利培酮
替扎尼定				文拉法辛	他汀类
三环类				伏硫西汀	三环类
华法林					丙戊酸盐
					文拉法辛
					维拉唑酮
					伏硫西汀
					Z-催眠药

　　药代动力学相互作用的临床后果在单个患者身上很难预测。有一些明显具有临床意义：如帕罗西汀（一种强 CYP2D6 酶抑制剂）和他莫昔芬同服时，在 20 个女性中 1 个以上会在 5 年内因停用他莫昔芬而死亡[3]。药物相互作用的结果取决于以下因素：酶被抑制或诱导的程度、受影响药物和其他合用药物的药代动力学性质、受影响药物的血浆浓度和药效动力学之间的关系、患者特异性因素（如主要和次要代谢途径的个体差异）以及伴发的躯体疾病[4]。

药效学相互作用

三环类抗抑郁药[7-10]

- 具有 H_1 受体阻滞效应（导致镇静）。这一作用可被其他镇静剂或者酒精加重。注意呼吸抑制。
- 具有抗胆碱能效应（导致口干、视物模糊、便秘）。这种效应可被其他抗胆碱能药（如抗组胺药或抗精神病药)加重。注意认知损害和胃肠道阻塞。

- 具有 α_1 肾上腺素受体阻滞效应(导致直立性低血压)。一般来说该作用可以被其他阻滞 α_1 受体的药物以及降压药加重。注意预防跌倒。肾上腺素与 α_1 受体阻滞剂合用可导致高血压。
- 导致心律失常。与其他可以直接或间接改变心脏传导的药物合用时,需要特别注意。见本章的"抗抑郁药诱发的心律失常"。
- 降低癫痫发作阈值。与其他可诱发癫痫的药物(如抗精神病药)合用时,尤其患者正在治疗癫痫时,需要慎重。见第 10 章的"癫痫"部分。
- 具有不同程度的 5-羟色胺再摄取抑制效应(尤其是丙米嗪和氯米帕明)。这些药物可能会与其他 5-HT 能药物(如曲马多、SSRI、MAOI、曲普坦类)发生相互作用,导致 5-HT 综合征。

SSRI/SNRI[7-9,11,12]

- 增加 5-HT 的神经传导。与其他 5-HT 能药物合用时,主要关注 5-HT 综合征。
- 抑制血小板聚集,增加出血风险,特别是上消化道。这一效应可被阿司匹林和 NSAID 加重(见本章"SSRI 与出血"部分)。
- 可能比其他抗抑郁药更容易引起低钠血症(见本章"抗抑郁药诱发的低钠血症"部分)。可能会加重其他药物(如利尿剂)引起的电解质紊乱。
- 可能会导致骨质减少。这会加重升高催乳素的药物对骨密度的负面影响,并增加患者摔倒受伤的风险。

单胺氧化酶抑制剂 [13,14]

- 阻止单胺类神经递质(如 5-羟色胺)的破坏。与 5-羟色胺能药物(尤其是再摄取抑制剂或促进释放剂)合用时,可增加致命性 5-羟色胺综合征的风险。这样的案例包括 SSRI 和一些相关的抗抑郁药,甚至某些非处方药(如氯苯那敏、右美沙芬)、阿片类药物(如曲马多、哌替啶)以及滥用药物(如去甲基苯丙胺 MDMA)。
- 阻止其他单胺类神经递质(如儿茶酚胺)的破坏。与可能升高血压的拟交感神经能药物(如兴奋剂)合用时,引起高血压危象。MAOI 也抑制膳食酪胺(陈旧或发酵食品中含量高)的降解,作为儿茶酚胺释放剂可引起类似的高血压反应。

总结

通过下述策略避免/减少问题:

- 如果需要抗抑郁药多药联合治疗,选择更安全的药物合用。第二种抗抑郁药开始治疗后,仔细监测不良反应。
- 避免合用有相似药理学特征但不是作为抗抑郁药被批准上市的其他药物(如托莫西汀、安非他酮)。
- **药效动力学相互作用**:指一种药物通过生理学机制改变另一种药物的作用,例如直接竞争受体部位(如多巴胺激动剂和多巴胺阻滞剂合用没有任何疗效)、增强同种神经递质通路(如氟西汀合用曲马多或者曲普坦可导致 5-HT 综合征)或者通过不同方式对一个器官/器官系统的生理功能产生影响[如 SSRI 可损害凝血功能,而非甾体抗炎药(NSAID)对胃黏膜具有刺激作用；当这些药物合用时，胃肠道出血的风险就会增加]。最新的药物间重要相互作用的列表可在线获得，大多数已知的药物相互作用在每一个药物的文献中进行了描述。

参考文献

1. Cashman JR. Human flavin-containing monooxygenase: substrate specificity and role in drug metabolism. *Curr Drug Metabol* 2000; **1**:181–191.
2. Anderson GD. A mechanistic approach to antiepileptic drug interactions. *Ann Pharmacother* 1998; **32**:554–563.
3. Kelly CM, et al. Selective serotonin reuptake inhibitors and breast cancer mortality in women receiving tamoxifen: a population based cohort study. *BMJ* 2010; **340**:c693.
4. Devane CL. Antidepressant-drug interactions are potentially but rarely clinically significant. *Neuropsychopharmacology* 2006; **31**:1594–1604.
5. Andrade C. Ketamine for depression, 5: potential pharmacokinetic and pharmacodynamic drug interactions. *J Clin Psychiatry* 2017; **78**:e858–e861.
6. Preskorn SH. Drug-drug interactions (DDIs) in psychiatric practice, part 9: interactions mediated by drug-metabolizing cytochrome P450 enzymes. *J Psychiatr Pract* 2020; **26**:126–134.
7. Medicines Complete. Stockley's drug interactions. 2020; https://www.medicinescomplete.com.
8. Preskorn SH. Drug-drug interactions (DDIs) in psychiatric practice, part 8: relative receptor binding affinity as a way of understanding the differential pharmacology of currently available antidepressants. *J Psychiatr Pract* 2020; **26**:46–51.
9. BNF Online. British national formulary. 2020; https://www.medicinescomplete.com/mc/bnf/current.
10. Gillman PK. Tricyclic antidepressant pharmacology and therapeutic drug interactions updated. *Br J Pharmacol* 2007; **151**:737–748.
11. Preskorn SH. Drug-drug interactions (DDIs) in psychiatric practice, part 6: pharmacodynamic considerations. *J Psychiatr Pract* 2019; **25**:290–297.
12. Williams LJ, et al. Selective serotonin reuptake inhibitor use and bone mineral density in women with a history of depression. *Int Clin Psychopharmacol* 2008; **23**:84–87.
13. Gillman PK. Advances pertaining to the pharmacology and interactions of irreversible nonselective monoamine oxidase inhibitors. *J Clin Psychopharmacol* 2011; **31**:66–74.
14. Grady MM, et al. Practical guide for prescribing MAOIs: debunking myths and removing barriers. *CNS Spectr* 2012; **17**:2–10.
15. Mitchell PB. Drug interactions of clinical significance with selective serotonin reuptake inhibitors. *Drug Saf* 1997; **17**:390–406.
16. Hedrich WD, et al. Insights into CYP2B6-mediated drug-drug interactions. *Acta Pharm Sin B* 2016; **6**:413–425.

第 3 章

第3章

抗抑郁药对心脏的影响——小结

抗抑郁药对心脏的影响，在表3.16进行了小结。

表3.16　抗抑郁药对心脏的影响

药物	心率	血压	Q-T间期	心律失常	传导紊乱	心肌梗死后许可限制	注解
阿戈美拉汀[1,2]	无改变的报道	无改变的报道	单例Q-T间期延长	无报告	不明	无特殊禁忌	谨慎推荐
安非他酮*[3-6]	轻度加快	轻度升高，有时明显升高。罕见直立性低血压（又称直立性低血压）	缩短，但过量服用时可能延长	没有影响。过量服用时亦罕见报道	无	心肌梗死后用于戒烟时耐受良好	注意相互作用。监测血压
西酞普兰[7-11]（假定艾司西酞普兰相同）	轻度加快	轻度的收缩压降低	剂量相关的延长	有报道可致尖端扭转型室性心动过速，主要见于过量服用时	无	近期心肌梗死或非代偿性心力衰竭患者慎用，但有证据支持该药对心血管病患者的安全性	次要代谢产物可能延长Q-T间期。没有明确证据表明会在治疗剂量范围内增加心律失常风险
度洛西汀[12-17]	轻度加快	重要影响（见产品特征概要）。高血压时慎重	个别报道延长	个别报道有毒性	个别报道有毒性	慎用于"其病情可能会因为心率加快或血压升高而受到影响"的患者	不推荐用于离子性心脏疾病
氟西汀[18-27]	平均心率轻度减慢	对血压的影响极小	无影响	无	无	慎用于急性心肌梗死患者或失代偿性心力衰竭患者。	证据表明心肌梗死后应用安全
氟伏沙明[22-23]	心率影响极小	收缩压稍降	无明显影响	无	无	慎用	发现心电图的有限变化
左米那普仑[24,25]	轻度加快	轻度增加	无影响	开始治疗前，应先治疗已有心律失常	无	心脏病患者慎用	监测心率和血压

续表

药物	心率	血压	Q-T 间期	心律失常	传导紊乱	心肌梗死后许可限制	注解
洛非帕明 [26,27]	轻度加快	和其他三环类相比,直立性血压下降程度较小	高剂量可延长	在高剂量可出现,但罕见	不明	近期心肌梗死者禁用	较其他 TCA 心脏毒性小,原因未明
MAOI [26-28]	心率减慢	直立性低血压,可能导致高血压危象	不详,但可缩短 Q-T 间期	可引起心律失常和降低左室功能	无明确影响	心血管病患者慎用	不推荐用于心血管病患者
米那普仑 [29,30]	轻度加快(c. 10 次/min)	轻微升高收缩压和舒张压	无影响	无	无	慎用	禁用于高血压和心力衰竭患者
米氮平 [31,32]	影响极小	影响极小	无影响	无	无	近期心肌梗死者慎用	有证据表明心肌梗死后使用安全,是 SSRI 好的替代药
吗氯贝胺 [33-35]	临界性心率减慢	影响极小。个别有高血压发作	常规剂量无影响。过量延长	无	无	通常慎用于有心脏病史的患者	过量可能导致致心律失常
帕罗西汀 [36,37]	轻度减慢	影响极小	无影响	无	无	心脏病患者通常慎用	心肌梗死后应用可能安全
瑞波西汀 [38-40]	明显加快	临界性收缩压和舒张压升高,高剂量时直立性低血压	无影响	可出现心律异常	心房心室异位搏动,特别是老年人	心脏病患者慎用	冠心病最好禁用
舍曲林 [41-45]	影响极小	影响极小	治疗剂量时无影响,在 400mg/d 剂量时轻度延长(<10ms) [46]	无	无	心肌梗死后患者的首选药,但正式说明书认为对 Q-T 间期有影响,告诫有 Q-T 间期延长额外风险因素者慎用	用于心肌梗死后和心力衰竭患者是安全的
曲唑酮 [26,47,48]	常见减慢,也可出现加快	可导致严重直立性低血压	可延长	有几例报道可致 Q-T 间期延长和心律不齐	不明	禁用于急性心肌梗死患者	在心脏病患者中可造成心律失常

第3章

续表

药物	心率	血压	Q-T间期	心律失常	传导紊乱	心肌梗死后允许可限制	注解
三环类 [26,49-51]	加快	直立性低血压	延长 Q-T 间期和 QRS 间期	过量使用常见。室性心律失常,也有报道发生尖端扭转型室性心动过速	减慢传导,阻滞心脏 Na/K 通道	近期心肌梗死患者禁用	影响心脏收缩性。有些与缺血性心脏病和心源性猝死相关。避免用于冠脉心病患者
文拉法辛 [15,52-56](假设去甲文拉法辛相同)	临界增加	直立性血压升高。高剂量导致血压升高	过量时可能延长,但很罕见	在过量时罕见心律失常的报道	罕见报告	尚未在心肌梗死后患者中进行评估。慎用	致心律失常的证据很少,但是冠脉疾病患者避免使用
维拉唑酮 [57-59]	过量时加快	过量时升高	即使过量,也无影响	即使过量,也无报道	无影响	无特殊禁忌	在临床剂量范围可能对心血管功能无影响
伏硫西汀 [60-62]	无影响	无影响	无影响	无影响	无影响	无特殊禁忌	试验数据显示对 Q-T 间期和凝血参数没有影响

一般来说,选择性 5-HT 再摄取抑制剂可推荐用于心脏病患者,但要注意抗血小板效应,以及与心血管药合用时经细胞色素酶系介导的相互作用。米氮平是合适的替代药物 [32],但是分析结果提示米氮平也和出血性疾病相关 [63]。

SSRI 可能防止心肌梗死 [64,65],未治疗的抑郁症会恶化心血管病的预后 [66]。对于心肌梗死患者,使用 SSRI 和米氮平不但不增加死亡率,甚至还可能降低死亡率 [67]。因此,心肌梗死后不应停用 SSRI 治疗抑郁症。心肌梗死后抑郁症治疗的保护作用,可能与抗抑郁药的抗凝作用或间接减少心律失常的频率有关 [43,68]。认知行为治疗(CBT)则没有这方面的作用 [69]。注意,SSRI 的抗血小板作用也可能导致不良后果(见本章 "SSRI 与出血" 部分)。

参考文献

1. Dolder CR, et al. Agomelatine treatment of major depressive disorder. *Ann Pharmacotheropy* 2008; 42:1822–1831.
2. Kozian R, et al. [QTc prolongation during treatment with agomelatine]. *Psychiatr Prax* 2010; 37:405–407.
3. Roose SP, et al. Pharmacologic treatment of depression in patients with heart disease. *Psychosom Med* 2005; 67 Suppl 1:S54–S57.
4. Dwoskin LP, et al. Review of the pharmacology and clinical profile of bupropion, an antidepressant and tobacco use cessation agent. *CNS Drug Rev* 2006; 12:178 207.
5. Castro VM, et al. QT interval and antidepressant use: a cross sectional study of electronic health records. *BMJ* 2013; 346:f288.
6. Eisenberg MJ, et al. Bupropion for smoking cessation in patients hospitalized with acute myocardial infarction: a randomized, placebo-controlled trial. *J Am Coll Cardiol* 2013; 61:524–532.
7. Rasmussen SL, et al. Cardiac safety of citalopram: prospective trials and retrospective analyses. *J Clin Psychopharmacol* 1999; 19:407–415.
8. Catalano G, et al. QTc interval prolongation associated with citalopram overdose: a case report and literature review. *Clin Neuropharmacol* 2001; 24:158–162.
9. Lesperance F, et al. Effects of citalopram and interpersonal psychotherapy on depression in patients with coronary artery disease: the Canadian Cardiac Randomized Evaluation of Antidepressant and Psychotherapy Efficacy (CREATE) trial. *JAMA* 2007; 297:367–379.
10. Astrom-Lilja C, et al. Drug-induced torsades de pointes: a review of the Swedish pharmacovigilance database. *Pharmacoepidemiol Drug Saf* 2008; 17:587–592.
11. Zivin K, et al. Evaluation of the FDA warning against prescribing citalopram at doses exceeding 40 mg. *Am J Psychiatry* 2013; 170:642–650.
12. Sharma A, et al. Pharmacokinetics and safety of duloxetine, a dual-serotonin and norepinephrine reuptake inhibitor. *J Clin Pharmacol* 2000; 40:161–167.
13. Schatzberg AF. Efficacy and tolerability of duloxetine, a novel dual reuptake inhibitor, in the treatment of major depressive disorder. *J Clin Psychiatry* 2003; 64 Suppl 13:30–37.
14. Detke MJ, et al. Duloxetine, 60 mg once daily, for major depressive disorder: a randomized double-blind placebo-controlled trial. *J Clin Psychiatry* 2002; 63:308–315.
15. Colucci VJ, et al. Heart failure worsening and exacerbation after venlafaxine and duloxetine therapy. *Ann Pharmacother* 2008; 42:882–887.
16. Stuhec M. Duloxetine-induced life-threatening long QT syndrome. *Wien Klin Wochenschr* 2013; 125:165–166.
17. Orozco BS, et al. Duloxetine: an uncommon cause of fatal ventricular arrhythmia. *Clin Toxicol* 2014; 51:672–672.
18. Fisch C. Effect of fluoxetine on the electrocardiogram. *J Clin Psychiatry* 1985; 46:42–44.
19. Ellison JM, et al. Fluoxetine-induced bradycardia and syncope in two patients. *J Clin Psychiatry* 1990; 51:385–386.
20. Roose SP, et al. Cardiovascular effects of fluoxetine in depressed patients with heart disease. *Am J Psychiatry* 1998; 155:660–665.
21. Strik JJ, et al. Efficacy and safety of fluoxetine in the treatment of patients with major depression after first myocardial infarction: findings from a double-blind, placebo-controlled trial. *Psychosom Med* 2000; 62:783–789.
22. Strik JJ, et al. Cardiac side-effects of two selective serotonin reuptake inhibitors in middle-aged and elderly depressed patients. *Int Clin Psychopharmacol* 1998; 13:263–267.
23. Stirnimann G, et al. Brugada syndrome ECG provoked by the selective serotonin reuptake inhibitor fluvoxamine. *Europace* 2010; 12:282–283.
24. Mago R, et al. Safety and tolerability of levomilnacipran ER in major depressive disorder: results from an open-label, 48-week extension study. *Clin Drug Investig* 2013; 33:761–771.
25. U.S. Food & Drug Administration. Highlights of Prescribing Information. Fetzima (levomilnacipran) extended-release capsules for oral use. 2019; https://www.accessdata.fda.gov/drugsatfda_docs/label/2019/204168s006lbl.pdf.
26. Warrington SJ, et al. The cardiovascular effects of antidepressants. *Psychol Med Monogr Suppl* 1989; 16:i-40.
27. Stern H, et al. Cardiovascular effects of single doses of the antidepressants amitriptyline and lofepramine in healthy subjects. *Pharmacopsychiatry* 1985; 18:272–277.
28. WS W, et al. Acute myocarditis after massive phenelzine overdose. *Eur J Clin Pharmacol* 2007; 63:1007–1009.
29. Periclou A, et al. Effects of milnacipran on cardiac repolarization in healthy participants. *J Clin Pharmacol* 2010; 50:422–433.

30. U.S Food & Drug Administration. Highlights of Prescribing Information. Savella (milnacipran HCl) Tablets. 2009; https://www.accessdata. fda.gov/drugsatfda_docs/label/2011/022256s011lbl.pdf.

31. Montgomery SA. Safety of mirtazapine: a review. *Int Clin Psychopharmacol* 1995; **10 Suppl 4**:37–45.

32. Honig A, et al. Treatment of post-myocardial infarction depressive disorder: a randomized, placebo-controlled trial with mirtazapine. *Psychosom Med* 2007; **69**:606–613.

33. Moll E, et al. Safety and efficacy during long-term treatment with moclobemide. *Clin Neuropharmacol* 1994; **17 Suppl 1**:S74–S87.

34. Hilton S, et al. Moclobemide safety: monitoring a newly developed product in the 1990s. *J Clin Psychopharmacol* 1995; **15**:76S–83S.

35. Downes MA, et al. QTc abnormalities in deliberate self-poisoning with moclobemide. *Intern Med J* 2005; **35**:388–391.

36. Kuhs H, et al. Cardiovascular effects of paroxetine. *Psychopharmacology (Berl)* 1990; **102**:379–382.

37. Roose SP, et al. Comparison of paroxetine and nortriptyline in depressed patients with ischemic heart disease. *JAMA* 1998; **279**:287–291.

38. Mucci M. Reboxetine: a review of antidepressant tolerability. *J Psychopharmacology* 1997; **11**:S33–S37.

39. KJ H, et al. Reboxetine: a review of its use in depression. *CNS Drugs* 1999; **12**:65–83.

40. Fleishaker JC, et al. Lack of effect of reboxetine on cardiac repolarization. *Clin Pharmacol Ther* 2001; **70**:261–269.

41. Shapiro PA, et al. An open-label preliminary trial of sertraline for treatment of major depression after acute myocardial infarction (the SADHAT Trial). Sertraline Anti-Depressant Heart Attack Trial. *Am Heart J* 1999; **137**:1100–1106.

42. Glassman AH, et al. Sertraline treatment of major depression in patients with acute MI or unstable angina. *JAMA* 2002; **288**:701–709.

43. Winkler D, et al. Trazodone-induced cardiac arrhythmias: a report of two cases. *Human Psychopharmacology* 2006; **21**:61–62.

44. Jiang W, et al. Safety and efficacy of sertraline for depression in patients with CHF (SADHART-CHF): a randomized, double-blind, placebo-controlled trial of sertraline for major depression with congestive heart failure. *Am Heart J* 2008; **156**:437–444.

45. Leftheriotis D, et al. The role of the selective serotonin re-uptake inhibitor sertraline in nondepressive patients with chronic ischemic heart failure: a preliminary study. *Pacing Clin Electrophysiol* 2010; **33**:1217–1223.

46. Abbas R, et al. A thorough QT study to evaluate the effects of a supratherapeutic dose of sertraline on cardiac repolarization in healthy subjects. *Clin Pharmacol Drug Develop* 2020; **9**:307–320.

47. JA S, et al. QT Prolongation and delayed atrioventricular conduction caused by acute ingestion of trazodone. *Clin Toxicol (Phila)* 2008; **46**:71–73.

48. Dattilo PB, et al. Prolonged QT associated with an overdose of trazodone. *J Clin Psychiatry* 2007; **68**:1309–1310.

49. Hippisley-Cox J, et al. Antidepressants as risk factor for ischaemic heart disease: case-control study in primary care. *BMJ* 2001; **323**:666–669.

50. Whyte IM, et al. Relative toxicity of venlafaxine and selective serotonin reuptake inhibitors in overdose compared to tricyclic antidepressants. *QJM* 2003; **96**:369–374.

51. van Noord C, et al. Psychotropic drugs associated with corrected QT interval prolongation. *J Clin Psychopharmacol* 2009; **29**:9–15.

52. Khawaja IS, et al. Cardiovascular effects of selective serotonin reuptake inhibitors and other novel antidepressants. *Heart Dis* 2003; **5**:153–160.

53. Pfizer Limited. Summary of product characteristics. Efexor XL 75 mg hard prolonged release capsules. https://www.medicines.org.uk/2013.

54. Letsas K, et al. QT interval prolongation associated with venlafaxine administration. *Int J Cardiol* 2006; **109**:116–117.

55. Taylor D, et al. Volte-face on venlafaxine–reasons and reflections. *Journal of Psychopharmacology* 2006; **20**:597–601.

56. Cooper JM, et al. Desvenlafaxine overdose and the occurrence of serotonin toxicity, seizures and cardiovascular effects. *Clin Toxicol (Phila)* 2017; **55**:18–24.

57. Edwards J, et al. Vilazodone lacks proarrhythmogenic potential in healthy participants: a thorough ECG study. *Int J Clin Pharmacol Ther* 2013; **51**:456–465.

58. Heise CW, et al. A review of vilazodone exposures with focus on serotonin syndrome effects. *Clin Toxicol (Phila)* 2017; **55**:1004–1007.

59. Gaw CE, et al. Evaluation of dose and outcomes for pediatric vilazodone ingestions. *Clin Toxicol (Phila)* 2018; **56**:113–119.

60. Citrome L. Vortioxetine for major depressive disorder: a systematic review of the efficacy and safety profile for this newly approved antidepressant – what is the number needed to treat, number needed to harm and likelihood to be helped or harmed? *Int J Clin Pract* 2014; **68**:60–82.

61. Takeda Pharmaceuticals America Inc. Highlights of prescribing information. BRINTELLIX (vortioxetine) tablets. 2014; http://www.us.brintellix.com.

62. Baldwin DS, et al. The safety and tolerability of vortioxetine: analysis of data from randomized placebo-controlled trials and open-label extension studies. *J Psychopharmacology* 2016; **30**:242–252.

63. Na K-S, et al. Can we recommend mirtazapine and bupropion for patients at risk for bleeding?: a systematic review and meta-analysis. *J Affect Disord* 2018; **225**:221–226.

64. Alqdwah-Fattouh R, et al. Differential effects of antidepressant subgroups on risk of acute myocardial infarction: a nested case-control study. *Br J Clin Pharmacol* 2020; **86**:2040–2050.

65. Sauer WH, et al. Selective serotonin reuptake inhibitors and myocardial infarction. *Circulation* 2001; **104**:1894–1898.

66. Davies SJ, et al. Treatment of anxiety and depressive disorders in patients with cardiovascular disease. *BMJ* 2004; **328**:939–943.

67. Taylor D, et al. Pharmacological interventions for people with depression and chronic physical health problems: systematic review and meta-analyses of safety and efficacy. *British J Psychiatry* 2011; **198**:179–188.

68. Chen S, et al. Serotonin and catecholaminergic polymorphic ventricular tachycardia: a possible therapeutic role for SSRIs? *Cardiovasc J Afr* 2010; **21**:225–228.

69. Berkman LF, et al. Effects of treating depression and low perceived social support on clinical events after myocardial infarction: the Enhancing Recovery in Coronary Heart Disease Patients (ENRICHD) Randomized Trial. *JAMA* 2003; **289**:3106–3116.

抗抑郁药引起的心律失常

抑郁症可使心血管病[1]和心源性猝死[2]风险增加,这可能与血小板激活[3]、心率变异性降低[4]、躯体活动减少[5]、糖尿病风险增加或其他因素有关。

三环类抗抑郁药(TCA)已确定具有致心律失常作用,该作用源于这类药物对心脏钠离子通道的强效阻滞作用和对钾离子通道的多种作用[6]。所产生的心电图改变为 PR、QRS 和Q-T 间期延长,以及 Brugada 综合征[7]。一项研究表明,去甲替林可增加心搏骤停的风险[8],但一项大样本队列研究却没有肯定这一发现[9]。不知为何,虽然洛非帕明的主要代谢物地昔帕明是一种强效钾通道阻断剂,但该药似乎没有其他三环类抗抑郁药的致心律失常作用[10]。奇怪的是,在一项研究中[11],临床应用洛非帕明引起心肌梗死风险升高,而其他的抗抑郁药无此效应。在服用三环类药物的患者中,心电图监测比血药浓度监测更有意义、更有用。

有限的证据表明,文拉法辛具有钠通道拮抗作用[12]和较弱的 hERG 钾通道拮抗作用。但该药即使在严重过量时亦罕见心律失常报道[13-16],并且心电图改变也不如 SSRI 类药物常见[17]。治疗剂量的文拉法辛不会导致心电图改变[18],其心源性猝死风险也并不大于氟西汀或西酞普兰[9,19]。去甲文拉法辛在过量时,也没有致 Q-T 间期延长[20]。

在抗抑郁药中[1],吗氯贝胺[21]、西酞普兰[22,23]、艾司西酞普兰[24]、安非他酮[25]、曲唑酮[26,27]和舍曲林[28]在过量时有引起 Q-T 间期延长的报道,但是其临床后果尚待明确。舍曲林在400mg/d 剂量时,可延长 Q-T 间期 5~10mg[29],但是大部分 SSRI 在常规剂量时通常不引起Q-T 间期改变[30,31]。然而,可能发现 SSRI(作为一组)在正常用药时与 Q-T 间期改变有关[32],但这似乎在很大程度上归因于西酞普兰和艾司西酞普兰的作用[33]。西酞普兰和艾司西酞普兰对 Q-T 间期的影响与剂量相关[33],但程度为轻度[32]。无论是大型数据库研究[9],还是大型队列研究[33],均未发现在常规临床实践中西酞普兰与心律失常或心源性死亡有任何联系。事实上,高剂量西酞普兰(>40mg)比低剂量的不良后果更少[34]。一项大样本研究也未发现西酞普兰或艾司西酞普兰会增加心搏骤停和猝死的风险[35],但是最近一项来自我国台湾的研究结果显示以这些药物治疗者死亡率略有升高[36]。

伏硫西汀对 Q-T 间期似乎没有什么影响[37-39]。类似地,阿戈美拉汀甚至在超过治疗剂量时也没有影响[40]。维拉唑酮对心脏传导没有影响[41],左米那普仑[42]和米那普仑[43]至少在治疗剂量范围可能对 Q-T 间期也没有影响。

在高危患者中的使用

对于因近期心肌梗死而存在心律失常风险的患者,现有证据明确支持舍曲林[44]和米氮平[45]的安全性(西酞普兰[45]、氟西汀[46]和安非他酮[47]的安全性证据稍逊)。一项研究发现SSRI 和曲唑酮可以降低患者的心肌梗死风险[48],另一项研究提示任何抗抑郁药均不能升高或降低 MI 的发生风险[49]。一项研究支持西酞普兰在冠状动脉疾病患者中的安全性[50](尽管西酞普兰与尖端扭转型室性心动过速的风险有关[51])。一项研究发现艾司西酞普兰未增加心力衰竭患者的死亡率[52],随后一个系统综述发现所有 SSRI 对心力衰竭患者的死亡率均无不良影响[53]。舍曲林有助于减少心血管风险因素[54],但在老年患者中,所有现代抗抑郁药均有升高心律失常风险的可能[55]。

相对心脏毒性

抗抑郁药的相对心脏毒性难以准确确定。监测数据显示，所有上市的抗抑郁药均与心律失常（程度从无临床意义到致命都有）和心源性猝死有关。对于大多数药物，这些数据反映的可能更多是巧合，而非因果关系。

致死性中毒指数（fatal toxicity index，FTI）可提供一种比较药物毒性的方法。该指数指的是每百万次处方中过量死亡的数量（FP10）。FTI 数字表明，三环类药物毒性较高（尤其是度硫平，而不是洛非帕明），文拉法辛和吗氯贝胺毒性中等，而 SSRI、米氮平和瑞波西汀毒性较低[56-60]。然而，FTI 并不只反映心脏毒性（抗抑郁药不同程度地导致 5-HT 综合征、癫痫发作和昏迷），还受其他因素影响。支持这一论断的最有力证据是 FTI 会随时间而变化。一个很好的例子就是去甲替林，它的 FTI 值估计在 $0.6^{16} \sim 39.2^{12,56,57-59}$。该数值的变化可能反映的是服用去甲替林的患者类型不同，但是尸检时"双倍计数"（去甲替林是阿米替林的代谢产物）也有一定的影响。有充分的证据表明，文拉法辛相对较多地用于抑郁程度较重且相对更容易尝试自杀的患者[61-63]。这一现象可能夸大了文拉法辛的 FTI 值，从而错误地得出其内在毒性更强的结论。另一方面，也可以假定，FTI 的药物致心律失常的风险也低。

对于西酞普兰和艾司西酞普兰的过量使用，有报道约 1/3 患者会出现 Q-T 间期延长，除此之外，这两种药物过量的毒性都非常低[64]。常规剂量的西酞普兰可能与心搏骤停的风险增加有关[8]，但其他数据表明，常规或被批准的更大剂量的西酞普兰和艾司西酞普兰并未增加心律失常或死亡的风险[34]。西酞普兰和艾司西酞普兰可能是心脏毒性最大的 SSRI 类药物，但其毒性即使在最坏的情况下仍是轻微的，也许没有意义。

小结

- 三环类药物（不含洛非帕明）与离子通道阻滞和心律失常明确相关。
- 非三环类药物诱发心律失常的风险通常很低。
- 心肌梗死后患者推荐使用舍曲林，但其他 SSRI 和米氮平也可能是安全的。
- 安非他酮、西酞普兰、艾司西酞普兰、吗氯贝胺、洛非帕明和文拉法辛应该慎用或禁用于有严重心律失常风险的患者（如心力衰竭、左心室肥大、以前有心律失常或心肌梗死的患者）。若高危患者要使用这些药物，应该在用药初始和每次增加剂量一周后检查心电图。
- 最好避免将三环类药物（不含洛非帕明）用于有严重心律失常风险的患者。若实在无法避免，则应在用药初始、每次增加剂量一周后进行心电图检查，并在整个治疗过程中定期复查心电图。检查频率取决于患者心脏病的稳定程度以及所用三环类药物的种类（和剂量）。此外，还应该寻求心内科建议。
- 三环类和其他抗抑郁药致心律失常的可能性与剂量有关。若患者用药接近最大许可剂量，或同时服用其他可能通过药代动力学（如氟西汀）或药效动力学（如利尿剂）机制增加三环类用药风险的药物，则应考虑进行心电图监测。

参考文献

1. Taylor D. Antidepressant drugs and cardiovascular pathology: a clinical overview of effectiveness and safety. *Acta Psychiatr Scand* 2008; 118:434–442.

2. Whang W, et al. Depression and risk of sudden cardiac death and coronary heart disease in women: results from the Nurses' Health Study. *J*

Am Coll Cardiol 2009; 53:950–958.

3. Ziegelstein RC, et al. Platelet function in patients with major depression. *Intern Med J* 2009; 39:38–43.

4. Glassman AH, et al. Heart rate variability in acute coronary syndrome patients with major depression: influence of sertraline and mood improvement. *Arch Gen Psychiatry* 2007; 64:1025–1031.

5. Whooley MA, et al. Depressive symptoms, health behaviors, and risk of cardiovascular events in patients with coronary heart disease. *JAMA* 2008; 300:2379–2388.

6. Thanacoody HK, et al. Tricyclic antidepressant poisoning: cardiovascular toxicity. *Toxicol Rev* 2005; 24:205–214.

7. Sicouri S, et al. Sudden cardiac death secondary to antidepressant and antipsychotic drugs. *Exp Opin Drug Saf* 2008; 7:181–194.

8. Weeke P, et al. Antidepressant use and risk of out-of-hospital cardiac arrest: a nationwide case-time-control study. *Clin Pharmacol Ther* 2012; 92:72–79.

9. Leonard CE, et al. Antidepressants and the risk of sudden cardiac death and ventricular arrhythmia. *Pharmacoepidemiol Drug Saf* 2011; 20:903–913.

10. Hong HK, et al. Block of the human ether-a-go-go-related gene (hERG) K+ channel by the antidepressant desipramine. *Biochem Biophys Res Commun* 2010; 394:536–541.

11. Coupland C, et al. Antidepressant use and risk of cardiovascular outcomes in people aged 20 to 64: cohort study using primary care database. *BMJ* 2016; 352:i1350.

12. Khalifa M, et al. Mechanism of sodium channel block by venlafaxine in guinea pig ventricular myocytes. *J Pharmacol Exp Ther* 1999; 291:280–284.

13. Colbridge MG, et al. Venlafaxine in overdose – experience of the National Poisons Information Service (London centre). *J Toxicol Clin Toxicol* 1999; 37:383.

14. Blythe D, et al. Cardiovascular and neurological toxicity of venlafaxine. *Hum Exp Toxicol* 1999; 18:309–313.

15. Combes A, et al. Conduction disturbances associated with venlafaxine. *Ann Intern Med* 2001; 134:166–167.

16. Isbister GK. Electrocardiogram changes and arrhythmias in venlafaxine overdose. *Br J Clin Pharmacol* 2009; 67:572–576.

17. Whyte IM, et al. Relative toxicity of venlafaxine and selective serotonin reuptake inhibitors in overdose compared to tricyclic antidepressants. *QJM* 2003; 96:369–374.

18. Feighner JP. Cardiovascular safety in depressed patients: focus on venlafaxine. *J Clin Psychiatry* 1995; 56:574–579.

19. Martinez C, et al. Use of venlafaxine compared with other antidepressants and the risk of sudden cardiac death or near death: a nested case-control study. *BMJ* 2010; 340:c249.

20. Cooper JM, et al. Desvenlafaxine overdose and the occurrence of serotonin toxicity, seizures and cardiovascular effects. *Clin Toxicol (Phila)* 2017; 55:18–24.

21. Downes MA, et al. QTc abnormalities in deliberate self-poisoning with moclobemide. *Intern Med J* 2005; 35:388–391.

22. Kelly CA, et al. Comparative toxicity of citalopram and the newer antidepressants after overdose. *J Toxicol Clin Toxicol* 2004; 42:67–71.

23. Grundemar L, et al. Symptoms and signs of severe citalopram overdose. *Lancet* 1997; 349:1602.

24. Mohammed R, et al. Prolonged QTc interval due to escitalopram overdose. *J MissState Med Assoc* 2010; 51:350–353.

25. Isbister GK, et al. Bupropion overdose: qTc prolongation and its clinical significance. *Ann Pharmacother* 2003; 37:999–1002.

26. Service JA, et al. QT Prolongation and delayed atrioventricular conduction caused by acute ingestion of trazodone. *Clin Toxicol (Phila)* 2008; 46:71–73.

27. Dattilo PB, et al. Prolonged QT associated with an overdose of trazodone. *J Clin Psychiatry* 2007; 68:1309–1310.

28. de Boer RA, et al. QT interval prolongation after sertraline overdose: a case report. *BMC Emerg Med* 2005; 5:5.

29. Abbas R, et al. A thorough QT study to evaluate the effects of a supratherapeutic dose of sertraline on cardiac repolarization in healthy subjects. *Clin Pharmacol Drug Develop* 2020; 9:307–320.

30. Maljuric NM, et al. Use of selective serotonin re-uptake inhibitors and the heart rate corrected QT interval in a real-life setting: the population-based Rotterdam Study. *Br J Clin Pharmacol* 2015; 80:698–705.

31. van Haelst IM, et al. QT interval prolongation in users of selective serotonin reuptake inhibitors in an elderly surgical population: a cross-sectional study. *J Clin Psychiatry* 2014; 75:15–21.

32. Beach SR, et al. Meta-analysis of selective serotonin reuptake inhibitor-associated QTc prolongation. *J Clin Psychiatry* 2014; 75:e441–e449.

33. Castro VM, et al. QT interval and antidepressant use: a cross sectional study of electronic health records. *BMJ* 2013; 346:f288.

34. Zivin K, et al. Evaluation of the FDA warning against prescribing citalopram at doses exceeding 40 mg. *Am J Psychiatry* 2013; 170:642–650.

35. Ray WA, et al. High-dose citalopram and escitalopram and the risk of out-of-hospital death. *J Clin Psychiatry* 2017; 78:190–195.

36. Lin YT, et al. Selective serotonin reuptake inhibitor use and risk of arrhythmia: a nationwide, population-based cohort study. *Clin Ther* 2019; 41:1128–1138.e1128.

37. Dubovsky SL. Pharmacokinetic evaluation of vortioxetine for the treatment of major depressive disorder. *Exp Opin Drug Metab Toxicol* 2014; 10:759–766.

38. Alam MY, et al. Safety, tolerability, and efficacy of vortioxetine (Lu AA21004) in major depressive disorder: results of an open-label, flexible-dose, 52-week extension study. *Int Clin Psychopharmacol* 2014; 29:36–44.

39. Wang Y, et al. Effect of vortioxetine on cardiac repolarization in healthy adult male subjects: results of a thorough QT/QTc study. *Clin Pharmacol Drug Develop* 2013; 2:298–309.

40. Donazzolo Y, et al. Evaluation of the effects of therapeutic and supra-therapeutic doses of agomelatine on the QT/QTc interval – A phase I, randomised, double-blind, placebo-controlled and positive-controlled, cross-over thorough QT/QTc study conducted in healthy volunteers. *J Cardiovasc Pharmacol* 2014; 64:440–451.

41. Edwards J, et al. Vilazodone lacks proarrhythmogenic potential in healthy participants: a thorough ECG study. *Int J Clin Pharmacol Ther*

2013; **51**:456–465.

42. Mago R, et al. Safety and tolerability of levomilnacipran ER in major depressive disorder: results from an open-label, 48-week extension study. *Clin Drug Investig* 2013; **33**:761–771.

43. Periclou A, et al. Effects of milnacipran on cardiac repolarization in healthy participants. *J Clin Pharmacol* 2010; **50**:422–433.

44. Glassman AH, et al. Sertraline treatment of major depression in patients with acute MI or unstable angina. *JAMA* 2002; **288**:701–709.

45. van Melle JP, et al. Effects of antidepressant treatment following myocardial infarction. *Br J Psychiatry* 2007; **190**:460–466.

46. Strik JJ, et al. Efficacy and safety of fluoxetine in the treatment of patients with major depression after first myocardial infarction: findings from a double-blind, placebo-controlled trial. *Psychosom Med* 2000; **62**:783–789.

47. Rigotti NA, et al. Bupropion for smokers hospitalized with acute cardiovascular disease. *Am J Med* 2006; **119**:1080–1087.

48. Alqdwah-Fattouh R, et al. Differential effects of antidepressant subgroups on risk of acute myocardial infarction: a nested case-control study. *Br J Clin Pharmacol* 2020; **86**:2040–2050.

49. Wu CS, et al. Use of antidepressants and risk of hospitalization for acute myocardial infarction: a nationwide case-crossover study. *J Psychiatr Res* 2017; **94**:7–14.

50. Lesperance F, et al. Effects of citalopram and interpersonal psychotherapy on depression in patients with coronary artery disease: the Canadian Cardiac Randomized Evaluation of Antidepressant and Psychotherapy Efficacy (CREATE) trial. *JAMA* 2007; **297**:367–379.

51. Astrom-Lilja C, et al. Drug-induced torsades de pointes: a review of the Swedish pharmacovigilance database. *Pharmacoepidemiol Drug Saf* 2008; **17**:587–592.

52. Angermann CE, et al. Effect of escitalopram on all-cause mortality and hospitalization in patients with heart failure and depression: the MOOD-HF randomized clinical trial. *JAMA* 2016; **315**:2683–2693.

53. Hedrick R, et al. The impact of antidepressants on depressive symptom severity, quality of life, morbidity, and mortality in heart failure: a systematic review. *Drugs Context* 2020; **9**.

54. Sherwood A, et al. Effects of exercise and sertraline on measures of coronary heart disease risk in patients with major depression: results from the SMILE-II randomized clinical trial. *Psychosom Med* 2016; **78**:602–609.

55. Biffi A, et al. Antidepressants and the risk of arrhythmia in elderly affected by a previous cardiovascular disease: a real-life investigation from Italy. *Eur J Clin Pharmacol* 2018; **74**:119–129.

56. Crome P. The toxicity of drugs used for suicide. *Acta Psychiatr Scand Suppl* 1993; **371**:33–37.

57. Cheeta S, et al. Antidepressant-related deaths and antidepressant prescriptions in England and Wales, 1998–2000. *Br J Psychiatry* 2004; **184**:41–47.

58. Buckley NA, et al. Fatal toxicity of serotoninergic and other antidepressant drugs: analysis of United Kingdom mortality data. *BMJ* 2002; **325**:1332–1333.

59. Buckley NA, et al. Greater toxicity in overdose of dothiepin than of other tricyclic antidepressants. *Lancet* 1994; **343**:159–162.

60. Morgan O, et al. Fatal toxicity of antidepressants in England and Wales, 1993–2002. *Health Stat Q* 2004; 18–24.

61. Egberts ACG, et al. Channeling of three newly introduced antidepressants to patients not responding satisfactorily to previous treatment. *J Clin Psychopharmacol* 1997; **17**:149–155.

62. Mines D, et al. Prevalence of risk factors for suicide in patients prescribed venlafaxine, fluoxetine, and citalopram. *Pharmacoepidemiol Drug Saf* 2005; **14**:367–372.

63. Chan AN, et al. A comparison of venlafaxine and SSRIs in deliberate self-poisoning. *J Med Toxicol* 2010; **6**:116–121.

64. Hasnain M, et al. Escitalopram and QTc prolongation. *J Psychiatry Neurosci* 2013; **38**:E11.

抗抑郁药引起的低钠血症

　　大多数抗抑郁药与低钠血症有关,通常在开始治疗后 30 天内(中位数是 11 天)出现[1-3],并且可能与剂量无关[1,4],也有一些案例报告提示和剂量相关[5,6]。这种不良反应最可能的机制是抗利尿激素分泌异常综合征(SIADH)。因低钠血症住院的风险,从一般人群的 1/1 600 到接受抗抑郁药治疗者的 1/300[7]。低钠血症是抗抑郁药可能出现的严重不良反应,需要注意监测[8],尤其是对于高风险的患者。各种严重程度的低钠血症均可能增加死亡率[9]。

抗抑郁药

　　目前,尚无哪种抗抑郁药明确与低钠血症无关,几乎所有抗抑郁药均有致低钠血症的报道[10]。有人提出 5-羟色胺能药物相比去甲肾上腺素能药物更容易引起低钠血症[11,12],但是该观点尚存在争议[13]。一篇综述提示,SSRI 比三环类药物和米氮平更容易引起低钠血症[14],合用其他已知降血钠药物的老年女性风险最高[15]。

　　近年上市的 5-羟色胺能药物中,尚未有哪种药物没有这种不良反应,案例报道的米氮平[16-19](尽管报告的发生率很低[15])、艾司西酞普兰[5,20-23]和度洛西汀[4,23-28]都有。伏硫西汀[29,30]和去甲文拉法辛[31]也和低钠血症有关。去甲肾上腺素能抗抑郁药也明确与低钠血症相关[32-38],尽管频率低于 SSRI。目前,关于单胺氧化酶抑制剂诱导低钠血症的报道非常少[39-40]。

　　一项法国药物警戒数据库研究发现低钠血症和阿戈美拉汀有关,这和大多数其他研究结果相反[41]。另一个数据库研究使用了 FDA 的数据,发现低钠血症和抗抑郁药关系最强的是米氮平,也与其他大多数报道相反[42]。基于法国数据库的进一步的研究发现度洛西汀的低钠血症风险最高[43]。但是从不良事件报告数据库外推,以此估计低钠血症的相对风险或绝对风险,仍然较为困难。存在的问题包括:不成比例地报告感觉有罕见不良反应的抗抑郁药,无法对适应证的混杂作用进行校正(更有可能将认为风险低的药物用于已是低钠血症高风险的患者)以及联合治疗药物的影响。

　　细胞色素 P2D6 慢代谢型患者服用抗抑郁药后,其低钠血症发生风险升高[44],但是证据稍有不一(表 3.17)[45]。

表 3.17　抗抑郁药低钠血症风险汇总[7,14,45-48]

药物/种类	低钠血症风险	支持证据的等级
SSRI	高	强
SNRI	高	强
三环类药	中	强
MAOI	低	弱
NaSSa(米氮平,米安色林)	低	强
安非他酮	低	中
阿戈美拉汀	低	弱

监测 [1,14,15,49-53]

所有服用抗抑郁药的患者都应该被告知并观察是否存在低钠血症的迹象(头晕、恶心、嗜睡、意识模糊、抽筋、癫痫发作)。该风险在抗抑郁药初始治疗的前2~4周最高,随着治疗时间延长逐渐减弱,治疗3~6个月后,风险和未服用抗抑郁药的患者相似[47,48]。对于存在药物所致低钠血症的高危人群,应该定期(基线、第2和4周、然后每3个月1次[54])监测血钠。高危因素如下:

- 高龄
- 女性
- 大手术
- 有低钠血症史或基线血钠浓度低
- 合用了其他已知与低钠血症相关的药物(例如:利尿剂、*NSAID*、抗精神病药、卡马西平、癌症化疗药物、钙拮抗剂、血管紧张素转换酶抑制剂)
- 肾功能减退(肾小球滤过率 <50mL/min)
- 存在躯体共病(如甲状腺功能减退、糖尿病、慢性阻塞性肺疾病、高血压、头部受伤、充血性心力衰竭、脑血管意外、各种癌症)
- 低体重者

年龄也许是最重要的风险因素,因此,对于老年人(尤其是女性),必须监测血钠[15,47,55,56]。

治疗 [56]

用限制液体的方法有可能控制轻度低钠血症[50]。有人建议增加钠的摄入[4],但是这可能有点不切实际。如果症状持续,则应停用抗抑郁药。

- 血清钠的正常范围是 136~145mmol/L。
- 若血清钠 >125mmol/L,应每天监测血钠直到正常。此时的症状包括头痛、恶心、呕吐、肌肉痉挛、不安、嗜睡、意识模糊和定向障碍。考虑停用相应的抗抑郁药。
- 若血清钠 <125mmol/L,应转诊到专科治疗。此时,出现危及生命的症状(如癫痫发作、昏迷和呼吸停止)的风险增加。应立即停用抗抑郁药(注意停药症状可能使临床表现变得复杂)。过快纠正低钠血症也可能有害[19]。

重新开始治疗

- 对于那些因使用 SSRI 而出现低钠血症的患者,有许多案例报道患者在重新使用同种或不同 SSRI 时,会再次出现低钠血症;但在换用其他类别的抗抑郁药后,再次引起低钠血症的报道则相对较少[16,17]。也有再次使用 SSRI 却未再出现低钠血症的报道[1]。
- 考虑停用与低钠血症相关的其他药物(当抗抑郁药和利尿剂等药物合用时,该风险呈指数增加[3])。
- 换用其他类别的药物。考虑去甲肾上腺素能药物(如去甲替林和洛非帕明)、米氮平或单胺氧化酶抑制剂(如吗氯贝胺)。也可考虑阿戈美拉汀或安非他酮[57]。换药时起始剂量宜低,加量宜慢,并应密切监测。若低钠血症复发,但仍需使用抗抑郁药,可考虑限水和/或谨慎使用地美环素(详见《英国国家药品集》)。

- 考虑电抽搐治疗（ECT）。

其他处方药

众所周知,卡马西平和抗利尿激素分泌异常综合征有关 [58]。注意抗精神病药也与低钠血症有关 [59-61]（见第 1 章中 "低钠血症" 部分）。其他常用药物,如噻嗪类利尿剂、阿片类药物、NSAID、曲马多、细胞毒素、奥美拉唑和甲氧苄啶,也会导致低钠血症 [2,51,58]。

参考文献

1. Egger C, et al. A review on hyponatremia associated with SSRIs, reboxetine and venlafaxine. *Int J Psychiatry Clin Pract* 2006; 10:17–26.
2. Liamis G, et al. A review of drug-induced hyponatremia. *Am J Kidney Dis* 2008; 52:144–153.
3. Letmaier M, et al. Hyponatraemia during psychopharmacological treatment: results of a drug surveillance programme. *Int J Neuropsychopharmacol* 2012; 15:739–748.
4. Kruger S, et al. Duloxetine and hyponatremia: a report of 5 cases. *J Clin Psychopharmacol* 2007; 27:101–104.
5. Naschitz JE. Escitalopram dose-dependent hyponatremia. *J Clin Pharmacol* 2018; 58:834–835.
6. Das S, et al. Dose dependent hyponatremia caused by Vilazodone: a case report. *Asian J Psychiatr* 2019; 43:213.
7. Gandhi S, et al. Second-generation antidepressants and hyponatremia risk: a population-based cohort study of older adults. *Am J Kidney Dis* 2017; 69:87–96.
8. Mohan S, et al. Prevalence of hyponatremia and association with mortality: results from NHANES *Am J Med* 2013; 126:1127–1137.e1121.
9. Selmer C, et al. Hyponatremia, all-cause mortality, and risk of cancer diagnoses in the primary care setting: a large population study. *Eur J Intern Med* 2016; 36:36–43.
10. Thomas A, et al. Hyponatraemia and the syndrome of inappropriate antidiuretic hormone secretion associated with drug therapy in psychiatric patients. *CNS Drugs* 1995; 5:357–369.
11. Movig KL, et al. Serotonergic antidepressants associated with an increased risk for hyponatraemia in the elderly. *Eur J Clin Pharmacol* 2002; 58:143–148.
12. Movig KL, et al. Association between antidepressant drug use and hyponatraemia: a case-control study. *Br J Clin Pharmacol* 2002; 53:363–369.
13. Kirby D, et al. Hyponatraemia and selective serotonin re-uptake inhibitors in elderly patients. *Int J Geriatr Psychiatry* 2001; 16:484–493.
14. De Picker L, et al. Antidepressants and the risk of hyponatremia: a class-by-class review of literature. *Psychosomatics* 2014; 55:536–547.
15. Dirks AC, et al. Recurrent hyponatremia after substitution of citalopram with duloxetine. *J Clin Psychopharmacol* 2007; 27:313.
16. Lim SY, et al. Hyponatraemia: the importance of obtaining a detailed history and corroborating point-of-care analysis with laboratory testing. *BMJ Case Rep* 2019; 12:e229221.
17. Bavbek N, et al. Recurrent hyponatremia associated with citalopram and mirtazapine. *Am J Kidney Dis* 2006; 48:e61–e62.
18. Ladino M, et al. Mirtazapine-induced hyponatremia in an elderly hospice patient. *J Palliat Med* 2006; 9:258–260.
19. Cheah CY, et al. Mirtazapine associated with profound hyponatremia: two case reports. *Am J Geriatr Pharmacother* 2008; 6:91–95.
20. Grover S, et al. Escitalopram-associated hyponatremia. *Psychiatry Clin Neurosci* 2007; 61:132–133.
21. Covyeou JA, et al. Hyponatremia associated with escitalopram. *N Engl J Med* 2007; 356:94–95.
22. Vidyasagar S, et al. Escitalopram induced SIADH in an elderly female: a case study. *Psychopharmacol Bull* 2017; 47:64–67.
23. Şahan E, et al. Duloxetine induced hyponatremia. *Turk Psikiyatri Dergisi* 2019; 30:287–289.
24. Sun CF, et al. Duloxetine-induced hyponatremia in an elderly male patient with treatment-refractory major depressive disorder. *Case Rep Psychiatry* 2019; 2019:4109150.
25. Hu D, et al. Hyponatremia induced by duloxetine: a case report. *Consult Pharm* 2018; 33:446–449.
26. Yoshida K, et al. Acute hyponatremia resulting from duloxetine-induced syndrome of inappropriate antidiuretic hormone secretion. *Intern Med* 2019; 58:1939–1942.
27. Wang D, et al. Rapid-onset hyponatremia and delirium following duloxetine treatment for postherpetic neuralgia: case report and literature review. *Medicine (Baltimore)* 2018; 97:e13178.
28. Takayama A, et al. Duloxetine and angiotensin II receptor blocker combination potentially induce severe hyponatremia in an elderly woman. *Intern Med* 2019; 58:1791–1794.
29. Pelayo-Terán JM, et al. Safety in the use of antidepressants: vortioxetine-induce hyponatremia in a case report. *Revista de psiquiatria y salud mental* 2017; 10:219–220.
30. Lundbeck Limited. Summary of product characteristics. Brintellix (vortioxetine) tablets 5, 10 and 20mg. 2020; https://www.medicines.org.uk/emc/medicine/30904.
31. Lee G, et al. Syndrome of inappropriate secretion of antidiuretic hormone due to desvenlafaxine. *Gen Hosp Psychiatry* 2013; 35:574.e571–573.
32. O'Sullivan D, et al. Hyponatraemia and lofepramine. *Br J Psychiatry* 1987; 150:720–721.
33. Wylie KR, et al. Lofepramine-induced hyponatraemia. *Br J Psychiatry* 1989; 154:419–420.
34. Ranieri P, et al. Reboxetine and hyponatremia. *N Engl J Med* 2000; 342:215–216.
35. Miller MG. Tricyclics as a possible cause of hyponatremia in psychiatric patients. *Am J Psychiatry* 1989; 146:807.

36. Colgate R. Hyponatraemia and inappropriate secretion of antidiuretic hormone associated with the use of imipramine. *Br J Psychiatry* 1993; 163:819–822.

37. Koelkebeck K, et al. A case of non-SIADH-induced hyponatremia in depression after treatment with reboxetine. *World J Biol Psychiatry* 2009; 10:609–611.

38. Kate N, et al. Bupropion-induced hyponatremia. *Gen Hosp Psychiatry* 2013; 35:681.e611–682.

39. Mercier S, et al. Severe hyponatremia induced by moclobemide (in French). *Therapie* 1997; 52:82–83.

40. Peterson JC, et al. Inappropriate antidiuretic hormone secondary to a monamine oxidase inhibitor. *JAMA* 1978; 239:1422–1423.

41. Rochoy M, et al. [Antidepressive agents and hyponatremia: a literature review and a case/non-case study in the French Pharmacovigilance database]. *Therapie* 2018; 73:389–398.

42. Mazhar F, et al. Association of hyponatraemia and antidepressant drugs: a pharmacovigilance-pharmacodynamic assessment through an analysis of the US food and drug administration adverse event reporting system (FAERS) database. *CNS Drugs* 2019; 33:581–592.

43. Revol R, et al. [Hyponatremia associated with SSRI/NRSI: descriptive and comparative epidemiological study of the incidence rates of the notified cases from the data of the French National Pharmacovigilance Database and the French National Health Insurance]. *Encephale* 2018; 44:291–296.

44. Kwadijk-de GS, et al. Variation in the CYP2D6 gene is associated with a lower serum sodium concentration in patients on antidepressants. *Br J Clin Pharmacol* 2009; 68:221–225.

45. Stedman CA, et al. Cytochrome P450 2D6 genotype does not predict SSRI (fluoxetine or paroxetine) induced hyponatraemia. *Human Psychopharmacology* 2002; 17:187–190.

46. Leth-Moller KB, et al. Antidepressants and the risk of hyponatremia: a Danish register-based population study. *BMJ Open* 2016; 6:e011200.

47. Lien YH. Antidepressants and hyponatremia. *Am J Med* 2018; 131:7–8.

48. Farmand S, et al. Differences in associations of antidepressants and hospitalization due to hyponatremia. *Am J Med* 2018; 131:56–63.

49. Jacob S, et al. Hyponatremia associated with selective serotonin-reuptake inhibitors in older adults. *Ann Pharmacother* 2006; 40:1618–1622.

50. Roxanas M, et al. Venlafaxine hyponatraemia: incidence, mechanism and management. *Aust N Z J Psychiatry* 2007; 41:411–418.

51. Reddy P, et al. Diagnosis and management of hyponatraemia in hospitalised patients. *Int J Clin Pract* 2009; 63:1494–1508.

52. Siegler EL, et al. Risk factors for the development of hyponatremia in psychiatric inpatients. *Arch Intern Med* 1995; 155:953–957.

53. Mannesse CK, et al. Characteristics, prevalence, risk factors, and underlying mechanism of hyponatremia in elderly patients treated with antidepressants: a cross-sectional study. *Maturitas* 2013; 76:357–363.

54. Arinzon ZH, et al. Delayed recurrent SIADH associated with SSRIs. *Ann Pharmacother* 2002; 36:1175–1177.

55. Fabian TJ, et al. Paroxetine-induced hyponatremia in the elderly due to the syndrome of inappropriate secretion of antidiuretic hormone (SIADH). *J Geriatr Psychiatry Neurol* 2003; 16:160–164.

56. Sharma H, et al. Antidepressant-induced hyponatraemia in the aged. Avoidance and management strategies. *Drugs Aging* 1996; 8:430–435.

57. Varela Piñón M, et al. Selective serotonin reuptake inhibitor-induced hyponatremia: clinical implications and therapeutic alternatives. *Clin Neuropharmacol* 2017; 40:177–179.

58. Shepshelovich D, et al. Medication-induced SIADH: distribution and characterization according to medication class. *Br J Clin Pharmacol* 2017; 83:1801–1807.

59. Ohsawa H, et al. An epidemiological study on hyponatremia in psychiatric patients in mental hospitals in Nara Prefecture. *Jpn J Psychiatry Neurol* 1992; 46:883–889.

60. Leadbetter RA, et al. Differential effects of neuroleptic and clozapine on polydipsia and intermittent hyponatremia. *J Clin Psychiatry* 1994; 55 Suppl B:110–113.

61. Collins A, et al. SIADH induced by two atypical antipsychotics. *Int J Geriatr Psychiatry* 2000; 15:282–283.

抗抑郁药与高催乳素血症

人体内催乳素的释放受内源性多巴胺控制,同时也间接受到 $5\text{-}HT_{1c}$ 和 $5\text{-}HT_2$ 受体[1,2] 的调控。在抗抑郁药[3] 的使用中,很少见到血清催乳素的持续升高(伴或不伴有相应症状)。即使抗抑郁药确实导致了高催乳素血症,其升高幅度一般也很小,而且持续时间很短[4],很少出现临床症状。乳腺癌[5] 的发生与 SSRI 类药物的使用无关。

一般不推荐常规监测催乳素,但有症状提示可能有高催乳素血症时,就需要监测血浆催乳素。一旦确定患者为有症状的高催乳素血症,宜将药物换为米氮平(详见下面内容),但是有证据表明换为另一种 SSRI 类药物可以改善症状[6,7]。

抗抑郁药与催乳素升高的关系见表 3.18。

表 3.18 已发现的抗抑郁药与催乳素升高的关联

药物/种类	前瞻性研究	病例报告/系列病例报告
阿戈美拉汀	在临床试验中[8] 没有提到催乳素改变 褪黑素本身可抑制催乳素的产生[9]	无
安非他酮	单次剂量高达 100mg 似乎对催乳素无影响[10] 可能会降低泌乳素[11]	无
单胺氧化酶抑制剂(MAOI)	发现苯乙肼[11] 和反苯环丙胺[12] 会引起轻度催乳素水平改变	非常偶然报道泌乳素升高[11]
米氮平	有力证据表明米氮平对催乳素无影响[13-15]	偶然报道溢乳[16] 和男子女性型乳房[17]
SNRI	观察到文拉法辛和度洛西汀与催乳素升高明确相关[18-20]	有报道显示溢乳与文拉法辛[21,22] 和度洛西汀[23,24] 的使用有关,度洛西汀引起的高催乳素血症可用阿立哌唑治疗[18]
SSRI	前瞻性研究普遍未发现催乳素改变[25-27]。来自处方事件监测的证据显示,SSRI 类药物与非产褥期泌乳的风险增高相关[28]。在一项法国的研究中,高催乳素血症占 SSRI 类药物不良反应的 1.6%[3]	有使用氟西汀[6,29] 和帕罗西汀[30,31] 溢乳的报告 有使用艾司西酞普兰[33] 和伏氟沙明[34] 出现正常泌乳素性溢乳和闭经[32] 的报告 有舍曲林可引起高催乳素血症的报告[7,35]
三环类	一些研究发现可致催乳素轻度改变[11,36,37],但其他研究则未发现任何改变[11,38]	丙米嗪[33]、度硫平[39] 及氯米帕明[40,41] 可引起有症状的高催乳素血症 去甲替林[42] 及曲唑酮联合西酞普兰[43] 治疗后,有溢乳的报道 催乳素水平升高可能和阿米替林疗效有关[36]
伏硫西汀	临床试验未提及催乳素变化[44-45]	无 一项综述显示"伏硫西汀和溢乳可能有关"[46]

参考文献

1. Emiliano AB, et al. From galactorrhea to osteopenia: rethinking serotonin-prolactin interactions. *Neuropsychopharmacology* 2004; 29:833–846.

2. Rittenhouse PA, et al. Neurons in the hypothalamic paraventricular nucleus mediate the serotonergic stimulation of prolactin secretion via 5-HT1c/2 receptors. *Endocrinology* 1993; 133:661–667.

3. Trenque T, et al. Serotonin reuptake inhibitors and hyperprolactinaemia: a case/non-case study in the French pharmacovigilance database. *Drug Saf* 2011; 34:1161–1166.

4. Voicu V, et al. Drug-induced hypo- and hyperprolactinemia: mechanisms, clinical and therapeutic consequences. *Exp Opin Drug Metab Toxicol* 2013; 9:955–968.

5. Ashbury JE, et al. Selective serotonin reuptake inhibitor (SSRI) antidepressants, prolactin and breast cancer. *Front Oncol* 2012; 2:177.

6. Mondal S, et al. A new logical insight and putative mechanism behind fluoxetine-induced amenorrhea, hyperprolactinemia and galactorrhea in a case series. *Ther Adv Psychopharmacol* 2013; 3:322–334.

7. Strzelecki D, et al. Hyperprolactinemia and bleeding following use of sertraline but not use of citalopram and paroxetine: a case report. *Arch Psychiatry Psychotherapy* 2012; 1:45–48.

8. Taylor D, et al. Antidepressant efficacy of agomelatine: meta-analysis of published and unpublished studies. *BMJ* 2014; 348:g1888.

9. Chu YS, et al. Stimulatory and entraining effect of melatonin on tuberoinfundibular dopaminergic neuron activity and inhibition on prolactin secretion. *J Pineal Res* 2000; 28:219–226.

10. Whiteman PD, et al. Bupropion fails to affect plasma prolactin and growth hormone in normal subjects. *Br J Clin Pharmacol* 1982; 13:745.

11. Meltzer HY, et al. Effect of antidepressants on neuroendocrine axis in humans. *Adv Biochem Psychopharmacol* 1982; 32:303–316.

12. Price LH, et al. Effects of tranylcypromine treatment on neuroendocrine, behavioral, and autonomic responses to tryptophan in depressed patients. *Life Sci* 1985; 37:809–818.

13. Laakmann G, et al. Effects of mirtazapine on growth hormone, prolactin, and cortisol secretion in healthy male subjects. *Psychoneuroendocrinology* 1999; 24:769–784.

14. Laakmann G, et al. Mirtazapine: an inhibitor of cortisol secretion that does not influence growth hormone and prolactin secretion. *J Clin Psychopharmacol* 2000; 20:101–103.

15. Schule C, et al. The influence of mirtazapine on anterior pituitary hormone secretion in healthy male subjects. *Psychopharmacology (Berl)* 2002; 163:95–101.

16. Schroeder K, et al. Mirtazapine-induced galactorrhea: a case report. *J Neuropsychiatry Clin Neurosci* 2013; 25:E13–E14.

17. Lynch A, et al. [Gynecomastia-galactorrhea during treatment with mirtazapine]. *Presse Med* 2004; 33:458.

18. Luo T, et al. Aripiprazole for the treatment of duloxetine-induced hyperprolactinemia: a case report. *J Affect Disord* 2019; 250:330–332.

19. Daffner-Bugia C, et al. The neuroendocrine effects of venlafaxine in healthy subjects. *Human Psychopharmacology* 1996; 11:1–9.

20. McGrane IR, et al. Probable galactorrhea associated with sequential trials of escitalopram and duloxetine in an adolescent female. *J Child Adolesc Psychopharmacol* 2019; 29:788–789.

21. Sternbach H. Venlafaxine-induced galactorrhea. *J Clin Psychopharmacol* 2003; 23:109–110.

22. Demir EY, et al. Hyperprolactinemia connected with venlafaxine: a case report. *Anatolian J Psychiatry* 2014; 15:S10–S14.

23. Ashton AK, et al. Hyperprolactinemia and galactorrhea induced by serotonin and norepinephrine reuptake inhibiting antidepressants. *Am J Psychiatry* 2007; 164:1121–1122.

24. Korkmaz S, et al. Galactorrhea during duloxetine treatment: a case report. *Turk Psikiyatri Dergisi* 2011; 22:200–201.

25. Sagud M, et al. Effects of sertraline treatment on plasma cortisol, prolactin and thyroid hormones in female depressed patients. *Neuropsychobiology* 2002; 45:139–143.

26. Schlosser R, et al. Effects of subchronic paroxetine administration on night-time endocrinological profiles in healthy male volunteers. *Psychoneuroendocrinology* 2000; 25:377–388.

27. Nadeem HS, et al. Comparison of the effects of citalopram and escitalopram on 5-Ht-mediated neuroendocrine responses. *Neuropsychopharmacology* 2004; 29:1699–1703.

28. Egberts AC, et al. Non-puerperal lactation associated with antidepressant drug use. *Br J Clin Pharmacol* 1997; 44:277–281.

29. Peterson MC. Reversible galactorrhea and prolactin elevation related to fluoxetine use. *Mayo Clin Proc* 2001; 76:215–216.

30. Morrison J, et al. Galactorrhea induced by paroxetine. *Can J Psychiatry* 2001; 46:88–89.

31. Evrensel A, et al. A case of galactorrhea during paroxetine treatment. *Int J Psychiatry Med* 2016; 51:302–305.

32. Selvaraj V, et al. Escitalopram-induced amenorrhea and false positive urine pregnancy test. *Korean J Fam Med* 2017; 38:40–42.

33. Mahasuar R, et al. Euprolactinemic galactorrhea associated with use of imipramine and escitalopram in a postmenopausal woman. *Gen Hosp Psychiatry* 2010; 32:341–343.

34. Vispute C, et al. Fluvoxamine-induced reversible euprolactinemic galactorrhea in a case of obsessive-compulsive disorder. *Ann Indian Psychiatry* 2017; 1:127–128.

35. Ekinci N, et al. Sertraline-related amenorrhea in an adolescent. *Clin Neuropharmacol* 2019; 42:99–100.

36. Fava GA, et al. Prolactin, cortisol, and antidepressant treatment. *Am J Psychiatry* 1988; 145:358–360.

37. Orlander H, et al. Imipramine induced elevation of prolactin levels in patients with HIV/AIDS improved their immune status. *West Indian Med J* 2009; 58:207–213.

38. Meltzer HY, et al. Lack of effect of tricyclic antidepressants on serum prolactin levels. *Psychopharmacology (Berl)* 1977; 51:185–187.

39. Gadd EM, et al. Antidepressants and galactorrhoea. *Int Clin Psychopharmacol* 1987; 2:361–363.

40. Anand VS. Clomipramine–induced galactorrhoea and amenorrhoea. *Br J Psychiatry* 1985; **147**:87–88.

41. Fowlie S, et al. Hyperprolactinaemia and nonpuerperal lactation associated with clomipramine. *Scott Med J* 1987; **32**:52.

42. Kukreti P, et al. Rising trend of use of antidepressants induced non- puerperal lactation: a case report. *JCDR* 2016; **10**:Vd01–vd02.

43. Arslan FC, et al. Trazodone induced galactorrhea: a case report. *Gen Hosp Psychiatry* 2015; **37**:373.e371–372.

44. Mahableshwarkar AR, et al. A randomized, double-blind, fixed-dose study comparing the efficacy and tolerability of vortioxetine 2.5 and 10 mg in acute treatment of adults with generalized anxiety disorder. *Human Psychopharmacology* 2014; **29**:64–72.

45. Baldwin DS, et al. Vortioxetine (Lu AA21004) in the long-term open-label treatment of major depressive disorder. *Curr Med Res Opin* 2012; **28**:1717–1724.

46. Verma A, et al. Risks associated with vortioxetine in the established therapeutic indication. *Curr Neuropharmacol* 2020. [Epub ahead of print].

抗抑郁药与糖尿病

抑郁症和糖尿病

　　糖尿病与抑郁症存在明确的相关性[1]。由于研究设计和筛查方法不同,不同研究报告,在糖尿病患者中,抑郁症共病率在 9%~60%[2]。患糖尿病后,共病抑郁症的概率将为正常人的 2 倍[2],患者被诊断糖尿病后,其抗抑郁药使用的可能性也随之增加[3,4]。抑郁症和糖尿病共病增加了心血管病的风险因素,并导致死亡风险增加 50%[5,6]。抑郁症会对人体的代谢调控造成负面影响。同样,如人体代谢调控较差,也会加重抑郁症的病情[7]。考虑到以上所有因素,对糖尿病患者共病的抑郁症进行治疗非常重要,药物的选择需要考虑到对人体内分泌代谢的可能影响(表 3.19)。Cochrane[8] 提示,抗抑郁药治疗有效,可中度改善血糖控制情况。但需要注意的是,使用抗抑郁药可能会降低患者对糖尿病药物的依从性[9]。

表 3.19　抗抑郁药对血糖平衡和体重的影响

抗抑郁药类别	对血糖平衡和体重的影响
SSRI[10-23]	■ 研究表明 SSRI 类药物对 2 型糖尿病患者的糖尿病指标有有利的影响,可降低胰岛素的用量 ■ 氟西汀可降低糖化血红蛋白(HbA_{1c})水平,降低胰岛素需要量,减轻体重,增加胰岛素敏感性。它对胰岛素敏感性的作用与对体重减轻的作用没有关系。舍曲林也可以降低糖化血红蛋白水平 ■ 艾司西酞普兰似乎也能改善血糖控制 ■ 一些证据提示,长期使用 SSRI 可增加一般人群[24] 患糖尿病的风险,尤其是增加妊娠糖尿病的风险[25],但是也有证据显示对两类人群均没有影响[26]
三环类 [16,17,27-29]	■ 三环类药物与食欲增加、体重增长及高血糖有关 ■ 在一项研究中,去甲替林可改善抑郁症,但对糖尿病患者的血糖控制有负面影响。抑郁症的全面改善对糖化血红蛋白有利。据报道,氯米帕明可促发糖尿病 ■ 长期使用三环类药物可增加罹患糖尿病的风险
单胺氧化酶抑制剂(MAOI)[30,31]	■ 不可逆性单胺氧化酶抑制剂有引起严重低血糖发作及体重增加的风险 ■ 吗氯贝胺没有影响
SNRI[28,32,33]	■ SNRI 类药物不干扰血糖的调控,对体重影响极小 ■ 在糖尿病神经病变治疗的研究中,度洛西汀对血糖调控几乎没有影响。度洛西汀用于糖尿病和抑郁症共病尚无资料 ■ 关于文拉法辛的资料有限 ■ 有一项去甲文拉法辛致高血糖的报道[34]
米氮平 [35,36]	■ 在非糖尿病性抑郁症患者中,米氮平似乎不损害糖耐量 ■ 短期治疗可改善 HbA_{1c},但是 HbA_{1c} 在随访 1 年后恶化 ■ 在糖尿病患者中,短期和长期米氮平治疗,可引起体重指数(BMI)增加
阿戈美拉汀 [22,23,37,38]	■ 一些研究提示阿戈美拉汀对血糖指标有一定程度的改善或不会恶化 ■ 阿戈美拉汀对体重影响极小
瑞波西汀、曲唑酮和伏硫西汀	■ 没有用于糖尿病患者的相关资料 ■ 一项研究显示,接受曲唑酮治疗的患者中,2 型糖尿病风险增高 20%[24]

建议

- 所有确诊为抑郁症的患者均应筛查糖尿病。

对共病糖尿病的患者：

- SSRI 类为一线用药，有数据支持选用舍曲林、艾司西酞普兰和氟西汀。
- SNRI 类也相对较安全，但支持性资料较少。
- 阿戈美拉汀是有希望的药物，可供参考的资料有限。
- 三环类及单胺氧化酶抑制剂影响体重和血糖平衡，应尽可能不用。
- 抗抑郁药开始使用、改变剂量及停药时，注意监测血糖和糖化血红蛋白。

参考文献

1. Katon WJ. The comorbidity of diabetes mellitus and depression. *Am J Med* 2008; **121 Suppl 2**:S8–S15.
2. Anderson RJ, et al. The prevalence of comorbid depression in adults with diabetes: a meta-analysis. *Diabetes Care* 2001; **24**:1069–1078.
3. Musselman DL, et al. Relationship of depression to diabetes types 1 and 2: epidemiology, biology, and treatment. *Biol Psychiatry* 2003; **54**:317–329.
4. Knol MJ, et al. Antidepressant use before and after initiation of diabetes mellitus treatment. *Diabetologia* 2009; **52**:425–432.
5. Katon WJ, et al. Cardiac risk factors in patients with diabetes mellitus and major depression. *J Gen Intern Med* 2004; **19**:1192–1199.
6. van Dooren FE, et al. Depression and risk of mortality in people with diabetes mellitus: a systematic review and meta-analysis. *PLoS One* 2013; **8**:e57058.
7. Lustman PJ, et al. Depression in diabetic patients: the relationship between mood and glycemic control. *J Diabetes Complications* 2005; **19**:113–122.
8. Baumeister H, et al. Psychological and pharmacological interventions for depression in patients with diabetes mellitus and depression. *Cochrane Database Syst Rev* 2012; **12**:Cd008381.
9. Lunghi C, et al. The association between depression and medication nonpersistence in new users of antidiabetic drugs. *Value Health* 2017; **20**:728–735.
10. Maheux P, et al. Fluoxetine improves insulin sensitivity in obese patients with non-insulin-dependent diabetes mellitus independently of weight loss. *Int J Obes Relat Metab Disord* 1997; **21**:97–102.
11. Gulseren L, et al. Comparison of fluoxetine and paroxetine in type II diabetes mellitus patients. *Arch Med Res* 2005; **36**:159–165.
12. Lustman PJ, et al. Sertraline for prevention of depression recurrence in diabetes mellitus: a randomized, double-blind, placebo-controlled trial. *Arch Gen Psychiatry* 2006; **63**:521–529.
13. Gray DS, et al. A randomized double-blind clinical trial of fluoxetine in obese diabetics. *Int J Obes Relat Metab Disord* 1992; **16 Suppl 4**:S67–S72.
14. Knol MJ, et al. Influence of antidepressants on glycaemic control in patients with diabetes mellitus. *Pharmacoepidemiol Drug Saf* 2008; **17**:577–586.
15. Briscoe VJ, et al. Effects of a selective serotonin reuptake inhibitor, fluoxetine, on counterregulatory responses to hypoglycemia in healthy individuals. *Diabetes* 2008; **57**:2453–2460.
16. Andersohn F, et al. Long-term use of antidepressants for depressive disorders and the risk of diabetes mellitus. *Am J Psychiatry* 2009; **166**:591–598.
17. Kivimaki M, et al. Antidepressant medication use, weight gain, and risk of type 2 diabetes: a population-based study. *Diabetes Care* 2010; **33**:2611–2616.
18. Rubin RR, et al. Antidepressant medicine use and risk of developing diabetes during the diabetes prevention program and diabetes prevention program outcomes study. *Diabetes Care* 2010; **33**:2549–2551.
19. Echeverry D, et al. Effect of pharmacological treatment of depression on A1C and quality of life in low-income Hispanics and African Americans with diabetes: a randomized, double-blind, placebo-controlled trial. *Diabetes Care* 2009; **32**:2156–2160.
20. Dhavale HS, et al. Depression and diabetes: impact of antidepressant medications on glycaemic control. *J Assoc Physicians India* 2013; **61**:896–899.
21. Mojtabai R. Antidepressant use and glycemic control. *Psychopharmacology (Berl)* 2013; **227**:467–477.
22. Salman MT, et al. Comparative effect of agomelatine versus escitalopram on glycemic control and symptoms of depression in patients with type 2 diabetes mellitus and depression. 2015; **6**:4304-09.
23. Kang R, et al. Comparison of paroxetine and agomelatine in depressed type 2 diabetes mellitus patients: a double-blind, randomized, clinical trial. *Neuropsychiatr Dis Treat* 2015; **11**:1307–1311.
24. Nguyen TTH, et al. Role of serotonin transporter in antidepressant-induced diabetes mellitus: a pharmacoepidemiological-pharmacodynamic study in VigiBase(®). *Drug Saf* 2018; **41**:1087–1096.

第 3 章

25. Dandjinou M, et al. Antidepressant use during pregnancy and the risk of gestational diabetes mellitus: a nested case-control study. *BMJ Open* 2019; 9:e025908.

26. Kuo HY, et al. Antidepressants and risk of type 2 diabetes mellitus: a population-based nested case-control study. *J Clin Psychopharmacol* 2020; 40:359–365.

27. Lustman PJ, et al. Effects of nortriptyline on depression and glycemic control in diabetes: results of a double-blind, placebo-controlled trial. *Psychosom Med* 1997; 59:241–250.

28. McIntyre RS, et al. The effect of antidepressants on glucose homeostasis and insulin sensitivity: synthesis and mechanisms. *Expert Opinion on Drug Safety* 2006; 5:157–168.

29. Mumoli N, et al. Clomipramine-induced diabetes. *Ann Intern Med* 2008; 149:595–596.

30. Goodnick PJ. Use of antidepressants in treatment of comorbid diabetes mellitus and depression as well as in diabetic neuropathy. *Ann Clin Psychiatry* 2001; 13:31–41.

31. McIntyre RS, et al. Mood and psychotic disorders and type 2 diabetes: a metabolic triad. *Canadian Journal of Diabetes* 2005; 29:122–132.

32. Raskin J, et al. Duloxetine versus routine care in the long-term management of diabetic peripheral neuropathic pain. *J Palliat Med* 2006; 9:29–40.

33. Crucitti A, et al. Duloxetine treatment and glycemic controls in patients with diagnoses other than diabetic peripheral neuropathic pain: a meta-analysis. *Curr Med Res Opin* 2010; 26:2579–2588.

34. Mekonnen AD, et al. Desvenlafaxine-associated hyperglycemia: a case report and literature review. *Ment Health Clin* 2020; 10:85–89.

35. Song HR, et al. Does mirtazapine interfere with naturalistic diabetes treatment? *J Clin Psychopharmacol* 2014; 34:588–594.

36. Song HR, et al. Effects of mirtazapine on patients undergoing naturalistic diabetes treatment: a follow-up study extended from 6 to 12 months. *J Clin Psychopharmacol* 2015; 35:730–731.

37. Karaiskos D, et al. Agomelatine and sertraline for the treatment of depression in type 2 diabetes mellitus. *Int J Clin Pract* 2013; 67:257–260.

38. Vasile D, et al. P.2.c.002 Agomelatine versus selective serotoninergic reuptake inhibitors in major depressive disorder and comorbid diabetes mellitus. *Eur Neuropsychopharmacol* 2011; 21:S383–S384.

第 3 章

抗抑郁药与性功能障碍

　　虽然缺乏可靠、准确的数据,但性功能障碍在一般人群中非常普遍[1]。报告的患病率差别很大,取决于如何定义和评估性功能障碍,以及资料收集的方法[1]。躯体疾病、精神疾病、物质滥用及处方药物治疗均可导致性功能障碍[2]。与一般人群相比,抑郁症患者更容易有肥胖[3]、糖尿病[4]及心血管病[5],因而更容易遭受性功能障碍的痛苦,甚至超过抑郁症本身带来的痛苦。

　　处方药物前,需要首先确定基线的性功能水平,因为治疗中发生的性功能障碍对患者的生活质量有负面影响,甚至因此降低患者对治疗的依从性[6]。调查问卷或评估量表可能有用(例如《亚利桑那性体验量表》[7])。如果没有使用量表,可以直接进行询问,主动询问要比单纯依靠患者的自发报告更有效[8]。患者抱怨性功能障碍,可能意味着其潜在躯体疾病或精神障碍加重或疗效不佳。也可能是药物治疗的结果,而对性功能障碍的干预可明显提高生活质量[6]。

抑郁症的影响

　　抑郁症本身及抗抑郁药均可导致性欲、性兴奋及性高潮的障碍。性功能障碍的具体性质可以表明主要原因是抑郁症本身还是抗抑郁药。例如,40%~50% 的抑郁症患者,在确定诊断之前的一个月内,就有过性欲减退及性唤起问题;但是在服用抗抑郁药之前,只有 15%~20% 的患者有性高潮问题[9]。性欲减退的患病率显然与抑郁症严重程度相关[10]。

　　虽然,很多患者在服用抗抑郁药后出现了性功能障碍,但是其他患者在抑郁症状减轻后,性欲和性满足可随之提高[6]。性功能障碍改善多见于抗抑郁治疗有效的患者[6]。例如,对"抑郁症的序贯治疗(STAR*D)"研究数据的事后分析发现,在服用西酞普兰治疗后抑郁症缓解的患者中性功能障碍的患病率为 21%,而未缓解的患者中患病率为 61%[11]。

抗抑郁药的影响

　　抗抑郁药可导致镇静、激素改变、胆碱能/肾上腺素能平衡紊乱、外周去甲肾上腺素能受体激动、一氧化氮抑制和 5-HT 神经传递增强,这些均可导致性功能障碍。虽然不同抗抑郁药引起性功能障碍的发生率差别很大(表 3.20),但是普遍认为性功能障碍是所有抗抑郁药的不良反应。个体易感性也有很大的差异,至少有一部分是由遗传决定的[12]。

　　抗抑郁药对性功能的影响具有剂量依赖性[12],通常是完全可逆的[12]。但是,也有报道抗抑郁药对性功能的影响长期存在,即使停用 SSRI/SNRI 治疗[13],这些症状还持续存在。有一个专门术语"SSRI 后性功能障碍(PSSD)就是用来描述这些症状的。其患病率和病生理机制目前尚不清楚"[14]。

　　在抗抑郁药对性功能所造成的影响中,并非所有都是不良反应:包括氯米帕明在内的 5-羟色胺能抗抑郁药可治疗早泄[6],对性偏好障碍也可能有利。短效 SSRI 达泊西汀对于早泄是有效的药物,在很多国家被批准用于治疗早泄[6,15]。一项针对曲唑酮 RCT 研究进行的系统综述显示,曲唑酮可有效地缓解"心因性勃起功能障碍"[6]。

通过谨慎选择抗抑郁药,可将性功能方面的不良反应降至最低。需要注意,在临床试验中,对性功能不良反应的评估通常是不够的,经常依靠患者的自我报告,并未使用有效的问卷进行评估,缺乏阳性对照[16]。对于有意且直接调查性功能不良反应的研究,应该尽可能从中获取信息。对于服用抗抑郁药发生性功能障碍的患者,其处置策略在表3.21中进行了汇总。没有一种方法被认为是"理想的"[6],因此建议逐个案例进行个体化评估。

表3.20　抗抑郁药致性功能障碍的相对频率 [10,12,17-19]

抗抑郁药	对性反应的影响			评论 [12]
	性欲 *	性唤起	性高潮	
阿戈美拉汀	–	–	–	发生率同安慰剂 [6]
安非他酮	–	+/–	–	发生率低于其他抗抑郁药 [20]。总体来说,大多证据显示发生率不高于安慰剂
度洛西汀	++	+	++	一项荟萃分析显示,发生率与SSRI和文拉法辛相似 [20]
左米那普仑	?	++	++	与其他抗抑郁药的对比研究不多 [21],因此相对发生率不确定。在RCT中,勃起功能障碍和射精障碍多于安慰剂
MAOI	++	++	++	发生率20%~40%,但资料有限。经皮司来吉兰的发生率与安慰剂相似
米氮平	+	–	–	低于SSRI [22]
吗氯贝胺	++	++	++	一致显示发生率较低
瑞波西汀	–	+	+	发生率低于SSRI/SNRI [23],但疗效一直有争议
SSRI	++	++	++	全部证据显示所有SSRI的发生率均高(但是不同SSRI差别很大) [12]。伏氟沙明的性高潮缺乏发生率较低 [24]
曲唑酮	–	+	+	案例报道中,有阴茎异常勃起发生,但是总体上发生率较低。较早的案例报道曾记录有性欲增强
三环类药	++	++	++	常见于氯米帕明(尤其是性高潮缺乏)、阿米替林和丙米嗪更常见,少见于仲胺类TCA(地昔帕明,去甲替林)
文拉法辛	++	++	++	发病率高。有性欲增强、性高潮增强和自发勃起的个别病例报告
维拉唑酮	+	+	+	在RCT研究中,发生率低于西酞普兰,与安慰剂相似。但不确定是否优于其他抗抑郁药 [21]
伏硫西汀	–	+	+	剂量低于10mg/d时,发生率和安慰剂相当 [23,25],但不确定是否优于其他抗抑郁药 [21,26]

注:++,常见;+,可能发生;–,无或罕见;?,未知/信息不足 *。

* 或冲动。

+ 易于性唤起,能够润滑或勃起。

± 轻松达到性高潮和性高潮满足感。

表 3.21　性相关不良反应的处置

策略	详解
1. 排除其他可能原因 [27]	■ 抑郁症状伴有性功能损害。将抗抑郁药治疗中的性功能与治疗前比较,不与抑郁症之前的性功能比较 ■ 考虑其他可能的原因(如酒精/物质滥用、糖尿病、动脉粥样硬化、心脏病以及中枢和外周神经系统疾病)。原因也可能是其他药物,包括非精神类药物(如利尿剂、β受体阻断剂)和其他精神药物(详见指南其他章节的汇总)
2. 换为低风险抗抑郁药 [23]	■ 低风险抗抑郁药有阿戈美拉汀、安非他酮、米氮平、维拉唑酮、伏硫西汀和吗氯贝胺 [12]。有充分证据表明,其中的阿戈美拉汀、安非他酮和伏硫西汀在性功能不良反应方面更有优势 [12]
非药物治疗	■ **等待自发缓解**:广泛使用但疗效最差的方法 [24]。可见于少数患者(5%~10%),需要等待 4~6 个月 [12] 对于许多患者不适用,但是轻症病例可考虑 [13] ■ **减量**:可用于接受抗抑郁药治疗获得完全缓解的患者 [6] ■ **药物假期**:在性活动前暂时停用 1~2 次药物可能有帮助,但有停药症状的风险 [12]。氟西汀半衰期长,此方法无效 [12]。在性活动前,连续两天将剂量降低 50% 可能是另一种策略 [24]
药物治疗	■ **磷酸二酯酶抑制剂**:西地那非和他达拉非可改善男性抗抑郁药相关勃起不能性功能障碍 [23,28]。女性证据有限,一项 RCT 发现有效 [23]。 ■ **安非他酮**:高剂量(300mg/d)可能对女性有用 [28]。低剂量时无效 [23],一项 RCT 研究数据显示对男性有效,后来被撤回 [29] ■ **米氮平**:证据混乱。开放性研究提示对有些抗抑郁药所致的 SD 有效,但是一项 RCT 研究得到的是阴性结果 [27] ■ **透皮睾酮**:RCT 提示在 SSRI/SNRI 所致性欲丧失的女性患者 [30],及持续服用 5-羟色胺能抗抑郁药且有较低或低于正常睾酮水平的患者男性中可能有效 [31] ■ **其他** [12]:很多其他药物也进行了研究,但有些药物几乎没有有效的证据。一项针对西酞普兰或帕罗西汀所致性功能障碍的研究,发现**丁螺环酮**有效,但是另一项针对氟西汀的研究未发现疗效。**赛庚啶**也成功治疗了一例 SSRI 所致的男性性功能障碍和性高潮缺乏的女性。一项小样本开放研究,发现**氯雷他定**可有效地治疗 SSRI 所致的男性勃起障碍。在早期的研究中,发现金刚烷胺治疗 SSRI 所致的性功能障碍有效,但是最近的研究得出了阴性结果。**育亨宾**治疗药物所致的 SD 更有效,两项小样本研究报告有改善(尽管结果未达到统计学显著性)。**贝沙奈酚**对 TCA 引起的性功能障碍有帮助,需要在性活动前服用。已有研究评价了**格拉司琼**的效果,但是现有数据未得出肯定结论。FDA 批准**氟班色林**和**布雷美拉肽**治疗绝经前女性 HSDD[32],但是没有资料支持其用于抗抑郁药所致的 SD ■ **难治性抑郁的增效剂**:有些药物用于难治性抑郁症的增效治疗,在次要分析中,发现可改善性功能。阿立哌唑可改善性功能和性欲,仅见于女性 [24]。一项研究提示依匹哌唑具有中度改善作用 [33]。匹莫范色林,用于 SSRI/SNRI 的增效治疗,另一项分析中发现可以改善性功能 [34]

参考文献

1. McCabe MP, et al. Incidence and prevalence of sexual dysfunction in women and men: a consensus statement from the fourth international consultation on sexual medicine 2015. *J Sex Med* 2016; **13**:144–152.

2. Chokka PR, et al. Assessment and management of sexual dysfunction in the context of depression. *Ther Adv Psychopharmacol* 2018; **8**:13–23.

3. Pereira-Miranda E, et al. Overweight and obesity associated with higher depression prevalence in adults: a systematic review and meta-analysis. *J Am Coll Nutr* 2017; **36**:223–233.

4. Semenkovich K, et al. Depression in type 2 diabetes mellitus: prevalence, impact, and treatment. *Drugs* 2015; **75**:577–587.

5. Cohen BE, et al. State of the art review: depression, stress, anxiety, and cardiovascular disease. *Am J Hypertens* 2015; **28**:1295–1302.

6. Montejo AL, et al. The impact of severe mental disorders and psychotropic medications on sexual health and its implications for clinical management. *World Psychiatry* 2018; **17**:3–11.

7. McGahuey CA, et al. The Arizona Sexual Experience Scale (ASEX): reliability and validity. *J Sex Marital Ther* 2000; **26**:25–40.

8. Papakostas GI. Identifying patients who need a change in depression treatment and implementing that change. *J Clin Psychiatry* 2016; **77**:e1009.

9. Kennedy SH, et al. Sexual dysfunction before antidepressant therapy in major depression. *J Affect Disord* 1999; **56**:201–208.

10. Clayton AH, et al. Antidepressants and sexual dysfunction: mechanisms and clinical implications. *Postgrad Med* 2014; **126**:91–99.

11. Ishak WW, et al. Sexual satisfaction and quality of life in major depressive disorder before and after treatment with citalopram in the STAR*D study. *J Clin Psychiatry* 2013; **74**:256–261.

12. Clayton AH, et al. Sexual dysfunction due to psychotropic medications. *Psychiatr Clin North Am* 2016; **39**:427–463.

13. Rothmore J. Antidepressant-induced sexual dysfunction. *Med J Aust* 2020; **212**:329–334.

14. Bala A, et al. Post-SSRI sexual dysfunction: a literature review. *Sex Med Rev* 2018; **6**:29–34.

15. McMahon CG. Dapoxetine: a new option in the medical management of premature ejaculation. *Ther Adv Urol* 2012; **4**:233–251.

16. Khin NA, et al. Regulatory and scientific issues in studies to evaluate sexual dysfunction in antidepressant drug trials. *J Clin Psychiatry* 2015; **76**:1060–1063.

17. Serretti A, et al. Treatment-emergent sexual dysfunction related to antidepressants: a meta-analysis. *J Clin Psychopharmacol* 2009; **29**:259–266.

18. Chiesa A, et al. Antidepressants and sexual dysfunction: epidemiology, mechanisms and management. *J Psychopathology* 2010; **16**:104–113.

19. Lew-Starowicz M, et al. *Impact of psychotropic medications on sexual functioning*. Cham: Springer; 2021:353–371.

20. Reichenpfader U, et al. Sexual dysfunction associated with second-generation antidepressants in patients with major depressive disorder: results from a systematic review with network meta-analysis. *Drug Saf* 2014; **37**:19–31.

21. Wagner G, et al. Efficacy and safety of levomilnacipran, vilazodone and vortioxetine compared with other second-generation antidepressants for major depressive disorder in adults: a systematic review and network meta-analysis. *J Affect Disord* 2018; **228**:1–12.

22. Watanabe N, et al. Mirtazapine versus other antidepressive agents for depression. *Cochrane Database Syst Rev* 2011; CD006528.

23. Cleare A, et al. Evidence-based guidelines for treating depressive disorders with antidepressants: a revision of the 2008 British Association for Psychopharmacology guidelines. *J Psychopharmacology* 2015; **29**:459–525.

24. Montejo AL, et al. Management strategies for antidepressant-related sexual dysfunction: a clinical approach. *J Clin Med* 2019; **8**:1640.

25. Jacobsen PL, et al. Treatment-emergent sexual dysfunction in randomized trials of vortioxetine for major depressive disorder or generalized anxiety disorder: a pooled analysis. *CNS Spectr* 2016; **21**:367–378.

26. Koesters M, et al. Vortioxetine for depression in adults. *Cochrane Database Syst Rev* 2017; **7**:Cd011520.

27. Francois D, et al. Antidepressant-induced sexual side effects: incidence, assessment, clinical implications, and management. *Psychiatric Ann* 2017; **47**:154–160.

28. Taylor MJ, et al. Strategies for managing sexual dysfunction induced by antidepressant medication. *CochraneDatabaseSystRev* 2013; **5**:CD003382.

29. Safarinejad MR. The effects of the adjunctive bupropion on male sexual dysfunction induced by a selective serotonin reuptake inhibitor: a double-blind placebo-controlled and randomized study. *BJU Int* 2010; **106**:840–847.

30. Montejo AL, et al. Sexual side-effects of antidepressant and antipsychotic drugs. *Curr Opin Psychiatry* 2015; **28**:418–423.

31. Amiaz R, et al. Testosterone gel replacement improves sexual function in depressed men taking serotonergic antidepressants: a randomized, placebo-controlled clinical trial. *J Sex Marital Ther* 2011; **37**:243–254.

32. Bitzer J, et al. *Female sexual dysfunctions*. Cham: Springer; 2021:109–134.

33. Clayton AH, et al. Effect of brexpiprazole on prolactin and sexual functioning: an analysis of short- and long-term study data in major depressive disorder. *J Clin Psychopharmacol* 2020; **40**:560–567.

34. Freeman MP, et al. Improvement of sexual functioning during treatment of MDD with adjunctive pimavanserin: a secondary analysis. *Depress Anxiety* 2020; **37**:485–495.

扩展阅读

Montejo, A.L., et al. Management strategies for antidepressant-related sexual dysfunction: a clinical approach. *Journal of clinical medicine* 2019; **8**:1640.

SSRI 与出血

发生血管损伤后,5-羟色胺从血小板释放,促进血管收缩,改变血小板的形态以促进其聚集[1]。5-羟色胺转运体负责将 5-羟色胺摄入血小板内,而 SSRI 类药物能抑制这一过程。SSRI 类药物耗竭血小板内的 5-羟色胺,使血小板凝集能力下降,从而增加出血的风险。广义上来讲,相比于未用 SSRI/SNRI 者,SSRI/SNRI 治疗者各类出血事件相对风险大约是 1.4 倍,绝对风险为 0.5%~6%[2](取决于多种因素,尤其是治疗时长)。

SSRI 类药物也可增加胃酸分泌,从而间接地刺激胃黏膜[3],增加消化性溃疡的风险[4]。SSRI 类药物引起各类异常出血的风险在治疗的前 30 天最高[5,6]。对出血的影响,可能但并未确定,与每种 SSRI 对 5-羟色胺转运体的亲和性相关(表 3.22)[7,8]。

表 3.22　抗抑郁药及其对 5-羟色胺再摄取抑制程度[6,9]

5-羟色胺再摄取抑制程度	抗抑郁药(SSRI)
强抑制	舍曲林,帕罗西汀,氟西汀,度洛西汀,氯米帕明
中等抑制	西酞普兰,艾司西酞普兰,伏氟沙明,维拉唑酮,伏硫西汀,文拉法辛 阿米替林,丙米嗪
弱或无抑制	阿戈美拉汀,度硫平,多塞平,洛非帕明,米氮平,吗氯贝胺,去甲替林,瑞波西汀,米安色林

SSRI 所致出血的风险因素
■ 年龄,尤其是超过 65 岁者
■ 酒精滥用
■ 冠状动脉疾病
■ 药物滥用
■ 高血压
■ GI 出血史
■ 卒中史
■ 大出血史
■ 肝脏疾病
■ 不稳定的国际标准化比值(INR)
■ 易致出血药物
■ 消化性溃疡
■ 肾脏疾病
■ 吸烟

在为患有痛风、哮喘、慢性阻塞性肺疾病(COPD)、狼疮、银屑病、干扰素治疗丙型病毒性肝炎[10] 和关节炎所诱发的抑郁等患者应慎用 5-羟色胺能类抗抑郁药,因为患者可能同时服

用皮质类固醇、阿司匹林或 NSAID。

胃肠道出血

使用 5-羟色胺能抗抑郁药是出血性事件的独立风险因素。一项基于人群的研究提示,控制所有相关风险因素后,服用 SSRI 类药物可以增加上消化道出血(风险比为 1.97)和下消化道出血(风险比为 2.96)的发生率[11]。在绝对值上,应用 SSRI 抗抑郁治疗,可使出血事件的发生率较正常背景增加 3 次/1 000 患者-年[7,12,13],但这个数据并没有体现不同患者群体发生风险的差异性。例如,在既往发生过消化道出血的患者中,使用 SSRI 将使 1/85 的患者再次出血[14]。

一项数据库研究表明,胃黏膜保护剂(质子泵抑制剂,PPI)可降低 SSRI(单用或联用 NSAID)相关的消化道出血的风险,但是还远未低到对照组水平[15]。2020 年一项研究发现,在因房颤而服用直接作用抗凝剂的患者中,使用 SSRI 治疗增加了胃肠道出血的风险,而这一风险在那些未服用 PPI 的患者中进一步升高[16](另一项研究未发现 SSRI 增加任何抗凝剂治疗患者的出血风险[17])。

其他的数据库研究也发现,与年龄、性别匹配的对照组相比,服用 SSRI 类药物可明显增加因上消化道出血而住院的风险[7,15,18,19]。在控制年龄、性别和其他药物,如阿司匹林、NSAID 的作用后,这种关系仍然成立[2]。此外,一个针对 22 项研究的荟萃分析得出结论,与未服用 SSRI 类药物的患者相比,正服用 SSRI 的患者发生上消化道出血的风险高出 55%。这一风险非常显著,并且会随着合用抗血小板药或 NSAID 进一步升高[5]。

与单独使用 SSRI 类药物相比,联合小剂量的阿司匹林发生上消化道出血的风险至少翻倍,而联合使用 NSAID 发生消化道出血的风险将接近 4 倍[20]。联合使用 SSRI 类和 NSAID 将会显著增加抑酸剂的使用[21]。老年人及既往有消化道出血病史的患者发生消化道出血的风险最大[14,15,19]。

早期的研究发现,SSRI 可使服用法华林的患者非消化道出血的发生率增加 2~3 倍(相当于 NSAID 的效应值),但消化道出血的风险并没有升高[22,23]。随后的一项研究[11]显示,联合使用华法林和 5-羟色胺能抗抑郁药(表 3.23),上消化道和下消化道出血风险均升高。然而,这与国际标准化比值(INR)的影响似乎无关,故尚无法确定出血风险最高的群体[23]。与这些研究结果一致,在使用抗凝剂治疗急性冠脉综合征的患者中,SSRI 的确可降低轻微心血管事件的发生率,代价是出血的风险升高[24]。因此,SSRI 虽然使上消化道出血的风险升高,但它或许也可以降低栓塞的发生率。一项数据库研究发现,SSRI 使用者首次心肌梗死的发生率较对照组并未降低[25];而另一项研究[26]则表明,服用 SSRI 的吸烟患者首次因心肌梗死而入院的风险降低。第二项研究的效应值很大:服用 SSRI 的患者因心肌梗死而住院的概率降低了 $1/10^{26}$。这与阿司匹林等抗血小板治疗的效应值相似[27]。

表 3.23　合用 SSRI 时胃肠道出血的近似绝对风险[28]

药物	上消化道出血的绝对风险	下消化道出血的绝对风险
阿司匹林 +SSRI	6%	3%
华法林 +SSRI	4%	3%
NSAID+SSRI	3%	1%
单用 SSRI	2%	1%

注:表中的百分比数字为四舍五入到最接近的整数。

很多研究并未陈述肠道出血绝对风险的改变,其中有些并未提供分母的细节(即治疗时长)。理想情况下,应该将风险定义为每 1 000 患者年额外发生的例数。表 3.23 列出了近似绝对风险(没有分母),来源于一项研究[11]和个人通讯(发表在 Psychiatric News 上)[28]。

既往用过 SSRI 类药物的患者发生消化道出血的风险与对照组无明显差异,表明与出血有关的主要是治疗本身,而非被治疗患者的固有特征[7]。它也意味着 SSRI 的影响在停药后消失了。

出血的风险升高不仅限于上消化道(见表 3.23)。使用 SSRI 后,下消化道出血[29]和子宫出血[12]的发生率也会增加。

颅内/脑内出血(ICH)

SSRI 使用与颅内/脑内出血明确相关,合用 NSAID 和抗凝剂出血风险则进一步增加。

所有 5-羟色胺能活性的抗抑郁药均增高颅内/脑内出血风险。一项含 1 363 990 例 SSRI 使用者的队列研究中[6],颅内/脑内出血的总发生率为 3.8/10 000 患者-年。相比于 TCA,现用 SSRI 药物可升高颅内/脑内出血的风险(RR 为 1.17),绝对调整发生率差异为 6.7/100 000 患者-年。在 SSRI 类药物中,相比于对 5-羟色胺再摄取系统抑制作用弱的抗抑郁药,抑制作用强的药物颅内/脑内出血风险高出 25%(表 3.24)。这相当于绝对调整发生率差异 9.5/100 000 患者-年。总体风险在用药的前 30 天最高。一项 2018 年对 12 项研究进行的荟萃分析证实,SSRI 使颅内/脑内出血风险增高(OR 值 0.8~2.42),意味着再摄取抑制越强的 SSRI,颅内/脑内出血风险越高[30]。此后,一项研究报道 SSRI 药物,无论是单用还是和与抗凝剂合用,均未升高颅内/脑内出血风险[31];而另一项研究[32]发现,SSRI 升高颅内/脑内出血复发的风险高达 31%。

一项数据库研究[33]还发现 SSRI 单用或与 NSAID 合用,均可升高颅内/脑内出血风险。该研究和其他研究提供的绝对风险数据在表 3.24 中进行了汇总。

表 3.24 列出了根据 3 项研究得出的颅内/脑内出血绝对风险估计值。

表 3.24　SSRI 合用或未合用抗凝剂或 NSAID 致颅内出血的绝对风险

研究	单用 SSRI 的风险	SSRI+NSAID 的风险	抗抑郁药 + 抗凝剂的风险
Shin et al. 2015[33]	1/632*(0.16%)	1/175*(0.57%)	—
Renoux et al. 2017[6]	1/450**(0.22%)	—	1/260**(0.38%)
Smoller et al. 2009[34]	1/240***(0.42%)	—	—

* 服用抗抑郁药的 30 天之内。
** 用药者中发生(没有时间限制)。
*** 每年风险(老年人)。

妇产科出血

一项多中心横断面研究[35]发现,抗抑郁药的使用和月经失调有关(异常出血或经血量多,月经不规律,月经过多,等)。该研究还发现,服用 SSRI、文拉法辛、米氮平合用 SSRI 或米氮平的研究组,其月经失调的发生率(24.6%)显著高于未服用任何抗抑郁药的对照组(12.2%)。

异常阴道出血

据报道,有一例年轻女性[36]、一例绝经后妇女[37]和一名 11 岁的青春期前女孩[38]服用 SSRI 发生了异常阴道出血。

产后出血(PPH)

一项研究[39]未发现使用 SSRI 或非 SSRI 抗抑郁药患者 PPH 的风险增高,但是一项大样本队列研究[40]发现 PPH 与各种抗抑郁药的使用相关,正在服用 SSRI 者 NNH(出现 1 例伤害的治疗例数)为 80,服用其他抗抑郁药者 NNH 为 97。一项基于医院的队列研究[41]发现,现用 SSRI 的女性,经非手术阴道分娩后,PPH 的绝对风险为 18%,产后贫血的绝对风险为 12.8%;而没有任何抗抑郁药暴露的女性,PPH 和产后贫血的绝对风险为 8.7%。有 SSRI 暴露的女性产后失血(484mL)也显著高于未服用 SSRI 者(398mL)。服用 SSRI 者住院时长明显增加。最近一项人群研究[42]发现,相比于未服用任何精神活性药物者,使用 5-羟色胺能药物的患者 PPH 风险升高 1.5 倍。该研究强调,已经在服用其他精神药物(如抗精神病药和心境稳定剂)的女性,其 PPH 的风险比未服用任何药物者增加了 3 倍多,提示 PPH 的发生并非完全因为 5-羟色胺能活性,还需要进一步研究来探明其他病理机制。

2021 年,英国 UHRA 签署了一项关于 SSRI 使用和产后失血的警示[43]。

手术和术后出血(表 3.25)

围手术期使用 SSRI 将会使住院患者的死亡率增加 20%(绝对死亡率为 1∶1 000),但不能排除由患者本身原因所致[44]。一项研究发现[45],服用 SSRI 者在骨科手术期间需要输血的可能性为不使用者的 4 倍。这相当于每 10 个服用 SSRI 的患者做手术,就有 1 个需要输血,这是单独服用 NSAID 发生出血风险的 2 倍。同时,需要注意的是,SSRI 治疗过程中,发生髋骨骨折[46]的风险增加 2.4 倍,老年人骨折[47]的风险增加 2 倍(米氮平[48]和 TCA[46]也会增高髋骨骨折的风险)。一项最近的研究发现,术前使用 SSRI、其他类抗抑郁药或抗精神病药,均是择期快速髋关节和膝关节成形术中输血的独立风险因素[49]。

高龄、SSRI 治疗、骨科手术和使用 NSAID 均构成很大的风险。然而,在冠状动脉旁路移植术中,出血的发生率未见明显改变[50]。

表 3.25　SSRI 使用者与未用者围手术期失血和输血的风险[51]

手术	SAD* 使用者和未用者因出血需要再次手术	SAD 使用者和未用者需要输入血制品或红细胞	SAD 使用者和未用者死亡风险的升高
冠状动脉搭桥手术	OR 1.07(0.66~1.74)	OR 1.06(0.90~1.24)	OR 1.53(1.15~2.04)
乳腺癌导向手术	OR 2.7(1.6~4.56)	—	—
骨科手术	—	OR 1.61(0.97~2.68)	OR 0.83(0.69~1.00)
大手术	—	OR 1.19(1.15~1.23)	OR 1.19(1.03~1.37)

*5-羟色胺能抗抑郁药。

OR,优势比。

　　一项对 10 年中接受乳房美容手术的女性进行的总结发现,SSRI 使用者术后出血风险是未服用者的 4.14 倍。作者强调,在择期手术前,权衡停用抗抑郁药的风险和获益非常重要,尤其是心理脆弱的患者[52]。

　　一篇纳入 13 项研究的系统综述发现,服用 SSRI 后围手术期出血的优势比有所增加(*OR* 为 1.21~4.14)[53]。一项研究表明,SSRI 会增加女性乳腺手术[54]过程中出血的风险,所以作者建议手术前 2 周内停用 SSRI。但另一些专家则认为,目前尚缺乏充分的证据支持术前常规停用 SSRI,呼吁这一问题还需随机对照试验进一步阐明[55]。文拉法辛也有类似的作用[53],但度洛西汀可能不会增加出血风险[56]。

SSRI/SNRI 的替代药物

　　非 SSRI 类抗抑郁药,如米氮平和安非他酮,被推荐作为 SSRI 和 SNRI 的安全替代药物[57]。初步研究显示,米氮平、安非他酮和去甲替林对可检测的凝血机制影响较小[58]。但是几乎没有证据证明这些药物更安全。一项荟萃分析发现,米氮平(相比于未接受治疗者)可升高上消化道出血的风险,米氮平或安非他酮与 SSRI 间的出血风险没有差异[59]。

小结

　　5-羟色胺能抗抑郁药会增加各种出血风险。SSRI 类药物的证据最强,出血风险可能与药物对 5-羟色胺转运体的亲和性相关。SSRI 增加消化道出血、出血性卒中、围手术期出血、产后出血和子宫出血等风险。合用阿司匹林、抗凝剂和 NSAID 会加重出血风险。在大多数情况下,使用 SSRI 可增加具临床意义的出血事件风险,尤其是合用其他影响凝血功能的药物时。

概要

- SSRI 会增加消化道出血、子宫出血、脑出血及围手术期出血的风险。
- 在同时服用阿司匹林、NSAID 或口服抗凝剂的患者中,出血的风险进一步增加。
- 正在接受 NSAID、阿司匹林、口服抗凝剂治疗,或既往有脑出血或消化道出血史的患者,尽量避免使用 SSRI/SNRI。
- 更安全的替代药物尚未确定,但是去甲肾上腺素能抗抑郁药(去甲替林、安非他酮)可以选择。
- 如果无法避免使用 SSRI,一定要密切监控,并给予有胃保护作用的 PPI。
- 有限的证据提示 5-羟色胺再摄取抑制作用弱的药物,出血风险可能较低。

参考文献

1. Skop BP, et al. Potential vascular and bleeding complications of treatment with selective serotonin reuptake inhibitors. *Psychosomatics* 1996; 37:12–16.

2. Laporte S, et al. Bleeding risk under selective serotonin reuptake inhibitor (SSRI) antidepressants: a meta-analysis of observational studies. *Pharmacol Res* 2017; 118:19–32.

3. Andrade C, et al. Serotonin reuptake inhibitor antidepressants and abnormal bleeding: a review for clinicians and a reconsideration of mechanisms. *J Clin Psychiatry* 2010; 71:1565–1575.

4. Dall M, et al. There is an association between selective serotonin reuptake inhibitor use and uncomplicated peptic ulcers: a population-based case-control study. *Aliment Pharmacol Ther* 2010; 32:1383–1391.

5. Jiang HY, et al. Use of selective serotonin reuptake inhibitors and risk of upper gastrointestinal bleeding: a systematic review and meta-

analysis. *Clin Gastroenterol Hepatol* 2015; 13:42–50.

6. Renoux C, et al. Association of selective serotonin reuptake inhibitors with the risk for spontaneous intracranial hemorrhage. *JAMA Neurology* 2017; 74:173–180.

7. Dalton SO, et al. Use of selective serotonin reuptake inhibitors and risk of upper gastrointestinal tract bleeding: a population-based cohort study. *Arch Intern Med* 2003; 163:59–64.

8. Verdel BM, et al. Use of serotonergic drugs and the risk of bleeding. *Clin Pharmacol Ther* 2011; 89:89–96.

9. Tatsumi M, et al. Pharmacological profile of antidepressants and related compounds at human monoamine transporters. *Eur J Pharmacol* 1997; 340:249–258.

10. Weinrieb RM, et al. A critical review of selective serotonin reuptake inhibitor-associated bleeding: balancing the risk of treating hepatitis C-infected patients. *J Clin Psychiatry* 2003; 64:1502–1510.

11. Cheng YL, et al. Use of SSRI, but not SNRI, increased upper and lower gastrointestinal bleeding: a nationwide population-based cohort study in Taiwan. *Medicine (Baltimore)* 2015; 94:e2022.

12. Meijer WE, et al. Association of risk of abnormal bleeding with degree of serotonin reuptake inhibition by antidepressants. *Arch Intern Med* 2004; 164:2367–2370.

13. Yuet WC, et al. Selective serotonin reuptake inhibitor use and risk of gastrointestinal and intracranial bleeding. *J Am Osteopath Assoc* 2019; 119:102–111.

14. van Walraven C, et al. Inhibition of serotonin reuptake by antidepressants and upper gastrointestinal bleeding in elderly patients: retrospective cohort study. *BMJ* 2001; 323:655–658.

15. de Abajo FJ, et al. Risk of upper gastrointestinal tract bleeding associated with selective serotonin reuptake inhibitors and venlafaxine therapy: interaction with nonsteroidal anti-inflammatory drugs and effect of acid-suppressing agents. *Arch Gen Psychiatry* 2008; 65:795–803.

16. Lee MT, et al. Concomitant use of NSAIDs or SSRIs with NOACs requires monitoring for bleeding. *Yonsei Med J* 2020; 61:741–749.

17. Quinn GR, et al. Selective serotonin reuptake inhibitors and bleeding risk in anticoagulated patients with atrial fibrillation: an analysis from the ROCKET AF trial. *J Am Heart Assoc* 2018; 7:e008755.

18. de Abajo FJ, et al. Association between selective serotonin reuptake inhibitors and upper gastrointestinal bleeding: population based case-control study. *BMJ* 1999; 319:1106–1109.

19. Lewis JD, et al. Moderate and high affinity serotonin reuptake inhibitors increase the risk of upper gastrointestinal toxicity. *Pharmacoepidemiol Drug Saf* 2008; 17:328–335.

20. Paton C, et al. SSRIs and gastrointestinal bleeding. *BMJ* 2005; 331:529–530.

21. de Jong JC, et al. Combined use of SSRIs and NSAIDs increases the risk of gastrointestinal adverse effects. *Br J Clin Pharmacol* 2003; 55:591–595.

22. Schalekamp T, et al. Increased bleeding risk with concurrent use of selective serotonin reuptake inhibitors and coumarins. *Arch Intern Med* 2008; 168:180–185.

23. Wallerstedt SM, et al. Risk of clinically relevant bleeding in warfarin-treated patients–influence of SSRI treatment. *Pharmacoepidemiol Drug Saf* 2009; 18:412–416.

24. Ziegelstein RC, et al. Selective serotonin reuptake inhibitor use by patients with acute coronary syndromes. *Am J Med* 2007; 120:525–530.

25. Meier CR, et al. Use of selective serotonin reuptake inhibitors and risk of developing first-time acute myocardial infarction. *Br J Clin Pharmacol* 2001; 52:179–184.

26. Sauer WH, et al. Selective serotonin reuptake inhibitors and myocardial infarction. *Circulation* 2001; 104:1894–1898.

27. Antiplatelet Trialists' Collaboration. Collaborative overview of randomised trials of antiplatelet therapy–I: prevention of death, myocardial infarction, and stroke by prolonged antiplatelet therapy in various categories of patients. *BMJ* 1994; 308:81–106.

28. Cheng YL Personal communication, 2017.

29. Wessinger S, et al. Increased use of selective serotonin reuptake inhibitors in patients admitted with gastrointestinal haemorrhage: a multicentre retrospective analysis. *Aliment Pharmacol Ther* 2006; 23:937–944.

30. Douros A, et al. Risk of intracranial hemorrhage associated with the use of antidepressants inhibiting serotonin reuptake: a systematic review. *CNS Drugs* 2018; 32:321–334.

31. Liu L, et al. Selective serotonin reuptake inhibitors and intracerebral hemorrhage risk and outcome. *Stroke* 2020; 51:1135–1141.

32. Kubiszewski P, et al. Association of selective serotonin reuptake inhibitor use after intracerebral hemorrhage with hemorrhage recurrence and depression severity. *JAMA Neurology* 2020; 78:1–8.

33. Shin JY, et al. Risk of intracranial haemorrhage in antidepressant users with concurrent use of non-steroidal anti-inflammatory drugs: nationwide propensity score matched study. *BMJ (Clinical Research Ed)* 2015; 351:h3517.

34. Smoller JW, et al. Antidepressant use and risk of incident cardiovascular morbidity and mortality among postmenopausal women in the Women's Health Initiative study. *Arch Intern Med* 2009; 169:2128–2139.

35. Uguz F, et al. Antidepressants and menstruation disorders in women: a cross-sectional study in three centers. *Gen Hosp Psychiatry* 2012; 34:529–533.

36. Andersohn F, et al. Citalopram-induced bleeding due to severe thrombocytopenia. *Psychosomatics* 2009; 50:297–298.

37. Durmaz O, et al. Vaginal bleeding associated with antidepressants. *Int J Gynaecol Obstet* 2015; 130:284.

38. Turkoglu S, et al. Vaginal bleeding and hemorrhagic prepatellar bursitis in a preadolescent girl, possibly related to fluoxetine. *J Child Adolesc Psychopharmacol* 2015; 25:186–187.

39. Salkeld E, et al. The risk of postpartum hemorrhage with selective serotonin reuptake inhibitors and other antidepressants. *J Clin Psychopharmacol* 2008; 28:230–234.

40. Palmsten K, et al. Use of antidepressants near delivery and risk of postpartum hemorrhage: cohort study of low income women in the United States. *BMJ* 2013; 347:f4877.

41. Lindqvist PG, et al. Selective serotonin reuptake inhibitor use during pregnancy increases the risk of postpartum hemorrhage and anemia: a hospital-based cohort study. *J Thromb Haemost* 2014; 12:1986–1992.

42. Heller HM, et al. Increased postpartum haemorrhage, the possible relation with serotonergic and other psychopharmacological drugs: a matched cohort study. *BMC Pregnancy Childbirth* 2017; 17:166.

43. Gov.UK. Drug Safety Update. SSRI/SNRI antidepressant medicines: small increased risk of postpartum haemorrhage when used in the month before delivery. 2021; https://www.gov.uk/drug-safety-update/ssri-slash-snri-antidepressant-medicines-small-increased-risk-of-postpartum-haemorrhage-when-used-in-the-month-before-delivery?utm_source=e-shot&utm_medium=email&utm_campaign=DSU_January2021split1.

44. Auerbach AD, et al. Perioperative use of selective serotonin reuptake inhibitors and risks for adverse outcomes of surgery. *JAMA Int Med* 2013; 173:1075–1081.

45. Movig KL, et al. Relationship of serotonergic antidepressants and need for blood transfusion in orthopedic surgical patients. *Arch Intern Med* 2003; 163:2354–2358.

46. Liu B, et al. Use of selective serotonin-reuptake inhibitors of tricyclic antidepressants and risk of hip fractures in elderly people. *Lancet* 1998; 351:1303–1307.

47. Richards JB, et al. Effect of selective serotonin reuptake inhibitors on the risk of fracture. *Arch Intern Med* 2007; 167:188–194.

48. Leach MJ, et al. The risk of hip fracture due to mirtazapine exposure when switching antidepressants or using other antidepressants as add-on therapy. *Drugs – Real World Outcomes* 2017; 4:247–255.

49. Gylvin SH, et al. Psychopharmacologic treatment and blood transfusion in fast-track total hip and knee arthroplasty. *Transfusion (Paris)* 2017; 57:971–976.

50. Andreasen JJ, et al. Effect of selective serotonin reuptake inhibitors on requirement for allogeneic red blood cell transfusion following coronary artery bypass surgery. *Am J Cardiovasc Drugs* 2006; 6:243–250.

51. Singh I, et al. Influence of pre-operative use of serotonergic antidepressants (SADs) on the risk of bleeding in patients undergoing different surgical interventions: a meta-analysis. *Pharmacoepidemiol Drug Saf* 2015; 24:237–245.

52. Basile FV, et al. Use of selective serotonin reuptake inhibitors antidepressants and bleeding risk in breast cosmetic surgery. *Aesthetic Plast Surg* 2013; 37:561–566.

53. Mahdanian AA, et al. Serotonergic antidepressants and perioperative bleeding risk: a systematic review. *Exp Opin Drug Saf* 2014; 13:695–704.

54. Jeong BO, et al. Use of serotonergic antidepressants and bleeding risk in patients undergoing surgery. *Psychosomatics* 2014; 55:213–220.

55. Mrkobrada M, et al. Selective serotonin reuptake inhibitors and surgery: to hold or not to hold, that is the question: comment on 'Perioperative use of selective serotonin reuptake inhibitors and risks for adverse outcomes of surgery'. *JAMA Int Med* 2013; 173:1082–1083.

56. Perahia DG, et al. The risk of bleeding with duloxetine treatment in patients who use nonsteroidal anti-inflammatory drugs (NSAIDs): analysis of placebo-controlled trials and post-marketing adverse event reports. *Drug Healthcare Patient Saf* 2013; 5:211–219.

57. Bixby AL, et al. Clinical management of bleeding risk with antidepressants. *Ann Pharmacother* 2019; 53:186–194.

58. Halperin D, et al. Influence of antidepressants on hemostasis. *Dialogues Clin Neurosci* 2007; 9:47–59.

59. Na K-S, et al. Can we recommend mirtazapine and bupropion for patients at risk for bleeding?: a systematic review and meta-analysis. *J Affect Disord* 2018; 225:221–226.

圣约翰草

圣约翰草（St John's Wort, SJW）是贯叶连翘（*Hypericum perforatum*）的俗名。它含有至少 10 种成分，包括金丝桃素、贯叶金丝桃素和黄酮类化合物[1]。圣约翰草制剂制备尚未标准化，这也加大了其临床试验结果的解释难度。圣约翰草的活性成分和作用机制尚不明确[1]。圣约翰草的成分可抑制单胺氧化酶，抑制去甲肾上腺素和 5-羟色胺再摄取，上调 5-羟色胺能受体水平，减少 5-羟色胺受体表达[1]。

一些圣约翰草制剂已经获得传统植物药登记证书[2]；注意它的使用是基于传统用法，而非根据已经证明的疗效和安全性数据。圣约翰草在德国被批准用于治疗抑郁症[2]。

圣约翰草治疗抑郁症的证据

多项研究已经检验了圣约翰草治疗抑郁症的疗效。这些结果已被广泛地审查[3-6]，大多数作者认为圣约翰草似乎对轻、中度抑郁症[3,5-7]有效。例如，Cochrane 的结论是，圣约翰草在治疗轻、中度抑郁症时，疗效优于安慰剂，与标准抗抑郁药相当，耐受性则优于标准抗抑郁药[4]。支持性证据也有不足。德语国家较其他地区的研究得出的结果更好[4]。在和 SSRI 进行的对照研究中，SSRI 的剂量不够，这一问题最近引起了关注[8,9]。有一项圣约翰草的大样本、随机对照试验结果为阴性，对其数据进行重新分析（共两项）发现，猜测自己被纳入活性治疗药物组的患者，其疗效优于认为自己被纳入安慰剂组的患者；患者和医师对接受活性药物的猜测与病情改善有关，但实际接受的治疗与病情改善无关[10,11]。该药对严重抑郁症的疗效仍不明确[4-6]。几乎没有圣约翰草治疗绝经后抑郁[12]和某些疼痛综合征[13]的证据。

需要指出的是：

- 圣约翰草治疗抑郁症的活性成分尚不明确。不同研究使用的圣约翰草制剂均是根据金丝桃素总含量进行标准化。但是研究证据提示，金丝桃素本身不能治疗抑郁症[5]。
- 通过互联网购买的圣约翰草制剂，许多是作为非管制食品添加剂进行销售，通常质量较差或者有掺假[3]。最近对 47 种不同圣约翰草制剂的分析发现，36% 掺入了其他金丝桃品种，19% 掺入了食用色素[2]。
- 所发表的研究一般是急性期治疗研究。只有一些初期的资料支持圣约翰草在中期使用的有效性，圣约翰草对抑郁症长期或预防复发的疗效数据尚不存在[14]。

总的说来，圣约翰草不应使用，因为我们不知道其活性成分是什么，治疗剂量是多少。大部分圣约翰草的制剂未获得批准。

不良反应

圣约翰草的耐受性较好[5,6]。一项对现有研究的系统综述显示，圣约翰草的不良反应明显少于老一代抗抑郁药，略少于 SSRI，与安慰剂相当[6]。其不良反应很少，最常见的是恶心、皮疹、疲乏、坐立不安和光过敏[15]。虽然严重的光毒性反应罕见，仍然应告知患者圣约翰草可增加光敏感性[15]。圣约翰草与 SSRI 类似，会增加出血风险。曾有一个病例报告提示，圣约翰草塞鼻后导致长期鼻衄[16]。案例报告还描述了圣约翰草治疗发生的躁狂、轻躁狂和混合状态[17]。躁狂症状发生于开始治疗后 3 天至 2 个月[17]。接受高剂量治疗以及原有双相障碍病史的患者需谨慎[18]。

药物相互作用

圣约翰草是肠道和肝内 CYP3A4、CYP2C9、CYP2C19、CYP2E1 和肠道 P-糖蛋白的强诱导剂[15,19]。贯叶金丝桃素是产生该效应的原因[20]。不同圣约翰草制剂中的贯叶金丝桃含量差异可达 50 倍，导致不同品牌药物的药物相互作用倾向存在差异。每天少于 1mg 贯叶金丝桃的制剂不太可能诱导细胞色素酶活性[20,21]。CYP3A4 活性在使用圣约翰草后 1~2 周被诱导出来，在停药大概 7 天后转为正常[22]。

研究显示，圣约翰草显著降低血浆华法林[23]、激素类避孕药[24]、地高辛和茚地那韦（一种治疗 HIV 的药物）浓度[15]。据病例报告，圣约翰草降低血浆氯氮平、茶碱、环孢素、格列齐特和他汀类药物浓度[15,19,25,26]。理论上，圣约翰草存在与抗癫痫药发生相互作用的风险[19]。圣约翰草能增强氯吡格雷（前体药物）的作用[19]。当圣约翰草与舍曲林、帕罗西汀、奈法唑酮和色胺类联用时，曾发生 5-羟色胺综合征[27,28]。圣约翰草不能与任何具有显著 5-羟色胺能作用的药物联用。

很多人认为植物药是"天然的"因而无害的[29]。许多人没有意识到这些治疗导致不良反应或与其他药物发生相互作用的潜在风险。在圣约翰草被注册为抗抑郁药的德国，曾经进行一项大样本研究（$n=588$），发现每开一张圣约翰草处方，就有一人在没有寻求医师指导的情况下购买了圣约翰草[30]。这些人中许多有严重或持久的抑郁症，但是很少有人告诉医师他们在服用圣约翰草。一项美国的小样本研究（$n=22$）发现，患者倾向于服用圣约翰草，因为它是容易获得的替代药物，而且认为该药比处方药更纯、更安全。很少有人会与传统的保健人员讨论该药[31]。临床医师应主动询问患者是否使用该类药物，并努力破除患者认为天然等于安全的迷信（框 3.3）。

框 3.3　患者应该知道的要点

- 现有证据提示圣约翰草治疗轻、中度抑郁症有效，但是我们不太了解应该服用多大剂量、其不良反应是什么。对重度抑郁的疗效证据较少。
- 圣约翰草不是获批的药物。
- 圣约翰草可与其他药物发生药物相互作用，导致严重不良反应。一些重要药物因此代谢增快，导致治疗无效，发生严重后果（如 HIV 载量增高、口服避孕药失败导致意外妊娠、降低华法林的抗凝作用导致血栓形成）。
- 抑郁症的症状有时候可由其他躯体疾病或精神障碍造成。必须调查这些可能的病因。
- 如果患者准备或已经使用植物药或者自然疗法进行治疗，最好首先咨询医师。

参考文献

1. Velingkar VS, et al. A current update on phytochemistry, pharmacology and herb–drug interactions of Hypericum perforatum. *Phytochemistry Rev* 2017; **16**:725–744.

2. Booker A, et al. St John's wort (Hypericum perforatum) products – an assessment of their authenticity and quality. *Phytomedicine* 2018; **40**:158–164.

3. National Institute for Clinical Excellence. Depression: the treatment and management of depression in adults. Clinical Guidance [CG90] 2009 (last reviewed December 2013); https://www.nice.org.uk/guidance/cg90.

4. Linde K, et al. St John's Wort for major depression. *Cochrane Database Syst Rev* 2008; CD000448.

5. Ng QX, et al. Clinical use of Hypericum perforatum (St John's wort) in depression: a meta-analysis. *J Affect Disord* 2017; 210:211–221.

6. Apaydin EA, et al. A systematic review of St. John's wort for major depressive disorder. *Syst Rev* 2016; 5:148.

7. Volz HP. Hypericum and Depression, in P Riederer, G Laux, T Nagatsu, W Le, C Riederer eds., *NeuroPsychopharmacotherapy*. Cham: Springer; 2020:1–8.

8. Asher GN, et al. Comparative benefits and harms of complementary and alternative medicine therapies for initial treatment of major depressive disorder: systematic review and meta-analysis. *J Altern Complement Med* 2017; 23:907–919.

9. Gartlehner G, et al. Pharmacological and non-pharmacological treatments for major depressive disorder: review of systematic reviews. *BMJ Open* 2017; 7:e014912.

10. Chen JA, et al. Association between patient beliefs regarding assigned treatment and clinical response: reanalysis of data from the Hypericum Depression Trial Study Group. *J Clin Psychiatry* 2011; 72:1669–1676.

11. Chen JA, et al. Association between physician beliefs regarding assigned treatment and clinical response: re-analysis of data from the Hypericum Depression Trial Study Group. *Asian J Psychiatr* 2015; 13:23–29.

12. Eatemadnia A, et al. The effect of Hypericum perforatum on postmenopausal symptoms and depression: a randomized controlled trial. *Complement Ther Med* 2019; 45:109–113.

13. Galeotti N. Hypericum perforatum (St John's wort) beyond depression: a therapeutic perspective for pain conditions. *J Ethnopharmacol* 2017; 200:136–146.

14. Cleare A, et al. Evidence-based guidelines for treating depressive disorders with antidepressants: a revision of the 2008 British Association for Psychopharmacology guidelines. *J Psychopharmacology* 2015; 29:459–525.

15. Russo E, et al. Hypericum perforatum: pharmacokinetic, mechanism of action, tolerability, and clinical drug-drug interactions. *Phytother Res* 2014; 28:643–655.

16. Crampsey DP, et al. Nasal insertion of St John's wort: an unusual cause of epistaxis. *J Laryngol Otol* 2007; 121:279–280.

17. Bostock E, et al. Mania associated with herbal medicines, other than cannabis: a systematic review and quality assessment of case reports. *Front Psychiatry* 2018; 9:280.

18. Sarris J. Herbal medicines in the treatment of psychiatric disorders: 10-year updated review. *Phytother Res* 2018; 32:1147–1162.

19. Soleymani S, et al. Clinical risks of St John's Wort (Hypericum perforatum) co-administration. *Exp Opin Drug Metab Toxicol* 2017; 13:1047–1062.

20. Chrubasik-Hausmann S, et al. Understanding drug interactions with St John's wort (Hypericum perforatum L.): impact of hyperforin content. *J Pharm Pharmacol* 2018; 71:129–138.

21. Nicolussi S, et al. Clinical relevance of St. John's wort drug interactions revisited. *Br J Pharmacol* 2020; 177:1212–1226.

22. Imai H, et al. The recovery time-course of CYP3A after induction by St John's wort administration. *Br J Clin Pharmacol* 2008; 65:701–707.

23. Choi S, et al. A systematic review of the pharmacokinetic and pharmacodynamic interactions of herbal medicine with warfarin. *PLoS One* 2017; 12:e0182794.

24. Berry-Bibee EN, et al. Co-administration of St. John's wort and hormonal contraceptives: a systematic review. *Contraception* 2016; 94:668–677.

25. Xu H, et al. Effects of St John's wort and CYP2C9 genotype on the pharmacokinetics and pharmacodynamics of gliclazide. *Br J Pharmacol* 2008; 153:1579–1586.

26. Andren L, et al. Interaction between a commercially available St. John's wort product (Movina) and atorvastatin in patients with hypercholesterolemia. *Eur J Clin Pharmacol* 2007; 63:913–916.

27. Anon. Reminder: St John's Wort (*Hypericum perforatum*) interactions. *Curr Problems Pharmacovigilance* 2000; 26:6–7.

28. Lantz MS, et al. St. John's wort and antidepressant drug interactions in the elderly. *J Geriatr Psychiatry Neurol* 1999; 12:7–10.

29. Barnes J, et al. Different standards for reporting ADRs to herbal remedies and conventional OTC medicines: face-to-face interviews with 515 users of herbal remedies. *Br J Clin Pharmacol* 1998; 45:496–500.

30. Linden M, et al. Self medication with St. John's wort in depressive disorders: an observational study in community pharmacies. *J Affect Disord* 2008; 107:205–210.

31. Wagner PJ, et al. Taking the edge off: why patients choose St. John's Wort. *J Fam Pract* 1999; 48:615–619.

抗抑郁药：相对不良反应——简略指南

表 3.26 非常粗略地列出了与标准抗抑郁药相关的少数不良反应的绝对和相对风险，未列出参考文献。

表 3.26　抗抑郁药的常见不良反应

药物	镇静	体位性低血压§	心脏传导紊乱§	抗胆碱能作用	恶心、呕吐	性功能障碍§
三环类						
阿米替林	+++	+++	+++	+++	+	+++
氯米帕明	++	+++	+++	++	++	+++
度硫平	+++	+++	+++	++	+	+
多塞平	+++	++	+++	+++	+	+
丙米嗪	++	+++	+++	++l	+	+
洛非帕明	+	+	+	++	+	+
去甲替林	+	++	++	+	+	+
曲米帕明	+++	+++	++	++	+	+
其他抗抑郁药						
阿戈美拉汀	+	−	−	−	−	−
度洛西汀	−	−*	−	−	++	++
左米那普仑（SNRI）	−	−*	−	−	++	++
米安色林	++	−	−	−	−	−
米氮平	+++	+	−	+	+	−
瑞波西汀	+	−*	−	+	+	+
曲唑酮	+++	+	+	+	+	+
文拉法辛（SNRI）	−	−*	+	−	+++	+++
选择性 5-羟色胺再摄取抑制剂						
西酞普兰	−	−	+	−	++	+++
艾司西酞普兰	−	−	+	−	++	+++
氟西汀	−	−	−	−	++	+++
氟伏沙明	+	−	−	−	+++	+++
帕罗西汀	+	−	−	+	++	+++
舍曲林	−	−	−	−	++	+++
维拉唑酮	−	−	−	−	++	++
伏硫西汀	−	+	−	−	++	+

续表

药物	镇静	体位性 低血压 [§]	心脏 传导紊乱 [§]	抗胆碱能 作用	恶心、 呕吐	性功能 障碍 [§]
单胺氧化酶抑制剂						
异卡波	+	++	+	++	+	+
苯已肼	+	+	+	+	+	+
反环苯丙胺	−	+	+	+	+	+
可逆性单胺氧化酶 A 抑制剂						
吗氯贝胺	−	−	−	−	+	+

注:

+++,高发生率/严重性;++,中度发生率/严重性;+,极低或无。

* 报告过高血压。

[§] 有时可在本章特定章节找到更详细的解释。

焦虑谱系障碍

　　焦虑障碍可独立发生,与其他精神障碍共病(尤其是抑郁症),继发于其他躯体疾病(如甲状腺功能亢进),或由药物(如咖啡因)所致。焦虑障碍与其他精神疾病共病很常见。

　　焦虑谱系障碍倾向于慢性化,治疗通常只是部分有效。值得注意的是,焦虑障碍患者可能对药物的不良反应特别敏感[1]。例如,初始高剂量的 SSRI 可能特别难以耐受。

苯二氮䓬类药物

　　苯二氮䓬类药物能够快速缓解急性焦虑状态[2]。所有的指南和共识声明均建议,这类药物只应用于治疗严重、致残性或使人极其痛苦的焦虑。因为这类药物可能造成躯体依赖和戒断症状,所以应该使用最低有效剂量,持续最短的时间(最长 4 周);而药物滥用的患者则应该慎重地使用更长期的治疗策略。这些建议对大多数患者都是合理的,需要遵守。只有极少数能力严重受损的焦虑患者可从苯二氮䓬类药物长期治疗中获益,对于这些患者不应拒绝长期苯二氮䓬类药物治疗。然而,众所周知,在焦虑[3]和抑郁[4]的治疗中,苯二氮䓬类药物长期过度使用非常普遍,尤其在美国,对苯二氮䓬类药物的态度明显不同于其他发达国家[5]。

　　NICE(英国国家卫生与临床优化研究所)建议苯二氮䓬类药物不应用于治疗惊恐障碍[6]。在其他国家,阿普唑仑被广泛地用于这一疾病。将苯二氮䓬类药物用于治疗创伤后应激障碍时应该特别小心[7]。

SSRI/SNRI

　　治疗广泛性焦虑障碍(GAD)时,SSRI 的初始剂量应为治疗抑郁症常规初始剂量的 50%(因治疗开始后可能出现焦虑症状加重[8]),并逐渐增加至患者可耐受的正常抗抑郁作用的剂量范围。该建议也适用于文拉法辛和度洛西汀。通常在 6 周内出现轻度药物疗效,且疗效随时间逐渐增加[9]。GAD 的最佳疗程尚无定论,但应该至少 1 年[10,11]。对广泛性焦虑障碍的有效治疗可预防患者发展为抑郁症[10]。

　　早期一项网络荟萃分析提示,在所有治疗 GAD 的 SSRI 类药物中,氟西汀可能最有效,舍曲林耐受性最好[12]。最近一项分析发现安非他酮[13]或阿戈美拉汀[14]是最有效的 GAD 治疗药物。两个分析均未发现劳拉西泮或伏硫西汀的疗效明确优于安慰剂。

　　治疗惊恐障碍时,初始剂量和加药原则与广泛性焦虑障碍相同。氯米帕明[15]、西酞普兰[16]和舍曲林[17]在抗抑郁药量范围下端时,可获得疗效和不良反应的最佳平衡,而帕罗西汀则需较高剂量($\geqslant 40$mg)[18]。当药物的标准剂量无效时,尝试使用较高剂量可能有效——SSRI 在批准的剂量范围内,随着剂量升高,治疗焦虑障碍的疗效增强(SNRI 没有该效应)[19]。药物起效时间最长可能达 6 周。SSRI 对女性的疗效优于男性[20]。有证据表明,合用氯硝西泮可更快起效(但不会提高整体有效率)[18]。最佳疗程尚无定论,但应该至少 8 个月[21]。一项大型自然研究发现令人信服的证据,支持用药 3 年以上是有益的[22]。停药后只有不到 50%的患者能维持良好的状态[23]。

　　治疗创伤后应激障碍时,SSRI 也需从低剂量起始,尽管要达到最佳疗效常常需要高剂量(如氟西汀 60mg)。起效时间通常在 8 周内,但也可能长达 12 周[23]。其治疗时间需持续至少 6 个月,甚至更长时间 [11,24,25]。

尽管 SSRI 被批准用于治疗强迫症的剂量高于被批准用于治疗抑郁症的剂量(如氟西汀 60mg,帕罗西汀 40~60mg),但较低的剂量(标准抗抑郁药量)也可能有效,尤其是用于维持治疗 [26]。通常,起效时间往往慢于抑郁症(可能需要 10~12 周)。应该增加到足够剂量以获得最佳疗效。治疗时间需持续至少 1 年 [11]。持续治疗 2 年的患者,其复发率是刚有效即停药者的 50%(25%~40% vs 80%)[27]。大多数强迫症患者病情迁延,症状严重程度随着时间而波动 [28]。二线治疗通常是加用阿立哌唑或利培酮。

躯体变形障碍(BDD)应首先用认知行为疗法治疗。若症状为中、重度,可使用 SSRI 增强疗效 [29]。丁螺环酮可以增强 SSRI 的疗效 [29],但尚未开展 RCT 研究。

社交恐惧症患者常常能耐受抗抑郁药的标准起始剂量 [30,31],有些患者增加剂量可能有益,但并非必须加量。药物通常在 8 周内起效,但治疗需持续至少 1 年 [31]。需要注意的是,NICE 推荐将认知行为治疗作为社交恐惧症的一线治疗 [32]。

使用 SSRI 类药物治疗的患者,均应密切监测其静坐不能、焦虑加重和自杀观念等不良反应的出现;年龄小于 30 岁、合并抑郁症和已知自杀风险高的患者出现上述症状的风险最大 [29,33]。

选择性 5-羟色胺再摄取抑制剂(SSRI)不宜突然停药,因为焦虑谱系障碍患者对停药症状(见本章关于 "抗抑郁药停药症状" 部分)特别敏感。在可耐受的情况下,缓慢减药的过程需要数月。

普瑞巴林

普瑞巴林已被批准用于广泛性焦虑障碍(GAD)的治疗。几项大型随机对照试验表明,其疗效和耐受性良好,起效速度可与苯二氮䓬类药物相媲美 [34]。普瑞巴林用于治疗广泛性焦虑障碍的初始剂量为 150mg,逐渐增加至最高剂量 600mg,分 2~3 次服用。普瑞巴林常被滥用(往往与阿片类药物合用 [35]),有显著的用于娱乐的风险 [36]。普瑞巴林不应突然停药,因为可能会引起严重的停药综合征,包括癫痫发作 [37]。

心理学方法

目前,已有充分证据支持心理干预对焦虑谱系障碍的疗效 [11,38]。如暴露疗法可用于治疗强迫症和社交恐惧症。治疗初期,可能需要药物治疗,以帮助患者提高对心理干预的接受度,但是支持这种假说的证据有限。一些研究表明,心理治疗和药物治疗结合可取得最佳疗效 [6,39],但也有研究结果为阴性 [40,41]。

对心理干预循证基础的讨论不在本指南的范围之内。人们普遍认为,对于多数患者而言,心理疗法是合适的一线治疗,这得到了 NICE 的支持 [6]。

NICE 指南中广泛性焦虑障碍 [6]、惊恐障碍 [6] 和强迫症 [29] 治疗概要

- 建议使用 "阶梯治疗" 方案,以便选择最有效的干预措施。
- 建议综合评估,考虑痛苦和功能损害的程度,合并精神疾病、物质滥用或躯体疾病的影响,以及既往用药的疗效。
- 首先治疗原发疾病。
- 心理治疗比药物治疗有效,应该尽可能将其作为一线治疗。NICE 指南中有关于所推荐心

理治疗的类型和疗程的详细说明。
- 药物治疗也是有效的。大多数证据支持使用 SSRI（舍曲林为一线用药）。
- 告知患者每种治疗方法可能的利弊。
- 难治性复杂性焦虑障碍应考虑联合治疗。

惊恐障碍

- 不宜使用苯二氮䓬类药物。
- SSRI 应作为一线用药。如有 SSRI 类药物禁忌证或治疗无效，可用丙米嗪或氯米帕明。
- 应鼓励患者自助（基于认知行为治疗原则），同样鼓励接受正规的认知行为治疗。

广泛性焦虑障碍

- 不宜使用苯二氮䓬类药物，除非危急情况。
- 一种 SSRI 应作为一线用药。
- SNRI 和普瑞巴林可分别作为二线和三线选择。
- 应鼓励高强度的心理干预和自助（基于认知行为治疗原则）。
- 不宜使用抗精神病药（包括喹硫平）。

强迫症（有中度或重度功能损害）

- 使用 SSRI 或强化认知行为治疗。
- 单一治疗方法不理想时，联合 SSRI 和认知行为治疗。
- SSRI 无效时换用氯米帕明。
- 若疗效仍欠佳，加用一种抗精神病药，或联合氯米帕明和西酞普兰（框 3.4~框 3.8）。

框 3.4 广泛性焦虑障碍

危机管理	
药物	评论
苯二氮䓬类药	通常仅短期使用，最长时间 2~4 周；但是也有人认为苯二氮䓬类药的风险被夸大了[42]
一线治疗药物（按优先顺序）[29]	
SSRI（最高剂量为批准的最大剂量）	治疗初期症状可能加重。建议小剂量起始。优先选择氟西汀和舍曲林[12]
SNRI[14]（最高剂量为批准的最大剂量）	治疗初期症状可能加重。建议小剂量起始
普瑞巴林，150~600mg/d，分次服用	治疗第一周即可起效[43]。滥用增多。明显的停药综合征
二线治疗药物（耐受性差或证据弱，没有优先顺序）	
阿戈美拉汀[44]：10~50mg/d	阿戈美拉汀治疗 6 个月可预防复发[45]
β 受体阻断剂 普萘洛尔 40~120mg/d，分次服用	40mg 起始，逐渐增加剂量到起效。对躯体症状有效，尤其是心动过速[46]
丁螺环酮 15~60mg/d，分次服用	起效延迟，需要 6 周时间获得和苯二氮䓬类药物相似疗效[47]

续框

危机管理	
药物	评论
羟嗪 50~100mg/d,分次服用	尚不清楚羟嗪的疗效是因为其抗焦虑作用还是镇静作用 [48]
喹硫平 (缓释剂,50~300mg/d)	推荐单药治疗。对于难治性患者,作为 SSRI/SNRI 的增效剂可能无效 [49]
三环类抗抑郁药 氯米帕明,50~250mg/d[50-52]	氯米帕明从 10mg/d 起始,逐渐增加剂量
丙米嗪 75~200mg/d,分次服用 [53]	丙米嗪每 4 天增加 25mg,达到 100mg 后,增量为 50mg[10]
MAOI 苯乙肼 45~90mg/d,分次服 [54]	用于治疗焦虑抑郁混合状态,患者需要禁食高酪胺食物
米氮平 15~30mg,晚上服 [55,56]	
实验性 母菊,220~1 500mg/d	两项 RCT,使用标准剂量母菊和安慰剂对照,一项阳性结果,一项阴性结果 [57]
银杏叶 240~480mg/d	一项 RCT 使用了标准剂量银杏叶和安慰剂对照,结果阳性 [58]
薰衣草油制剂 80~160mg/d	一项 RCT,使用了标准剂量薰衣草油制剂与安慰剂和帕罗西汀对照,结果阳性 [59]
利鲁唑 50~100mg/d[60]	需要监测肝功能

框 3.5　惊恐障碍

危机管理	
药物	评论
苯二氮䓬类药	快速起效,如果停药惊恐症状会很快反复 [61]。NICE 不推荐 [6]。Cochrane 也不推荐 [62]
一线治疗药物(按优先顺序)[6,63]	
SSRI (最高剂量为批准的最大剂量)	疗效延迟(所有抗抑郁药均有这种特征 [64]),治疗初期惊恐症状可能加重 [6]。得到 Cochrane 支持 [65]
文拉法辛 MR 75~225mg[63]	从 37.5mg 起始,治疗 7 天
二线治疗药物(耐受性差或证据弱,没有优先顺序)	
米氮平 15~60mg/d[66]	一项荟萃分析提示米氮平对惊恐症状没有效果,但是对其焦虑症状有效 [63]。总体而言,资料相当有限 [67]

续框

危机管理	
药物	**评论**
吗氯贝胺 300~500mg/d [68]	一项使用 450mg/d 的固定剂量研究和一项可变剂量研究支持其有效 [68,69]
MAOI 苯乙肼 10~60mg/d [64]	没有长期治疗的研究,由于耐受性较差,仅用于难治性病例 [64]
三环类抗抑郁药 氯米帕明 25~250mg/d [64] 丙米嗪 25~300mg/d [64] 洛非帕明 70~140mg/d,分次服用 [70]	小剂量起始,根据疗效和安全性逐渐增加剂量
实验性	
D-环丝氨酸 50mg/d	一项 RCT 研究提示可提高对 CBT 的疗效,但在随访时,疗效消失 [71]
加巴喷丁 600~3 600mg/d	一项 RCT 研究发现加巴喷丁和安慰剂没有区别。但是能显著改善严重患者的症状 [72]
肌醇 12g/d [73]	一项含 21 例受试者的安慰剂对照研究结果为阳性。在一项研究中疗效和伏氟沙明相似 [74]。耐受性良好
左乙拉西坦 250mg,每天两次 [67]	通常耐受性良好
吲哚洛尔 7.5mg/d	一项含 21 例患者的双盲安慰剂对照研究显示,吲哚洛尔 2.5mg,每天 3 次作为氟西汀的增效剂,治疗难治性惊恐障碍有效 [75]
丙戊酸盐 500~2 250mg/d	两项小样本的开放性研究得到阳性结果 [76,77]
氢化可的松	仅仅在急性期治疗证明可以预防 PTSD 发生 [78]

框 3.6　创伤后应激障碍(PTSD)

一线治疗药物(按优先顺序) (注意:在药物治疗前,应该先使用心理方法 [79,80])	
SSRI (最高剂量为批准的最大剂量)	帕罗西汀、舍曲林或者氟西汀是优先选用的 SSRI [81,82]。NICE 推荐 [79]
文拉法辛 MR 37.5~300mg [83]	NICE 推荐 [79]
二线治疗药物(耐受性差或证据弱,没有优先顺序)	
抗精神病药 奥氮平 5~20mg 利培酮 0.5~6 mg 喹硫平 50~800mg [85]	抗精神病药对 PTSD 的闯入性症状(闪回和梦魇)有效,但是对回避和过度唤醒症状无效。作为单一治疗或辅助治疗进行了研究 [84]。 NICE 特别提到了利培酮 [79]

续框

米氮平 15~45mg/d[86]	NICE 指南推荐 [79]。一项网络荟萃分析提示为第二个最有效的药物 [87]
MAOI	NICE 指南推荐 [79]。一项网络荟萃分析提示为最有效的药物 [87]
苯乙肼 15~75mg/d[88]	
哌唑嗪 2~15mg,晚上服 [89]	治疗梦魇和睡眠紊乱。从晚上服 1mg 起始,逐渐加量以减少低血压的风险。一项系统综述支持该疗效 [90]
三环类抗抑郁药	NICE 指南推荐阿米替林 [79]
阿米替林 50~300mg/d[91]	所有 TCA 都需从小剂量起始,根据耐受性逐渐加量
丙米嗪 50~300mg/d	最好的支持性证据是去甲丙米嗪,但是该药没有广泛提供 [87]
IV 氯胺酮 [92,93]	可快速减轻症状。高质量 RCT 显示其急性和长期疗效 [94]
实验性	
度洛西汀 60~120mg/d	两项小样本开放研究显示其疗效。起始剂量 30mg,1 周 [95,96]
拉莫三嗪 最高到 500mg/d	一项 15 例患者的小样本双盲研究 [97]
苯妥英 血浆浓度 10~20ng/mL[98]	12 例患者的开放性研究
丙戊酸盐,最高 2.5g[99]	可能无效 [87]

框 3.7   强迫性障碍

一线治疗药物(按优先顺序)	
药物	**评论**
所有 SSRI[39] (最高剂量为批准的最大剂量)	若第一个 SSRI 不能耐受或者疗效差,可以尝试换用另一个 SSRI[29]
氯米帕明(最高 250mg)	由于耐受性差,推荐至少是在一个 SSRI 治疗失败后再用 [29]
二线治疗药物(耐受性差或证据弱)	
在 SSRI 基础上加用抗精神病药(研究中用了低至中等剂量)[100,101]	大部分证据支持用阿立哌唑或利培酮 [100],也有些证据支持氟哌啶醇 [101]
西酞普兰 40mg 联合氯米帕明 150mg	根据一项小样本随机开放研究 [102]。NICE 推荐 [29]。需要监测 ECG
乙酰半胱氨酸 [103] 最高 2 400mg/d, 在 SSRI 或氯米帕明基础上合用	胃肠道不良反应可能成问题。5 项对照研究中,2 项为阴性结果。汇总分析显示治疗有效 [104]
拉莫三嗪 100mg+SSRI[105]	拉莫三嗪必须按照说明书逐渐增加剂量。对有些患者可能加重 OCD 症状 [106]
托吡酯 最高 400mg[107,108],SSRI 基础上加用	托吡酯耐受性差,对强迫思维有效,但对强迫行为效果差 [107]。两项试验发现托吡酯无效 [109,110]

续框

药物	评论
实验性	
高剂量 SSRI： 艾司西酞普兰 25~50mg[111] 舍曲林 250~400mg[112]	根据耐受性逐渐增加剂量。建议监测 ECG
美金刚 20mg/d	在 SSRI 基础上加用，有良好的证据[113]
NSAID 如塞来昔布 400mg/d	有一些支持证据[110]
金刚烷胺 200mg/d	一项 RCT 获得阳性结果[114]
SNRI 文拉法辛，最高 375mg[115] 度洛西汀 60mg[116]	
米氮平 30~60mg[117]	30 例患者的小样本研究[120]
5-HT₃ 拮抗剂 格拉司琼 1mg+ 伏氟沙明 200mg[118] 昂丹司琼 4mg+ 氟西汀 20mg[119]	每个药都有证据，昂丹司琼可能效果更好[120]
普瑞巴林 75~225mg/d，在舍曲林治疗基础上加用	一项 RCT 获得阳性结果[121]
利鲁唑 50mg，每天 2 次，在原有药物治疗基础上加用[122]	早期研究结果不一致[110]
抗雄激素，曲普瑞林 3.75mg 肌内注射，4 周一次，在原有药物治疗基础上加用[123]	在 6 例男性患者中进行的开放研究
氯米帕明静脉注射[124] 氯胺酮静脉注射[125,126]	相比于口服剂型，起效快。 一项氯米帕明研究提示，口服氯米帕明治疗无效后，静脉给药有效。 氯胺酮——证据资料正在积累中[110]
吗啡，每周一次 15~45mg，在原有药物治疗基础上加用[127]	含 23 例难治性患者的小样本研究。疗效持续时间短暂。

框 3.8 社交焦虑障碍

一线治疗药物 [128] (按优先顺序)	
SSRI (最高剂量为批准的最大剂量)	如果第一个 SSRI 疗效差,可以尝试换到另一个 SSRI [29] 荟萃分析支持伏氟沙明 [129] 和西酞普兰 [130] 维拉唑酮的资料逐渐积累 [131]
文拉法辛缓释剂 75~225mg/d	
二线治疗药物(耐受性差或证据弱,没有优先顺序)	
奥氮平 5~20mg [132]	几乎没有关于抗精神病药的研究。大部分证据是奥氮平
阿替洛尔 25~100mg/d	可以减轻表演场景的自主神经症状 [132]
苯二氮䓬类药 氯硝西泮 0.3~6mg/d [132] 舍曲林 + 氯硝西泮 (最高 3mg/d) [133]	按需使用苯二氮䓬类药物有效,大部分证据是氯硝西泮或溴西泮治疗 由一种 SSRI 换用文拉法辛,不如在 SSRI 治疗基础上加氯硝西泮 有效 [133]
加巴喷丁 900mg+3 600mg/d [132]	
左乙拉西坦 300~3 000mg/d,分次服用 [134]	
吗氯贝胺 600mg/d 分次服	起始剂量 300mg/d,分次服。在英国吗氯贝胺有社交焦虑障碍的适 应证。NICE 指南推荐 [128]
苯乙肼 15~90mg/d [135]	必须避免食用含酪胺食品。 NICE 指南推荐 [128]
普瑞巴林 150~600mg/d [132]	600mg/d 优于安慰剂 [132]
实验性	
氯胺酮 0.5mg/kg 静脉注射	一项设计严格的 RCT 试验 [136]
托吡酯 25~400mg/d [137]	一项含 23 例患者的开放研究提示有效,但是耐受性差
丙戊酸盐 500~2 500mg/d [138]	一项含 17 例患者的开放研究提示有效

参考文献

1. Nash JR and Nutt DJ. Pharmacotherapy of anxiety. *Handb Exp Pharmacol* 2005; 469–501.
2. Martin JL, et al. Benzodiazepines in generalized anxiety disorder: heterogeneity of outcomes based on a systematic review and meta-analysis of clinical trials. *J Psychopharmacology* 2007; 21:774–782.
3. Benitez CI, et al. Use of benzodiazepines and selective serotonin reuptake inhibitors in middle-aged and older adults with anxiety disorders: a longitudinal and prospective study. *Am J Geriatr Psychiatry* 2008; 16:5–13.
4. Demyttenaere K, et al. Clinical factors influencing the prescription of antidepressants and benzodiazepines: results from the European study of the epidemiology of mental disorders (ESEMeD). *J Affect Disord* 2008; 110:84–93.
5. Hirschtritt ME, et al. Balancing the risks and benefits of benzodiazepines. *JAMA* 2021; 325:347–348.
6. National Institute for Health and Clinical Excellence. Generalised anxiety disorder and panic disorder in adults: management. Clinical Guideline [CG113]. 2011 (last updated July 2019); http://guidance.nice.org.uk/CG113.
7. Davidson JR. Use of benzodiazepines in social anxiety disorder, generalized anxiety disorder, and posttraumatic stress disorder. *J Clin Psychiatry* 2004; 65 Suppl 5:29–33.
8. Scott A, et al. Antidepressant drugs in the treatment of anxiety disorders. *Adv Psychiatric Treatment* 2001; 7:275–282.
9. Ballenger JC. Remission rates in patients with anxiety disorders treated with paroxetine. *J Clin Psychiatry* 2004; 65:1696–1707.

10. Davidson JR, et al. A psychopharmacological treatment algorithm for generalised anxiety disorder (GAD). *J Psychopharmacology* 2010; 24:3–26.

11. Baldwin DS, et al. Evidence-based pharmacological treatment of anxiety disorders, post-traumatic stress disorder and obsessive-compulsive disorder: a revision of the 2005 guidelines from the British Association for Psychopharmacology. *J Psychopharmacol* 2014; 28:403–439.

12. Baldwin D, et al. Efficacy of drug treatments for generalised anxiety disorder: systematic review and meta-analysis. *BMJ* 2011; 342:d1199.

13. Slee A, et al. Pharmacological treatments for generalised anxiety disorder: a systematic review and network meta-analysis. *Lancet* 2019; 393:768–777.

14. Kong W, et al. Comparative remission rates and tolerability of drugs for generalised anxiety disorder: a systematic review and network meta-analysis of double-blind randomized controlled trials. *Front Pharmacol* 2020; 11:580858.

15. Caillard V, et al. Comparative effects of low and high doses of clomipramine and placebo in panic disorder: a double-blind controlled study. French University Antidepressant Group. *Acta Psychiatr Scand* 1999; 99:51–58.

16. Wade AG, et al. The effect of citalopram in panic disorder. *Br J Psychiatry* 1997; 170:x549–x553.

17. Londborg PD, et al. Sertraline in the treatment of panic disorder. A multi-site, double-blind, placebo-controlled, fixed-dose investigation. *Br J Psychiatry* 1998; 173:54–60.

18. Pollack MH, et al. Combined paroxetine and clonazepam treatment strategies compared to paroxetine monotherapy for panic disorder. *J Psychopharmacology* 2003; 17:276–282.

19. Jakubovski E, et al. Systematic review and meta-analysis: dose-response curve of SSRIs and SNRIs in anxiety disorders. *Depress Anxiety* 2019; 36:198–212.

20. Clayton AH, et al. Sex differences in clinical presentation and response in panic disorder: pooled data from sertraline treatment studies. *Arch Women's Mental Health* 2006; 9:151–157.

21. Rickels K, et al. Panic disorder: long-term pharmacotherapy and discontinuation. *J Clin Psychopharmacol* 1998; 18:12S-18S.

22. Choy Y, et al. Three-year medication prophylaxis in panic disorder: to continue or discontinue? A naturalistic study. *Compr Psychiatry* 2007; 48:419–425.

23. Michelson D, et al. Continuing treatment of panic disorder after acute response: randomised, placebo-controlled trial with fluoxetine. The Fluoxetine Panic Disorder Study Group. *Br J Psychiatry* 1999; 174:213–218.

24. Davidson J, et al. Efficacy of sertraline in preventing relapse of posttraumatic stress disorder: results of a 28-week double-blind, placebo-controlled study. *Am J Psychiatry* 2001; 158:1974–1981.

25. Stein DJ, et al. Pharmacotherapy for post traumatic stress disorder (PTSD). *Cochrane Database Syst Rev* 2006; CD002795.

26. Martenyi F, et al. Fluoxetine v. placebo in prevention of relapse in post-traumatic stress disorder. *Br J Psychiatry* 2002; 181:315–320.

27. The Expert Consensus Panel for obsessive-compulsive disorder. Treatment of obsessive-compulsive disorder. *J Clin Psychiatry* 1997; 58 Suppl 4:2–72.

28. Catapano F, et al. Obsessive-compulsive disorder: a 3-year prospective follow-up study of patients treated with serotonin reuptake inhibitors OCD follow-up study. *J Psychiatr Res* 2006; 40:502–510.

29. National Institute for Clinical Excellence. Surveillance decision. Evidence: obsessive-compulsive disorder and body dysmorphic disorder: treatment. Clinical Guidance [CG31]. 2005 (last updated February 2019); https://www.nice.org.uk/guidance/cg31/resources/2019-surveillance-of-obsessivecompulsive-disorder-and-body-dysmorphic-disorder-treatment-nice-guideline-cg31-6713804845/chapter/Surveillance-decision?tab=evidence.

30. Blomhoff S, et al. Randomised controlled general practice trial of sertraline, exposure therapy and combined treatment in generalised social phobia. *Br J Psychiatry* 2001; 179:23–30.

31. Hood SD and Nutt DJ. 'Psychopharmacological treatments: an overview,' in WR Crozier and LE Alden, eds., *International handbook of social anxiety concepts, research and interventions relating to the self and shyness*. Oxford: John Wiley and Sons Ltd; 2001.

32. Mayo-Wilson E, et al. Psychological and pharmacological interventions for social anxiety disorder in adults: a systematic review and network meta-analysis. *Lancet Psychiatry* 2014; 1:368–376.

33. National Institute for Clinical Excellence. Depression: the treatment and management of depression in adults. Clinical Guidance [CG90]. 2009 (last reviewed December 2013); https://www.nice.org.uk/guidance/cg90.

34. Pollack MH. Refractory generalized anxiety disorder. *J Clin Psychiatry* 2009; 70 Suppl 2:32–38.

35. Lancia M, et al. Pregabalin abuse in combination with other drugs: monitoring among methadone patients. *Front Psychiatry* 2019; 10:1022.

36. Hägg S, et al. Current evidence on abuse and misuse of gabapentinoids. *Drug Saf* 2020; 43:1235–1254.

37. Naveed S, et al. Pregabalin-associated discontinuation symptoms: a case report. *Cureus* 2018; 10:e3425.

38. Roberts NP, et al. Early psychological interventions to treat acute traumatic stress symptoms. *Cochrane Database Syst Rev* 2010; CD007944.

39. Skapinakis P, et al. Pharmacological and psychotherapeutic interventions for management of obsessive-compulsive disorder in adults: a systematic review and network meta-analysis. *Lancet Psychiatry* 2016; 3:730–739.

40. van Apeldoorn FJ, et al. Is a combined therapy more effective than either CBT or SSRI alone? Results of a multicenter trial on panic disorder with or without agoraphobia. *Acta Psychiatr Scand* 2008; 117:260–270.

41. Marcus SM, et al. A comparison of medication side effect reports by panic disorder patients with and without concomitant cognitive behavior therapy. *Am J Psychiatry* 2007; 164:273–275.

42. Offidani E, et al. Efficacy and tolerability of benzodiazepines versus antidepressants in anxiety disorders: a systematic review and meta-analysis. *Psychother Psychosom* 2013; 82:355–362.

43. Generoso MB, et al. Pregabalin for generalized anxiety disorder: an updated systematic review and meta-analysis. *Int Clin Psychopharmacol* 2017; 32:49–55.

44. Wang SM, et al. Agomelatine for the treatment of generalized anxiety disorder: a meta-analysis. *Clin Psychopharmacol Neurosci* 2020; 18:423–433.

45. Stein DJ, et al. Agomelatine prevents relapse in generalized anxiety disorder: a 6-month randomized, double-blind, placebo-controlled discontinuation study. *J Clin Psychiatry* 2012; 73:1002–1008.

46. Hayes PE, et al. Beta-blockers in anxiety disorders. *J Affect Disord* 1987; 13:119–130.

47. Chessick CA, et al. Azapirones for generalized anxiety disorder. *Cochrane Database Syst Rev* 2006; 3:CD006115.

48. Guaiana G, et al. Hydroxyzine for generalised anxiety disorder. *Cochrane Database Syst Rev* 2010; Cd006815.

49. Khan A, et al. Extended-release quetiapine fumarate (quetiapine XR) as adjunctive therapy in patients with generalized anxiety disorder and a history of inadequate treatment response: a randomized, double-blind study. *Ann Clin Psychiatry* 2014; 26:3–18.

50. Wingerson D, et al. Clomipramine treatment for generalized anxiety disorder. *J Clin Psychopharmacol* 1992; 12:214–215.

51. den Boer JA, et al. Effect of serotonin uptake inhibitors in anxiety disorders; a double-blind comparison of clomipramine and fluvoxamine. *Int Clin Psychopharmacol* 1987; 2:21–32.

52. Kahn RS, et al. Effect of a serotonin precursor and uptake inhibitor in anxiety disorders; a double-blind comparison of 5-hydroxytryptophan, clomipramine and placebo. *Int Clin Psychopharmacol* 1987; 2:33–45.

53. Rickels K, et al. Antidepressants for the treatment of generalized anxiety disorder. A Placebo-controlled Comparison of Imipramine, Trazodone, and Diazepam. *Arch Gen Psychiatry* 1993; 50:884–895.

54. Robinson DS, et al. The monoamine oxidase inhibitor, phenelzine, in the treatment of depressive –anxiety states. A Controlled Clinical Trial. *Arch Gen Psychiatry* 1973; 29:407–413.

55. Gambi F, et al. Mirtazapine treatment of generalized anxiety disorder: a fixed dose, open label study. *J Psychopharmacology* 2005; 19:483–487.

56. Sitsen JMA, et al. Mirtazapine, a Novel Antidepressant, in the Treatment of Anxiety Symptoms. *Drug Invest* 1994; 8:339–344.

57. Amsterdam JD, et al. A randomized, double-blind, placebo-controlled trial of oral Matricaria recutita (chamomile) extract therapy for generalized anxiety disorder. *J Clin Psychopharmacol* 2009; 29:378–382.

58. Woelk H, et al. Ginkgo biloba special extract EGb 761 in generalized anxiety disorder and adjustment disorder with anxious mood: a randomized, double-blind, placebo-controlled trial. *J Psychiatr Res* 2007; 41:472–480.

59. Kasper S, et al. Lavender oil preparation Silexan is effective in generalized anxiety disorder–a randomized, double-blind comparison to placebo and paroxetine. *Int J Neuropsychopharmacol* 2014; 17:859–869.

60. Mathew SJ, et al. Open-label trial of riluzole in generalized anxiety disorder. *Am J Psychiatry* 2005; 162:2379–2381.

61. Otto MW, et al. Discontinuation of benzodiazepine treatment: efficacy of cognitive-behavioral therapy for patients with panic disorder. *Am J Psychiatry* 1993; 150:1485–1490.

62. Breilmann J, et al. Benzodiazepines versus placebo for panic disorder in adults. *Cochrane Database Syst Rev* 2019; 3:Cd010677.

63. Andrisano C, et al. Newer antidepressants and panic disorder: a meta-analysis. *Int Clin Psychopharmacol* 2013; 28:33–45.

64. Batelaan NM, et al. Evidence-based pharmacotherapy of panic disorder: an update. *Int J Neuropsychopharmacol* 2012; 15:403–415.

65. Bighelli I, et al. Antidepressants versus placebo for panic disorder in adults. *Cochrane Database Syst Rev* 2018; 4:Cd010676.

66. Boshuisen ML, et al. The effect of mirtazapine in panic disorder: an open label pilot study with a single-blind placebo run-in period. *Int Clin Psychopharmacol* 2001; 16:363–368.

67. Zulfarina MS, et al. Pharmacological therapy in panic disorder: current guidelines and novel drugs discovery for treatment-resistant patient. *Clin Psychopharmacol Neurosci* 2019; 17:145–154.

68. Tiller JW, et al. Moclobemide for anxiety disorders: a focus on moclobemide for panic disorder. *Int Clin Psychopharmacol* 1997; **12 Suppl** 6:S27–S30.

69. Kruger MB, et al. The efficacy and safety of moclobemide compared to clomipramine in the treatment of panic disorder. *Eur Arch Psychiatry Clin Neurosci* 1999; **249 Suppl** 1:S19–S24.

70. Fahy TJ, et al. The galway study of panic disorder. I: clomipramine and lofepramine in DSM III-R panic disorder: a placebo controlled trial. *J Affect Disord* 1992; 25:63–75.

71. Otto MW, et al. Randomized trial of D-cycloserine enhancement of cognitive-behavioral therapy for panic disorder. *Depress Anxiety* 2016; 33:737–745.

72. Pande AC, et al. Placebo-controlled study of gabapentin treatment of panic disorder. *J Clin Psychopharmacol* 2000; 20:467–471.

73. Benjamin J, et al. Double-blind, placebo-controlled, crossover trial of inositol treatment for panic disorder. *Am J Psychiatry* 1995; 152:1084–1086.

74. Palatnik A, et al. Double-blind, controlled, crossover trial of inositol versus fluvoxamine for the treatment of panic disorder. *J Clin Psychopharmacol* 2001; 21:335–339.

75. Hirschmann S, et al. Pindolol augmentation in patients with treatment-resistant panic disorder: a double-blind, placebo-controlled trial. *J Clin Psychopharmacol* 2000; 20:556–559.

76. Woodman CL, et al. Panic disorder: treatment with valproate. *J Clin Psychiatry* 1994; 55:134–136.

77. Primeau F, et al. Valproic acid and panic disorder. *Can J Psychiatry* 1990; 35:248–250.

78. Astill Wright L, et al. Pharmacological prevention and early treatment of post-traumatic stress disorder and acute stress disorder: a systematic review and meta-analysis. *Trans Psychiatry* 2019; 9:334.

79. National Institute for Clinical Excellence. Post-traumatic stress disorder. NICE Guideline [NG116]. 2018; https://www.nice.org.uk/guidance/NG116.

80. Moore BA, et al. Management of post-traumatic stress disorder in veterans and military service members: a review of pharmacologic and psychotherapeutic interventions since 2016. *Curr Psychiatry Rep* 2021; 23:9.

81. Hoskins M, et al. Pharmacotherapy for post-traumatic stress disorder: systematic review and meta-analysis. *Br J Psychiatry* 2015; 206:93–100.

第3章

82. Lee DJ, et al. Psychotherapy versus pharmacotherapy for posttraumatic stress disorder: systematic review and meta-analyses to determine first-line treatments. *Depress Anxiety* 2016; 33:792–806.

83. Davidson J, et al. Treatment of posttraumatic stress disorder with venlafaxine extended release: a 6-month randomized controlled trial. *Arch Gen Psychiatry* 2006; 63:1158–1165.

84. Han C, et al. The potential role of atypical antipsychotics for the treatment of posttraumatic stress disorder. *J Psychiatr Res* 2014; 56:72–81.

85. Villarreal G, et al. Efficacy of quetiapine monotherapy in posttraumatic stress disorder: a randomized, placebo-controlled trial. *Am J Psychiatry* 2016; 173:1205–1212.

86. Davidson JR, et al. Mirtazapine vs. placebo in posttraumatic stress disorder: a pilot trial. *Biol Psychiatry* 2003; 53:188–191.

87. Cipriani A, et al. Comparative efficacy and acceptability of pharmacological treatments for post-traumatic stress disorder in adults: a network meta-analysis. *Psychol Med* 2018; 48:1975–1984.

88. Kosten TR, et al. Pharmacotherapy for posttraumatic stress disorder using phenelzine or imipramine. *J Nerv Ment Dis* 1991; 179:366–370.

89. George KC, et al. Meta-analysis of the efficacy and safety of prazosin versus placebo for the treatment of nightmares and sleep disturbances in adults with posttraumatic stress disorder. *J Trauma & Dissoc* 2016; 17:494–510.

90. Coventry PA, et al. Psychological and pharmacological interventions for posttraumatic stress disorder and comorbid mental health problems following complex traumatic events: systematic review and component network meta-analysis. *PLoS Med* 2020; 17:e1003262.

91. Davidson J, et al. Treatment of posttraumatic stress disorder with amitriptyline and placebo. *Arch Gen Psychiatry* 1990; 47:259–266.

92. Albott CS, et al. Efficacy, safety, and durability of repeated ketamine infusions for comorbid posttraumatic stress disorder and treatment-resistant depression. *J Clin Psychiatry* 2018; 79:17m11634.

93. Feder A, et al. Efficacy of intravenous ketamine for treatment of chronic posttraumatic stress disorder: a randomized clinical trial. *JAMA Psychiatry* 2014; 71:681–688.

94. Feder A, et al. A randomized controlled trial of repeated ketamine administration for chronic posttraumatic stress disorder. *Am J Psychiatry* 2021; 178:193–202.

95. Walderhaug E, et al. Effects of duloxetine in treatment-refractory men with posttraumatic stress disorder. *Pharmacopsychiatry* 2010; 43:45–49.

96. Villarreal G, et al. Duloxetine in military posttraumatic stress disorder. *Psychopharmacol Bull* 2010; 43:26–34.

97. Hertzberg MA, et al. A preliminary study of lamotrigine for the treatment of posttraumatic stress disorder. *Biol Psychiatry* 1999; 45:1226–1229.

98. Bremner DJ, et al. Treatment of posttraumatic stress disorder with phenytoin: an open-label pilot study. *J Clin Psychiatry* 2004; 65:1559–1564.

99. Adamou M, et al. Valproate in the treatment of PTSD: systematic review and meta analysis. *Curr Med Res Opin* 2007; 23:1285–1291.

100. Veale D, et al. Atypical antipsychotic augmentation in SSRI treatment refractory obsessive-compulsive disorder: a systematic review and meta-analysis. *BMC Psychiatry* 2014; 14:317.

101. Dold M, et al. Antipsychotic augmentation of serotonin reuptake inhibitors in treatment-resistant obsessive-compulsive disorder: an update meta-analysis of double-blind, randomized, placebo-controlled trials. *Int J Neuropsychopharmacol* 2015; 18.

102. Pallanti S, et al. Citalopram for treatment-resistant obsessive-compulsive disorder. *Eur Psychiatry* 1999; 14:101–106.

103. Costa DLC, et al. Randomized, double-blind, placebo-controlled trial of n-acetylcysteine augmentation for treatment-resistant obsessive-compulsive disorder. *J Clin Psychiatry* 2017; 78:e766–e773.

104. Couto JP, et al. Oral N-acetylcysteine in the treatment of obsessive-compulsive disorder: a systematic review of the clinical evidence. *Prog Neuropsychopharmacol Biol Psychiatry* 2018; 86:245–254.

105. Bruno A, et al. Lamotrigine augmentation of serotonin reuptake inhibitors in treatment-resistant obsessive-compulsive disorder: a double-blind, placebo-controlled study. *J Psychopharmacology* 2012; 26:1456–1462.

106. Sharma V, et al. Lamotrigine-induced obsessive-compulsive disorder in patients with bipolar disorder. *CNS Spectr* 2019; 24:390–394.

107. Berlin HA, et al. Double-blind, placebo-controlled trial of topiramate augmentation in treatment-resistant obsessive-compulsive disorder. *J Clin Psychiatry* 2011; 72:716–721.

108. Mowla A, et al. Topiramate augmentation in resistant OCD: a double-blind placebo-controlled clinical trial. *CNS Spectr* 2010; 15:613–617.

109. Afshar H, et al. Topiramate augmentation in refractory obsessive-compulsive disorder: a randomized, double-blind, placebo-controlled trial. *J Res Med Sci* 2014; 19:976–981.

110. Grassi G, et al. Investigational and experimental drugs to treat obsessive-compulsive disorder. *J Exp Pharmacol* 2020; 12:695–706.

111. Rabinowitz I, et al. High-dose escitalopram for the treatment of obsessive-compulsive disorder. *Int Clin Psychopharmacol* 2008; 23:49–53.

112. Ninan PT, et al. High-dose sertraline strategy for nonresponders to acute treatment for obsessive-compulsive disorder: a multicenter double-blind trial. *J Clin Psychiatry* 2006; 67:15–22.

113. Modarresi A, et al. A systematic review and meta-analysis: memantine augmentation in moderate to severe obsessive-compulsive disorder. *Psychiatry Res* 2019; 282:112602.

114. Naderi S, et al. Amantadine as adjuvant therapy in the treatment of moderate to severe obsessive-compulsive disorder: a double-blind randomized trial with placebo control. *Psychiatry Clin Neurosci* 2019; 73:169–174.

115. Dell'Osso B, et al. Serotonin-norepinephrine reuptake inhibitors in the treatment of obsessive-compulsive disorder: a critical review. *J Clin Psychiatry* 2006; 67:600–610.

116. Mowla A, et al. Duloxetine augmentation in resistant obsessive-compulsive disorder: a double-blind controlled clinical trial. *J Clin*

第 3 章

Psychopharmacol 2016; 36:720–723.

117. Koran LM, et al. Mirtazapine for obsessive-compulsive disorder: an open trial followed by double-blind discontinuation. *J Clin Psychiatry* 2005; 66:515–520.

118. Askari N, et al. Granisetron adjunct to fluvoxamine for moderate to severe obsessive-compulsive disorder: a randomized, double-blind, placebo-controlled trial. *CNS Drugs* 2012; 26:883–892.

119. Soltani F, et al. A double-blind, placebo-controlled pilot study of ondansetron for patients with obsessive-compulsive disorder. *Human Psychopharmacology* 2010; 25:509–513.

120. Sharafkhah M, et al. Comparing the efficacy of ondansetron and granisetron augmentation in treatment-resistant obsessive-compulsive disorder: a randomized double-blind placebo-controlled study. *Int Clin Psychopharmacol* 2019; 34:222–233.

121. Mowla A, et al. Pregabalin augmentation for resistant obsessive-compulsive disorder: a double-blind placebo-controlled clinical trial. *CNS Spectr* 2020; 25:552–556.

122. Coric V, et al. Riluzole augmentation in treatment-resistant obsessive-compulsive disorder: an open-label trial. *Biol Psychiatry* 2005; 58:424–428.

123. Eriksson T. Anti-androgenic treatment of obsessive-compulsive disorder: an open-label clinical trial of the long-acting gonadotropin-releasing hormone analogue triptorelin. *Int Clin Psychopharmacol* 2007; 22:57–61.

124. Fallon BA, et al. Intravenous clomipramine for obsessive-compulsive disorder refractory to oral clomipramine: a placebo-controlled study. *Arch Gen Psychiatry* 1998; 55:918–924.

125. Rodriguez CI, et al. Randomized controlled crossover trial of ketamine in obsessive-compulsive disorder: proof-of-concept. *Neuropsychopharmacology* 2013; 38:2475–2483.

126. Bloch MH, et al. Effects of ketamine in treatment-refractory obsessive-compulsive disorder. *Biol Psychiatry* 2012; 72:964–970.

127. Koran LM, et al. Double-blind treatment with oral morphine in treatment-resistant obsessive-compulsive disorder. *J Clin Psychiatry* 2005; 66:353–359.

128. National Institute for Health and Clinical Excellence. Social anxiety disorder: recognition, assessment and treatment. Clinical Guidance [CG159]. 2013 (Last updated March 2020); https://www.nice.org.uk/guidance/cg159

129. Liu X, et al. Efficacy and tolerability of fluvoxamine in adults with social anxiety disorder: a meta-analysis. *Medicine (Baltimore)* 2018; 97:e11547.

130. Baldwin DS, et al. Efficacy of escitalopram in the treatment of social anxiety disorder: a meta-analysis versus placebo. *Eur Neuropsychopharmacol* 2016; 26:1062–1069.

131. Careri JM, et al. A 12-week double-blind, placebo-controlled, flexible-dose trial of vilazodone in generalized social anxiety disorder. *Primary Care Companion CNS Disord* 2015; 17:10.4088/PCC.15m01831.

132. Blanco C, et al. The evidence-based pharmacotherapy of social anxiety disorder. *Int J Neuropsychopharmacol* 2013; 16:235–249.

133. Pollack MH, et al. A double-blind randomized controlled trial of augmentation and switch strategies for refractory social anxiety disorder. *Am J Psychiatry* 2014; 171:44–53.

134. Simon NM, et al. An open-label study of levetiracetam for the treatment of social anxiety disorder. *J Clin Psychiatry* 2004; 65:1219–1222.

135. Blanco C, et al. A placebo-controlled trial of phenelzine, cognitive behavioral group therapy, and their combination for social anxiety disorder. *Arch Gen Psychiatry* 2010; 67:286–295.

136. Taylor JH, et al. Ketamine for social anxiety disorder: a randomized, placebo-controlled crossover trial. *Neuropsychopharmacology* 2018; 43:325–333.

137. Van Ameringen M, et al. An open trial of topiramate in the treatment of generalized social phobia. *J Clin Psychiatry* 2004; 65:1674–1678.

138. Kinrys G, et al. Valproic acid for the treatment of social anxiety disorder. *Int Clin Psychopharmacol* 2003; 18:169–172.

苯二氮䓬类药物在精神障碍治疗中的应用

苯二氮䓬类药物在治疗某些类型的癫痫和严重的肌肉痉挛,或作为一些手术的术前用药,起着重要的作用。但是,大多数处方还是用于催眠和抗焦虑。它们也用于快速镇静,或者作为辅助药物治疗抑郁症和精神分裂症。苯二氮䓬类药物处方和滥用均很常见。欧洲一项研究发现,大约 10% 成年人曾在一年内使用过苯二氮䓬类药物[1],2019 年,美国一项研究报道 12.6% 的成年人过去一年使用苯二氮䓬类药物[2]。总体上,过去几十年越来越不支持在精神疾病中应用苯二氮䓬类药物[3]。

苯二氮䓬类药物通常可根据半衰期长短分为两组:催眠药(半衰期短)或抗焦虑药(半衰期长),但是也有很多例外(如硝西泮和阿普唑仑)。

抗焦虑作用

苯二氮䓬类药物可以缓解病理性焦虑、激越和紧张症状。苯二氮䓬类药物无论是单用,还是联合 SSRI 类,用于广泛性焦虑障碍的短期治疗都有效[4],但是有明确的成瘾性;许多患者持续使用这些药物多年[5],却没有明确获益,且可能有许多危害。如果处方苯二氮䓬类药物,一般不应超过一个月。

NICE 建议,苯二氮䓬类药物不应作为广泛性焦虑障碍的常规用药,除非在紧急情况下短期使用[6]。在其他类型的焦虑障碍中,证据比较混乱,应权衡苯二氮䓬类药物使用的风险和获益。少数临床研究报道苯二氮䓬类药物在社交焦虑障碍中有效[7]。苯二氮䓬类药物可以用于惊恐障碍[8],但尚需进一步研究,才能对其长期应用的疗效和安全性得出可靠结论[8,9]。苯二氮䓬类药物治疗 PTSD[10] 或恐怖[11] 无效,甚至可能有伤害。

对于有严重人格问题,且困难不大可能得到解决的患者,尤其是药物治疗无效者,应避免重复使用苯二氮䓬类药物。同样,苯二氮䓬类药物也应尽量避免用于有物质滥用史的患者。

催眠作用

苯二氮䓬类药物抑制 REM 睡眠,停药后会出现 REM 反跳[11]。关于这一属性的临床意义尚有争论[12]。

苯二氮䓬类药物是有效的催眠药,至少在短期内有效[13]。随机对照试验证实了 Z 类催眠药在长达 6 个月内的有效性[13,14],但目前尚不清楚苯二氮䓬类药物是否也如此。间歇使用可以延长苯二氮䓬类药物作为催眠药的有效时长。

使用催眠药之前,应先排除躯体原因(如疼痛、呼吸困难等)或物质滥用(最常见的是咖啡因摄取过量)所致睡眠障碍。如有可能,在处方催眠药之前先实施行为治疗(如 CBT 治疗失眠)[14,15]。住院患者使用催眠药的比例很高[16]。应注意避免出院后常规使用催眠药。

用于抑郁症

苯二氮䓬类药物并非抑郁症的治疗药物。唯一一项荟萃分析发现,苯二氮䓬类药物对抑郁症的疗效并不好于安慰剂[17]。但也有些证据支持苯二氮䓬类药物有助于预防精神病性

抑郁的复发 [18]。

在英国,国家心理健康服务体系(National Service Framework for Mentalhealth)[19] 曾一度特别强调这一点,并要求全科医师登记在临床实践中苯二氮䓬类药物和抗抑郁药处方量的比值。NICE 建议,苯二氮䓬类药物在抑郁症开始治疗的前 2 周是有效的,尤其是在联用 SSRI 时(可改善睡眠,并减轻 SSRI 所致的激越)[6]。不鼓励使用时间超过此范围。限制初始处方量在短期内(1~7 天),可减少患者长期使用苯二氮䓬类药物的风险 [20]。

用于精神病

苯二氮䓬类药物单用或者与抗精神病药联用,通常用于快速镇静 [21]。然而,一项 Cochrane 系统评价认为,目前尚无确切证据支持抗精神病药与苯二氮䓬类药物联用优于抗精神病药或苯二氮䓬类药物单用 [22]。

另一项 Cochrane 系统评价认为,除了短期镇静作用,苯二氮䓬类药物对精神分裂症患者并无确切疗效 [23]。相反,另一项系统综述采用不同的结局指标,发现在总体功能、精神科和行为结局方面,苯二氮䓬类药物优于安慰剂,但是在长期总体结局方面不如抗精神病药 [24]。极少数精神病患者单独使用抗精神病药时疗效不充分,这可能导致苯二氮䓬类药物的长期使用 [25]。然而,无证据支持苯二氮䓬类药物作为抗精神病药增加治疗精神分裂症的疗效,它们应当被限制用于急性激越患者的短期镇静 [26]。支持苯二氮䓬类药物治疗迟发性运动障碍的证据较弱 [27],这些药物仍然是迟发性运动障碍的治疗选择之一。

不良反应

头痛、意识模糊、共济失调、构音障碍、视物模糊、胃肠功能紊乱、黄疸和反常兴奋(paradoxical excitement)都是可能出现的不良反应。苯二氮䓬类药物损害认知,长期治疗可致一系列认知(如记忆、注意和处理速度)障碍,即使是停药后,这些影响依然持续 [28]。老年患者使用苯二氮䓬类药物可致髋骨骨折风险增加至少 50% [29],可能是因为苯二氮䓬类药物可增加跌倒的风险 [30]。用药的最初几天风险最高 [29]。大剂量时特别容易出现问题 [30]。这种风险可能是苯二氮䓬类药物的共同效应(即便使用半衰期短的药物,其风险并没有降低 [30])。苯二氮䓬类药物常导致顺行性遗忘,并可能影响驾驶操作 [31,32]。苯二氮䓬类药物还会导致脱抑制(见本章"苯二氮䓬类药物与脱抑制"部分)。苯二氮䓬类药物也可引起攻击性行为,但是这种相关性仅为轻度,可能与剂量和人格因素有关 [33]。

流行病学研究显示,苯二氮䓬类药物使用与严重躯体疾病关联,包括痴呆、感染和癌症 [34-36]。但尚未确定因果关系,证据互相矛盾 [35]。虽然苯二氮䓬类药物使用和痴呆有关 [37],但是没有剂量-反应关系,使得人们反对这种因果联系 [38]。所有该领域的研究均未包含苯二氮䓬类药物的非法使用,使得情况变得复杂。

呼吸抑制在口服治疗时较少出现,但在静脉注射时有可能发生。口含和鼻内给药也可以引起呼吸抑制 [39,40]。若出现呼吸抑制,使用苯二氮䓬类特异性拮抗剂氟马西尼治疗有效,但也有风险(如惊厥,尤其是混合 TCA 且过量服用时),因此建议选择性使用 [41]。氟马西尼的半衰期比地西泮短得多,故在给药后几小时内需对患者密切观察。

苯二氮䓬类药物的水溶性低,静脉注射时可产生疼痛,导致血栓性静脉炎,故在准备注射制剂时需加入溶剂。地西泮乳剂(Diazemuls,在英国上市)可克服上述问题。

药物相互作用

苯二氮䓬类药物不能诱导微粒体酶的活性,故与其他药物的药代动力学相互作用并不常见。大多数苯二氮䓬类药物被 CYP3A4 代谢,而后者可被红霉素、某些 SSRI 和酮康唑所抑制。在理论上,苯二氮䓬类药物与这些药物合用时,会导致苯二氮䓬类药物血浆浓度升高。药效学相互作用(通常是镇静作用增强)也可能发生。苯二氮䓬类药物与美沙酮有重要的药效学相互作用,应慎用于服用氯氮平的患者(增加心肺抑制的风险),禁止用于接受肌内注射奥氮平的患者。

参考文献

1. Demyttenaere K, et al. Clinical factors influencing the prescription of antidepressants and benzodiazepines: results from the European study of the epidemiology of mental disorders (ESEMeD). *J Affect Disord* 2008; **110**:84–93.
2. Maust DT, et al. Benzodiazepine use and misuse among adults in the United States. *Psychiatr Serv* 2019; **70**:97–106.
3. Hirschtritt ME, et al. Balancing the risks and benefits of benzodiazepines. *JAMA* 2021; **325**:347–348.
4. Baldwin DS, et al. Evidence-based pharmacological treatment of anxiety disorders, post-traumatic stress disorder and obsessive-compulsive disorder: a revision of the 2005 guidelines from the British Association for Psychopharmacology. *J Psychopharmacol* 2014; **28**:403–439.
5. Kurko TA, et al. Long-term use of benzodiazepines: definitions, prevalence and usage patterns – a systematic review of register-based studies. *Eur Psychiatry* 2015; **30**:1037–1047.
6. National Institute for Health and Clinical Excellence. Generalised anxiety disorder and panic disorder in adults: management Clinical Guideline [CG113] 2011 (last updated July 2019); https://www.nice.org.uk/guidance/cg113.
7. Williams T, et al. Pharmacotherapy for social anxiety disorder (SAnD). *Cochrane Database Syst Rev* 2017; **10**:Cd001206.
8. Perna G, et al. Long-term pharmacological treatments of anxiety disorders: an updated systematic review. *Curr Psychiatry Rep* 2016; **18**:23.
9. Bighelli I, et al. Antidepressants and benzodiazepines for panic disorder in adults. *Cochrane Database Syst Rev* 2016; **9**:Cd011567.
10. Guina J, et al. Benzodiazepines for PTSD: a systematic review and meta-analysis. *J Psychiatr Pract* 2015; **21**:281–303.
11. Guina J, et al. Benzodiazepines I: upping the care on downers: the evidence of risks, benefits and alternatives. *J Clin Med* 2018; **7**.
12. Roehrs T, et al. Drug-related sleep stage changes: functional significance and clinical relevance. *Sleep Med Clin* 2010; **5**:559–570.
13. Winkler A, et al. Drug treatment of primary insomnia: a meta-analysis of polysomnographic randomized controlled trials. *CNS Drugs* 2014; **28**:799–816.
14. Riemann D, et al. European guideline for the diagnosis and treatment of insomnia. *J Sleep Res* 2017; **26**:675–700.
15. Qaseem A, et al. Management of chronic insomnia disorder in adults: a clinical practice guideline from the American College of Physicians. *Ann Intern Med* 2016; **165**:125–133.
16. Mahomed R, et al. Prescribing hypnotics in a mental health trust: what consultants say and what they do. *Pharm J* 2002; **268**:657–659.
17. Benasi G, et al. Benzodiazepines as a monotherapy in depressive disorders: a systematic review. *Psychother Psychosom* 2018; **87**:65–74.
18. Shiwaku H, et al. Benzodiazepines reduce relapse and recurrence rates in patients with psychotic depression. *J Clin Med* 2020; **9**:1938.
19. Gov.UK. Guidance: national service framework for mental health: modern standards and service models. 1999. https://www.gov.uk/government/publications/quality-standards-for-mental-health-services.
20. Bushnell GA, et al. Simultaneous antidepressant and benzodiazepine new use and subsequent long-term benzodiazepine use in adults with depression, United States, 2001–2014. *JAMA Psychiatry* 2017; **74**:747–755.
21. Baldwin DS, et al. Benzodiazepines: risks and benefits. A reconsideration. *J Psychopharmacology* 2013; **27**:967–971.
22. Zaman H, et al. Benzodiazepines for psychosis-induced aggression or agitation. *Cochrane Database Syst Rev* 2017; **12**:Cd003079.
23. Dold M, et al. Benzodiazepines for schizophrenia. *Cochrane Database Syst Rev* 2012; **11**:Cd006391.
24. Sim F, et al. Re-examining the role of benzodiazepines in the treatment of schizophrenia: a systematic review. *J Psychopharmacology* 2015; **29**:212–223.
25. Paton C, et al. Benzodiazepines in schizophrenia. Is there a trend towards long-term prescribing? *Psychiatric Bull* 2000; **24**:113–115.
26. Dold M, et al. Benzodiazepine augmentation of antipsychotic drugs in schizophrenia: a meta-analysis and Cochrane review of randomized controlled trials. *Eur Neuropsychopharmacol* 2013; **23**:1023–1033.
27. Bergman H, et al. Benzodiazepines for antipsychotic-induced tardive dyskinesia. *Cochrane Database Syst Rev* 2018; **1**:Cd000205.
28. Crowe SF, et al. The residual medium and long-term cognitive effects of benzodiazepine use: an updated meta-analysis. *Arch Clin Neuropsychol* 2018; **33**:901–911.
29. Donnelly K, et al. Benzodiazepines, Z-drugs and the risk of hip fracture: a systematic review and meta-analysis. *PLoS One* 2017; **12**:e0174730.
30. Diaz-Gutierrez MJ, et al. Relationship between the use of benzodiazepines and falls in older adults: a systematic review. *Maturitas* 2017; **101**:17–22.
31. Barbone F, et al. Association of road-traffic accidents with benzodiazepine use. *Lancet* 1998; **352**:1331–1336.
32. Rudisill TM, et al. Medication use and the risk of motor vehicle collisions among licensed drivers: a systematic review. *Accid Anal Prev* 2016; **96**:255–270.
33. Albrecht B, et al. Benzodiazepine use and aggressive behaviour: a systematic review. *Aust N Z J Psychiatry* 2014; **48**:1096–1114.

34. Kim DH, et al. Use of hypnotics and risk of cancer: a meta-analysis of observational studies. *Korean J Fam Med* 2018; 39:211–218.

35. Brandt J, et al. Benzodiazepines and Z-drugs: an updated review of major adverse outcomes reported on in epidemiologic research. *Drugs in R&D* 2017; 17:493–507.

36. Peng TR, et al. Hypnotics and risk of cancer: a meta-analysis of observational studies. *Medicina (Kaunas)* 2020; 56.

37. Lee J, et al. Use of sedative-hypnotics and the risk of Alzheimer's dementia: a retrospective cohort study. *PLoS One* 2018; 13:e0204413.

38. Gray SL, et al. Benzodiazepine use and risk of incident dementia or cognitive decline: prospective population based study. *BMJ* 2016; 352:i90.

39. Mula M. The safety and tolerability of intranasal midazolam in epilepsy. *Expert Rev Neurother* 2014; 14:735–740.

40. Midazolam oral transmucosal route. An alternative to rectal diazepam for some children. *Prescrire Int* 2013; 22:173–177.

41. Penninga EI, et al. Adverse events associated with flumazenil treatment for the management of suspected benzodiazepine Intoxication–A systematic review with meta-analyses of randomised trials. *Basic Clin Pharmacol Toxicol* 2016; 118:37–44.

苯二氮䓬类药物、Z 类药物和加巴喷丁类药：依赖、脱毒和停药

在大多数发达国家，苯二氮䓬类药物或 Z 类药物限制最长用 2~4 周[1-3]。但在英国，长期使用仍很普遍，约 300 000 成年人服用苯二氮䓬类药物或 Z 类药物长达 12 个月以上[4]。包括 NICE 在内的大多数指南建议，长期使用苯二氮䓬类药物或 Z 类药物的人群应停药，因为对药物产生耐受（用药 2~4 周后可能发生）意味着长期用药对失眠或焦虑无效，还因为可能会产生依赖，意味着继续用药仅仅是为了防止戒断症状（表 3.27）[5]。

加巴喷丁类药物（GABA 类似物），有着与苯二氮䓬类药物相似的作用机制，在同时的时段内也可能引起成瘾、躯体依赖和戒断症状[6-8]。总体上，150 万英国人在使用加巴喷丁类药物[9]，过去 10 年这些药物的处方量增加了 7 倍[10]。

表 3.27 苯二氮䓬类药物不良反应

认知 [*11-13]	可能被误认为精神障碍的反应 [14]
■ 记忆损害	■ 激越
■ 注意损害	■ 情感不稳
■ 反应时延长	■ 坐卧不安
■ 运动不协调	■ 服药间歇期撤药症状
■ 困倦	
■ 梦魇/闯入性思维	
■ 判断力受损	
■ 错觉/妄想	
躯体 [15]	**情感 [15]**
■ 运动不协调/共济失调	■ 抑郁/心境恶劣
■ 头晕	■ 麻木/情绪麻痹
■ 言语不清	■ 焦虑/恐怖/惊恐
■ 感觉异常（耳鸣/奇怪味觉/感觉异常/麻木/灼烧感）	■ 愤怒/易激惹/情绪不稳
■ 皮疹	■ 兴奋/欣快
■ 自主神经功能异常（心动过速/心动过缓/多汗/低血压/高血压）	
发生率增高 [12,13]	**行为表现 [15]**
■ 交通事故发生风险升高	■ 失眠
■ 跌倒风险升高（老年人）	■ 回避/场所恐惧
■ 谵妄（老年人）	■ 食欲/体重（厌食/体重增加）
■ ? 痴呆	■ 冲动/脱抑制
■ ? 癌症	■ 自杀
■ ? 感染	■ 攻击

* 有些损害持续到停药后。

大多数对这些药物依赖的人群并不是通过非法途径获得药品，而是通过医师的处方获得药品（所谓的"医源性依赖"）。

长期使用苯二氮䓬类药物存在许多问题（表 3.27），患者对此并不了解，只是停药后才体

会到 [16]。长期使用 Z 类药物有类似的风险 [17]。加巴喷丁类药可能增加自杀、非蓄意过量、交通事故、头部和躯体伤害等风险 [18],建议谨慎限制这些药物的长期使用。

戒断症状

这些药物通常很难停用(表 3.28)。一项研究发现 90% 的患者会出现戒断症状,其中 32% 使用长半衰期药物和 42% 使用短半衰期药物的人群因为戒断症状而无法停药 [19]。与长效药(如地西泮)相比,短效药(如劳拉西泮)在停药时会出现更多的问题 [20,21]。由于这些药物长期使用对焦虑和失眠无效,因此停药后出现的症状为戒断症状,而不是复发(尽管症状可能相似) [22]。精神状态会随着戒断症状缓解而改善 [23]。

为避免或减少这些问题,最佳实践要求将苯二氮䓬类药物(以及 Z 类药物)用于催眠或抗焦虑时,时间不应超过 4 周。此外,以最低可能剂量间断使用(即不是每天都用)是明智的。该原则也适用于加巴喷丁类药。

表 3.28　苯二氮䓬类药物戒断症状 [24,25]

躯体	心理
■ 肌肉僵硬	■ 焦虑/失眠
■ 疲乏、虚弱	■ 恐怖/惊恐发作
■ 胃肠不适	■ 噩梦
■ 感觉异常	■ 人格解体/现实解体
■ 流感样症状	■ 妄想和幻觉
■ 视力障碍	■ 抑郁
■ 感觉过敏	■ 精神病 *
■ 惊厥 *	■ 情绪不稳
■ 认知损害	■ 妄想
■ 记忆损害	■ 强迫症状
■ 震颤	■ 自杀观念
■ 头晕	■ 躁狂
■ 肌肉痉挛/抽筋	
■ 胸痛	
■ 高血压	
■ 心动过速	
■ 怕光	
■ 意识模糊、谵妄 *	

* 常仅见于非常快速戒断。

关于戒断症状持续时间的正规研究有限,有些报道会持续数周,但也有报道持续超过 1 年,尤其是长期用药的患者 [20,23]。极少数案例,戒断症状持续存在超过数年,有时被称为"急性期后戒断综合征" [26]。

停用苯二氮䓬类药物

若患者同意,应该停用苯二氮䓬类药物。逐渐减量可能会很困难,不应违背患者的意愿强制减药。一项整群随机试验证实了面对面教育干预的有效性[27]。可能需要给予持续的支持,以便帮助患者做好停药的准备,完成整个过程(如心理治疗或自助小组)[28]。

逐渐减量

逐渐减少苯二氮䓬类药物,可以减少戒断症状的程度,其原理是让这些戒断症状分散在更长的时间内(并使中枢神经对药物的适应消退)[22]。荟萃分析已经证实,相比于常规的临床治疗,逐渐减量可以提高苯二氮䓬类药物的停药率[29]。大部分研究发现,在至少10周内逐渐撤药,最有可能成功实现长期停药[30],但是很多患者需要更长时间(有时是几年)。突然停用苯二氮䓬类药物有致命风险,因此逐渐停药始终是合理的。

直接减量还是换为地西泮

服用短效、中效苯二氮䓬类药物的患者,可直接逐渐减量直至停药,但可能需要一天多次给药。

另一种替代方案是换为等效剂量的地西泮(地西泮半衰期较长,因而较少引起严重的戒断反应)[20,24],值得注意的是,有些患者突然换成地西泮后会出现戒断症状,因此,逐步换药更明智。Cochrane 不热衷于换成地西泮这种方法[30]。近似的"地西泮等效"剂量[31]见表 3.29。由于个体间差异,一些患者可能需要更多或较少的地西泮来控制戒断症状。

表 3.29　近似的"地西泮等效"剂量[31]

氯氮䓬	25mg	洛美西泮	1~2mg
氯硝西泮	0.5mg	硝西泮	10mg
地西泮	**10mg**	奥沙西泮	20mg
劳拉西泮	1mg	替马西泮	20mg

苯二氮䓬类药物的半衰期相差较大,各药物诱导的镇静程度也不同,因而很难计算精确的等效剂量。表 3.28 仅是一个近似的指南。另外,对于肝功能异常的患者,应该格外小心,因为地西泮和其他长效药物可蓄积到中毒水平。

减量方法

苯二氮䓬类药物剂量与其对主要靶点 GABA-A 受体的效应呈双曲线模式,具有下列意义:

- 按固定剂量减量(图 3.6a 的 12.5mg),将导致 GABA-A 受体占有率下降幅度越来越大。
- 与临床观察相似,戒断症状和减量呈非线性关系(如从 20mg 地西泮减量 1mg 可以耐受,但是从 5mg 地西泮减量 1mg 则不能耐受[32])。
- 地西泮从 50mg 减少 5mg,会导致 GABA-A 受体占有率减少 2.3%;但是从 5mg 减少 5mg,则使 GABA-A 受体占有率减少 18.3%。

　　减少苯二氮䓬类药物剂量时,为了使其对主要靶点的作用等量减少,需要采用双曲线法减量(图 3.6b):

- 这就意味着随着总剂量减少,减量的幅度也应越来越小。
- 在临床实践中,最容易计算减量幅度的方法,是根据最近的剂量按比例折算(指数法)。
- 患者经常报告每 2~4 周减量 10% 可以耐受(根据末次剂量计算,因此减量幅度越来越小),但是一些长期用药者可能需要更慢地减量。
- 停药前的末次剂量需要非常小(经常低于 1mg 地西泮等效剂量)。

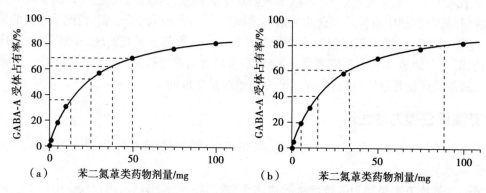

图 3.6　(a) 剂量呈线性减少时,引起 GABA-A 受体效应下降的幅度越来越大。(b) 为使 GABA-A 受体效应等量减少,需要采用双曲线法减少地西泮剂量。注意,为了防止最后一步降幅太大,需要使用的终末剂量非常小。改编自 Brouillet 等(1991)[33]

上述原则的实际应用

逐渐减药之前

- 应告知所有患者,停用苯二氮䓬类药物、Z 类药物或加巴喷丁类药物时,有出现戒断症状的风险(阿普唑仑和劳拉西泮的风险高)。
- 应该警示患者不要突然停用苯二氮䓬类药物,因为突然停药可能会引起癫痫发作,甚至死亡,而且这种方法极有可能产生严重而持久的戒断症状。
- 尽管停用苯二氮䓬类药物可以产生不舒服的症状,但是如果逐渐而小心地减量,减药过程也可耐受;对于过去有快速减药经历的人,可能需要给予保证。
- 大部分患者需要几个月或几年时间来逐渐减量。但是,减量速度应由患者的耐受性如何而定,而不是由外部强加的时间表来定。
- 过去的减药经历有助于预测再次减药后可能发生戒断症状。
- 逐渐减少苯二氮䓬类药物,可能需要做些准备,如:减轻工作或家庭责任,或提高非药物应对技能(包括接纳、呼吸练习、锻炼、业余爱好、记日记和去创伤化)[28,34]。
- 在减量期间,失眠患者可加用褪黑素辅助治疗,惊恐障碍患者可加用认知行为治疗[24,35,36]。与单用监督下减量法或单用心理干预相比,逐渐减量联合心理干预(放松、认知行为治疗)的成功率更高[37]。
- 患者和医师熟悉各种戒断症状(上述),可有助于在戒断症状发生时减轻不必要的焦虑。

戒断症状并不意味着需要使用该药,而是应该降低减药速度。

逐渐减药的过程

- 可以根据发生风险将患者大致分层:
  - 低风险患者(用药时间 <6 个月,长半衰期苯二氮䓬类药,过去未出现明显戒断症状)可试验减量 25%。
  - 高风险患者(用药时长 >6 个月,短半衰期苯二氮䓬类药,曾有戒断症状)建议试验减量 5%~10%。
- 应该根据末次剂量按比例(如 10%)减量。这意味着,随着总剂量减少,建议的减量幅度越来越小。大部分患者能够每个月减少最近一次剂量的 5%~10%。
- 减量后,应该监测戒断症状 2~4 周,或者直到戒断症状缓解。监测方法可简单地每天评估症状(如十分之几),或者使用标准化的苯二氮䓬类药戒断量表。
- 应该根据患者对症状的耐受程度进一步减量。如果戒断症状不能耐受,需要增加剂量,稳定一段时间,然后更缓慢地减量。轻度、可耐受的症状,说明可以同样比例继续减量。

问题解决

- 若在任何时候发生了明显的戒断症状,或者维持现有剂量直至症状缓解,或者如果无法耐受,加回到症状可以忍受的上一个剂量,并且维持该剂量直到症状缓解。稳定后,需要以慢的速度减量:降低减量幅度,或延长减药间隔时间。
- 出现令人感到苦恼的戒断症状,并非说明患者不能停苯二氮䓬类药,而是提示患者减药的速度要更慢一些(有些患者每月减药的幅度要低于最近剂量的 5%)。
- 剂量很低时,可能需要液体剂型,现有地西泮和劳拉西泮液体剂型。因此换成液体剂型可能有用;其他选择包括专门配制的液体制剂。很多患者报告把片剂切开、称重,或者研成粉末自己配制液体,但不推荐这种方法。
- 停药前最后的剂量必须很小,以免对大脑的作用大幅减弱。例如,若每月地西泮减量 10%,最后的剂量可能是 0.25mg[33]。

减药日程

简单的地西泮减药指南:

- 每 2~4 周减少 5~10mg/d,减至每天剂量为 50mg。
- 每 2~4 周减少 2~5mg/d,减至每天剂量为 20mg。
- 每 2~4 周减少 1~2mg/d,减至每天剂量为 10mg。
- 每 2~4 周减少 0.5~1mg/d,减至每天剂量为 5mg
- 每 2~4 周减少 0.25~0.5mg/d,减至每天剂量为 2.5mg
- 每 2~4 周减少 0.1~0.25mg/d,直到停药。

其他药物的减量方案

同样的原则也适用于 Z 类药物和加巴喷丁类药。加巴喷丁类药可引起严重的戒断反应,但是存在较大的个体间差异。虽然 Z 类药物每天使用一次,也有耐受和戒断的报告,甚至短暂或间断使用后也可发生 [38,39]。根据类似的指数法减药(或者有时交叉滴定到地西泮)。主要戒断症状是失眠和焦虑。在理想情况下,逐渐减量的速度以保持正常睡眠为准。

参考文献

1. BNF Online. British national formulary. 2020; https://www.medicinescomplete.com/mc/bnf/current.
2. National Institute for Clinical Excellence. Guidance on the use of zaleplon, zolpidem and zopiclone for the short-term management of insomnia. Technical Appraisal [TA77]. 2004 (reviewed August 2010); https://www.nice.org.uk/guidance/ta77.
3. National Institute for Health and Clinical Excellence. Generalised anxiety disorder and panic disorder in adults: management. Clinical Guideline [CG113]. 2011 (last updated July 2019); https://www.nice.org.uk/guidance/cg113.
4. Davies J, et al. Long-term benzodiazepine and Z-drugs use in the UK: a survey of general practice. *Br J Gen Pract* 2017; 67:e609–e613.
5. National Institute for Health and Care Excellence. Benzodiazepine and z-drug withdrawal. 2019; https://cks.nice.org.uk/topics/benzodiazepine-z-drug-withdrawal/?_escaped_fragment_=topicsummary.
6. Schifano F, et al. An insight into Z-drug abuse and dependence: an examination of reports to the European Medicines Agency Database of Suspected Adverse Drug Reactions. *Int J Neuropsychopharmacol* 2019; 22:270–277.
7. Evoy KE, et al. Abuse and misuse of pregabalin and gabapentin. *Drugs* 2017; 77:403–426.
8. Public Health England. Advice for prescribers on the risk of the misuse of pregabalin and gabapentin. 2014; https://assets.publishing.service.gov.uk/government/uploads/system/uploads/attachment_data/file/385791/PHE-NHS_England_pregabalin_and_gabapentin_advice_Dec_2014.pdf.
9. Marsden J, et al. Medicines associated with dependence or withdrawal: a mixed-methods public health review and national database study in England. *Lancet Psychiatry* 2019; 6:935–950.
10. Gov.UK. Dependence and withdrawal associated with some prescribed medicines. An evidence review. 2020; https://www.gov.uk/government/publications/prescribed-medicines-review-report.
11. Crowe SF, et al. The residual medium and long-term cognitive effects of benzodiazepine use: an updated meta-analysis. *Arch Clin Neuropsychol* 2018; 33:901–911.
12. Brandt J, et al. Benzodiazepines and Z-drugs: an updated review of major adverse outcomes reported on in epidemiologic research. *Drugs in R&D* 2017; 17:493–507.
13. Donnelly K, et al. Benzodiazepines, Z-drugs and the risk of hip fracture: a systematic review and meta-analysis. *PLoS One* 2017; 12:e0174730.
14. Gutierrez MA, et al. Paradoxical reactions to benzodiazepines. *Am J Nurs* 2001; 101:34–39; quiz 39–40.
15. Guina J, et al. Benzodiazepines I: upping the care on downers: the evidence of risks, benefits and alternatives. *J Clin Med* 2018; 7:17.
16. Golombok S, et al. Cognitive impairment in long-term benzodiazepine users. *Psychol Med* 1988; 18:365–374.
17. Finkle WD, et al. Risk of fractures requiring hospitalization after an initial prescription for zolpidem, alprazolam, lorazepam, or diazepam in older adults. *J Am Geriatr Soc* 2011; 59:1883–1890.
18. Molero Y, et al. Associations between gabapentinoids and suicidal behaviour, unintentional overdoses, injuries, road traffic incidents, and violent crime: population based cohort study in Sweden. *BMJ* 2019; 365:l2147.
19. Schweizer E, et al. Long-term therapeutic use of benzodiazepines. II. Effects of gradual taper. *Arch Gen Psychiatry* 1990; 47:908–915.
20. Schweizer E, et al. Benzodiazepine dependence and withdrawal: a review of the syndrome and its clinical management. *Acta Psychiatr Scand* 1998; 98 Suppl 393:95–101.
21. Uhlenhuth EH, et al. International study of expert judgment on therapeutic use of benzodiazepines and other psychotherapeutic medications: IV. Therapeutic dose dependence and abuse liability of benzodiazepines in the long-term treatment of anxiety disorders. *J Clin Psychopharmacol* 1999; 19:23S–29S.
22. Ashton H. The diagnosis and management of benzodiazepine dependence. *Curr Opin Psychiatry* 2005; 18:249–255.
23. Ashton H. Benzodiazepine withdrawal: outcome in 50 patients. *Br J Addict* 1987; 82:665–671.
24. Soyka M. Treatment of benzodiazepine dependence. *N Engl J Med* 2017; 376:1147–1157.
25. Petursson H. The benzodiazepine withdrawal syndrome. *Addiction* 1994; 89:1455–1459.
26. Ashton H. Protracted Withdrawal From Benzodiazepines: The Post-Withdrawal Syndrome. *Psychiatr Ann* 1995; 1:174–179.
27. Tannenbaum C, et al. Reduction of inappropriate benzodiazepine prescriptions among older adults through direct patient education: the empower cluster randomized trial. *JAMA Int Med* 2014; 174:890–898.
28. Guy A, et al. *Guidance for psychological therapists: enabling conversations with clients taking or withdrawing from prescribed psychiatric drugs.* London: APPG for Prescribed Drug Dependence; 2019.
29. Parr JM, et al. Effectiveness of current treatment approaches for benzodiazepine discontinuation: a meta-analysis. *Addiction* 2009; 104:13–24.
30. Denis C, et al. Pharmacological interventions for benzodiazepine mono-dependence management in outpatient settings. *Cochrane Database Syst Rev* 2006; CD005194.
31. Ashton H. Benzodiazepines: how they work & how to withdraw, the Ashton Manual. 2002; http://www.benzo.org.uk/manual/bzcha01.htm.
32. Ashton H. Benzodiazepine dependence. *Adv Syndrom Psychiatric Drugs* 2004; 239–260.
33. Brouillet E, et al. In vivo bidirectional modulatory effect of benzodiazepine receptor ligands on GABAergic transmission evaluated by positron emission tomography in non-human primates. *Brain Res* 1991; 557:167–176.

34. Inner Compass Initiative Inc. The withdrawal project. 2019; https://withdrawal.theinnercompass.org.

35. Voshaar RCO, et al. Strategies for discontinuing long-term benzodiazepine use: meta-analysis. *Br J Psychiatry* 2006; **189**:213–220.

36. Fluyau D, et al. Challenges of the pharmacological management of benzodiazepine withdrawal, dependence, and discontinuation. *Ther Adv Psychopharmacol* 2018; **8**:147–168.

37. Gould RL, et al. Interventions for reducing benzodiazepine use in older people: meta-analysis of randomised controlled trials. *Br J Psychiatry* 2014; **204**:98–107.

38. Pollmann AS, et al. Deprescribing benzodiazepines and Z-drugs in community-dwelling adults: a scoping review. *BMC Pharmacol & Toxicol* 2015; **16**:19.

39. Kales A, et al. Rebound insomnia after only brief and intermittent use of rapidly eliminated benzodiazepines. *Clin Pharmacol Ther* 1991; **49**:468–476.

苯二氮䓬类药物与脱抑制

通常将继发于药物治疗的攻击或冲动行为意外增加称为脱抑制或矛盾反应。这些反应包括急性兴奋、活动过度、焦虑增加、生动梦境、性行为脱抑制、攻击、敌意和愤怒。造成脱抑制的物质包括苯丙胺、哌甲酯、苯二氮䓬类药和乙醇。苯二氮䓬类药的矛盾反应是一个重要的因素，因为使用这些药物的目的本来是镇静和安宁，而矛盾性反应适得其反。这些反应在大内科也是一个重要问题，因为米达唑仑等药被广泛地用于意识清醒状态下的镇静。在重症医学科，苯二氮䓬类药相关的脱抑制反应很难和多动型谵妄相鉴别[1]。

苯二氮䓬类药物脱抑制反应普遍吗？

脱抑制反应的发生率在不同人群中差异很大（见下文中"谁具有高风险"部分）。例如，对苯二氮䓬类药物随机对照试验的一项荟萃分析发现，在数百名诊断各异的患者中，苯二氮䓬类药物脱抑制反应发生率低于1%（与安慰剂相似）[2]。类似地，一项在精神科病房进行的行为脱抑制频率分析发现，不管是否接受苯二氮䓬类药物治疗，脱抑制的发生频率没有区别[3]。但是，挪威一项研究报道了415个"在药物影响下驾驶"的案例，他们使用的主要是氟硝西泮，发现6%的不良反应可被描述为脱抑制反应[4]。一项以惊恐障碍患者为研究对象的随机对照试验报道其发生率为13%[5]。病例系列（往往报告的是高危患者的用药情况）研究者报道的发生率为10%~20%[2]；一项以边缘型人格障碍患者为研究对象的随机对照试验则报道其发生率高达58%[6]。

脱抑制很难定义，因此发生率难以确定。攻击可以看作是一种脱抑制反应，但本质上并未定义为脱抑制。攻击很明显地与苯二氮䓬类药物使用相关，包括长期使用以及仅单次用药[7,8]。

其他GABA能激动剂，尤其是唑吡坦，也与睡行症、自动症、遗忘和躁狂发作等脱抑制反应相关[9-12]。

谁容易发生脱抑制？

有下述因素者出现脱抑制反应的风险增高：存在学习障碍、神经系统疾病或中枢神经系统退行性疾病[13]、年轻（儿童或青少年）或年老[13-16]、既往有过攻击/冲动控制能不良[6,17]。若苯二氮䓬类药物的效价强、半衰期短、剂量大或经静脉给药（导致血浆水平很高并快速波动），则风险进一步增加[13,18-20]。某些患者的风险可能存在遗传基础[21]。

不同风险因素的组合非常重要：低风险长效苯二氮䓬类药物可导致儿童等高危人群发生脱抑制[16]，高风险短效药物静脉给药极有可能导致人格障碍患者发生脱抑制。

可能的机制[18,22-24]

目前，已有多种理论试图解释脱抑制反应的发生机制。第一，苯二氮䓬类药物的抗焦虑和记忆损害作用可能导致对正常社交行为的控制减弱；第二，其镇静和记忆损害可能导致患者对指引正确行为的外部社交线索的关注能力减退；第三，苯二氮䓬类药物介导的GABA神经传导增加可能引起大脑皮质抑制作用的下降，导致不受约束的兴奋、焦虑和敌意。

　　氟马西尼常用于逆转苯二氮䓬类药物的镇静和呼吸抑制,它也可以有效治疗脱抑制反应[25]。

主观报告

　　与服用安慰剂者相比,服用苯二氮䓬类药物者自我评价更为宽容和友好,但对挑衅刺激的反应却更强烈[26]。存在冲动控制问题的苯二氮䓬类药物服用者,常自觉充满力量,并表现出过强的自尊心[27]。心理评定量表证明,他们的暗示性增强,不能识别他人的怒气,识别社交线索的能力也降低了。该研究者的体验(曾在手术前静脉注射咪达唑仑)是,患者可能完全没有意识到他们的行为奇怪,也不知道这是药物所致脱抑制的结果。

临床意义

　　苯二氮䓬类药物常用于快速镇静和行为紊乱的短期治疗。在大多数治疗中,苯二氮䓬类药物产生镇静、减轻了焦虑和攻击。但是必须知道,它们可能会引起的反常的脱抑制反应。

　　苯二氮䓬类药物使用中的矛盾性脱抑制/攻击行为:
- 在一般人群中罕见,但在冲动控制障碍、中枢神经系统损害、年幼或老年者中更常见。
- 在胃肠外给予高剂量、高效价药物时发生率最高。
- 通常发生在患者遭遇(往往非常轻微的)刺激时,他人往往不知道患者究竟受什么刺激了。
- 能被他人识别,但患者本人常常意识不到,常常认为自己是友好、宽容的。

　　可疑的矛盾反应应明确记录在临床记录中。在极端情况下,可使用氟马西尼逆转这种反应。如果使用苯二氮䓬类药物的目的是控制急性行为紊乱,将来再次发作时,治疗应该使用抗精神病药[27]或其他非苯二氮䓬类镇静剂。

（李清伟　张燕 译　田成华 审校）

参考文献

1. Schieveld JNM, et al. On benzodiazepines, paradoxical agitation, hyperactive delirium, and chloride homeostasis. *Crit Care Med* 2018; **46**:1558–1559.
2. Dietch JT, et al. Aggressive dyscontrol in patients treated with benzodiazepines. *J Clin Psychiatry* 1988; **49**:184–188.
3. Rothschild AJ, et al. Comparison of the frequency of behavioral disinhibition on alprazolam, clonazepam, or no benzodiazepine in hospitalized psychiatric patients. *J Clin Psychopharmacol* 2000; **20**:7–11.
4. Bramness JG, et al. Flunitrazepam: psychomotor impairment, agitation and paradoxical reactions. *Forensic Sci Int* 2006; **159**:83–91.
5. O'Sullivan GH, et al. Safety and side-effects of alprazolam. Controlled study in agoraphobia with panic disorder. *Br J Psychiatry* 1994; **165**:79–86.
6. Gardner DL, et al. Alprazolam-induced dyscontrol in borderline personality disorder. *Am J Psychiatry* 1985; **142**:98–100.
7. Albrecht B, et al. Motivational drive and alprazolam misuse: a recipe for aggression? *Psychiatry Res* 2016; **240**:381–389.
8. Albrecht B, et al. Benzodiazepine use and aggressive behaviour: a systematic review. *Aust N Z J Psychiatry* 2014; **48**:1096–1114.
9. Sabe M, et al. Zolpidem stimulant effect: induced mania case report and systematic review of cases. *Prog Neuropsychopharmacol Biol Psychiatry* 2019; **94**:109643.
10. Poceta JS. Zolpidem ingestion, automatisms, and sleep driving: a clinical and legal case series. *J Clin Sleep Med* 2011; **7**:632–638.
11. Pressman MR. Sleep driving: sleepwalking variant or misuse of z-drugs? *Sleep Med Rev* 2011; **15**:285–292.
12. Daley C, et al. 'I did what?' Zolpidem and the courts. *J Am Acad Psychiatry Law* 2011; **39**:535–542.
13. Bond AJ. Drug-induced behavioural disinhibition incidence, mechanisms and therapeutic implications. *CNS Drugs* 1998; **9**:41–57.
14. Hakimi Y, et al. Paradoxical adverse drug reactions: descriptive analysis of French reports. *Eur J Clin Pharmacol* 2020; **76**:1169–1174.
15. Hawkridge SM, et al. A risk-benefit assessment of pharmacotherapy for anxiety disorders in children and adolescents. *Drug Saf* 1998;

第 3 章

19:283–297.

16. Kandemir H, et al. Behavioral disinhibition, suicidal ideation, and self-mutilation related to clonazepam. *J Child Adolesc Psychopharmacol* 2008; 18:409.

17. Daderman AM, et al. Flunitrazepam (Rohypnol) abuse in combination with alcohol causes premeditated, grievous violence in male juvenile offenders. *J Am Acad Psychiatry Law* 1999; 27:83–99.

18. van der Bijl P, et al. Disinhibitory reactions to benzodiazepines: a review. *J Oral Maxillofac Surg* 1991; 49:519–523.

19. McKenzie WS, et al. Paradoxical reaction following administration of a benzodiazepine. *J Oral MaxillofacSurg* 2010; 68:3034–3036.

20. Wilson KE, et al. Complications associated with intravenous midazolam sedation in anxious dental patients. *Prim Dent Care* 2011; 18:161–166.

21. Short TG, et al. Paradoxical reactions to benzodiazepines–a genetically determined phenomenon? *Anaesth Intensive Care* 1987; 15:330–331.

22. Weisman AM, et al. Effects of clorazepate, diazepam, and oxazepam on a laboratory measurement of aggression in men. *Int Clin Psychopharmacol* 1998; 13:183–188.

23. Blair RJ, et al. Selective impairment in the recognition of anger induced by diazepam. *Psychopharmacology (Berl)* 1999; 147:335–338.

24. Wallace PS, et al. Reduction of appeasement-related affect as a concomitant of diazepam-induced aggression: evidence for a link between aggression and the expression of self-conscious emotions. *Aggress Behav* 2009; 35:203–212.

25. Tae CH, et al. Paradoxical reaction to midazolam in patients undergoing endoscopy under sedation: incidence, risk factors and the effect of flumazenil. *Dig Liver Dis* 2014; 46:710–715.

26. Bond AJ, et al. Behavioural aggression in panic disorder after 8 weeks' treatment with alprazolam. *J Affect Disord* 1995; 35:117–123.

27. Paton C. Benzodiazepines and disinhibition: a review. *Psychiatric Bull* 2002; 26:460–462.

第 3 章

成瘾与物质滥用

背景介绍

由使用精神活性物质所致的精神和行为障碍非常普遍。世界卫生组织（WHO）《国际疾病分类第 10 版》（ICD-10)[1] 中提到物质相关障碍包括急性中毒、有害使用、依赖综合征、戒断状态、伴有谵妄的戒断状态、精神病性障碍、遗忘综合征、残留和迟发性精神病性障碍、其他精神和行为障碍和未指定的精神和行为障碍等。许多精神活性物质都可能导致健康问题，包括酒精、阿片类、苯二氮䓬类、γ-羟基丁酸（GHB）/γ-丁内酯（GBL）、兴奋剂、新型精神活性物质（NPS）（包括卡西酮、合成大麻素和苯乙胺）、阿拉伯茶（khat）、硝酸盐类、致幻剂、合成类固醇和烟草等。

物质滥用常见于严重精神疾病（所谓共病诊断）和人格障碍患者。在许多成人精神科中，共病是常态，不是例外。在全球许多地方，物质滥用服务可能是在一般精神科服务机构之外单独提供的。大多数成瘾治疗机构的治疗模式意味着，若是患者缺乏治疗动机，将不能保证对其进行诊疗和随访。由于普遍缺乏共病诊治的医疗团队，这些患者得不到最佳治疗[2]。

根据 ICD-10，依赖综合征是一组生理、行为和认知症状的综合征，即个体使用某种或某类精神活性物质极大地优先于其他曾经比较重要的活动。确诊物质依赖需要在过去一年内至少满足以下 3 条：

- 强迫性使用精神活性物质
- 难以控制使用精神活性物质的行为
- 生理戒断状态
- 耐受性的证据
- 忽视其他兴趣
- 尽管有害，但仍继续使用

物质使用障碍的治疗通常应将药物治疗与心理社会综合干预相结合。本章内容将侧重介绍对酒精、阿片类物质和尼古丁使用的药物治疗，而对苯二氮䓬类、GHB/GBL、兴奋剂、新型精神活性物质（包括卡西酮、合成大麻素和苯乙胺）、阿拉伯茶、硝酸盐类、致幻剂和合成代谢类固醇的治疗仅作简要介绍。注意，英国卫生研究所与临床最佳实践（NICE）的指南和技术评估、英国卫生部物质滥用指南（橙皮书)[3]、英国公共卫生部[2] 和近期即将更新的英国精神药理协会共识指南（BAP)[4] 等也提供了详细的治疗方法概述。

参考文献

1. World Health Organisation. International statistical classification of diseases and related health problems. Online version. 2016; http://apps. who.int/classifications/icd10/browse/2016/en.

2. Public Health England. Better care for people with co-occurring mental health and alcohol/drug use conditions. A guide for commissioners and service providers. 2017; https://www.gov.uk/government/uploads/system/uploads/attachment_data/file/625809/Co-occurring_mental_health_and_alcohol_drug_use_conditions.pdf.

3. Department of Health and Social Care. Drug misuse and dependence: UK guidelines on clinical management. 2017; https://www.gov.uk/government/publications/drug-misuse-and-dependence-uk-guidelines-on-clinical-management.

4. Lingford-Hughes AR, et al. Evidence-based guidelines for the pharmacological management of substance abuse, harmful use, addiction and comorbidity: recommendations from BAP. *J Psychopharmacol* 2012; 26:899–952.

酒依赖

酒精

什么叫标准单位酒精(unit of alcohol)

一个标准单位酒精相当于 10mL 酒精,或 1L 1% 酒精饮料。例如,250mL 含 10% 酒精的葡萄酒为 2.5 个单位酒精 [2]。

饮多少酒算多?

最大限度地减少饮酒所带来的健康风险,英国卫生部提出了以下忠告和建议 [1]:

- 经常饮酒时,每周不应超过 140mL 纯酒精,男女均适用。
- 用 3 天或 3 天以上时间饮用该数量的酒精时,危害会降到最低。
- 单次大量饮酒与伤害、受伤和事故发生的风险有关。
- 无论饮酒多少均与许多疾病相关,例如喉癌、口腔癌和乳腺癌。
- 妊娠期间没有绝对安全的饮酒量,建议孕妇避免饮酒,降低对婴儿伤害的风险。

评估与简短结构化咨询

英国 NICE 关于有害性饮酒及酒依赖的诊断、评估和处理的指南提出,在可能会遇到问题饮酒者的治疗机构,工作人员应该有能力识别和评估有害饮酒和酒依赖 [2]。NICE 关于减少有害饮酒的公共卫生指南提出,对于饮酒相关问题风险较高的每个人,都要进行一次简短的结构化咨询 [3],该咨询基于 FRAMES 原则(反馈 feedback、责任 responsibility、建议 advice、选择菜单 menu、共情 empathy、自我效能 self-efficacy),是一种有效的干预方法。

若发现饮酒量超过建议的水平,则需要进行更全面的临床评估。评估内容包括以下方面:

- 饮酒史,包括每天饮酒量和近期的饮酒模式。
- 既往酒精戒断发作史。
- 最近一次饮酒时间。
- 家族成员或照料者提供的病史。
- 其他药物(非法和处方药)使用情况。
- 依赖和戒断症状的严重程度。
- 其他躯体或精神科问题共病情况。
- 体格检查,包括认知功能检查。
- 呼气酒精检测:检测呼气中的绝对酒精水平。注意:需要在最后一口酒后 20min 及 1h 进行检测,以避免检测的是口腔中的酒精浓度而出现偏高的错误结果。
- 实验室检查:全血细胞检查、尿素氮、电解质、肝功能、国际标准化比值(INR)、凝血酶原时间和尿毒检。

推荐使用以下结构化评估工具 [2]。

- 酒精使用障碍筛查问卷(AUDIT) [4]:该问卷包括 10 个问题,对于被确定为酒精使用障碍高风险者,是有用的筛查工具。其中问题 1~3 是关于具体饮酒量,问题 4~6 是关于依赖的症状和体征,问题 7~10 是关于有害性饮酒的行为和症状。每个问题的分值范围为 0~4 分,总分最高为 40 分。得分≥8 分提示存在危险性饮酒或有害性饮酒。危险性饮酒,即饮酒有可能造成损害。有害性饮酒,即饮酒已经造成精神或躯体问题。

- 酒依赖严重程度问卷(SADQ)[5]:该问卷更详细,包括 20 个条目,每个问题的得分范围为 0~3 分,总分最高 60 分。

酒依赖严重度
轻度:SADQ 得分≤15 分
中度:SADQ 得分 16~30 分[①]
重度:SADQ 得分≥31 分

酒精戒断

酒精依赖患者的中枢神经系统已经适应了体内持续存在的酒精(神经适应)。当血液酒精浓度(BAC)突然下降时,大脑仍处于过度兴奋状态,导致戒断综合征(表 4.1)。

表 4.1　轻、重度酒精戒断的临床表现及并发症

轻度酒精戒断——表现	末次饮酒后症状通常出现的时间	其他信息
■ 激越/焦虑/易怒 ■ 手、舌及眼睑震颤 ■ 出汗 ■ 恶心、呕吐、腹泻 ■ 发热 ■ 心动过速 ■ 收缩期高血压 ■ 全身不适	3~12h 起病 24~48h 达到高峰 持续 14 天	■ 症状是非特异性的 ■ 症状的缺乏并不能排除戒断 ■ 可能在血液酒精水平降至 0 之前出现

管理
戒断症状可能是自限性的,使用足量苯二氮䓬类药物与对症支持治疗可使其得到缓解
监测生命体征。使用戒断评估量表
* 见下文所推荐的苯二氮䓬类药物

重度酒精戒断——并发症	末次饮酒后症状通常出现的时间	其他信息
全身性大发作	12~18h	■ 可能在血液酒精水平降至 0 之前出现

管理
- 在药物辅助戒酒期间,如首次出现癫痫发作,需要进行全面检查,以排除器质性疾病或特发性癫痫
- 一项关于评估药物预防酒精戒断性癫痫发作疗效试验的荟萃分析表明,苯二氮䓬类药物,特别是地西泮等长效制剂,可显著减少新的癫痫发作[6,7]
- 对于既往有癫痫发作史的患者,推荐使用长效苯二氮䓬类药物作为预防性治疗[8]
- 某些抗癫痫药与苯二氮䓬类药物疗效相同,有些病房建议对未治疗的癫痫患者使用卡马西平,或在服用足量苯二氮䓬类药物后仍有癫痫发作的患者可使用卡马西平
- 苯妥英单独使用或与苯二氮䓬类药物联合使用,均不能预防与酒精戒断相关的癫痫发作。[9] 使用抗癫痫药预防酒精戒断的癫痫发作时,没必要长期使用[9]

① 原文中是 15 分,译者参考其他文献修改。

重度酒精戒断——并发症	末次饮酒后症状通常出现的时间	其他信息和管理
震颤性谵妄(详见本章具体章节) ■ 意识混浊/模糊 ■ 鲜明的幻觉,尤其是视幻觉和触幻觉 ■ 明显的震颤 其他临床特征还包括自主神经功能亢进(心动过速、高血压、出汗和发热)、妄想、激越和失眠 前驱症状包括夜间失眠、不安、恐惧和精神错乱 危险因素:严重酒精依赖、非医疗性干预的自我戒酒、多次因酒精戒断入院、合并躯体疾病、震颤谵妄和酒精性癫痫发作史、低钾、低镁、维生素 B_1 缺乏、戒断治疗不充分 震颤性谵妄的正确识别十分重要,因为其治疗不同于其他原因引起的谵妄。震颤性谵妄**需要使用更大剂量的苯二氮䓬类药物,而且使用抗精神病药需更加谨慎** 管理 ■ 这是一种医疗急症,需要立即将患者转入综合医院救治[9],最好是高依赖病房[10,11] ■ 必须亲自检查患者(见本章"震颤谵妄")	3~4 天 (72~96h)	■ 因戒酒住院的患者中发生率为 3%~5% ■ 医疗急症 ■ 未治疗者死亡率为 10%~20%

药物辅助戒酒(酒精戒断治疗)

处理不当时,酒精戒断可出现较高的发病率及死亡率。

需要药物辅助戒酒的情况包括:

■ 每天规律饮酒 >150mL 纯酒精。

■ AUDIT 总分 >20 分。

■ 以前有过明显的戒断症状。

症状量表有助于确定控制戒断症状所需的药物剂量。临床机构酒精戒断评估量表修订版(CIWA-Ar,图 4.1)[12] 和简明酒精戒断量表(SAWS,表 4.2)[13] 均只有 10 个条目,约 5min 完成。CIWA-Ar 是他评量表,而 SAWS 则是自评工具。当 CIWA-Ar 得分 >10 分或 SAWS 得分 >12 分时,提示应该采用药物辅助戒酒。

以下情况可在社区戒酒:

■ 有一个照料者(最好 24h)能够全程监督戒酒过程。

■ 与患者、他们的照料者和全科医师达成一致的治疗计划。

■ 与患者、他们的照料者和全科医师达成一致的应急计划。

■ 戒酒治疗过程中,患者可以每天来取药,以便专业人员定期进行评估。

■ 已有包括心理社会支持治疗在内的门诊/社区戒酒方案。

患者：_____ 日期：_____

时间_____ (24 小时制,午夜 =00:00)：_____

脉搏或心率,计数 1 分钟：_____

血压：_____

恶心和呕吐——问"你胃里有恶心的感觉吗？有没有呕吐？"观察

0 无恶心,无呕吐
1 轻度恶心,无呕吐
2
3
4 间断恶伴干呕
5
6
7 持续恶心,频繁的干呕和呕吐

震颤——两臂伸展,手指分开。观察
0 无震颤
1 不可见,指尖对指尖可感受到
2
3
4 中度,患者两臂延展
5
6
7 重度,即使两臂不伸展也有

阵发性出汗——观察
0 看不见出汗
1 勉强察觉出汗,手掌潮湿
2
3
4 前额有明显的汗珠
5
6
7 汗水湿透

焦虑——询问"你觉得紧张吗？"观察
0 无焦虑,自由自在
1 轻度焦虑
2
3
4 中度焦虑,或谨慎,因此推测有焦虑
5
6
7 相当于严重谵妄或急性精神病性反应所见的急性惊恐状态

激越——观察
0 正常活动
1 比正常活动略多
2
3
4 中度烦躁不安
5
6
7 访谈期间多半来回走动或辗转反侧

触觉障碍——询问"你有发痒、发麻、烧灼、麻木、皮肤上或皮下虫子爬的感觉吗？"观察
0 无
1 很轻的瘙痒、针刺、烧灼或麻木感
2 轻度瘙痒、针刺、烧灼或麻木感
3 中度瘙痒、针刺、烧灼或麻木感
4 中度幻觉
5 重度幻觉
6 极严重的幻觉
7 持续的幻觉

听觉障碍——询问"你对周围的声音更敏感吗？声音刺耳吗？声音是否吓着你？你听到什么烦人的声音了？你知道你听到的声音是不存在的吗？"观察
0 不存在
1 很轻的刺耳或令你害怕
2 轻度刺耳或令人害怕
3 中度刺耳或令人害怕
4 中度幻觉
5 重度幻觉
6 极严重的幻觉
7 持续的幻觉

视觉障碍——询问"光线是否看起来太亮？颜色有什么不同？光线刺疼了你的眼睛吗？你看到什么让你困扰的东西吗？你知道你看到的东西是不存在的吗？"观察
0 不存在
1 很轻的敏感
2 轻度敏感
3 中度敏感
4 中度幻觉
5 重度幻觉
6 极严重的幻觉
7 持续的幻觉

头痛头胀——问"你是否感觉头部不一样？感觉像一条带子缠在头上？头晕或头昏？"评分。否则评定严重程度
0 没有
1 很轻
2 轻度
3 中度
4 中重度
5 重度
6 很重
7 极重

定向障碍和意识模糊——询问："今天的日期是什么？你在哪里？我是谁？"
0 定向力存在,可做连加法
1 不会做连加法,或不确定日期
2 日期错误最多 2 天
3 日期错误超过 2 天
4 地点/人物定向障碍

分数
≤10 分,轻度戒断(不需要其他药物)
≤15 分,中度戒断
>15 分,重度戒断

总 CIWA-Ar 得分_____
评估者姓名首字母缩写_____
最高可能得分:67 分

图 4.1 临床机构酒精戒断评估量表(修订版)[12](CIWA-Ar 无版权,可免费复制)

若患者再次饮酒,或未能按照商定的治疗计划进行,应停止社区戒酒治疗。

若有下列情况者,可能需要住院治疗:

- 每天规律饮酒量 >300mL 纯酒精。
- SADQ>30 分(重度依赖)。
- 有癫痫发作或震颤谵妄史。
- 非常年轻或年纪很大。
- 存在苯二氮䓬类药物与酒精合用。
- 除酒之外,存在其他物质滥用。
- 共病其他精神或躯体、学习困难或认知障碍。
- 妊娠。
- 无家可归或无社会支持。
- 社区戒酒失败。

在某些情况下,上述患者在临床上可能有理由进行社区戒酒(表 4.3);但是,这些理由必须非常明确,并由经验丰富的临床医师作出决定。

表 4.2　简明酒精戒断量表(SAWS)[13]

	无(0)	轻度(1)	中度(2)	重度(3)
焦虑				
睡眠障碍				
记忆障碍				
恶心				
不安				
震颤(手抖)				
混乱感				
出汗				
痛苦感				
心跳加速				

表 4.3　酒精戒断的治疗:总结

严重程度	支持性/内科治疗	药物治疗逆转神经适应性变化	硫胺素补充	治疗场所
轻度 CIWA-Ar≤10 分	中、高水平支持性治疗,很少需要内科治疗	很少需要,简单治疗即可(见下文)	营养状况良好的患者,口服给药即可	家中
中度 CIWA-Ar≤15 分	中、高水平支持性治疗,很少需要内科治疗	很少需要,仅需要对症治疗(见下文)	营养不良患者,肌内注射硫胺素制剂,然后口服补充	家中或社区团队
重度 CIWA-Ar>15 分	高水平支持性治疗+医疗监护	对症治疗,可能需要替代治疗(氯氮䓬)	肌内注射硫胺素制剂,然后口服补充	社区团队或医院
CIWA-Ar>10 分合并酒精相关躯体疾病	高水平支持性治疗+专业内科治疗	通常需要对症治疗和替代治疗	肌内注射硫胺素制剂,然后口服补充	医院

苯二氮䓬类药物是治疗酒精戒断症状的首选药物。它们与酒精有交叉耐受,并有抗癫痫作用。它们也得到 NICE 指南 [2,14]、Cochrane 系统综述 [7] 及英国精神药学协会(BAP)指南 [9] 等支持。**肠胃外维生素 B_1 作为另一种**维生素替代疗法,是重要的辅助治疗,可以预防或治疗韦尼克-科尔萨科夫综合征及其他维生素相关神经精神疾病。

氯氮䓬是英国大多数治疗中心用于多数患者的苯二氮䓬类药物,因其依赖性较低。也有些治疗机构使用地西泮。对于肝功能受损者,可用短效苯二氮䓬类药物,如奥沙西泮或劳拉西泮。

目前,有三种类型的辅助戒酒方案:**固定剂量减药**(常用于非专业机构中),根据症状**给药**(通常使用的苯二氮䓬类药物剂量较小,但最好由戒酒治疗专业人员实施),最后是**冲击给药**(不常用,限于严重酒精戒断症状)[2,9]。如果血液酒精浓度很高或仍在上升阶段,则不宜进行药物辅助戒酒治疗。需监测患者是否存在过度镇静或呼吸抑制。

固定剂量减量方案

固定剂量减量方案可在社区、非专业机构的病房或住宿治疗项目中使用。可根据患者酒依赖严重度(临床病史、每天饮酒量及 SADQ 得分)开始使用某一剂量的苯二氮䓬类药物。以氯氮䓬为例,一般的经验是根据当前酒精摄入量来估算起始剂量。若每天饮酒相当于 200mL 纯酒精,则起始剂量应是 20mg,4 次/d。该剂量在接下来的 5~10 天内逐渐停用。应该采用经过验证的评估工具(如 CIWA-Ar[12] 或 SAWS[13])来监测酒精戒断症状。

轻度酒依赖患者通常仅需很低剂量的氯氮䓬,也可以不用药。

对于**中度**酒依赖患者,典型的方案可以是氯氮䓬 10~20mg,4 次/d,5~7 天内逐渐停用。需要注意的是,疗程通常 5~7 天足够,不必延长治疗时间,因更长治疗时间获益极小。建议每天给药之前,监测戒断症状和血液酒精浓度。在社区进行药物辅助戒酒治疗时,通常应该从周一开始,持续 5 天。中度酒依赖固定剂量氯氮䓬治疗方案的示例如表 4.4 所示。

表 4.4　中度酒依赖:固定剂量氯氮䓬治疗方案示例

时间	剂量	每天总剂量/mg
第 1 天	20mg,4 次/d	80
第 2 天	15mg,4 次/d	60
第 3 天	10mg,4 次/d	40
第 4 天	5mg,4 次/d	20
第 5 天	5mg,2 次/d	10

重度酒依赖患者通常需要住院进行药物辅助的戒酒治疗,因为有发生致命并发症的风险。然而,极少的情况下也会采用社区治疗的方式。但在这种情况下,关于在社区进行药物辅助的戒酒治疗的决定,必须由经验丰富的临床医师向患者和照料者说明。建议在最初 2~3 天进行严密监测。在周末可能需要做出特别的安排。重度酒依赖固定剂量氯氮䓬治疗方案的示例如表 4.5 所示。

患者醉酒时不宜开始用药。在这种情况下,告诉患者醒酒后尽早复诊。在这类患者中,苯二氮䓬类药物剂量减完可能需要 7~10 天(若依赖非常严重,或既往戒酒期间出现过并发症,则疗程偶尔可能更长)。

根据症状给药方案

该方案适用于在专门戒酒的病房或养老院(residential settings)住宿治疗项目中进行药物辅助戒酒。需要定期监测,如:脉搏、血压、体温、意识水平。只有在出现戒断症状(以 CIWA-Ar、SAWS 或其他有效量表来评估)时,才能给药。根据症状给药方案一般仅在无并发症史的患者中使用。典型的方案是根据需要,每小时给予氯氮䓬 20~30mg。注意:每天的总剂量应从第 2 天开始减少。根据症状给药方案通常维持 24~48h 后,就换成个体化的固定剂量减量方案。**根据症状给药**方案偶尔可能需要超过 24h,如在震颤谵妄时。

表 4.5　重度酒依赖:固定剂量氯氮䓬治疗方案示例

时间	剂量	每天总剂量/mg
第 1 天(第一个 24h)	40mg,4 次/d,需要时加 40mg	200
第 2 天	40mg,4 次/d	160
第 3 天	30mg,4 次/d	120
第 4 天	25mg,4 次/d	100
第 5 天	20mg,4 次/d	80
第 6 天	15mg,4 次/d	60
第 7 天	10mg,4 次/d	40
第 8 天	10mg,3 次/d	30
第 9 天	5mg,4 次/d	20
第 10 天	10mg,每晚	10

根据症状给予氯氮䓬 的方案示例[2]

第 1~5 天:根据患者症状,间隔最长每小时按需给予氯氮䓬 20~30mg。

韦尼克脑病

韦尼克脑病是一种因维生素 B_1 缺乏导致的急性神经精神疾病。在酒依赖中,维生素 B_1 缺乏继发于食物的摄入和吸收均减少。

酒精依赖患者发生韦尼克脑病的危险因素如下[14]:

- 急性戒断
- 营养不良
- 失代偿性肝病
- 急诊科就诊
- 因共病住院
- 无家可归

临床表现

虽然韦尼克脑病的典型三联征(眼肌麻痹、共济失调和意识错乱)并不多见,但该综合征还是比人们普遍的印象要多见。因此,戒酒患者凡有下列体征,应推断诊断为韦尼克脑病:

- 共济失调
- 体温过低
- 低血压
- 意识错乱
- 眼肌麻痹/眼球震颤
- 记忆障碍
- 意识丧失/昏迷

同时应注意了解营养不良、近期体重减轻、呕吐、腹泻或周围神经病等病史[15]。

预防性使用维生素 B_1

饮食正常且无神经精神科并发症的低风险饮酒者,可于药物辅助戒酒期间或连续饮酒期间口服维生素 B_1,每天最低剂量为300mg[9]。

注意:维生素 B_1 是利用葡萄糖所必需的,在维生素 B_1 缺乏的患者中,葡萄糖负荷可导致韦尼克脑病。

对于出现精神异常的所有患者,在补充葡萄糖前,应给予肠外复合 B 族维生素(在英国,商品名为 Pabrinex)。

对于住院戒酒的患者,通常建议预防性给予胃肠外维生素 B_1[2,9,14,16,17],但是随机对照试验未提供足够证据说明最佳剂量、频率和疗程。指南根据"专家意见"提出的标准建议是,每天 1 次给予两支高效 **Pabrinex 肌内注射**(每剂含维生素 B_1 250mg),持续治疗 5 天;然后口服维生素 B_1 或复合维生素 B(进食不足,或再次饮酒者),服药时间长短根据需要确定[9]。所有住院患者均应实施方案。

维生素 B_1 肌内注射剂的过敏反应发生率低于静脉注射剂,发生率约为 500 万对安瓿出现一例,远低于许多没有过敏警示的常用药物。然而,这种风险却导致害怕使用胃肠外制剂,以及不适当地使用口服制剂(未提供足够保护)。考虑到韦尼克脑病的风险,其风险收益比提示应该使用胃肠外维生素 B_1[9,16,18]。使用胃肠外制剂时,应准备好应对过敏反应的措施[19]。

一旦怀疑韦尼克脑病,患者应当转入可以静脉注射维生素 B_1 的内科病房。若不治疗,韦尼克脑病可发展为科萨科夫氏综合征(表现为持久的记忆障碍、虚构、意识错乱和人格改变)。

可疑或确诊为韦尼克脑病患者的治疗(急诊内科病房):

至少 2 对 Pabrinex 静脉注射高效制剂(即 4 支安瓿),每天 3 次,持续 3~5 天;此后减量至 2 支/次,每天 1 次,持续 3~5 天或更长时间,直至病情稳定[2,9]。

躯体症状的治疗

在药物辅助戒酒过程中,躯体症状很常见。一些简单的治疗建议见**表 4.6**。

表 4.6 躯体症状的治疗

症状	治疗建议
脱水	保证充分液体摄入,以保持水电解质平衡 脱水可引起致命的心律失常
疼痛	对乙酰氨基酚
恶心、呕吐	每 4~6h 给予甲氧氯普胺 10mg 或丙氯拉嗪 5mg
腹泻	地芬诺酯、阿托品或洛哌丁胺
皮肤瘙痒	常见,不仅发生于酒精性肝病患者:口服抗组胺药

预防复发

度过急性酒精戒断期之后,不需要继续使用苯二氮䓬类药物。英国已经批准使用阿坎酸、监护下使用双硫仑结合心理社会干预来治疗酒依赖[2]。应由专业机构开始治疗,12 周后可转给全科医师治疗,但是可能还需要继续专科治疗(共同治疗)。中、重度酒依赖也推荐使用纳曲酮作为辅助治疗[2]。英国目前未批准该药用于治疗酒依赖,开始治疗前应获取知情同意,并加以记录。

阿坎酸

阿坎酸是合成的牛磺酸类药物,为谷氨酸 NMDA 受体拮抗剂,还具有增加 GABA 能的作用。其 NNT 为 9~11 人[9],即每治疗 9~11 个患者会有 1 个保持守戒。其戒酒疗效在 6 个月时最佳,复饮风险比(与安慰剂相比)降至 0.83,但是其疗效最长可持续 12 个月[2,20,21]。应在戒酒后尽早给予阿坎酸(BAP 共识指南建议应在戒酒期间使用阿坎酸[9],因为它有潜在的神经保护作用)。NICE 建议阿坎酸应维持治疗最长达 6 个月[2],并定期(每月)监测。产品特征概要(Summary of Product Charateristics,SPC)或药品说明书建议维持治疗时间为一年。

阿坎酸具有相对较好的耐受性,不良反应包括腹泻、腹部疼痛、恶心、呕吐和瘙痒[2]。禁忌证为严重肝、肾损害,治疗前应做肝、肾功能检测。孕期及哺乳期禁用。

阿坎酸:NICE 临床指南 115,2011[2,20]

阿坎酸联合心理治疗适用于预防中、重度酒依赖的复发。对于治疗有效并希望继续服用阿坎酸的患者,用药时间最长可达 6 个月,甚至更长。体重 60kg 以上的患者,剂量为 666mg,3 次/d;体重 60kg 以下者,剂量为 1 332mg/d。开始使用该药治疗后,若患者继续饮酒 4~6 周,应停止该治疗。

纳曲酮

阿片受体拮抗剂可在摄入酒精后,通过阻止多巴胺能活动增加来降低奖赏效应。非选择性的阿片受体拮抗剂纳曲酮,可显著减少再次重度饮酒[2,22]。早期试验使用的药物剂量为50mg/d,近来美国的研究将剂量增加到100mg/d。英国常用剂量仍为50mg/d,试验剂量为25mg使用2天,以评估不良反应。

纳曲酮的耐受性良好,不良反应包括恶心(特别是在治疗早期)、头痛、腹痛、食欲降低和疲劳。进行纳曲酮治疗前,应进行综合医学评估,包括基线的肝肾功能检查。纳曲酮可在患者饮酒或药物辅助戒酒时开始使用。关于最佳疗程没有确切的证据,一般认为随访6个月可能比较合适,其间包括监测肝功能[9]。

纳曲酮治疗期间,患者选择镇痛药物时应避免阿片受体激动剂,应使用非阿片类镇痛药。若必须使用阿片类受体激动剂进行镇痛,应在停用纳曲酮48~72h后再使用。高剂量纳曲酮有肝毒性,因此应该避免用于急性肝功能衰竭的患者[23]。

> **纳曲酮:NICE临床指南115,2011[2,22]**
>
> 预防中、重度酒依赖复发,应给予纳曲酮50mg/d,并结合心理治疗。对于治疗有效并希望继续服用该药的患者,疗程最长应该达到6个月,甚至更长。开始治疗后,若患者继续饮酒4~6周,或服药时感觉不适,应该停止治疗。

目前,已经研发出纳曲酮长效针剂用于提高治疗依从性,其不良反应与口服制剂类似[24]。NICE认为初步证据令人鼓舞,但是尚不足以支持常规使用。

纳美芬

纳美芬同样是阿片类受体拮抗剂,NICE推荐其作为酒精依赖患者减少饮酒的一种治疗选择[2,22]。一项间接荟萃分析显示,它在减少重度饮酒方面优于纳曲酮[25]。然而,对纳美芬的使用仍然存在争议。另一项荟萃分析表明,纳美芬在减少饮酒方面的效果有限,其在治疗酒精成瘾和预防复发方面的价值尚未被完全确定[26]。

双硫仑(戒酒硫)

双硫仑抑制乙醛脱氢酶,从而阻止酒精在肝脏中的完全代谢。这导致有毒的中间产物乙醛蓄积,从而引起酒精-双硫仑反应。

因此,双硫仑的治疗效果是因为它与酒精不相容,导致患者厌恶酒精。监督用药可优化依从性,有助于提高疗效。

不耐受反应的程度呈剂量依赖性,与酒精摄入量和双硫仑剂量有关。然而,目前认为治疗效果主要是由心理上对厌恶反应的预期所致,并非药物本身的作用。若剂量超过1 000mg,更易发生猝死[27]。因此,必须慎重考虑使用高剂量双硫仑的价值。

首次使用剂量为800mg/d,最后减量至100~200mg/d维持治疗。酒精和可卡因双重依赖的患者曾用过500mg/d的剂量。口臭是双硫仑常见的不良反应。若发生突发性黄疸(肝中毒的罕见并发症),应立即停药,并需要寻求紧急医疗关注。

轻度酒精-双硫仑反应

- 颜面潮红
- 出汗
- 恶心
- 过度换气
- 呼吸困难
- 心动过速
- 低血压

禁忌证

- 之前 24h 内摄入过酒精
- 心力衰竭
- 冠心病
- 高血压
- 脑血管病
- 妊娠
- 母乳喂养
- 肝脏疾病
- 周围神经病
- 严重精神疾病

重度酒精-双硫仑反应

- 急性心力衰竭
- 心肌梗死
- 心律失常
- 心动过缓
- 呼吸抑制
- 重度低血压

双硫仑的证据比阿坎酸和纳曲酮要少[2]。在英国,NICE 建议将其"作为中、重度酒依赖患者不适用阿坎酸或纳曲酮时的二线药物,或者用于对双硫仑有特定偏好及治疗目标为长期戒酒的患者"[2]。

双硫仑:NICE 临床指南 115,2011[2]

对于不适合使用阿坎酸或纳曲酮,但希望戒酒的患者,应该考虑使用双硫仑并结合心理干预。应该在末次饮酒后至少 24h 开始治疗,并有家人或照料者监护。建议监测频率为:前 2 个月每两周 1 次,后 4 个月每月 1 次。治疗 6 个月之后,应该继续进行医学监测,每 6 个月 1 次。患者服用双硫仑时不能饮酒。

巴氯酚

巴氯酚是一种 GABA-β 激动剂,未被批准用于酒依赖治疗,但是有一些临床医师在用。最近一项荟萃分析发现巴氯芬无效,也不支持将其作为酒精使用障碍的一线治疗药物[28]。巴氯酚的使用也与较高的不良反应发生率有关,包括抑郁、眩晕、嗜睡、麻木和肌肉强直。

抗癫痫药

现有证据不足以支持在临床上使用抗癫痫药治疗酒精依赖;但是研究发现,与安慰剂组相比,使用抗癫痫药与每天饮酒量减少和平均饮酒程度下降呈高度相关[29]。大多数的研究都是关于托吡酯的。对加巴喷丁[30]、丙戊酸和左乙拉西坦的研究较少。

妊娠与饮酒

有证据表明,在妊娠期间饮酒可能会对胎儿造成伤害。英国卫生部建议女性孕期不宜摄入任何酒精[1]。妊娠期间每天摄入 10~20mL 纯酒精会增加早产、低出生体重儿或孕龄偏小的风险。NICE 参考《英国首席医务官指南》,于 2018 年 12 月对 NICE 指南进行了修订。

对有戒断症状的酒依赖孕妇,应使用药物进行戒酒,最好能住院治疗。在不同孕期中戒酒时机的选择,应该根据继续饮酒的风险和对胎儿的风险评估来决定[9]。氯氮䓬被认为不大可能造成很大的风险,但也有剂量依赖性畸形的报道[9]。英国畸胎信息服务机构[31] 为全国保健专业人士提供相关建议,并希望随访需要戒酒治疗的孕妇。始终应该征求专家建议(见第 7 章)。尚未在孕期对预防复发的药物进行评估[9]。

儿童和青少年

儿童和青少年(10~17 岁)应该根据 NICE 的临床指南 CG115(2011 年发布)的描述进行评估[2]。

虽然需要药物治疗的酒依赖青少年人数较少,但是对于酒依赖者,住院门槛应该降低。进行药物辅助戒酒时,氯氮䓬剂量可能需要调整,但是对酒精戒断的处理原则与成年人相同。所有青少年都需要做全面的健康检查,以确认躯体和精神问题。阿坎酸、纳曲酮和双硫仑治疗 16~19 岁青少年的证据仍在积累之中[9],但是有很充分的证据支持将纳曲酮用于此年龄段[32,33]。

老年人

对于老年人,药物辅助戒酒的入院门槛应该降低[2]。首选苯二氮䓬类药物,治疗时宜用低剂量,有些情况下可能需要首选短效制剂[9]。酒精使用障碍的老人均需要做全面的常规体格检查,以确认躯体和精神问题。有关老年人酒精使用障碍的药物治疗,研究证据有限。

酒药合用障碍

酒精和其他药物使用障碍共存时,应该同时积极治疗酒精和药物使用障碍[2]。

酒精和苯二氮䓬类药物依赖共病

无论是使用氯氮䓬还是地西泮,最好单一用药。起始剂量应该考虑药物辅助戒酒的需要量,以及相关苯二氮䓬类药物的等效剂量[2]。一般需要住院治疗 2~3 周,甚至更长[2]。

酒精和可卡因依赖共病

可卡因与酒精共同依赖患者中,每天给予 150mg 纳曲酮,可降低男性的酒精与可卡因用量,但对女性没有影响[34]。

酒精和阿片类物质依赖共病

两种病均应治疗,需要注意的是停用两种药物均会增加死亡率。

酒精和尼古丁依赖共病

鼓励患者戒烟。参阅初级预防保健及其他机构的戒烟方案。在药物辅助戒酒期间,在门诊提供尼古丁贴片/吸入器具。应始终宣传电子烟是比烟草更安全的选择。

共病精神障碍

酒精使用障碍的患者往往伴有其他精神障碍,尤其是焦虑和抑郁症。英国公共卫生部将其描述为"一种常态,而不是例外",并鼓励一线诊疗中心之间采取合作的、有效的和灵活的方式,称这是"每个人的工作","杜绝推诿"[35]。

包括酒精滥用在内的物质使用障碍不应成为拒绝为患者提供下列服务的理由:
- 精神科危机干预服务。
- 脱瘾后的情绪、焦虑、人格问题服务。

抑郁

抑郁和焦虑症状在戒酒过程中经常出现,但是通常在戒酒后 3~4 周消失。荟萃分析表明,对于酒依赖者的抑郁症状,多通路的抗抑郁药(曲米帕明或丙米嗪)的疗效优于选择性5-羟色胺再摄取抑制剂(SSRI 类药物,如氟西汀、舍曲林),但其疗效一般[2,9,36,37]。若抑郁症发生在戒酒至少 1 周后,排除戒酒引起的情感症状,则抗抑郁效果更好。有更强的证据表明抑郁症是独立的,而不是精神活性物质诱发的[36]。由于治疗效果可被相对较大的安慰剂效应所掩盖,即安慰剂效应掩盖了药物疗效,因此有必要开展更大规模的临床随机对照试验。三环类抗抑郁药尽管有支持的证据,但是由于有潜在的心脏毒性和过量中毒,不推荐在临床使用。

预防复发药物应与抗抑郁药联合使用。Pettinati[38]等发现,舍曲林(200mg/d)与纳曲酮(100mg/d)联合使用,比安慰剂或两药单用效果更佳,对改善饮酒结果及情绪有利。相比之下,西酞普兰合用纳曲酮后,没有显示出任何益处[39]。

对阿坎酸和纳曲酮试验的二次分析表明:
- 阿坎酸可通过延长戒酒时间,间接地产生轻度的抗抑郁作用。
- 对于酒依赖共病抑郁的患者,纳曲酮和抗抑郁药物合用比单用的效果好[9],但各种研究结果不一致[39]。

双相障碍

双相障碍患者往往通过饮酒来减轻焦虑症状。存在共病时,必须按照双相障碍指南治疗不同的疾病时相。两项临床研究显示,与单药锂盐相比,丙戊酸盐和锂盐合用能更好地改善饮酒后果,因此值得推荐。但是与单用锂盐相比,合用不能进一步改善情感症状(参见2012年英国精神药理学会的共识)[9]。需注意,继续饮酒的患者可因电解质紊乱诱发锂中毒。酗酒者最好不用锂盐。

应该尽早给予纳曲酮帮助双相障碍患者减少饮酒量[9]。纳曲酮无效时可换用阿坎酸。若两种药物对于戒酒都无效,需要考虑双硫仑治疗,并将风险告知患者。

焦虑

酒依赖患者在醉酒、戒酒和守戒早期常出现焦虑症状。酒精常常被患者本人用于缓解焦虑,尤其是社交焦虑。对酒依赖者来说,很难确定其焦虑究竟在多大程度上是由酒精引起,还是一个独立的疾病。通常需要药物辅助及支持下戒酒后8周才能进行全面评估。如果无法进行药物辅助戒酒,也应尝试治疗焦虑障碍,具体可参考焦虑障碍治疗指南。

苯二氮䓬类药物因其潜在的滥用和依赖可能性,目前对其使用存在争议[9]。只有经过成瘾专业机构评估后才考虑使用。

一项荟萃分析表明,丁螺环酮可有效地减轻焦虑症状,但不能降低饮酒量[9,40]。研究还发现,帕罗西汀(最大剂量60mg/d)对共病社交焦虑的患者比安慰剂疗效好,但不能减少饮酒量[9,40]。

在创伤后应激障碍和酒依赖共病的患者中,无论是纳曲酮还是双硫仑,单用还是合用,对改善饮酒结局都比安慰剂要好。对酒依赖临床试验的事后分析表明,阿坎酸和巴氯芬均对减轻焦虑有益(参见英国精神药理学会共识)[9]。因此,确保患者守戒并给予预防复发药物治疗十分重要。随后可根据NICE相应指南对焦虑进行治疗。

精神分裂症

对于精神分裂症和酒精使用障碍共病的患者,应该进行评估,并针对酒精使用障碍的复发给予预防药物,如纳曲酮或阿坎酸。应优化抗精神病药治疗[9],可考虑使用氯氮平。然而,目前没有足够证据表明具体哪种抗精神病药效果更好。

参考文献

1. Department of Health and Social Care. UK chief medical officers' guidelines on how to keep health risks from drinking alcohol to a low level. 2016; https://www.gov.uk/government/publications/alcohol-consumption-advice-on-low-risk-drinking.

2. National Institute for Health and Clinical Excellence. Alcohol use disorders: diagnosis, assessment and management of harmful drinking and alcohol dependence. Clinical Guidance [CG115]. 2011 (last checked July 2019); https://www.nice.org.uk/guidance/cg115.

3. National Institute for Health and Care Excellence. Alcohol-use disorders: prevention. Public health guideline [PH24]. 2010; (last checked July 2019). https://www.nice.org.uk/guidance/ph24.

4. Babor T, et al. AUDIT: the alcohol use disorders identification test guidelines for use in primary care. 2nd edition. 2001; http://whqlibdoc.who.int/hq/2001/WHO_MSD_MSB_01.6a.pdf?ua=1.

5. Stockwell T, et al. The severity of alcohol dependence questionnaire: its use, reliability and validity. *Br J Addict* 1983; 78:145–155.

6. Minozzi S, et al. Anticonvulsants for alcohol withdrawal. *Cochrane Database Syst Rev* 2010; CD005064.

7. Amato L, et al. Efficacy and safety of pharmacological interventions for the treatment of the Alcohol Withdrawal Syndrome. *Cochrane Database Syst Rev* 2011; CD008537.

8. Brathen G, et al. EFNS guideline on the diagnosis and management of alcohol-related seizures: report of an EFNS task force. *Eur J Neurol* 2005; 12:575–581.

9. Lingford-Hughes AR, et al. Evidence-based guidelines for the pharmacological management of substance abuse, harmful use, addiction and comorbidity: recommendations from BAP. *J Psychopharmacol* 2012; 26:899–952.

10. NSW Government. Drug and alcohol withdrawal clinical practice guidelines. 2008; https://www1.health.nsw.gov.au/pds/ActivePDSDocuments/

GL2008_011.pdf.

11. Schuckit MA. Recognition and management of withdrawal delirium (delirium tremens). *N Engl J Med* 2014; **371**:2109–2113.

12. Sullivan JT, et al. Assessment of alcohol withdrawal: the revised clinical institute withdrawal assessment for alcohol scale (CIWA-Ar). *Br J Addict* 1989; **84**:1353–1357.

13. Gossop M, et al. A Short Alcohol Withdrawal Scale (SAWS): development and psychometric properties. *Addict Biol* 2002; **7**:37–43.

14. National Institute for Health and Clinical Excellence. Alcohol-use disorders: physical complications. Clinical Guidance [CG100] 2010 (last updated April 2017); https://www.nice.org.uk/guidance/cg100.

15. Thomson AD, et al. Time to act on the inadequate management of Wernicke's encephalopathy in the UK. *Alcohol Alcohol* 2013; **48**:4–8.

16. Thomson AD, et al. The Royal College of Physicians report on alcohol: guidelines for managing Wernicke's encephalopathy in the accident and Emergency Department. *Alcohol Alcohol* 2002; **37**:513–521.

17. Day E, et al. Thiamine for prevention and treatment of Wernicke-Korsakoff Syndrome in people who abuse alcohol. *Cochrane Database Syst Rev* 2013; **7**:CD004033.

18. Thomson A, et al. Incidence of adverse reactions to parenteral thiamine in the treatment of Wernicke's encephalopathy, and recommendations. *Alcohol Alcohol* 2019; **54**:609–614.

19. BNF Online. British national formulary. 2020; https://www.medicinescomplete.com/mc/bnf/current.

20. Rösner S, et al. Acamprosate for alcohol dependence. *Cochrane Database Syst Rev* 2010; Cd004332.

21. Donoghue K, et al. The efficacy of acamprosate and naltrexone in the treatment of alcohol dependence, Europe versus the rest of the world: a meta-analysis. *Addiction* 2015; **110**:920–930.

22. Rösner S, et al. Opioid antagonists for alcohol dependence. *Cochrane Database Syst Rev* 2010; Cd001867.

23. Accord Healthcare Limited. Summary of Product Characteristics. Naltrexone Hydrochloride 50 mg Film-coated Tablets. 2014; https://www.medicines.org.uk/emc/medicine/25878.

24 Krupitsky E, et al. Injectable extended-release naltrexone (XR-NTX) for opioid dependence: long-term safety and effectiveness. *Addiction* 2013; **108**:1628–1637.

25. Soyka M, et al. Comparing nalmefene and naltrexone in alcohol dependence: are there any differences? Results from an indirect meta-analysis. *Pharmacopsychiatry* 2016; **49**:66–75.

26. Palpacuer C, et al. Risks and benefits of nalmefene in the treatment of adult alcohol dependence: a systematic literature review and meta-analysis of published and unpublished double-blind randomized controlled trials. *PLoS Med* 2015; **12**:e1001924.

27. Mutschler J, et al. Current findings and mechanisms of action of disulfiram in the treatment of alcohol dependence. *Pharmacopsychiatry* 2016; **49**:137–141.

28. Minozzi S, et al. Baclofen for alcohol use disorder. *Cochrane Database Syst Rev* 2018; **11**:Cd012557.

29. Pani PP, et al. Anticonvulsants for alcohol dependence. *Cochrane Database Syst Rev* 2014; Cd008544.

30. Kranzler HR, et al. A meta-analysis of the efficacy of gabapentin for treating alcohol use disorder. *Addiction* 2019; **114**:1547–1555.

31. UK Teratology Information Service (UKTIS). 2020; www.uktis.org.

32. O'Malley SS, et al. Reduction of alcohol drinking in young adults by naltrexone: a double-blind, placebo-controlled, randomized clinical trial of efficacy and safety. *J Clin Psychiatry* 2015; **76**:e207–e213.

33. Miranda R, et al. Effects of naltrexone on adolescent alcohol cue reactivity and sensitivity: an initial randomized trial. *Addict Biol* 2014; **19**:941–954.

34. Pettinati HM, et al. Gender differences with high-dose naltrexone in patients with co-occurring cocaine and alcohol dependence. *J Subst Abuse Treat* 2008; **34**:378–390.

35. Public Health England. Better care for people with co-occurring mental health and alcohol/drug use conditions. A guide for commissioners and service providers. 2017; https://www.gov.uk/government/uploads/system/uploads/attachment_data/file/625809/Co-occurring_mental_health_and_alcohol_drug_use_conditions.pdf.

36. Agabio R, et al. Antidepressants for the treatment of people with co-occurring depression and alcohol dependence. *Cochrane Database Syst Rev* 2018; **4**:Cd008581.

37. Stokes PRA, et al. Pharmacological treatment of mood disorders and comorbid addictions: a systematic review and meta-analysis: traitement pharmacologique des troubles de L'humeur et des Dépendances Comorbides: une Revue Systématique et une Méta-Analyse. *Can J Psychiatry* 2020; **65**:749–769.

38. Pettinati HM, et al. A double-blind, placebo-controlled trial combining sertraline and naltrexone for treating co-occurring depression and alcohol dependence. *Am J Psychiatry* 2010; **167**:668–675.

39. Adamson SJ, et al. A randomized trial of combined citalopram and naltrexone for nonabstinent outpatients with co-occurring alcohol dependence and major depression. *J Clin Psychopharmacol* 2015; **35**:143–149.

40. Ipser JC, et al. Pharmacotherapy for anxiety and comorbid alcohol use disorders. *Cochrane Database Syst Rev* 2015; **1**:Cd007505.

扩展阅读

Cheng HY, et al. Treatment interventions to maintain abstinence from alcohol in primary care: systematic review and network meta-analysis. BMJ 2020; **371**:m3934

酒精戒断性谵妄：震颤谵妄

在因戒酒入院的患者中，震颤谵妄的发生率为 3%~5%，所以从事联络会诊精神科的医师很可能会遇到这种情况[1]。它是一种激越性谵妄，在末次饮酒后 72h 左右发生。既往癫痫发作或谵妄史、低钾血症、低镁血症、硫胺素缺乏和全身性疾病，以及治疗欠充分的酒精戒断，均易导致谵妄。因其死亡率高，而且治疗方法与其他原因引起的谵妄不同，如需要更大剂量苯二氮䓬类药物治疗，谨慎使用抗精神病药等，识别震颤谵妄至关重要。

虽然这是一本处方指南书，但需要再次强调的是，震颤谵妄是一种医疗紧急情况，需要由医师亲自检查患者。患者应该在综合医院接受护理[2]，最好是在重症监护病房[1,3]，尽管在临床实践中可能很难实施。恰当的处理需要精神科、内科和护理团队密切合作，识别和纠正致病的躯体因素，如电解质失衡、硫胺素缺乏和败血症等，并通过社会心理干预[安排在办公室附近刺激很少的病室、一对一护理观察、频繁的重新定向（reorientation）和安慰] 和药物治疗尽量减轻患者的行为紊乱。应尽早通知重症监护室提供外联服务或随叫随到。如果患者不接受口服药物治疗，需要注射高剂量苯二氮䓬类药物，则重症监护室应该直接参与治疗。

治疗震颤性谵妄的证据不足，大多来自 1979 年以前[1,4]。荟萃分析比较了镇静催眠药（地西泮、戊巴比妥和副醛）和抗精神病药，发现使用抗精神病药治疗的患者死亡率增加了 6 倍[4]。最近的研究比较了静脉注射劳拉西泮合用或不合用苯巴比妥，或加用右美托咪定。研究都是在 ICU 环境中进行的，因此对一般病房的适用性有限[5]。

NICE 指南 CG100（更新于 2017 年）建议在综合医院进行护理，并口服或静脉使用劳拉西泮，但没有进一步详细说明[2]。澳大利亚新南威尔士指南推荐地西泮，并且给出了更详细的说明（表 4.7）。《新英格兰医学杂志》（NEJM）最近一篇综述建议"最好是静脉注射苯二氮䓬类药物，剂量要高到足以使人轻微嗜睡，但仍可唤醒，同时监测生命体征，直到谵妄缓解"，并列出了来自早期临床随机对照试验的劳拉西泮和地西泮的使用方案[1]（见表 4.7）。

表 4.7　震颤谵妄的详细给药方案

新南威尔士指南[3]	《新英格兰医学杂志》地西泮[1]	《新英格兰医学杂志》劳拉西泮[1]
方案 1： 每小时口服 20mg 地西泮直至达到浅镇静； 最大剂量 80mg； 如果仍激越，则舌下含服 10mg 奥氮平 方案 2： 若不能接受地西泮，在重症病房可静脉注射 5mg 咪达唑仑，然后为 2mg/h	方案 1： 每 1~4h 10~20mg 地西泮口服，或静脉注射 方案 2： 5mg 静脉推注； 然后每 10min 10mg 静脉推注，共 2 次； 必要时继续 20mg 静脉推注； 然后每小时 5~20mg 静脉注射	方案 1： 每 15min 8mg 劳拉西泮口服、肌内注射或静脉注射，共 2 次；若需要第 3 次给药，则再静脉注射 8mg；达到镇静状态后，每小时给药 10~30mg 方案 2： 每 30~60min 肌内注射劳拉西泮 1~4mg，直至到达镇静状态，此后每小时按需给药 方案 3： 根据需要每 5~15min 静脉注射劳拉西泮 1~4mg

下面几点总结了这些方法：

- 以密集"冲击"方式给予地西泮或劳拉西泮治疗,每次给药间隔不超过 1h。
- 允许使用高剂量药物。
- 不使用抗精神病药,或者只在大剂量苯二氮䓬类药无效后使用。

因此,现有的研究证据和详细的官方指南均支持对震颤谵妄进行治疗,所用方法与通常的快速镇静或其他谵妄治疗方案不同。这可能需要明确告知重症监护团队,否则他们可能(错误地)采取标准快速镇静方案,包括氟哌啶醇,使用苯二氮䓬类药物的剂量也相对较低。

所有震颤谵妄的患者应按治疗剂量静脉注射硫胺素(如英国的 Pabrinex),因为营养不良是已知的震颤谵妄的易感因素。在给予此治疗和静脉补液前,应使患者达到足够的镇静状态。

首先,临床经验表明,内科和重症监护团队对新南威尔士方案 1(口服地西泮)或《新英格兰医学杂志》方案 2(肌内注射劳拉西泮)接受度最高。NICE 建议氟哌啶醇可用于治疗震颤性谵妄患者的行为紊乱,但其他人员强调应该慎用,因氟哌啶醇有心脏毒性和诱发癫痫的可能性 [1,2]。NICE 和新南威尔士指南均建议,对于苯二氮䓬类药物治疗无效的行为紊乱,可选择奥氮平 [2,3]。

慢性阻塞性肺疾病(COPD)患者或其他呼吸道疾病患者,不能采用苯二氮䓬类药物负荷给药法;这些患者更可能需要呼吸支持来耐受药物辅助的戒酒,因此重症监护团队早期参与非常重要。应注意监测呼吸频率(RR)和血氧饱和度,特别是对吸烟者和可能患有隐匿性呼吸系统疾病者。"必要时"可使用氟马西尼对苯二氮䓬类药物进行解毒治疗。

参考文献

1. Schuckit MA. Recognition and management of withdrawal delirium (delirium tremens). *N Engl J Med* 2014; 371:2109–2113.

2. National Institute for Health and Clinical Excellence. Alcohol-use disorders: physical complications. Clinical Guidance [CG100]. 2010 (last updated April 2017); https://www.nice.org.uk/guidance/cg100.

3. NSW Government. Drug and alcohol withdrawal clinical practice guidelines. 2008; https://www1.health.nsw.gov.au/pds/ActivePDSDocuments/GL2008_011.pdf.

4. Mayo-Smith MF, et al. Management of alcohol withdrawal delirium. An evidence-based practice guideline. *Arch Intern Med* 2004; 164:1405–1412.

5. Nguyen TA, et al. Phenobarbital and symptom-triggered lorazepam versus lorazepam alone for severe alcohol withdrawal in the intensive care unit. *Alcohol* 2020; 82:23–27.

阿片类物质依赖

阿片类物质依赖的处方用药

> **重要提示：**
>
> 阿片类物质依赖治疗通常需要专科干预，不具备专科经验的全科医师在治疗前需和物质滥用机构获取联系。除非由专业人员直接指导，否则强烈建议普通成人精神科医师不要进行阿片类物质替代治疗。所有阿片类药物都是呼吸抑制剂。处方阿片类药物，如美沙酮和丁丙诺啡，对未用药个体的致死剂量很低，而且难以评估其耐受性。
>
> **阿片戒断本身不会致命，但阿片中毒可导致死亡。**
>
> 患者若无法忍受阿片类药物的戒断反应，可能会不遵医嘱自行出院，这也会带来风险。因此，应该先使用非阿片类药物治疗阿片类药物戒断反应（见有关住院的部分），直到获得适当的其他建议。

在英国，用于阿片类药物依赖患者的药物干预包括减少药物危害的措施（如提供带回家的纳洛酮），使用阿片类替代的维持治疗（如美沙酮或丁丙诺啡），以及使用纳曲酮预防复吸。药物治疗与心理治疗均是康复治疗的重要组成部分。本章对心理治疗不做介绍，读者可参考"康复路线"和《药物滥用和依赖：英国临床管理指南》（或更常被称为"橙色指南"）的心理社会一章，以了解成瘾治疗的相关内容 [1,2]。

阿片类药物过量的治疗

在阿片类药物使用人群中，阿片类药物过量是一种可预防的死亡原因。这包括过量服用非法阿片类药物（如海洛因、芬太尼和羟考酮），以及过量服用处方阿片类药物（如美沙酮或丁丙诺啡）。

阿片类药物过量的临床表现为：

- 意识丧失
- 呼吸频率降低（RR<12 次/min）
- 针尖样瞳孔
- 发绀
- 皮肤湿冷

纳洛酮是一种阿片类受体拮抗剂，可逆转阿片类药物过量。可用预装注射器，并且应在叫救护车和进行第一轮胸部按压后进行肌内注射。建议初始剂量为 400μg，可在 3 个周期（各30 次胸外按压）后重复使用，直到救护车到达或呼吸恢复 [3]。可能需要更高剂量的纳洛酮来取代高亲和力阿片类药物，如丁丙诺啡或芬太尼 [4]。

应"按需"为任何疑似有阿片类药物有害使用或依赖的住院患者给予"纳洛酮 400μg 肌内注射或静脉注射"的处方，并应在病房的苏醒袋（resuscitation bag）中备用。任何人都可以用纳洛酮来防止药物过量引起的死亡。应该告知出院患者他们对药物的耐受性可能会消失，为患者及其家人提供带回家的纳洛酮并进行使用培训[1]。图 4.2 总结了在阿片类药物过量情况下应采取的流程,带回家的纳洛酮培训包括这些流程。

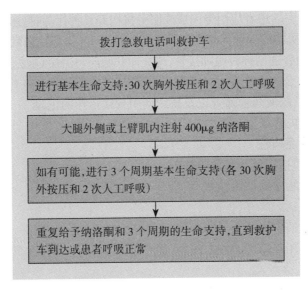

图 4.2　纳洛酮给药流程图(改编自 WHO[3])

鼻喷纳洛酮

最近,开发了浓缩鼻喷(IN)纳洛酮替代肌内注射纳洛酮[5]。由于外行或旁观者可能因害怕、缺乏注射相关知识或者有被针头刺伤的风险而难以完成注射,因此研发了带回家的纳洛酮的替代剂型[6]。

1mg、2mg 和 4mg 鼻喷纳洛酮的血药浓度峰值(C_{max})均超过肌内注射 400μg 纳洛酮,但达峰时间(T_{max})晚于肌内注射(15~30min vs 10min)。在起效时间方面,2mg 鼻喷相当于 400μg IM。鼻喷给药比肌内注射或静脉注射更能持久维持纳洛酮血浆水平[7]。

阿片类替代治疗(OST)

阿片类药物依赖的药物治疗主要是替代治疗。替代治疗可用于脱毒治疗,即给予一定剂量的替代药物以控制戒断症状,然后逐步减量与停用。**替代治疗**也可被用于"维持治疗",即较长时间使用稳定剂量的**替代治疗**,从数月至数年。

替代治疗的目标如下:
- 减少或预防戒断症状
- 减少或消除非处方用药
- 稳定药物入量和生活方式
- 减少药物有关的伤害(尤其是注射行为)
- 吸引并创造机会帮助患者康复

治疗取决于:
- 可获得何种药物疗法或其他干预措施

- 患者既往用药和治疗史
- 患者目前的药物使用和环境
- 开始治疗的场所/机构

　　大多数有精神疾病的患者应由专门成瘾服务机构开具替代药物处方,但是他们应继续接受来自精神健康服务机构的专业治疗[8]。一些同时存在阿片类药物依赖和精神疾病的患者应被收入精神科病房,由普通精神科医师接管,或立即开始药物治疗(参见后面专门章节)[1]。

　　临床医师应注意确认患者在开始替代治疗前对阿片类药物存在生理依赖,例如阿片类药物戒断的临床证据、尿液药物筛查以及持续使用替代治疗的记录。

　　评估应包括以下内容:

- 患者使用何种阿片类药物
- 使用的其他药物,包括酒精和其他镇静剂
- 所用全部精神活性物质的使用频率、用量及给药途径
- 最后一次用药时间
- 可能影响用药选择的躯体共病,如 COPD
- 可与替代药物发生相互作用的处方药物,如呼吸抑制剂、延长 Q-T 间期的药物
- 既往治疗经历
- 既往的过量用药
- 是否有带回家的纳洛酮
- 使用经过验证的量表,如客观阿片类药物戒断量表(OOWS)或临床阿片类药物戒断量表(COWS),评估是否存在阿片类物质戒断的客观体征,见表 4.8
- 检查注射部位
- 向成瘾服务机构和药房了解其替代药物的常规剂量和最近发放的药物剂量

　　未经治疗的海洛因戒断症状通常在最后一次注射后 4~6h 开始出现,32~72h 达到高峰。5 天后症状会明显消退。未经治疗的美沙酮戒断症状通常在最后一次给药后 4~6 天达到高峰,症状在 10~12 天内不会消退。未经治疗的丁丙诺啡戒断症状通常持续长达 10 天。特定的阿片类药物戒断量表(如 COWS[9] 或 OOWS[10])可用于帮助评估依赖和戒断症状。

如何安全地处方替代药物

- 使用已批准用于治疗海洛因依赖的药物(美沙酮及丁丙诺啡)。
- 确定患者依赖阿片类药物。
- 给予一个安全的初始剂量(见后文)并谨慎滴定。
- 在治疗的前几个月或达到稳定(稳定 = 戒除非法阿片类药物)之前,每天在监督下服药。
- 在治疗的前几个月或达到稳定之前,尽量减少外带药物剂量。

替代药物维持治疗的诱导和稳定

　　美沙酮和丁丙诺啡是 NICE 推荐用于维持治疗的替代药物。美沙酮和丁丙诺啡维持疗法对治疗戒断症状和减少非法阿片类药物的使用均有效[11]。最近指南和系统综述显示,并无证据支持两者孰优孰劣[1]。美沙酮和丁丙诺啡的药理学特性不同。美沙酮是 μ 阿片受体的完全激动剂,而丁丙诺啡是部分激动剂。药理学上的不同与每种药物的优缺点相关,如

表 4.8 临床阿片类药物戒断量表（COWS）

静息脉率：_____ 次/min

患者坐位或卧位 1min 后测量：

0——脉率 80 次/min 以下

1——脉率 81~100 次/min

2——脉率 101~120 次/min

4——脉率大于 120 次/min

消化系统紊乱——过去 30min：

0——无消化系统症状

1——胃痉挛

2——恶心或便溏

3——呕吐或腹泻

5——多次腹泻或呕吐

出汗——过去 30min 内，且不受室温及患者活动影响：

0——没有寒战或潮红

1——主观报告的寒战或潮红

2——面部潮红或可见湿润

3——眉毛或脸上有汗珠

4——汗水从脸上淌下

震颤——观察伸出的双手：

0——无震颤

1——可以感觉到震颤，但不能被观察到

2——可观察到细微震颤

4——剧烈震颤或肌肉抽搐

坐立不安——观察期间评估：

0——可以静坐

1——报告有静坐困难，但仍能做到

3——手臂或腿频繁移动或不必要的运动

5——几秒都不能静坐

打哈欠——观察期间评估：

0——无

1——评估过程中 1~2 次

2——评估过程中 ≥3 次

4——每分钟多次

瞳孔大小：

0——室光下瞳孔固定或正常大小

1——室光下瞳孔可能比正常大

2——瞳孔中度扩大

5——瞳孔扩大到只能看到虹膜边缘

焦虑或易怒：

0——无

1——患者报告易怒或焦虑加重

2——患者明显易怒或焦虑

4——患者易怒或焦虑明显，以致难以完成评估

骨或关节疼痛——若患者既往有过疼痛，则只评定由阿片戒断导致的疼痛：

0——无

1——轻度、弥漫的不适

2——患者报告严重弥漫性关节或肌肉疼痛

4——患者一直揉搓关节或肌肉，并由于疼痛无法静坐

起鸡皮疙瘩：

0——皮肤光滑

3——可触及皮肤凸起感或汗毛竖立

5——明显的鸡皮疙瘩

流涕或流泪——与感冒或过敏无关：

0——无

1——鼻塞或眼睛异常湿润

2——流涕或流泪

4——持续流涕，或眼泪顺脸颊流下来

总分 _____

（总分为 11 项得分之和）

得分：5~12 分为轻度，13~24 分为中度，25~36 分为中度严重，大于 36 分为严重戒断。

表 4.9 所示。具体使用何种药物需基于以下因素：患者个人偏好，既往治疗经历，多物质使用（特别是共病苯二氮䓬类药物依赖或酒精依赖），被挪用的风险（患者开药但自己不用，出售或给予他人）等，长期治疗计划（包括选择其中一种用于脱毒治疗），在使用丁丙诺啡时是否可保持长时间不用海洛因来避免戒断症状等。美沙酮似乎比丁丙诺啡的治疗维持率更佳，至少在低剂量时如此[7]。

表 4.9　美沙酮和丁丙诺啡的选择

	美沙酮	丁丙诺啡
戒断综合征	更明显且时间更长，最好用于维持治疗	戒断综合征轻于美沙酮，适用于脱毒治疗[14,15]
起始的不同	在药物加量阶段死亡率升高 需要逐步加量，数周后达到治疗范围（60~100mg/d）	在药物加量阶段，死亡率不升高 可在数天达到治疗剂量（12~16mg/d） 如果患者尚未停用阿片类药物，则有引发戒断症状的风险
治疗保持率的差别	与低剂量（<7mg）丁丙诺啡相比，美沙酮的治疗保持率更高	低剂量（<7mg）及不固定剂量的丁丙诺啡治疗脱失率更高
不良反应的区别	美沙酮可能与 Q-T 间期延长与尖端扭转性室性心动过速相关，患者使用可延长 Q-T 间期的抗精神病药或合并可卡因滥用时尤其令人担心	丁丙诺啡通常被认为比美沙酮镇静作用弱，故不受患者欢迎[1]
慢性疼痛	对于需要使用额外阿片类药物镇痛的慢性疼痛患者，丁丙诺啡因有"阻断"作用，难以用于治疗；但这在临床中并非主要问题	丁丙诺啡比美沙酮（剂量 <60mg 时）具有更强的"阻断"作用[16-18]。正在使用丁丙诺啡治疗的患者如出现急性疼痛，可加用其他阿片类药物，并根据反应调整剂量[19]
与其他药物合用	美沙酮可能与抑制/诱导 CYP3A4 的药物（如红霉素、某些 SSRI、利巴韦林、部分抗癫痫药和 HIV 药物）发生相互作用，从而改变其血浆浓度。若患者不规律使用 CYP3A4 抑制剂/诱导剂，则美沙酮剂量难以评估	丁丙诺啡较少受药物相互作用影响，对某些患者更合适
孕妇	广泛应用于孕妇	丁丙诺啡与不太严重的新生儿戒断症状有关[20]。然而，丁丙诺啡不应在妊娠期开始使用或把美沙酮换成丁丙诺啡，因为有诱导胎儿出现戒断症状的风险
挪用	用药物风险较大（如既往有挪用药物史、在监狱内治疗）的患者最好使用美沙酮治疗	丁丙诺啡舌下含片更容易被挪用，且有将片剂变成注射剂的风险。与纳洛酮的合剂（赛宝松）可预防被挪用注射
用药保障		如果不能监督患者每天服用，那么最好使用丁丙诺啡

患者的躯体健康也是需要考虑的重要因素。例如,有证据表明,对于躯体健康、使用阿片类药物的患者,丁丙诺啡引起呼吸抑制的可能性小于美沙酮[12]。在戒毒机构中,大约 1/3 患者的肺活量相当于 COPD[13]。然而,并无公开证据显示此类患者对丁丙诺啡耐受性更好。

在极少数情况下,患者可能对美沙酮、丁丙诺啡或配方中的某些成分过敏。

美沙酮

临床疗效

美沙酮是一种长效阿片受体激动剂。已经证实美沙酮维持治疗有助于海洛因依赖者坚持治疗,减少海洛因用量,而且其疗效优于非阿片类药物替代治疗[11]。英国卫生部指南建议在治疗维持率、降低海洛因和可卡因使用量方面,高剂量美沙酮(60~100mg/d)的疗效优于低剂量。

根据目前的小规模开放性研究,美沙酮能够有效地减少处方阿片类药物依赖者的药物滥用,使患者继续接受治疗,其效果与丁丙诺啡相同[21]。美沙酮还减少了与 HIV 传播有关的吸毒行为。2017 年,美国的 POATS(n=653)发现,丁丙诺啡与纳洛酮合剂作为维持(即持续)用药而不是逐渐减量时,能够有效地治疗处方阿片类药物依赖[22]。

处方信息:美沙酮和丁丙诺啡是具有高度依赖性的管制药物。美沙酮的致死剂量特别低,因此对其有特殊的管理要求,包括在处方上注明患者的姓名、出生日期和地址,并以数字和文字书写每天剂量和总剂量。比如,须在监督下服药的要求,亦应加以说明,例如"每天监督服药"。

对于新开的处方,建议每天在监督下进行服药,至少持续几个月[1]。如果不能做到,应使用分期处方,以供每天配药和取药。除特殊情况外,每次发放的药量不得超过一周[1]。在新型冠状病毒感染流行期间,英国公共卫生部决定,在疫情期间监督下用药时,社交接触的风险超过挪用和药物过量的风险,因此在大多数情况下放松了管理。目前,还不清楚这种改变在实践中产生的后果,以及这种改变是否会持续或恢复到既往管理规定。

美沙酮的常用剂型为 1mg/mL 的口服液[1]。表中应注明患者的住址和出生日期,并用数字和文字书写每天处方剂量和处方总剂量。应明确注明需要监督服药。因片剂可被压碎和注射使用,通常不用片剂[1,23]。

> **重要提示:**必须告知所有开始美沙酮治疗的患者,该药有中毒和过量的风险,对于带回家的药物要安全存放[1,24-26]。安全保存药物至关重要,尤其是家中有儿童时。已有儿童服用美沙酮致死的案例报道。开药医师在给药物依赖者制订全部评估和治疗计划时,应该考虑药物对儿童的风险。

对于目前没有使用美沙酮的海洛因或其他阿片类物质依赖患者,为了避免潜在的阿片类物质中毒,在确定美沙酮治疗**起始剂量**时需考虑以下因素:

- 对阿片类物质的耐受性受多种因素影响,并可显著影响个体中毒的风险[27]。其中尤为重要的是评估者自我报告的目前药物使用剂量、频率和途径,要注意患者偏高的自我报告。一般在停用阿片类物质 3~4 天后,对美沙酮的耐受性明显降低,此后要特别谨慎,再次从起始剂量逐渐加量。

- 使用其他中枢神经系统抑制剂,如酒精、苯二氮䓬类药物和精神药物(如普瑞巴林),会增加中毒风险。
- 在45岁以上的患者中,药物相关死亡的风险增加了2.9倍[28]。
- 合并的躯体疾病(如COPD)导致基线氧饱和度低。
- 美沙酮半衰期较长,可在3~10天内发生蓄积中毒[29,30]。因此,应定期评估其中毒症状,若有嗜睡或其他中毒迹象,应及时中断用药。
- 如果剂量不当可能危及生命,尤其是在用药最初几天[24,25,31,32]。已有起始剂量低于30mg/d的致死病例报道[1]。

比较安全的用药方案是从低剂量开始。如果后来发现剂量不够,可以间隔一段后增加剂量。应谨慎使用阿片类物质和美沙酮的直接换算表,因为有多种因素影响其使用价值,如街头海洛因的质量。根据出现的戒断症状来调整剂量要安全得多。

根据耐受情况,美沙酮**起始剂量**大多数为10~30mg/d[1,33]。如果不确定,建议10~20mg。在急性期内科病房或精神科病房,通常建议的起始剂量为20mg/d,因为在内科病房患者有可能躯体情况不佳,在精神科病房患者往往使用其他精神活性药物。

注意:给药后30min内可明显起效,给药后2~4h达血药峰浓度。

美沙酮在社区的诱导和稳定

适用于在过去3天内没有服用处方药的患者(包括一直服用替代药物但3天内没有领取处方药的患者)。美沙酮治疗的最初两周会显著增加药物过量死亡的风险[1,23,34-36]。在此期间进行适当的评估、剂量调整和监测是很重要的。通常在专业机构中由具备专业能力的人进行治疗,治疗之前需进行全面评估及尿毒检,确定有阿片类物质使用和戒断的明确证据。

- **第一周**

门诊患者每周应就诊3次,由开药医师进行评估,并根据戒断症状调整药物剂量。每次增加的药物剂量不超过5~10mg,第一周总剂量不能比起始剂量多出30mg[33]。注意末次剂量增加后5天才能达到稳态血药浓度。一旦患者使用充足剂量的美沙酮且病情稳定,应改为每天1次给药。不宜临时给药或者剂量不固定。最好监测最初几个月的用药情况。

- **后期治疗**

经过第一周的治疗后,可继续增加美沙酮剂量5~10mg,每次增加剂量需间隔至少一周[1]。可能需要几周方能达到60~120mg/d的治疗剂量[1]。一般需要6周甚至更长时间才能到达稳定。然而,有时必须考虑有些患者可能需要更快达到稳定。此时需要增加监督和观察的强度,以便能更快地增加药物剂量。治疗剂量指可缓解阿片类药物戒断症状,有效地预防海洛因使用,但不会导致过度镇静[37]。医师应考虑可能影响美沙酮剂量的相关因素,例如合并使用可卡因(可卡因可降低美沙酮水平)和年龄的增加(因年龄>45岁人群使用较低剂量的美沙酮也有过量的风险)[28]。

美沙酮注意事项

- **中毒**

对任何怀疑有中毒迹象的患者不应给予美沙酮治疗,尤其是酒精或其他中枢神经系统抑制剂(如苯二氮䓬类药物)中毒[27,38]。美沙酮与酒精或其他呼吸抑制剂(包括苯二氮䓬类药物和普瑞巴林)使用时,会大大增加过量致死风险[39,40]。因为与多药滥用相关的过量风险增加,在考虑后续美沙酮治疗时,必须牢记要警惕患者同时饮酒,或者处方药与毒品合用的情况[25,31,38,41]。

■ 严重肝、肾功能不全

这将影响美沙酮的代谢与消除,应根据临床表现调整给药剂量和间隔时间。由于美沙酮的半衰期延长,在给药初期也需要适当延长评估的间隔时间。

美沙酮过量

万一美沙酮过量,应参照"阿片类药物过量"章节给予**纳洛酮**治疗。

美沙酮与尖端扭转型室性心动过速/Q-T 间期延长的风险

美沙酮单用或联合其他可延长 Q-T 间期的药物,可增加 Q-T 间期延长的风险。Q-T 间期延长与尖端扭转型室性心动过速相关,可危及生命[42-44]。

关于心电图监测的建议

2006 年,药物和保健管理部门(MHRA)建议,存在下列 Q-T 间期延长危险因素的患者服用美沙酮时应密切监测:心脏或肝脏疾病、电解质紊乱、合并 CYP3A4 抑制剂治疗、服用可能造成 Q-T 间期延长的药物(如某些抗精神病药、红霉素等)。可卡因和合成大麻素受体激动剂(SCRA)或"香料(spice)",可能会延长 Q-T,所以应该密切监测服用可卡因或香料的患者[45,46]。此外,美沙酮剂量超过 100mg/d 的患者应密切监测心电图[47],因为这可增加 Q-T 间期延长风险[42]。其他增加 Q-T 延长风险的个体因素包括共病进食障碍、心脏病或卒中史、肝病、代谢紊乱(如低钾血症、低钙血症和 HIV 阳性)(不考虑用药情况)[48]。

因此,存在上述危险因素的个体,都应该做基线心电图和后续心电图监测。具体复查的时间间隔尚无严格证据支持,但对于没有心脏症状者,至少应每年检查一次。同样重要的是,检查与美沙酮合用的药物对 CYP3A4 的抑制作用;在开始美沙酮治疗时,需告知患者风险获益情况[49]。丁丙诺啡似乎较少引起 Q-T 间期延长,因此在这方面可能是更为安全的选择[50],然而,目前尚缺乏相关研究。选择合适的阿片类替代药物时,需要考虑许多其他因素。

表 4.10 记录了简要的指导方针。出现 Q-T 间期延长时,常常需要寻求专家建议。最近关于心电图监测的评论表明,在美沙酮维持治疗的患者中,Q-T 筛查策略预防心脏病和死亡的效果证据并不充分;有人担心在某些治疗机构中,心电图监测相关的程序烦琐,可能足以阻止患者参加或留在美沙酮项目中[51]。在内科或精神科病房接受或准备接受美沙酮治疗的患者都应该进行心电图监测。社区内使用高剂量美沙酮或有其他风险因素的患者也尽可能进行心电图监测,但是如果社区患者拒绝做心电图监测,需要考虑其风险与获益。

丁丙诺啡

丁丙诺啡是一种合成的阿片类受体部分激动剂,内在活性低,对 μ 阿片类受体具有高亲和力。这意味着,即使在受体饱和的剂量下,它也几乎不会产生兴奋作用,同时还会阻止其他阿片类药物的作用。若使用固定剂量,它对海洛因成瘾是一种有效的治疗,但足剂量时其疗效并不比美沙酮好[11]。丁丙诺啡的治疗保持率低于美沙酮;使用丁丙诺啡的临床经验

表 4.10　对 ECG 监测的建议

	Q-T 间期临界性延长	处理	Q-T 间期延长	处理	Q-T 间期明显延长	处理
女性 男性	≥470ms ≥440ms	■ 重测 EEG ■ 调节电解质平衡 ■ 纠正 Q-T 间期风险因素,如使用可卡因、合成大麻素受体激动剂、美沙酮剂量、精神药物 ■ 定期复查心电图至正常	≥500ms	■ 重测 ECG ■ 调节电解质平衡 ■ 纠正 Q-T 间期风险因素 ■ 寻求心内科和成瘾科专家帮助 ■ 减少美沙酮剂量 ■ 若美沙酮减量后 Q-T 间期仍持续延长,计划改用丁丙诺啡 ■ 定期复查心电图至正常	≥550ms	■ 心内科和成瘾科专家急会诊 ■ 复查心电图 ■ 调节电解质平衡 ■ 纠正 Q-T 间期风险因素 ■ 减少美沙酮剂量并在一周内重新评估。住院患者计划改用丁丙诺啡

表明,开始丁丙诺啡治疗可能比较困难,因为开始使用丁丙诺啡之前必须充分停用阿片类物质,但是戒断症状又不能影响患者到治疗中心就医,很难平衡二者之间的关系。它还被发现可有效地减少处方阿片类药物依赖者的药物使用,并提高治疗依从性[21]。丁丙诺啡和美沙酮在脱毒治疗的完成率上无显著差别,但使用丁丙诺啡时戒断症状缓解更快[52]。

舌下含服丁丙诺啡

丁丙诺啡最常用的剂型是通过舌下含服而吸收。每片药需要 5~10min 分解和吸收。它能够治疗阿片类物质依赖是因为:

- 可减轻/预防阿片类物质戒断症状和渴求。
- 对阿片类受体的亲和力高,可降低阿片类物质使用效果[16-18]。
- 作用时间长,可每天用药 1 次(或更少)。作用持续时间与剂量相关:低剂量(如 2mg)可维持最长 12h,高剂量(如 16~32mg)可持续 48~72h,允许每周给药 3 次。

丁丙诺啡长效针剂

一种皮下缓释丁丙诺啡注射剂(在英国和欧盟的商品名为 Buvidal,在美国的商品名为 Sublocade 等),其周注射和月注射剂型在英国获得许可(表 4.11)。某些患者可能更偏向/受益于每周或每月的给药,例如,工作或学习任务重、需要经常旅行(每天取药困难)以及难以坚持每天遵医嘱服药者。

缓释丁丙诺啡注射剂与丁丙诺啡舌下含服效果相同,即抑制戒断症状和渴求,同时阻断阿片类受体(服用其他阿片类药物时)。它有一个持续释放的过程,一些患者发现它减少了舌下丁丙诺啡带来的明显的波峰和波谷的体验。反过来,这可能会减少阿片类药物的"顶格"(on-top)使用。丁丙诺啡缓释注射剂的禁忌证为对活性物质或辅料高度敏感或过敏、严重肝损害、酒精依赖和震颤谵妄。

表 4.11 常规舌下丁丙诺啡每天治疗剂量及建议每周、每月 Buvidal 相应给药剂量

舌下丁丙诺啡每天剂量	Buvidal 每周	Buvidal 每月
2~6mg	8mg	32mg
8~10mg	16mg	64mg
12~16mg	24mg	96mg
18~24mg	32mg	128mg

不同品牌的口服丁丙诺啡和生物利用度

Espranor 是丁丙诺啡的一个品牌,在英国社区成瘾服务机构中使用越来越多。Espranor 要放在舌上,而不是舌下。丁丙诺啡的药代动力学表现出相当大的个体间差异[53];根据患者个人的治疗反应缓慢增加剂量,由此可以适应药代动力学的变异。然而,根据临床经验,对于从丁丙诺啡或其他品牌的丁丙诺啡换成 Espranor,制定了以下转换表:

舌下丁丙诺啡	Espranor 口崩剂
8mg	6mg
10mg	8mg
12mg	10mg
14/16mg	12mg
18mg	14mg
20/22mg	16mg
>26mg	18mg

鉴于剂量等效性的不确定性,在没有充分理由的情况下应谨慎更换不同品牌药物。

丁丙诺啡的起始剂量

丁丙诺啡的起始治疗原则与美沙酮相同。在药物依赖服务中心以外工作的医师应该意识到,丁丙诺啡不会像美沙酮、可待因或海洛因那样包括在标准的尿毒检套餐中。通常需要单独的 UDS 试剂盒进行检测,且在成瘾服务中心之外的机构没有。因此,为了及时确认其使用情况,应该考虑向药房确认患者的药物使用情况,或请特定实验室对尿样进行检测。然而,丁丙诺啡特别令人感兴趣的是其促戒断作用。促戒断作用的原因是丁丙诺啡为一种部分激动剂,受体亲和力高。如果它在有完全激动剂(如美沙酮或海洛因)存在时进入大脑,它就会竞争结合阿片受体,取代完全激动剂。因此,一些先前完全激动的受体变成部分激动。这种改变使患者出现阿片类物质戒断症状。然而,如果患者已处于戒断状态,他们将体验到部分激动效应,在一定程度上激动阿片受体,缓解戒断症状。减少诱导过程中问题的重要措施是进行患者教育。

　　第一剂丁丙诺啡应在患者出现阿片类戒断症状（激动剂活性下降的迹象）时给予，以降低促戒断作用的风险。与美沙酮一样，在开始使用丁丙诺啡之前，必须有明确的每天使用阿片类药物（包括毒物检测）和戒断症状的证据。

　　初始剂量的建议如下：

患者目前情况	丁丙诺啡剂量
有戒断症状，无危险因素	8mg
无戒断症状，无危险因素	4mg
伴发危险因素（躯体疾病、多种药物滥用、依赖的严重程度低或不明确、使用其他精神药物）	2~4mg

　　在非专业机构，第一天服用丁丙诺啡不应超过 8mg。在某些情况下，8mg 可能就足够了，但如果有持续的戒断迹象，而没有中毒迹象，第二天可能会增加到 12~16mg。可以分次给药，以便发生中毒时可以迅速查明，但是在实践中没有现场配药的情况下很难做到这一点。《药物滥用和成瘾：英国临床治疗指南》推荐的维持剂量是每天 12~24mg。如果考虑可能需要超过 16mg 的剂量，应寻求专科医师的建议，只有在成瘾专家的建议下才能够增加剂量。

　　如果患者正在服用其他呼吸抑制药物，如苯二氮䓬类药物，则应使用较低剂量，并监测中毒和呼吸抑制情况。

从美沙酮换成丁丙诺啡

　　通常应在有经验的专家指导下进行。从美沙酮换成丁丙诺啡治疗时，有可能引起促戒断症状，轻度戒断症状可持续 1~2 周。影响促戒断症状的因素见表 4.12。

表 4.12　从美沙酮换用丁丙诺啡是影响促戒断症状的风险因素

因素	讨论	建议
美沙酮剂量	美沙酮剂量高于 30mg 易发生。一般来说，剂量越高，促戒断症状越严重[54]	尝试从美沙酮剂量 <40mg（最好 30mg）换药；若之前使用剂量 >60mg，不宜换药
末次使用美沙酮和首次使用丁丙诺啡的间隔时间	至少间隔 24h。延长间隔会减少戒断症状的发生率和严重程度[55,56]	停用美沙酮，直到出现美沙酮戒断症状时，再首次给予丁丙诺啡
丁丙诺啡剂量	很低剂量丁丙诺啡（2mg）通常不足以替代美沙酮；首次剂量高（8mg）时易引起促戒断反应	首次剂量一般为 4mg；2~3h 后评估患者情况
患者期望	对促戒断反应无心理准备者，更易感到痛苦和困惑	提前告知患者；对严重症状有应急方案
其他药物使用	对症处理药物（洛非西定）可能有助于缓解症状	按照治疗计划使用

从美沙酮剂量 <40mg/d(最好≤30mg)换成丁丙诺啡

美沙酮应该突然停用,至少 24h 后首次给予丁丙诺啡。建议起始剂量的转换如下,根据临床表现,以后可能需要增加药物剂量。

美沙酮末次使用剂量	丁丙诺啡第 1 天起始剂量	丁丙诺啡第 2 天剂量
20~40mg	4mg	6~8mg
10~20mg	4mg	4~8mg
1~10mg	2mg	2~4mg

从美沙酮剂量 40~60mg 换成丁丙诺啡

- 只要患者没有变得病情不稳或吵闹,美沙酮剂量应尽可能减少,然后突然停用;
- 首次使用丁丙诺啡的时间是患者出现明确的戒断症状时,通常是美沙酮末次给药 48~96h 后。
- 起始剂量为 2~4mg。2~3h 后进行评估。
- 如果促发了戒断反应,可进一步对症用药。
- 若未促发或加重戒断反应,当天可增加 2~4mg。
- 第 2 天进行评估后,剂量增加至 8~12mg。

从美沙酮剂量 >60mg 换成丁丙诺啡

除非特殊情况下由有经验的医师处理,否则不宜在门诊进行换药。通常患者经过部分脱毒,将美沙酮剂量调整至 30mg/d 以下时,才换成丁丙诺啡。然而,如果需要从高剂量美沙酮换成丁丙诺啡,应尽可能考虑将患者转诊到专用的成瘾病房。

其他阿片类处方药物换成丁丙诺啡

使用丁丙诺啡治疗处方阿片类药物依赖的证据越来越多,已经发现丁丙诺啡可以改善药物治疗的依从性,并减少处方阿片类药物滥用[21]。在英国,《药物滥用和成瘾:英国临床治疗指南》建议小剂量分次服用,以确定稳定时所需剂量[1]。

从患者控制镇痛开始使用丁丙诺啡

患者控制镇痛(PCA)通常用于严重急性疼痛的管理。患者可在设定的限度内按需静脉注射阿片类药物(如吗啡或芬太尼)[57]。

对于在接受 PCA 治疗前已开始使用丁丙诺啡的患者,建议在接受 PCA 治疗的同时,舌下含服 0.4mg 丁丙诺啡,每天 4 次,开始阿片类药物替代治疗。交错给药很重要,可以避免通常的峰值浓度,后者会增加促戒断反应的风险。

在不再需要 PCA 的第 1 天(表 4.13 中第 1 天),丁丙诺啡舌下含服可增加到 2mg,每天 2 次。次日剂量可增至 4mg,每天 2 次。第 3 天,丁丙诺啡可每天 1 次,每次 8mg。如果使用丁丙诺啡后戒断症状立即加重,可能必须调整剂量。在这种情况下,停用丁丙诺啡,并联系成瘾专家咨询。

表 4.13   患者控制镇静到重新使用丁丙诺啡

日期	患者在用 PCA?	舌下丁丙诺啡剂量	频率
0	是	0.4mg	4 次/d
1	否	1mg	2 次/d
2	否	2mg	2 次/d
3	否	4mg	1 次/d

丁丙诺啡稳定期剂量

患者在治疗后头几天应定期看门诊,以便医师能进行评估和调整药物剂量。每次增加剂量 2~4mg,必要时每天增加 1 次,最高单日剂量为 32mg。建议的有效维持剂量通常为 12~16mg/d[1],患者一般在开始丁丙诺啡治疗 1~2 周内到达维持剂量,通常比服用美沙酮更快。

丁丙诺啡用药低于每天 1 次

丁丙诺啡在英国被批准为每天使用。国际证据和经验表明,许多患者 2~3 天用一次药可保持较好的状态[58-61]。对某些有挪用风险、不符合"带药回家"条件者,可考虑采用此种治疗方案。

转换率建议如下:

2 天的丁丙诺啡剂量 = 丁丙诺啡每天剂量(最大剂量为 32mg)× 2
3 天的丁丙诺啡剂量 = 丁丙诺啡每天剂量(最大剂量为 32mg)× 3

注:如果患者使用丁丙诺啡时无法保持稳定状态(通常是从美沙酮换药的患者),可以考虑换回美沙酮治疗。在末次使用丁丙诺啡 24h 后给予美沙酮。根据临床反应慎重调整美沙酮剂量,注意丁丙诺啡残留的"阻断"效应可能会持续几天,这意味着美沙酮中毒可能会延迟发生。

丁丙诺啡的注意事项

- **肝功能**:有证据表明,高剂量丁丙诺啡可导致肝病患者的肝功能变化[62]。该类患者开始丁丙诺啡治疗前应做肝功能检查,6~12 周后复查。对某些伴严重肝脏疾病的患者,应该考虑增加检测频率。然而,若没有具备临床意义的肝病,肝酶升高不一定是丁丙诺啡的禁忌证。
- **中毒**:对有任何中毒迹象的患者,尤其是酒精或其他中枢抑制剂(如苯二氮䓬类、镇静性抗精神病药和普瑞巴林[39])所致者,禁止使用丁丙诺啡。丁丙诺啡与其他镇静药物合用可导致呼吸抑制、镇静、昏迷,甚至死亡。由于与多种物质滥用相关的过量风险增加,在考虑以后使用丁丙诺啡时,必须注意合用酒精和非法药物的情况。

丁丙诺啡过量

单用丁丙诺啡过量,比美沙酮或海洛因过量相对安全,因为它的呼吸抑制作用较轻,与过量死亡相关的可能性更小[63]。但与呼吸抑制剂合用时,药物过量则难以处理。可能需要很高剂量的纳洛酮(如 10~15mg),才能逆转丁丙诺啡作用(一般低剂量,如 0.8~2mg 就够了)[4]。因此,如果丁丙诺啡导致呼吸抑制(如多种药物过量),常常需要呼吸机支持。

丁丙诺啡与纳洛酮合剂(赛宝松)

为了减少药物被挪用的风险,医师可考虑使用丁丙诺啡/纳洛酮合剂。丁丙诺啡和纳洛酮舌下和胃肠外吸收的特点不同,这是关键因素:当舌下含服时,纳洛酮的作用可以忽略。但是,若注射这种混合制剂,则纳洛酮的作用很强,短期内可减轻丁丙诺啡的作用,在使用阿片受体完全激动剂的阿片类物质依赖者中,它可能促发戒断症状[64]。

其他口服阿片类制剂

美沙酮和丁丙诺啡的口服制剂仍是主要治疗手段[1];其他口服制剂,如吗啡口服缓释剂和双氢可待因,在英国尚未获得治疗阿片类物质依赖的许可[1]。

但是若患者对美沙酮或丁丙诺啡不能耐受,或者在其他特殊情况下,专科医师在充分考虑半衰期短、监管要求和挪用风险等相关困难的情况下,可以使用口服双氢可待因来进行维持治疗[1]。

在欧洲的其他地方,有证据显示,吗啡口服缓释剂对不能耐受美沙酮维持治疗者有效,但也只能由专科医师开具处方[1]。近期一篇综述显示,没有充足证据可评估吗啡口服缓释剂的疗效[65]。

二醋吗啡注射剂维持治疗

有可靠的证据支持,对于一线阿片类药物替代治疗无效的患者,可以注射二醋吗啡进行维持治疗[66]。不同于早年无监督地注射阿片类药物,现在使用注射制剂的患者必须做到以下几点:

- 根据治疗计划,亲自参加处方阿片类药物注射维持治疗——每天或更频繁。
- 在有能力的工作人员直接监督下进行注射。
- 不得外带注射药品。

在英国,处方医师必须有内政部(Home Office)颁发的执照,才能为阿片类药物依赖者开二醋吗啡处方。如果实施注射的诊所不是每天运营,当不能在监督下注射药物时,可以给予几天的口服阿片类药物替代治疗。这种治疗是辅以心理社会干预的整体护理方案的组成部分,因此不同于"注射室",即为静脉注射毒品(通常不接受治疗)的人提供的配有无菌设备的安全场所。虽然它的成本效益已经得到证明,但是建设成本高限制了它的实施[67]。

目前,注射阿片类药物与心理社会干预相结合,只是总体治疗方案中一个环节。对于口服阿片类药物替代治疗效果不佳者,若所在地区有监督下用药的必需条件,则支持使用这种方法[1,68]。患者通常在专业机构监管下每天注射 2 次。对于因使用处方二醋吗啡而被急症医院收治的患者,医师需要咨询当地的政策。通常情况下,与在社区开处方的成瘾精神科医师沟通并进行记录后,就可以继续开处方。

精神科病房阿片类药物依赖的治疗

　　阿片类药物使用过量也可发生在医院。所有阿片类药物依赖的住院患者在"必要时"都应该使用纳洛酮。

　　在住院情况下,必须控制阿片类药物戒断症状,以便让患者留在病房,并根据其在精神科住院的原因进行针对性的干预。在急性精神科住院期间,最有效的预防阿片类药物戒断的方法是继续使用他们现有的阿片类药物替代治疗。为了继续开相同剂量的阿片类药物替代药物,需要分别确认以下几点:

- 成瘾服务机构对处方剂量的确认。
- 从药房确认其最近监督下用药的剂量,是否给予了外带的剂量。如果最近监督下用药的时间是 3 天以前,患者需要重新开始阿片类药物替代治疗,以避免过量(见"起始治疗"部分)。周末入院的患者可能有外带回家的药物,如果不直接询问他们,那么他们可能不一定披露这些。如果患者最后一次使用阿片类药物替代治疗后超过 3 天,他们将失去耐受性,需要根据成瘾科医师的建议重新用药。

　　只有在上述信息得到证实且满足以下情况时,才应继续按报告剂量使用阿片类药物替代治疗:

- 在此剂量下,患者表现清醒和舒适。
- 患者没有出现其他物质中毒。

> 　　如果对前面列出的任何因素存在疑问或担忧,则不应使用阿片类药物替代治疗。

　　低年资医师可能会发现,他们在照顾阿片类药物戒断的患者时,无法立即确认上述所有信息,因此无法安全地使用阿片类药物替代治疗。阿片类药物戒断,虽然不是致命的,但是是非常负面的,并且在患者需要住院治疗时,如果自行出院则存在很大的风险。在寻求此类帮助之前,其他药物可能也有助于处理阿片类药物戒断症状。但是一旦使用阿片类药物替代治疗,其他药物就没有多大用处了。由于与多种药物和多种物质使用相关的风险,不鼓励在阿片类药物替代治疗诱导期间使用它们。以下是英国现行药物依赖治疗临床指南针对特定症状的建议[1](表 4.14):

表 4.14　针对特定症状的药物依赖治疗(改编自《药物滥用和依赖:英国临床管理指南 2017》[1])

症状	治疗
腹泻	洛哌丁胺 4mg,每次稀便后 2mg,每天最多 16mg,持续 5 天
恶心和呕吐	甲氧氯普胺 10mg,每天 3 次,持续最多 5 天;丙氯拉嗪 5mg,每天 3 次,或 12.5mg 肌内注射,每天 2 次
腹部绞痛	甲苯凡林 135mg,每天 3 次
激越、焦虑和失眠	有苯二氮䓬类药物依赖史的患者,必要时可服用地西泮 5~10mg,每天 3 次,或佐匹克隆 7.5mg,每晚
肌肉疼痛和头痛	对乙酰氨基酚、阿司匹林或非甾体抗炎药。外用发红药可有效地缓解美沙酮戒断引起的肌肉疼痛

因精神科急症住院治疗的患者不应对阿片类药物替代治疗进行脱毒治疗,应考虑对尚未接受治疗的阿片类药物依赖患者开始阿片类药物替代治疗(在当地成瘾专家的建议下)。

急性住院患者的美沙酮起始治疗(或在非成瘾机构中由非专业人员使用)

诱导期——第 1 天:

患者必须表现出客观的阿片类戒断症状,以阿片类戒断量表(如 COWS)进行评估(表 4.3):

- 根据戒断症状的严重程度,给予 10mg 美沙酮(1mg/ 1mL),每天仅用 1 次。美沙酮会在 20~30min 后开始起作用,在 4h 达到峰值。
- 继续每 4h 监测 1 次戒断症状,并根据需要进一步给药 5~10mg,同时观察中毒症状。
- 最初的每天剂量(24h)通常不会超过 30mg。
- 如果过量,"按需"给予纳洛酮。注意药物蓄积,即反复的小剂量逐渐蓄积达中毒剂量。

第 2 天:

- 按患者第 1 天所需的剂量单次或分次使用。
- 继续监测戒断症状和镇静作用。

维持用药

- 咨询成瘾专家后,考虑进一步增加剂量,每 3~4 天增加 5~10mg,直至戒断症状完全缓解。
- 一旦达到稳定,继续使用所需药物剂量。

在急诊住院情况下,通常建议患者保持稳定的治疗剂量,而不是尝试脱瘾。

由每天 2 次给药改为每天给药 1 次

患者通常从急诊医院转到精神科医院,并分次服用美沙酮。在社区中分开给药会带来药物被挪用的风险,所以除怀孕期间外,不鼓励分次给药。在出院前一天,应将给药方式改为每天 1 次,注意美沙酮浓度达到峰值时可出现镇静和呼吸抑制。

> 所有离开病房的患者都应该接受家用纳洛酮的使用培训,发放家用纳洛酮[1],并在戒瘾服务机构预约,以便在出院前继续开具处方。

给阿片类药物依赖患者处方精神药物

普通精神科医师经常为成瘾患者提供治疗,以治疗精神疾病的共病。关于共病精神疾病的药物治疗指南,见《英国精神药理协会物质滥用指南》[69]。一般来说,医师应该谨慎地开具经许可的用于治疗共病精神疾病的镇静剂,因为它会增加呼吸抑制的风险,例如普瑞巴林,它的过量与死亡有关[39]。普瑞巴林和奥氮平在阿片类药物依赖人群中也有滥用的倾向[70,71]。阿片类物质依赖患者更容易患抑郁症——参加治疗的患者中约 50% 符合抑郁症的标准。他们稳定病情所需的美沙酮剂量可能会比非抑郁症患者多 20%~50%[72],但在大多数情况下,病情稳定可促进药物滥用的缓解[73]。关于抗抑郁药在阿片类药物依赖中的使用,有少数低到中等质量的临床试验证据,表明其对情绪或药物滥用的益处均有限[69,73]。结果为阳性的研究大多使用的是有多种药理作用的药物,如三环类抗抑郁药[74]。然而,由于其心脏毒性,不推荐在共病药物滥用的患者中使用[75]。基于证据推荐的抗抑郁治疗方法包括:首先稳定使用阿片类药物替代治疗的患者;如果抑郁症状持续,则考虑使用SSRI,因为它们相对安全;但是如果患者没有反应,则考虑使用混合药理机制的抗抑郁药作为二线药物[74]。舍曲林是美沙酮治疗患者的首选药物,因为它很少存在潜在的药物间相互作用。

阿片类物质脱毒和减量方案

阿片类药物维持治疗可持续数周以上,取决于临床需要。一些患者喜欢在短期稳定后便脱毒,另一些则选择在较长时期的维持治疗后脱毒。整体治疗计划应该包括脱毒计划。脱毒后有出现严重致死性药物过量的风险,因此提供脱毒治疗的机构应对患者进行健康教育,告知这些风险,提供纳洛酮,并培训患者药物过量时如何使用纳洛酮急救。

关于脱毒时间的长短,NICE指南认为"减量可在数天至数月内完成,起始稳定剂量越大,减量时间越长",并指出"美沙酮减量一般需要3个月,丁丙诺啡一般需14天至数周"[76]。在实践中,社区脱毒治疗时间应适当延长,这有助于让患者顺利度过减药过程,提高治疗依从性,在脱毒过程中坚持不用非法药物,及减少其脱毒后复吸的可能性。

对于住院脱毒治疗,NICE指南指出:"因支持性的环境有助于患者耐受戒断反应",其脱毒时间可以比社区短些(建议美沙酮14~21天,丁丙诺啡7~21天)[77]。与社区脱毒一样,首先要使阿片类药物替代治疗的剂量达到稳定,接下来逐渐减量;如果需要,可适量增加合法处方的药物以减轻戒断症状。

脱毒治疗后有复发和过量致死的风险。因此,患者接受脱毒时,需要准备充分的后续服务,如康复计划和社区支持等。对于因紧急躯体或精神问题住院的患者,除非有专业支持及后续服务准备,一般不考虑脱毒治疗。

社区环境下停用阿片类物质

美沙酮

美沙酮治疗达到稳定状态或者维持治疗一段时间后,作为整体治疗计划的一部分,患者和医师商议进行药物减量。一般每1~2周减5~10mg,但可以酌情调整减量幅度和速度。在社区中,患者意愿是影响减药幅度和速度的最重要因素。应定期回顾脱毒计划,并根据情况进行适当调整和改变,如患者复吸非法药物或担心减药速度等。当患者增加海洛因或其他毒品剂量,或身体、心理、社会生活状况恶化时,可暂时增加或停止减量,或放慢减药速度。在脱毒末期,减药速度可以减慢,为每周1~2mg。近期研究显示,维持治疗时状态稳定的时间长短以及长期的减药计划(可达1年)可显著增加守戒成功率[78]。

丁丙诺啡

丁丙诺啡脱毒方案及原则与美沙酮类似。应逐渐减量以减少撤药反应。推荐的减药方案见下表:

丁丙诺啡每天剂量	减量速度
大于 16mg	每 1~2 周 4mg
8~16mg	每 1~2 周 2~4mg
2~8mg	每 1~2 周 2mg
小于 2mg	每周 0.4~0.8mg

在成瘾专科住院部停用阿片类物质

美沙酮

在 48h 内,专科团队应该对患者进行美沙酮起始剂量评估。接下来 4 周内对美沙酮进行逐渐减药。

丁丙诺啡

住院环境下,可使用丁丙诺啡进行短期脱毒治疗,脱毒原则与美沙酮相同。

纳曲酮对预防复发的作用

有关纳曲酮对阿片类物质依赖者预防复发的研究结果并不十分一致[79]。如果患者愿意参加戒毒项目、全面了解其治疗效果及可能的不良反应、具有较强的治疗动机、选择戒毒为治疗目标、具有较好的社会支持,那么,NICE 认为纳曲酮有助于戒除阿片类物质滥用,是比较经济的治疗策略[80]。目前,虽然纳曲酮植入剂在英国尚未批准使用,但对于有治疗动机患者,也可能会起一定的作用[81]。

开始使用纳曲酮后需进行严密监测,因为在此阶段发生过量中毒致死的风险较高。纳曲酮停药也会增加非法阿片药物意外过量的风险。因此,监测用药情况,并谨慎选择患者(如具有较强的治疗动机并以戒断为目标)非常重要。此外,使用纳曲酮的患者经常出现烦躁(心境恶劣)、抑郁、失眠等不良反应,可能导致患者在纳曲酮治疗期间重新使用非法药物,或者终止纳曲酮治疗。心境恶劣可能是非法药物的戒断反应,也可能是纳曲酮本身所致,因此必须强调纳曲酮治疗只是治疗方案的一部分,治疗方案还包括心理社会干预和常规的支持治疗[80]。

开始纳曲酮治疗

对于目前正在使用阿片类物质,或者既往使用过阿片类物质但还没有经过充分"清洗期"的患者,使用纳曲酮有可能引起严重戒断反应。

停止阿片类物质与开始纳曲酮治疗之间的最短间隔时间,取决于所用阿片药物的种类、使用的时间长短及末次用量。长半衰期的阿片激动剂(如美沙酮)需要 10 天的清洗期,而短效阿片药物(如海洛因、吗啡或芬太尼)可能只需 7 天的清洗期。对于丁丙诺啡使用者(末次用量大于 2mg,使用时间大于 2 周),需要 7 天的清洗期。有时候停药 2~3 天后便可开始纳曲酮治疗(如末次用量小于 2mg,使用时间短于 2 周)。

在开始纳曲酮治疗前,可以试验性肌内注射纳洛酮 0.2~0.8mg(其半衰期较纳曲酮短)。纳洛酮诱发的戒断反应持续时间比纳曲酮短。

患者在接受治疗前必须被告知戒断反应的风险。必须仔细询问患者是否无意中服用过含阿片类物质的制剂(如非处方止痛药)。

纳曲酮治疗要点

- 确保患者充分了解治疗可增加致死性阿片过量的风险。
- 在脱毒后或防止复吸的任何阶段,个体对阿片类物质的耐受性会显著降低,此时使用阿片类物质出现过量中毒的风险大大地增加。
- 停用纳曲酮也可导致阿片药物意外过量的风险增加,因此进行密切监测及提供支持非常重要。

纳曲酮剂量

停用阿片类药物适当时间后,才能给予起始剂量的纳曲酮 25mg(适当情况下可进行纳洛酮催瘾实验)。在首次用药后 4h 内,要监测阿片类物质戒断反应。必要时,在纳曲酮治疗首日,应准备戒断反应的对症治疗药物洛非西定(戒断症状可持续 4~8h)。当患者对低剂量的纳曲酮耐受以后,可增加至 50mg/d 维持治疗。

纳曲酮禁用于肝功能异常者,纳曲酮治疗过程中需监测肝功能。

阿片类药物替代治疗患者的疼痛处理

美沙酮治疗患者的镇痛

合适的情况下首选非阿片类镇痛药(例如对乙酰氨基酚、非甾体抗炎药)。疼痛的类型和严重程度提示需要使用阿片类药物(如可待因、二氢可待因、吗啡等),可按照常规镇痛原则,根据疼痛缓解情况来逐步增加剂量。

如果患者正在使用美沙酮,在适合使用阿片类镇痛剂情况下,可以合用美沙酮之外的阿片类药物,即不必拘泥于用一种药物满足全部的阿片类作用需求[82]。在某些情况下,可以逐步增加美沙酮剂量来产生镇痛作用,但仅限于有经验的专家使用。

正如本章其他部分介绍过,服用丁丙诺啡或纳曲酮的患者对阿片类药物的镇痛作用相对不敏感;但在临床实践中,使用丁丙诺啡的患者需要治疗急性疼痛时,可选择其他阿片类药物,并根据反应调整剂量[19]。如果为了使用阿片类药物镇痛需要停用纳曲酮,必须注意密切监测患者,因为复发和过量的风险都增加了[35,82]。

药物滥用患者可能还会因手术、外伤或其他疾病需要在医院进行急性镇痛处理。在此期间的主要目标是控制疼痛、预防戒断症状,因此提供足够的药物支持对两个目标都十分重要。应与住院疼痛处理团队及成瘾治疗机构联系,并与患者共同讨论。成瘾治疗机构在了解患者的情况之后,可以提供信息协助制订治疗计划,帮助患者从非法药物(如果他们正在使用非法药物)换成处方镇痛药物,并帮助患者在经过急性疼痛处理后,顺利换成对药物滥用的持续管理[35]。详见英国疼痛协会、皇家精神科医师协会、皇家全科医师学会及药物滥用顾问委员会的共识[82]。

　　如姑息治疗的共识所述,给物质滥用患者提供镇痛治疗的原则,"与需要姑息治疗的其他成年人基本相同",当然必须加强与物质滥用治疗机构的联系。阿片类物质依赖者可在药物滥用治疗机构接受维持治疗,"其处方应该单独的,与疼痛门诊患者的镇痛处方是分开的"(见上文慢性非癌症疼痛)。在住院期间,所有药物通常都应该从医院获得,"除非是在疾病终末期,出院时应该对药物滥用和疼痛缓解分别制订明确的随访计划"[82]。详细信息可参考共识[82]。共识发布之后,人们开始关注普瑞巴林(一种用于慢性疼痛的非阿片类药物[70])滥用的可能性,以及普瑞巴林和阿片类药物处方增加过量使用的可能性。建议在为慢性疼痛患者开具普瑞巴林时要谨慎。

孕期阿片类物质使用(也可见本章"妊娠期的药物滥用")

> 孕期可随时改用替代治疗,其风险低于继续吸毒。治疗应在稳定药物使用和减少替代阿片类药物剂量之间取得平衡,以预防新生儿戒断综合征。

　　在妊娠任何时期都可能出现阿片类物质依赖,稳定使用美沙酮替代治疗是首选治疗。在妊娠头 3 个月禁止进行脱毒治疗,因为会增加自发流产的风险;在妊娠最后 3 个月也禁止进行脱毒治疗,因为可能与早产、胎儿窘迫和死产有关。如要求进行脱毒治疗,则在妊娠中期脱毒比较安全,但须在具有专业能力的专科医师指导下进行,同时严密监测不稳定的证据。脱毒处方的减量应小而频繁,例如每3~5 天减少美沙酮2~3mg[l]。禁止进行强制脱毒治疗,因为这会使部分求治的患者望而却步,也会使大部分患者在孕期某个阶段复吸[83];间断吸毒会引起母体血内阿片类物质浓度波动,进而引起胎儿戒断反应或药物过量[84,85]。丁丙诺啡与较轻的新生儿戒断症状有关[14]。然而,丁丙诺啡不应在妊娠期间使用,也不应换用美沙酮,因为有诱导胎儿戒断反应的风险。

孕期替代处方

　　应在一个多学科团队(包括产科团队、麻醉师、新生儿医师和成瘾专家)内进行,提供全面的系列照料。有关治疗的证据较少[86]。目前,美沙酮和丁丙诺啡在安全性方面似乎没有任何区别。美沙酮与较好的治疗保持率有关,而丁丙诺啡则与较轻的新生儿戒断综合征有关[86]。因此,最新的指南建议,当患者妊娠时,允许患者选择其中之一,或继续服用原来的药物[1]。在妊娠期间应避免使用赛宝松(suboxone)。然而,也不建议将美沙酮换成丁丙诺啡,因为胎儿有发生戒断反应的风险。在妊娠最后 3 个月,机体对美沙酮的代谢可能增加,需要分次给药。

新生儿戒断综合征

　　母亲使用美沙酮维持治疗时,所分娩的新生儿大多数需要接受戒断综合征的治疗。该病以各种自主神经系统、胃肠道、呼吸系统症状和体征为特征[84]。婴儿可能会发出尖锐的哭声,如饥似渴地吃奶却吃不进去多少,而且呈过度觉醒状态。严重新生儿戒断综合征常伴有过度紧张和癫痫发作,但并不常见。美沙酮治疗后的新生儿戒断综合征通常在 48h 后出

现 [87]，但也可能延迟 7~10 天 [1]。若母亲吸毒或接受阿片类药物替代治疗，必须有条件接受熟练的新生儿护理服务，以监测新生儿并根据情况进行处理。母乳喂养可降低新生儿戒断综合征的严重程度（见下文）。

对于孕期使用阿片类止痛药治疗的妇女，需要重视由此带来的潜在问题：因为增加了相关的风险，此类患者需要在产前专科诊所进行治疗。针对预期的麻醉风险、止痛需求、静脉通路等问题，建议由麻醉科医师进行产前评估。

母乳喂养

出于以下原因，应鼓励服用美沙酮或丁丙诺啡的妇女进行母乳喂养，即使她们继续使用非法阿片类药物：

■ 对母亲和婴儿的总体健康有益。

■ 减少住院时间和需要新生儿戒断综合征干预的确切益处 [88]。

■ 低浓度的美沙酮和丁丙诺啡被转移给婴儿 [88]。

应告知患者逐渐停止母乳喂养，因为突然停止母乳喂养可能会导致迟发的新生儿戒断综合征 [88]。使用精制可卡因或大剂量苯二氮䓬类药物的患者不宜母乳喂养 [1]。

参考文献

1. Department of Health and Social Care. Drug misuse and dependence: UK guidelines on clinical management. 2017; https://www.gov.uk/government/publications/drug-misuse-and-dependence-uk-guidelines-on-clinical-management.

2. Ellis K, et al. Routes to recovery. 2007; http://americanradioworks.publicradio.org/features/nola/transcript.html.

3. World Health Organization. Community management of opioid overdose. 2014; http://www.who.int/substance_abuse/publications/management_opioid_overdose/en.

4. FDA. FDA advisory committee on the most appropriate dose or doses of naloxone to reverse the effects of life-threatening opioid overdose in the community settings. 2016; https://www.fda.gov/downloads/AdvisoryCommittees/CommitteesMeetingMaterials/Drugs/AnestheticAndAnalgesicDrugProductsAdvisoryCommittee/UCM522688.pdf.

5. Strang J, et al. Naloxone without the needle – systematic review of candidate routes for non-injectable naloxone for opioid overdose reversal. *Drug Alcohol Depend* 2016; 163:16–23.

6. Beletsky L, et al. Prevention of fatal opioid overdose. *JAMA* 2012; 308:1863–1864.

7. McDonald R, et al. Pharmacokinetics of concentrated naloxone nasal spray for opioid overdose reversal: phase I healthy volunteer study. *Addiction* 2018; 113:484–493.

8. National Institute for Health and Care Excellence. Coexisting severe mental illness and substance misuse: community health and social care services. NICE Guidance NG58. 2016; https://www.nice.org.uk/guidance/ng58.

9. Wesson DR, et al. The Clinical Opiate Withdrawal Scale (COWS). *J Psychoactive Drugs* 2003; 35:253–259.

10. Handelsman L, et al. Two new rating scales for opiate withdrawal. *Am J Drug Alcohol Abuse* 1987; 13:293–308.

11. Mattick RP, et al. Buprenorphine maintenance versus placebo or methadone maintenance for opioid dependence. *Cochrane Database Syst Rev* 2014; 2:CD002207.

12. Comer SD, et al. Abuse liability of prescription opioids compared to heroin in morphine-maintained heroin abusers. *Neuropsychopharmacology* 2008; 33:1179–1191.

13. Jolley CJ, et al. P214 The prevalence of respiratory symptoms and lung disease in a South London 'lung health in addictions' service. *Thorax* 2016; 71:A201.

14. Seifert J, et al. Detoxification of opiate addicts with multiple drug abuse: a comparison of buprenorphine vs. methadone. *Pharmacopsychiatry* 2002; 35:159–164.

15. Jasinski DR, et al. Human pharmacology and abuse potential of the analgesic buprenorphine: a potential agent for treating narcotic addiction. *Arch Gen Psychiatry* 1978; 35:501–516.

16. Bickel WK, et al. Buprenorphine: dose-related blockade of opioid challenge effects in opioid dependent humans. *J Pharmacol Exp Ther* 1988; 247:47–53.

17. Walsh SL, et al. Acute administration of buprenorphine in humans: partial agonist and blockade effects. *J Pharmacol Exp Ther* 1995; 274:361–372.

18. Comer SD, et al. Buprenorphine sublingual tablets: effects on IV heroin self-administration by humans. *Psychopharmacology* 2001; 154:28–37.

19. Alford DP, et al. Acute pain management for patients receiving maintenance methadone or buprenorphine therapy. *Ann Intern Med* 2006;

144:127–134.

20. Jones HE, et al. Neonatal abstinence syndrome after methadone or buprenorphine exposure. *N Engl J Med* 2010; 363:2320–2331.

21. Nielsen S, et al. Opioid agonist treatment for pharmaceutical opioid dependent people. *Cochrane Database Syst Rev* 2016; Cd011117.

22. Weiss RD, et al. The prescription opioid addiction treatment study: what have we learned. *Drug Alcohol Depend* 2017; 173 Suppl 1:S48–S54.

23. Department of Health Task Force to Review Services for Drug Misusers. Report of an independent review of drug treatment services in England. 1996; http://www.dh.gov.uk.

24. Caplehorn JR. Deaths in the first two weeks of maintenance treatment in NSW in 1994: identifying cases of iatrogenic methadone toxicity. *Drug Alcohol Rev* 1998; 17:9–17.

25. Zador D, et al. Deaths in methadone maintenance treatment in New South Wales, Australia 1990–1995. *Addiction* 2000; 95:77–84.

26. Hall W. Reducing the toll of opioid overdose deaths in Australia. *Drug Alcohol Rev* 1999; 18:213–220.

27. White JM, et al. Mechanisms of fatal opioid overdose. *Addiction* 1999; 94:961–972.

28. Gao L, et al. Risk-factors for methadone-specific deaths in Scotland's methadone-prescription clients between 2009 and 2013. *Drug Alcohol Depend* 2016; 167:214–223.

29. Wolff K, et al. The pharmacokinetics of methadone in healthy subjects and opiate users. *Br J Clin Pharmacol* 1997; 44:325–334.

30. Rostami-Hodjegan A, et al. Population pharmacokinetics of methadone in opiate users: characterization of time-dependent changes. *Br J Clin Pharmacol* 1999; 48:43–52.

31. Harding-Pink D. Methadone: one person's maintenance dose is another's poison. *Lancet* 1993; 341:665–666.

32. Drummer OH, et al. Methadone toxicity causing death in ten subjects starting on a methadone maintenance program. *Am J Forensic Med Pathol* 1992; 13:346–350.

33. National Institute for Clinical Excellence. Methadone and buprenorphine for the management of opioid dependence. Technology Appraisal guidance [TA114]. 2007 (last checked February 2016). https://www.nice.org.uk/guidance/ta114.

34. Amato L, et al. Methadone at tapered doses for the management of opioid withdrawal. *Cochrane Database Syst Rev* 2013; 2:CD003409.

35. Cornish R, et al. Risk of death during and after opiate substitution treatment in primary care: prospective observational study in UK General Practice Research Database. *BMJ* 2010; 341:c5475.

36. Strang J, et al. Loss of tolerance and overdose mortality after inpatient opiate detoxification: follow up study. *BMJ* 2003; 326:959–960.

37. Bell J. Pharmacological maintenance treatments of opiate addiction. *Br J Clin Pharmacol* 2014; 77:253–263.

38. Farrell M, et al. Suicide and overdose among opiate addicts. *Addiction* 1996; 91:321–323.

39. Abrahamsson T, et al. Benzodiazepine, z-drug and pregabalin prescriptions and mortality among patients in opioid maintenance treatment-A nation-wide register-based open cohort study. *Drug Alcohol Depend* 2017; 174:58–64.

40. Pierce M, et al. Impact of treatment for opioid dependence on fatal drug-related poisoning: a national cohort study in England. *Addiction* 2016; 111:298–308.

41. Neale J. Methadone, methadone treatment and non-fatal overdose. *Drug Alcohol Depend* 2000; 58:117–124.

42. Krantz MJ, et al. Torsade de pointes associated with very-high-dose methadone. *Ann Intern Med* 2002; 137:501–504.

43. Kornick CA, et al. QTc interval prolongation associated with intravenous methadone. *Pain* 2003; 105:499–506.

44. Martell BA, et al. The impact of methadone induction on cardiac conduction in opiate users. *Ann Intern Med* 2003; 139:154–155.

45. Mayet S, et al. Methadone maintenance, QTc and torsade de pointes: who needs an electrocardiogram and what is the prevalence of QTc prolongation? *Drug Alcohol Rev* 2011; 30:388–396.

46. Hancox JC, et al. Synthetic cannabinoids and potential cardiac arrhythmia risk: an important message for drug users. *Ther Adv Drug Saf* 2020; 11:2042098620913416.

47. Medicines and Healthcare Products Regulatory Agency. Risk of QT interval prolongation with methadone. *Curr Prob Pharmacovigilance* 2006; 31:6.

48. Isbister GK, et al. Drug induced QT prolongation: the measurement and assessment of the QT interval in clinical practice. *Br J Clin Pharmacol* 2013; 76:48–57.

49. Cruciani RA. Methadone: to ECG or not to ECG … that is still the question. *J Pain Symptom Manage* 2008; 36:545–552.

50. Wedam EF, et al. QT-interval effects of methadone, levomethadyl, and buprenorphine in a randomized trial. *Arch Intern Med* 2007; 167:2469–2475.

51. Pani PP, et al. QTc interval screening for cardiac risk in methadone treatment of opioid dependence. *Cochrane Database Syst Rev* 2013; 6:CD008939.

52. Gowing L, et al. Buprenorphine for managing opioid withdrawal. *Cochrane Database Syst Rev* 2017; 2:Cd002025.

53. Strain EC, et al. Relative bioavailability of different buprenorphine formulations under chronic dosing conditions. *Drug Alcohol Depend* 2004; 74:37–43.

54. Walsh SL, et al. Effects of buprenorphine and methadone in methadone-maintained subjects. *Psychopharmacology* 1995; 119:268–276.

55. Strain EC, et al. Acute effects of buprenorphine, hydromorphone and naloxone in methadone-maintained volunteers. *J Pharmacol Exp Ther* 1992; 261:985–993.

56. Strain EC, et al. Buprenorphine effects in methadone-maintained volunteers: effects at two hours after methadone. *J Pharmacol Exp Ther* 1995; 272:628–638.

57. Grass JA. Patient-controlled analgesia. *Anesth Analg* 2005; 101:S44–S61.

58. Amass L, et al. Alternate-day buprenorphine dosing is preferred to daily dosing by opioid-dependent humans. *Psychopharmacology* 1998; 136:217–225.

59. Amass L, et al. Alternate-day dosing during buprenorphine treatment of opioid dependence. *Life Sci* 1994; 54:1215–1228.

60. Johnson RE, et al. Buprenorphine treatment of opioid dependence: clinical trial of daily versus alternate-day dosing. *Drug Alcohol Depend*

1995; **40:**27–35.

61. Eissenberg T, et al. Controlled opioid withdrawal evaluation during 72 h dose omission in buprenorphine-maintained patients. *Drug Alcohol Depend* 1997; **45:**81–91.

62. Berson A, et al. Hepatitis after intravenous buprenorphine misuse in heroin addicts. *J Hepatol* 2001; **34:**346–350.

63. Paone D, et al. Buprenorphine infrequently found in fatal overdose in New York City. *Drug Alcohol Depend* 2015; **155:**298–301.

64. Stoller KB, et al. Effects of buprenorphine/naloxone in opioid-dependent humans. *Psychopharmacology* 2001; **154:**230–242.

65. Ferri M, et al. Slow-release oral morphine as maintenance therapy for opioid dependence. *Cochrane Database Syst Rev* 2013; **6:** CD009879.

66. Strang J, et al. Heroin on trial: systematic review and meta-analysis of randomised trials of diamorphine-prescribing as treatment for refractory heroin addiction dagger. *Br J Psychiatry* 2015; **207:**5–14.

67. Byford S, et al. Cost-effectiveness of injectable opioid treatment v. oral methadone for chronic heroin addiction. *Br J Psychiatry* 2013; **203:**341–349.

68. Strang J, et al. Supervised injectable heroin or injectable methadone versus optimised oral methadone as treatment for chronic heroin addicts in England after persistent failure in orthodox treatment (RIOTT): a randomised trial. *Lancet* 2010; **375:**1885–1895.

69. Lingford-Hughes AR, et al. Evidence-based guidelines for the pharmacological management of substance abuse, harmful use, addiction and comorbidity: recommendations from BAP. *J Psychopharmacol* 2012; **26:**899–952.

70. Baird CR, et al. Gabapentinoid abuse in order to potentiate the effect of methadone: a survey among substance misusers. *Eur Addict Res* 2014; **20:**115–118.

71. James PD, et al. Non-medical use of olanzapine by people on methadone treatment. *B J Psych Bull* 2016; **40:**314–317.

72. Tenore PL. Psychotherapeutic benefits of opioid agonist therapy. *J Addict Dis* 2008; **27:**49–65.

73. Nunes EV, et al. Treatment of depression in patients with alcohol or other drug dependence: a meta-analysis. *JAMA* 2004; **291:**1887–1896.

74. Nunes EV, et al. Treatment of co-occurring depression and substance dependence: using meta-analysis to guide clinical recommendations. *Psychiatr Ann* 2008; **38:**nihpa128505.

75. Lingford-Hughes AR, et al. BAP updated guidelines: evidence-based guidelines for the pharmacological management of substance abuse, harmful use, addiction and comorbidity: recommendations from BAP. *J Psychopharmacol* 2012; **26:**899–952.

76. National Institute for Clinical Excellence. Drug misuse in over 16s: opioid detoxification. Clinical Guidance 52. 2007; https://www.nice.org.uk/guidance/cg52.

77. National Institute for Clinical Excellence. Drug misuse in over 16s: psychosocial interventions. Clinical Guidance [CG51]. 2007; (last checked July 2016). https://www.nice.org.uk/guidance/cg51.

78. Nosyk B, et al. Defining dosing pattern characteristics of successful tapers following methadone maintenance treatment: results from a population-based retrospective cohort study. *Addiction* 2012; **107:**1621–1629.

79. Minozzi S, et al. Oral naltrexone maintenance treatment for opioid dependence. *Cochrane Database Syst Rev* 2011; **4:**CD001333.

80. National Institute for Clinical Excellence. Naltrexone for the management of opioid dependence. Technology Appraisal [TA115]. 2007 (reviewed November 2010); https://www.nice.org.uk/guidance/ta115.

81. Kunoe N, et al. Naltrexone implants after in-patient treatment for opioid dependence: randomised controlled trial. *Br J Psychiatry* 2009; **194:**541–546.

82. The British Pain Society, et al. Pain and substance misuse: improving the patient experience. A consensus statement prepared by The British Pain Society in collaboration with The Royal College of Psychiatrists, The Royal College of General Practitioners and The Advisory Council on the Misuse of Drugs. 2007; http://www.britishpainsociety.org/book_drug_misuse_main.pdf.

83. Winklbaur B, et al. Treating pregnant women dependent on opioids is not the same as treating pregnancy and opioid dependence: a knowledge synthesis for better treatment for women and neonates. *Addiction* 2008; **103:**1429–1440.

84. Finnegan LP. Neonatal abstinence syndrome. in RA Hoekelman, et al., ed. Primary pediatric care. St Louis: Mosby 1992; 1367–1378.

85. Winklbaur B, et al. Opioid dependence and pregnancy. *Curr Opin Psychiatry* 2008; **21:**255–259.

86. Minozzi S, et al. Maintenance agonist treatments for opiate-dependent pregnant women. *Cochrane Database Syst Rev* 2013; **12:**CD006318.

87. Fischer G, et al. Methadone versus buprenorphine in pregnant addicts: a double-blind, double-dummy comparison study. *Addiction* 2006; **101:**275–281.

88. Holmes AP, et al. Breastfeeding considerations for mothers of infants with neonatal abstinence syndrome. *Pharmacotherapy* 2017; **37:**861–869.

尼古丁和戒烟

吸烟是导致世界上可预防疾病和过早死亡的主要原因。戒烟干预对患有精神疾病和没有精神疾病者均具有临床和成本效益。

在英国,NICE 建议每个吸烟者,包括接受社区和住院精神健康照顾者,都应该得到戒烟支持;对于那些不能或不愿意戒烟的人,他们应该在住院治疗期间暂时性戒烟[1]。

对于那些希望尝试戒烟者,NICE 推荐了三种戒烟首选药物:尼古丁替代疗法(NRT)、伐尼克兰和安非他酮,这些药物使戒烟成功率至少增加一倍。如果吸烟者得到有戒烟治疗经验的医师支持,那么戒烟成功率还会增加[2]。

那些不愿意或感觉无法戒烟的人,应该鼓励他们尽量减少伤害,以尼古丁替代疗法或电子烟替代烟草的尼古丁[3,4]。

在有各种精神健康问题的患者中,戒烟治疗的有效性似乎并没有降低[5]。

尼古丁替代疗法(NRT)

NRT 被许可应用于 12 岁以上的吸烟者,以帮助那些想戒烟的人戒烟,以及完全戒烟前或不能吸烟的临时强制戒毒期间减少吸烟。它也适用于试图戒烟的孕妇和哺乳期妇女。

NRT 的目的是帮助戒烟者从吸烟向完全戒烟过渡。用 NRT 产品暂时替代从烟草中获得的尼古丁,尽量减少尼古丁戒断症状和吸烟动机,以此实现戒烟。已经戒烟的人如果希望继续使用尼古丁或防止复吸,可以安全地使用 NRT。

NRT 是一种多功能戒烟药物。目前,英国有八种获得许可的 NRT 产品:透皮贴、锭剂(lozenge)、口香糖、舌下片、吸入剂、鼻喷雾、口腔喷雾和口腔贴。

所有产品都是常规销售清单上的药品,可以在柜台购买(英国)。NRT 是为全身吸收而制定的,在贴片的情况下通过皮肤吸收,或其他情况下通过口腔或鼻腔黏膜吸收。这意味着从 NRT 中吸收尼古丁的速度比从香烟中吸入要慢得多,对 NRT 成瘾的风险也更低[6]。

临床疗效

NRT 是研究最多的戒烟药物。有超过 150 个试验,包括 5 万多名吸烟者。与安慰剂相比,以任何形式的 NRT 戒烟率的比值比是 1.84。NRT 合剂(即合并两种类型,例如贴剂联合口腔/鼻腔制剂)比使用单一的 NRT 产品更有效。联合 NRT 产品与单一 NRT 产品戒烟率的比值比为 1.43。NRT 合剂的疗效与伐尼克兰相似,优于安非他酮(表 4.15)[7]。

表 4.15 剂型和剂量

	吸烟少于 20 支/d	吸烟多于 20 支/d,或起床后 30min 内吸烟
外用透皮贴 24h 剂型(21mg、14mg 和 7mg) 16h 剂型(25mg、15mg、10mg)	如果每天吸烟超过 20 支,使用 21mg(24h)或 25mg(16h)贴剂 16h 剂型和 24h 剂型的效果没有区别 16h 贴剂应在就寝时摘除	
鼻喷剂(0.5mg/喷)	想吸烟时,在每个鼻孔里喷一下,每小时不超过 2 次;最多 64 喷/d	

续表

	吸烟少于 20 支/d	吸烟多于 20 支/d,或起床后 30min 内吸烟
口腔黏膜喷雾剂(1mg/喷)	想吸烟时喷 1~2 次;每次不超过 2 喷;每小时不超过 24 喷;最多 64 喷/d	
锭剂(1mg、2mg 和 4mg)	每小时 1mg 以控制吸烟渴求	每小时用 2mg 或 4mg 以控制吸烟渴求,通常每天不超过 15mg
尼古丁口香糖(2mg、4mg 和 6mg)	每小时用一片 2mg 以控制吸烟渴求	每小时用 4mg 或 6mg 以控制吸烟渴求,通常每天不超过 15 片 4mg
吸入剂(15mg)	15mg 规格每天不超过 6 管	
舌下含片(2mg)	每小时用 1~2 片以控制吸烟渴求	每小时用 2 片以控制吸烟渴求,每天不超过 40 片
口胶带(2.5mg)	每小时用一条 2.5mg 以控制吸烟渴求	每小时用 1 条以控制吸烟渴求,每天不超过 15 条

对普通人群吸烟者的研究表明,根据吸烟的频率和强度,每支香烟为吸烟者提供 1~2.9mg 的尼古丁[8]。对精神分裂症患者的研究发现,与没有精神疾病的人相比,他们在更短的时间内更频繁地吸烟,他们从香烟中摄入的尼古丁更多[9]。因此,有理由认为,这些吸烟者可能需要更高剂量的尼古丁替代品。

口服产品中的尼古丁必须通过颊黏膜、牙龈和嘴唇后部来吸收。正确的方法是咀嚼口香糖或吮吸含片,直到味道变浓,然后把它放在颊黏膜和牙龈之间。当味道开始变淡时,建议重复这个过程 20~30min。许多口香糖使用者将口香糖压在(口腔的)牙龈上,以增加接触的表面积,从而提高尼古丁的吸收率。锭剂还能通过舌下吸收尼古丁,但其尺寸通常不允许使用这种方法,除非打成更小的碎片。舌下药片的体积要小得多。

饮用咖啡和碳酸饮料可能会妨碍口服尼古丁产品的吸收[10]。

不良反应

使用 NRT 的不良反应与产品类型有关,包括贴片对皮肤的刺激,以及口服产品对口腔内部的刺激和咳嗽。如果患者仍然吸烟,可能会发生恶心。在治疗早期可能会出现一些睡眠障碍,但是这也是尼古丁戒断的症状。NRT 与精神药物不存在已知的相互作用。

伐尼克兰

伐尼克兰是一种选择性烟碱型乙酰胆碱受体部分激动剂。它模仿尼古丁的作用,在中脑边缘通路中引起多巴胺的持续释放。它还能阻止尼古丁摄入导致的多巴胺释放。这意味着,如果按照处方使用,那么任何尝试吸烟的行为都将在药理学层面上失去意义,也不会让吸烟者感到满足。伐尼克兰适用于年龄超过 18 岁、有戒烟动机的吸烟者。

临床疗效

在最近的 Cochrane 综述中,与安慰剂相比,伐尼克兰持续戒断率的比值比为 2.24。与安非他酮(比值比 1.39)和单剂型 NRT(比值比 1.25)相比,伐尼克兰更有效,与联合剂型 NRT 疗效类似[11,12]。对于大多数合并严重精神疾病的吸烟者而言,与安慰剂相比,伐尼克兰可将戒烟概率提高 4~5 倍[13,14]。

制剂和剂量

吸烟者开始伐尼克兰治疗后,应该在 1~2 周内设定戒烟的目标日期。那些不愿意或不能在 1~2 周内设定目标日期者,可以先开始治疗,然后在 5 周内选择一个戒烟日期。试图戒烟者的治疗程序及剂量方案可参见本章末内容。对于在 12 周后成功戒烟的人,可以考虑再进行 12 周的疗程,每天两次,每次 1mg,以维持戒烟[15]。

不良反应

常见不良反应包括恶心、怪梦、睡眠障碍和头痛,其发生率超过 1/10。伐尼克兰与精神药物不存在已知的药代动力学相互作用。

直到 2016 年,伐尼克兰在英国还带有一个黑色三角形符号,表示需要对有精神健康问题的人进行额外的安全监测。然而,在"全球戒烟研究不良事件评估"(EAGLES)研究发表后,欧洲药品管理局取消了这一规定;该研究发现,与安慰剂或尼古丁贴片相比,不论有无精神障碍史,伐尼克兰和安非他酮均未显著增加神经精神不良事件(包括焦虑、抑郁、攻击行为、精神病和自杀行为)的风险[16]。

安非他酮

安非他酮是一种抗抑郁药,具有多巴胺能和肾上腺素能作用,同时也是烟碱型乙酰胆碱受体的拮抗剂。适用于年龄超过 18 岁、有戒烟动机的吸烟者。

临床疗效

在最近的考克兰综述中,与安慰剂相比,安非他酮戒烟的相对危险度为 1.64[12]。安非他酮与单剂型 NRT 相比疗效类似(*RR* 为 0.99),但其效果不如伐尼克兰(尽管一项研究结果表明二者效果相同[17])以及联合剂型 NRT[7]。在患有严重精神疾病的吸烟者中,安非他酮相比安慰剂,成功戒烟的概率提高了 3~4 倍[13,14]。

制剂和剂量

吸烟者应该在开始安非他酮治疗的前两周设定一个"戒烟日期"。关于试图戒烟者的用药方案,其治疗程序可以在本章末找到。

不良反应

安非他酮禁用于癫痫、进食障碍和酒精依赖者。临床医师应该警惕双相障碍患者的潜在转躁风险(风险很低,但可能发生[18])。常见不良反应包括头晕、味觉变化、肠胃功能紊乱和失眠,为了减少这些反应可以避免睡前用药。与 NRT 和伐尼克兰不同,安非他酮已知与精神药物存在相互作用。它由细胞色素 CYP2B6 代谢。当安非他酮与已知可诱导细胞色素代谢(如卡马西平、苯妥英)或抑制细胞色素代谢(如丙戊酸盐)的药物同时服用时,应当谨慎,因为临床疗效可能受到影响。安非他酮也可抑制 CYP2B6 途径,因此应避免与由该酶代谢的药物(如利培酮和氟哌啶醇)共同服用。

电子烟

电子烟是一种尼古丁输送装置,不含烟草,也不产生烟雾。它们受《欧盟烟草产品指令》管控(即对原料、包装和广告都有控制)。电子烟制造商可向药品和保健产品管理局(MHRA)申请医药许可证。迄今为止,MHRA 只批准了一种电子烟,但制造商没有生产,这意味着在本报告撰写之时,还不能开电子烟处方。英国公共卫生部、英国国民医疗服务体系和护理质量委员会支持精神卫生住院患者使用电子烟和电子烟设备 [19-21]。

临床疗效

在最近关于电子烟戒烟效果的考克兰综述中,使用含有尼古丁的电子烟的人,其戒烟率显著高于那些使用不含尼古丁的电子烟的人(*RR* 为 1.7)或 NRT(*RR* 为 1.69)[22]。自 2013 年以来,它们一直是英国最受欢迎的戒烟方式;据估计,在 2017 年,有 50 700~69 930 名吸烟者用电子烟成功戒烟,否则他们还会继续吸烟 [23]。有少量证据表明,电子烟也能有效地帮助有心理健康问题的人减少吸烟 [24]。

制剂和剂量

在欧洲,一次性预充电子烟液体的容器上都标有每毫升中的尼古丁含量(mg)或每单位体积的百分比重量(w/V)。尼古丁含量范围从零(0%)到最大值 20mg/mL(或 2%)。尼古丁盐(作为电子烟液体的替代品)最近在电子烟用户中很受欢迎;盐具有较低的 pH,可以更顺畅地入喉,一些使用者用户说它提供了一种更类似于吸烟的感觉。此外,尼古丁盐可以在较低的温度下蒸发,使吸入的尼古丁含量更高,这可能有助于从吸烟换为电子烟 [24]。表 4.16 列出了尝试戒烟者的治疗程序,表 4.17 列出了不想戒烟者的治疗程序。

电子烟有多种类型和形状。下面是一些类型的电子烟:

- 一次性产品(通常称为 "cigalikes")
- 可重复使用、可充电的烟具,设计有可更换的药盒或药囊。
- 可重复使用、可充电的烟具,设计由用户填充药液(通常称为烟罐,但现在也有可填充的烟盒)。
- 可重复使用、可充电的烟具,通常被称为 "模组"(可修改的),允许用户定制他们的产品,例如调节从电池到加热元件的功率。

不良反应

口咽刺激、咳嗽、头痛和恶心是使用电子烟最常见的症状,这些症状会随着时间的推移而消退[22]。英国皇家医师学会[4]、英格兰公共卫生部[25]和食品、消费品和环境化学物质毒性委员会[26]建议,对于烟草依赖者和旁观者来说,受监管的电子烟/电子烟具是一种危害小得多的烟草替代品。皇家医师学会认为,长期吸入电子烟造成的危害不太可能超过吸烟造成危害的 5%。同时,吸烟和使用电子烟(双重途径)可能降低不了对健康的有害风险,应该鼓励使用电子烟的人完全戒烟,而从不吸烟的人应该不吸烟,也不要使用电子烟[24,26]。

表 4.16　尝试戒烟者的治疗程序

戒烟的一线药物治疗是**联合剂型的** NRT 或**伐尼克兰**。

所有戒烟的尝试均应得到有经验的烟草依赖治疗医师的支持,至少每周 1 次。

联合剂型 NRT 戒烟	伐尼克兰戒烟
每天吸烟超过 20 支,或起床后 30min 内吸烟者: 开始使用 21mg(24h 贴剂)或 25mg(16h 贴剂),自行选择口服或鼻喷 NRT 产品 继续使用贴剂达 12 周,旨在每 4 周减少 1 次贴剂的用量 当烟瘾来袭时,继续使用口服或鼻喷 NRT 产品 每天吸烟不到 20 支,或起床后 30min 内不吸烟者: 开始使用 14mg(24h 贴剂)或 15mg(16h 贴剂),和一个自行选择的口服或鼻喷 NRT 产品 继续使用贴剂达 12 周,旨在每 4 周减少 1 次贴剂的用量 当烟瘾来袭时,继续使用口服或鼻喷 NRT 产品	在开始伐尼克兰治疗后的 1~2 周内设定一个戒烟目标日期 1~3 天:伐尼克兰 0.5mg,每天 1 次,口服 4~7 天:伐尼克兰 0.5mg,每天 2 次,口服 8~84 天:伐尼克兰 1mg 每天 2 次,口服 对于在最初 12 周伐尼克兰疗程结束后成功戒烟的人,考虑再延长 12 周伐尼克兰 1mg 每天 2 次口服,以持续戒烟

安非他酮可以考虑作为二线治疗使用,或者在吸烟者表示喜欢安非他酮治疗时使用

安非他酮

在开始安非他酮治疗的前两周设定一个"戒烟日期"

1~6 天:安非他酮 150mg,每天 1 次,口服

7~49 天:安非他酮加至 150mg,每天 2 次,口服(两次服药间隔至少 8h)

50~63 天:安非他酮维持 150mg,口服(如果戒烟失败,则停用)

在患有严重精神疾病的吸烟者中,与安慰剂相比,伐尼克兰和安非他酮成功戒烟的概率增加了 4 倍以上。在稳定期精神疾病患者中,也发现 NRT 贴剂成功戒烟的概率是安慰剂的 2 倍。与安慰剂或 NRT 相比,不论吸烟者有无精神疾病,伐尼克兰和安非他酮均未显著增加神经精神科不良事件(包括焦虑、抑郁、攻击行为、精神病和自杀行为)的风险。

当患者尝试戒烟时,监测患者的心理健康总是正确的

希望使用**电子烟**戒烟的人通常应该设定一个戒烟日期,并使用电子烟一次性戒烟,尽快用电子烟代替所有的烟草。他们也可以在几周内逐渐减少烟草用量,增加电子烟的用量,直到完全换成电子烟。和使用 NRT 一样,建议使用者从尼古丁含量较高的电子烟开始

表 4.17　不想戒烟（即暂时戒烟者或只想减少烟量）者的治疗程序

对于不愿意或觉得无法戒烟的人，应该鼓励他们尽量降低对健康的损害，并使用**联合剂型的** NRT 或**电子烟**来替代烟草中的尼古丁。

联合剂型的 NRT	电子烟或电子烟设备
每天吸烟超过 20 支，或起床后 30min 内吸烟者： 开始使用 21mg（24h 贴剂）或 25mg（16h 贴剂），和一个自行选择的口服或鼻喷 NRT 产品 即使患者一开始拒绝，也应继续提供 NRT 产品 当烟瘾来袭时，吸烟者应使用指尖控制 NRT 每天吸烟不到 20 支，或起床后 30min 内不吸烟者： 开始使用 14mg（24h 贴剂）或 15mg（16h 贴剂），和一个自行选择的口服或鼻喷 NRT 产品 即使患者一开始拒绝，也应继续提供 NRT 产品 当烟瘾来袭时，吸烟者应使用指尖控制的 NRT	吸烟者从电子烟中吸取的尼古丁剂量取决于设备、电子烟液的容积、液体中的其他成分、吸入的频率、大小和吸入深度。吸烟者的依赖度越高，建议所用尼古丁的浓度也越高 一个大致的指南是： 每天吸烟 20 支可能每天需要 20mg 尼古丁 当烟瘾来袭时，患者应当有可以使用指尖控制的电子烟。 与 NRT 类似，应鼓励吸烟者在吸烟草期间经常使用电子烟，以延长不吸烟草的间隔时间

　　目前，不可能在 NHS 中开具电子烟处方。从业者应该咨询当地的无烟政策，以确定哪种类型的电子烟允许在精神病住院患者中使用，以及如何获得它们。

参考文献

1. National Institute for Health and Care Excellence. Smoking cessation – acute, maternity and mental health services. Public Health Guidance 48. 2013 (last checked March 2017); http://guidance.nice.org.uk/PH48.
2. National Institute for Health and Clinical Excellence. Stop smoking interventions and services. NICE Guideline [NG92]. 2018; https://www.nice.org.uk/guidance/ng92.
3. National Institute for Health and Care Excellence. Smoking: harm reduction. Public Health Guidance [PH45]. 2013 (last checked March 2017); https://www.nice.org.uk/guidance/ph45.
4. Royal College of Physicians. Nicotine without smoke: tobacco harm reduction. A report by the Tobacco Advisory Group of the Royal College of Physicians. 2016; https://www.rcplondon.ac.uk/projects/outputs/nicotine-without-smoke-tobacco-harm-reduction-0.
5. Tidey JW, et al. Smoking cessation and reduction in people with chronic mental illness. *BMJ* 2015; 351:h4065.
6. Hajek P, et al. Dependence potential of nicotine replacement treatments: effects of product type, patient characteristics, and cost to user. *Prev Med* 2007; 44:230–234.
7. Cahill K, et al. Pharmacological interventions for smoking cessation: an overview and network meta-analysis. *Cochrane Database Syst Rev* 2013; Cd009329.
8. Henningfield JE, et al. Pharmacotherapy for nicotine dependence. *CA Cancer J Clin* 2005; 55:281–299; quiz 322–283, 325.
9. Williams JM, et al. Increased nicotine and cotinine levels in smokers with schizophrenia and schizoaffective disorder is not a metabolic effect. *Schizophr Res* 2005; 79:323–335.
10. Henningfield JE, et al. Drinking coffee and carbonated beverages blocks absorption of nicotine from nicotine polacrilex gum. *JAMA* 1990; 264:1560–1564.
11. Cahill K, et al. Nicotine receptor partial agonists for smoking cessation. *Cochrane Database Syst Rev* 2016; Cd006103.
12. Howes S, et al. Antidepressants for smoking cessation. *Cochrane Database Syst Rev* 2020; 4:Cd000031.
13. Roberts E, et al. Efficacy and tolerability of pharmacotherapy for smoking cessation in adults with serious mental illness: a systematic review and network meta-analysis. *Addiction* 2016; 111:599–612.
14. Siskind DJ, et al. Pharmacological interventions for smoking cessation among people with schizophrenia spectrum disorders: a systematic review, meta-analysis, and network meta-analysis. *Lancet Psychiatry* 2020; 7:762–774.
15. Hajek P, et al. Varenicline in prevention of relapse to smoking: effect of quit pattern on response to extended treatment. *Addiction* 2009; 104:1597–1602.
16. Anthenelli RM, et al. Neuropsychiatric safety and efficacy of varenicline, bupropion, and nicotine patch in smokers with and without psychiatric disorders (EAGLES): a double-blind, randomised, placebo-controlled clinical trial. *Lancet* 2016; 387:2507–2520.
17. Benli AR, et al. A comparison of the efficacy of varenicline and bupropion and an evaluation of the effect of the medications in the context of the smoking cessation programme. *Tob Induc Dis* 2017; 15:10.
18. Giasson-Gariepy K, et al. A case of hypomania during nicotine cessation treatment with bupropion. *Addict Sci Clin Pract* 2013; 8:22.
19. Care Quality Commission. Brief guide: the use of 'blanket restrictions' in mental health wards. 2020; https://www.cqc.org.uk/sites/default/

files/20191125_900767_briefguide-blanket_restrictions_mental_health_wards_v3.pdf.

20. Health and Social Care. Using electronic cigarettes in NHS mental health organisations. 2020; https://www.gov.uk/government/publications/e-cigarettes-use-by-patients-in-nhs-mental-health-organisations/using-electronic-cigarettes-in-nhs-mental-health-organisations.

21. NHS England. Long Term Plan. 2020; https://www.longtermplan.nhs.uk/wp-content/uploads/2019/08/nhs-long-term-plan-version-1.2.pdf.

22. Hartmann-Boyce J, et al. Electronic cigarettes for smoking cessation. *Cochrane Database Syst Rev* 2020; 10:Cd010216.

23. Beard E, et al. Association of prevalence of electronic cigarette use with smoking cessation and cigarette consumption in England: a time-series analysis between 2006 and 2017. *Addiction* 2020; 115:961–974.

24. McNeill A, et al. *Vaping in England: an evidence update including mental health and pregnancy, March 2020: a report commissioned by Public Health England*. London: Public Health England. 2020; https://assets.publishing.service.gov.uk/government/uploads/system/uploads/attachment_data/file/869401/Vaping_in_England_evidence_update_March_2020.pdf.

25. McNeill A, et al. *Evidence review of ecigarettes and heated tobacco products 2018. A report commissioned by Public Health England*. London: Public Health England. 2018; https://assets.publishing.service.gov.uk/government/uploads/system/uploads/attachment_data/file/684963/Evidence_review_of_e-cigarettes_and_heated_tobacco_products_2018.pdf.

26. Committee on Toxicity of Chemicals in Food Consumer Products and the Environment (COT). Statement on the potential toxicological risks from electronic nicotine (and non-nicotine) delivery systems (E(N)NDS – e-cigarettes). 2020; https://cot.food.gov.uk/sites/default/files/2020-09/COT%20E%28N%29NDS%20statement%202020-04.pdf.

兴奋剂依赖的药物治疗

经常被滥用的兴奋剂包括可卡因（盐酸盐或游离碱）、硫酸苯丙胺和盐酸甲基苯丙胺。使用方式通常为粉末吸入（如盐酸可卡因、硫酸苯丙胺）、烟雾吸入（可卡因碱）或注射。兴奋剂的使用、滥用和依赖在世界上大部分地区都比较普遍。它们可以被单独使用，也可以与其他药物一起使用，如海洛因和强效可卡因、粉状可卡因和酒，或者甲基苯丙胺和 GBL[1]。

在兴奋剂滥用和依赖的治疗中，目前已评估了多种药物的药理学作用。尽管一些药物已经显示出了初步前景，但迄今为止还没有发现任何有益的研究证据[2,3]。对许多人来说，除了提供最小化伤害的建议和心理教育之外，兴奋剂的使用是自限性的。对于那些与酒精、海洛因或 GBL 联合使用的患者，对合并的物质依赖进行有效干预可能会减少兴奋剂的使用。研究表明，对于那些依赖兴奋剂的人来说，结合意外事件管理的方法疗效最大。对许多人来说，戒断的途径是通过互助和同伴支持，比如可卡因匿名戒毒会、冰毒匿名戒毒会或理性康复会。关于有效治疗可卡因依赖的更多信息可在英国临床指南中找到[1]。

可卡因

脱毒

戒断症状包括抑郁情绪、激越和失眠，通常是自限性的。由于可卡因具有半衰期短和间断性大量使用的特点，很多患者实际上常用不借助药物进行自我脱毒。短期使用镇静催眠药可部分缓解症状，但这些药物本身就可能成为依赖的物质[1]。

替代治疗

很少有证据表明替代治疗对可卡因滥用有效，因此通常不应使用[1-3]。

苯丙胺类

被滥用苯丙胺类物质有许多种类，包括"街头"苯丙胺、甲基苯丙胺和药用的右苯丙胺。所有该类药物都存在滥用潜力。

脱毒

戒断综合征在依赖者中十分常见。治疗应着眼于缓解症状，尽管苯丙胺的许多戒断症状（情绪低落、精神萎靡、乏力等）持续时间较短，且用药物治疗不一定有效。失眠可短期使用催眠药治疗，但应警惕对其产生依赖的风险[1-3]。

维持治疗

不宜使用右苯丙胺（或其他兴奋剂）进行苯丙胺依赖的维持治疗，因其有效性证据不足[1]。

持续使用右苯丙胺的患者

在英国，仍有一些患者多年来一直使用右苯丙胺作为药物依赖的维持治疗。在理想情况下,这些患者应该在几个月内逐渐脱毒。然而,对一些人来说,强制脱毒的后果可能比继续使用右苯丙胺更糟糕。在这种情况下,可能最好的决定是继续开药。只有成瘾专家才能决定是否继续给患者开右苯丙胺[1]。

多种物质滥用

对于同时依赖阿片类物质和可卡因的患者,使用美沙酮或丁丙诺啡作为阿片依赖的有效替代治疗,也可减少可卡因使用[3]。

兴奋剂相关精神疾病

甲基苯丙胺相关的精神病性症状与其使用频率和依赖的严重程度有关[4]。在大多数情况下,精神病性症状可以随着中毒症状的消失而消失,即持续 1 天左右的时间。在紧急情况下,大多数近期服用过甲基苯丙胺且存在急性精神病性症状的患者,可以通过简单的镇静治疗来控制病情[5]。例如,在激越时,可根据需要每 4~6h 用地西泮 5~10mg,以及治疗性质的休息。然而,有些患者可能需要更严格的治疗,请参阅第 2 章。

值得注意的是,在使用兴奋剂的情况下,精神病性症状随着兴奋剂的持续使用而逐渐加重;他们往往在每次大量吸食时更早出现,持续的时间也更长。平均 25% 的患者报告在使用甲基苯丙胺 1 个月后还有症状[6]。中毒时的精神病性症状与被害妄想和幻触有关,而更长期的甲基苯丙胺相关精神病的特征是被害妄想和幻听,大多很难与原发性精神病区分[6]。在急诊科,很难做出明确的诊断。最初被诊断为甲基苯丙胺所致精神病的患者中,16%~38% 后来被诊断为精神分裂症[6]。

在兴奋剂或 GBL 等多种药物合用较普遍的地区的急诊室,对于甲基苯丙胺使用者表现出的激越性精神病,另一个重要的鉴别诊断是 GBL 戒断性谵妄。兴奋剂中毒(自主神经过敏、激越、幻觉)和 GBL 戒断性谵妄之间有症状的重叠。后者需要更高剂量的苯二氮䓬类药物和更长的治疗时间(见本章 "GHB 和 GBL 依赖")。

如前所述,在紧急情况下,最初使用苯二氮䓬类药物进行简单的镇静通常就足够了。如果需要使用抗精神病药,使用甲基苯丙胺的患者出现锥体外系不良反应的概率会增加 4 倍,这一点应得到重视[7]。应该使用引起锥体外系不良反应倾向低的药物,有证据表明奥氮平有较好的疗效。阿立哌唑可能是快速镇静的首选药物,因为奥氮平和苯二氮䓬类药物不应合用。不应使用氟哌啶醇。对于是否需要继续用药,早期和持续评估至关重要,因为大多数患者的症状在 2~3 周内就会消失,并且没有证据支持在甲基苯丙胺相关精神病中可以预防性地使用抗精神病药[8]。

兴奋剂相关抑郁

一些患者在兴奋剂戒断早期可出现明显的快感缺乏。许多患者的这种情绪低落会随着戒断时间延长和支持性心理社会干预而消失[1]。对于症状持续存在者,心理治疗有效,但是由于存在管理体制方面的问题,成瘾患者很难获得心理治疗服务。

抗抑郁药的评估主要是将其作为物质依赖的治疗药物,其次才是将其作为抑郁的治疗药物。一些证据(主要是关于三环类抗抑郁药的)表明,抗抑郁药可以减轻抑郁症状[10]。然而,由于三环类抗抑郁药的心脏毒性,不推荐将其用于共病的药物滥用者[11]。没有证据支持

SSRI 类药物的临床使用,事实上它们与兴奋剂存在显著的相互作用,且伴有治疗脱落率升高的风险[9]。

参考文献

1. Department of Health and Social Care. Drug misuse and dependence: UK guidelines on clinical management. 2017; https://www.gov.uk/government/publications/drug-misuse-and-dependence-uk-guidelines-on-clinical-management.

2. Siefried KJ, et al. Pharmacological treatment of methamphetamine/amphetamine dependence: a systematic review. *CNS Drugs* 2020; 1–29.

3. Ronsley C, et al. Treatment of stimulant use disorder: a systematic review of reviews. *PloS One* 2020; 15:e0234809.

4. Arunogiri S, et al. A systematic review of risk factors for methamphetamine-associated psychosis. *Aust N Z J Psychiatry* 2018; 52:514–529.

5. Isoardi KZ, et al. Methamphetamine presentations to an emergency department: management and complications. *Emerg Med Aust* 2019; 31:593–599.

6. Voce A, et al. A systematic review of the symptom profile and course of methamphetamine-associated psychosis: substance use and misuse. *Subst Use Misuse* 2019; 54:549–559.

7. Temmingh HS, et al. Methamphetamine use and antipsychotic-related extrapyramidal side-effects in patients with psychotic disorders. *J Dual Diag* 2020; 16:208–217.

8. Shoptaw SJ, et al. Treatment for amphetamine psychosis. *Cochrane Database Syst Rev* 2009; CD003026.

9. Farrell M, et al. Responding to global stimulant use: challenges and opportunities. *The Lancet* 2019; 394:1652–1667.

10. Pani PP, et al. Antidepressants for cocaine dependence and problematic cocaine use. *Cochrane Database Syst Rev* 2011.

11. Lingford-Hughes AR, et al. BAP updated guidelines: evidence-based guidelines for the pharmacological management of substance abuse, harmful use, addiction and comorbidity: recommendations from BAP. *J Psychopharmacol* 2012; 26:899–952.

第 4 章

γ-羟基丁酸和 γ-丁内酯依赖

γ-羟基丁酸(GHB)和 γ-丁内酯(GBL)使用较少,但临床上很重要,因为依赖者停用会很快进展到激越性谵妄,进而危及生命。并发症包括癫痫发作、心动过缓、心搏骤停和肾衰竭。急诊室和精神科病房的医师应该能够识别并处理急性戒断症状。

GHB 和 GBL(GHB 的前体药物)在口语中经常被称为"G"。它们主要通过对 GABA-B 受体的作用来减少焦虑,产生脱抑制和镇静作用。这些药物用于娱乐社交,偶尔也用于帮助睡眠。在男性之间的性行为中,它们通常与兴奋剂(甲氧麻黄酮和甲基苯丙胺晶体等)合用,在潜在高风险的性行为("化学性行为")中促进性行为。依赖很少见,但在依赖者中戒断症状发生快,可产生严重的谵妄,伴有妄想和危及生命的并发症[1]。

戒断综合征 [1,2]

依赖者会"24h"使用药物(每隔 1~3h 或更频繁)。戒断症状通常在最后一次使用后几个小时内出现。戒断综合征类似于酒精戒断,可能包括心动过速、失眠、焦虑、出汗和细微震颤等症状[1]。若不治疗,可发展为激越性谵妄,通常伴有精神病性症状(包括妄想和幻觉),随后出现严重的震颤、肌强直和癫痫发作[1]。肌强直严重可引起发热、横纹肌溶解和急性肾功能衰竭。停药 4~6 天后,为了控制症状而对药物的需求会减轻,但是有的患者戒断症状持续时间更长。

戒断管理

脱瘾治疗的证据基础有限。戒断管理的核心原则是早期治疗,从而防止发展为谵妄和其他并发症。谵妄一旦产生,很难控制[3]。早期需要使用苯二氮䓬类药物治疗,使用巴氯酚(GABA-B 受体激动剂)和苯巴比妥作为辅助药物也有效[1,4]。巴氯酚在网上很容易获得,使用者可在没有监督的情况下将其用于戒断[5];这在戒药过程中存在危险,应该明确劝阻。

GHB 戒药也获得成功,方法是每 3h 减量 1 次,持续 2 周[6]。药用 GHB 管理戒断可能比苯二氮䓬类药物更有效[7]。

现有的酒精戒断量表不太可能有助于评估戒断的严重程度。关于 GHB/GBL 撤药管理的最新指导意见(英国),建议向国家毒物管理信息服务(NPIS)寻求信息,特别是其 24h 电话服务和毒物信息数据库 TOXBASE®。

临床医师应该熟悉两种情况:药物依赖者计划外的急性戒药和有计划的戒药(表 4.18 和表 4.19)。

表 4.18　急性非计划性戒断的处理

场所	■ 急性突发性戒断是一种紧急医疗情况,应在急性住院环境下进行处理 ■ 严重的戒断可能需要进入重症监护病房
初始药物治疗	■ 当观察到早期戒断症状时,开始使用地西泮 20mg 口服 ■ 地西泮可每 30min 至 4h 重复服用 1 次,直到症状消失 ■ 大多数 GBL 戒断的病例在最初 24h 内需要 60~80mg 地西泮 ■ 可能需要更高的每天剂量,最高可达地西泮 300mg 口服 ■ 如果患者嗜睡,暂停地西泮,并复核诊断 ■ 一对一的护理可能有助于重症者的管理 ■ 根据需要使用氟马西尼逆转作用
辅助药物治疗	■ 在苯二氮䓬类药物疗效不足的情况下,采用巴氯酚 10mg,每天 3 次口服联合苯二氮䓬类药物的戒断方案 ■ 在持续焦虑和烦躁的情况下,可加到巴氯酚 20mg,每天 3 次,口服 ■ 在严重戒断情况下,可考虑加苯巴比妥,剂量为 150~450mg/d,静脉滴注(仅限 ICU) ■ 在严重戒断反应仍无法控制的情况下,可能需要静脉麻醉,如异丙酚(仅限 ICU)。硫喷妥钠 * 也用于严重而难治的戒断综合征 [8]

　* 苯巴比妥、硫喷妥钠和异丙酚的呼吸抑制作用不可逆转,应配备机械通气设施。

表 4.19　计划性选择性戒断的处理

场所	■ 所有的计划戒断均应在医学监督下进行 ■ 社区门诊脱毒只有在没有谵妄或精神病史的情况下方可尝试。需要有第三者在身边观察及支持戒断过程。如果症状没有得到很好的控制,应该选择将患者送到住院部
戒断前	■ 与患者和其支持者讨论治疗计划 ■ 鼓励患者保持记录 1 周 GBL 使用的日记,包括使用剂量、频率和数量 ■ 在选择性戒断前,鼓励患者停用"顶级"药物,如甲氧麻黄酮和甲基苯丙胺 ■ 在目标停药日期前 3~7 天开始服用巴氯酚 10mg,每天 3 次,口服 ■ 鼓励患者将 GBL 剂量减少到可耐受的程度,做法是每 1~2 天将每次剂量减少 0.1mL,或者增加用药间隔时间
戒断期	■ 计划性门诊戒药的第 1 天,让患者完全停用 GBL 至少 2h,并建议他们处理掉手中剩余的 GBL ■ 第 1 天建议患者在诊所观察 4h,戒断期间不能驾驶机动车,禁止饮酒或服用其他镇静剂 ■ 增加巴氯酚至 20mg,每天 3 次,口服 ■ 一旦出现心动过速、手心出汗、细小震颤、焦虑等戒断症状和体征,开始苯二氮䓬类药物治疗。首次给予地西泮 20mg,2h 后复查,监测焦虑/镇静/呼吸抑制。如有必要,再次予地西泮最多 20mg,口服 ■ 末次使用 GBL 6h 后,可再给予患者最多 40mg 地西泮,然后,在接下来的 2 天进行观察 ■ 每天复查地西泮剂量,并根据症状加量。超过 7 天很少再需要地西泮。初始剂量通常为 40~60mg/d
戒断后	■ 停用苯二氮䓬类药物后,继续予巴氯酚 20mg,每天 3 次 口服,持续 4~6 周。相关少数试验中有一项试验每天成功使用 45~60mg 剂量,持续 3 个月 [9] ■ 戒断后,持续焦虑和失眠是常见的,且复发风险高。在开始选择性戒断治疗前,应制订治疗计划,对患者进行至少 4 周的随访和支持,将复发风险降到最低

参考文献

1. Kamal RM, et al. Pharmacological treatment in gamma-hydroxybutyrate (GHB) and gamma-butyrolactone (GBL) Dependence: detoxification and relapse prevention. *CNS Drugs* 2017; 31:51–64.

2. Bell J, et al. Gamma-butyrolactone (GBL) dependence and withdrawal. *Addiction* 2011; 106:442–447.

3. Novel Psychoactive Treatment UK Network (NEPTUNE). Guidance on the clinical management of acute and chronic harms of club drugs and novel psychoactive substances. 2015; http://neptune-clinical-guidance.co.uk/wp-content/uploads/2015/03/NEPTUNE-Guidance-March-2015.pdf.

4. LeTourneau JL, et al. Baclofen and gamma-hydroxybutyrate withdrawal. *Neurocrit Care* 2008; 8:430–433.

5. Floyd CN, et al. Baclofen in gamma-hydroxybutyrate withdrawal: patterns of use and online availability. *Eur J Clin Pharmacol* 2018; 74:349–356.

6. Dijkstra BA, et al. Detoxification with titration and tapering in gamma-hydroxybutyrate (GHB) dependent patients: the Dutch GHB monitor project. *Drug Alcohol Depend* 2017; 170:164–173.

7. Beurmanjer H, et al. Tapering with pharmaceutical GHB or benzodiazepines for detoxification in GHB-dependent patients: a matched-subject observational study of treatment-as-usual in Belgium and the Netherlands. *CNS Drugs* 2020; 34:651–659.

8. Vos CF, et al. Successful treatment of severe, treatment resistant GHB withdrawal through thiopental-coma. *Subst Abus* 2020; 1–6.

9. Beurmanjer H, et al. Baclofen to prevent relapse in gamma-hydroxybutyrate (GHB)-dependent patients: a multicentre, open-label, non-randomized, controlled trial. *CNS Drugs* 2018; 32:437–442.

苯二氮䓬类药物滥用

在20世纪60—70年代,苯二氮䓬类药物的处方量增加,主要是因为它们的安全性相对于巴比妥类药物有所提高。然而,人们很快注意到苯二氮䓬类药物极有可能导致依赖。最初用于治疗其他疾病的处方往往会持续很长时间,并导致依赖。无论过去还是现在,在老年患者和焦虑症或抑郁症患者中均很常见。在英国,苯二氮䓬类的处方从2015—2016年的1 630万降至2018—2019年的1 490万张。

有一些新型或"设计"的苯二氮䓬类药物(例如依替唑仑、氟哌唑仑、氟硝唑仑和诺氟地西泮)。目前,有关这些物质对健康和社会危害的信息有限,但它们可能与现有的苯二氮䓬类药物相似,甚至更严重[1]。其中一些苯二氮䓬类药物(氟哌唑仑、氟硝唑仑和诺氟地西泮)在英国被列管为1类,而处方苯二氮䓬类药物被列管为3类或4类。除处方外,苯二氮䓬类药物还可通过非法市场、挪用处方和互联网等方式购买(据悉这是一个上升趋势)[2]。

苯二氮䓬类药物依赖被认为是医源性(多年来每天使用低剂量)或非医源性(大剂量、非法获得、间断性使用)。

停药

此前发表的考克兰综述(现已撤稿)评估了对单一苯二氮䓬类药物依赖进行药物干预的证据,结论是逐步减少苯二氮䓬类的剂量比突然停用更佳[3]。最近的一篇综述证实,对大多数患者来说,6个月以内的戒断时间较合适[4],英国药物滥用和依赖指南建议每两周减少约1/8的剂量[5]。澳大利亚全科医师指南评论其"缺乏最佳减药速度的证据","确切的减药速度应该根据药物、剂量和治疗时间进行个体化设定"[6]。

一项荟萃分析指出了针对老年患者减少苯二氮䓬类使用的综合干预(通常包括心理干预/支持)的有效性[7]。一项随机对照试验表明,基于自我效能理论单纯使用教育法,即使约1/4的长期苯二氮䓬类使用者自愿减量或停止使用[8]。2018年考克兰综述发现,没有任何附加药物可以帮助停药过程。有些药物似乎表现出一些有益的效果,但证据质量太差,无法提出任何临床建议[9]。

许多接受成瘾治疗的患者除主要的滥用物质外,可能还使用非法苯二氮䓬类药物。患有非医源性苯二氮䓬类药物依赖的人每天服用的剂量往往超过100mg地西泮。尽管一些治疗机构会开具苯二氮䓬类药物处方,但并没有证据表明苯二氮䓬类药物替代治疗最终会减少苯二氮䓬类药物滥用。若开具苯二氮䓬类药物处方,应该最后是短期的、有时限性的(2~3周)处方,并以脱毒为目的。

如果患者已经服用苯二氮䓬类药物很长时间,最好改用等效的地西泮,因为它的作用时间更长,产生戒断症状的可能性更小。苯二氮䓬类药物依赖作为多物质依赖的组成部分,也应该采取逐步停药来治疗。每天超过与30mg地西泮等效的苯二氮䓬类药物可能会造成伤害[5],因此应尽量避免(此剂量在医源性依赖中很少见[10])。包括意外事故管理(contingency management)在内的心理社会干预在减少苯二氮䓬类药物的使用方面取得了一些效果。一篇考克兰综述发现,有证据支持认知行为治疗(CBT)结合BZD逐渐减量治疗的短期疗效。目前尚无证据支持动机性访谈(MI)的临床应用。此外,最新证据表明,简要干预如结构化咨询和家庭医师写的个性化信件,值得进一步研究[11]。

妊娠和苯二氮䓬类药物滥用

苯二氮䓬类药物并非主要人类致畸原,但在计划妊娠前最好逐渐停用。使用苯二氮
类药物的女性一旦妊娠,应尽量在短时间内停药,注意戒断性癫痫发作及对孕妇和胎儿的潜
在风险。需权衡利弊并咨询专家(见第 7 章)。在减少剂量之前,建议所有依赖苯二氮䓬类
药物的女性换用地西泮以稳定病情[5]。

小结

- 苯二氮䓬类药物应以每两周减约 1/8 剂量的速度戒断。
- 停药通常应在 6 个月内完成。
- 在停药前改用等效地西泮是很常见的。
- 苯二氮䓬类药物滥用常见于多种物质滥用,阿片类药物可能是主要的依赖药物。

医源性依赖的标准地西泮戒断方案

基线	30mg/d
第 2 周	25mg/d
第 4 周	20mg/d
第 6 周	18mg/d
第 8 周	16mg/d
第 10 周	14mg/d
第 12 周	12mg/d
第 14 周	10mg/d

此后,如果可以耐受,每两周减少 2mg/d。

参考文献

1. Advisory Council on the Misuse of Drugs (ACMD). *A review of the evidence of use and harms of Novel Benzodiazepines*. London: Home Office. 2020; https://assets.publishing.service.gov.uk/government/uploads/system/uploads/attachment_data/file/881969/ACMD_report_-_a_review_of_the_evidence_of_use_and_harms_of_novel_benzodiazepines.pdf.
2. Manchester KR, et al. The emergence of new psychoactive substance (NPS) benzodiazepines: A review. *Drug Test Anal* 2018; 10:392–393.
3. Denis C, et al. Pharmacological interventions for benzodiazepine mono-dependence management in outpatient settings. *Cochrane Database Syst Rev* 2006; CD005194.
4. Lader M, et al. Withdrawing benzodiazepines in primary care. *CNS Drugs* 2009; 23:19–34.
5. Department of Health (DoH). *Drug misuse and dependence: UK guidelines on clinical management*. London: Department of Health. 2017; https://assets.publishing.service.gov.uk/government/uploads/system/uploads/attachment_data/file/673978/clinical_guidelines_2017.pdf.
6. Royal Australian College of General Practitioners (RACGP). Prescribing drugs of dependence in general practice, Part B – benzodiazepines. Melbourne, Australia. 2015; https://www.racgp.org.au/FSDEDEV/media/documents/Clinical%20Resources/Guidelines/Drugs%20of%20dependence/Prescribing-drugs-of-dependence-in-general-practice-Part-B-Benzodiazepines.pdf.
7. Gould RL, et al. Interventions for reducing benzodiazepine use in older people: meta-analysis of randomised controlled trials. *Br J Psychiatry* 2014; 204:98–107.
8. Tannenbaum C, et al. Reduction of inappropriate benzodiazepine prescriptions among older adults through direct patient education: the EMPOWER cluster randomized trial. *JAMA Inter Med* 2014; 174:890–898.
9. Baandrup L, et al. Pharmacological interventions for benzodiazepine discontinuation in chronic benzodiazepine users. *Cochrane Database Syst Rev* 2018; 3:Cd011481.

10. Vicens C, et al. Comparative efficacy of two interventions to discontinue long-term benzodiazepine use: cluster randomised controlled trial in primary care. *Br J Psychiatry* 2014; 204:471–479.

11. Darker CD, et al. Psychosocial interventions for benzodiazepine harmful use, abuse or dependence. *Cochrane Database Syst Rev* 2015; Cd009652.

合成大麻素受体激动剂

合成大麻素受体激动剂(SCRA)的临床重要性在于有急性毒性(潜在的生命威胁),与精神病相关,以及有依赖性。在急诊科、精神科和成瘾服务机构工作的医生应该能够识别和处理合成大麻素急性中毒。

SCRA 是一组结构多样、作为大麻素受体 CB1 受体激动剂的化学物质。其命名复杂,大量的化学结构难以分类[1]。经常出现新型的 SCRA 类别[2]。

在英国,SCRA 使用者主要是无家可归者和囚犯等弱势群体。然而,最近的尸检毒理学证据表明,其大多数后代生活在稳定的住所,使用 SCRA 是多物质使用模式的一部分[3]。

最常见的情况是把 SCRA 溶解在酒精中,喷洒在植物材料上,然后烟熏。在一个草药包中可能含有一种以上的SCRA化合物,在撰写本书时,SCRA 有 700 多个俗称,最常见的是"香料(spice)"和"K2"[4]。尽管许多患者最近使用了 SCRA,但他们可能并不承认[5]。与大麻的主要精神活性成分四氢大麻酚(THC)相比,SCRA 对 CB1 受体的作用更强、持久。它们也有不同的非 CB1 的反应,这可能会影响其临床效应[6]。

急性中毒不同于四氢大麻酚中毒,比四氢大麻酚中毒更严重,可出现致命的躯体损害[7,8]。在英国,与 SCRA 相关的死亡人数正在上升,尽管绝大多数人摄入了多种物质[3];相反,全球报告的 SCRA 相关死亡中,通常只是使用 SCRA[9]。

英国 SCRA 死亡情况:

- 因心脏或呼吸骤停引起突然摔倒
- 大多数没有目击者
- 多数发生在既往无躯体健康问题者
- 超过 40% 死后检测出阿片类药物

SCRA 与心脏毒性有关,至少有一些可诱发 Q-T 间期延长[10]。因此,应当为使用 SCRA 的人做心电图检查,特别是那些处方美沙酮的人。有一个案例报道,使用纳洛酮成功抢救了 SCRA 过量,有人猜测这可能与阿片类和大麻素系统相互作用有关[11]。

据估计,需要急救的风险比大麻高出 30 倍[12]。SCRA 中毒后可导致持续性精神病。约 15% 的服用者报告有依赖症状和类似于大麻戒断的戒断综合征。

急性 SCRA 中毒

急性 SCRA 中毒需要根据临床表现加以识别,因为 SCRA 的结构多样,在紧急情况下不可能做尿液药物检测[13]。实验室检测可能会有帮助,但不可能在有临床意义的时间内给出结果。基于急诊的系列病例报告,SCRA 中毒的特征详见表 4.20[5,7,8,14]。具体表现和发生率差异很大,这可能反映出其化学结构的多样性。最常见的症状是激越、恶心和心动过速。中毒通常是短暂的,78% 患者 8h 内症状消退[5]。通常会促发精神病发作,看急诊的急性中毒患者中,41% 出现精神病性症状[14]。

表 4.20 急性 SCRA 中毒的特征

对系统的影响		
	心血管系统	心动过速
		高血压
		心动过缓
		低血压
		胸痛——可诱发心肌缺血
		心搏骤停
	消化系统和腹部器官	恶心
		呕吐——经常是大量呕吐
		腹痛
		肝毒性
		急性肾损伤——急性肾小管坏死和急性间质肾炎
	神经系统	激越
		焦虑
		攻击性
		意识模糊
		精神病性症状——中毒后会持续存在
		癫痫发作
		昏迷
		紧张性姿势
	其他	结膜充血
		横纹肌溶解

急性 SCRA 中毒的处理

- 患者应该在适当的机构中进行治疗。
- 心电图监测,以发现心肌缺血和心律失常。
- 血化验:血气分析、尿素氮、电解质、肌酸激酶和肝功能。
- 用苯二氮䓬类药物进行支持治疗。
- 静脉补液、吸氧和止吐药。
- 很少使用抗精神病药或麻醉剂。

令人欣慰的是,在 SCRA 中毒中使用抗精神病药或苯二氮䓬类均与心血管不良反应无关,抗精神病药与癫痫发作发生率增加亦无关 [15]。

SCRA 相关精神病的管理

精神病性症状是 SCRA 中毒的常见表现,在 30% 患者中急性中毒期后仍持续存在 [16]。SCRA 相关精神病:

- 阳性症状比大麻相关精神病更突出。
- 阴性症状比大麻相关精神病更不明显。

- 不太可能有躁狂表现。
- 通常伴有自杀想法。
- 可能需要在精神科住院，以治疗行为障碍。
- 需要比大麻相关精神病更高剂量的抗精神病药（平均剂量相当于 11mg 氟哌啶醇，而大麻使用者的平均剂量为 6mg/d，而无共病者为 3mg/d）[17]。
- 需要比大麻相关的精神病治疗更长时间。

关于 SCRA 引起的急性行为紊乱（ABD）的治疗，请见本章"急性行为（ABD）的急性住院"。

SCRA 依赖与戒断的治疗

SCRA 的依赖性在病例研究和调查中都有报道，鉴于 SCRA 的作用更强，估计 SCRA 依赖的发生率高于大麻。建议使用动机访谈技术和药物日记对 SCRA 依赖进行一般心理社会治疗，逐渐减少对 SCRA 的依赖。应慎用低效应（因而有害性更低）的大麻替代治疗方案，因相关研究显示大麻并不减轻 SCRA 的戒断[18]，而且患者完全了解二者在法律上的意义不同，即持久大麻是犯罪行为，而持有大多数 SCRA 并不违法。

持续数月每天使用者会出现生理戒断综合征，包括：

- 睡眠紊乱
- 怪梦
- 不安
- 焦虑
- 渴求
- 寒战
- 肌肉抽搐
- 心率和血压升高

据报道，苯二氮䓬类药物治疗结果不一致。对苯二氮䓬类治疗无效的病例，低剂量喹硫平（50mg）有效[19]。

参考文献

1. Potts AJ, et al. Synthetic cannabinoid receptor agonists: classification and nomenclature. *Clin Toxicol (Phila)* 2020; 58:82–98.
2. Alam RM, et al. Adding more 'spice' to the pot: A review of the chemistry and pharmacology of newly emerging heterocyclic synthetic cannabinoid receptor agonists. *Drug Test Anal* 2020; 12:297–315.
3. Yoganathan P, et al. Synthetic cannabinoid-related deaths in England, 2012–2019. *OSF* 2020.
4. European Monitoring Centre for Drugs and Drug Addiction. Synthetic cannabinoids. 2020; https://www.emcdda.europa.eu/topics/synthetic-cannabinoids_en.
5. Abouchedid R, et al. Analytical confirmation of synthetic cannabinoids in a cohort of 179 presentations with acute recreational drug toxicity to an Emergency Department in London, UK in the first half of 2015. *Clin Toxicol (Phila)* 2017; 55:338–345.
6. Fattore L. Synthetic cannabinoids – further evidence supporting the relationship between cannabinoids and psychosis. *Biol Psychiatry* 2016; 79:539–548.
7. Tait RJ, et al. A systematic review of adverse events arising from the use of synthetic cannabinoids and their associated treatment. *Clin Toxicol (Phila)* 2016; 54:1–13.
8. Hoyte CO, et al. A characterization of synthetic cannabinoid exposures reported to the National Poison Data System in 2010. *Ann Emerg Med* 2012; 60:435–438.
9. Giorgetti A, et al. Post-mortem toxicology: a systematic review of death cases involving synthetic cannabinoid receptor agonists. *Front Psychiatry* 2020; 11:464.
10. Hancox JC, et al. Synthetic cannabinoids and potential cardiac arrhythmia risk: an important message for drug users. *Ther Adv Drug Saf* 2020; 11:2042098620913416.
11. Jones JD, et al. Can naloxone be used to treat synthetic cannabinoid overdose? *Biol Psychiatry* 2017; 81:e51–e52.

12. Winstock A, et al. Risk of emergency medical treatment following consumption of cannabis or synthetic cannabinoids in a large global sample. *J Psychopharmacol* 2015; 29:698–703.

13. Novel Psychoactive Treatment UK Network (NEPTUNE). Guidance on the clinical management of acute and chronic harms of club drugs and novel psychoactive substances 2015; http://neptune-clinical-guidance.co.uk/wp-content/uploads/2015/03/NEPTUNE-Guidance-March-2015.pdf.

14. Monte AA, et al. Characteristics and treatment of patients with clinical illness due to synthetic cannabinoid inhalation reported by medical toxicologists: a toxic database study. *J Med Toxicol* 2017; 13:146–152.

15. Gurney SM, et al. Pharmacology, toxicology, and adverse effects of synthetic cannabinoid drugs. *Forensic Sci Rev* 2014; 26:53–78.

16. Hobbs M, et al. Spicing it up – synthetic cannabinoid receptor agonists and psychosis - a systematic review. *Eur Neuropsychopharmacol* 2018; 28:1289–1304.

17. Bassir Nia A, et al. Psychiatric comorbidity associated with synthetic cannabinoid use compared to cannabis. *J Psychopharmacol* 2016; 30:1321–1330.

18. Nacca N, et al. The synthetic cannabinoid withdrawal syndrome. *J Addict Med* 2013; 7:296–298.

19. Castaneto MS, et al. Synthetic cannabinoids: epidemiology, pharmacodynamics, and clinical implications. *Drug Alcohol Depend* 2014; 144:12–41.

第 4 章

药物诱发急性行为障碍的急性住院

药物诱发急性行为障碍（drug-induced acute behavioural disturbance, ABD）或"激越性谵妄"是一种识别率低、可能致死的综合征，包括谵妄、攻击行为和生理反应失调[1]。使用非法药物是最常见的原因，尤其是可卡因和新型兴奋剂（NPS），包括合成大麻素（"香料"）和麻黄碱等兴奋剂。物质戒断和躯体原因也可以产生 ABD[2]。

本节的目的是提醒人们注意，当非法物质的急性作用导致患者行为对自己或他人构成危险时，需要采取的措施。"急性行为障碍"与"激越性谵妄"这两个术语均颇具争议，也都不是公认的诊断。本节中使用这些术语，并不意味着它们可能包含预期的病程及处境。具体来说，不一定发生躯体情况恶化，而且躯体情况恶化与急性使用非法物质本身所致的行为改变并无必然联系，也不一定会导致使用这些物质。早期干预和降阶治疗（de-escalation）是有效和安全治疗的关键。应尽可能地避免物理约束，因为这种约束对患者的生命存在很大的危险。

病理生理学

谵妄导致定向障碍和"战斗或逃跑（fight or flight）"反应，而试图"逃跑"时，体力消耗会导致体温升高和儿茶酚胺释放[3]。体温过高会导致横纹肌溶解（肌酸激酶升高）[4]，并使谵妄恶化[5]。交感神经兴奋时儿茶酚胺过量可延长心脏 Q-T 间期，并可致心源性晕厥[6]。过度的肌肉活动、升高的儿茶酚胺、高温和脱水，会导致代谢性酸中毒和二氧化碳的产生，出现呼吸急促，预示即将发生心血管系统衰竭。

识别

并不存在特征性症状，但一项前瞻性研究发现，最常见的症状是暴力行为、对疼痛的耐受性增强和持续活动[7]。呼吸急促、不知疲倦、高热和可触及的体温升高是经常被报道的表现[8]。

管理

好言相劝，并努力保证患者和他人的环境安全——常规用于谵妄患者的定向力提示可能会有所帮助。**尽量减少身体接触**，并要意识到约束可能会加剧高温和儿茶酚胺释放，使结果恶化[9]。镇静对于缓解攻击行为、减少持续性发热和儿茶酚胺释放非常重要。有证据支持肌内注射的药物有：苯二氮䓬类药物（包括地西泮、劳拉西泮、咪达唑仑）[10]、抗精神病药（包括氟哌啶醇、氟哌利多、奥氮平和氯丙嗪）[10,11] 以及二者联合使用[12]。需要警惕神经阻滞剂可能导致恶性综合征的风险。

确保安全情况下记录脉搏、血压和体温。尿检筛查通常对新型兴奋剂的效果有限，但许多临床实验室检测可识别致病化合物。在患者镇静下来之前，可能无法进行心电图检查。需要救护车将患者转到急诊室（ED）进行全面评估与治疗[13]。可能需要精神科护理来保护和支持患者。在急诊科，氯胺酮肌内注射是首选的镇静剂，在 2~4mg/kg 的剂量范围内[14]，因有量效关系可预测其效果。退热剂是无效的降温剂，可能需要冷却静脉输液、水喷雾和全身冰敷等物理降温。

结果

死亡率不详,仅有的数据来源是不科学的观察报道[15]。有时会忽略或没有考虑到与新型兴奋剂使用相关的躯体情况恶化。死亡风险与发热的持续时间及最高体温相关:温度超过 42℃通常提示预后很差。体重指数 >25kg/m^2 与预后较差相关。在非致命性情况下,大多数病例病程较短,48h 内可完全恢复,但可发生心脏、肾脏和肝脏的长期损害。

参考文献

1. Tracy DK, et al. Acute behavioural disturbance: a physical emergency psychiatrists need to understand. *B J Psych Advances* 2020:1–10

2. Kennedy DB, et al. Delayed in-custody death involving excited delirium. *J Correct Health Care* 2018; 24:43–51.

3. Bunai Y, et al. Fatal hyperthermia associated with excited delirium during an arrest. *Leg Med (Tokyo)* 2008; 10:306–309.

4. Borek HA, et al. Hyperthermia and multiorgan failure after abuse of 'bath salts' containing 3,4-methylenedioxypyrovalerone. *Ann Emerg Med* 2012; 60:103–105.

5. Otahbachi M, et al. Excited delirium, restraints, and unexpected death: a review of pathogenesis. *Am J Forensic Med Pathol* 2010; 31:107–112.

6. Wittstein IS, et al. Neurohumoral features of myocardial stunning due to sudden emotional stress. *N Engl J Med* 2005; 352:539–548.

7. Hall CA, et al. Frequency of signs of excited delirium syndrome in subjects undergoing police use of force: descriptive evaluation of a prospective, consecutive cohort. *J Forensic Leg Med* 2013; 20:102–107.

8. Baldwin S, et al. Distinguishing features of excited delirium syndrome in non-fatal use of force encounters. *J Forensic Leg Med* 2016; 41:21–27.

9. Stratton SJ, et al. Factors associated with sudden death of individuals requiring restraint for excited delirium. *Am J Emerg Med* 2001; 19:187–191.

10. Isbister GK, et al. Randomized controlled trial of intramuscular droperidol versus midazolam for violence and acute behavioral disturbance: the DORM study. *Ann Emerg Med* 2010; 56:392–401 e391.

11. Page CB, et al. A prospective study of the safety and effectiveness of droperidol in children for prehospital acute behavioral disturbance. *Prehosp Emerg Care* 2019; 23:519–526.

12. O'Connor N, et al. Pharmacological management of acute severe behavioural disturbance: a survey of current protocols. *Aust Psychiatry* 2017; 25:395–398.

13. Wetli CV, et al. Cocaine-associated agitated delirium and the neuroleptic malignant syndrome. *Am J Emerg Med* 1996; 14:425–428.

14. Li M, et al. Evaluation of ketamine for excited delirium syndrome in the adult emergency department. *J Emerg Med* 2019.

15. Baldwin S, et al. Excited delirium syndrome (ExDS): situational factors and risks to officer safety in non-fatal use of force encounters. *Int J Law Psychiatry* 2018; 60:26–34.

"街头非法药物"和处方精神药物的相互作用

"街头非法药物"和精神药物之间的潜在相互作用很常见,尤其是因为这类患者开精神药物处方的比例很高[1]。目前,尚缺乏系统研究,资料多来源于个案报道或理论推测。重要相互作用的概要见表 4.21。

对滥用街头非法药物的所有患者:

- 乙型和丙型病毒性肝炎感染常见。相关肝功能损害可能导致对其他药物的代谢能力下降,对不良反应的敏感性增加。
- HIV 感染常见[2,3]。抗反转录病毒药可能与许多处方和非处方药发生药代动力学相互作用[4]。例如,利托那韦可以减少摇头丸的代谢,促发中毒;许多抗反转录病毒药物可增加或减少美沙酮代谢[5]。
- 处方药可能像非法药物那样使用(即不规律且不按医嘱使用)。不应给门诊患者提供大量处方药物。
- 在美沙酮或其他阿片受体激动剂过量致死病例中,有呼吸抑制作用的药物之间存在叠加或协同作用是重要原因[6]。给予镇静剂(如苯二氮䓬类)时应谨慎。

表 4.21　"街头非法药物"与精神药物的相互作用

一般注意事项	大麻	海洛因/美沙酮[6]	可卡因、苯丙胺、摇头丸、MDA、6-APD	酒精	氯胺酮[7]
一般注意事项	■ 常将香烟吸入(诱导 CYP1A2) ■ 可镇静 ■ 剂量相关心动过速 ■ THC/CBD 抑制 CYP3A4、CYP2C19 和 CYP2D6[8,9]	■ 可致镇静/呼吸抑制 ■ 美沙酮也与 Q-T 同期延长相关(见本章"美沙酮")	■ 兴奋剂(可卡因高剂量可镇静) ■ 可能心律不齐 ■ 可卡因可致大脑/心脏缺血,可能致死 ■ MDMA(3,4-亚甲基二氧甲基苯丙胺抑制 CYP 2D6/3A4 ■ 摇头丸可致高热/脱水[10]	■ 镇静 ■ 肝脏损害可能 ■ 诱导多种酶	■ 镇静易导致意识丧失 ■ 鼻喷或静脉注射很快起效
第一代抗精神病药	■ 抗精神病药通过阻断多巴胺受体降低几乎所有滥用药物的精神作用(多巴胺是与"奖赏"相关的神经递质,如氟哌啶醇和 MDMA[11])	■ 服用抗精神病药的患者为了代偿,可能会增加非法物质的摄入 ■ 服用摇头丸的患者更易发生锥体外系反应 ■ 至少起始阶段避免使用有心脏毒性或镇静作用很强的抗精神药的风险[12] ■ 使用甲氧基二苯丙胺可增加氟哌啶醇使锥体外系反应(舒必利是相对安全的首选药物)			
第二代抗精神病药	■ 可增加镇静 ■ 大麻烟可诱导 CYP1A2,降低奥氮平和氯氮平的血药浓度[13] ■ 氯氮平可减少大麻和酒精摄入[14] ■ THC/CBD 对 CYP1A2 的抑制是未知的	■ 可增加镇静 ■ 有利培酮促发美沙酮戒断反应的个案报道[15] ■ 少数报道显示氯氮平增加美沙酮水平,尤其是肝脏 CYP2D6 代谢缓慢患者[16]	■ 抗精神病药可减少渴求及可卡因所致欣快[17-21] ■ 奥氮平可加重可卡因依赖[22] ■ 氯氮平可增加可卡因水平,但降低主观反应[23]	■ 增加奥氮平(及其他 β 受体阻滞剂)所致高血压的风险	■ 增加镇定
抗抑郁药	■ 有心动过速报道(监测脉搏,注意三环类抗抑郁药)[24] ■ 复杂且无法预测的 CYP 诱导(烟草)和 CYP 抑制(THC/CBD)作用	■ 避免镇静作用强的抗抑郁药 ■ 有些 SSRI 可增加美沙酮血浆水平[25](可选西酞普兰,但要注意可轻度增加 Q-T 同期延长的风险) ■ 舍曲林和美沙酮合用于缓和医疗患者时,有发生 5-羟色胺综合征的个案报道[26]	■ 避免镇静作用强的抗抑郁药(心律失常风险) ■ 禁用单胺氧化酶抑制剂类(高血压) ■ 吗氯贝丙胺和 MDMA 合用可能致命[27] ■ SSRI 类抗抑郁药可增加 MDMA 的血药浓度[28],但降低主观反应[29] ■ SSRI 类药物(尤其是氟西汀)有升高可卡因水平的风险[30] ■ SSRI 类抗抑郁药,阿立哌唑和其他兴奋性药(尤其是 MDA 和 6-APD)合用可促发 5-羟色胺综合征[31,32] ■ SSRI 类可增强对卡因的主观反应[33]	■ 避免镇静作用强的抗抑郁药 ■ 避免使用过量时有毒的抗抑郁药 ■ 损害精神运动技能(非 SSRI)	■ CYP3A4 抑制剂(例如氟西汀/帕罗西汀)会延长氯胺酮的半衰期 ■ 注意 SNRI 和瑞波西汀所致的高血压

续表

	大麻	海洛因/美沙酮[6]	可卡因、苯丙胺、摇头丸、MDA、6-APD	酒精	氯胺酮[7]
抗胆碱能药物	■ 可能滥用。尽可能避免使用(必须使用抗精神病药时,可选用第二代抗精神病药) ■ 可导致幻觉,情感高涨及认知损害				
锂盐	■ 不规律使用时毒性很大 ■ 时刻考虑到脱水的影响(尤其在合并酒精或摇头丸时)				
卡马西平/丙戊酸钠	■ CBZ 可通过诱导 CYP3A4 降低 THC 浓度[34]	■ 卡马西平(CBZ)降低美沙酮水平(突然停用卡马西平有危险)[35] ■ 丙戊酸钠发生药物相互作用可能性低	■ 卡马西平诱导 CYP 3A4,导致更快地形成去甲可卡因(比可卡因的心脏和肝脏毒性更大)[36]	■ 肝功能检测	■ CBZ 通过诱导 CYP3A4 降低氯胺酮血药浓度
苯二氮䓬类药物	■ 监测镇静水平	■ 过度镇静(可能有呼吸抑制) ■ 合用可导致意外过量 ■ 可能有药代动力学相互作用(增加美沙酮水平)	■ 过度镇静(使用高剂量可卡因时) ■ 可卡因中毒后使用较普遍 ■ 脱毒后将来有滥用可能	■ 可能过度镇静(和呼吸抑制) ■ 广泛用于波酒	■ 可能过度镇静(和呼吸抑制)

注:6-APD,6-(2-氨基丙基)苯并呋喃或 1-苯并呋喃-6-基丙-2-胺;CBZ,卡马西平;MDA,3,4-亚甲基二氧苯丙胺;SSRI,选择性 5-羟色胺再摄取抑制剂。

第 4 章

参考文献

1. Zapelini Do Nascimento D, et al. Potential psychotropic drug interactions among drug-dependent people. *J Psychoactive Drugs* 2020; 1–9.

2. Vocci FJ, et al. Medication development for addictive disorders: the state of the science. *Am J Psychiatry* 2005; 162:1432–1440.

3. Tsuang J, et al. Pharmacological treatment of patients with schizophrenia and substance abuse disorders. *Addict Disord Their Treatment* 2005; 4:127–137.

4. Bracchi M, et al. Increasing use of 'party drugs' in people living with HIV on antiretrovirals: a concern for patient safety. *AIDS* 2015; 29:1585–1592.

5. Gruber VA, et al. Methadone, buprenorphine, and street drug interactions with antiretroviral medications. *Curr HIV/AIDS Rep* 2010; 7:152–160.

6. Department of Health and Social Care. Drug misuse and dependence: UK guidelines on clinical management. 2017; https://www.gov.uk/government/publications/drug-misuse-and-dependence-uk-guidelines-on-clinical-management.

7. Pfizer Limited. Summary of product characteristics. Ketalar 10 mg/ml Injection. 2020; https://www.medicines.org.uk/emc/medicine/12939.

8. Arellano AL, et al. Neuropsychiatric and general interactions of natural and synthetic cannabinoids with drugs of abuse and medicines. *CNS Neurol Disord Drug Targets* 2017; 16:554–566.

9. Abbott KL, et al. Adverse pharmacokinetic interactions between illicit substances and clinical drugs. *Drug Metab Rev* 2020; 52:44–65.

10. Gowing LR, et al. The health effects of ecstasy: a literature review. *Drug Alcohol Rev* 2002; 21:53–63.

11. Liechti ME, et al. Acute psychological and physiological effects of MDMA ("Ecstasy") after haloperidol pretreatment in healthy humans. *Eur Neuropsychopharmacol* 2000; 10:289–295.

12. Matthew BJ, et al. Drug-induced parkinsonism following chronic methamphetamine use by a patient on haloperidol decanoate. *Int J Psychiatry Med* 2015; 50:405–411.

13. Zullino DF, et al. Tobacco and cannabis smoking cessation can lead to intoxication with clozapine or olanzapine. *Int Clin Psychopharmacol* 2002; 17:141–143.

14. Green AI, et al. Alcohol and cannabis use in schizophrenia: effects of clozapine vs. risperidone. *Schizophr Res* 2003; 60:81–85.

15. Wines JD, Jr., et al. Opioid withdrawal during risperidone treatment. *J Clin Psychopharmacol* 1999; 19:265–267.

16. Uehlinger C, et al. Increased (R)-methadone plasma concentrations by quetiapine in cytochrome P450s and ABCB1 genotyped patients. *J Clin Psychopharmacol* 2007; 27:273–278.

17. Poling J, et al. Risperidone for substance dependent psychotic patients. *Addict Disord Treat* 2005; 4:1–3.

18. Albanese MJ, et al. Risperidone in cocaine-dependent patients with comorbid psychiatric disorders. *J Psychiatr Pract* 2006; 12:306–311.

19. Sattar SP, et al. Potential benefits of quetiapine in the treatment of substance dependence disorders. *J Psychiatry Neurosci* 2004; 29:452–457.

20. Grabowski J, et al. Risperidone for the treatment of cocaine dependence: randomized, double-blind trial. *J Clin Psychopharmacol* 2000; 20:305–310.

21. Kishi T, et al. Antipsychotics for cocaine or psychostimulant dependence: systematic review and meta-analysis of randomized, placebo-controlled trials. *J Clin Psychiatry* 2013; 74:e1169–e1180.

22. Kampman KM, et al. A pilot trial of olanzapine for the treatment of cocaine dependence. *Drug Alcohol Depend* 2003; 70:265–273.

23. Farren CK, et al. Significant interaction between clozapine and cocaine in cocaine addicts. *Drug Alcohol Depend* 2000; 59:153–163.

24. Benowitz NL, et al. Effects of delta-9-tetrahydrocannabinol on drug distribution and metabolism. Antipyrine, pentobarbital, and ethanol. *Clin Pharmacol Ther* 1977; 22:259–268.

25. Hemeryck A, et al. Selective serotonin reuptake inhibitors and cytochrome P-450 mediated drug-drug interactions: an update. *Curr Drug Metabol* 2002; 3:13–37.

26. Bush E, et al. A case of serotonin syndrome and mutism associated with methadone. *J Palliat Med* 2006; 9:1257–1259.

27. Vuori E, et al. Death following ingestion of MDMA (ecstasy) and moclobemide. *Addiction* 2003; 98:365–368.

28. Rietjens SJ, et al. Pharmacokinetics and pharmacodynamics of 3,4-methylenedioxymethamphetamine (MDMA): interindividual differences due to polymorphisms and drug-drug interactions. *Crit Rev Toxicol* 2012; 42:854–876.

29. Papaseit E, et al. MDMA interactions with pharmaceuticals and drugs of abuse. *Expert Opin Drug Metab Toxicol* 2020; 16:357–369.

30. Fletcher PJ, et al. Fluoxetine, but not sertraline or citalopram, potentiates the locomotor stimulant effect of cocaine: possible pharmacokinetic effects. *Psychopharmacology* 2004; 174:406–413.

31. Silins E, et al. Qualitative review of serotonin syndrome, ecstasy (MDMA) and the use of other serotonergic substances: hierarchy of risk. *Aust N Z J Psychiatry* 2007; 41:649–655.

32. Kotwal A, et al. Serotonin syndrome in the setting of lamotrigine, aripiprazole, and cocaine use. *Case Rep Med* 2015; 2015:769531.

33. Soto PL, et al. Citalopram enhances cocaine's subjective effects in rats. *Behav Pharmacol* 2009; 20:759–762.

34. GW Pharma Ltd. Summary of product characteristics. Sativex oromucosal spray. 2020; https://www.medicines.org.uk/emc/product/602.

35. Miller BL, et al. Neuropsychiatric effects of cocaine: SPECT measurements. in A Paredes, Gorelick, eds. Cocaine: physiological and physiopathological effects. 1st edition. New York: Haworth Press 1993; 47–58.

36. Roldan CJ, et al. Toxicity, cocaine. 2004. http://www.emedicine.com/med/topic400.htm.

药物滥用：总结

在许多精神科病房、门诊和医师办公室,尿液毒品筛查是常规检测。必须注意各种非法药物的检测时间窗有限,以及导致尿检假阳性的其他物质或药物的使用情况。有些假阳性很难预测(即与化学相似性无关),例如使用氨磺必利的患者可出现丁丙诺啡假阳性结果[1]。使用现场免疫测试盒时易出现假阳性。如果尿检阳性事关患者的人身自由,且患者否认使用过非法药物,应将第二份样本送实验室,用液相色谱和质谱(LC-MS)进行最终测试。药物滥用的基本情况总结见表 4.22。

表 4.22　药物滥用的基本情况总结

药物	躯体症状/中毒症状	最常见精神状态改变[2]	戒断症状	戒断持续时间	尿检时限[3,4]	可致尿检假阳性结果的其他物质[5-7]
安非他明类兴奋剂[8]	心动过速 血压升高 厌食 颤动 坐立不安	幻视/幻触/幻嗅/幻听 偏执 情感高涨	疲劳 饥饿 抑郁 易激惹 渴求 社交退缩	7~34h 达到高峰；最长持续 5 天	取决于半衰期，大多 48~72h	止咳剂和减充血剂 安非他酮 氯噻 氯丙嗪 拉贝洛尔 异丙嗪 雷尼替丁 司来吉兰 大量酪胺 反苯环丙胺 曲唑酮等多种物质 去甲文拉法辛可导致苯环己哌啶检测结果为阳性[9]
GHB/GBL		社交增强自信	震颤心动 过速 偏执 谵妄 精神病 幻视/幻触/幻嗅/幻听	3~4 天	难以检测，不常规筛查	未知 通常（且可信）用 LC-MS 检测[10]
苯二氮䓬类	镇静 脱抑制	放松 幻视 定向障碍 睡眠紊乱	焦虑 失眠 谵妄 癫痫发作 幻视/幻触/幻嗅/幻听 精神病	通常持续时间较短，但也有持续数周至数月者	最长 28 天，取决于所服药物的半衰期	奈福泮 舍曲林 佐匹克隆 依非韦伦

续表

药物	躯体症状/中毒症状	最常见精神状态改变[2]	戒断症状	戒断持续时间	尿检时限[3,4]	可致尿检阳性结果的其他物质[5-7]
大麻[11-17]	心动过速 协调障碍 红眼 直立性低血压	情感高涨 精神病 视物变形 记忆/判断障碍 患精神分裂症风险增加 2 倍	坐立不安 易激惹 失眠 焦虑	不确定；可能少于 1 个月 (重度依赖者可更长)	单次使用：3 天；长期大量使用：长达 30 天	被动"吸入"大麻 依非韦伦 布洛芬 萘普生
合成大麻素受体激动剂 (SCRA)	心动过速 高血压 眼睛红肿 激越	焦虑 烦躁 攻击行为 精神病性症状 意识模糊	焦虑 失眠 头痛	未知	由于化学成分不同，使用常规筛选方法难以检测	对于尿液筛检而言，化学成分过于多样化，例如 AB-fubinaca, ADB-fubinaca, AB-chminaca, 3-甲基丁酸，DB-chminaca 和 5-氟-PB-22 都被归类为 SCRA LC-MS 的检测效果最好[18]
可卡因	心动过速 呼吸急促 血压增高 头痛 呼吸抑制 胸痛	欣快 偏执狂 精神病 惊恐发作 焦虑 失眠 激动	疲劳 饥饿 抑郁 易怒 渴求 社交退缩	12~18h	长达 96h	含有古柯叶的食物/茶 可待因 麻黄碱/伪麻黄碱
海洛因	针尖样瞳孔 皮肤湿冷 呼吸抑制	困倦 欣快 幻觉	瞳孔散大 恶心 腹泻 全身疼痛 鸡皮疙瘩 流涕 流泪	36~72h 达到高峰	长达 72h	苯甲酸乙酯 纳曲酮 纳洛酮 阿片类镇痛药 含罂粟籽食物 苯海拉明 4-喹诺酮类 曲马多
美沙酮	针尖样瞳孔 呼吸抑制 肺水肿	同上	同上，症状较轻，持续时间较长	4~6 天达到高峰，可持续 6 周	长期使用长达 7 天	喹硫平

第 4 章

续表

药物[19-22]	躯体症状/中毒症状	最常见精神状态改变[2]	戒断症状	戒断持续时间	尿检时限[3,4]	可致尿检假阳性结果的其他物质[5-7]
氯胺酮	心率增快 血压升高 心悸 头晕 腹部不适 下尿路症状 共济失调	意识受损 分离 幻觉 自我同一性'扩'散	疲劳 食欲不振 嗜睡 渴求 焦虑 烦躁 不安 心悸 震颤 出汗	48h	氯胺酮—最长 2 天 去甲氯胺酮—最长 14 天	喹硫平
致幻剂(LSD)[23]	表现多样 瞳孔扩大 血压和心率中度升高 脸红 出汗 唾液分泌增加 腱反射亢进	欣快、内省、错觉、假性幻觉、时间感改变、思维过程改变、对身体的感知改变、对重要记忆的生动回忆	无	不适用	最长 14 天	氨溴索 阿米替林 溴苯那敏 安非他酮 丁螺环酮 头孢霉素 氯丙嗪 地西帕明 地尔硫草 多塞平 麦角新碱 芬太尼 氟西汀 氯哌啶醇 丙米嗪 拉贝洛尔 麦普替林 哌甲酯 甲氧氯普胺 丙氯拉嗪 利培酮 舍曲林 硫利达嗪 曲唑酮 维拉帕米

注:此表为基本总结。

关于尿检中物质交叉反应的更多细节,可参见 Moeller 的文献[24]。

GHB,γ-羟基丁酸;GBL,γ-丁内酯。

参考文献

1. Couchman L, et al. Amisulpride and sulpiride interfere in the C&DIA DAU buprenorphine test. *Ann Clin Psychiatry* 2008; 45 Suppl 1.
2. Truven Health Analytics. Micromedex 2.0. 2017; https://www.micromedexsolutions.com/home/dispatch.
3. Substance Abuse and Mental Health Services Administration (US). Substance abuse: clinical issues in intensive outpatient treatment. Treatment Improvement Protocol (TIP) Series, No. 47. 2006.
4. Mayo Medical Laboratories. Approximate Detection Times. 2016; http://www.mayomedicallaboratories.com/test-info/drug-book/viewall. html.
5. Brahm NC, et al. Commonly prescribed medications and potential false-positive urine drug screens. *Am J Health Syst Pharm* 2010; 67:1344–1350.
6. Saitman A, et al. False-positive interferences of common urine drug screen immunoassays: a review. *J Anal Toxicol* 2014; **38**:387–396.
7. Liu CH, et al. False positive ketamine urine immunoassay screen result induced by quetiapine: A case report. *J Formos Med Assoc* 2017; **116**:720–722.
8. Shoptaw SJ, et al. Treatment for amphetamine psychosis. *Cochrane Database Syst Rev* 2009; CD003026.
9. Farley TM, et al. False-positive phencyclidine (PCP) on urine drug screen attributed to desvenlafaxine (Pristiq) use. *BMJ Case Rep* 2017; 2017:bcr-2017-222106.
10. Busardò FP, et al. Ultra-high performance liquid chromatography tandem mass spectrometry (UHPLC-MS/MS) for determination of GHB, precursors and metabolites in different specimens: application to clinical and forensic cases. *J Pharm Biomed Anal* 2017; **137**:123–131.
11. Johns A. Psychiatric effects of cannabis. *Br J Psychiatry* 2001; **178**:116–122.
12. Hall W, et al. Long-term cannabis use and mental health. *Br J Psychiatry* 1997; **171**:107–108.
13. Murray RM, et al. Traditional marijuana, high-potency cannabis and synthetic cannabinoids: increasing risk for psychosis. *World Psychiatry* 2016; **15**:195–204.
14. Marconi A, et al. Meta-analysis of the association between the level of cannabis use and risk of psychosis. *Schizophr Bull* 2016; **42**:1262–1269.
15. Arseneault L, et al. Causal association between cannabis and psychosis: examination of the evidence. *Br J Psychiatry* 2004; **184**:110–117.
16. Budney AJ, et al. Review of the validity and significance of cannabis withdrawal syndrome. *Am J Psychiatry* 2004; **161**:1967–1977.
17. Bonnet U, et al. The cannabis withdrawal syndrome: current insights. *Subst Abuse Rehabil* 2017; **8**:9–37.
18. Tebo C, et al. Suspected synthetic cannabinoid receptor agonist intoxication: does analysis of samples reflect the presence of suspected agents? *Am J Emerg Med* 2019; **37**:1846–1849.
19. Novel Psychoactive Treatment UK Network (NEPTUNE). Guidance on the clinical management of acute and chronic harms of club drugs and novel psychoactive substances. 2015; http://neptune-clinical-guidance.co.uk/wp-content/uploads/2015/03/NEPTUNE-Guidance-March-2015.pdf.
20. Chen WY, et al. Gender differences in subjective discontinuation symptoms associated with ketamine use. *Subst Abuse Treatment Prev Policy* 2014; **9**:39.
21. Critchlow DG. A case of ketamine dependence with discontinuation symptoms. *Addiction* 2006; **101**:1212–1213.
22. Adamowicz P, et al. Urinary excretion rates of ketamine and norketamine following therapeutic ketamine administration: method and detection window considerations. *J Anal Toxicol* 2005; **29**:376–382.
23. Passie T, et al. The pharmacology of lysergic acid diethylamide: a review. *CNS Neurosci Ther* 2008; **14**:295–314.
24. Moeller KE, et al. Clinical interpretation of urine drug tests: what clinicians need to know about urine drug screens. *Mayo Clin Proc* 2017; **92**:774–796.

妊娠期的药物滥用 [1]

妊娠期间药物滥用会产生许多不良影响,包括低出生体重儿、早产 [2]、各种新生儿戒断综合征,以及后代一系列发育、情绪和行为问题 [3]。

酒精

众所周知,妊娠期间饮酒会对后代产生深远的影响。应鼓励滥用酒精的孕妇停止饮酒,并用苯二氮䓬类药物治疗戒断症状,最好住院治疗 [4]。

并没有证据表明阿坎酸、双硫仑和纳曲酮在妊娠期的使用是安全的,但是未接受治疗的个体复饮风险更高,相比之下人们更喜欢合用它们(也可见本章"酒依赖")。

烟草

应该鼓励患者完全停止吸烟,因为继续吸烟会增加流产、早产和死胎的风险 [5]。电子烟可作为首选,但其安全性尚未确定。NICE 推荐使用 NRT [6],不推荐安非他酮和伐尼克林。

阿片类药物(见本章"阿片类药物依赖")

妊娠期间使用阿片类药物可能不会直接致畸,但经常使用者中发生新生儿戒断综合征的风险超过 70% [7]。

使用处方美沙酮或丁丙诺啡,要好于滥用非法阿片类药物,因为这提供了减量治疗的可能性,并降低了与非法使用物质相关的危害性。即使不能减少剂量,使用这些替代药物也可以降低早产的风险。

在妊娠晚期,可能因为分布容积增加,对美沙酮的需求量也会增加。越来越多的证据表明,使用丁丙诺啡产生的新生儿戒断综合征比美沙酮程度轻 [8,9]。

大多数专家建议,孕妇一般情况下不应尝试停用阿片类药物 [4,10]。一般应鼓励正在接受稳定阿片类药物替代治疗的妇女进行母乳喂养,并在几周后谨慎地断奶。

大麻和合成大麻素受体激动剂

妊娠期间使用大麻与妊娠和后代的一系列不良后果有关 [11]。应该鼓励停止使用。目前,没有可用的药物治疗方法。

苯二氮䓬类药物

苯二氮䓬类药物在妊娠期的安全性尚不明确(见第 7 章)。众所周知,妊娠晚期使用苯二氮䓬类药物会导致婴儿软瘫综合征。

大多数指南 [3,9] 建议使用地西泮等长效药物慢慢停用苯二氮䓬类药物,并考虑让患者住院接受戒断治疗。

兴奋剂

使用可卡因和安非他明与一系列先天性畸形、早产和低出生体重有关。然而,尚无有效的药物治疗,脱毒是主要目标,可让患者住院接受治疗[4]。

(司昱琪 译　赵敏 校　田成华 审校)

参考文献

1. Wilson CA, et al. Alcohol, smoking, and other substance use in the perinatal period. *BMJ* 2020; **369**:m1627–m1627.

2. Mayet S, et al. Drugs and pregnancy – outcomes of women engaged with a specialist perinatal outreach addictions service. *Drug Alcohol Rev* 2008; **27**:497–503.

3. Kaltenbach K, et al. Neonatal abstinence syndrome, pharmacotherapy and developmental outcome. *Neurobehav Toxicol Teratol* 1986; **8**:353–355.

4. World Health Organisation. WHO guidelines approved by the guidelines review committee. Guidelines for the identification and management of substance use and substance use disorders in pregnancy. Geneva. 2014.

5. Cohen A, et al. Substance misuse in pregnancy. *Obstetr Gynaecol Reprod Med* 2017; **27**:316–321.

6. National Institute for Clinical Excellence. Pregnancy and complex social factors: a model for service provision for pregnant women with complex social factors. Clinical guideline [CG110]. 2010 (last checked August 2018); https://www.nice.org.uk/Guidance/CG110.

7. Winklbaur B, et al. Treating pregnant women dependent on opioids is not the same as treating pregnancy and opioid dependence: a knowledge synthesis for better treatment for women and neonates. *Addiction* 2008; **103**:1429–1440.

8. Jones HE, et al. Maternal Opioid Treatment: Human Experimental Research (MOTHER)–approach, issues and lessons learned. *Addiction* 2012; **107** Suppl 1:28–35.

9. U.S. Department of Health & Human Services. Substance Abuse and Mental Health Services Administration (SAMHSA). 2020; https://www.samhsa.gov.

10. McAllister-Williams RH, et al. British Association for Psychopharmacology consensus guidance on the use of psychotropic medication preconception, in pregnancy and postpartum 2017. *J Psychopharmacol* 2017; **31**:519–552.

11. Jansson LM, et al. Perinatal marijuana use and the developing child. *JAMA* 2018; **320**:545–546.

特殊患者的药物治疗

第5章

儿童与青少年

儿童与青少年用药原则

- **针对症状而不是诊断**。对儿童来说,诊断可能很困难,且共病很常见。治疗应该针对关键症状。尽管一个明确的诊断有利于做出对疾病的预期,也有助于同父母和患者沟通,但应该牢记,疾病的发展演变需要时间。

- **儿童用药的技术层面**。1968年的医药法案以及欧洲立法规定,医师可以"超适应证"或"超说明书"使用药物,或者使用未被批准的药物。但是,医师在使用某种药物之前,应当负责任地确保有足够的信息,来支持该药物的质量、疗效、安全性和预期用途。在儿科实践中,在知情同意的情况下使用未经批准的药物,或者将已经批准的药物用于未批准的用途(即"超说明书"使用)经常是必要的。

  - 英国的处方书写:为12岁以下儿童开具仅凭处方的药物时,法律要求必须注明年龄,但是最好在所有儿童处方中都注明年龄。

- **小剂量开始,缓慢加量,并监测疗效和不良反应**。在门诊实践中,药物剂量按每千克体重每天的毫克数计算,儿童患者的起始剂量通常小于成年人。根据需要逐渐增加剂量,最终剂量应当能充分缓解症状,并能将不良反应控制到最低(不良反应在儿童和青少年中更为常见)。在常规的临床护理中,定期监测疗效和不良反应至关重要,以确保继续治疗是必要的。

- **重病患者往往需要多种药物治疗**。单药治疗是最理想的。但是,儿童期起病的疾病可能很严重,因此可能需要将心理社会治疗方法与一种以上药物合用。联合用药是针对不同的疾病或症状使用不同的药物,多重用药是使用多种药物来处理同一病症。儿童常有多种共病,因此联合用药很常见。

- **足疗程治疗**。儿童的疾病通常比成年人严重,通常需要治疗更长时间才能起效。对需要住院治疗的抑郁症或者精神分裂症患者而言,充分的治疗可能需要8周。

- **如果有可能,一次只调整一种药物**。在可能的情况下,一次只调整一种药物,并在添加新药物时尝试撤掉一种药物。

- **多个情境下监测治疗结局**。需要牢记,在对症治疗时(比如使用兴奋剂治疗注意缺陷多动障碍),在不同情境中(比如家庭和学校),疾病的表现可能不同。根据父母报告增加的药物剂量,相对于白天在学校的情景而言可能就过高了。

- **对患者和家庭进行用药教育是必要的**。对于一些儿童和青少年精神障碍患者,药物治疗可能需要维持终身。因此,对于长期的治疗结局和治疗依从性来说,最初的用药体验非常关键。应针对具体问题、药物治疗、不良反应和药物依从性进行教育。在治疗方案发生改变时,应当鼓励患者及其监护人对此进行问询。

扩展阅读

For detailed description of prescribing and adverse effects of CNS Drugs in Children and Adolescents, see:

British Medical Association et al. *British National Formulary for Children 2020/2021* (September 2020). London: Pharmaceutical Press; 2020.

Elbe D, et al. *Clinical Handbook of Psychotropic Drugs for Children and Adolescents.* 4th revised edn. Oxford, UK: Hogrefe Publishing; 2019.

Gerlach M, et al. *Psychiatric Drugs in Children and Adolescents. Basic Pharmacology and Practical Applications.* Vienna: Springer-Verlag Wien; 2014.

Martin A, et al. *Pediatric Psychopharmacology: Principles and Practice.* Second Edition. New York, USA: Oxford University Press; 2011.

儿童与青少年抑郁症

诊断问题

大约 15% 的儿童和青少年在 18 岁之前经历过抑郁症,并且这些年轻人常会出现显著的功能损害以及伤害的风险 [1]。与患抑郁症的成年人相比,患有抑郁症的儿童和青少年更容易出现易怒、精力减退、失眠和体重变化,较少出现快感缺失和注意力集中的问题 [1]。抑郁症的这些症状与其他精神障碍的一些症状相似,甚至重叠,或者可能被忽视,并错误地归因于青少年特有的发育问题,使得诊断具有挑战性。因此,儿童和青少年的抑郁评估应当交由了解发育差异并能准确识别青少年抑郁症的临床医师负责 [2]。

临床指南

对于儿童和青少年的轻度抑郁症,英国卫生与临床优化研究所(NICE)指南 [4] 及美国儿童和青少年精神病学学会(AACAP)实践指南 [3] 建议,应该考虑将支持治疗或心理干预作为一线治疗,不应开具抗抑郁药物。

对于中、重度抑郁症,NICE 指南建议单用心理治疗,或者抗抑郁药物与心理治疗合用。此外,ACAPP 实践指南建议:如果患者病情严重而无法进行谈话治疗,或者暂时无法实施心理干预,或者患者及其家属喜欢用药,可考虑单用抗抑郁药物。

这些指南主要来自三项大型随机对照试验:青少年抑郁症治疗研究(TADS)[5]、青少年难治性抑郁症治疗研究(TORDIA)[6],以及青少年抑郁症抗抑郁药物和心理治疗试验(ADAPT)[7]。这些试验证实了选择性 5-羟色胺再摄取抑制剂(SSRI)治疗青少年抑郁症的有效性。例如,TADS 发现,在急性期(12 周内),氟西汀的有效率为 61%,明显高于安慰剂的有效率 35%,需要治疗人数(number needed to treat,NNT)为 4[5]。后续的系统综述和荟萃分析进一步证实了 SSRI 治疗青少年抑郁症的有效性和可接受性 [8,9]。大多数研究发现抗抑郁药物的疗效相对一般,有一项荟萃分析得出的 NNT 为 10[10],可能是因为安慰剂有效率较高 [11]。

对治疗儿童和青少年抑郁症,现有证据尚不能明确单用 SSRI 药物、单独进行心理治疗、两者联合,这三种方案何者最优。TADS 发现,单用氟西汀或者氟西汀联合 CBT 可加快起效时间,并且联合 CBT 可减少包括自杀在内的药物不良反应,从而提高氟西汀的安全性 [5,12]。然而,其他研究并没能得到相同的结论 [7],并且荟萃分析认为仅有限的证据表明联合治疗比单用抗抑郁药物对青少年患者更有效 [13,14]。

儿童和青少年抑郁症用药

开处方之前

- 进行综合评估:明确抑郁症的临床诊断。排除其他诊断,包括精神障碍(如双相情感障碍)、躯体疾病(如内分泌失调)和药物相关影响(如类固醇不良反应)。识别是否存在其他精神或躯体方面的共病。考虑 SSRI 的禁忌证以及潜在的药物相互作用。评估自伤和伤人的风险。考虑诱发、促成和延续抑郁症的可能因素,例如精神障碍(包括抑郁症和双相情感障碍)的家族史和环境压力因素(包括受害和其他不良经历)。如果发现同时出现其他问题,则应综合评估,确定处理的优先顺序,并解决这些问题。

- 评估基线期的严重程度:抑郁症状的评估工具包括医师用的儿童抑郁量表修订版(CDRS-R)[15,16]、父母版和儿童版的情绪问卷(MFQ)[17]或者儿童焦虑抑郁量表修订版(RCADS)[18],功能损害的评估工具主要是儿童大体评定量表(CGAS)[19]。
- 获得知情同意:讨论抑郁症的性质、病程和治疗、药物的潜在不良反应、治疗效果的延迟现象、监测和维持药物治疗的计划,以及潜在的停药反应。
- 制订安全计划:除特殊情况外,父母或其看护者应负责为儿童或青少年安全存放药物。同时,建议青少年及其父母或看护者在遇到严重不良反应、伤害风险或症状恶化时应及时联系专业人员或服务机构。

处方什么药物

- 氟西汀是治疗儿童和青少年抑郁症的一线药物[3,4]。目前为止,氟西汀疗效的支持证据是最有力的[8,20-22],并且 NICE 认为氟西汀是唯一一种临床试验表明益处大于风险的抗抑郁药[4]。氟西汀应当从 10mg/d 的低剂量开始服用,一周后可增加到最低有效剂量 20mg/d。高剂量(40~60mg/d)的氟西汀也可以考虑使用,尤其是对于高体重的大龄儿童,或因病情严重而期待获得早期疗效的患儿[4-7]。氟西汀的长半衰期对青少年可能是有益的,因为即使出现晚服或漏服,也不会出现停药反应[23]。氟西汀被美国食品药品管理局(FDA)批准用于 8 岁及以上儿童。
- 相比于安慰剂,舍曲林和艾司西酞普兰也能有效地治疗青少年抑郁症[8,22],如果患者不能耐受氟西汀,可以考虑舍曲林和艾司西酞普兰。舍曲林和艾司西酞普兰也应从小剂量开始(舍曲林 25~50mg/d、艾司西酞普兰 5~10mg/d),然后逐渐增加剂量,直到有效剂量(舍曲林 50~200mg/d、艾司西酞普兰 10~20mg/d)。舍曲林、艾司西酞普兰和其他一些抗抑郁药,其半衰期在青少年中可能要比成年人短,因此在使用时应当考虑一天 2 次,特别是在低剂量的情况下,以防出现停药反应[24]。艾司西酞普兰被 FDA 批准用于治疗 12 岁以上患者的抑郁症。
- 单用 SSRI 无效或者仅部分有效时:对于有明显抑郁症状的儿童和青少年,尽管进行了充分的 SSRI 单药治疗,仍有明显的抑郁症状,导致身心痛苦或功能损害,此时可以考虑合用 SSRI 和心理治疗[21,25]。
- 难治性抑郁症的药物治疗(SSRI 和心理治疗无效或仅部分有效):对于有明显抑郁症状的儿童和青少年,尽管进行了充分的 SSRI(氟西汀)药物治疗和心理治疗,仍有明显的抑郁症状,可以考虑改用不同的 SSRI(舍曲林、西酞普兰[4]或艾司西酞普兰)[25]。这是基于 TORDIA 试验的指导,该试验是唯一一项在青少年中比较不同治疗策略对 SSRI 耐药抑郁症的疗效的随机对照试验[6]。这项试验发现,当换用另一种 SSRI 或文拉法辛时,许多被试者的病情[27]得到了改善;若同时合并 CBT,则改善更加完全。换用 SSRI 与文拉法辛一样有效,且前者不良反应较轻,因此首选换用 SSRI。
- 如果使用上述药物充分治疗仍没有足够的疗效,应当考虑加用另一种药物(如第二代抗精神病药物或锂盐),来为 SSRI 增效;尤其是当 SSRI 能部分改善病情时,应考虑使用增效剂。或者,考虑换用不同类别的抗抑郁药,例如米氮平(尤其适用于伴有睡眠问题的患者)。

如果上述药物无效,抑郁症又非常严重,可考虑其他治疗,例如重复经颅磁刺激、电休克疗法以及艾司氯胺酮。但是因为缺乏对儿童和青少年的相关研究,所以不建议对儿童进行这些治疗。除换用不同的 SSRI 外,其他所有的建议都是基于成年人研究的证据 [25]。

- NICE 不建议使用帕罗西汀、文拉法辛、三环类抗抑郁药或圣约翰草来治疗青少年的抑郁症,因为它们有潜在的不良反应和药物相互作用 [4]。
- ω-3 脂肪酸对治疗成年人抑郁症几乎没有益处 [25];先前在青少年中进行的一项随机对照试验表明 ω-3 脂肪酸对治疗抑郁症有效 [26],但随后的一项更大规模的试验却并没有证明其有效性 [27]。因此,不建议青少年服用 ω-3 脂肪酸治疗抑郁症。
- 框 5.1 总结了儿童和青少年抑郁症的药物治疗。

框 5.1 儿童和青少年抑郁症的药物治疗总结 [3,4,21,25]

	药物	起始剂量	治疗剂量范围
一线	氟西汀(FDA 批准用于 8 岁以上患儿)	10mg/d	20~60mg/d
二线	舍曲林 或 西酞普兰 *	25~50mg/d 5~10mg/d	50~200mg/d 10~40mg/d
三线	艾司西酞普兰(FDA 批准用于 12 岁以上患儿)	5~10mg/d	10~20mg/d
四线	考虑在抗抑郁药治疗的基础上增加第二代抗精神病药或锂盐 ** 考虑米氮平 **(需要镇静时)		

* 建议心脏病或肝病患者慎用。
** 该治疗没有针对青少年的随机对照试验证据(仅存在来自成年人试验的证据)支持。

用药以后

急性期

- 定期监测不良反应,例如前 4 周每周监测一次。儿童和青少年对 SSRI 的耐受性一般都很好。可能的不良反应类似成年人,如第 3 章所述。此外,服用 SSRI 的青少年出现自杀行为和转为躁狂的风险略有增加(见下文"特殊事项")。因此,应密切监测并妥善处理伤害风险、情绪和行为状况 [3,4,21,25]。
- 使用治疗剂量的 SSRI 治疗 4 周后,使用基线时完成的量表评估疗效,包括抑郁症的严重程度。大多数治疗效果在 4 周后显现 [9]。
- 若部分有效或无效,需考虑治疗依从性差、诊断不准确、共病以及疾病维持因素发生改变的可能性。
- 如果这些因素都不能解释持续的抑郁症状,并且青少年并未出现不良反应,可考虑增加剂量。每 4 周评估一次 [3,25]。
- 如果出现不良反应,应当考虑将剂量降低至最高耐受剂量。
- 如果在 SSRI 的最大推荐剂量(或最高耐受剂量)治疗 8 周后无效或者仅部分有效,应考虑替换前述药物。

维持期

■ 病情缓解后继续服药 6~12 个月，以降低复发风险。如果抑郁症反复发作或慢性发作，可以考虑更长时间的维持治疗[3,4,21,25]。

停药期

■ 在维持期治疗结束后，可以考虑停药，最好在患者压力较小的时候进行。应缓慢减少药物剂量（见第 3 章），以尽量降低出现撤药症状的风险[3,4,21,25]。

特殊事项

■ 年龄：上述建议的证据来源青少年多于儿童，因此为儿童患者开药时应更加慎重。目前，还没有研究调查抗抑郁药物在学龄前儿童中的使用情况，故暂不推荐该年龄组使用[4,8]。

■ 自杀倾向：抗抑郁药物治疗与年轻人自杀风险的增加有关，因此美国 FDA、英国药品和保健品管理局以及欧洲药品管理局在 2003 年发布了黑框警告。同时，一些荟萃分析发现了抗抑郁药物与自杀倾向相关的证据[8,10]（特别是文拉法辛[20,22]），以及与攻击行为关系的证据[28]。但是，自杀意念或自杀行为的风险很小。例如，一项荟萃分析发现，抗抑郁药物组自杀率为 2%，而安慰剂组为 1%，需治疗人数（number needed to harm，NNH）为 112[10]。此外，抗抑郁药物的使用与自杀致死之间没有联系。相反，未经治疗的抑郁症才是自杀的重要危险因素。在 FDA 对儿童使用抗抑郁药物发出警告后，抗抑郁药物的使用率下降，未经治疗的抑郁症患者增加，以致自杀率上升[29,30]。考虑到抑郁症患者不经治疗可能发生自杀和功能损伤，并且使用 SSRI 收获的益处远大于可能出现的严重不良反应。因此，对于中、重度抑郁症，使用抗抑郁药物（尤其是氟西汀），其潜在收益超过相关风险。尽管如此，还是应当仔细监测潜在风险[3,4,21,25]。

■ 转躁：据估计，每年服用抗抑郁药物的青少年中有 6% 会转为躁狂，而且儿童的风险似乎比成年人更高[31]。然而，没有明确的证据表明这种转变是由抗抑郁药物引起的。躁狂症状应与具有激活性质的不良反应相区别，后者是开始服用抗抑郁药物或增加剂量时出现的短暂的脱抑制反应，以冲动、烦躁和易怒为特征[3]。

参考文献

1. Avenevoli S, et al. Major depression in the national comorbidity survey-adolescent supplement: prevalence, correlates, and treatment. *J Am Acad Child Adolesc Psychiatry* 2015; 54:37–44.e32.

2. Rice F, et al. Adolescent and adult differences in major depression symptom profiles. *J Affect Disord* 2019; 243:175–181.

3. Birmaher B, et al. Practice parameter for the assessment and treatment of children and adolescents with depressive disorders. *J Am Acad Child Adolesc Psychiatry* 2007; 46:1503–1526.

4. National Institute for Health and Care Excellence (NICE). Depression in children and young people: identification and management. NICE Guideline [NG134]. 2019; www.nice.org.uk/guidance/ng134.

5. March J, et al. Fluoxetine, cognitive-behavioral therapy, and their combination for adolescents with depression: Treatment for Adolescents with Depression Study (TADS) randomized controlled trial. *JAMA* 2004; 292:807–820.

6. Brent D, et al. Switching to another SSRI or to venlafaxine with or without cognitive behavioral therapy for adolescents with SSRI-resistant depression: the TORDIA Randomized Controlled Trial. *JAMA: The Journal of the American Medical Association* 2008; 299:901–913.

7. Goodyer I, et al. Selective Serotonin Reuptake Inhibitors (SSRIs) and routine specialist care with and without cognitive behaviour therapy in adolescents with major depression: randomised controlled trial. *BMJ* 2007; 335:142.

8. Hetrick SE, et al. Newer generation antidepressants for depressive disorders in children and adolescents. *Cochrane Database Syst Rev* 2012; 11:CD004851.

9. Varigonda AL, et al. Systematic review and meta-analysis: early treatment responses of selective serotonin reuptake inhibitors in pediatric major depressive disorder. *J Am Acad Child Adolesc Psychiatry* 2015; 54:557–564.

10. Bridge JA, et al. Clinical response and risk for reported suicidal ideation and suicide attempts in pediatric antidepressant treatment: a meta-analysis of randomized controlled trials. *JAMA* 2007; 297:1683–1696.

11. Walkup JT Antidepressant efficacy for depression in children and adolescents: industry- and NIMH-funded studies. *Am J Psychiatry* 2017; 174:430–437.

12. Treatment for Adolescents With Depression Study (TADS) Team. The Treatment for Adolescents With Depression Study (TADS): long-term effectiveness and safety outcomes. *Arch Gen Psychiatry* 2007; 64:1132–1143.

13. Cox GR, et al. Psychological therapies versus antidepressant medication, alone and in combination for depression in children and adolescents. *Cochrane Database Syst Rev* 2014; Cd008324.

14. Dubicka B, et al. Combined treatment with cognitive-behavioural therapy in adolescent depression: meta-analysis. *Br J Psychiatry* 2010; 197:433–440.

15. Poznanski EO, et al. *Children's Depression Rating Scale, Revised (CDRS-R)*. Los Angeles, Calif.: Western Psychological Services 1996.

16. Mayes TL, et al. Psychometric properties of the Children's Depression Rating Scale-Revised in adolescents. *J Child Adolesc Psychopharmacol* 2010; 20:513–516.

17. Angold A, et al. Development of a short questionnaire for use in epidemiological studies of depression in children and adolescents. *Int J Methods Psychiatr Res* 1995; 5:237–249.

18. Chorpita BF, et al. Assessment of symptoms of DSM-IV anxiety and depression in children: a revised child anxiety and depression scale. *Behav Res Ther* 2000; 38:835–855.

19. Shaffer D, et al. A children's global assessment scale (CGAS). *Arch Gen Psychiatry* 1983; 40:1228–1231.

20. Cipriani A, et al. Comparative efficacy and tolerability of antidepressants for major depressive disorder in children and adolescents: a network meta-analysis. *Lancet* 2016; 388:881–890.

21. Goodyer IM, et al. Practitioner review: therapeutics of unipolar major depressions in adolescents. *J Child Psychol Psychiatry* 2019; 60:232–243.

22. Zhou X, et al. Comparative efficacy and acceptability of antidepressants, psychotherapies, and their combination for acute treatment of children and adolescents with depressive disorder: a systematic review and network meta-analysis. *Lancet Psychiatry* 2020; 7:581–601.

23. Wilens TE, et al. Fluoxetine pharmacokinetics in pediatric patients. *J Clin Psychopharmacol* 2002; 22:568–575.

24. Findling RL, et al. The relevance of pharmacokinetic studies in designing efficacy trials in juvenile major depression. *J Child Adolesc Psychopharmacol* 2006; 16:131–145.

25. Dwyer JB, et al. Annual research review: defining and treating pediatric treatment-resistant depression. *J Child Psychol Psychiatry* 2020; 61:312–332.

26. Nemets H, et al. Omega-3 treatment of childhood depression: a controlled, double-blind pilot study. *Am J Psychiatry* 2006; 163:1098–1100.

27. Marangell LB, et al. A double-blind, placebo-controlled study of the omega-3 fatty acid docosahexaenoic acid in the treatment of major depression. *Am J Psychiatry* 2003; 160:996–998.

28. Sharma T, et al. Suicidality and aggression during antidepressant treatment: systematic review and meta-analyses based on clinical study reports. *BMJ* 2016; 352:i65.

29. Gibbons RD, et al. Early evidence on the effects of regulators' suicidality warnings on SSRI prescriptions and suicide in children and adolescents. *Am J Psychiatry* 2007; 164:1356–1363.

30. Libby AM, et al. Decline in treatment of pediatric depression after FDA advisory on risk of suicidality with SSRIs. *Am J Psychiatry* 2007; 164:884–891.

31. Baldessarini RJ, et al. Antidepressant-associated mood-switching and transition from unipolar major depression to bipolar disorder: a review. *J Affect Disord* 2013; 148:129–135.

儿童和青少年双相障碍

临床指南

用药之前

- 建立临床诊断,如果可能,最好建立在结构化评估工具的基础之上。通过心情日志或睡眠日志前瞻性地监测症状模式。若有疑问,及早咨询相关专家。
- 向患者和家属解释诊断,并投入时间和精力进行心理教育。这样做有可能改善依从性,减少复发率,至少在成年人中有支持证据[1]。
- 评估基线期的躁狂症状(如用杨氏躁狂评定量表[2],YMRS)、抑郁症状(如儿童抑郁量表[3],CDRS)以及缺陷程度(如临床大体印象量表-双相情感障碍版[4])。借助这些评估工具,建立明确且可行的治疗目标。
- 测量基线的身高、体重、腰围、脉搏、心电图、血压和血液检查(包括空腹血糖、糖化血红蛋白、空腹血脂、全血细胞计数、尿素和电解质、肌酸激酶、肝功能、催乳素)。

处方什么药物

- 对于青少年躁狂和轻躁狂的治疗,NICE 指南建议:可以与成年人一样,将第二代抗精神病药物作为一线用药,在两种第二代抗精神病药物治疗失败后添加心境稳定剂[5]。
- 根据一项荟萃分析,第二代抗精神病药(相比安慰剂,效应值为 0.65)的短期疗效优于心境稳定剂(相比安慰剂,效应值为 0.20)[6]。
- 与成年人相比,青少年使用第二代抗精神病药似乎更容易引起体重增加和嗜睡[6],但是,对这个年龄层的青少年进行体重评估,会因为生长发育而变得相对棘手。
- 青少年女性应禁用丙戊酸盐。
- 坚持使用锂盐和监测血锂水平对于青少年可能是困难的。
- 总之,我们建议使用第二代抗精神病药作为儿童和青少年躁狂急性期治疗的一线药物(表 5.1),这与对成年人的建议类似。

用药以后

- 定期评估和监测症状以确定疗效。
- 每一次访视都监测体重与身高;3 个月时复查血检(以后每 6 个月 1 次);提供关于健康生活方式和锻炼的建议。
- 大多数药物的试用时间都是 3~5 周。这应该指导医师来决定单药治疗多长时间为宜。如果治疗 1~2 周完全无效,提示应该换用另一种第二代抗精神病药。
- 如果治疗无效,检查依从性,(如果可能)监测血药浓度,并考虑增加剂量。考虑合用第二代抗精神病药和心境稳定剂。
- 由于青少年双相情感障碍的证据非常有限,将成年人证据推导到儿童时宜谨慎[7],这包括治疗时间长短和预防复发[5,6,8]。

表 5.1　在双相躁狂青少年患者中药物治疗的 RCT 证据总结

药物	述评
锂盐	锂盐在儿童体内清除相对较快,因此需要每天给药两次,尤其在使用液体剂型或非调释制剂时[20]。一项双盲安慰剂对照随机试验[21]显示,25 例双相情感障碍合并物质滥用的青少年患者,经过 6 周治疗,物质使用显著减少,临床评分显著改善。在一项为期 2 周的安慰剂对照、双盲停药试验($n=40$)中,锂盐组与安慰剂组的复发率没有显著差异[22]
	随后的一项为期 8 周的双盲安慰剂对照研究($n=81$)发现,接受锂盐治疗的青少年患者,YMRS 评分明显改善,但与安慰剂组的差异在治疗 6 周后才开始出现。同时服用锂盐后促甲状腺素显著增加,但体重增加没有差别[23]
	在一项为期 18 个月的青少年患者的维持试验中($n=60$),合用锂盐和双丙戊酸盐病情稳定以后开始进行试验,结果发现锂盐维持治疗组和双丙戊酸盐维持治疗组之间没有差异[24]。但是,鉴于有充分的证据表明锂盐在成年患者中有良好的维持和预防效果,我们建议针对青少年患者,临床医师应当优先考虑使用锂盐,而不是丙戊酸盐
	一项荟萃分析[25]发现,在躁狂症患者中,锂盐疗效"明显劣于"利培酮。同时,一项为期 6 个月的小样本研究发现,与维持服用锂盐的患者相比,停用锂盐的患者复发率较高[26]。另一项为期 8 个月的自然研究表明,锂盐治疗有效且耐受性良好[27]
丙戊酸盐	在一项随机对照试验中($n=150$)[28],双丙戊酸盐缓释剂(渐加到临床有效或 80~125mg/L)治疗第 4 周时,在 YMRS 评分上并不优于安慰剂(另见下面的利培酮和喹硫平部分)
奥卡西平	一项双盲安慰剂对照研究($n=116$)发现,在治疗第 7 周减少躁狂评分上,奥卡西平(平均剂量 1 515mg/d)与安慰剂无明显差异[29]
奥氮平	一项双盲安慰剂对照研究($n=161$)[30]发现,治疗 3 周之后,在 YMRS 平均分减少值上,奥氮平(5~20mg/d)显著优于安慰剂。注意:治疗组体重增加较多(奥氮平组 3.7kg,安慰剂组 0.3kg),伴有空腹血糖、总胆固醇、AST、ALT 和尿酸等明显升高
利培酮	一项双盲安慰剂对照研究($n=169$)发现,在 3 周随访期间,YMRS 平均分减少值上,利培酮(0.5~2.5mg 或 3~6mg)显著优于安慰剂[31]。低剂量组疗效与高剂量组相同,但不良反应的风险较低。治疗组嗜睡和乏力比较常见。同时,值得注意的是,治疗组平均体重增加(安慰剂组 0.7kg,低剂量组 1.7kg,高剂量组 1.4kg)
	在早发躁狂治疗研究(the treatment of early age mania,TEAM)中,利培酮(平均剂量 2.57mg)有效率和代谢不良反应发生率高于锂盐组(平均血锂浓度 1.09mmol/L)和丙戊酸组(平均血药浓度 113.6mg/L)[32]。这项研究的随机随访再次表明,作为对锂盐和双丙戊酸盐无反应者的替代治疗,以及两种心境稳定剂的辅助治疗,利培酮具有优越性[33]。但是,该研究对躁狂症的定义比较宽泛,且不同于大多数英国临床医师对双相情感障碍的定义,因此解释研究结果时应当慎重。在另一项双盲安慰剂对照试验中,由于类似的原因,利培酮组(平均剂量 0.5mg)和丙戊酸组(平均血药浓度 81mg/L)在被诊断为躁狂症的 3~7 岁儿童中明显表现出更好疗效[34]
喹硫平	一项双盲安慰剂对照试验($n=277$)[35]发现,在治疗第 3 周时的 YMRS 平均分减少值上,喹硫平(400mg/d 或 600mg/d)显著优于安慰剂。最常见的不良反应包括嗜睡和镇静。喹硫平组体重增加 1.7kg,安慰剂组为 0.4kg
	喹硫平作为丙戊酸盐的增效剂合用时,其疗效相似于单用丙戊酸盐($n=30$,6 周)[36];在一项双盲试验中,喹硫平与丙戊酸盐疗效相同($n=50$,4 周)[37]

第 5 章

续表

药物	述评
阿立哌唑	一项双盲安慰剂对照研究[38,39]发现，在治疗第 4 周(n=296)[38]时和第 30 周(n=210)[39]时，在 YMRS 平均分减少值上，阿立哌唑(10mg/d 或 30mg/d)显著优于安慰剂。治疗组较易发生锥体外系不良反应(尤其是高剂量组)。治疗组体重增加在第 30 周(而不是第 4 周)明显高于安慰剂组(安慰剂组 3.0kg，低剂量组 6.5kg，高剂量组 6.6kg)
齐拉西酮	一项双盲安慰剂对照试验(n=237)[40]发现，在治疗第 4 周时，在 YMRS 平均分减少值上，齐拉西酮(可变剂量 40~160mg/d)显著优于安慰剂。镇静和嗜睡是最常见的不良反应，代谢不受影响，也没有 Q-T 间期延长
阿塞那平	一项为期 3 周的双盲安慰剂对照研究(n=350)发现，在不同剂量(2.5mg、5mg 或 10mg，每天两次)下，阿塞那平疗效均优于安慰剂，并且这种显著差异在治疗的第 4 天就已出现。然而，许多不良反应也被报道，包括体重较正常增加 7% 以上(阿塞那平组发生率为 8%~12%，安慰剂组发生率为 1.1%)、代谢改变(空腹胰岛素、血脂、血糖升高)，以及嗜睡、镇静、口腔感觉减退和感觉异常[41]

ALT，谷丙转氨酶；AST，谷草转氨酶；ER，缓释剂；MS，情绪稳定剂；RCT，随机对照试验；YMRS，杨氏躁狂评定量表。

- 维持治疗应遵循成年人指南。在治疗过程中可考虑早期使用锂盐，既可单用锂盐进行预防，也可在急性期用药的基础上将锂盐作为辅助药物。

特殊事项

- 双相抑郁是一个常见的临床挑战，并且与成年人相比，对年轻人群的治疗研究要少得多(表 5.2)。抗抑郁药物的使用应当慎重，且只能在抗躁狂药物治疗的背景下使用[5]。在成年人中，尚无证据表明抗抑郁药物可以使双相抑郁患者从中受益[9]。由于在儿童中的药物试验极度缺乏，我们建议谨慎地根据成年人研究结果进行推论[5]，并且建议将奥氮平/氟西汀合剂或喹硫平作为一线用药，还可使用鲁拉西酮，因为实验证据支持鲁拉西酮用于 10~17 岁儿童[10-12]。
- 目前，ADHD 与双相情感障碍之间的确切关系仍存在争议。有证据提示，针对儿童 ADHD 和躁狂症状，兴奋剂的耐受性可能较好，在情绪平稳后可以安全且有效地使用[13]。但处方这类药物需要谨慎和经验(表 5.3 和表 5.4)。
- DSM-5 引入一个新的分类"破坏性情绪失调障碍(DMDD)"来描述严重易激惹的儿童(过去在美国经常被误诊为双相情感障碍)。对于破坏性情绪失调障碍，目前尚没有能被证实的治疗方法。锂盐无效[14]，但是可以考虑 SSRI 和心理治疗，例如育儿干预[15]。

其他治疗

- 在成年人与儿童都有证据表明，辅助心理教育、认知行为治疗和聚焦于家庭的干预可以提高双相障碍的治疗效果，预防双相抑郁复发[16]。
- 目前，高频重复经颅磁刺激(rTMS)在青少年难治性单相抑郁中的应用仅得到开放试验的支持[17]，尚未在单相或双相抑郁的青少年中进行随机对照试验。因此，rTMS 的应用仍被认为处于试验阶段。一项右侧前额叶皮质重复经颅磁刺激的随机伪治疗(sham)对照(n=26)研究显示，作为标准药物的辅助治疗措施，rTMS 对青少年急性躁狂发作无效[18]。

表 5.2　在双相抑郁青少年患者中药物治疗的 RCT 证据总结

药物	述评
喹硫平	在成年人中,存在有效治疗的良好证据(参阅"双相抑郁"),如喹硫平[42,43]。在一项小样本研究(32 名青少年)[44] 以及随后的一项大样本随机对照试验(n=193)[45] 中,却发现没有什么疗效。这项最新研究具有很高的安慰剂效应,而在成年人喹硫平研究中并不存在这一问题[46],并且这可能反映了之前已经注意到的关于情感障碍表型和多中心研究的问题[47]
奥氮平/氟西汀合剂	唯一一项在治疗青少年双相抑郁症方面取得阳性结果的双盲随机安慰剂对照试验,是一项为期 8 周的奥氮平/氟西汀合剂(每天 6/25mg 或 12/50mg)治疗青少年双相抑郁的大型研究(n=255)[48]。在第 1 周和所有的后续随访中,组间差异显著。最常见的不良反应是体重增加(奥氮平/氟西汀合剂组为 4.4kg,安慰剂组为 0.5kg)、嗜睡和高脂血症。NICE 指南推荐奥氮平/氟西汀合剂[5] 与喹硫平作为青少年双相抑郁的一线治疗,与成年人一样。虽然奥氮平/氟西汀合剂目前在英国没有生产出单一制剂,但可以通过组合使用奥氮平和氟西汀(例如 5/20mg 或 10/40mg)来实现其效果
鲁拉西酮	鲁拉西酮已被证明对 49~51 岁成年人的双相抑郁症有效[49-51],并且它似乎不会导致体重增加和其他代谢紊乱。它在治疗青少年精神分裂症方面是安全有效的[52],且已被证实对儿童(10~17 岁)患者急性期[10] 和随访 2 年的治疗有效[12]。剂量范围为 18.5(20)mg~74(80)mg,但多数患者使用最低剂量。由于其良好的耐受性,鲁拉西酮可能是儿童首选的抗精神病药物[53]
拉莫三嗪	拉莫三嗪在成年双相抑郁中仅有(如果有)轻微的疗效[54];在儿童和青少年中还没有进行随机对照试验,因此不推荐作为一线用药。此外,在一项持续超过 36 周的安慰剂随机对照治疗青年双相情感障碍研究中,停用辅助药物拉莫三嗪并未能推迟发病时间[55]

RCT,随机对照试验。

表 5.3　建议用于急性期躁狂的一线治疗 *

药物	剂量	药物	剂量
阿立哌唑	10mg/d	喹硫平	最高 400mg/d
利培酮	0.5~2.5mg/d	阿塞那平	2.5~10mg bid
奥氮平	5~20mg/d		

* 急性期的有效剂量继续使用,作为预防复发的措施,并考虑是否应用锂盐。

表 5.4　建议用于双相抑郁的一线治疗 *

药物	剂量
鲁拉西酮	18.5~74mg/d 或 20~80mg/d
奥氮平/氟西汀合剂	6/25~12/50mg/d
喹硫平	最高 300mg/d

* 急性期的有效剂量继续使用,作为预防复发的措施,并考虑是否应用锂盐。

■ 一项小样本试验支持在患有躁狂症的成年人中辅助使用褪黑素(6mg/d)[19]。虽然现有证据不足以推荐在儿童中使用褪黑素,但是足以支持在儿童躁狂发作期服用褪黑素是安全的。

参考文献

1. Colom F, et al. A randomized trial on the efficacy of group psychoeducation in the prophylaxis of recurrences in bipolar patients whose disease is in remission. *Arch Gen Psychiatry* 2003; 60:402–407.

2. Young RC, et al. A rating scale for mania: reliability, validity and sensitivity. *Br J Psychiatry* 1978; 133:429–435.

3. Poznanski EO, et al. Preliminary studies of the reliability and validity of the children's depression rating scale. *J Am Acad Child Psychiatry* 1984; 23:191–197.

4. Spearing MK, et al. Modification of the Clinical Global Impressions (CGI) Scale for use in bipolar illness (BP): the CGI-BP. *Psychiatry Res* 1997; 73:159–171.

5. National Institute for Health and Care Excellence. Bipolar disorder: assessment and management: Clinical Guidance [CG185] 2014 (last updated February 2020); https://www.nice.org.uk/guidance/cg185.

6. Correll CU, et al. Antipsychotic and mood stabilizer efficacy and tolerability in pediatric and adult patients with bipolar I mania: a comparative analysis of acute, randomized, placebo-controlled trials. *Bipolar disorders* 2010; 12:116–141.

7. Geddes JR, et al. Treatment of bipolar disorder. *Lancet* 2013; 381:1672–1682.

8. Diaz-Caneja CM, et al. Practitioner review: Long-term pharmacological treatment of pediatric bipolar disorder. *J Child Psychol Psychiatry* 2014; 55:959–980.

9. Pacchiarotti I, et al. The International Society for Bipolar Disorders (ISBD) task force report on antidepressant use in bipolar disorders. *AmJPsychiatry* 2013; 170:1249–1262.

10. DelBello MP, et al. Efficacy and Safety of Lurasidone in Children and Adolescents With Bipolar I Depression: A Double-Blind, Placebo-Controlled Study. *J Am Acad Child Adolesc Psychiatry* 2017; 56:1015–1025.

11. Singh MK, et al. Lurasidone in children and adolescents with bipolar depression presenting with mixed (subsyndromal hypomanic) features: post hoc analysis of a randomized placebo-controlled trial. *J Child Adolesc Psychopharmacol* 2020; 30:590–598.

12. DelBello MP, et al. 159 Safety and efficacy of lurasidone in children and adolescents with bipolar depression: results from a 2-year open-label extension study. *CNS Spectr* 2020; 25:301–302.

13. Goldsmith M, et al. Antidepressants and psychostimulants in pediatric populations: is there an association with mania? *PaediatrDrugs* 2011; 13:225–243.

14. Dickstein DP, et al. Randomized double-blind placebo-controlled trial of lithium in youths with severe mood dysregulation. *J Child Adolesc Psychopharmacol* 2009; 19:61–73.

15. Vidal-Ribas P, et al. The status of irritability in psychiatry: a conceptual and quantitative review. *J Am Acad Child Adolesc Psychiatry* 2016; 55:556–570.

16. Miklowitz DJ. Evidence-based family interventions for adolescents and young adults with bipolar disorder. *J Clin Psychiatry* 2016; 77 Suppl E1:e5.

17. Wall CA, et al. Magnetic resonance imaging-guided, open-label, high-frequency repetitive transcranial magnetic stimulation for adolescents with major depressive disorder. *J Child Adolesc Psychopharmacol* 2016; 26:582–589.

18. Pathak V, et al. Efficacy of adjunctive high frequency repetitive transcranial magnetic stimulation of right prefrontal cortex in adolescent mania: a randomized sham-controlled study. *Clinical psychopharmacology and neuroscience : the official scientific journal of the Korean College of Neuropsychopharmacology* 2015; 13:245–249.

19. Moghaddam HS, et al. Efficacy of melatonin as an adjunct in the treatment of acute mania: a double-blind and placebo-controlled trial. *Int Clin Psychopharmacol* 2020; 35:81–88.

20. Grant B, et al. Using Lithium in Children and Adolescents with bipolar disorder: efficacy, tolerability, and practical considerations. *Paediatr Drugs* 2018; 20:303–314.

21. Geller B, et al. Double-blind and placebo-controlled study of lithium for adolescent bipolar disorders with secondary substance dependency. *J Am Acad Child Adolesc Psychiatry* 1998; 37:171–178.

22. Kafantaris V, et al. Lithium treatment of acute mania in adolescents: a placebo-controlled discontinuation study. *J Am Acad Child Adolesc Psychiatry* 2004; 43:984–993.

23. Findling RL, et al. Lithium in the acute treatment of bipolar I disorder: a double-blind, placebo-controlled study. *Pediatrics* 2015; 136:885–894.

24. Findling RL, et al. Double-blind 18-month trial of lithium versus divalproex maintenance treatment in pediatric bipolar disorder. *J Am Acad Child Adolesc Psychiatry* 2005; 44:409–417.

25. Duffy A, et al. Efficacy and tolerability of lithium for the treatment of acute mania in children with bipolar disorder: a systematic review: a report from the ISBD-IGSLi joint task force on lithium treatment. *Bipolar disorders* 2018; 20:583–593.

26. Findling RL, et al. Lithium for the maintenance treatment of bipolar I disorder: a double-blind, placebo-controlled discontinuation study. *J Am Acad Child Adolesc Psychiatry* 2019; 58:287–296.e284.

27. Masi G, et al. Lithium treatment in bipolar adolescents: a follow-up naturalistic study. *Neuropsychiatr Dis Treat* 2018; 14:2749.

28. Wagner KD, et al. A double-blind, randomized, placebo-controlled trial of divalproex extended-release in the treatment of bipolar disorder in children and adolescents. *J Am Acad Child Adolesc Psychiatry* 2009; 48:519–532.

29. Wagner KD, et al. A double-blind, randomized, placebo-controlled trial of oxcarbazepine in the treatment of bipolar disorder in children and adolescents. *Am J Psychiatry* 2006; 163:1179–1186.

30. Tohen M, et al. Olanzapine versus placebo in the treatment of adolescents with bipolar mania. *Am J Psychiatry* 2007; 164:1547–1556.

31. Haas M, et al. Risperidone for the treatment of acute mania in children and adolescents with bipolar disorder: a randomized, double-blind,

placebo-controlled study. *Bipolar Disorders* 2009; **11**:687–700.

32. Geller B, et al. A randomized controlled trial of risperidone, lithium, or divalproex sodium for initial treatment of bipolar I disorder, manic or mixed phase, in children and adolescents. *Arch Gen Psychiatry* 2012; **69**:515–528.

33. Walkup JT, et al. Treatment of early-age mania: outcomes for partial and nonresponders to initial treatment. *J Am Acad Child Adolesc Psychiatry* 2015; **54**:1008–1019.

34. Kowatch RA, et al. Placebo-controlled trial of valproic acid versus risperidone in children 3–7 years of age with bipolar I disorder. *J Child Adolesc Psychopharmacol* 2015; **25**:306–313.

35. Pathak S, et al. Efficacy and safety of quetiapine in children and adolescents with mania associated with bipolar I disorder: a 3-week, double-blind, placebo-controlled trial. *JClinPsychiatry* 2013; **74**:e100–e109.

36. Delbello MP, et al. A double-blind, randomized, placebo-controlled study of quetiapine as adjunctive treatment for adolescent mania. *J Am Acad Child Adolesc Psychiatry* 2002; **41**:1216–1223.

37. Delbello MP, et al. A double-blind randomized pilot study comparing quetiapine and divalproex for adolescent mania. *J Am Acad Child Adolesc Psychiatry* 2006; **45**:305–313.

38. Findling RL, et al. Acute treatment of pediatric bipolar I disorder, manic or mixed episode, with aripiprazole: a randomized, double-blind, placebo-controlled study. *J Clin Psychiatry* 2009; **70**:1441–1451.

39. Findling RL, et al. Aripiprazole for the treatment of pediatric bipolar I disorder: a 30–week, randomized, placebo-controlled study. *BipolarDisord* 2013; **15**:138–149.

40. Findling RL, et al. Ziprasidone in adolescents with schizophrenia: results from a placebo-controlled efficacy and long-term open-extension study. *J Child Adolesc Psychopharmacol* 2013; **23**:531–544.

41. Findling RL, et al. Asenapine for the acute treatment of pediatric manic or mixed episode of bipolar I disorder. *J Am Acad Child Adolesc Psychiatry* 2015; **54**:1032–1041.

42. Calabrese JR, et al. A randomized, double-blind, placebo-controlled trial of quetiapine in the treatment of bipolar I or II depression. *Am J Psychiatry* 2005; **162**:1351–1360.

43. Thase ME, et al. Efficacy of quetiapine monotherapy in bipolar I and II depression: a double-blind, placebo-controlled study (the BOLDER II study). *J Clin Psychopharmacol* 2006; **26**:600–609.

44. Delbello MP, et al. A double-blind, placebo-controlled pilot study of quetiapine for depressed adolescents with bipolar disorder. *Bipolar disorders* 2009; **11**:483–493.

45. Findling RL, et al. Efficacy and safety of extended-release quetiapine fumarate in youth with bipolar depression: an 8 week, double-blind, placebo-controlled trial. *J Child Adolesc Psychopharmacol* 2014; **24**:325–335.

46. Suttajit S, et al. Quetiapine for acute bipolar depression: a systematic review and meta-analysis. *Drug Des Devel Ther* 2014; **8**:827–838.

47. Bridge JA, et al. Clinical response and risk for reported suicidal ideation and suicide attempts in pediatric antidepressant treatment: a meta-analysis of randomized controlled trials. *JAMA* 2007; **297**:1683–1696.

48. Detke HC, et al. Olanzapine/fluoxetine combination in children and adolescents with bipolar I depression: a randomized, double-blind, placebo-controlled trial. *J Am Acad Child Adolesc Psychiatry* 2015; **54**:217–224.

49. Loebel A, et al. Lurasidone monotherapy in the treatment of bipolar I depression: a randomized, double-blind, placebo-controlled study. *AmJPsychiatry* 2014; **171**:160–168.

50. Suppes T, et al. Lurasidone adjunctive with lithium or valproate for bipolar depression: A placebo-controlled trial utilizing prospective and retrospective enrolment cohorts. *J Psychiatr Res* 2016; **78**:86–93.

51. Suppes T, et al. Lurasidone for the treatment of major depressive disorder with mixed features: a randomized, double-blind, placebo-controlled study. *Am J Psychiatry* 2016; **173**:400–407.

52. Goldman R, et al. Efficacy and safety of lurasidone in adolescents with schizophrenia: a 6–week, randomized placebo-controlled study. *J Child Adolesc Psychopharmacol* 2017:516–525.

53. Solmi M, et al. Safety of 80 antidepressants, antipsychotics, anti-attention-deficit/hyperactivity medications and mood stabilizers in children and adolescents with psychiatric disorders: a large scale systematic meta-review of 78 adverse effects. *World psychiatry* 2020; **19**:214–232.

54. Calabrese JR, et al. Lamotrigine in the acute treatment of bipolar depression: results of five double-blind, placebo-controlled clinical trials. *Bipolar disorders* 2008; **10**:323–333.

55. Findling RL, et al. Adjunctive Maintenance Lamotrigine for Pediatric Bipolar I Disorder: A Placebo-Controlled, Randomized Withdrawal Study. *J Am Acad Child Adolesc Psychiatry* 2015; **54**:1020-1031.e1023.

儿童与青少年精神病

精神分裂症在儿童中罕见,但在青少年中发病率迅速升高。在做出诊断之前,通常需要进行详细的发育和躯体评估[1,2]。早发精神分裂症谱系障碍经常是慢性的,大多数需要长期的抗精神病药治疗[3]。

关于第一代抗精神病药,已有几项随机对照试验,其中许多使用非常高的剂量,均发现锥体外系反应发生率高,且有明显的镇静作用[4]。即便是使用较小的剂量[5],治疗中出现的急性运动障碍也相当麻烦[6]。第一代抗精神病药一般应当避免用于儿童和青少年。

针对早发精神分裂症谱系障碍,已有许多关于第二代抗精神病药的随机对照试验。这些研究证明,奥氮平[7-9]、利培酮[7,8,10,11]、阿立哌唑[12,13]、喹硫平[13,14]、帕利哌酮[15]、阿塞那平[16]、齐拉西酮[17]、鲁拉西酮[18]治疗精神病均有效。来自系统综述和网络荟萃分析的证据表明,除齐拉西酮(疗效较差)和阿塞那平(疗效不明)外[19],大多数第二代抗精神病药的疗效相当。齐拉西酮可以延长 Q-T 间期,因此增加了心脏安全性的担忧[20,21]。阿立哌唑似乎对青少年的 Q-T 间期没有影响[22]。

与成年人相比,儿童和青少年有更大的风险发生不良反应,如锥体外系症状、催乳素升高、镇静(即便是阿立哌唑[13])、体重增加和代谢异常[23]。

证据显示,氯氮平对青少年难治性精神病有效,但是相比于成年人,青少年容易出现粒细胞缺乏和癫痫发作[24-27]。从较年轻成年人的治疗中获得的数据显示,尽管已经明确在青少年中氯氮平比奥氮平更有效[25,26],但在换用氯氮平之前,应当尝试使用奥氮平,因为奥氮平可能有效[28]。

总之,对儿童和青少年精神病的治疗,其程序与成年人相同(见第 2 章)。NICE[29] 推荐口服抗精神病药联合家庭干预和个体 CBT。起始剂量应在成年人剂量范围的下限或更低。

在为儿童和青少年开具抗精神病药处方时,始终按照精神分裂症章节中的指导来测量基线参数并进行监测。对于儿童和青少年,检测和评估还包括:腰围和臀围、运动障碍、营养状况、饮食和身体活动水平[29]。

参考文献

1. Pina-Camacho L, et al. Autism spectrum disorder and schizophrenia: boundaries and uncertainties. *Br J Psych Adv* 2016; 22:316–324.
2. Hayes D, et al. Dilemmas in the treatment of early-onset first-episode psychosis. *Ther Adv Psychopharmacol* 2018; 8:231–239.
3. Kumra S, et al. Efficacy and tolerability of second-generation antipsychotics in children and adolescents with schizophrenia. *Schizophr Bull* 2008; 34:60–71.
4. Lee ES, et al. Psychopharmacologic treatment of schizophrenia in adolescents and children. *Child Adolesc Psychiatr Clin N Am* 2020; 29:183–210.
5. Connor DF, et al. Neuroleptic-related dyskinesias in children and adolescents. *J Clin Psychiatry* 2001; 62:967–974.
6. Campbell M, et al. Neuroleptic-related dyskinesias in autistic children: a prospective, longitudinal study. *J Am Acad Child Adolesc Psychiatry* 1997; 36:835–843.
7. Sikich L, et al. A pilot study of risperidone, olanzapine, and haloperidol in psychotic youth: a double-blind, randomized, 8-week trial. *Neuropsychopharmacology* 2004; 29:133–145.
8. Sikich L, et al. Double-blind comparison of first- and second-generation antipsychotics in early-onset schizophrenia and schizo-affective disorder: findings from the treatment of early-onset schizophrenia spectrum disorders (TEOSS) study. *Am J Psychiatry* 2008; 165:1420–1431.
9. Kryzhanovskaya L, et al. Olanzapine versus placebo in adolescents with schizophrenia: a 6-week, randomized, double-blind, placebo-controlled trial. *J Am Acad Child Adolesc Psychiatry* 2009; 48:60–70.
10. Haas M, et al. A 6-week, randomized, double-blind, placebo-controlled study of the efficacy and safety of risperidone in adolescents with

schizophrenia. *J Child Adolesc Psychopharmacol* 2009; 19:611–621.

11. Haas M, et al. Efficacy, safety and tolerability of two dosing regimens in adolescent schizophrenia: double-blind study. *Br J Psychiatry* 2009; 194:158–164.

12. Findling RL, et al. A multiple-center, randomized, double-blind, placebo-controlled study of oral aripiprazole for treatment of adolescents with schizophrenia. *Am J Psychiatry* 2008; 165:1432–1441.

13. Pagsberg AK, et al. Quetiapine extended release versus aripiprazole in children and adolescents with first-episode psychosis: the multicentre, double-blind, randomised tolerability and efficacy of antipsychotics (TEA) trial. *Lancet Psychiatry* 2017; 4:605–618.

14. Findling RL, et al. Efficacy and safety of quetiapine in adolescents with schizophrenia investigated in a 6-week, double-blind, placebo-controlled trial. *J Child Adolesc Psychopharmacol* 2012; 22:327–342.

15. Singh J, et al. A randomized, double-blind study of paliperidone extended-release in treatment of acute schizophrenia in adolescents. *Biol Psychiatry* 2011; 70:1179–1187.

16. Findling RL, et al. Safety and efficacy from an 8 week double-blind trial and a 26 week open-label extension of asenapine in adolescents with schizophrenia. *J Child Adolesc Psychopharmacol* 2015; 25:384–396.

17. Findling RL, et al. Ziprasidone in adolescents with schizophrenia: results from a placebo-controlled efficacy and long-term open-extension study. *J Child Adolesc Psychopharmacol* 2013; 23:531–544.

18. Arango C, et al. Lurasidone compared to other atypical antipsychotic monotherapies for adolescent schizophrenia: a systematic literature review and network meta-analysis. *Eur Child Adolesc Psychiatry* 2020; 29:1195–1205.

19. Pagsberg AK, et al. Acute antipsychotic treatment of children and adolescents with schizophrenia-spectrum disorders: a systematic review and network meta-analysis. *J Am Acad Child Adolesc Psychiatry* 2017; 56:191–202.

20. Scahill L, et al. Sudden death in a patient with Tourette syndrome during a clinical trial of ziprasidone. *J Psychopharmacol* 2005; 19:205–206.

21. Blair J, et al. Electrocardiographic changes in children and adolescents treated with ziprasidone: a prospective study. *J Am Acad Child Adolesc Psychiatry* 2005; 44:73–79.

22. Jensen KG, et al. Change and dispersion of QT interval during treatment with quetiapine extended release versus aripiprazole in children and adolescents with first-episode psychosis: results from the TEA trial. *Psychopharmacology (Berl)* 2018; 235:681–693.

23. Correll CU Addressing adverse effects of antipsychotic treatment in young patients with schizophrenia. *J Clin Psychiatry* 2011; 72:e01.

24. Kumra S, et al. Childhood-onset schizophrenia. A double-blind clozapine-haloperidol comparison. *Arch Gen Psychiatry* 1996; 53:1090–1097.

25. Shaw P, et al. Childhood-onset schizophrenia: a double-blind, randomized clozapine-olanzapine comparison. *Arch Gen Psychiatry* 2006; 63:721–730.

26. Kumra S, et al. Clozapine and "high-dose" olanzapine in refractory early-onset schizophrenia: a 12-week randomized and double-blind comparison. *Biol Psychiatry* 2008; 63:524–529.

27. Schneider C, et al. Systematic review of the efficacy and tolerability of clozapine in the treatment of youth with early onset schizophrenia. *Eur Psychiatry* 2014; 29:1–10.

28. Agid O, et al. An algorithm-based approach to first-episode schizophrenia: response rates over 3 prospective antipsychotic trials with a retrospective data analysis. *J Clin Psychiatry* 2011; 72:1439–1444.

29. National Institute for Health and Care Excellence. Psychosis and schizophrenia in children and young people: recognition and management. Clinical Guidance 155 [CG155]. 2013 (last updated October 2016). https://www.nice.org.uk/guidance/cg155.

儿童和青少年焦虑障碍

诊断问题

大约 15% 的年轻人在 18 岁时经历过抑郁,而且这些年轻人往往存在明显的功能受损和伤害风险。与患有抑郁症的成年人相比,年轻人倾向于体验到更多易激惹、精力体力不足、失眠和体重改变,以及快感缺失和注意力不集中。这些症状可能与其他障碍下的表现重叠或者相似,或者会被最小化及间接归因为典型的青少年发展表现,这导致诊断困难。因此评估应由了解发育变异的医生进行,并能够准确识别年轻人的抑郁情绪。

临床指南

儿童和青少年的焦虑症状常随年龄增长而改善,可能与前额叶发育水平(尤其是执行功能)相平行。但是,焦虑障碍是一种痛苦并导致功能损害的疾病,需要尽快进行治疗。慢性压力可能对大脑发育产生明显的影响[4],焦虑症状导致的功能损害可能妨碍了年轻人获得正常的体验,后者对其社交、情感和认知发展至关重要。早期和有效的治疗可防止精神病理改变延续到成年期,例如,与不焦虑的年轻人相比,有焦虑障碍的年轻人在成年期患焦虑和抑郁的风险要高出 3 倍[5]。

目前,儿童和青少年焦虑障碍治疗指南在英国和美国可以获得。NICE 指南侧重儿童与青少年社交焦虑障碍的治疗,建议开展认知行为治疗(CBT),并且告诫在儿童和青少年中,不该将药物作为常规治疗[6]。美国儿童和青少年精神病学学会(AACAP)的指南则包含了对所有非强迫、非创伤后应激障碍的焦虑障碍的治疗[7]。AACAP 指南建议多模式治疗,包括心理教育、心理治疗(例如 12 次基于暴露的 CBT)以及药物治疗。对于中、重度焦虑症状,当功能损害导致难以参加心理治疗,或者心理治疗仅部分有效时,赞同使用药物。

儿童和青少年焦虑障碍的用药

用药以前

- **排除其他诊断**。焦虑症状可能与一系列精神障碍的症状相仿,包括抑郁症(注意力不集中、睡眠问题)、双相障碍(易激惹、睡眠问题、坐立不安)、对立违抗障碍(易激惹、对抗行为),精神病性障碍(社会退缩、坐立不安)、ADHD(注意涣散、坐立不安)、阿斯伯格综合征(社会退缩、社交技能不足、重复行为与活动),以及学习障碍。焦虑症状也可以与一系列内分泌疾病(甲状腺功能亢进、低血糖症、嗜铬细胞瘤)、神经系统疾病(偏头痛、癫痫发作、谵妄、脑肿瘤)、心血管病(心律失常)、呼吸系统疾病(哮喘)和铅中毒等症状类似。焦虑样症状可见于一些药物或者精神活性物的反应,包括抗哮喘药、拟交感神经药、类固醇、SSRI、抗精神病药(静坐不能不良反应)、减肥药、感冒药、咖啡因和能量饮料。
- **小心 SSRI 的禁忌证和潜在的相互作用**。
- **评估基线的严重程度**。结构化的访谈,包括焦虑障碍访谈量表(ADIS)和情感障碍与精神分裂症的 Kiddie 量表(Kiddie SADS);问卷,包括修订版儿童抑郁与焦虑量表(RCADS)、儿童焦虑和相关情感障碍筛查问卷(SCARED)或儿童多维焦虑量表(MASC);功能损害的评估工具包括儿童总体评估量表(CGAS)。

- **获得同意**。与儿童及其家人讨论治疗方案(如药物名称、起始剂量、估计的终末剂量、加药时间表、可能的不良反应及其监测或减轻策略,监测进展情况的方法、对难治性病例的干预方案)。书面记录同意情况。

处方什么药物

- **SSRI 是儿童和青少年焦虑障碍治疗的可选药物**。一项荟萃分析,纳入了 7 个随机对照试验(<16 周;治疗组 446 例,对照组 386 例),检验 SSRI(氟西汀、氟伏沙明、帕罗西汀、舍曲林)对年轻焦虑障碍患者功能损害的影响(CGI-I)。结果提示,相对于安慰剂,治疗反应的总体比值比为 4.6(95% CI=3.1~7.5),焦虑症状的平均改善为 5.2(95% CI=2.8~8.8)[8]。儿童焦虑多模式研究(CAMS)显示,舍曲林单药治疗的有效率为 55%,CBT 的有效率为 60%,均高于安慰剂的有效率 24%;舍曲林联合 CBT 是最成功的,其有效率为 81%[9]。一项网络荟萃分析发现,SSRI 可以显著减少临床医师和父母(但不包括儿童)报告的焦虑症状,并增加缓解率[10]。一项网络荟萃分析显示,与其他药物相比,SSRI 治疗有效的可能性更高。另有荟萃分析表明,显著的临床治疗效果通常在治疗的第 6 周出现,并且与其他药物相比,SSRI 可以提供更快、更大的改善[11]。在耐受性方面,SSRI 是耐受性最好的一类药物,尤其是艾司西酞普兰和氟西汀[12]。

  舍曲林、氟西汀、氟伏沙明已被美国 FDA 批准治疗儿童强迫症,氟西汀和艾司西酞普兰被批准治疗儿童抑郁症。2004 年,美国 FDA 发布了黑框警告,提醒关注与 SSRI 相关的抑郁、激越和自杀观念的恶化现象。这些关注是基于青少年抑郁的研究综述,而不是基于年轻焦虑障碍患者。

- **SNRI**。2 个短期随机对照试验对文拉法辛进行了研究(治疗组 294 例,对照组 311 例),1 项短期随机对照试验(治疗组 135 例,对照组 137 例)对度洛西汀进行了测试,2 项短期随机对照试验对托莫西汀进行了测试。与安慰剂相比,SNRI 治疗有效的总体优势比为 2.4(95% CI=1.7~3.6)[8]。与安慰剂相比,SNRI 确实对焦虑症状的改善具有统计学意义,平均差异为 2.5(95% CI=0.1~5.1)[8]。前述网络荟萃分析发现,SNRI 显著减少了临床医师报告的(但不是父母或儿童报告的)焦虑症状[10]。因为 SSRI 更有效,耐受性更好[8],所以当使用两种 SSRI 试验治疗无效时,SNRI 可以作为焦虑障碍的三线治疗。

- $5HT_{1A}$ 受体部分激动剂,1 项短期随机对照试验(治疗组 334 例,对照组 225 例)发现,丁螺环酮的疗效不显著[OR 1.3(95% CI=0.7~3.4)],与焦虑症状改善无关[OR 0.8(95% CI=-3.1~4.8)][13]。

- α_2 受体激动剂,胍法辛在 1 项短期 RCT 中被评估(治疗组 62 例,对照组 21 例),发现与治疗反应的优势比相关[5.6(95% CI=1.4~26.8)],但与安慰剂相比,焦虑症状的平均改善程度不高[3.4(95% CI=-3.2~10)][14]。

- 苯二氮䓬类药物和三环类抗抑郁药的使用均未得到儿童对照试验的支持[8]。苯二氮䓬类药物还可能导致一些儿童出现矛盾性的脱抑制反应。尽管如此,在临床实践中有时会考虑使用长效苯二氮䓬类药物缓解 SSRI 初始加量期间的失能焦虑,以及获得快速镇静(表 5.5)。

表 5.5 总结了焦虑障碍的治疗药物和剂量。

表 5.5　儿童和青少年焦虑障碍治疗药物的常用剂量

药物	起始剂量/mg	剂量范围/mg·d^{-1}
SSRI		
舍曲林	12.5~25	25~200
氟西汀	5~10	10~60
氟伏沙明	12.5~25	50~200(若 >50,分 2 次服)
帕罗西汀	5~10	10~40
西酞普兰 *	5~10	10~40
SNRI		
文拉法辛缓释剂	37.5	37.5~225
度洛西汀	30	30~120
α$_2$ 受体激动剂		
胍法辛	1	1~6
5-HT$_{1A}$ 部分激动剂		
丁螺环酮 *	5,每天 3 次	15~60
苯二氮䓬类 *(需要时)		
氯硝西泮	0.25~0.5	
罗拉	0.5~1	

* 该治疗没有随机对照试验证据支持。

注:剂量始终要对照最新正式指南,如《英国国家处方集(儿童部分)》。

■ 用药以后

■ 急性期

- 最低剂量起始。
- 监测不良反应。SSRI 治疗焦虑年轻焦虑障碍患者时往往耐受性好。精神不良反应包括焦虑症状加重、易怒和脱抑制反应。躯体不良反应包括胃肠道症状(如恶心、呕吐、消化不良、腹痛、腹泻、便秘)、头痛、活动增多、失眠。这些不良反应往往轻微而短暂。
- 在 SSRI 治疗 1 周后(SNRI 为 2 周),若儿童的服药依从性好,不良反应轻微,则每周加量 1 次,至最低治疗剂量。
- 经常且系统地监测不良反应(请参照上面列出的内容)和疗效(如 RCADS、SCARED MASC、CGAS、CGI-I)。
- 由于儿童代谢较快,SSRI 的治疗剂量通常与成年人剂量相当。
- 疗效将在治疗的 6~8 周开始出现。向家属交代这一点非常重要。
- 若部分有效或无效,应当考虑诊断的准确性,药物是否足量、足疗程以及患者依从性。
- 改善疗效可以考虑:增加 CBT,换药(如换用 SSRI、其他类药物),或者联用药物(如治疗共病、不良反应、增效的药物)。有人提出了丁螺环酮、苯二氮䓬类、非典型抗精神病药和兴奋剂的增效策略,但缺乏经验支持 [7]。

- 维持期
  - 在保持稳定进步的前提下,继续维持治疗 1 年以上。
  - 定期监测疗效和不良反应。
- 停药期
  - 由于不了解药物长期安全性的信息,以及随着年龄和学习阶段症状改善的可能性,经过一定时间的稳定改善以后可以考虑停止治疗。尝试停药的时机应当选择压力和要求较低的时期。若药物不再起效,或者不良反应过于严重,也应考虑停药。逐渐减少 SSRI 剂量(每周 25%~50%),以降低撤药症状的风险。密切监测症状的复燃或复发;若注意到症状恶化,应立即重启药物治疗。

特殊事项

对学龄前儿童,焦虑障碍的治疗应当常规地以心理治疗为中心。在罕见情况下,低龄儿童有极其严重的持续的症状和功能损害,此时医师应当重新考虑诊断和个案概念化,重新评估心理治疗是否充分。对于学龄前儿童焦虑障碍,没有药物治疗的随机对照试验,但个案报告提示氟西汀和丁螺环酮有潜在的益处[15]。因此,给学龄前儿童开具的任何处方都属于超说明书用药[16]。

参考文献

1. Kessler RC, et al. Lifetime prevalence and age-of-onset distributions of DSM-IV disorders in the National Comorbidity Survey Replication. *Arch Gen Psychiatry* 2005; 62:593–602.

2. Merikangas KR, et al. Lifetime prevalence of mental disorders in U.S. adolescents: results from the National Comorbidity Survey Replication–Adolescent Supplement (NCS-A). *J Am Acad Child Adolesc Psychiatry* 2010; 49:980–989.

3. Simonoff E, et al. Psychiatric disorders in children with autism spectrum disorders: prevalence, comorbidity, and associated factors in a population-derived sample. *J Am Acad Child Adolesc Psychiatry* 2008; 47:921–929.

4. Danese A, et al. Adverse childhood experiences, allostasis, allostatic load, and age-related disease. *Physiol Behav* 2012; 106:29–39.

5. Pine DS, et al. The risk for early-adulthood anxiety and depressive disorders in adolescents with anxiety and depressive disorders. *Arch Gen Psychiatry* 1998; 55:56–64.

6. National Institute for Health and Clinical Excellence. Social anxiety disorder: recognition, assessment and treatment. Clinical Guidance 159 2013 (last checked June 2017); https://www.nice.org.uk/guidance/cg159.

7. Connolly SD, et al. Practice parameter for the assessment and treatment of children and adolescents with anxiety disorders. *J Am Acad Child Adolesc Psychiatry* 2007; 46:267–283.

8. Dobson ET, et al. Efficacy and tolerability of pharmacotherapy for pediatric anxiety disorders: a network meta-analysis. *J Clin Psychiatry* 2019; 80:17r12064.

9. Walkup JT, et al. Cognitive behavioral therapy, sertraline, or a combination in childhood anxiety. *N Engl J Med* 2008; 359:2753–2766.

10. Wang Z, et al. Comparative effectiveness and safety of cognitive behavioral therapy and pharmacotherapy for childhood anxiety disorders: a systematic review and meta-analysis. *JAMA Pediatrics* 2017; 171:1049–1056.

11. Strawn JR, et al. The impact of antidepressant dose and class on treatment response in pediatric anxiety disorders: a meta-analysis. *J Am Acad Child Adolesc Psychiatry* 2018; 57:235–244.e232.

12. Solmi M, et al. Safety of 80 antidepressants, antipsychotics, anti-attention-deficit/hyperactivity medications and mood stabilizers in children and adolescents with psychiatric disorders: a large scale systematic meta-review of 78 adverse effects. *World Psychiatry Off J World Psychiatric Assoc (WPA)* 2020; 19:214–232.

13. Strawn JR, et al. Buspirone in children and adolescents with anxiety: a review and Bayesian analysis of abandoned randomized controlled trials. *J Child Adolesc Psychopharmacol* 2018; 28:2–9.

14. Strawn JR, et al. Extended release guanfacine in pediatric anxiety disorders: a pilot, randomized, placebo-controlled trial. *J Child Adolesc Psychopharmacol* 2017; 27:29–37.

15. Gleason MM, et al. Psychopharmacological treatment for very young children: contexts and guidelines. *J Am Acad Child Adolesc Psychiatry* 2007; 46:1532–1572.

16. Mohatt J, et al. Treatment of separation, generalized, and social anxiety disorders in youths. *Am J Psychiatry* 2014; 171:741–748.

儿童和青少年强迫症和躯体变形障碍

儿童和青少年强迫症(OCD)和躯体变形障碍(BDD)的治疗原则与成年人相同(见第 3 章)。躯体变形障碍现在被 DSM-5 和 ICD-11 认定为强迫症谱系障碍的一种。CBT 对这两种疾病均有效,被 NICE 推荐为首选治疗方法[1,2],但是可合并药物治疗[3]。至少 2% 的青少年患有躯体变形障碍,但一直诊断不足[4]。NICE 建议对高风险人群进行躯体变形障碍的常规筛查,例如企图自杀或自伤者,或患有抑郁症、社交恐惧症、酒精或物质滥用、强迫症或进食障碍症状者,或者有轻度面部缺陷或瑕疵、寻求美容或皮肤科手术者[5]。

药物治疗

舍曲林[6-8](从 6 岁开始)和**氟伏沙明**(从 8 岁开始)在英国是被批准用于治疗儿童强迫症的 SSRI。历经 20 年的安慰剂对照研究已经确定了 SSRI 在儿童患者中的疗效。纳入 12 项随机对照试验的荟萃分析发现,在年轻人中,药物的疗效始终明显优于安慰剂[9]。舍曲林和氟西汀疗效相当,氟伏沙明可能逊色一些[9]。最初的荟萃分析表明,SSRI 治疗年轻人的强迫症具有中至大的效应值,但是最新的分析提出的效应值约为 0.43(介于"小"和"中度"之间)[9]。帕罗西汀不推荐用于儿童和年轻人。

氯米帕明对于一些患者仍然是有用的药物,尽管它的不良反应(镇静、口干、便秘、心血管潜在不良反应)往往限制了它在该人群中的使用。关于氯米帕明治疗年轻人的强迫症是否比 SSRI 有效一直存在争论。对于患强迫症的青年人,SSRI 通常仍然是推荐的首选药物。在英国,没有许可治疗成年人或儿童躯体变形障碍的药物。现有证据表明,SSRI 可显著改善躯体变形障碍症状和经常伴发的抑郁症状[10]。NICE 推荐氟西汀用于治疗儿童和青少年的躯体变形障碍。

尽管 50% 的躯体变形障碍病例对其外表存在妄想强度的信念,但使用抗精神病药并无益处。对成年人的研究表明,有这种信念的患者与非妄想患者一样,SSRI 单药治疗有效[10]。

开始药物治疗

最早在开始治疗 1~2 周后,SSRI 都类似地对症状产生缓慢而逐渐增强的效果,且相对于安慰剂的进步持续 24 周以上。在某些病例中,药物对情绪的积极影响可能先于强迫症或躯体变形障碍的症状改善[11]。对强迫症或躯体变形障碍核心症状的影响,可能需要几周到几个月才能显现。因此,在英国 NICE 建议对强迫症或躯体变形障碍进行为期三个月的 SSRI 治疗试验,逐渐增加至最大有效耐受剂量。向患者仔细解释药物的时间效应,对于维持依从性非常重要。另外,病情改善的最早迹象可能先由知情人发现,后由患者本人察觉。因此,在临床中使用他评定量评估工具,如儿童耶鲁-布朗强迫量表[12](CY-BOCS)或体象障碍评定量表(BDD-YBOCS)[13],可以帮助监测病情进展情况。英国精神药理协会建议,从最低有效剂量开始,持续治疗 12 周再评估其疗效[14]。此时如果临床疗效不充分,建议增加剂量。

给儿童处方 SSRI

2004 年,因为有可能增加自杀观念的风险,英国医疗保健品监管机构(MHRA)对 SSRI

在儿童和年轻人中的使用提出警告[15]。在强迫症和躯体变形障碍中,风险收益比明显不同于抑郁症。对治疗数据的仔细再分析显示,SSRI 对强迫症患者的疗效明显优于对儿童和年轻的中度抑郁症患者的疗效[16]。研究者认为,在所有研究中,儿童强迫症患者中自杀观念和自杀未遂的总风险低于 1%。这是一个确切的重要风险,应该向家属解释,并进行细心的监测。未经治疗的强迫症和身体变形障碍,在自然病程中往往不会自发缓解,而且会导致严重的疾病。现在已经明确,未经治疗的强迫症和躯体变形障碍伴有非常明显的疾病,包括与一般人群相比,其自杀死亡的风险增加了 10 倍[10,17]。在做出有关治疗的知情选择时,需要仔细考虑这些因素,并与患者及其照顾者或家人讨论。

有些情况下,舍曲林、氟伏沙明以外的药物可以作为"超说明书"的药物谨慎适当地使用。NICE 的强迫症治疗指南建议[5],在使用氯米帕明之前,应当尝试 SSRI,因为氯米帕明容易出现不良反应,并需要进行心脏监测。选择其他药物时需考虑的因素包括合并其他障碍(如氟西汀治疗伴发抑郁的强迫症)、某种药物对其他家庭成员疗效良好、存在其他疾病,以及药物的价格和可获得性。一些年轻人可能有药物依从性的问题,在某些情况下,这可能影响制剂的选择。例如,与其他 SSRI 相比,氟西汀半衰期较长,依从性较差的年轻人可能更适合接受氟西汀治疗。有些儿童会觉得片剂或胶囊难以吞咽,但液体制剂在大多数国家难以获得许可。

一些年轻人不愿意接受 CBT。虽然 CBT 是强迫症和躯体变形障碍的主要治疗方案,但在某些情况下,单用药物治疗可能是唯一可行的选择。有些儿童的自知力很差,或者进行 CBT 特别困难,这通常包括那些有学习问题或者与自闭症谱系障碍的患者。躯体变形障碍的自知力通常比强迫症差,这反过来会影响患者参与心理治疗的动机。如果将药物用作唯一的循证治疗,则必须对这一决定保持审慎,以便定期重新评估患者参与 CBT 的动机和能力。

NICE 关于强迫症与躯体变形障碍的评估与治疗指南

2005 年,NICE 出版了年轻人和成年强迫症和躯体变形障碍的循证治疗指南。NICE 推荐一种"阶梯治疗"模式,依据临床严重程度和复杂程度递增治疗的强度[5]。评估强迫症的严重程度和影响,可以借助 CY-BOCS、BDD-YBOCS 或其他定量评估工具,既可以在基线时用,也可以作为有用的监测工具[12]。

儿童强迫症和躯体变形障碍的 CBT 和药物治疗

现有的研究令人信服地证实,CBT 优于安慰剂,故应当努力为强迫症和躯体变形障碍儿童找合适的有经验的认知行为治疗师。

直接对比 CBT、舍曲林以及二者联合治疗儿童和青少年的主要研究认为,开始治疗儿童强迫症时,应该单用 CBT,或者 CBT 与 SSRI 合用[2]。关于开始治疗时是单用 CBT,还是采用联合治疗,一直存在争论。在国际上,心理治疗和药物治疗相结合的趋势越来越明显,尤其是针对躯体变形障碍患者。有经验和经验不足的治疗师使用 CBT 的效果存在差异,而合用 SSRI 则被证明可以弥补这种差异[6]。

对一些儿童,尤其是发育障碍的儿童,CBT 是极具挑战性的。在许多情况下,调整治疗方案可能是有效的。然而,对于一些孩子来说,在暴露疗法中的焦虑体验可能是难以承受的。有时需要使用普萘洛尔等 β 受体阻滞剂,将焦虑伴随的躯体症状减轻到可以进行 CBT 的程度。

图 5.1 总结了 NICE 指南的治疗流程。

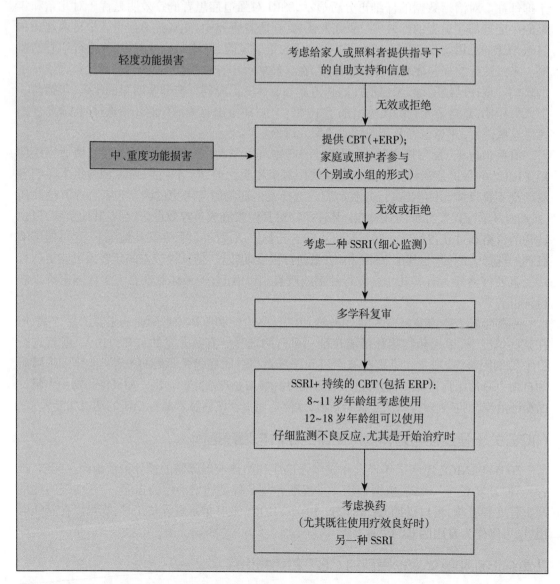

图 5.1   儿童和年轻强迫症或躯体变形障碍患者的治疗选择。CBT，认知行为治疗；ERP，暴露反应预防；
SSRI，5-羟色胺再摄取抑制剂（据 NICE 指南改编[5]，经允许复制[18]）

难治性儿童强迫症和躯体变形障碍

随机试验的证据提示，在接受药物治疗的患者中，3/4 有充分的疗效。因此，约 1/4 的儿童强迫症患者首次用 SSRI 治疗无效，尽管使用最大耐受剂量 12 周以上，且联合 CBT 和暴露反应预防。对这些儿童应当重新评估，明确其治疗依从性，并确保没有漏诊共病。这些儿童通常应当尝试至少一种其他 SSRI。研究提示，第二种 SSRI 会对约 40% 的强迫症[19]或躯体变形障碍[10]患者产生疗效。此后，如果疗效有限，通常应将儿童转诊到专科治疗中心。可以考虑尝试氯米帕明，或者合并小剂量利培酮或阿立哌唑以增强疗效[18,20]。研究提示，在两种

SSRI 充分治疗都无效以后,使用作用机制不同的药物(如利培酮或者氯米帕明)可能有益[11]。有证据表明,以可耐受的最高剂量 SSRI 治疗至少 3 个月疗效仍不充分的患者,"超说明书"使用抗精神病药作为增效剂,可能对患者有益。遗憾的是,在难治性成年患者中,只有 1/3 对这种增效治疗策略出现有意义的反应。因此,这些数据提示,对儿童和年轻的强迫症患者,应当慎用增效治疗策略。评估疗效时,为期 6 周低剂量抗精神病药物增效试验是必要的。如果发现无效,则必须停用。躯体变形障碍的治疗不存在相同的证据基础。如上所述,需要注意到,躯体变形障碍患者如果存在妄想程度的信念,则预示使用抗精神病药物会产生更好的疗效。

难治性儿童强迫症或躯体变形障碍患者通常会有共病,如孤独症谱系障碍、ADHD 或抽动障碍。这些共病对药物的疗效有不同的影响。例如,共病抽动症的患者以第二代抗精神病药增效治疗可能获益更多。未经治疗的 ADHD 患者由于注意力不集中,一般也会影响 CBT 的参与度。通常,通过适当治疗 ADHD(包括药物治疗),可以显著提高 CBT 的参与度。对于难治性强迫症或躯体变形障碍,仔细的临床评估以及重新个案概念化非常重要。应当考虑共病以及更广泛的心理社会因素对总体疗效的影响。临床经验往往表明,在治疗期间对家庭和护理人员的广泛支持至关重要。这通常需要帮助患者家庭放弃围绕强迫症或躯体变形障碍所形成的既定家庭模式。

疗程与长期随访

未治疗的强迫症将会呈现慢性病程。一系列成年人的研究显示,停药往往导致症状复发。一些作者提出,有共病者复发风险最高。考虑到研究中经常排除共病的情况,复发率很可能被低估了。NICE 指南建议,若某种药物对年轻患者有效,在完全缓解后,治疗应该持续至少 6 个月。临床经验提示,若打算终止治疗,应当缓慢、小心、以透明的方式与患者和家属一起进行。停药时,应当再次考虑仔细使用临床结局评估工具。停药通常与强迫症或躯体变形障碍的症状恶化相关。越来越多的成年人和年轻人被建议考虑长期服用 SSRI 药物以降低复发风险。成功地进行 CBT 后,有发育障碍的人常常难以概括治疗后的经验。因此,治疗后随访时,共同且贴切的回顾对此类人群是有益的。重要的是,在整个儿童期、青少年期直到成年期,强迫症或躯体变形障碍患者在需要时应该可以找到专业人员,获得治疗的机会以及其他支持。NICE 建议,若强迫症或躯体变形障碍复发,患者应当尽快就诊,而不是放在常规等待名单中。

参考文献

1. O'Kearney RT, et al. Behavioural and cognitive behavioural therapy for obsessive compulsive disorder in children and adolescents. *Cochrane Database Syst Rev* 2006:CD004856.

2. Freeman JB, et al. Cognitive behavioral treatment for young children with obsessive-compulsive disorder. *Biol Psychiatry* 2007; **61**:337–343.

3. Mancuso E, et al. Treatment of pediatric obsessive-compulsive disorder: a review. *J Child Adolesc Psychopharmacol* 2010; **20**:299–308.

4. National & Specialist OCD BDD and Related Disorders Service for Young People Maudsley Hospital. *Appearance Anxiety: A book on BDD for Young People, Families and Professionals*. Jessica Kingsley Publications; 2019.

5. National Institute for Clinical Excellence. Obsessive-compulsive disorder: core interventions in the treatment of obsessive-compulsive disorder and body dysmorphic disorder. *Clinical Guidance* 2005; **31** [CG31]. https://www.nice.org.uk/guidance/cg31.

6. The Pediatric OCD Treatment Study Team (POTS). Cognitive-behavior therapy, sertraline, and their combination for children and adolescents with obsessive-compulsive disorder: the Pediatric OCD Treatment Study (POTS) randomized controlled trial. *JAMA* 2004; **292**:1969–1976.

7. Geller DA, et al. Which SSRI? A meta-analysis of pharmacotherapy trials in pediatric obsessive-compulsive disorder. *Am J Psychiatry* 2003; 160:1919–1928.

8. March JS, et al. Treatment benefit and the risk of suicidality in multicenter, randomized, controlled trials of sertraline in children and adolescents. *J Child Adolesc Psychopharmacol* 2006; 16:91–102.

9. Kotapati VP, et al. The effectiveness of selective serotonin reuptake inhibitors for treatment of obsessive-compulsive disorder in adolescents and children: a systematic review and meta-analysis. *Frontiers Psychiatry* 2019; 10:523.

10. Phillips KA, et al. Treating body dysmorphic disorder with medication: evidence, misconceptions, and a suggested approach. *Body Image* 2008; 5:13–27.

11. Bloch MH, et al. Assessment and management of treatment-refractory obsessive-compulsive disorder in children. *J Am Acad Child Adolesc Psychiatry* 2015; 54:251–262.

12. Scahill L, et al. Children's Yale-Brown Obsessive Compulsive Scale: reliability and validity. *J Am Acad Child Adolesc Psychiatry* 1997; 36:844–852.

13. Phillips KA, et al. A severity rating scale for body dysmorphic disorder: development, reliability, and validity of a modified version of the Yale-Brown Obsessive Compulsive Scale. *Psychopharmacol Bull* 1997; 33:17–22.

14. Baldwin DS, et al. Evidence-based pharmacological treatment of anxiety disorders, post-traumatic stress disorder and obsessive-compulsive disorder: a revision of the 2005 guidelines from the British Association for Psychopharmacology. *J Psychopharmacol* 2014; 28:403–439.

15. Medicines and Healthcare Products Regulatory Agency. Report of the CSM expert working group on the safety of selective serotonin reuptake inhibitor antidepressants. 2005; https://www.neuroscience.ox.ac.uk/publications/474047.

16. Garland J, et al. Update on the use of SSRIs and SNRIs with children and adolescents in clinical practice. *J Can Acad Child Adolesc Psychiatry* 2016; 25:4–10.

17. Fernandez de la Cruz L, et al. Suicide in obsessive-compulsive disorder: a population-based study of 36 788 Swedish patients. *Mol Psychiatry* 2017; 22:1626–1632.

18. Heyman I, et al. Obsessive-compulsive disorder. *BMJ* 2006; 333:424–429.

19. Grados M, et al. Pharmacotherapy in children and adolescents with obsessive-compulsive disorder. *Child Adolesc Psychiatr Clin N Am* 1999; 8:617–634, x.

20. Bloch MH, et al. A systematic review: antipsychotic augmentation with treatment refractory obsessive-compulsive disorder. *Mol Psychiatry* 2006; 11:622–632.

扩展阅读

Nazeer A, et al. Obsessive-compulsive disorder in children and adolescents: epidemiology, diagnosis and management. *Translational Pediatrics* 2020; 9:S76–S93.

儿童与青少年创伤后应激障碍

诊断问题

创伤事件和创伤后应激障碍(PTSD)在年轻人中很常见。在 18 岁之前,1/3 的儿童经历过创伤性事件,接近 1/13 的儿童出现 PTSD[1]。在高危人群(如急诊患者、接受法医鉴定者、难民和寻求庇护者)中,青少年 PTSD 的发病率要高得多。患有 PTSD 的年轻人,自伤(近 50%)和自杀未遂(20%)的风险较高,并且通常出现社会功能受损,例如不升学、不就业且不接受职业培训(NEET,啃老)(超过 25%)[1]。值得注意的是,超过 3/4 的年轻 PTSD 患者同时患有精神疾病,最常见的是抑郁症、品行障碍、酒精依赖以及广泛性焦虑症[1]。此外,PTSD 并不是遭受创伤的年轻人最常见的诊断——在一般人群中常见的疾病(例如抑郁症、品行障碍和酒精依赖)在遭受创伤的年轻人中也更常见[1]。

诊断 PTSD 的基础是三联征:侵入性再体验,回避创伤相关的刺激,以及创伤暴露后的高唤醒症状。由于对创伤记忆的异常处理,PTSD 的年轻患者会通过噩梦或难忍的、令人痛苦的记忆持续地重新体验创伤事件,这些体验往往就像发生在"此时此地"一样,但在儿童和青少年身上一般不会出现明显的分离症状或闪回。为了尽量减少再体验症状,PTSD 的年轻患者通常会形成或公开或隐蔽的回避策略,让自己忙碌或分心,或远离引发回想创伤事件的人或地方。由于上述症状,PTSD 年轻患者经常感受到持续的威胁,因此表现出生理性的过度觉醒,对危险表现出警觉、易怒,并且难以专注于日常工作。由于临床表现多种多样,评估与治疗儿童和青少年 PTSD 的医师,应当对暴露于创伤的儿童的临床表现富有经验,而且能够从症状表现中理解发育的变异。

临床指南

NICE 指南[2]建议:儿童与青少年的创伤后应激障碍治疗应侧重于心理治疗。针对单一创伤事件导致的创伤后应激障碍,进行 12 次以创伤为焦点的认知行为治疗(TF-CBT);针对慢性或复发事件导致的 PTSD,进行更长时间的心理治疗。如果 TF-CBT 无效,根据年轻人的喜好,治疗还可以包括眼动脱敏和再加工(EMDR)。

根据目前的 NICE 指南[2]、美国儿童和青少年精神病学学会[3]和国际创伤应激研究学会[4](ISTSS)的证据,不推荐使用药物治疗儿童与青少年 PTSD。目前,关于成年人药物治疗(SSRI 和第二代抗精神病药)有效性的证据也有限[5,6]。然而,由于合并症的发生率很高[1],针对同时发生的精神疾病可能需要药物治疗。在成年人 PTSD 中,最受支持的治疗方法是氟西汀、帕罗西汀和文拉法辛[7]。MDMA[8]和致幻剂也有应用前景[9]。这些药物目前都没有在儿童和青少年中得到任何使用。

参考文献

1. Lewis SJ, et al. The epidemiology of trauma and post-traumatic stress disorder in a representative cohort of young people in England and Wales. *Lancet Psychiatry* 2019; 6:247–256.
2. National Institute for Clinical Excellence. Post-traumatic stress disorder. NICE guideline [NG116] 2018; https://www.nice.org.uk/guidance/NG116.

3. Cohen JA, et al. Practice parameter for the assessment and treatment of children and adolescents with posttraumatic stress disorder. *J Am Acad Child Adolesc Psychiatry* 2010; 49:414–430.

4. International Society for Traumatic Stress Studies (ISTSS). Posttraumatic stress disorder prevention and treatment guidelines: methodology and recommendations 2019; https://istss.org/getattachment/Treating-Trauma/New-ISTSS-Prevention-and-Treatment-Guidelines/ISTSS_PreventionTreatmentGuidelines_FNL-March-19-2019.pdf.aspx.

5. Cipriani A, et al. Comparative efficacy and acceptability of pharmacological treatments for post-traumatic stress disorder in adults: a network meta-analysis. *Psychol Med* 2018; 48:1975–1984.

6. Huang ZD, et al. Comparative efficacy and acceptability of pharmaceutical management for adults with post-traumatic stress disorder: a systematic review and meta-analysis. *Front Pharmacol* 2020; 11:559.

7. Ehret M. Treatment of posttraumatic stress disorder: focus on pharmacotherapy. *Ment Health Clin* 2019; 9:373–382.

8. Jerome L, et al. Long-term follow-up outcomes of MDMA-assisted psychotherapy for treatment of PTSD: a longitudinal pooled analysis of six phase 2 trials. *Psychopharmacology (Berl)* 2020; 237:2485–2497.

9. Krediet E, et al. Reviewing the potential of psychedelics for the treatment of PTSD. *Int J Neuropsychopharmacol* 2020; 23:385–400.

第 5 章

注意缺陷多动障碍

儿童注意缺陷多动障碍（ADHD）

- 儿童 ADHD 的诊断只能在经过专家的全面评估以后方能做出 [1]。对 ADHD 应该实施合适的心理、社会和行为干预。药物治疗应该只是整个治疗计划的一部分。
- 药物治疗的适应证：在环境改良、家长培训（如果合适）、提出养育策略的建议以及与学校联络之后，ADHD 造成的功能损害仍然存在。
- **哌甲酯**通常是有用药适应证时的首选药物。它是一种中枢神经系统兴奋性药物，有大量研究证据的支持。最常见的不良反应包括失眠、抑制食欲、血压升高、脉搏加快以及生长速度减慢。根据不良反应情况，通常可以通过对症处理、中断治疗或减少剂量进行处理。在英国，有几种不同释放特性的缓释制剂可以选用，包括仿制药（框 5.2）。

框 5.2 NICE 儿童注意缺陷多动障碍指南概要 [1]

- 药物治疗应该仅由专科医师在综合评估患者的精神、躯体健康状况以及社会功能影响后开始使用。对于 5 岁以下的儿童，应该在 ADHD 卫生服务机构（最好是三级服务机构）提供第二份专家意见后开始用药，该机构应当具备管理幼儿 ADHD 的专业背景。
- 对于 5 岁以下 ADHD 儿童，应当向其父母或照顾者提供以 ADHD 为焦点的家长培训方案。在所有情况下都需要实施环境改良。如果在环境改良之后，ADHD 症状仍然在至少一个领域造成持续性的显著损害，可以在基线评估后提供药物治疗。
- 建议按已被批准的适应证使用哌甲酯、赖右苯丙胺、右苯丙胺、托莫西汀和胍法辛。
- 短效或长效的哌甲酯是首选药物。
- 5 岁及以上儿童和年轻人，若已经试用 6 周的足量哌甲酯，但在减轻 ADHD 症状和相关损害方面没有获得足够益处，可以考虑改用赖右苯丙胺。
- 5 岁及以上儿童和年轻人，若使用赖右苯丙胺后改善了 ADHD，但是却不能长期耐受其不良反应，可以考虑右苯丙胺。
- 5 岁及以上儿童和年轻人，若不能耐受哌甲酯或赖右苯丙胺，或者分别进行 6 周的哌甲酯和赖右苯丙胺后没有反应，那么在考虑替代制剂和足够剂量后，可以提供托莫西汀或胍法辛。
- 监测指标应该包括测量身高和体重（输入生长图中），以及血压和心率。开始服用兴奋剂、托莫西汀或胍法辛之前，检查心电图（ECG）并非必须的，除非患者有下列情况之一：
  - 先天性心脏病史、既往心脏手术史
  - 40 岁以下一级亲属猝死病史，提示心脏病
  - 与同龄人相比，劳累时呼吸急促
  - 因劳累而晕倒，或因惊吓、噪声而晕倒
  - 快速、规律出现且突发突止的心悸
  - 心源性胸痛
  - 心力衰竭的症状
  - 心脏检查时听到杂音
  - 成年人高血压
  - 正在使用可能会增加心脏病风险的药物
  如果存在上述任何一种情况，应咨询心血管内科医师的意见。

第 5 章

- **右苯丙胺**是另一种可选的中枢神经系统兴奋性药物。其疗效和不良反应大体与哌甲酯相同，但疗性和安全性的证据要比哌甲酯少得多，且更有可能被挪用和滥用。哌甲酯和右苯丙胺均属于附表 2 管制药品，处方应当准确书写（总量用文字和数字表示），且最大的处方供应量为 30 天（在英国）。

- **赖右苯丙胺**是一种"前体药"——右苯丙胺与赖氨酸结合时没有活性。在红细胞里逐渐分解以后，右苯丙胺被逐渐释放出来。它与哌甲酯缓释制剂有类似的作用机制，所以二者类似，不太可能用于娱乐，或者被依赖症驱使而被滥用。几项随机对照试验证明，它对儿童[2,3]和青少年[4]的疗效优于安慰剂。初期的研究表明，其效应值至少和哌甲酯口崩片[3]一样大，不良反应也类似[5,6]。近期的网络荟萃分析发现，赖右苯丙胺比哌甲酯[7,8]有效，而且长期治疗的数据提示，可以考虑将它作为哌甲酯缓释制剂的替代药物[9]。

- **托莫西汀**[10-13]是一种非兴奋性替代药物。它尤其适合以下情况的儿童：兴奋剂无效、兴奋剂被挪用到非医疗领域成为棘手的问题，以及兴奋剂引起的"多巴胺能"不良反应（如抽动、焦虑和刻板）成为问题。应当告诫父母，使用该药可能出现自杀想法和肝脏疾病，并叮嘱他们注意其他可能发生的问题。托莫西汀不如兴奋剂有效[7,8,11,14,15]。

- 其他药物包括 α_2 激动剂可乐定[16]和胍法辛。2016 年 1 月，英国批准了一种胍法辛缓释制剂[17]，用于 ADHD 儿童，可被视为托莫西汀的非兴奋性替代药物。

- 有一些证据支持**三环类抗抑郁药**[18,19]的疗效，但在临床实践中不推荐使用。

- **安非他酮**[8,20,21]似乎有效，且耐受性良好。**莫达非尼**似乎在儿童中也似乎有效，但在患有 ADHD 的成年人中则没有作用[8,22,23]。与标准疗法相比，支持使用这些药物的证据有限[8]。

- 不推荐使用**第二代抗精神病药**[24,25]治疗 ADHD。这些药物可以减少孤独症谱系障碍[26]患者的多动症状，但不宜用于 ADHD。

- 共病精神疾病在 ADHD 儿童中常见。在总体上，兴奋剂常是有帮助的，但不太适合用于有精神病性障碍的儿童。在 ADHD 治疗[27]的同时，对物质滥用问题应该进行处理，而且需要谨慎地选择治疗方案。

- 虽然兴奋剂和托莫西汀联合治疗已经被使用，但是很少有临床试验，也没有明确的证据表明疗效有所改善[28]。

- 一旦确定兴奋剂治疗，后续可以由全科医师开处方[1]。

成年人 ADHD

在成年人中首次诊断 ADHD，既符合 ICD-11，也符合 DSM-5。NICE 指南把药物治疗作为一线治疗，治疗原则与儿童患者相同（表 5.6）。

- 大约 65% 的 ADHD 患者在成年后仍符合全部标准或只达到部分缓解[29]。对于成年期症状仍然损害其功能的患者，应该继续使用始于儿童期的治疗。

- 首次诊断成年人 ADHD 之前，需要进行综合评估。应该尽可能包括向其他知情者收集信息，以及向熟悉患者童年情况的成年人收集信息。在评估 ADHD 的症状和功能损害时，建议使用有效的诊断性访谈工具，例如，DSM-Ⅳ ADHD 诊断性访谈（DIVA）[30]。

- 在童年有 ADHD 但未被发现的成年人中，物质滥用和反社会人格障碍的患病率较高[31]。哌甲酯对该人群可能有效[32]，但是开药和监测时应该慎重。

表 5.6 注意缺陷多动障碍的用药

药物	起效和持续时间	剂量	述评	推荐的监测/一般注意事项
哌甲酯速释剂 品牌产品(利他林、Medikinet, Tranquilyn)和各种仿制药[33-35]	起效:20~60min 持续:2~4h	开始5~10mg/d, 每周增加5~10mg, 渐增到最高2.1mg/(kg·d), 分次服用。许可的最大剂量每天60mg(或经专家审查后每天最多90mg。注:未经许可)[1]	通常是一线治疗。一般耐受性好[36]	对于哌甲酯、右苯丙胺和赖右苯丙胺: 右苯丙胺: ■ 血压[37] ■ 脉搏 ■ 身高 ■ 体重 监测失眠、心境、食欲改变和抽动[38],但是一些证据表明抽动与兴奋剂无关[39] 1个月内无效则停药 属于管制药品
哌甲酯缓释剂*			一些儿童下午可能需要用哌甲酯速释剂以达到最佳疗效	
专注达 XL[33,34,40-42] 专注达 XL 的生物等效产品: Matoride XL, Xenidate XL, Xenidate XL, Delmosart缓释剂	起效:30min~2h 持续:12h	开始时18mg 晨服, 渐增到最高54mg(或在专家审查后, 每天最高可达108mg。注:未经许可) 18mg专注达=15mg哌甲酯速释剂	由22%速释成分和78%缓释成分组成	
Equasym XL[43,44]	起效:20~60min 持续:8h	开始时10mg 晨服, 渐增到许可的最高剂量60mg	由30%速释成分和70%缓释成分组成 胶囊可以打开后服用药物[45]	
Medikinet XL	起效:20~60min 持续:最长8h	剂量与Equasym XL相同	由50%速释成分和50%缓释成分组成。胶囊可以打开后服用药物	
利他林 XL(参考 SPC, 公开的评估报告)	起效:60min 持续:8~12h	剂量与Equasym XL相同	由50%速释成分和50%缓释成分组成	
右苯丙胺 速释剂[36,46]	起效:20~60min 持续:3~6h	2.5~10mg/d起始, 每周增加2.5~5mg, 最高到20mg/d(偶尔40mg/d), 分次服用	耐受性不如哌甲酯好[36]	
赖右苯丙胺 (Elvanse)[2-4]	起效:20~60min 持续:13h以上	开始时20mg 晨服, 渐增到许可的最高70mg	前体药, 逐渐水解为右苯丙胺 胶囊可以打开后服用药物[47] 许可用于成年人	

第 5 章

续表

药物	起效和持续时间	剂量	述评	推荐的监测/一般注意事项
托莫西汀[48,49]	4~6w（托莫西汀是去甲肾上腺素再摄取抑制剂）	若从兴奋剂换成该药，治疗头 4 周需继续使用兴奋剂 <70kg 儿童：从 0.5mg/(kg·d) 开始，持续 7 天，然后根据疗效增加 推荐维持剂量为 1.2mg/(kg·d)（单次或分次服用），最高剂量为 1.8mg/(kg·d)，必要时最高 120mg/d[1] >70kg 儿童：40mg/d 开始，持续 7 天，然后根据疗效增加。建议维持剂量 80mg/d	疗效不如兴奋剂（见"ADHD"）[11,15] 若兴奋剂转为非医疗用途成为问题，此药可能有用[50] 许可用于成年人	血压[51] 脉搏 身高 体重 监测失眠、情绪、食欲改变和抽动 监测患有 ADHD 的年轻人和成年人是否有性功能障碍（即勃起和射精功能障碍），这是托莫西汀的潜在不良反应。 非管制药物
胍法辛缓释剂[8,52]	1~5w[53]（胍法辛是一种中枢 α_{2A} 肾上腺素能受体激动剂）	6~12 岁儿童（体重≥25kg） 开始 1mg/d；如有必要且可耐受，每周调整 1mg；维持剂量为 0.05~0.12mg/(kg·d)（最大每剂 4mg） 13~17 岁儿童（体重 34~41.4kg） 开始 1mg/d；如有必要且可耐受，每周调整 1mg；维持剂量为 0.05~0.12mg/(kg·d)（最大每剂 4mg） 13~17 岁儿童（体重 41.5~49.4kg） 开始 1mg/d；如有必要且可耐受，每周调整 1mg；维持剂量为 0.05~0.12mg/(kg·d)（最大每剂 5mg） 13~17 岁儿童（体重 49.5~58.4kg） 开始 1mg/d；如有必要且可耐受，每周调整 1mg；维持剂量为 0.05~0.12mg/(kg·d)（最大每剂 6mg） 13~17 岁儿童（体重≥58.5kg） 开始 1mg/d；如必要且可耐受，每周调整 1mg；维持剂量为 0.05~0.12mg/(kg·d)（最大每剂 7mg）	疗效和耐受性数据应谨慎解读[8]	监测与其他治疗 ADHD 的药物类似

* 有关英国以外可用的其他制剂的详细信息，请参考 Cortese 等（2017）[54]。

第 5 章

- 治疗同时患有 ADHD 以及药物、酒精依赖的成年人时，ADHD 和成瘾障碍的专业人员应该保持密切联系。
- **哌甲酯**或**赖右苯丙胺**是成年人的首选药物[1]。
- 右苯丙胺可用于赖右苯丙胺治疗有效，但不能长期耐受其不良反应的 ADHD 成年患者
- 使用**托莫西汀**时，建议监测肝功能异常和自杀观念。
- **托莫西汀、赖右苯丙胺和两种哌甲酯缓释制剂**(Medikinet XL、Ritalin XL)已首次获准用于 ADHD 成年患者。如果在 18 岁之前使用 Concerta XL(哌甲酯的一种缓释制剂)，则允许成年后继续治疗使用。

NICE 成年人注意缺陷多动障碍指南概要[1]

- 仅应由专科医师在综合评估患者的精神、躯体健康状况以及社会功能影响后开始药物治疗。
- 如果在环境改良之后，成年人 ADHD 在至少一个方面仍然导致显著的功能损害，则应提供药物治疗。
- 若患者选择、依从性差或不良反应无法耐受，可以考虑非药物治疗(支持性治疗、CBT、定期复查)。在药物治疗部分有效时，也可以考虑联合药物治疗与非药物治疗。
- 建议将哌甲酯或赖右苯丙胺作为治疗 ADHD 成年患者的首选药物。在充足剂量试用 6 周后，若治疗效果欠佳，可以考虑在这两种药物之间切换。
- 右苯丙胺可用于赖右苯丙胺治疗有效，但无法长期耐受的 ADHD 成年患者。
- 如果符合以下条件，可以向成年人提供托莫西汀：
  - 不能耐受赖右苯丙胺或哌甲酯。
  - 赖右苯丙胺和哌甲酯试用 6 周无效，并考虑了替代制剂和足够的剂量后。
- 应该监测体重、血压和心率。与前述儿童和青少年的情况一致，应该考虑心内科的意见和心电图。

参考文献

1. National Institute for Health and Clinical Excellence. Attention deficit hyperactivity disorder: diagnosis and management. NICE guideline [NG87] 2018 (Last updated September 2019); https://www.nice.org.uk/guidance/NG87.

2. Biederman J, et al. Lisdexamfetamine dimesylate and mixed amphetamine salts extended-release in children with ADHD: a double-blind, placebo-controlled, crossover analog classroom study. *Biol Psychiatry* 2007; 62:970–976.

3. Coghill D, et al. European, randomized, phase 3 study of lisdexamfetamine dimesylate in children and adolescents with attention-deficit/hyperactivity disorder. *Eur Neuropsychopharmacol* 2013; 23:1208–1218.

4. Findling RL, et al. Efficacy and safety of lisdexamfetamine dimesylate in adolescents with attention-deficit/hyperactivity disorder. *J Am Acad Child Adolesc Psychiatry* 2011; 50:395–405.

5. Heal DJ, et al. Amphetamine, past and present – a pharmacological and clinical perspective. *J Psychopharmacol* 2013; 27:479–496.

6. Coghill DR, et al. Long-term safety and efficacy of lisdexamfetamine dimesylate in children and adolescents with ADHD: a phase IV, 2-year, open-label study in Europe. *CNS Drugs* 2017; 31:625–638.

7. Joseph A, et al. Comparative efficacy and safety of attention-deficit/hyperactivity disorder pharmacotherapies, including guanfacine extended release: a mixed treatment comparison. *Eur Child Adolesc Psychiatry* 2017; 26:875–897.

8. Cortese S, et al. Comparative efficacy and tolerability of medications for attention-deficit hyperactivity disorder in children, adolescents, and adults: a systematic review and network meta-analysis. *Lancet Psychiatry* 2018; 5:727–738.

9. Findling RL, et al. Long-term effectiveness and safety of lisdexamfetamine dimesylate in school-aged children with attention-deficit/hyperactivity disorder. *CNS Spectr* 2008; 13:614–620.

10. Michelson D, et al. Once-daily atomoxetine treatment for children and adolescents with attention deficit hyperactivity disorder: a randomized, placebo-controlled study. *Am J Psychiatry* 2002; 159:1896–1901.

11. Kratochvil CJ, et al. Atomoxetine and methylphenidate treatment in children with ADHD: a prospective, randomized, open-label trial. *J Am Acad Child Adolesc Psychiatry* 2002; **41**:776–784.

12. Weiss M, et al. A randomized, placebo-controlled study of once-daily atomoxetine in the school setting in children with ADHD. *J Am Acad Child Adolesc Psychiatry* 2005; **44**:647–655.

13. Kratochvil CJ, et al. A double-blind, placebo-controlled study of atomoxetine in young children with ADHD. *Pediatrics* 2011; **127**:e862–e868.

14. Catala-Lopez F, et al. The pharmacological and non-pharmacological treatment of attention deficit hyperactivity disorder in children and adolescents: a systematic review with network meta-analyses of randomised trials. *PLoS One* 2017; **12**:e0180355.

15. Liu Q, et al. Comparative efficacy and safety of methylphenidate and atomoxetine for attention-deficit hyperactivity disorder in children and adolescents: meta-analysis based on head-to-head trials. *J Clin Exp Neuropsychol* 2017; **39**:854–865.

16. Connor DF, et al. A meta-analysis of clonidine for symptoms of attention-deficit hyperactivity disorder. *J Am Acad Child Adolesc Psychiatry* 1999; **38**:1551–1559.

17. National Institute for Health and Care Excellence. Attention deficit hyperactivity disorder in children and young people: guanfacine prolonged-release. Evidence summary [ESNM70] 2016; https://www.nice.org.uk/advice/esnm70/chapter/Key-points-from-the-evidence.

18. Hazell P. Tricyclic antidepressants in children: is there a rationale for use? *CNS Drugs* 1996; **5**:233–239.

19. Otasowie J, et al. Tricyclic antidepressants for attention deficit hyperactivity disorder (ADHD) in children and adolescents. *Cochrane Database Syst Rev* 2014:Cd006997.

20. Gorman DA, et al. Canadian guidelines on pharmacotherapy for disruptive and aggressive behaviour in children and adolescents with attention-deficit hyperactivity disorder, oppositional defiant disorder, or conduct disorder. *Can J Psychiatry* 2015; **60**:62–76.

21. Ng QX. A systematic review of the use of bupropion for attention-deficit/hyperactivity disorder in children and adolescents. *J Child Adolesc Psychopharmacol* 2017; **27**:112–116.

22. Biederman J, et al. A comparison of once-daily and divided doses of modafinil in children with attention-deficit/hyperactivity disorder: a randomized, double-blind, and placebo-controlled study. *J Clin Psychiatry* 2006; **67**:727–735.

23. Wang SM, et al. Modafinil for the treatment of attention-deficit/hyperactivity disorder: a meta-analysis. *J Psychiatr Res* 2017; **84**:292–300.

24. Einarson TR, et al. *Novel antipsychotics for patients with attention-deficit hyperactivity disorder: a systematic review.* Ottawa: Canadian Coordinating Office for Health Technology Assessment (CCOHTA) 2001: Technology Report No 17.

25. Pringsheim T, et al. The pharmacological management of oppositional behaviour, conduct problems, and aggression in children and adolescents with attention-deficit hyperactivity disorder, oppositional defiant disorder, and conduct disorder: a systematic review and meta-analysis. Part 2: antipsychotics and traditional mood stabilizers. *Can J Psychiatry* 2015; **60**:52–61.

26. Ji N, et al. An update on pharmacotherapy for autism spectrum disorder in children and adolescents. *Current Opinion Psychiatry* 2015; **28**:91–101.

27. Humphreys KL, et al. Stimulant medication and substance use outcomes: a meta-analysis. *JAMA Psychiatry* 2013; **70**:740–749.

28. Treuer T, et al. A systematic review of combination therapy with stimulants and atomoxetine for attention-deficit/hyperactivity disorder, including patient characteristics, treatment strategies, effectiveness, and tolerability. *J Child Adolesc Psychopharmacol* 2013; **23**:179–193.

29. Thapar A, et al. Attention deficit hyperactivity disorder. *Lancet* 2016; **387**:1240–1250.

30. DIVA Foundation. DIVA-5: diagnostic interview for ADHD in adults (DIVA) 2019; https://www.divacenter.eu/DIVA.aspx?id=461.

31. Cosgrove PVF. Attention deficit hyperactivity disorder. *Primary Care Psychiatry* 1997; **3**:101–114.

32. Spencer T, et al. A double-blind, crossover comparison of methylphenidate and placebo in adults with childhood-onset attention-deficit hyperactivity disorder. *Arch Gen Psychiatry* 1995; **52**:434–443.

33. Wolraich ML, et al. Pharmacokinetic considerations in the treatment of attention-deficit hyperactivity disorder with methylphenidate. *CNS Drugs* 2004; **18**:243–250.

34. BNF Online. British National Formulary 2020; https://www.medicinescomplete.com/mc/bnf/current.

35. Janssen-Cilag Ltd. Summary of product characteristics. Concerta XL 18 mg 27 mg 36 mg and 54 mg prolonged-release tablets. 2020; https://www.medicines.org.uk/emc/product/6872/smpc.

36. Efron D, et al. Side effects of methylphenidate and dexamphetamine in children with attention deficit hyperactivity disorder: a double-blind, crossover trial. *Pediatrics* 1997; **100**:662–666.

37. Hennissen L, et al. Cardiovascular effects of stimulant and non-stimulant medication for children and adolescents with ADHD: a systematic review and meta-analysis of trials of methylphenidate, amphetamines and atomoxetine. *CNS Drugs* 2017; **31**:199–215.

38. Gadow KD, et al. Efficacy of methylphenidate for attention-deficit hyperactivity disorder in children with tic disorder. *Arch Gen Psychiatry* 1995; **52**:444–455.

39. Cohen SC, et al. Meta-analysis: risk of tics associated with psychostimulant use in randomized, placebo-controlled trials. *J Am Acad Child Adolesc Psychiatry* 2015; **54**:728–736.

40. Hoare P, et al. 12-month efficacy and safety of OROS MPH in children and adolescents with attention-deficit/hyperactivity disorder switched from MPH. *Eur Child Adolesc Psychiatry* 2005; **14**:305–309.

41. Remschmidt H, et al. Symptom control in children and adolescents with attention-deficit/hyperactivity disorder on switching from immediate-release MPH to OROS MPH results of a 3-week open-label study. *Eur Child Adolesc Psychiatry* 2005; **14**:297–304.

42. Wolraich ML, et al. Randomized, controlled trial of OROS methylphenidate once a day in children with attention-deficit/hyperactivity disorder. *Pediatrics* 2001; **108**:883–892.

43. Findling RL, et al. Comparison of the clinical efficacy of twice-daily ritalin and once-daily equasym XL with placebo in children with attention deficit/hyperactivity disorder. *Eur Child Adolesc Psychiatry* 2006; **15**:450–459.

44. Anderson VR, et al. Spotlight on methylphenidate controlled-delivery capsules (equasym XL™) in the treatment of children and adolescents with attention-deficit hyperactivity disorder. *CNS Drugs* 2007; **21**:173–175.

第 5 章

45. Flynn Pharma Ltd. Summary of Product Characteristics. Medikinet XL 5 mg 10 mg 20 mg 30 mg 40 mg 50 mg 60 mg modified release capsules 2019; https://www.medicines.org.uk/emc/product/313/smpc.

46. Cyr M, et al. Current drug therapy recommendations for the treatment of attention deficit hyperactivity disorder. *Drugs* 1998; **56**:215–223.

47. Shire Pharmaceuticals Limited. Summary of Product Characteristics. Elvanse 20 mg, 30 mg, 40 mg, 50 mg, 60 mg & 70 mg capsules, hard (lisdexamfetamine) 2019; https://www.medicines.org.uk/emc/medicine/27442.

48. Kelsey DK, et al. Once-daily atomoxetine treatment for children with attention-deficit/hyperactivity disorder, including an assessment of evening and morning behavior: a double-blind, placebo-controlled trial. *Pediatrics* 2004; **114**:e1-e8.

49. Wernicke JF, et al. Cardiovascular effects of atomoxetine in children, adolescents, and adults. *Drug Saf* 2003; **26**:729–740.

50. Heil SH, et al. Comparison of the subjective, physiological, and psychomotor effects of atomoxetine and methylphenidate in light drug users. *Drug Alcohol Depend* 2002; **67**:149–156.

51. Reed VA, et al. The safety of atomoxetine for the treatment of children and adolescents with attention-deficit/hyperactivity disorder: a comprehensive review of over a decade of research. *CNS Drugs* 2016; **30**:603–628.

52. Childress A, et al. Evaluation of the current data on guanfacine extended release for the treatment of ADHD in children and adolescents. *Expert Opin Pharmacother* 2020; **21**:417–426.

53. Takeda UK ltd. Guanfacine modified-release. Personal Communication, 2020.

54. Cortese S, et al. New formulations of methylphenidate for the treatment of attention-deficit/hyperactivity disorder: pharmacokinetics, efficacy, and tolerability. *CNS Drugs* 2017; **31**:149–160.

第 5 章

孤独症谱系障碍

孤独症谱系障碍(ASD)是以社交、行为(刻板行为、狭窄和非同寻常的兴趣模式)缺陷和感觉障碍为核心特征的一种复杂疾病。ASD 包括孤独症、阿斯伯格综合征及未在他处注明的广泛性发育障碍,在 ICD-10 里被归类于广泛性发育障碍,而 DSM-5 将孤独症谱系障碍定义为单一类别。

ASD 的异质性使得评估和治疗具有挑战性。ASD 的共病现象非常普遍[1],69%~79% 的ASD 患者一生中至少有过一种共病[2,3],包括注意缺陷多动障碍(ADHD)、破坏性行为障碍、焦虑症、强迫症和心境障碍。其他相关的异常还包括智力障碍、癫痫、睡眠紊乱、自伤、易激惹和攻击他人。与 ASD 相关的神经发育、躯体疾病和精神障碍使症状特征复杂化,并影响整体预后。因此,评估并以最佳方式治疗共病和异常行为至关重要。

目前,在缓解和治疗 ASD 的核心症状方面,尚没有验证有效的或被批准的药物[4,5]。但是,针对异常行为和共病的精神疾病,进行药物干预是常见的做法。

在 ASD 中,药物治疗常被用于辅助心理干预。迄今为止[4,6]的证据表明,利培酮、阿立哌唑对易激惹和攻击行为有一定的疗效,并支持使用哌甲酯、托莫西汀和胍法辛治疗 ADHD,使用褪黑素治疗睡眠问题,但 SSIR 对焦虑、抑郁和重复行为的疗效有限。抗癫痫药物的证据仍然不一致。α_2 激动剂、胆碱能激动剂、谷氨酸能、γ-氨基丁酸(GABA)能药和催产素都有潜在的作用,但需要进一步研究[4,6]。

相比于健康发育的人,ASD 患者可能会出现更严重的不良反应[4-6]。因此,达到有效剂量并保持最低的不良反应,很有挑战性。治疗应该从小剂量开始,大约每 5 个半衰期增加一次剂量,可能需要 4~6 周的滴定来确定每个个体的治疗剂量[7]。使用精神药物治疗问题行为之前,必须优先考虑排除躯体疾病、疼痛或任何其他身体不适(如胃食管反流)。全面的体检应当是标准治疗的一部分。

考虑到 ASD 患者沟通障碍,并且更容易出现不良反应,应该系统监测药物疗效和不良反应。标准化的行为量表和不良反应清单是必要的监测工具[8]。

孤独症谱系障碍核心症状的药物治疗

迄今为止,临床试验的证据还没有证明任何一种精神药物在常规治疗 ASD 核心症状方面有明确的疗效[4,6]。

局限、重复的行为和兴趣(RRBI)

RRBI 令人烦恼,并影响功能,因此是改善 ASD 总体结局的一个重要治疗目标[9]。行为治疗应该作为一线的治疗选择。若这些行为非常严重且对功能有显著影响,或给他人或自己造成危险,则应当考虑药物治疗。

Cochrane 综述发现(最近一次更新在 2013 年),尽管有数据支持 SSRI 在成年人中的使用,但"在儿童中没有证据表明 SSRI 对减少 RRBI 有效,相反,有害的证据却正在出现"[10]。有研究表明,利培酮能有效地降低易怒或攻击性高的儿童 RRBI[11],而对重复行为的任何具体疗效都是可疑的。也有报道称刻板行为有所减少[12-15],但是研究方法有局限性[6]。2020 年的一项荟萃分析对目前可用的主要药物进行了研究,结果认为只有抗精神病药物有效[16],而最近纳入 9 项研究的荟萃分析则认为,没有任何药物可以减少 RRBI[17]。考虑到多巴胺受体阻滞剂的不良反应,英国精神药理学协会[6]最新的指南告诫不要将其常规用于治疗 RRBI。如果使用这些药物,应使用低剂量,并在整个治疗进程中,做到慎重考虑、限定用药时间以及加以监测。

社交和沟通损害

目前为止,始终未发现有药物能改善 ASD 的社交和沟通损害[7]。利培酮可能通过改善易激惹而产生继发效应[18]。两个多中心试验的数据分析表明,利培酮治疗 ASD 的社会功能缺陷是有效的[19]。谷氨酸能药物和催产素是当下最有希望的药物[20]。然而,最近一项对 12 个随机对照试验的荟萃分析表明,尽管个别随机对照试验报告催产素有改善作用,但催产素对社交没有显著的影响[21]。因此,需要采用更好的研究方法进行更大规模的研究[22]。萝卜硫素[23]、胰岛素生长因子-1(IGF-1)[24] 和谷氨酸能药[25] 一样,在改善 ASD 核心症状方面的功效有待进一步证明。乙酰半胱氨酸[26] 可能无效。

尽管不一致,但越来越多的证据表明饮食干预可以减轻 ASD 的核心症状[27,28]。最近针对肠道微生物群的治疗,包括益生菌治疗和粪便微生物群移植,作为 ASD 的新型潜在疗法也引起了人们的广泛兴趣[29]。然而,几乎没有证据支持对 ASD 儿童使用营养补充剂或饮食疗法[27],甚至没有证据表明母亲的食物摄入和儿童的饮食与 ASD 症状严重程度的发展之间有任何关系[28]。

孤独症谱系障碍伴发疾病和问题行为的药物治疗

孤独症谱系障碍的注意缺陷、多动和冲动(ADHD 症状)

ASD 患者注意缺陷、多动和冲动的比率很高,大约 1/3 的人可以诊断为 ADHD[1,30]。

目前为止,最大的对照试验是由儿童精神药物孤独症网络的研究小组(RUPP)主持的关于哌甲酯的研究[31,32]。先前在对 ASD 儿童进行的回顾性和前瞻性研究中,Santosh 等[33] 报告了使用哌甲酯治疗的阳性结果。总体上,在兼有 ASD 和 ADHD 症状的儿童患者中,哌甲酯的疗效差别巨大,从显著有效且不良反应很少,到疗效不好且伴或不伴成问题的不良反应。对兼有智力残疾和 ADHD 儿童进行的一项大型双盲、安慰剂对照试验表明,最佳剂量的哌甲酯有时是有效的[34]。但是相对于单纯 ADHD 儿童,其不良反应的报道更常见[35-37]。不过,如果 ADHD 症状严重或者严重影响患者功能,尝试哌甲酯治疗是合理的。建议告知父母治疗有效的可能性较小,并且可能有不良反应。治疗从小剂量开始(大约 0.125mg/kg,每天 3 次,根据制剂而定),缓慢小幅加量。如果出现行为的恶化,或不可接受的不良反应,则应立即停药。最近的系统综述[6]证实,尽管哌甲酯对 ASD 患者的 ADHD 治疗有效,但其疗效不如仅有 ADHD 的患者,而且 ASD 患者预计会出现更多的不良反应(食欲下降、睡眠困难、腹部不适、社交退缩、易怒和情绪暴发)。

目前,还没有关于苯丙胺治疗儿童 ASD 的疗效的公开数据,尽管它们已经被用来治疗 ASD 患者和一般发育儿童的 ADHD。已发现赖右苯丙胺(含有与赖氨酸结合的 d-苯丙胺的前体药物)在治疗儿童和年轻人[38] 的 ADHD 方面具有疗效和耐受性,但没有关于 ASD 的具体数据。

托莫西汀是一种去甲肾上腺素能再摄取抑制剂,被批准用于治疗 ADHD,其疗效与哌甲酯相似[6]。来自小样本开放性试验和少数随机双盲试验[39,40]的初步证据表明,该药对患有 ASD 儿童可能有作用,最常见的不良反应是恶心、疲劳和睡眠困难,紧随的一项更大规模的试验证实托莫西汀(单独或与父母培训相结合)显著减少了 ADHD 症状[41]。该研究的 24 周延伸试验表明,托莫西汀联合父母培训在减少 ADHD 症状方面优于单独使用托莫西汀[42]。

有证据表明,α_2 受体激动剂(可乐定和胍法辛)可用作替代治疗。最近一项关于缓释胍法辛的随机对照试验,对患有 ASD 的儿童(平均年龄 8.5 岁)进行了为期 8 周的安慰剂对照研究,结果显示它可以安全有效地控制这一群体的多动症状[43]。除嗜睡、疲劳和食欲下降外,没有严重不良事件的报道。

有对照研究报告支持使用利培酮或阿立哌唑治疗 ADHD 症状。然而,这些不是研究的主要结果,因此需要进一步研究。

易激惹(攻击、自伤、严重破坏行为)

易激惹往往强调的是攻击他人和自我攻击,是 ASD 患者常见的问题。尽管建议使用行为方法和环境方法作为一线治疗,但是较严重和危险的行为常常必须使用药物治疗[44]。根据已发表证据难以建议合适的疗程,但治疗 6~12 个月似乎有益[45]。在疗程末,强烈建议减少药物剂量,或者若有可能,停止治疗[44,45]。

对于伴有易激惹的儿童和青少年 ASD,第二代抗精神病药是一线治疗[45-48]。利培酮[49,50]和阿立哌唑[51]已被可靠地证明有助于缓解 ASD 的易激惹和破坏性行为[5],并已被美国 FDA 批准使用。纳入 46 个随机对照试验[52]的荟萃分析比较了利培酮、阿立哌唑和其他化合物与安慰剂的疗效,结果显示利培酮和阿立哌唑的疗效最好,具有中等和较大的效应值。另一项荟萃分析显示,与安慰剂相比,阿立哌唑短期(8 周)治疗 6~17 岁 ASD 儿童的易激惹时也有类似的疗效[53]。最新的 Cochrane 综述[54]是对前一篇综述[55]的更新,其结论是阿立哌唑可能有助于治疗儿童 ASD 的易激惹、多动和刻板行为。通常推荐的阿立哌唑临床维持剂量为 5~15mg/d[45]。阿立哌唑起始为 2mg/d。利培酮的剂量相当复杂,FDA 推荐的利培酮剂量见框 5.3。

框 5.3　FDA 儿童和青少年使用利培酮的指南[68]

ASD 儿童患者使用利培酮的剂量/mg·d^{-1}				
体重	1~3d	4~18d	若需要,增加剂量	剂量范围
<20kg*	0.25mg	0.5mg	+0.25mg;间隔≥2w	0.5~3mg**
≥20kg	0.5mg	1.0mg	+0.5mg;间隔≥2w	1.0~3mg***

* 对于体重<15kg 的儿童应谨慎用药——暂时还没有可用的剂量数据。

** 治疗剂量达到 1mg/d 时,疗效达到平台期。

*** 体重超过 45kg 可能需要更高的剂量——在 3mg 时疗效达到平台期。

一般原则

- 利培酮每天可用 1 次或 2 次。
- 嗜睡患者可以睡前顿服一天的剂量。

续框

- 一旦达到并维持充分的临床疗效,可考虑逐渐减少剂量,以达到最佳的疗效-安全性平衡。
- 没有对照试验能够提供充分证据指明治疗应该持续多长时间。

不良反应

需要监测体重增加、嗜睡、高催乳素血症。儿童和青少年孤独症谱系障碍长期使用利培酮的安全性仍有待完全确定。

尽管有很好的疗效,体重增加、代谢改变、食欲增加和嗜睡(即使是阿立哌唑)等不良反应,也可能成为问题[15,56-59]。一项长期的安慰剂停用研究发现,继续服用阿立哌唑与随机改用安慰剂后,两组患者的复发率没有差别,这表明在易激惹症状稳定一段时间后,有必要重新评估阿立哌唑的使用[54]。只有一项头对头研究[60]结果提示,利培酮和阿立哌唑的耐受性和疗效相似。利培酮通常会导致高催乳素血症,虽然可能没有症状,但可能出现长期影响,因此需要密切监测;而阿立哌唑则不会,这使其成为优先的选择。另一方面,阿立哌唑可能对自伤行为无效[6]。

奥氮平[61]、喹硫平、齐拉西酮和氯氮平等第二代抗精神病药的效果目前尚未得到随机对照试验的有力验证。虽然有对照研究支持使用心境稳定剂(如锂盐[62,63]和丙戊酸钠[64])来治疗儿童的持续攻击行为,但它们治疗 ASD 的易激惹时,疗效不如第二代抗精神病药[65]。有限的数据支持利培酮和托吡酯合用比单用利培酮效果好[66]。至于脑源性神经营养因子刺激剂,如洛沙平和阿米替林[67],需要进一步进行随机对照试验。

利培酮在儿童和青少年中的使用

在英国、欧盟和美国,5 岁以上孤独症儿童和青少年出现易激惹,可以使用利培酮进行治疗。治疗剂量应根据患者的治疗反应个体化。

不建议使用苯二氮䓬类药物来处理 ASD 的易激惹和攻击行为。但是,苯二氮䓬类药物可以用于处理急性攻击行为。脱抑制行为可能使攻击行为恶化,必须考虑到这种可能性。

在随机双盲对照试验提供更好的证据之前,最近英国精神药理协会的指南不推荐使用米诺环素、(R)-巴氯芬、金刚烷胺来治疗易激惹[6]。

睡眠障碍

ASD 患儿有严重的睡眠问题[69],典型的问题有入睡困难、睡眠维持困难以及睡眠-觉醒节律紊乱。在开始治疗之前,了解睡眠问题的病因至关重要。褪黑素系统的异常引起了一些关注[70]。

已有 17 项研究表明褪黑素对 ASD 儿童有益[71]。纳入 5 项研究的荟萃分析[72]显示,按照 1~10mg 的剂量,治疗 14 天至 4 年,有较好的疗效。褪黑素的耐受性通常很好[72,73]。一项随机对照试验表明,虽然褪黑素改善了睡眠,但是儿童白天的行为并没有改善[74]。

也有证据表明,在减少失眠症状方面,褪黑素联合 CBT 优于单用褪黑素、单用 CBT 以及安慰剂[75]。

利培酮可能对那些极度易激惹儿童的睡眠困难有益。对于焦虑或抑郁的儿童,抗抑郁药可能有益;可乐定或氯硝西泮对过度觉醒导致的失眠有益[76]。

焦虑症、强迫症和抑郁症

SSRI 类药物对 ASD 的疗效有待证明。最近一项随机对照双盲临床试验的初步数据显示,氟西汀在减少 ASD 儿童的强迫症状方面有作用,但是试验的混杂因素导致无法得出肯定的结论[77]。最近的系统综述[6]显示,虽然一些研究认为利培酮可以减少 ASD 青少年的强迫和焦虑症状,但是最初选择的受试者均有高水平的易激惹,并不能得出利培酮对强迫症和焦虑症有效的确切结论。该综述认为,总体上很少或几乎没有证据表明利培酮、氯米帕明或 SSRI 类药物可以治疗焦虑或强迫症状。最近的 BAP 指南[6]与既往的 BAP 指南在治疗焦虑症和强迫症的方法上基本一致[78]。有数据显示,丁螺环酮对 ASD 患者的焦虑症状有效[79],而且普萘诺尔对改善 ASD 患者的认知有积极的作用[80],但是,还需要进一步评估。关于氟西汀剂量的指导见框 5.4。

氟西汀用于儿童和青少年

使用氟西汀治疗 ASD 的重复行为时,剂量一般比治疗抑郁症低得多。建议使用液体剂型,从尽可能低的剂量开始,并监测不良反应。框 5.4 列出的是适宜的用药方案。

框 5.4　氟西汀在儿童和青少年中的应用

液体氟西汀:(盐酸氟西汀)20mg/5mL

2.5mg/d 持续 1 周,注意:2.5mg=0.625mL,难以精确测量。

根据体重、耐受性、不良反应等,灵活调整加药方案,逐渐加到最高 0.8mg/(kg·d)[第 2 周,0.3mg/(kg·d);第 3 周,0.5mg/(kg·d);以后 0.8mg/(kg·d)]。若不良反应突出,应该减量。

不良反应

- 监测治疗中出现的**自杀**行为、自伤与敌意,尤其在治疗开始阶段。
- 低钠血症也可能出现——见第 3 章。

参考文献

1. Lai MC, et al. Prevalence of co-occurring mental health diagnoses in the autism population: a systematic review and meta-analysis. *Lancet Psychiatry* 2019; 6:819–829.
2. Lever AG, et al. Psychiatric co-occurring symptoms and disorders in young, middle-aged, and older adults with autism spectrum disorder. *J Autism Dev Disord* 2016; 46:1916–1930.
3. Buck TR, et al. Psychiatric comorbidity and medication use in adults with autism spectrum disorder. *J Autism Dev Disord* 2014; 44:3063–3071.
4. Goel R, et al. An update on pharmacotherapy of autism spectrum disorder in children and adolescents. *Int Rev Psychiatry (Abingdon, England)* 2018; 30:78–95.
5. Accordino RE, et al. Psychopharmacological interventions in autism spectrum disorder. *Expert Opin Pharmacother* 2016; 17:937–952.
6. Howes OD, et al. Autism spectrum disorder: consensus guidelines on assessment, treatment and research from the British Association for Psychopharmacology. *J Psychopharmacol* 2018; 32:3–29.
7. Santosh P. Medication in autism spectrum disorder. *Cut Edge Psychiatry Pract* 2014; 1:143–155.
8. Greenhill LL. Assessment of safety in pediatric psychopharmacology. *J Am Acad Child Adolesc Psychiatry* 2003; 42:625–626.
9. Leekam SR, et al. Restricted and repetitive behaviors in autism spectrum disorders: a review of research in the last decade. *Psychol Bull* 2011; 137:562–593.

10. Williams K, et al. Selective serotonin reuptake inhibitors (SSRIs) for autism spectrum disorders (ASD). *Cochrane Database Syst Rev* 2013; **8**:CD004677.

11. McDougle CJ, et al. A double-blind, placebo-controlled study of risperidone addition in serotonin reuptake inhibitor-refractory obsessive-compulsive disorder. *Arch Gen Psychiatry* 2000; **57**:794–801.

12. McDougle CJ, et al. Risperidone for the core symptom domains of autism: results from the study by the autism network of the research units on pediatric psychopharmacology. *Am J Psychiatry* 2005; **162**:1142–1148.

13. McCracken JT, et al. Risperidone in children with autism and serious behavioral problems. *N Engl J Med* 2002; **347**:314–321.

14. Arnold LE, et al. Parent-defined target symptoms respond to risperidone in RUPP autism study: customer approach to clinical trials. *J Am Acad Child Adolesc Psychiatry* 2003; **42**:1443–1450.

15. Dinnissen M, et al. Clinical and pharmacokinetic evaluation of risperidone for the management of autism spectrum disorder. *Expert Opin Drug Metab Toxicol* 2015; **11**:111–124.

16. Zhou MS, et al. Meta-analysis: pharmacologic treatment of restricted and repetitive behaviors in autism spectrum disorders. *J Am Acad Child Adolesc Psychiatry* 2020:Epub ahead of print.

17. Yu Y, et al. Pharmacotherapy of restricted/repetitive behavior in autism spectrum disorder: a systematic review and meta-analysis. *BMC Psychiatry* 2020; **20**:121.

18. Canitano R, et al. Risperidone in the treatment of behavioral disorders associated with autism in children and adolescents. *Neuropsychiatr Dis Treat* 2008; **4**:723–730.

19. Scahill L, et al. Brief report: social disability in autism spectrum disorder: results from Research Units on Pediatric Psychopharmacology (RUPP) Autism Network trials. *J Autism Dev Disord* 2013; **43**:739–746.

20. Posey DJ, et al. Developing drugs for core social and communication impairment in autism. *Child Adolesc Psychiatr Clin N Am* 2008; **17**:787–801.

21. Ooi YP, et al. Oxytocin and autism spectrum disorders: a systematic review and meta-analysis of randomized controlled trials. *Pharmacopsychiatry* 2017, **50**:5–13.

22. Alvares GA, et al. Beyond the hype and hope: critical considerations for intranasal oxytocin research in autism spectrum disorder. *Autism Res Off Int Soc Autism Res* 2017; **10**:25–41.

23. Singh K, et al. Sulforaphane treatment of autism spectrum disorder (ASD). *Proc Natl Acad Sci USA* 2014; **111**:15550–15555.

24. Riikonen R. Treatment of autistic spectrum disorder with insulin-like growth factors. *Eur J Paediatr Neurol* 2016; **20**:816–823.

25. Fung LK, et al. Developing medications targeting glutamatergic dysfunction in autism: progress to date. *CNS Drugs* 2015; **29**:453–463.

26. Dean OM, et al. A randomised, double blind, placebo-controlled trial of a fixed dose of N-acetyl cysteine in children with autistic disorder. *Aust N Z J Psychiatry* 2017; **51**:241–249.

27. Sathe N, et al. Nutritional and dietary interventions for autism spectrum disorder: a systematic review. *Pediatrics* 2017; **139**:e20170346.

28. Peretti S, et al. Diet: the keystone of autism spectrum disorder? *Nutr Neurosci* 2019; **22**:825–839.

29. Yang Y, et al. Targeting gut microbiome: a novel and potential therapy for autism. *Life Sci* 2018; **194**:111–119.

30. Lee YJ, et al. Advanced pharmacotherapy evidenced by pathogenesis of autism spectrum disorder. *Clin Psychopharmacol Neurosci Off Sci J Korean College Neuropsychopharmacol* 2014; **12**:19–30.

31. Research Units on Pediatric Psychopharmacology (RUPP) Autism Network. Randomized, controlled, crossover trial of methylphenidate in pervasive developmental disorders with hyperactivity. *Arch Gen Psychiatry* 2005; **62**:1266–1274.

32. Posey DJ, et al. Positive effects of methylphenidate on inattention and hyperactivity in pervasive developmental disorders: an analysis of secondary measures. *Biol Psychiatry* 2007; **61**:538–544.

33. Santosh PJ, et al. Impact of comorbid autism spectrum disorders on stimulant response in children with attention deficit hyperactivity disorder: a retrospective and prospective effectiveness study. *Child Care Health Dev* 2006; **32**:575–583.

34. Simonoff E, et al. Randomized controlled double-blind trial of optimal dose methylphenidate in children and adolescents with severe attention deficit hyperactivity disorder and intellectual disability. *J Child Psychol Psychiatry* 2013; **54**:527–535.

35. Sung M, et al. What's in the pipeline? Drugs in development for autism spectrum disorder. *Neuropsychiatr Dis Treat* 2014; **10**:371–381.

36. Siegel M, et al. Psychotropic medications in children with autism spectrum disorders: a systematic review and synthesis for evidence-based practice. *J Autism Dev Disord* 2012; **42**:1592–1605.

37. Williamson ED, et al. Psychotropic medications in autism: practical considerations for parents. *J Autism Dev Disord* 2012; **42**:1249–1255.

38. Coghill D, et al. European, randomized, phase 3 study of lisdexamfetamine dimesylate in children and adolescents with attention-deficit/hyperactivity disorder. *Eur Neuropsychopharmacol* 2013; **23**:1208–1218.

39. Arnold LE, et al. Atomoxetine for hyperactivity in autism spectrum disorders: placebo-controlled crossover pilot trial. *J Am Acad Child Adolesc Psychiatry* 2006; **45**:1196–1205.

40. Harfterkamp M, et al. A randomized double-blind study of atomoxetine versus placebo for attention-deficit/hyperactivity disorder symptoms in children with autism spectrum disorder. *J Am Acad Child Adolesc Psychiatry* 2012; **51**:733–741.

41. Handen BL, et al. Atomoxetine, parent training, and their combination in children with autism spectrum disorder and attention-deficit/hyperactivity disorder. *J Am Acad Child Adolesc Psychiatry* 2015; **54**:905–915.

42. Smith T, et al. Atomoxetine and parent training for children with autism and attention-deficit/hyperactivity disorder: a 24-week extension study. *J Am Acad Child Adolesc Psychiatry* 2016; **55**:868–876.e862.

43. Scahill L, et al. Extended-release guanfacine for hyperactivity in children with autism spectrum disorder. *Am J Psychiatry* 2015; **172**:1197–1206.

44. National Institute for Health and Care Excellence. Autism spectrum disorder in under 19s: support and management. Clinical Guidance 170 [CG170] 2013 (Reviewed September 2016); https://www.nice.org.uk/Guidance/CG170.

45. Kaplan G, et al. Psychopharmacology of autism spectrum disorders. *Pediatr Clin North Am* 2012; 59:175–187, xii.

46. McDougle CJ, et al. Atypical antipsychotics in children and adolescents with autistic and other pervasive developmental disorders. *J Clin Psychiatry* 2008; 69 Suppl 4:15–20.

47. Parikh MS, et al. Psychopharmacology of aggression in children and adolescents with autism: a critical review of efficacy and tolerability. *J Child Adolesc Psychopharmacol* 2008; 18:157–178.

48. DeVane CL, et al. Pharmacotherapy of autism spectrum disorder: results from the randomized BAART clinical trial. *Pharmacotherapy* 2019; 39:626–635.

49. Jesner OS, et al. Risperidone for autism spectrum disorder. *Cochrane Database Syst Rev* 2007:CD005040.

50. Scahill L, et al. Risperidone approved for the treatment of serious behavioral problems in children with autism. *J Child Adolesc Psychiatr Nurs* 2007; 20:188–190.

51. Curran MP. Aripiprazole: in the treatment of irritability associated with autistic disorder in pediatric patients. *Paediatr Drugs* 2011; 13:197–204.

52. Fung LK, et al. Pharmacologic treatment of severe irritability and problem behaviors in autism: a systematic review and meta-analysis. *Pediatrics* 2016; 137 Suppl 2:S124–135.

53. Douglas-Hall P, et al. Aripiprazole: a review of its use in the treatment of irritability associated with autistic disorder patients aged 6-17. *J Cent Nerv Syst Dis* 2011; 3:1–11.

54. Hirsch LE, et al. Aripiprazole for autism spectrum disorders (ASD). *Cochrane Database Syst Rev* 2016:Cd009043.

55. Ching H, et al. Aripiprazole for autism spectrum disorders (ASD). *Cochrane Database Syst Rev* 2012; 5:CD009043.

56. Caccia S. Safety and pharmacokinetics of atypical antipsychotics in children and adolescents. *Paediatr Drugs* 2013; 15:217–233.

57. Sharma A, et al. Efficacy of risperidone in managing maladaptive behaviors for children with autistic spectrum disorder: a meta-analysis. *J Pediatr Health Care* 2012; 26:291–299.

58. Kent JM, et al. Risperidone dosing in children and adolescents with autistic disorder: a double-blind, placebo-controlled study. *J Autism Dev Disord* 2013; 43:1773–1783.

59. Maayan L, et al. Weight gain and metabolic risks associated with antipsychotic medications in children and adolescents. *J Child Adolesc Psychopharmacol* 2011; 21:517–535.

60. Ghanizadeh A, et al. A head-to-head comparison of aripiprazole and risperidone for safety and treating autistic disorders, a randomized double blind clinical trial. *Child Psychiatry Hum Dev* 2014; 45:185–192.

61. Hollander E, et al. A double-blind placebo-controlled pilot study of olanzapine in childhood/adolescent pervasive developmental disorder. *J Child Adolesc Psychopharmacol* 2006; 16:541–548.

62. Campbell M, et al. Lithium in hospitalized aggressive children with conduct disorder: a double-blind and placebo-controlled study. *J Am Acad Child Adolesc Psychiatry* 1995; 34:445–453.

63. Malone RP, et al. A double-blind placebo-controlled study of lithium in hospitalized aggressive children and adolescents with conduct disorder. *Arch Gen Psychiatry* 2000; 57:649–654.

64. Donovan SJ, et al. Divalproex treatment for youth with explosive temper and mood lability: a double-blind, placebo-controlled crossover design. *Am J Psychiatry* 2000; 157:818–820.

65. Stigler KA, et al. Pharmacotherapy of irritability in pervasive developmental disorders. *Child Adolesc Psychiatr Clin N Am* 2008; 17:739–752.

66. Rezaei V, et al. Double-blind, placebo-controlled trial of risperidone plus topiramate in children with autistic disorder. *Prog Neuropsychopharmacol Biol Psychiatry* 2010; 34:1269–1272.

67. Hellings JA, et al. Dopamine antagonists for treatment resistance in autism spectrum disorders: review and focus on BDNF stimulators loxapine and amitriptyline. *Expert Opin Pharmacother* 2017; 18:581–588.

68. Janssen Pharmaceutical Companies. Highlights of Prescribing Information: RISPERDAL® (risperidone) tablets, RISPERDAL® (risperidone) oral solution, RISPERDAL® M-TAB® (risperidone) orally disintegrating tablets 2019; https://www.accessdata.fda.gov/drugsatfda_docs/label/2019/020272s082,020588s070,021444s056lbl.pdf.

69. Krakowiak P, et al. Sleep problems in children with autism spectrum disorders, developmental delays, and typical development: a population-based study. *J Sleep Res* 2008; 17:197–206.

70. Sanchez-Barcelo EJ, et al. Clinical uses of melatonin in pediatrics. *Int J Pediatr* 2011; 2011:892624.

71. Doyen C, et al. Melatonin in children with autistic spectrum disorders: recent and practical data. *Eur Child Adolesc Psychiatry* 2011; 20:231–239.

72. Rossignol DA, et al. Melatonin in autism spectrum disorders: a systematic review and meta-analysis. *Dev Med Child Neurol* 2011; 53:783–792.

73. Andersen IM, et al. Melatonin for insomnia in children with autism spectrum disorders. *J Child Neurol* 2008; 23:482–485.

74. Gringras P, et al. Melatonin for sleep problems in children with neurodevelopmental disorders: randomised double masked placebo controlled trial. *BMJ* 2012; 345:e6664.

75. Cortesi F, et al. Controlled-release melatonin, singly and combined with cognitive behavioural therapy, for persistent insomnia in children with autism spectrum disorders: a randomized placebo-controlled trial. *J Sleep Res* 2012; 21:700–709.

76. Johnson KP, et al. Sleep in children with autism spectrum disorders. *Curr Treat Options Neurol* 2008; 10:350–359.

77. Reddihough DS, et al. Effect of fluoxetine on obsessive-compulsive behaviors in children and adolescents with autism spectrum disorders: a randomized clinical trial. *JAMA* 2019; 322:1561–1569.

78. Baldwin DS, et al. Evidence-based guidelines for the pharmacological treatment of anxiety disorders: recommendations from the British Association for Psychopharmacology. *J Psychopharm* 2005; 19:567–596.

第 5 章

79. Buitelaar JK, et al. Buspirone in the management of anxiety and irritability in children with pervasive developmental disorders: results of an open-label study. *J Clin Psychiatry* 1998; 59:56–59.

80. Narayanan A, et al. Effect of propranolol on functional connectivity in autism spectrum disorder–a pilot study. *Brain Imaging and Behavior* 2010; 4:189–197.

抽动障碍与抽动秽语综合征

5%~20% 的儿童会出现一过性抽动。1% 的儿童会发生以持续的运动抽动和发声抽动为特征的抽动秽语综合征（TS）。65% 的 TS 儿童在成年后没有或者仅有轻微的抽动。因个体不同，抽动症状会随着时间而时好时坏，因应激、低活动或疲劳等外界因素而不同程度地加重。TS 在男孩中比女孩要多 2~3 倍 [1]。

共病的识别和治疗

TS 合并强迫症、ADHD、抑郁症、焦虑症和行为问题的发生率高于偶发概率，往往导致患者出现严重功能损害 [2]。在评估抽动所导致的失能水平之前，应该首先治疗这些共病 [3]。

教育和行为治疗

大多数 TS 患者不需药物治疗；对患者本人、家人、与之交往的人，尤其是学校人员，进行教育至关重要。如果抽动导致患者感到痛苦或功能损害，就应该提供以减少抽动为主的治疗。已经证实，行为干预与抗精神病药疗效相当 [4,5]。习惯反转、全面的行为干预、暴露和反应阻止是可选择的行为治疗方法 [6]。

药物治疗

对于 TS 的药物治疗研究难以解释，原因如下：

- 抽动频率和严重程度存在较大的个体差异。小样本随机研究的患者在基线水平上可能大不相同。
- 某一个体的抽动程度在不同时间变异很大，难以区分药物作用和自然变化。
- 大量文献由个案报告、病例系列报道、开放研究以及说服力小的对照研究组成。发表偏倚也可能是个问题。
- 抽动障碍患者合并其他精神障碍的比率也很高。难以区分药物对抽动的直接影响和对共病的影响，因而难以解释研究所报告的整体功能改善，而不是特定的抽动减少。
- 许多就诊的抽动秽语综合征患者使用补充治疗或者替代治疗，大多数人表示自己从中受益，多达 50% 的人发现这些方法比药物治疗更有帮助 [7]。但是，关于补充疗法和替代疗法的疗效以及不良反应，仍然缺乏可靠的研究 [8]。

在抽动障碍的临床试验中，安慰剂效应不如以前所认为的那样大 [9]。

α₂ 肾上腺素受体激动剂

在开放性研究中发现，可乐定可以减少抽动的程度和频率，但在一项研究中，该效应未能令人信服地显示超过安慰剂 [10]。其他研究显示抽动显著减少 [11-14]。可乐定的治疗剂量为 3~5μg/kg，应该缓慢加量。经皮贴剂也有效 [15]。主要不良反应是镇静、直立性低血压和抑郁。应该告诉患者及其家人不要突然停药，因为有导致反弹性高血压的风险。胍法辛对抽动障碍的治疗也有效 [16,17]，值得在特定个体（如伴有 ADHD 的患者）进行治疗试验。

抗精神病药

抗精神病药治疗抽动症时,其不良反应可能会超出有益的作用,因此建议首先尝试可乐定。但对于一些个体,与可乐定相比,抗精神病药能更有效地缓解抽动症状。

许多第一代抗精神病药被用来治疗抽动秽语综合征。在最近的 Cochrane 综述中,6 项试验的荟萃分析分析显示,匹莫齐特显示强大的疗效[19]。在这些试验中,匹莫齐特被用来和氟哌啶醇(1 项)、安慰剂(1 项),氟哌啶醇和安慰剂(2 项)以及利培酮(2 项)等对照,发现在减少抽动方面,比安慰剂有效,与利培酮相当,但稍弱于氟哌啶醇。匹莫齐特的不良反应比氟哌啶醇少,但与利培酮差不多。使用匹莫齐特和氟哌啶醇的患者有必要监测心电图。氟哌啶醇往往耐受性差。由于不良反应方面的特点,大多数作者建议使用第二代而不是第一代抗精神病药治疗抽动秽语综合征[18]。

最近的研究提示,阿立哌唑治疗儿童抽动秽语综合征(还有抽动症[20])有效且耐受性好。一项为期 10 周的多中心双盲安慰剂对照试验($n=61$)显示,阿立哌唑可以有效地减少抽动秽语综合征的抽动症状。阿立哌唑治疗与血清催乳素浓度明显下降以及平均体重(约增加 1.6kg)、体重指数(BMI)和腰围的增加有关[21]。在另一项随机双盲安慰剂对照试验($n=133$)中也发现阿立哌唑有效,该试验设置了为期 8 周的低剂量阿立哌唑组(如果体重<50kg,5mg/d;如果体重≥50kg,10mg/d)、高剂量阿立哌唑组(如果体重<50kg,10mg/d;如果体重≥50kg,20mg/d)和安慰剂组[22]。在第 8 周,根据耶鲁综合抽搐程度量表测量的抽搐总评分,高剂量组(-9.9;95% CI:-13.8~-5.9)和低剂量组(-6.3;95% CI:-10.2~-2.3)的得分均减少;进步非常大和进步较大的比例低剂量组为 69%(29/42),高剂量组为 74%(26/35),而安慰剂组为 38%(16/42)。令人惊讶的是,低剂量组体重显著增加(增重≥7%)的比例(18.2%)多于高剂量组(9.3%)和安慰剂组(9.1%),可能是因为该组在基线时平均体重比其他两组低>3kg。一些病例报告也同样支持使用阿立哌唑[23-26]。一项研究对阿立哌唑($n=25$)和匹莫齐特($n=25$)治疗抽动障碍 24 个月的代谢不良反应进行了评估,表明治疗未引起体重指数显著增加。然而,匹莫齐特治疗与血糖升高有关,且在第 12~24 个月时血糖也未进入平台期;阿立哌唑治疗与胆固醇升高有关;两种药物均与甘油三酯升高有关[27]。有两项荟萃分析分析支持阿立哌唑的疗效[28,29]。一项研究表明[30],每周给药两次的耐受性可能比每天给药更好。一项小型随机对照试验($n=24$)比较了阿立哌唑与丙戊酸钠对抽动障碍患儿的治疗效果,结果显示在减少抽动方面两药之间有显著的统计学差异[31],阿立哌唑占优势。

除上述提到的研究外,利培酮还在一项小样本($n=34$)随机对照试验中显示比安慰剂有效[32]。疲劳和食欲增加问题在利培酮组较多,且在为期 8 周的试验中,平均体重增加了 2.8kg。一项小样本随机对照研究发现,利培酮与可乐定一样有效[33]。一项小样本双盲交叉研究显示,奥氮平[34] 可能比匹莫齐特有效。舒必利与齐拉西酮[36] 治疗有效且耐受性良好[35]。开放性研究支持喹硫平[37]和奥氮平[38,39]的疗效。一项很小样本的交叉试验($n=7$)发现氯氮平无效[40]。

总之,第二代抗精神病药在代谢方面的不良反应和体重增加常见,甚至阿立哌唑也是如此,因此使用时应当充分考量收益/风险比[18]。

其他药物

一项小样本、双盲、安慰剂对照的交叉试验提示，巴氯酚对总体功能损害有效，对抽动症状无影响[41]。该研究中发现数值变化没有统计学意义。同样，一项双盲、安慰剂对照试验发现，以尼古丁作为氟哌啶醇的增效剂，也对总体功能损害有效，对抽动症状无影响[42]。这些效应甚至在停用尼古丁贴剂后数周仍然保持。尼古丁贴片与恶心(71%)和呕吐(40%)的发生率高有关。作者建议该药可能适合"需要时"使用。一项针对儿童和青少年抽动的双盲、安慰剂对照、交叉研究显示，小剂量培高利特(Pergolide，一种 D_1-D_2-D_3 受体激动剂)可以显著减少抽动症状[43]。其不良反应包括镇静、头昏、恶心和易激惹。在患慢性抽动与抽动秽语综合征的儿童和青少年中进行了一项随机试验，结果表明培高利特减少抽动症状的疗效明显优于安慰剂[44]。氟他胺(flutamide)是一种抗雄激素药，曾在小样本抽动秽语综合征成年患者的随机对照试验中做过研究[45]。该药对运动抽动有轻微而短期的疗效，但对发声抽动无效。小样本、随机对照试验也分别显示甲氧氯普胺[46]与托吡酯[47]均优于安慰剂。近期一项荟萃分析纳入了 14 项随机对照试验(均来自中国)，将托吡酯与氟哌啶醇或硫必利进行比较。其结论是，鉴于这些试验的研究设计总体质量很低，没有足够的证据支持托吡酯在临床上的常规使用[48]。最近，单胺递质消耗剂氘代丁苯那嗪被证明是有效的[49]。四苯嗪也可以作为一种辅助治疗[50]。依考匹泮(ecopipam)是一种 D_1 受体拮抗剂，在最近一项抽动秽语综合征患儿和青少年的随机安慰剂对照交叉试验中，发现它对抽动有效[51]。

关于昂丹司琼[52]、氯米芬[53]、曲马多[54]、酮色林[55]、环丙孕酮[56]、左乙拉西坦[57]、普瑞巴林[58]和大麻[59]的疗效，已经有病例报告和病例系列报告发表。一项 Cochrane 综述认为，大麻酚类(cannabinoids)目前几乎没有有效的证据[60]；虽然使用大麻素有可靠的生物学依据，但是大麻素的总体有效性和安全性在很大程度上仍不清楚[61]。其他许多药物在个案报告中有效。在这些报告中，患者均合并其他精神疾病，因此很难确定这些药物对单独的抽动秽语综合征的疗效。

肉毒毒素曾被用于治疗令人烦恼或痛苦的局灶性运动抽动，尤其是涉及颈部肌肉的抽动[18]。但是，最近一篇 Cochrane 综述表示，由于现有证据的质量较低，其在抽搐治疗中的地位尚不确定[62]。

可能有一亚型的儿童会发生与链球菌或其他感染有关的抽动或强迫症。与链球菌感染有关的该亚型群体缩写是 PANDAS(与链球菌感染有关的儿童自身免疫神经精神疾病)[63]，或者更宽泛的 PANS(儿童急性发作神经精神综合征)[64]。它被认为是自身免疫介导的效应，因此已经有许多针对该类儿童的免疫调节治疗试验，对活动性感染的抗生素治疗，以及预防性抗生素治疗。在这一领域需要进行更多研究(图 5.2)。

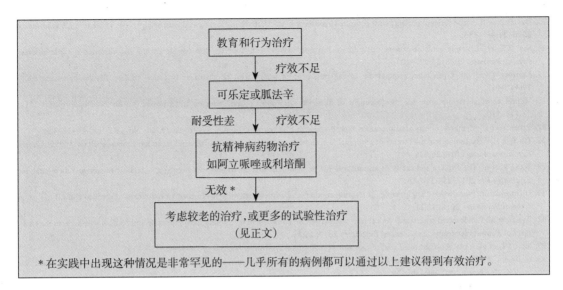

图 5.2　建议概要

参考文献

1. Murphy TK, et al. Practice parameter for the assessment and treatment of children and adolescents with tic disorders. *J Am Acad Child Adolesc Psychiatry* 2013; **52**:1341–1359.
2. Cath DC, et al. European clinical guidelines for Tourette syndrome and other tic disorders. Part I: Assessment. *Eur Child Adolesc Psychiatry* 2011; **20**:155–171.
3. Singer HS Treatment of tics and Tourette syndrome. *Curr Treat Options Neurol* 2010; **12**:539–561.
4. McGuire JF, et al. A meta-analysis of behavior therapy for Tourette syndrome. *J Psychiatr Res* 2014; **50**:106–112.
5. Rizzo R, et al. A randomized controlled trial comparing behavioral, educational, and pharmacological treatments in youths with chronic tic disorder or Tourette syndrome. *Frontiers Psychiatry* 2018; **9**:100.
6. Fründt O, et al. Behavioral therapy for Tourette syndrome and chronic tic disorders. *Neurol Clin Practice* 2017; **7**:148–156.
7. Patel H, et al. Use of complementary and alternative medicine in children with Tourette syndrome. *J Child Neurol* 2020; **35**:512–516.
8. Kumar A, et al. A comprehensive review of Tourette syndrome and complementary alternative medicine. *Current Dev Disorders Rep* 2018; **5**:95–100.
9. Cubo E, et al. Impact of placebo assignment in clinical trials of tic disorders. *Mov Disord* 2013; **28**:1288–1292.
10. Goetz CG, et al. Clonidine and Gilles de la Tourette's syndrome: double-blind study using objective rating methods. *Ann Neurol* 1987; **21**:307–310.
11. Leckman JF, et al. Clonidine treatment of Gilles de la Tourette's syndrome. *Arch Gen Psychiatry* 1991; **48**:324–328.
12. Group TsSS. Treatment of ADHD in children with tics: a randomized controlled trial. *Neurology* 2002; **58**:527–536.
13. Du YS, et al. Randomized double-blind multicentre placebo-controlled clinical trial of the clonidine adhesive patch for the treatment of tic disorders. *Aust N Z J Psychiatry* 2008; **42**:807–813.
14. Hedderick EF, et al. Double-blind, crossover study of clonidine and levetiracetam in Tourette syndrome. *Pediatr Neurol* 2009; **40**:420–425.
15. Song PP, et al. The efficacy and tolerability of the clonidine transdermal patch in the treatment for children with tic disorders: a prospective, open, single-group, self-controlled study. *Front Neurol* 2017; **8**:32.
16. Scahill L, et al. A placebo-controlled study of guanfacine in the treatment of children with tic disorders and attention deficit hyperactivity disorder. *Am J Psychiatry* 2001; **158**:1067–1074.
17. Cummings DD, et al. Neuropsychiatric effects of guanfacine in children with mild Tourette syndrome: a pilot study. *Clin Neuropharmacol* 2002; **25**:325–332.
18. Roessner V, et al. Pharmacological treatment of tic disorders and Tourette syndrome. *Neuropharmacology* 2013; **68**:143–149.
19. Pringsheim T, et al. Pimozide for tics in Tourette's syndrome. *Cochrane Database Syst Rev* 2009:CD006996.
20. Yoo HK, et al. An open-label study of the efficacy and tolerability of aripiprazole for children and adolescents with tic disorders. *J Clin Psychiatry* 2007; **68**:1088–1093.
21. Yoo HK, et al. A multicenter, randomized, double-blind, placebo-controlled study of aripiprazole in children and adolescents with Tourette's disorder. *J Clin Psychiatry* 2013; **74**:e772–e780.
22. Sallee F, et al. Randomized, double-blind, placebo-controlled trial demonstrates the efficacy and safety of oral aripiprazole for the treatment of Tourette's disorder in children and adolescents. *J Child Adolesc Psychopharmacol* 2017; **27**:771–781.

23. Davies L, et al. A case series of patients with Tourette's syndrome in the United Kingdom treated with aripiprazole. *Human Psychopharmacol* 2006; 21:447–453.

24. Seo WS, et al. Aripiprazole treatment of children and adolescents with Tourette disorder or chronic tic disorder. *J Child Adolesc Psychopharmacol* 2008; 18:197–205.

25. Murphy TK, et al. Open label aripiprazole in the treatment of youth with tic disorders. *J Child Adolesc Psychopharmacol* 2009; 19:441–447.

26. Wenzel C, et al. Aripiprazole for the treatment of Tourette syndrome: a case series of 100 patients. *J Clin Psychopharmacol* 2012; 32:548–550.

27. Rizzo R, et al. Metabolic effects of aripiprazole and pimozide in children with Tourette syndrome. *Pediatr Neurol* 2012; 47:419–422.

28. Liu Y, et al. Effectiveness and tolerability of aripiprazole in children and adolescents with Tourette's disorder: a meta-Analysis. *J Child Adolesc Psychopharmacol* 2016; 26:436–441.

29. Wang S, et al. The efficacy and safety of aripiprazole for tic disorders in children and adolescents: a systematic review and meta-analysis. *Psychiatry Res* 2017; 254:24–32.

30. Ghanizadeh A Twice-weekly aripiprazole for treating children and adolescents with tic disorder, a randomized controlled clinical trial. *Ann General Psychiatry* 2016; 15:21.

31. Tao D, et al. Randomized controlled clinical trial comparing the efficacy and tolerability of aripiprazole and sodium valproate in the treatment of Tourette syndrome. *Ann General Psychiatry* 2019; 18:24.

32. Scahill L, et al. A placebo-controlled trial of risperidone in Tourette syndrome. *Neurology* 2003; 60:1130–1135.

33. Gaffney GR, et al. Risperidone versus clonidine in the treatment of children and adolescents with Tourette's syndrome. *J Am Acad Child Adolesc Psychiatry* 2002; 41:330–336.

34. Onofrj M, et al. Olanzapine in severe Gilles de la Tourette syndrome: a 52-week double-blind cross-over study vs. low-dose pimozide. *J Neurol* 2000; 247:443–446.

35. Robertson MM, et al. Management of Gilles de la Tourette syndrome using sulpiride. *Clin Neuropharmacol* 1990; 13:229–235.

36. Sallee FR, et al. Ziprasidone treatment of children and adolescents with Tourette's syndrome: a pilot study. *J Am Acad Child Adolesc Psychiatry* 2000; 39:292–299.

37. Mukaddes NM, et al. Quetiapine treatment of children and adolescents with Tourette's disorder. *J Child Adolesc Psychopharmacol* 2003; 13:295–299.

38. Budman CL, et al. An open-label study of the treatment efficacy of olanzapine for Tourette's disorder. *J Clin Psychiatry* 2001; 62:290–294.

39. McCracken JT, et al. Effectiveness and tolerability of open label olanzapine in children and adolescents with Tourette syndrome. *J Child Adolesc Psychopharmacol* 2008; 18:501–508.

40. Caine ED, et al. The trial use of clozapine for abnormal involuntary movement disorders. *Am J Psychiatry* 1979; 136:317–320.

41. Singer HS, et al. Baclofen treatment in Tourette syndrome: a double-blind, placebo-controlled, crossover trial. *Neurology* 2001; 56:599–604.

42. Silver AA, et al. Transdermal nicotine and haloperidol in Tourette's disorder: a double-blind placebo-controlled study. *J Clin Psychiatry* 2001; 62:707–714.

43. Gilbert DL, et al. Tourette's syndrome improvement with pergolide in a randomized, double-blind, crossover trial. *Neurology* 2000; 54:1310–1315.

44. Gilbert DL, et al. Tic reduction with pergolide in a randomized controlled trial in children. *Neurology* 2003; 60:606–611.

45. Peterson BS, et al. A double-blind, placebo-controlled, crossover trial of an antiandrogen in the treatment of Tourette's syndrome. *J Clin Psychopharmacol* 1998; 18:324–331.

46. Nicolson R, et al. A randomized, double-blind, placebo-controlled trial of metoclopramide for the treatment of Tourette's disorder. *J Am Acad Child Adolesc Psychiatry* 2005; 44:640–646.

47. Jankovic J, et al. A randomised, double-blind, placebo-controlled study of topiramate in the treatment of Tourette syndrome. *J Neurol Neurosurg Psychiatry* 2010; 81:70–73.

48. Yang CS, et al. Topiramate for Tourette's syndrome in children: a meta-analysis. *Pediatr Neurol* 2013; 49:344–350.

49. Jankovic J, et al. 152 development of deutetrabenazine as a potential new non-antipsychotic treatment for Tourette syndrome in children and adolescents. *CNS Spectr* 2020; 25:297.

50. Porta M, et al. Tourette's syndrome and role of tetrabenazine: review and personal experience. *Clin Drug Invest* 2008; 28:443–459.

51. Gilbert DL, et al. Ecopipam, a D1 receptor antagonist, for treatment of Tourette syndrome in children: a randomized, placebo-controlled crossover study. *Mov Disord* 2018; 33:1272–1280.

52. Toren P, et al. Ondansetron treatment in patients with Tourette's syndrome. *Int Clin Psychopharmacol* 1999; 14:373–376.

53. Sandyk R Clomiphene citrate in Tourette's syndrome. *Int J Neurosci* 1988; 43:103–106.

54. Shapira NA, et al. Novel use of tramadol hydrochloride in the treatment of Tourette's syndrome. *J Clin Psychiatry* 1997; 58:174–175.

55. Bonnier C, et al. Ketanserin treatment of Tourette's syndrome in children. *Am J Psychiatry* 1999; 156:1122–1123.

56. Izmir M, et al. Cyproterone acetate treatment of Tourette's syndrome. *Can J Psychiatry* 1999; 44:710–711.

57. Awaad Y, et al. Use of levetiracetam to treat tics in children and adolescents with Tourette syndrome. *Mov Disord* 2005; 20:714–718.

58. Hienert M, et al. Pregabalin in Tourette's syndrome: a case series. *Am J Psychiatry* 2016; 173:1242–1243.

59. Sandyk R, et al. Marijuana and Tourette's syndrome. *J Clin Psychopharmacol* 1988; 8:444–445.

60. Curtis A, et al. Cannabinoids for Tourette's syndrome. *Cochrane Database Syst Rev* 2009:CD006565.

61. Artukoglu BB, et al. The potential of cannabinoid-based treatments in Tourette syndrome. *CNS Drugs* 2019; 33:417–430.

62. Pandey S, et al. Botulinum toxin for motor and phonic tics in Tourette's syndrome. *Cochrane Database Syst Rev* 2018; 1:Cd012285.

63. Martino D, et al. The PANDAS subgroup of tic disorders and childhood-onset obsessive-compulsive disorder. *J Psychosom Res* 2009; 67:547–557.
64. Chang K, et al. Clinical evaluation of youth with pediatric acute-onset neuropsychiatric syndrome (PANS): recommendations from the 2013 PANS Consensus Conference. *J Child Adolesc Psychopharmacol* 2015; 25:3–13.

褪黑素治疗儿童和青少年失眠

失眠是儿童期常见症状。潜在的原因可能是行为的（不当的睡眠联想或睡眠抵触）、生理的（睡眠时相延迟综合征）或潜在的情感障碍（焦虑症、抑郁症、双相障碍）。各种形式的失眠都更常见于学习困难、孤独症、ADHD 和感觉缺陷（特别是视觉缺陷）的儿童。尽管行为干预应该是主要的干预方法，并且具有坚实的证据基础，但是外源性褪黑素目前是用于儿童失眠的"一线"药物[1]。

褪黑素是由松果体按昼夜节律分泌的一种激素。黑暗促使褪黑素在傍晚时升高，这一般发生在进入自然睡眠之前两个小时[2]。褪黑素诱导睡眠，并且与昼夜节律系统同步。

市面上有各种各样未经批准的褪黑素速释、缓释和液体剂型。许多产品被归类于食品级而非药品级，有些价格不菲。褪黑素缓释剂（Circadin）于 2008 年 4 月在英国获批，用于短期治疗 55 岁以上患者的失眠。许多儿童无法吞咽这些药片，虽然可以将它们研碎（同时成为速释剂），但是药品许可证限制儿童获得这种长效制剂。然而，一种名为"Slenyto"的长效褪黑素迷你型片剂在英国已获批用于孤独症儿童，该药模拟夜间该激素的内源性释放模式。一项针对孤独症儿童的Ⅲ期多中心、随机、安慰剂对照研究对该药进行了评估。该研究先进行了 13 周的双盲治疗期，随后进入延伸开放治疗期，持续监测疗效和安全性。结果显示，护理日志报告的睡眠启动和维持（睡眠潜伏期、总睡眠时间、最长睡眠时间）有显著的改善[3]。治疗效果可以长期维持。该药的耐受性良好，没有发生意外的安全事故。在美国神经病学会最新出版的儿童和青少年孤独症患者失眠和睡眠紊乱的治疗实践指南中，该研究是唯一一项被评为 1 级的研究[4]。对次要结果的分析发现，儿童的社会功能和行为改善了，护理者的幸福感也增加了。

由于缺少头对头研究，对于是否应该使用、何时使用速释褪黑素制剂，目前没有可靠的数据。还有另外一些褪黑素类似物已经生产出来，或者正在研发中[5]，但是它们实际上从未用于儿童人群。也没有等效研究证据表明它们优于褪黑素本身。

疗效

一项关于褪黑素治疗成年人和儿童原发性睡眠障碍的荟萃分析显示，褪黑素缩短了入睡潜伏期，增加了总睡眠时间，且提高了整体睡眠质量。褪黑素对睡眠的作用适度，而且不会随着褪黑素的持续使用而消失[6]。

不良反应

在随机对照试验和发表的病例系列报道中，许多接受褪黑素治疗的儿童都有发育问题或感觉缺陷。在该人群中监测细微的不良反应有一定的局限性。并非所有的研究都会进行常规的不良反应监测。早期报告中包括一些小样本病例系列，发现褪黑素在短期内加剧癫痫[7]和哮喘[8,9]发作。其他报道的不良反应包括头痛、抑郁、不安、精神错乱、恶心、心动过速和瘙痒[10,11]。最近的大型安慰剂对照研究以及最近的微型片剂研究（PedPRM）发现，在学习困难、孤独症和癫痫儿童中[12-14]，与安慰组相比，治疗组没有发现过多的不良反应，尤其是癫痫发作没有加重。一项 Cochrane 综述发现，癫痫患者服用褪黑素后，癫痫发作频率没有增

加 [15]。最近一篇论文未发现褪黑素对青春期发育有明显影响 [16]。

剂量

对于儿童群体,生理剂量和药理剂量的界值为 500μg。生理剂量的褪黑素可以导致很高的受体占有率。在随机对照试验和病例报告中,使用的褪黑素剂量变异很大,500μg~5mg 最为普遍,但是也使用过更低或者更高的剂量。最佳剂量仍未可知,也没有证据显示量效之间的关系 [17]。在一项大样本随机对照试验中,18% 的儿童对 500μg 的剂量就有反应,但其他儿童需要更高的剂量(12mg) [14]。增加剂量超过 5mg 时,引起的很可能是褪黑素的镇静效应,而不是其改变睡眠时相的特点。对于一些有严重的双侧脑损伤的儿童,这可能是必要而且有帮助的。

睡液褪黑素测定价格很高,但是对识别严重睡眠时相延迟的儿童很重要,他们使用外源性褪黑素可能最有效;对识别褪黑素慢代谢型患者也很重要,因为白天褪黑素在血清中的蓄积(尤其高剂量情况下),最终导致失去疗效(图 5.3)。

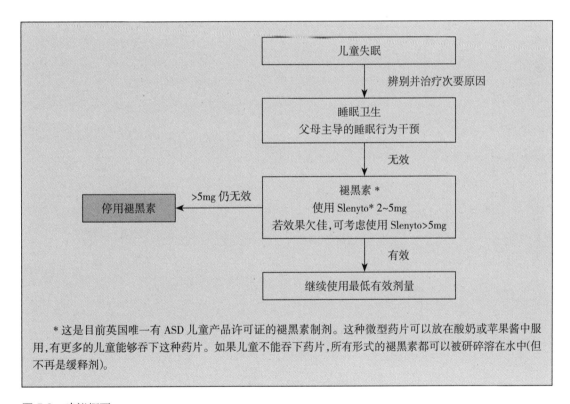

图 5.3 建议概要

参考文献

1. Gringras P. When to use drugs to help sleep. *Arch Dis Child* 2008; 93:976–981.
2. Macchi MM, et al. Human pineal physiology and functional significance of melatonin. *Front Neuroendocrinol* 2004; 25:177–195.
3. Gringras P, et al. Efficacy and safety of pediatric prolonged-release melatonin for insomnia in children with autism spectrum disorder. *J Am Acad Child Adolescent Psychiatry* 2017; 56:948–957.e944.
4. Williams Buckley A, et al. Practice guideline: treatment for insomnia and disrupted sleep behavior in children and adolescents with autism

spectrum disorder: report of the Guideline Development, Dissemination, and Implementation Subcommittee of the American Academy of Neurology. *Neurology* 2020; 94:392–404.

5. Arendt J, et al. Melatonin and its agonists: an update. *Br J Psychiatry* 2008; 193:267–269.

6. Ferracioli-Oda E, et al. Meta-analysis: melatonin for the treatment of primary sleep disorders. *PLoS One* 2013; 8:e63773.

7. Sheldon SH Pro-convulsant effects of oral melatonin in neurologically disabled children. *Lancet* 1998; 351:1254.

8. Maestroni GJ The immunoneuroendocrine role of melatonin. *J Pineal Res* 1993; 14:1–10.

9. Sutherland ER, et al. Elevated serum melatonin is associated with the nocturnal worsening of asthma. *J Allergy Clin Immunol* 2003; 112:513–517.

10. Chase JE, et al. Melatonin: therapeutic use in sleep disorders. *Ann Pharmacother* 1997; 31:1218–1226.

11. Jan JE, et al. Melatonin treatment of sleep-wake cycle disorders in children and adolescents. *Dev Med Child Neurol* 1999; 41:491–500.

12. Coppola G, et al. Melatonin in wake-sleep disorders in children, adolescents and young adults with mental retardation with or without epilepsy: a double-blind, cross-over, placebo-controlled trial. *Brain Dev* 2004; 26:373–376.

13. Garstang J, et al. Randomized controlled trial of melatonin for children with autistic spectrum disorders and sleep problems. *Child Care Health Dev* 2006; 32:585–589.

14. Gringras P, et al. Melatonin for sleep problems in children with neurodevelopmental disorders: randomised double masked placebo controlled trial. *BMJ* 2012; 345:e6664.

15. Brigo F, et al. Melatonin as add-on treatment for epilepsy. *Cochrane Database Syst Rev* 2016:Cd006967.

16. Malow BA, et al. Sleep, growth, and puberty after 2 years of prolonged-release melatonin in children with autism spectrum disorder. *J Am Acad Child Adolesc Psychiatry* 2020:S0890-8567(0820)30034-30034.

17. Sack RL, et al. Sleep-promoting effects of melatonin: at what dose, in whom, under what conditions, and by what mechanisms? *Sleep* 1997; 20:908–915.

第5章

儿童和青少年的快速镇静

与成年人一样,减少强制性非胃肠道给药的关键在于全面的精神状态评估、正确实施的治疗计划、在降低兴奋方面有丰富经验的工作人员以及对患者的妥当安置。

对儿童和青少年实施快速镇静或限制性医疗措施的卫生专业人员应当受过专业培训,有能力在该群体中采取这些措施,并且应当清楚所用限制性措施的法律背景。考虑使用高效价抗精神病药(如氟哌啶醇)时,应该特别慎重,尤其是那些从未服用过抗精神病药物的人,因为该年龄组患者出现急性肌张力障碍的风险较高[1]。儿童使用精神药物或躯体疾病药物治疗时,极易出现锥体外系反应[2]。NICE 推荐肌内注射劳拉西泮(不推荐其他药物)[3]。最近的一项综述表明,劳拉西泮有效(中位剂量为 1mg),且很少引起氧饱和度下降[4]。在处理严重病例时,注射奥氮平或口服阿立哌唑是安全的,但超过 50% 的患者可能需要使用第二种药物来达到镇静[5]。

此处给出的快速镇静药物的剂量范围很宽。用药宜谨慎,尤其对于低龄儿童;但对大龄青少年,可以考虑使用成年人剂量,尤其是非初次用药者,以及使用剂量范围低端的剂量无效的患者(表 5.7)。

表 5.7 口服药物被拒绝或者无效时推荐用于快速镇静的药物

药物	剂量	起效时间	评述
奥氮平肌内注射[6,7]	2.5~10mg	15~30min	与苯二氮䓬类合用可能增加呼吸抑制的风险,尤其是饮酒后。应该间隔 1h 以上使用
氟哌啶醇肌内注射[8]	<12 岁:每次 0.025~0.075mg/kg(最高 2.5mg)>12 岁青少年可以接受成年人剂量(2.5~5mg)	20~30min	必须常备注射用抗胆碱能药,以防喉肌痉挛或其他肌张力障碍(儿童更容易出现严重的肌张力障碍)成年人的资料显示,同时给予异丙嗪可以减少 EPS 风险[9]**心电图监测是必要的**
劳拉西泮 * 肌内注射[10,11]	<12 岁:0.5~1mg;>12 岁:0.5~2mg	20~40min	比咪达唑仑起效慢NICE 推荐的唯一治疗氟马西尼是所有苯二氮䓬类药物的逆转剂
咪达唑仑 * 肌内注射、静脉注射或口服液[11,12]	0.1~0.15mg/kg(肌内注射)咪达唑仑口服液,300~500µg/kg 或6~10 岁:7.5mg>10 岁:10mg	10~20min肌内注射(1~3min,静脉注射)	比劳拉西泮或地西泮起效快,但持续时间短只有在非常慎重且备好心肺复苏设备时才应静脉给药(通常是最后一招)比氟哌啶醇起效快,持续时间也短若用口服液,起效时间为 15~30min[13]。有一些发表的精神卫生数据,但仅见于成年人[14]。口服液未批准该用途
地西泮 * 静脉注射(不适合肌内注射)[15]	每次 0.1mg/kg 缓慢静脉注射。<12 岁最高日剂量 40mg>12 岁最高日剂量 60mg	1~3min	半衰期长与镇静作用时间长无关。有蓄积的可能**绝对不要肌内注射**

续表

药物	剂量	起效时间	评述
齐拉西酮肌内注射[16-19]（英国不用）	10~20mg	15~30min 肌内注射	效果显著。Q-T 间期延长在该患者群体里值得关注 **心电图监测是必要的**
阿立哌唑肌内注射[20,21]	9.75mg	15~30min	有证据对成年人有效，但对儿童和青少年尚无数据
异丙嗪肌内注射	<12 岁：5~25mg，最高量 50mg/d；>12 岁：25~50mg，最高量 100mg/d	最长 60min	尽管起效较慢，但是有效的镇静剂。若行为紊乱的原因不明，且对儿童和青少年使用抗精神病药有顾虑，可以使用

* 注意年轻人使用苯二氮䓬类药物时尤其容易出现脱抑制反应。

　　在采取注射治疗之前，无例外地应当给予口服药物（如果儿童愿意服用，必要时可以重复使用）。在撰写本文时，口服咪达唑仑[14] 和吸入性洛沙平[22] 在儿童快速镇静中尚未得到广泛研究，而且供应有限。口服咪达唑仑常用于儿童癫痫发作。快速镇静后的监测与成年人相同（见第 3 章）。

参考文献

1. National Institute for Health and Care Excellence. Psychosis and schizophrenia in children and young people: recognition and management. Clinical Guidance 155 2013 (last updated October 2016); https://www.nice.org.uk/guidance/cg155.
2. Chang MY, et al. Drug-induced extrapyramidal symptoms at the pediatric emergency department. *Pediatr Emerg Care* 2020; 36:468–472.
3. National Institute for Health and Care Excellence. Violence and aggression: short-term management in mental health, health and community settings. *Clinical Guidance* 10 [CG10]. 2015 (Last checked December 2019); https://www.nice.org.uk/guidance/ng10.
4. Kendrick JG, et al. Pharmacologic management of agitation and aggression in a pediatric emergency department – a retrospective cohort study. *J Pediatric Pharmacol Therapeutics* 2018; 23:455–459.
5. Rudolf F, et al. A retrospective review of antipsychotic medications administered to psychiatric patients in a tertiary care pediatric emergency department. *J Pediatric Pharmacol Therapeutics* 2019; 24:234–237.
6. Breier A, et al. A double-blind, placebo-controlled dose-response comparison of intramuscular olanzapine and haloperidol in the treatment of acute agitation in schizophrenia. *Arch Gen Psychiatry* 2002; 59:441–448.
7. Lindborg SR, et al. Effects of intramuscular olanzapine vs. haloperidol and placebo on QTc intervals in acutely agitated patients. *Psychiatry Res* 2003; 119:113–123.
8. Powney MJ, et al. Haloperidol for psychosis-induced aggression or agitation (rapid tranquillisation). *Cochrane Database Syst Rev* 2012; 11:CD009377.
9. TREC Collaborative Group. Rapid tranquillisation for agitated patients in emergency psychiatric rooms: a randomised trial of midazolam versus haloperidol plus promethazine. *BMJ* 2003; 327:708–713.
10. Sorrentino A Chemical restraints for the agitated, violent, or psychotic pediatric patient in the emergency department: controversies and recommendations. *Curr Opin Pediatr* 2004; 16:201–205.
11. Nobay F, et al. A prospective, double-blind, randomized trial of midazolam versus haloperidol versus lorazepam in the chemical restraint of violent and severely agitated patients. *Acad Emerg Med* 2004; 11:744–749.
12. Kennedy RM, et al. The "ouchless emergency department". Getting closer: advances in decreasing distress during painful procedures in the emergency department. *Pediatr Clin North Am* 1999; 46:1215–1247.
13. Schwagmeier R, et al. Midazolam pharmacokinetics following intravenous and buccal administration. *Br J Clin Pharmacol* 1998; 46:203–206.
14. Taylor D, et al. Buccal midazolam for agitation on psychiatric intensive care wards. *Int J Psychiatry Clin Pract* 2008; 12:309–311.
15. Nunn K, et al. Medication Table. in K N, C D, ed. *The Clinician's Guide to Psychotropic Prescribing in Children and Adolescents*. 1. Sydney: Glad Publishing 2003:383–452.
16. Khan SS, et al. A naturalistic evaluation of intramuscular ziprasidone versus intramuscular olanzapine for the management of acute agitation and aggression in children and adolescents. *J Child Adolesc Psychopharmacol* 2006; 16:671–677.
17. Staller JA Intramuscular ziprasidone in youth: a retrospective chart review. *J Child Adolesc Psychopharmacol* 2004; 14:590–592.
18. Hazaray E, et al. Intramuscular ziprasidone for acute agitation in adolescents. *J Child Adolesc Psychopharmacol* 2004; 14:464–470.

19. Barzman DH, et al. A retrospective chart review of intramuscular ziprasidone for agitation in children and adolescents on psychiatric units: prospective studies are needed. *J Child Adolesc Psychopharmacol* 2007; **17**:503–509.

20. Sanford M, et al. Intramuscular aripiprazole: a review of its use in the management of agitation in schizophrenia and bipolar I disorder. *CNS Drugs* 2008; **22**:335–352.

21. National Institute for Health and Clinical Excellence. Aripiprazole for schizophrenia in people aged 15 to 17 years. Technology Appraisal 13 [TA213] 2011; https://www.nice.org.uk/guidance/ta213.

22. Lesem MD, et al. Rapid acute treatment of agitation in individuals with schizophrenia: multicentre, randomised, placebo-controlled study of inhaled loxapine. *Br J Psychiatry* 2011; **198**:51–58.

儿童和青少年常用精神药物的剂量

常用药物的剂量见表 5.8。

表 5.8　儿童和青少年常用精神药物的起始剂量 [1,2]*

药物	起始剂量 **	述评
抗精神病药		
阿立哌唑	2mg	根据疗效和不良反应调节剂量
氯氮平	6.25~12.5mg	根据血药浓度确定维持剂量
奥氮平	2.5~5mg	根据疗效和不良反应调节剂量
喹硫平	25mg	有效剂量范围通常在 150~200mg/d
利培酮	0.25~2mg	根据疗效和不良反应调节剂量
抗抑郁药		
氟西汀	5~10mg/d	根据疗效和不良反应调节剂量
舍曲林	25~50mg/d	有效剂量通常为 50~100mg/d
西酞普兰	10mg/d	有效剂量为 10~40mg（注意 Q-T 间期）
其他药物		
锂盐	碳酸锂 100~200mg/d	根据血药浓度确定维持剂量
丙戊酸盐	10~20mg/(kg·d) 分次服	根据血药浓度确定维持剂量。不要给女孩或者有生育能力的年轻女性使用丙戊酸盐，除非有适当的避孕措施[3]。
褪黑素	夜间 2mg	有效剂量 2~10mg

　* 我们已经将氟哌啶醇、阿米替林、艾司西酞普兰和卡马西平从该表中删除，因为这些药物都不推荐用于儿童。

　** 推荐大致的口服起始剂量（对具体适应证的剂量参考原始文献）。推荐剂量范围的下限是为体重低于 25kg 的儿童所设。

（张玉龙　译　刘寰忠　校　田成华　审校）

参考文献

1. BNF Online. British National Formulary 2020; https://www.medicinescomplete.com/mc/bnf/current.
2. BNFC Online. British National Formulary for Children 2020; https://www.medicinescomplete.com/#/browse/bnfc.
3. GOV.UK Guidance. Valproate use by women and girls 2020; https://www.gov.uk/guidance/valproate-use-by-women-and-girls.

老年人精神药物的应用

一般原则

在老年人中,大多数药物的药代动力学和药效动力学会有较大程度的改变。若想治疗有效,且不良反应最少,则须考虑药物处置和药物作用中的这些变化。老年人经常同时罹患多种疾病,可能需要同时使用几种药物治疗。这会导致由药物相互作用引起的问题增多,以及整体上药源性问题增多[1]。有理由推测所有的药物在老年患者中比年轻患者更容易产生不良反应。

药物如何影响衰老的身体(药效动力学变化)

随着年龄增长,我们对反射作用(如血压和体温调节)的控制下降。受体可能变得更敏感,导致药物不良反应发生率和严重程度增加。例如,减弱肠蠕动的药物更容易引起便秘(如抗胆碱药和阿片类药物),影响血压的药物更容易导致跌倒(如三环类抗抑郁药和利尿剂)。老年人会对苯二氮䓬类和阿片类药物等中枢神经系统活性药物表现出过度反应,其中一部分原因是年龄相关的中枢神经系统功能下降,另一部分原因是个体药效学敏感性增加[2]。药物的治疗反应也可能会延迟。例如,老年人对抗抑郁药的反应时间可能长于年轻人[3]。

对于一些药物,老年人可能更容易发生严重不良反应,例如,氯氮平导致的粒细胞缺乏症[4]和中性粒细胞减少症[5],抗精神病药[6]导致的脑卒中,以及选择性 5-羟色胺再摄取抑制剂导致的出血。

衰老如何影响药物治疗(药代动力学变化)[7]

吸收

随着年龄的增长,肠蠕动减弱,胃酸分泌减少。这将导致药物吸收的速度变慢,进而起效更慢。与年轻人相比,老年人吸收的药量相同,但吸收速度较慢。

分布

与年轻人相比,老年人的身体脂肪比例增多,水分和白蛋白比例减少。这会导致一些脂溶性药物(如地西泮)的分布容积增加,作用持续时间延长,某些药物在作用部位浓度更高(如地高辛),与白蛋白结合的药量变少(游离的活性成分增加,如华法林、苯妥英)。

代谢

多数药物在肝脏代谢。老年人肝脏体积缩小,如果无肝脏疾病或肝血流量无显著减少,代谢能力并不会明显降低。药代动力学相互作用改变不大,但这些相互作用的药效学结果可能被放大。

排泄

肾功能随年龄的增长而下降:到 65 岁时肾功能将丧失 35%,80 岁时将丧失 50%。

如果同时具有多种疾病,如心脏病、糖尿病或高血压,肾功能会丧失更多。老年人血清肌酐或尿素的测量结果会误导人,因为肌肉量减少,相应地产生的肌酐就少了。用肾小球滤过率估计值(eGFR)[8]测量老年人群的肾功能是非常重要的措施。最好假设所有老年患者的肾功能最多是正常值的 2/3。

大多数药物最终(代谢后)由肾脏排泄。少数药物排泄前不经过生物转化,锂盐和舒必利就是重要的例子。主要通过肾脏排泄的药物在老年人身上会积聚,进而产生毒性反应和不良反应。因此,可能需要减少剂量(见"肾衰竭与精神药物"一节)。

药物相互作用

有些药物治疗指数小(少量增加可引起中毒,轻微减少会导致治疗作用丧失)。最常用的处方药有:地高辛、华法林、茶碱、苯妥英和锂盐。老年人身体处理这些药物的方式发生变化,且与其他药物更容易发生相互作用,因而更可能出现药物中毒和治疗失败。这些药物可以安全使用,但必须多加小心,并且应该在可能的情况下监测血药浓度。

有些药物抑制或诱导肝代谢酶。重要的例子包括一些 SSRI、红霉素和卡马西平。这可能会导致另一种药物的代谢改变。许多药物间发生相互作用正是通过这种机制。具体的药物相互作用及其后果参见《英国国家药典》(BNF 网络版)[9]。大部分也可以通过扎实的药理学知识进行推测。

降低老年人药物相关风险

遵守以下原则,会降低药物相关的发病率和死亡率。

- 只有在绝对必要的时才使用药物。
- 尽可能避免使用阻滞 α_1 受体、具有抗胆碱能不良反应、镇静作用强、半衰期长或是肝代谢酶强效抑制剂的药物。
- 开始使用低剂量,缓慢增加,但不能治疗不足。一些药物仍然需要充分的成人剂量。
- 治疗药物不良反应时,尽量不用另外的药物。找到一个更好耐受的药物来替代。
- 保持治疗药物用法简单,即尽可能每天用药 1 次。

药物加在食物中暗服 [10-12]

有时患者会拒绝药物治疗,即使这种治疗可以使其获得最大利益。在英国,患者有精神疾病或有能力时,应遵守精神卫生法。但是,如果患者缺乏能力,则可能不必做出该选择。如果未与多学科团队和患者家属充分讨论,不宜给老年痴呆症患者暗服药物。这一讨论的结果应该清楚地记录在患者病历中。只有当目标明确而清楚地是为了减轻患者痛苦时,才可以暗服药物。(有关进一步的信息,请参阅"在食品和饮料中隐蔽给药"部分。)

关于老年人使用精神药物的建议,参照本章的"老年人常用精神药物剂量指南"。

参考文献

1. Royal College of Physicians. Medication for older people. Summary and recommendations of a report of a working party of The Royal College of Physicians. *J R Coll Physicians Lond* 1997; **31**:254–257.

2. Bowie MW, et al. Pharmacodynamics in older adults: a review. *Am J Geriatr Pharmacother* 2007; **5**:263–303.

3. Baldwin R, et al. Management of depression in later life. *Adv Psychiatr Treatment* 2004; **10**:131–139.

4. Munro J, et al. Active monitoring of 12,760 clozapine recipients in the UK and Ireland. Beyond Pharmacovigilance. *Br J Psychiatry* 1999; **175**:576–580.

5. O'Connor DW, et al. The safety and tolerability of clozapine in aged patients: a retrospective clinical file review. *World J Biol Psychiatry* 2010; **11**:788–791.

6. Douglas IJ, et al. Exposure to antipsychotics and risk of stroke: self-controlled case series study. *BMJ* 2008; **337**:a1227.

7. Mayersohn M. Special pharmacokinetic considerations in the elderly. In W Evans, J Schentage, J Jusko, eds. *Applied pharmacokinetics: principles of therapeutic drug monitoring*. Vancouver, WA: Applied Therapeutics Inc, 1992.

8. Morriss R, et al. Lithium and eGFR: a new routinely available tool for the prevention of chronic kidney disease. *Br J Psychiatry* 2008; **193**:93–95.

9. National Institute for Health and Care Excellence. British National Formulary (BNF). 2020; https://bnf.nice.org.uk

10. Royal College of Psychiatrists. College statement on covert administration of medicines. *Psychiatric Bulletin* 2004; **28**:385–386.

11. Haw C, et al. Administration of medicines in food and drink: a study of older inpatients with severe mental illness. *Int Psychogeriatr* 2010; **22**:409–416.

12. Haw C, et al. Covert administration of medication to older adults: a review of the literature and published studies. *J Psychiatr Ment Health Nurs* 2010; **17**:761–768.

痴呆

　　痴呆是一种进展性、退行性、神经系统综合征,65 岁以上的人中约 5% 受此影响,而 80 岁以上者则上升到 20%。这种年龄相关疾病的特点是认知功能下降、记忆力和思维受损、逐渐丧失日常生活所需的技能。情绪、人格和社交行为的变化也是常见表现[1]。

　　根据影响大脑的疾病过程不同,将痴呆分为不同类型。痴呆最常见的原因是阿尔茨海默病,占所有痴呆患者的 60% 左右。其他主要是血管性痴呆和路易小体痴呆。阿尔茨海默病和血管性痴呆可能并存,在临床上往往难以分开。30%~70% 帕金森病患者也有痴呆[1](见本章"帕金森病"部分)。

阿尔茨海默病

用于阿尔茨海默病的认知增强剂的作用机制

乙酰胆碱酯酶(AChE)抑制剂

　　阿尔茨海默病的胆碱能假说是基于观察——与该病相关的认知功能恶化源于胆碱能神经元逐渐丧失和大脑乙酰胆碱(ACh)水平下降[2]。然而,人们不再普遍认为阿尔茨海默病症状仅是由于胆碱能耗竭[3]。

　　目前,在英国和其他国家已许可三种乙酰胆碱酯酶抑制剂用于治疗轻、中度阿尔茨海默病性痴呆,它们是多奈哌齐、卡巴拉汀和加兰他敏。这三种药物现在也被推荐用于重度阿尔茨海默病性痴呆。此外,已许可卡巴拉汀治疗轻、中度帕金森病性痴呆。

　　乙酰胆碱酯酶(AChE)和丁酰胆碱酯酶(BuChE)在乙酰胆碱酯酶降解中都起着重要的作用[4]。这几个胆碱酯酶抑制剂的药理作用不同:多奈哌齐选择性抑制 AChE,卡巴拉汀影响 AChE 和 BuChE,加兰他敏选择性抑制 AChE 并有烟碱受体激动剂特点[5]。至目前为止,并未发现这些差异导致疗效或耐受性的差异(AChE 抑制剂的比较见表 6.1)。

美金刚

　　英国和其他国家已许可美金刚用于治疗中、重度阿尔茨海默病性痴呆。它是一种低至中等亲和力的非竞争性 N-甲基-D-天冬氨酸(NMDA)谷氨酸受体拮抗剂,通过优先结合打开 NMDA 受体介导的钙通道,从而发挥其治疗作用。这种依赖于活性的结合阻断了 NMDA 受体介导的离子通量,可以减轻持续异常升高的谷氨酸水平(及其兴奋毒性)导致的神经元功能障碍[6](表 6.1)。

抗痴呆药的疗效

　　目前,没有任何治疗方法可以改变或逆转痴呆的疾病进展。因此,治疗干预针对的是特定的症状,以及改善或减缓认知功能下降。胆碱酯酶抑制剂(ACE-Is)可能会给轻、中度 AD 患者带来认知、功能和整体状况的获益。[15]

　　简易精神状态检查(MMSE)是基本认知功能量表,总分 30 分。阿尔茨海默病评估量表——认知分量表(ADAS-cog)总分 70 分,主要评定认知功能障碍。采用这两个量表

表 6.1　认知增强剂的特点 [7~14]

特点	多奈哌齐	卡巴拉汀	加兰他敏	美金刚
主要作用机制	AChE-I（选择性的+可逆的）	AChE-I（可逆的,非竞争性抑制剂）	AChE-I（选择性的+可逆的）	NMDA 受体拮抗剂
其他作用机制	无	BuChE-I	烟碱受体激动剂	5-HT$_3$ 受体拮抗剂
初始剂量	每天 5mg	1.5mg,每天 2 次（口服）（或每 24h 4.6mg 贴剂）	缓释片,每天 8mg（或口服液 4mg,每天 2 次）（速释片剂在一些国家已经停产）	每天 5mg
常规治疗剂量（最大剂量）	每天 10mg	3~6mg,每天 2 次（口服）或每 24h 9.5mg 贴剂	每天最大量缓释剂 16~24mg（或口服液 8~12mg,每天 2 次）	每天 20mg 或（10mg,每天 2 次）
推荐增加剂量的最小间隔	4 周（每天按 5mg 增加）	口服 2 周（增加 1.5mg,每天 2 次）贴剂 4 周（增加到每 24h 9.5mg）（如果 9.5mg/24h 可耐受,且出现有意义的认知/功能下降,6 个月后可考虑增到每 24h 13.3mg）	4 周（增加缓释剂 8mg,每天 1 次,或口服液 4mg,每天 2 次）	1 周（每天增加 5mg）
不良反应 [7~13] *很常见：≥1/10 常见：≥1/100	腹泻*,恶心*,头痛*,感冒,厌食,幻觉,激越,攻击行为,异常的梦和噩梦,晕厥,头晕,失眠,呕吐,腹部不适,皮疹,皮肤瘙痒,肌肉痉挛,尿失禁,疲劳,疼痛	厌食*,头晕*,恶心*,呕吐*,腹泻*,腹痛*,意识模糊,焦虑,食欲下降,噩梦,震颤,嗜睡,腹痛和消化不良,出汗,疲倦乏力,不适,体重下降（使用贴剂和胶囊出现不良反应的频率可能不同）	恶心*,呕吐*,食欲下降,幻觉,抑郁,晕厥,头晕,震颤,昏睡,心动过缓,高血压,腹痛和腹部不适,腹泻,消化不良,疲劳,乏力,身体不适,体重下降	药物过敏,嗜睡,头晕,平衡失调,高血压,呼吸困难,便秘,肝功能指标升高,头痛

第 6 章

续表

特点	多奈哌齐	卡巴拉汀	加兰他敏	美金刚
半衰期 (h)	~70	~1 (口服) 3.4 (贴剂)	7~8 (口服液) 8~10 (缓释胶囊)	60~100
代谢	CYP 3A4 CYP 2D6 (次要途径)	极少涉及 CYP 同工酶	CYP 3A4 CYP 2D6	主要是非肝途径
药物相互作用	有 (见单独的表)	相互作用不大可能	有 (见单独的表)	有 (见单独的表)
食物对吸收影响	无	降低吸收速度和程度	降低速度,但不降低吸收程度	无
药品费用 [7~14] (英国常用最大剂量治疗 1 个月)	片剂:£1.52 口崩片:£10.43 口服液 (1mg/mL):£100.22	胶囊:£66.10 口服液 (2mg/mL):£135.55 贴剂 9.5mg:£19.97 4.6mg 和 13.3mg:£77.97	缓释胶囊 £79.80 口服液 (4mg/mL):£201.60	片剂:£8.46 口崩片:£49.98 口服液 (10mg/mL):£61.77 注意:带给药泵的药瓶每次按压压出 5mg/0.5mL
相对成本	$	$$	$$	$
专利状况	有非专利药	有非专利药	有专利药	有非专利药

第 6 章

进行评定,这三种乙酰胆碱酯酶抑制剂似乎临床效果相似。估计需要治疗的人数(NNT)(ADAS-cog 改善>4 分)为 4~12[16]。

美金刚

分析结果显示美金刚改善认知功能的 NNT 为 3~8[17]。Cochrane 的美金刚综述显示,在中、重度阿尔茨海默病中,用美金刚治疗 6 个月具有较小的获益。在轻度至中度痴呆患者中,认知功能的小幅获益在血管性痴呆患者中检测不到,在 AD 患者也几乎检测不到。[17]

2020 年的一项研究[18]考察了胆碱酯酶抑制剂和美金刚的"真实世界"有效性。研究发现,总体而言,MMSE 和蒙特利尔认知评估量表(MoCA)得分的最初下降大约发生在开始用药的 2 年前。使用药物后的 2~5 个月,认知功能基本稳定。在认知功能受损更严重的患者服药时,这种效果会增强,而在服用抗精神病药时,这种效果会减弱。重要的是,至少换药一次的患者往往会以用药前的速度继续下降,可见,这类患者显然没有从药物干预中受益。总体而言,68% 的患者对治疗有反应,在一段时间内认知功能稳定,而后认知功能以治疗前的速度继续下降。

抗痴呆药的换用

当 AChE-I 治疗中断后,原治疗效果很快消失[19],重新开始药物治疗时,疗效可能无法完全恢复[20]。一种药物耐受性差,不能排除另一个耐受性好[21]。最近修订的英国精神药理协会抗痴呆药指南证实,既往比较性试验未能一致证明三种 AChE-I 之间的疗效存在任何显著差异,主要差异在于不良事件的频率和类型。因此,患者若不能耐受一种药物,则换用不同的 AChE-I 后,相当一部分患者(高达 50%)不仅能耐受,而且也可从中获益,该指南的这个建议仍然合理[22]。

据报道,有数例停用多奈哌齐后出现撤药综合征[23,24],提示应该尽可能地逐步减药。然而,一项研究比较突然和逐步从多奈哌齐转换到美金刚的不良反应,结果发现差异没有临床意义,尽管突然停药组的不良反应发生率较高(分别为 46% 与 32%)[25]。(关于换用卡巴拉汀贴剂的内容见下面"耐受性"。)

根据文献的系统性综述[26],有人提出一种实用的方法来换用 AChE-I:若对药物不耐受,只有在停用原来药物且不良反应完全缓解后,才能换成另外一种药物。若缺乏疗效,可以突然换药,之后快速加量。在开始治疗几年后丧失疗效的患者不推荐换用另一种 AChE-I。

其他影响

AChE 抑制剂也可能影响阿尔茨海默病和其他痴呆的非认知方面。一些研究已经调查了药物对于痴呆非认知症状的安全性和有效性。关于治疗这些症状的更多信息,参见本章"痴呆的精神行为症状(BPSD)治疗"部分。

剂量与剂型

剂量信息见表 6.1。

在一项为期 6 个月的双盲、安慰剂对照随机对照试验(RCT)中,**卡巴拉汀贴剂**(9.5mg/24h)已被证明与最高剂量胶囊的效果一样,但具有更好的耐受性[27],中国的一项研究也证实了这一点[28]。现在也已研制出了一种鼻腔喷雾剂[29]。

根据Ⅲ期临床试验的阳性结果，FDA 批准了更高剂量的**多奈哌齐缓释剂(23mg)**治疗中度至重度 AD 患者。目前，多奈哌齐 23mg/d 已在美国和亚洲部分地区上市。在一项针对中度至重度 AD 患者的全球Ⅲ期试验中，多奈哌齐 23mg/d 比多奈哌齐 10mg /d 对认知功能的改善更好，严重障碍量表(SIB)评分在整个研究人群中平均变化值的治疗组间差异为 2.2 分，晚期 AD 患者中为 3.1 分。由于多奈哌齐剂量从每天 10mg 增加到 23mg 时，观察到胃肠道(GI)不良反应发生率增加，因此，剂量增加在一定程度上具有挑战性。但这些不良反应很少持续 1 个月以上。采用逐步加量策略可能会解决这些胃肠道不良反应问题，可用以下方法在 1~2 个月内将多奈哌齐的剂量从 10mg 逐步增加到 23mg：每天 1 次服用 10mg 片剂和 5mg 片剂各 1 片，持续 1 个月，然后每天服用 23mg，或隔日服用 10mg 片剂和 23mg 片剂。韩国设计了一项研究，确定成功滴定至 23mg/d 的最佳剂量递增策略[30]。临床建议强调了选择患者(AD 严重程度、低剂量多奈哌齐的耐受性和无禁忌证)、逐步增加剂量，以及在 AD 患者管理中对患者和照护者进行适宜的监测和咨询等的重要性[30]。

美金刚缓释胶囊(ER)28mg，每天 1 次，于 2010 年在美国获批，现已广泛销售。其疗效在一项大型、跨国、Ⅲ期试验中得到证实。该试验表明，与胆碱酯酶抑制剂单药治疗相比，胆碱酯酶抑制剂加用美金刚缓释剂(ER)可改善关键疗效结局，包括认知功能和整体状态。最常见的不良事件为头痛、腹泻和头晕[31]。

值得注意的是，这些高剂量的多奈哌齐和美金刚还没有在英国和其他国家得到批准。此外，与临床试验中的患者相比，临床实践中大多数老年 AD 患者可能更虚弱，共病更多，因此，也许不太可能耐受更高的剂量。

联合治疗

虽然联合使用乙酰胆碱酯酶抑制剂和美金刚的疗效研究结果仍有争议，欧洲神经病学会(EAN)指南和英国卫生和保健研究所(NICE)[1] 都推荐在中度至重度 AD 患者中联合使用乙酰胆碱酯酶抑制剂和美金刚，而不是单独使用乙酰胆碱酯酶抑制剂。支持这一建议的证据相当薄弱[32]。研究证实，AChE-I 与美金刚之间不存在药代动力学或药效学相互作用[33,34]。

耐受性

AChE-I 药物之间耐受性可能不同，但是在没有充分直接比较的情况下，很难得出明确的结论。根据临床试验中脱落患者的数量可以大致评估总体耐受性。在多奈哌齐试验中的脱落率[35,36]为 4%~16%(安慰剂组 1%~7%)。卡巴拉汀[37,38]脱落率为 7%~29%(安慰剂组 7%)。加兰他敏[39-41]脱落率为 7%~23%(安慰剂组 7%~9%)。这些数字与明确由不良反应引起的脱落相关。已报道其伤害的 NNH 为 12[16]。法国药物监测数据库研究发现，年龄、抗精神病药、降压药和针对消化道和代谢的药物，是 AChE-I引起严重反应的相关因素[42]。

耐受性似乎受加药速度影响，可能也受剂量影响。在临床试验中，大多数不良反应发生在加药过程中，建议在临床上缓慢加药。这可能意味着这些药物在实践中均具有良好的耐受性。

卡巴拉汀贴剂使用方便，耐受性优于卡巴拉汀胶囊[27,28]。三个试验的数据发现，卡巴拉汀贴剂比胶囊耐受性好，胃肠道不良反应及其导致的脱落也少[43]。有数据支持下述建议：使用高剂量卡巴拉汀胶囊(>6mg/d) 者,直接换成 9.5mg/24h 的贴剂;使用低剂量胶囊(≤6mg/d)者,开始时使用 4.6mg/24h 的贴剂 4 周,然后增至 9.5mg/24h 的贴剂。后一换药方法也适用于从其他口服胆碱酯酶抑制剂换成卡巴拉汀贴剂(对不良反应较为敏感、体重较轻或有心动过缓病史的患者,需要 1 周的洗脱期)[44]。经过 6 个月 9.5mg/24h 贴剂治疗,如果耐受性好且认知或功能出现有意义的下降时,可以考虑增加剂量到 13.3mg/24h[49]。一项为期 48 周的随机对照试验发现,相比 9.5mg/24h 的贴剂,大规格的贴剂(13.3mg)能显著减轻工具性日常生活活动的恶化,并且耐受性好[45]。

患者和照护者应该被告知卡巴拉汀贴剂的重要使用细节[9]:

- 经皮贴剂不适用于红肿、发炎或有伤口的皮肤。
- 应避免 14 天内重复贴在同处皮肤,以尽量减少皮肤刺激的潜在风险。
- 在每天使用新的贴片之前,必须将前一天的贴片取下。
- 一次只能贴一片贴剂。
- 不能把贴剂切割成小片。

使用 AChE-I 时应注意以下疾病:哮喘、慢性阻塞性肺疾病(COPD)、病态窦房结综合征、室上性传导异常、易患消化性溃疡、癫痫发作史和膀胱流出道梗阻。在使用卡巴拉汀贴剂时,存在贴剂误用导致致命性过量的风险[46]。

美金刚具有良好的耐受性[47,48],唯一与警告相关的情况包括肝脏损伤和癫痫/癫痫发作[49](肾功能损害所需的剂量调整见《英国国家处方集》或同等资料)。据报道,当美金刚与华法林联合使用时,个别病例的国际标准化比值(INR)升高。

不良反应

胆碱酯酶抑制剂

当 AChE-I 出现不良反应时,它们在很大程度上是可预测的:过度胆碱能兴奋导致恶心、呕吐、头晕、失眠和腹泻[50]。这些反应往往发生在开始治疗或增加剂量时。它们是剂量相关的,往往是短暂的。也有研究报道过尿失禁[51]。虽然临床试验表明多奈哌齐的不良事件发生频率相对较低,但在不良事件的类型或频率上,不同药物之间似乎没有显著的区别。这可能是其他药物试验中加药方法较激进的反映。在临床试验中,口服卡巴拉汀比其他胆碱酯酶抑制剂引起胃肠道反应似乎更常见,但是通过缓慢加药、与食物同服或使用贴剂,可降低出现胃肠道反应的风险。

对来自 VigiBase 数据库 16 年个体病例安全报告的分析发现,AChE-I 最常见的不良反应为神经精神症状(31.4%)、胃肠道疾病(15.9%)、全身性紊乱和给药部位疾病(11.9%)。心血管药物不良反应占 11.7%[52]。

根据药理作用,AChE-I 可能对心率有迷走神经紧张性作用(即心动过缓)(图 6.1)。这种作用可能对某些患者特别重要,如患有病态窦房结综合征或其他室上性心脏传导障碍(如窦房或房室传导阻滞)者[7-12]。

加兰他敏治疗轻度认知损害(MCI)对照试验结果显示,加兰他敏相关的死亡率比安慰剂组高(分别为 1.5% 和 0.5%),这提示我们需要注意 AChE-I 相关的心脏不良反应[55]。虽然没有占优势的具体死亡原因,所报告的死亡病例 50% 死于心血管病。因此,FDA 发布了一

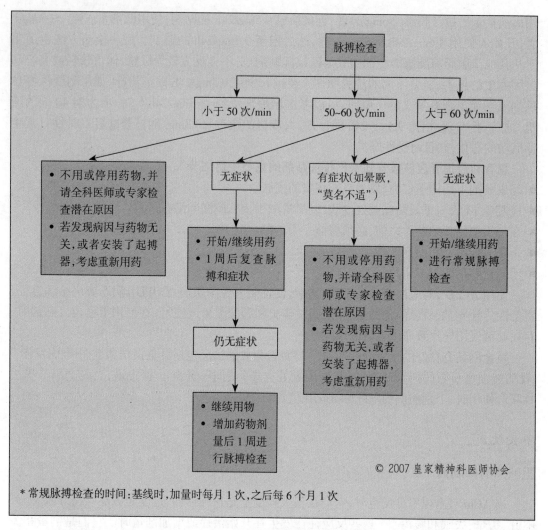

脉搏检查

小于 50 次/min　　50~60 次/min　　大于 60 次/min

- 不用或停用药物,并请全科医师或专家检查潜在原因
- 若发现病因与药物无关,或者安装了起搏器,考虑重新用药

无症状

- 开始/继续用药
- 1 周后复查脉搏和症状

仍无症状

- 继续用物
- 增加药物剂量后 1 周进行脉搏检查

有症状(如晕厥,"莫名不适")

- 不用或停用药物,并请全科医师或专家检查潜在原因
- 若发现病因与药物无关,或者安装了起搏器,考虑重新用药

无症状

- 开始/继续用药
- 进行常规脉搏检查

© 2007 皇家精神科医师协会

* 常规脉搏检查的时间:基线时,加量时每月 1 次,之后每 6 个月 1 次

图 6.1　AD 患者 AChE-ls 治疗前和治疗期间心血管风险管理建议指南 [53,54]。"药物"是指选定的乙酰胆碱酯酶抑制剂。经允许复制

项限制 MCI 患者使用加兰他敏的警告。心血管病与阿尔茨海默病的关联性依旧不清楚 [56]。对 AChE-I 随机对照试验数据进行汇总的 Cochrane 综述发现,与安慰剂组相比,AChE-I 组晕厥发生率较高(3.43% vs 1.87%)。一项基于人群的研究,使用病例-时间-对照(case-time-control design)设计,调查了安大略省 140 万老年人的健康记录,发现用 AChE-I 治疗者因心动过缓住院的风险增加 1 倍,50% 以上病例在出院时会重新使用这些药物,提示临床医师低估了 AChE-I 的心血管毒性 [57]。似乎路易体痴呆患者更容易出现这些药物导致的心动过缓,这与该病所致的自主神经功能不全有关 [58]。相似的研究发现,服用 AChE-I 人群比对照组因晕厥就诊者更多:比例分别为 31.5/1 000 人-年和 18.6/1 000 人-年(校正 HR 1.76)[59]。

因此,三种药物的制造商建议,对有心血管病或合用降低心率药物(如地高辛或 β 受体阻滞剂)的患者,用药应谨慎。虽然建议在治疗前需要强制检查心电图 [56],但是已发表的证据显示,心血管不良反应的发生率低,严重不良反应更是罕见。此外,治疗前筛查和常规心

电图检查的价值受到质疑。目前,英国卫生和保健研究所(NICE)并未做此推荐。然而,对有心血管病史或合用负性心率药物的患者,建议检查心电图。(见 2016 年约克郡和亨伯临床网络指南——痴呆患者处方乙酰胆碱酯酶抑制剂前的心脏状况评估。)

一项 204 例阿尔茨海默病患者的研究评估了 AChE-I 治疗前、后的心电图和血压。有人指出,没有哪一种 AChE-I 与负性心率、心律失常或降压作用的增多有关,因此在迷走神经紧张作用方面,不能确定首选哪种药物[60]。同样,丹麦的回顾性队列研究[61]发现,在心肌梗死或心力衰竭的风险上,使用多奈哌齐或其他 AChE-I 之间没有实质性差异。实际上美金刚组不同原因死亡的风险最高,然而美金刚治疗选择的都是病情较重者。一项瑞典的队列研究发现,对于阿尔茨海默病患者,AChE-I 与心肌梗死或死亡的风险下降相关性为 35%[62]。随着 AChE-I 剂量增加,相关性增强。为了证实这项观察性研究的结果,需要进行随机对照试验,但它们与其他降低死亡率的观察结果很吻合。

一项关于痴呆药物心血管作用的综述发现,尽管与 AChE-I 有关的心血管不良事件罕见,但有证据表明,与 AChE-I 相关的晕厥和心动过缓风险呈现小幅度但有统计学意义的增加。也有一些报告指出,这些药物有时可能与 Q-T 间期延长和尖端扭转性室性心动过速有关。

美金刚

虽然对美金刚的心血管影响了解很少,但有报道称,使用美金刚会导致心动过缓和心血管事件存活率降低[63]。

美金刚汇总数据分析表明,在安慰剂对照临床试验中,最常报道的不良反应包括激越(美金刚和安慰剂组分别为 7.5% 和 12%)、跌倒(6.8% 和 7.1%)、头晕(6.3% 和 5.7%)、意外损伤(6.0% 和 7.2%)、流感样症状(6% 和 5.8%)、头痛(5.2% 和 3.7%)和腹泻(5% 和 5.6%)[64]。

一项法国药物监测数据库研究比较了**多奈哌齐**与**美金刚**的不良反应。单用多奈哌齐与单用美金刚后最常见的药物不良反应分别为:心动过缓(10% 和 7%)、虚弱(5% 和 6%)和抽搐(4% 和 3%)。虽然普遍认为多奈哌齐与心动过缓有关,美金刚与癫痫发作相关,但是这一分析提示,美金刚也可以引起心动过缓,多奈哌齐也可以诱发癫痫发作。因此,在治疗具有心动过缓或癫痫病史的痴呆患者时,需要特别注意[65]。

相互作用

潜在的相互作用也可以协助区分现有的胆碱酯酶抑制剂。多奈哌齐[66]和加兰他敏[67]由细胞色素 2D6 和 3A4 代谢,因此,其药物浓度可能会受影响这些酶的药物所改变。胆碱酯酶抑制剂本身也可能干扰其他药物代谢,虽然这也许是一个理论上的考虑。卡巴拉汀几乎没有潜在的相互作用,因为它在作用部位代谢,不影响肝细胞色素酶。在一项前瞻性分析中,调查了卡巴拉汀与老年人常用药物(22 种不同的治疗类别)的药效学相互作用,比较卡巴拉汀和安慰剂之间不良反应的比值比。与安慰剂相比,卡巴拉汀未增加药物相互作用相关的不良反应[68]。药物相互作用是一个重要因素,因为老年人群容易出现多药合用的情况,而卡巴拉汀似乎极少导致药物相互作用(表 6.2)。

法国药物监测数据库分析发现,大多数关于 AChE-I 药物相互作用的报道属于药效学相互作用,最常见的问题见于 AChE-I 合用导致心动过缓的药物(β 受体阻滞剂、地高辛、胺碘

表 6.2　药物相互作用 [8-12,74,75]

药物	代谢	升高血药浓度的药物	降低血药浓度的药物	药效动力学相互作用
多奈哌齐 (安理申®)	3A4 和 2D6 的底物	酮康唑 伊曲康唑 红霉素 奎尼丁 氟西汀 帕罗西汀	利福平 苯妥英 卡马西平 酒精	与抗胆碱能药和竞争性神经肌肉阻滞剂(如筒箭毒碱)有拮抗作用; 与拟胆碱药、如去极化神经肌肉阻滞剂的胆碱酯酶抑制剂(如新斯的明)可能有协同作用; β 受体阻滞剂、胺碘酮或钙通道阻滞剂可能对心脏传导导致叠加作用。肌肉阻断剂(如琥珀酰胆碱)、胆碱能受体激动剂和外周作用; 谨慎与导致 Q-T 间期延长或尖端扭转性室性心动过速的药物合用; 抗精神病药和胆碱酯酶抑制剂合用, 可发生运动障碍和神经阻滞剂恶性综合征; 与降低癫痫发作阈值的药物合用, 可降低癫痫发作的阈值
卡巴拉汀 (艾斯能®)	非肝代谢	代谢性相互作用似乎不太可能	卡巴拉汀可抑制丁酰胆碱酯酶介导导的其他物质的代谢, 如可卡因 吸烟可增加卡巴拉汀的清除	与抗胆碱能药和竞争性神经肌肉阻滞剂(如筒箭毒碱)有拮抗作用; 与拟胆碱药、如去极化神经肌肉肉阻断剂(如琥珀酰胆碱)肉阻断剂或外周作用的胆碱酯酶抑制剂(如新斯的明)可能有协同作用; 与 β 受体阻滞剂、胺碘酮和钙通道阻滞剂对心脏传导导致协同效应; 谨慎与导致 Q-T 间期延长或尖端扭转性室性心动过速的药物合用; 抗精神病药和胆碱酯酶抑制剂合用, 可发生运动障碍和神经阻滞剂恶性综合征; 与甲氧氯普胺合用, 可增加锥体外系症状的风险
加兰他敏 (Reminyl®)	3A4 和 2D6 的底物	酮康唑 红霉素 利托那韦 奎尼丁 帕罗西汀 氟伏沙明 阿米替林	不详	与抗胆碱能药和竞争性神经肌肉阻滞剂(如筒箭毒碱)有拮抗作用; 与拟胆碱药、如去极化神经肌肉肉阻断剂(如琥珀酰胆碱)、胆碱能受体激动剂和外周作用; 用的胆碱酯酶抑制剂(如新斯的明)可能有协同作用; 与显著降低心率的药物(如地高辛、β 受体阻滞剂、钙通道阻滞剂和胺碘酮)可能有相互作用; 谨慎与可引起足 Q-T 间期延长或尖端扭转性室速的药物合用(厂家建议在这种情况下做心电图); 抗精神病药和胆碱酯酶抑制剂合用, 可发生运动障碍和神经阻滞剂恶性综合征

第 6 章

续表

药物	代谢	升高血药浓度的药物	降低血药浓度的药物	药效动力学相互作用
美金刚 (Exiba®)	主要是非肝代谢,经肾脏消除	西咪替丁 雷尼替丁 普鲁卡因胺 奎尼丁 尼古丁 甲氧苄氨嘧啶 据报道,合用华法林时,个别病例标准化比值升高(建议密切监测凝血酶原时间或 INR) 碱化尿液的药物(pH~8)(如碳酸酐酶抑制剂、碳酸氢钠)可降低肾脏对美金刚的清除率	不详 同时给予美金刚可能降低血清氯噻嗪水平	左旋多巴、多巴胺受体激动剂,司米吉兰和抗胆碱能药的效果可被增强 巴比妥类药物和抗精神病药的效果可能会减弱。 避免合用金刚烷胺、氯胺酮和右美沙芬——有导致中枢神经系统中毒的风险。已出版的一份病例报告提示苯妥英与美金刚联用可能有风险; 当给予美金刚时,解痉剂、丹曲林或巴氯芬的剂量可能需要调整; 单个病例报告,与复方新诺明或甲氧苄氨苄啶合用时,会出现肌阵挛和意识模糊

注:这个列表并不详尽,注意抑制或增强 CYP 3A4 和 2D6 酶的其他药物。
ECG,心电图;INR,国际标准化比值。

酮、钙通道拮抗剂)。这些相互作用几乎有 1/3 导致心血管不良反应,如心动过缓、房室传导阻滞和低血压。其次见于 AChE-I 与抗胆碱能药物合用时,导致药理学拮抗作用[69]。

近期一篇全面的综述总结了抗痴呆药的药效动力学、药代动力学和药物遗传学特点[70,71]。

何时停止治疗

对居住在社区的中重度 AD 患者的一项大型多中心研究[72]调查了多奈哌齐超过 12 个月的长期疗效,并与 3 个月后停用多奈哌齐换为美金刚,或多奈哌齐与美金刚联合使用的疗效进行了比较。多奈哌齐的持续治疗与认知功能长期获益有关,MMSE 评分低至 3 分的患者也能从中获益。这表明患者应该尽可能长时间地使用 AChE-I 治疗,而不应该设定停止治疗的 MMSE 界限分。此外,该研究的二次分析和事后多重比较发现,中重度 AD 患者停用多奈哌齐后 12 个内,入住疗养院的风险增加,但在接下来的 3 年随访期间并没有差异。这一研究结果强调,即使持续治疗的可感知获益不够明确,作出停药或继续治疗的决定时仍应告知可能的停药风险[73]。

AChE-I 在痴呆进程中的疗效尚不完全清楚。一方面,有证据表明,最初处方这些药物时,认知功能可以在 2~5 个月内保持稳定[18]。另一方面,前文所引用的研究表明,即使是在疾病病程较晚时停药,也可能会产生不利影响。现实情况是,治疗反应可能存在个体差异,目前,这些差异尚未被充分了解,也无法预测。因此,要根据每个患者的情况来决定是否停用 AChE-I,并要考虑家人和照护者的意见。然而,人们的共识是,如果药物耐受性好,患者的身体状况稳定,那么最好继续用药。停用抗痴呆药物的风险与继续治疗的不良反应和费用之间应该进行权衡[95]。

此外,一项荟萃分析评估了三种 AChE-I 和美金刚与 AD 严重程度的关系,发现除了美金刚,其他药物的疗效与痴呆各维度的严重程度无关。美金刚对功能损害的效果事实上在重度患者中更好。研究结果表明,不同阶段的 AD 患者对 AChE-I 和美金刚的治疗仍有反应。因此,药物治疗的效果基本上与疾病的严重程度无关,严重程度不同的患者均可以从药物治疗中获益。这表明患者病情的严重程度不应该妨碍这些药物的治疗[76]。

以下章节总结了在临床实践中停用抗痴呆药物的指导[77]。

停止治疗的原因

- 当患者/照护者决定停止治疗时(应在被告知停止治疗的风险和获益后)
- 当患者拒绝服药时(但可参阅有关暗服药的部分)
- 当患者的依从性出现问题,而又无法合理解决时
- 当患者的认知、功能和行为下降因为治疗而加重时
- 当有无法忍受的不良反应时
- 当共患疾病使治疗有风险或无效时(例如绝症)
- 在继续治疗没有临床意义的情况下(当患者在认知测查结果上达到特定分数,或被送到机构照护时,应该根据临床情况作出判断,而不是停止治疗)
- 当痴呆发展到严重受损阶段[总体衰退量表(GDS)第 7 阶段:出现吞咽困难]

当决定停止治疗(不是因为耐受性差时),建议逐渐减少剂量,并监测患者在接下来 1~3 个月是否出现显著衰退的证据。如果出现显著衰退,应考虑恢复治疗。

NICE 建议

NICE 在 2018 年 6 月更新了关于痴呆的指南 [78]。

NICE 阿尔茨海默病治疗指南概要 [1,81]

- 建议将多奈哌齐、加兰他敏和卡巴拉汀三种 AChE-I 用于轻、中度阿尔茨海默病。
- 建议将美金刚用于对 AChE-I 不能耐受或有禁忌证的中度阿尔茨海默病患者,或用于重度阿尔茨海默病。
- 对于已在服用 AChE-I 的 AD 确诊患者:
  - 如果是中度 AD 患者,考虑在 AChE-I 基础上加用美金刚。
  - 如果是重度 AD 患者,在 AChE-I 的基础上加用美金刚。
- 治疗需符合以下条件:
  对于没有服用过 AChE-I 或美金刚的患者,只能在有充足知识和技能的临床医师的建议下才处方药物。
  包括:
  - 二级医疗专科医师,如精神科医师、老年科医师和神经科医师。
  - 其他有诊断和治疗 AD 专业知识的医疗卫生专业人员(如全科医师、护士顾问和高级护理从业者)
- 一旦决定开始 AChE-I 或美金刚治疗,可以在初级保健机构首次处方。
- 对于已经服用过 AChE-I 的患者,初级保健机构的处方者可以在不征求专科医师建议的情况下开始使用美金刚治疗。
- 确保当地的处方、供应和治疗审查等安排符合 NICE 药物优化指南 [80]。
- 不要单纯因为疾病严重程度而停止 AD 患者的 AChE-I 使用。
- AChE-I 治疗应从价格最低的药物开始(一旦开始部分自费治疗,考虑每天所需的剂量及该剂量的价格)。根据药物不良反应特点、依从性估计、躯体共病、药物相互作用可能性和用药特点,可能需要考虑替代药物。

NICE 非 AD 型痴呆治疗指南概要 [78,79]

- 轻、中度的路易体痴呆(DLB)患者用多奈哌齐或卡巴拉汀治疗。
- 对多奈哌齐和卡巴拉汀不耐受的轻中度 DLB 患者,只考虑加兰他敏。
- 重度的 DLB 患者考虑使用多奈哌齐或卡巴拉汀治疗。
- 对 AChE-I 不耐受或者禁忌的 DLB 患者,考虑使用美金刚治疗。
- 血管性痴呆患者如果怀疑合并 AD、帕金森病痴呆或 DLB,只考虑 AChE-I 或美金刚。
- 额颞叶痴呆患者不使用 AChE-I 和美金刚。
- 多发性硬化症引起的认知障碍不使用 AChE-I 和美金刚。
- 帕金森病痴呆的药物治疗指导,见 NICE 帕金森病痴呆指南。

可能导致认知损害的药物 [1]

- 注意一些常用的处方药会增加抗胆碱能负担,从而导致认知障碍。
- 考虑尽量少用增加抗胆碱能负担的药物,并尽可能寻找替代药物:
  - 在评估是否将疑似痴呆患者转诊进行诊断时。
  - 在对痴呆患者的用药进行审查时。
- 注意使用有效的评估抗胆碱能负担的工具,但尚无足够的证据推荐任何一种(请参阅"躯体疾病药物在痴呆中的安全使用"部分)。
- 进行药物审查的指导意见,见 NICE 药物优化指南中的药物审查。
  注意:《抗胆碱能药对认知功能影响》(AEC)量表可在 www.medichec.com 查询。

其他治疗(证据尚不确定)

银杏叶制剂

Cochrane 综述发现,虽然与安慰剂相比银杏叶制剂是安全的,不良反应不多于安慰剂,但是尚无令人信服的证据表明其对于痴呆和认知损害是有效的。许多试验样本量都太小,使用的方法不理想,并且发表偏倚不能排除。该综述的结论是,银杏叶制剂治疗痴呆或认知障碍的临床获益结果不一,且缺乏说服力[81]。对几项系统综述的回顾发现,当剂量大于200mg/d(通常为240mg/d),并持续至少 5 个月时,它具有潜在的益处。但是证据质量较低,需要做进一步严格设计、多中心、大规模随机对照试验[82]。几份报告指出,银杏叶制剂可能会增加出血的风险[83]。这种药物在德国被广泛使用,但在其他地方却用得较少。

维生素 E

关于维生素 E 治疗阿尔茨海默病和轻度认知障碍(MCI),Cochrane 综述核查了三项研究。作者的结论是,没有证据表明维生素 E 对阿尔茨海默病或 MCI 的预防和治疗有效,需要进一步研究以确定其在这方面的作用[84]。最近的一项 RCT 研究(TEAM-AD),考察了维生素 E 2 000IU/d 治疗 613 例轻、中度阿尔茨海默病患者的疗效。研究结果表明,维生素 E 组主要结局指标,即日常生活活动功能,其年衰退率下降了 19%,作者认为这相当于病情进展被推迟 6 个月。对于次要结果,安慰剂组需照护的时间比维生素 E 组多了 2h;认知能力或其他次要结局未见显著获益[85]。AD 患者的维生素 E 试验中,使用的 α-生育酚的剂量远远高于每天推荐的 22.4IU,这与出血性卒中、前列腺癌、心力衰竭和死亡率增高等不良反应有关。由于维生素 E 对 AD 患者的疗效证据有限,在推荐维生素 E 之前,必须权衡其效果和这些潜在的不良影响。[86]

叶酸

一项 Cochrane 综述发现,没有证据表明叶酸(合用或不合用维生素 B)可以改善患有或无痴呆的未经选择的老年人的认知功能[87]。但是,根据最近一篇综述的数据,似乎叶酸补充剂可以改善认知功能,其机制是降低同型半胱氨酸、改善血管功能、减轻炎症状态、调节大脑叶酸缺乏和抗氧化反应等。半胱氨酸水平高的人对叶酸补充剂有更好的反应,这可能是因为血清叶酸浓度低。目前,还不知道可能改善认知功能所需的最佳叶酸剂量[88]。

血清同型半胱氨酸含量升高被证明是认知损害的一种潜在危险因素。一些证据表明,补充维生素 B 可以通过降低同型半胱氨酸水平来缓解认知功能下降。最近的一项荟萃分析研究评估了叶酸合用维生素 B_{12} 和/或维生素 B_6 降低同型半胱氨酸,从而减轻老年 AD 或痴呆患者认知能力下降的疗效。补充维生素 B 可有效地降低血清同型半胱氨酸水平,然而,这并没有转化为改善认知功能的作用。这一结果表明,现有的有关维生素 B 通过降低同型半胱氨酸水平来改善认知的数据是矛盾的[89]。

ω-3 脂肪酸

Cochrane 综述回顾了 ω-3 治疗痴呆的三项试验,共包括 632 例轻、中度 AD 患者。该综述研究发现,连续服用 6 个月的 ω-3 多不饱和脂肪酸补充剂对认知(学习和理解)、日常功能、生活质量或心理健康没有作用。它对疾病的总体严重程度评分也没有作用。这些试验未充分报告不良反应,但没有研究报告其会对健康造成明显有害的影响[90]。

人参

一项前瞻性开放性研究评估了人参对阿尔茨海默病认知功能的作用。97 例患者随机使用人参或安慰剂治疗 12 周后,以及停止人参治疗 12 周后,测量认知功能。人参治疗后,ADAS 认知分量表和 MMSE 分数开始显示好转,持续到 12 周;但是停用人参后,分数下降到对照组的水平[91]。最近的一项系统综述和荟萃分析(包括 4 项共 259 例受试者的随机对照试验)表明,人参对 AD 的作用尚未得到证实。现有研究的主要局限性是样本量小、方法学质量差和未设置安慰剂对照。将来还需要更大规模的、精心设计的研究来评估人参对 AD 的作用[92]。

Dimebon(拉曲吡啶)

Dimebon,非选择性抗组胺药,以前在俄罗斯获批准,后来由于商业原因停产。该药治疗轻、中度阿尔茨海默病的安全性、耐受性和疗效得到了评估。它是弱的丁酰胆碱酯酶和乙酰胆碱酯酶抑制剂,轻度阻断 NMDA 受体信号通路,抑制线粒体通透性转换孔开放[93]。最近一项 Cochrane 综述得出结论,Dimebon 对轻、中度 AD 患者的认知和功能状况无益,但对行为似乎略有益处。[94]。

水蛭素

天然水蛭素是从药用水蛭唾液腺中分离出来的,是凝血酶的直接抑制剂,在中国已应用多年。在一项为期 20 周的开放随机对照试验中,84 例患者接受多奈哌齐或多奈哌齐加水蛭素(3g /d),结果发现,与单用多奈哌齐相比,联合用药者的 ADAS-cog 评分下降和 ADL 评分增加更明显。然而,与多奈哌齐单用组相比,联合组多见出血和过敏反应(分别为 2.4% 和 2.4% 对应 11.9% 和 7.1%)[95]。水蛭素可能会引起出血,在考虑临床应用之前,还需对此进一步探讨。

石杉碱甲

石杉碱甲是从中草药蛇足石杉中分离出的一种生物碱,是一种强效、高选择性、可逆的 AChE-I,自 1994 以来在中国用于治疗阿尔茨海默病,在美国作为保健品。最近一项荟萃分析发现,石杉碱甲 300~500μg/d 持续 8~24 周用于阿尔茨海默病治疗,显著改善 MMSE(平均变化 3.5)和 ADL,效应值随着治疗时间而增加。大多数不良反应是胆碱能性的,未发生严重不良反应[96]。后来一项荟萃分析也得出了类似的阳性结果(也许不确定)[97]。然而,一项关于石杉碱甲用于血管性痴呆的 Cochrane 综述发现,它在血管性痴呆中的价值并没有令人信服的证据[98]。同样,Cochrane 综述关于石杉碱甲对轻度认知功能障碍的作用尚缺乏足够的证据,因为尚未找到合格的临床试验[99]。然而,最近的一项网状荟萃分析表明,石杉碱甲在轻、中度认知功能下降组中取得了良好的疗效[100]。

藏红花

有越来越多的证据表明,藏红花治疗阿尔茨海默病可能有效。最近对随机对照试验的一项系统综述和荟萃分析显示,与安慰剂组相比,藏红花显著改善了 ADAS-cog 和临床痴呆评定量表测量的认知功能。此外,藏红花与常规药物(多奈哌齐和美金刚)无显著差异。藏红花改善了日常生活功能,但结果无统计学意义。纳入的研究中未报告严重的不良事件。藏红花可能有利于改善轻度认知障碍和 AD 患者的认知功能,但没有证据表明它对其他类型的痴呆也有作用[101]。需要更多高质量的随机安慰剂对照试验来进一步证实藏红花对轻度认知障碍和痴呆患者的疗效和安全性[101]。

脑活素

脑活素是肠胃外给药的、来源于猪脑的肽类制剂,具有类似内源性神经营养因子的药效学作用。一项荟萃分析,包含了 6 项脑活素(30mg/d)与安慰剂治疗轻、中度 AD 的随机对照试验。结果发现,与安慰剂相比,在第 4 周时,脑活素改善了认知能力;在第 4 周和 6 个月时,脑活素改善了总体临床变化和"总体改善";安全性两者相当。此外,一项为期 28 周的比较脑活素、多奈哌齐或联合治疗的大型随机对照试验显示,脑活素和联合治疗的整体结局改善明显高于多奈哌齐;而在认知、功能和行为方面三组没有明显差异;在全部随访中,联合治疗组的认知改善得分均最高[102]。

2019 年更新的 Cochrane 综述评估了脑活素对血管性痴呆的疗效,发现静脉注射脑活素可以改善血管性痴呆患者的认知功能和总体功能,且没有不良反应。但是,这些数据不是确定的。这项分析受异质性的限制,且纳入的文献有较高的偏倚。脑激素对血管性痴呆即使有疗效,其效应也是微小的,不具有临床意义。脑活素仍然被作为血管性痴呆的治疗药物使用和推广,但是其支持证据薄弱。报告最多的非严重不良反应有头痛、乏力、头晕、高血压和低血压[103]。

他汀类药物

在阿尔茨海默病中,淀粉样蛋白以细胞外斑块的形式沉积;研究已经确定,淀粉样蛋白的生成是胆固醇依赖性的。高胆固醇血症也参与了血管性痴呆的发病机制。他汀类药物有降低胆固醇的作用,因此已经对其作为治疗痴呆的一种手段进行研究。然而,Cochrane 综述发现,仍然没有足够的证据来推荐他汀类药物用于治疗痴呆。对现有研究的分析表明,它们对 ADAS-cog 或 MMSE 测量结果没有益处[104]。进一步的 Cochrane 综述评估了他汀类药物是否可以预防痴呆。只有 2 项随机试验适合纳入分析,共 26 340 名患者。结果显示,与安慰剂相比,服用他汀类药物的患者其 AD 或痴呆的发生率并未明显降低[105]。随后一项纳入 25 个研究的系统综述和荟萃分析表明,使用他汀类药物可降低所有类型的痴呆、AD 和轻度认知障碍的风险,但不能降低血管性痴呆的发生率[106]。同样,一项荟萃分析(包括 30 个观察性研究,共 9 162 509 名患者)提示,他汀类药物的使用与痴呆风险的降低有关。使用他汀类药物患者的 AD 风险比(RR)为 0.69(95% CI 0.60~0.80,$P<0.000\ 1$),使用他汀类药物患者的血管性痴呆风险比(RR)为 0.93(95% CI 0.74~1.136,$P=0.54$)。然而,在得到进一步的证据之前,临床医师应仅在心血管疾病的治疗中使用他汀类药物[107]。

可可

纵向前瞻性研究调查了健康老年人群中巧克力摄入量与认知能力下降的关系。对 531

例年龄≥65 岁、MMSE 评分正常的受试者随访了 48 个月。基线时评估饮食习惯,在基线和随访时采用 MMSE 评估整体认知功能。校正混杂因素后,巧克力摄入量与认知功能下降风险较低相关($RR=0.59$, 95% CI 0.38~0.92)。这种保护作用仅在咖啡因平均日摄入量低于 75mg 的受试者中观察到[108]。

Souvenaid(智敏捷®)

Souvenaid 是保健食品,用于早期阿尔茨海默病的饮食管理。这种饮料中的混合营养成分被认为能改善认知功能,但是其作为保健食品的健康声明并未经过政府机构的评估。在对 259 例轻度 AD 患者进行为期 24 周的试验中,主要结局——记忆复合评分支持其显著获益。但在一项 AD 生物标志物阳性受试者为期 24 个月的试验中,情景记忆损害并无获益。虽然这些保健食品可能是安全的,但总的来说它们对 AD 有效的证据还很薄弱[86]。

伊达洛吡啶(idalopirdine)

伊达洛吡啶是一种 5-HT$_6$ 受体拮抗剂。5-HT$_6$ 受体在中枢神经系统和记忆有关的脑区表达,并有证据表明,阻断这些受体可诱导乙酰胆碱的释放,因此,在功能退化的胆碱能系统中,该化合物有可能通过 5-HT$_6$ 拮抗作用来恢复乙酰胆碱水平[109]。最近的一项系统综述和荟萃分析,纳入 4 项随机对照试验,共 2803 名受试者,发现伊达洛吡啶对 AD 患者无效,且与转氨酶升高、呕吐等风险有关。虽然伊达洛吡啶高剂量在中度 AD 亚组中可能更有效,但是其效应值较小,且临床意义非常有限[110]。

抗炎类药物

大量的随机对照试验都未能证实抗炎药物对 AD 患者的主要结局有作用。非甾体抗炎药(NSAID)(包括吲哚美辛、萘普生和罗非昔布)治疗 AD 的大规模研究均告失败。其他抗炎药物(如泼尼松龙、羟氯喹、辛伐他汀、阿托伐他汀、阿司匹林和罗格列酮)的随机对照试验,也未证明其对 AD 的认知结局产生具有临床意义的变化[22]。2020 年的 Cochrane 综述评估了阿司匹林和其他 NSAID 预防痴呆的作用,发现并没有证据支持使用低剂量的阿司匹林或其他 NSAID(如塞来昔布、罗非考昔和萘普生)可以预防痴呆。然而,与安慰剂相比,有证据表明阿司匹林增加死亡风险和大出血的发生率。其中,还有一项研究发现,NSAID 组罹患痴呆人数更多。NSAID 组还出现了更多的胃出血和其他胃病,如疼痛、恶心、胃炎[111]。

曲唑酮和二苯甲酰甲烷

这两种化合物已被发现在神经退行性变小鼠模型中,长时间使用临床相关剂量干预,具有显著的神经保护作用,而且无全身毒性。曲唑酮是 5-羟色胺拮抗剂和再摄取抑制剂类的抗抑郁药,还具有抗焦虑和催眠作用,已被证明能减少 AD 患者的精神和行为症状(BPSD)。最近一项小型的回顾性研究考察了长期使用曲唑酮(一种慢波睡眠增强剂)是否与延迟认知衰退有关。结果表明,未使用曲唑酮者的 MMSE 分数下降(主要结局)比使用曲唑者快 2.6 倍。事后多重比较分析(post-hoc)发现,这种效果与受试者睡眠问题减少相关。结果表明,曲唑酮的使用与认知功能下降延迟之间存在关联,但还需要通过前瞻性研究来证实曲唑酮与认知功能之间是因果关系,还是间接表现了其他作用,如(通过增加慢波睡眠)使睡眠中断现象得到治疗[112]。

二苯甲酰甲烷(DBM)是甘草中的一种次要成分,具有抗肿瘤作用(如前列腺和乳腺肿瘤)。在朊蛋白病小鼠模型中,曲唑酮和 DBM 治疗均可恢复其记忆缺陷,消除神经系统体征,预防神经退行性变,并显著延长生存时间。在 tau 蛋白病-额颞叶痴呆小鼠模型中,两种药物都具有神经保护作用,改善记忆缺陷和海马萎缩。此外,曲唑酮降低了磷酸化 tau 蛋白的负担。这些化合物代表了潜在的改善痴呆疾病进程的新疗法[113]。目前尚无证据表明曲唑酮能降低痴呆的风险,但有些数据表明其在老年人中有重要的不良结局[114]。

新型治疗方法

数种 AD 新药的三期临床试验均未发现其能显著改善临床结局,包括:

- **司马西特**(semagacestat),一种 γ-分泌酶抑制剂[115];临床试验纳入了 3 000 例患者。由于与对照组相比,研究组的认知功能未得到改善,高剂量组认知功能恶化,该试验在 2010 年终止。另外,研究组中皮肤癌的发病率也较高[116]。
- **索拉奈珠单抗**(solanezumab),一种人源单克隆抗体,可结合可溶性淀粉样蛋白,促进其从大脑清除[117]。一项对 2 129 例轻度 AD 患者的随机对照试验(EXPEDITION3)发现,Solanezumab 400mg 剂量,每 4 周给药 1 次,对认知功能下降无显著影响[118]。
- **巴匹组单抗**(Bapineuzumab),一种人源抗淀粉样蛋白单克隆抗体[119]。2017 年一项针对 Bapineuzumab 随机对照试验进行的荟萃分析证实其缺乏临床疗效,并与严重的不良反应(血管源性水肿)相关。由于淀粉样蛋白相关影像学异常伴渗出或水肿发生率较高,这些研究中 Bapineuzumab 的剂量受限。不推荐用于轻至中度 AD 患者[120]。

阿杜卡奴单抗(Aducanumab)是一种靶向 Aβ 的抗体。其优先与聚集的 Aβ 结合,通过这种作用,可以减少 β 淀粉样蛋白的蓄积,减少大脑中淀粉样斑块的数量,从而有可能减缓神经退行性变和疾病进展。2019 年初,生产商(Biogen)宣布阿杜卡奴单抗在两个相同设计的 Ⅲ 期 AD 试验中无效,停止了研发,但是在今年宣布正在申请美国 FDA 的上市批准。他们解释说,他们重新分析了上述有效性分析截止后,继续参加研究的患者的数据,发现一个重要的结果,并且第二项试验的亚组数据支持了这些阳性结果[121]。最近外部专家小组对数据进行审查的结果并不乐观,FDA 将于 2021 年 3 月宣布是否批准阿杜卡奴单抗的最终结果。

针对 β 淀粉样蛋白的治疗是近 30 年的研究重点。然而,非常有前景的药物在Ⅲ期临床试验中均未显示获益。即使 Biogen 报告的阿杜卡奴单抗阳性结果也不够完全明确,需要进一步的数据来证实其有效性。因此,研究人员开始转向研究以 tau-蛋白为靶点的治疗方法,因为 tau 蛋白似乎比 β 淀粉样蛋白与认知能力下降的严重程度更相关。目前,大多数临床试验中抗 tau 蛋白药物都是免疫疗法,正处于临床研究的早期阶段。到目前为止,四种抗 tau 蛋白单克隆抗体(gosuranemab,tilavonemab,semorinemab 和 zagotenemab)和一种抗 tau 疫苗(AADvacl))已经进入Ⅱ期临床试验阶段[122]。

血管性痴呆(VaD)

据报道,血管性痴呆占所有痴呆的 10%~50%,是继阿尔茨海默病后第二种最常见的痴呆类型。它是由脑缺血损伤引起,与认知功能障碍和行为异常相关。目前的处理措施非常有限,集中在控制脑血管病的危险因素方面[123]。

请注意,要明确诊断血管性痴呆或阿尔茨海默性痴呆是不可能的,许多痴呆的原因是混合性的。这也许可以解释为什么某些 AChE-I 在可能是血管性痴呆患者中并非总能产生一致的结果,而显示认知结局疗效的数据多来自老年患者,这些患者可能伴发阿尔茨海默病[124]。

目前,在英国没有一种药物被正式批准用于治疗血管性痴呆。关于血管性痴呆的处理措施,已有专门的总结[125,126]。不同于脑卒中的情况,没有确凿的证据表明,用他汀类药物治疗高脂血症,或者用阿司匹林治疗凝血异常,会对血管性痴呆的发病率或疾病进展有影响[127]。类似地,Cochrane 综述发现,没有研究支持他汀类药物在治疗血管性痴呆中的作用[105]。关于多奈哌齐治疗血管性认知损害的 Cochrane 综述发现,有证据支持治疗 6 个月后,可在改善认知功能、临床总体印象和日常生活活动方面获益[128]。关于加兰他敏治疗血管性认知损害的 Cochrane 综述发现[129,130],有限的数据表明在认知和总体临床症状方面,该药比安慰剂有一些优势。加兰他敏的临床试验报告,该药引起的胃肠道不良反应发生率较高。关于卡巴拉汀治疗血管性认知损害的 Cochrane 综述发现一些有益的证据,其结论是基于一项大型研究,而且卡巴拉汀的不良反应导致很大比例患者退出试验[105,131]。此外,对随机对照试验的荟萃分析发现,胆碱酯酶抑制剂和美金刚可以轻度改善认知,这种获益的临床意义尚未确定。结论是目前的数据不足以支持这些药物在血管性痴呆中的广泛使用[111]。最近,一项系统综述和贝叶斯网络荟萃分析比较了促认知药物治疗血管性痴呆的疗效和安全性,发现多奈哌齐、加兰他敏和美金刚对认知功能有显著疗效。美金刚在总体状况上获得显著疗效。这三种药物安全性和耐受性良好[132]。一项新的关于胆碱酯酶抑制剂治疗血管性痴呆和其他血管性认知障碍的 Cochrane 系统综述正在进行中。

路易体痴呆

有人提出路易体痴呆占痴呆的 15%~25%(尽管尸检表明其比率要低得多)。其特征性症状为痴呆伴有认知功能波动、早期和持续的幻视以及帕金森综合征的自发运动。跌倒、晕厥、短暂意识障碍、对抗精神病药敏感和其他感觉通道的幻觉也常见[133]。

2018 年更新的 NICE 指南,推荐在 DLB 中使用胆碱酯酶抑制剂和美金刚(见 NICE 指南概要)。

卡巴拉汀和多奈哌齐临床试验的荟萃分析,支持将胆碱酯酶抑制剂用于路易体痴呆,改善认知、整体功能和生活能力。证据表明,患者使用 AChE-I 后,病情即使没有改善,也不太可能恶化。美金刚对 DLB 的疗效尚不明确,但它的耐受性好,无论是单一治疗还是作为 AChE-I 的辅助治疗,都有可能有益[134]。

管理 DLB 患者具有复杂性。其临床表现因人而异,同一患者也会随时发生变化。治疗解决一种症状的同时,也会使另一种症状恶化,这也加大了疾病管理的困难。症状经常由多名专家各自独立地处理,因而难以实现高质量的照护。现在,临床试验和荟萃分析为治疗路易体痴呆患者的认知、神经精神、运动症状提供了证据基础。此外,专家共识支持对路易体痴呆相关疾病(例如帕金森病)进行治疗,从而管理其常见症状(例如自主神经功能障碍)。然而,证据仍相当不足,未来的临床试验需要关注路易体痴呆患者特定症状的治疗[135]。关于 DLB 特定症状管理的指南,请参阅"路易体痴呆管理概要——钻石路易"[136]。

轻度认知损害（MCI）

轻度认知功能损害被假设为痴呆的临床前阶段，但是是一个预后不同的异质性组。评价 AChE-I 治疗轻度认知损害的安全性和有效性的 Cochrane 综述发现，几乎没有证据表明它们能影响痴呆进展或认知测试评分。这微弱的证据被不良反应增加的风险抵消，特别是胃肠道反应，这意味着无法建议使用 AChE-I 治疗轻度认知损害[137]。最近的一项系统综述[138] 发现，没有可重复证据表明哪种干预，包括 AChE-I 和 NSAID 罗非昔布，对轻度认知损害是有效的。进一步的系统综述和荟萃分析发现，尽管 AChE-I 对 MCI 有些许疗效，但仍存在许多安全性问题。因此，难以推荐用于 MCI 的治疗[139]。不同国家的专家最近总结了 MCI 的药物和非药物治疗的证据[140]。

其他痴呆

一项对额颞叶痴呆随机对照试验的系统综述显示，某些药物可有效地减少行为症状（如 SSRI 和曲唑酮），但对认知没有影响[141]。

Cochrane 综述评估了 AChE-I 对神经系统疾病相关罕见痴呆的疗效和安全性。大多数试验的样本量都非常小，对认知功能和肌萎缩脊髓侧索硬化的疗效不明确，但是与安慰剂相比，AChE-I 与胃肠道不良反应增多有关[142]。

英国精神药理协会抗痴呆药临床实践指南概要[22]

AChE-I 和美金刚适用于不同程度的阿尔茨海默病。不推荐其他药物，包括他汀类药物、抗炎药物、维生素 E 和银杏叶制剂，用于治疗或预防阿尔茨海默病。轻度认知损害用 AChE-I 和美金刚均无效。AChE-I 对额颞叶痴呆无效，且可能导致激越。AChE-I 可用于路易体痴呆（既有帕金森病性痴呆也有路易体痴呆），美金刚也可能有益。没有药物对血管性痴呆明确有效，但是 AChE-I 对混合性痴呆有效。早期证据表明，多因素干预有可能预防或延缓痴呆的发病。很多针对 AD 患者或 AD 高危人群的新型药物治疗方法仍在研发过程中，包括减少淀粉样蛋白和 tau 蛋白的策略。尽管，我们还在期待早期（前驱期/轻度）AD 关键研究的结果，但到目前为止，明确诊断的（轻、中度）AD 的研究结果仍模棱两可，也尚无疾病修饰疗法的药物获批，或可以推荐用于临床。英国精神药理协会的建议概要见表 6.3。

表 6.3 英国精神药理协会建议概要

	首选	次选
阿尔茨海默病	AChE-I	美金刚
血管性痴呆	无	无
混合性痴呆	AChE-I	美金刚
路易体痴呆	AChE-I	美金刚
轻度认知损害	无	无
帕金森病性痴呆	AChE-I	美金刚
额颞叶痴呆	无	无

参考文献

1. National Institute for Clinical Excellence. Dementia: assessment, management and support for people living with dementia and their carers. NICE guideline [NG97] 2018; www.nice.org.uk/guidance/ng97.

2. Francis PT, et al. The cholinergic hypothesis of Alzheimer's disease: a review of progress. *J Neurol Neurosurg Psychiatry* 1999; 66:137–147.

3. Craig LA, et al. Revisiting the cholinergic hypothesis in the development of Alzheimer's disease. *Neurosci Biobehav Rev* 2011; 35:1397–1409.

4. Mesulam M, et al. Widely spread butyrylcholinesterase can hydrolyze acetylcholine in the normal and Alzheimer brain. *Neurobiol Dis* 2002; 9:88–93.

5. Weinstock M. Selectivity of cholinesterase inhibition: clinical implications for the treatment of Alzheimer's disease. *CNS Drugs* 1999; 12:307–323.

6. Matsunaga S, et al. Memantine monotherapy for Alzheimer's disease: a systematic review and meta-analysis. *PLoS One* 2015; 10:e0123289.

7. BNF Online. British National Formulary. 2020; https://www.medicinescomplete.com/mc/bnf/current.

8. Eisai Ltd. Summary of product characteristics. Aricept tablets (donepezil hydrochloride). 2018; https://www.medicines.org.uk/emc/product/3776/smpc.

9. Novartis Pharmaceuticals UK Limited. Summary of product characteristics. Exelon 4.6 mg/24h, 9.5 mg/24h, 13.3 mg/24h transdermal patch. 2020; https://www.medicines.org.uk/emc/product/7764/smpc.

10. Sandoz Limited. Summary of product characteristics. Rivastigmine Sandoz 1.5 mg, 3 mg, 4.5 mg, 6 mg hard capsules. 2016; https://www.medicines.org.uk/emc/product/8407/smpc.

11. Shire Pharmaceuticals Limited. Summary of product characteristics. Reminyl XL 8mg, 16mg and 24mg prolonged release capsules. 2019; https://www.medicines.org.uk/emc/product/3934/smpc.

12. Shire Pharmaceuticals Limited. Summary of product characteristics. Reminyl Oral Solution. 2020; https://www.medicines.org.uk/emc/medicine/10337.

13. Lundbeck Limited. Summary of product characteristics. Ebixa 5mg/pump actuation oral solution, 20mg and 10 mg Tablets and Treatment Initiation Pack. 2019; https://www.medicines.org.uk/emc/product/8222/smpc.

14. NHS Prescription Services. Drug tariff. 2020; http://www.drugtariff.nhsbsa.nhs.uk/#/00791628-DD/DD00791615/Home.

15. Buckley JS, et al. A risk-benefit assessment of dementia medications: systematic review of the evidence. *Drugs Aging* 2015; 32:453–467.

16. Lanctot KL, et al. Efficacy and safety of cholinesterase inhibitors in Alzheimer's disease: a meta-analysis. *CMAJ* 2003; 169:557–564.

17. McShane R, et al. Memantine for dementia. *Cochrane Database Syst Rev* 2006; CD003154.

18. Vaci N, et al. Real-world effectiveness, its predictors and onset of action of cholinesterase inhibitors and memantine in dementia: retrospective health record study. *Br J Psychiatry* 2020:1–7. [Epub ahead of print].

19. Burns A, et al. Efficacy and safety of donepezil over 3 years: an open-label, multicentre study in patients with Alzheimer's disease. *Int J Geriatr Psychiatry* 2007; 22:806–812.

20. Doody RS, et al. Open-label, multicenter, phase 3 extension study of the safety and efficacy of donepezil in patients with Alzheimer disease. *Arch Neurol* 2001; 58:427–433.

21. Farlow MR, et al. Effective pharmacologic management of Alzheimer's disease. *Am J Med* 2007; 120:388–397.

22. O'Brien JT, et al. Clinical practice with anti-dementia drugs: A revised (third) consensus statement from the British Association for Psychopharmacology. *J Psychopharmacol* 2017; 31:147–168.

23. Singh S, et al. Discontinuation syndrome following donepezil cessation. *Int J Geriatr Psychiatry* 2003; 18:282–284.

24. Bidzan L, et al. Withdrawal syndrome after donepezil cessation in a patient with dementia. *Neurol Sci* 2012; 33:1459–1461.

25. Waldemar G, et al. Tolerability of switching from donepezil to memantine treatment in patients with moderate to severe Alzheimer's disease. *Int J Geriatr Psychiatry* 2008; 23:979–981.

26. Massoud F, et al. Switching cholinesterase inhibitors in older adults with dementia. *Int Psychogeriatr* 2011; 23:372–378.

27. Winblad B, et al. A six-month double-blind, randomized, placebo-controlled study of a transdermal patch in Alzheimer's disease–rivastigmine patch versus capsule. *Int J Geriatr Psychiatry* 2007; 22:456–467.

28. Zhang ZX, et al. Rivastigmine patch in Chinese Patients with Probable Alzheimer's disease: A 24-week, randomized, double-blind parallel-group study comparing rivastigmine patch (9.5 mg/24 h) with Capsule (6 mg Twice Daily). *CNS Neurosci Ther* 2016; 22:488–496.

29. Morgan TM, et al. Absolute bioavailability and safety of a novel rivastigmine nasal spray in healthy elderly individuals. *Br J Clin Pharmacol* 2017; 83:510–516.

30. Sabbagh M, et al. Clinical recommendations for the use of donepezil 23 mg in moderate-to-severe Alzheimer's disease in the Asia-Pacific region. *Dementia Geriatr Cogn Disord Extra* 2016; 6:382–395.

31. Plosker GL. Memantine extended release (28 mg once daily): a review of its use in Alzheimer's disease. *Drugs* 2015; 75:887–897.

32. Schmidt R, et al. EFNS-ENS/EAN guideline on concomitant use of cholinesterase inhibitors and memantine in moderate to severe Alzheimer's disease. *Eur J Neurol* 2015; 22:889–898.

33. Periclou AP, et al. Lack of pharmacokinetic or pharmacodynamic interaction between memantine and donepezil. *Ann Pharmacother* 2004; 38:1389–1394.

34. Grossberg GT, et al. Rationale for combination therapy with galantamine and memantine in Alzheimer's disease. *J Clin Pharmacol* 2006; 46:17S-26S.

35. Rogers SL, et al. Donepezil improves cognition and global function in Alzheimer disease: a 15-week, double-blind, placebo-controlled study. Donepezil Study Group. *Arch Intern Med* 1998; 158:1021–1031.

36. Rogers SL, et al. A 24-week, double-blind, placebo-controlled trial of donepezil in patients with Alzheimer's disease. Donepezil Study Group. *Neurology* 1998; 50:136–145.

37. Corey-Bloom J, et al. A randomized trial evaluating the efficacy and safety of ENA 713 (rivastigmine tartrate), a new acetylcholinesterase inhibitor, in patients with mild to moderately severe Alzheimer's disease. *International Journal of Geriatric Psychopharmacology* 1998; 1:55–64.

38. Rosler M, et al. Efficacy and safety of rivastigmine in patients with Alzheimer's disease: international randomised controlled trial. *BMJ* 1999; 318:633–638.

39. Tariot PN, et al. A 5-month, randomized, placebo-controlled trial of galantamine in AD. The Galantamine USA-10 Study Group. *Neurology* 2000; 54:2269–2276.

40. Raskind MA, et al. Galantamine in AD: A 6-month randomized, placebo-controlled trial with a 6-month extension. The Galantamine USA-1 Study Group. *Neurology* 2000; 54:2261–2268.

41. Wilcock GK, et al. Efficacy and safety of galantamine in patients with mild to moderate Alzheimer's disease: multicentre randomised controlled trial. Galantamine International-1 Study Group. *BMJ* 2000; 321:1445–1449.

42. Pariente A, et al. Factors associated with serious adverse reactions to cholinesterase inhibitors: a study of spontaneous reporting. *CNS Drugs* 2010; 24:55–63.

43. Sadowsky CH, et al. Safety and tolerability of rivastigmine transdermal patch compared with rivastigmine capsules in patients switched from donepezil: data from three clinical trials. *Int J Clin Pract* 2010; 64:188–193.

44. Sadowsky C, et al. Switching from oral cholinesterase inhibitors to the rivastigmine transdermal patch. *CNS Neurosci Ther* 2010; 16:51–60.

45. Cummings J, et al. Randomized, double-blind, parallel-group, 48-week study for efficacy and safety of a higher-dose rivastigmine patch (15 vs. 10 cm(2)) in Alzheimer's disease. *Dement Geriatr Cogn Disord* 2012; 33:341–353.

46. National Institute for Health and Care Excellence. British National Formulary (BNF). 2020; https://bnf.nice.org.uk.

47. Parsons CG, et al. Memantine is a clinically well tolerated N-methyl-D-aspartate (NMDA) receptor antagonist–a review of preclinical data. *Neuropharmacology* 1999; 38:735–767.

48. Reisberg B, et al. Memantine in moderate-to-severe Alzheimer's disease. *N Engl J Med* 2003; 348:1333–1341.

49. Jones RW. A review comparing the safety and tolerability of memantine with the acetylcholinesterase inhibitors. *Int J Geriatr Psychiatry* 2010; 25:547–553.

50. Dunn NR, et al. Adverse effects associated with the use of donepezil in general practice in England. *J Psychopharmacol* 2000; 14:406–408.

51. Hashimoto M, et al. Urinary incontinence: an unrecognised adverse effect with donepezil. *Lancet* 2000; 356:568.

52. Kroger E, et al. Adverse drug reactions reported with cholinesterase inhibitors: an analysis of 16 years of individual case safety reports from VigiBase. *Ann Pharmacother* 2015; 49:1197–1206.

53. NHS Yorkshire and Humber Clinical Networks. The assessment of cardiac status before prescribing acetyl cholinesterase inhibitors for dementia. Version 1. 2016; http://www.yhscn.nhs.uk/media/PDFs/mhdn/Dementia/ECG%20Documents/ACHEIGuidance%20V1_Final.pdf.

54. Rowland JP, et al. Cardiovascular monitoring with acetylcholinesterase inhibitors: a clinical protocol. *Adv Psychiatr Treatment* 2007; 13:178–184.

55. FDA Alert for Healthcare Professionals. Galantamine hydrobromide (marketed as Razadyne, formerly Reminyl). 2005; https://www.fda.gov/Drugs/DrugSafety/ucm109350.htm.

56. Malone DM, et al. Cholinesterase inhibitors and cardiovascular disease: a survey of old age psychiatrists' practice. *Age Ageing* 2007; 36:331–333.

57. Park-Wyllie LY, et al. Cholinesterase inhibitors and hospitalization for bradycardia: a population-based study. *PLoS Med* 2009; 6:e1000157.

58. Rosenbloom MH, et al. Donepezil-associated bradyarrhythmia in a patient with dementia with Lewy bodies (DLB). *Alzheimer Dis Assoc Disord* 2010; 24:209–211.

59. Gill SS, et al. Syncope and its consequences in patients with dementia receiving cholinesterase inhibitors: a population-based cohort study. *Arch Intern Med* 2009; 169:867–873.

60. Isik AT, et al. Which cholinesterase inhibitor is the safest for the heart in elderly patients with Alzheimer's disease? *Am J Alzheimers Dis Other Demen* 2012; 27:171–174.

61. Fosbol EL, et al. Comparative cardiovascular safety of dementia medications: a cross-national study. *J Am Geriatr Soc* 2012; 60:2283–2289.

62. Nordstrom P, et al. The use of cholinesterase inhibitors and the risk of myocardial infarction and death: a nationwide cohort study in subjects with Alzheimer's disease. *Eur Heart J* 2013; 34:2585–2591.

63. Howes LG. Cardiovascular effects of drugs used to treat Alzheimer's disease. *Drug Saf* 2014; 37:391–395.

64. Farlow MR, et al. Memantine for the treatment of Alzheimer's disease: tolerability and safety data from clinical trials. *Drug Saf* 2008; 31:577–585.

65. Babai S, et al. Comparison of adverse drug reactions with donepezil versus memantine: analysis of the French Pharmacovigilance Database. *Therapie* 2010; 65:255–259.

66. Dooley M, et al. Donepezil: a review of its use in Alzheimer's disease. *Drugs Aging* 2000; 16:199–226.

67. Scott LJ, et al. Galantamine: a review of its use in Alzheimer's disease. *Drugs* 2000; 60:1095–1122.

68. Grossberg GT, et al. Lack of adverse pharmacodynamic drug interactions with rivastigmine and twenty-two classes of medications. *Int J Geriatr Psychiatry* 2000; 15:242–247.

69. Tavassoli N, et al. Drug interactions with cholinesterase inhibitors: an analysis of the French pharmacovigilance database and a comparison of two national drug formularies (Vidal, British National Formulary). *Drug Saf* 2007; 30:1063–1071.

70. Noetzli M, et al. Pharmacodynamic, pharmacokinetic and pharmacogenetic aspects of drugs used in the treatment of Alzheimer's disease. *Clin Pharmacokinet* 2013; 52:225–241.

71. Pasqualetti G, et al. Potential drug-drug interactions in Alzheimer patients with behavioral symptoms. *Clin Interv Aging* 2015; 10:1457–1466.
72. Howard R, et al. Donepezil and memantine for moderate-to-severe Alzheimer's disease. *N Engl J Med* 2012; 366:893–903.
73. Howard R, et al. Nursing home placement in the Donepezil and Memantine in Moderate to Severe Alzheimer's Disease (DOMINO-AD) trial: secondary and post-hoc analyses. *Lancet Neurol* 2015; 14:1171–1181.
74. Medicines Complete. Stockley's drug interactions. 2020; https://www.medicinescomplete.com.
75. Truven Health Analytics. Micromedex 2.0. 2017; https://www.micromedexsolutions.com/home/dispatch.
76. Di Santo SG, et al. A meta-analysis of the efficacy of donepezil, rivastigmine, galantamine, and memantine in relation to severity of Alzheimer's disease. *J Alzheimers Dis* 2013; 35:349–361.
77. Parsons C. Withdrawal of antidementia drugs in older people: who, when and how? *Drugs Aging* 2016; 33:545–556.
78. National Institute for Health and Clinical Excellence. Dementia: assessment, management and support for people living with dementia and their carers. NICE Guideline [NG97]. 2018; https://www.nice.org.uk/guidance/ng97.
79. National Institute for Health and Clinical Excellence. Donepezil, galantamine, rivastigmine and memantine for the treatment of Alzheimer's disease. Technology Appraisal Guidance TA217. 2011 (last updated June 2018); https://www.nice.org.uk/Guidance/TA217.
80. National Institute for Health and Clinical Excellence. Medicines optimisation: the safe and effective use of medicines to enable the best possible outcomes. National Guidance [NG5]. 2015 (last checked March 2019); https://www.nice.org.uk/guidance/ng5.
81. Birks J, et al. Ginkgo biloba for cognitive impairment and dementia. *Cochrane Database Syst Rev* 2009; CD003120.
82. Yuan Q, et al. Effects of Ginkgo biloba on dementia: an overview of systematic reviews. *J Ethnopharmacol* 2017; 195:1–9.
83. Bent S, et al. Spontaneous bleeding associated with ginkgo biloba: a case report and systematic review of the literature: a case report and systematic review of the literature. *J Gen Intern Med* 2005; 20:657–661.
84. Farina N, et al. Vitamin E for Alzheimer's dementia and mild cognitive impairment. *Cochrane Database Syst Rev* 2017; 1:Cd002854.
85. Dysken MW, et al. Effect of vitamin E and memantine on functional decline in Alzheimer disease: the TEAM-AD VA cooperative randomized trial. *JAMA* 2014; 311:33–44.
86. Joe E, et al. Cognitive symptoms of Alzheimer's disease: clinical management and prevention. *BMJ* 2019; 367:l6217.
87. Malouf R, et al. Folic acid with or without vitamin B12 for the prevention and treatment of healthy elderly and demented people. *Cochrane Database Syst Rev* 2008; CD004514.
88. Enderami A, et al. The effects and potential mechanisms of folic acid on cognitive function: a comprehensive review. *Neurol Sci* 2018; 39:1667–1675.
89. Zhang DM, et al. Efficacy of Vitamin B supplementation on cognition in elderly patients with cognitive-related diseases. *J Geriatr Psychiatry Neurol* 2017; 30:50–59.
90. Burckhardt M, et al. Omega-3 fatty acids for the treatment of dementia. *Cochrane Database Syst Rev* 2016; 4:Cd009002.
91. Lee ST, et al. Panax ginseng enhances cognitive performance in Alzheimer disease. *Alzheimer Dis Assoc Disord* 2008; 22:222–226.
92. Wang Y, et al. Ginseng for Alzheimer's disease: a systematic review and meta-analysis of randomized controlled trials. *Curr Top Med Chem* 2016; 16:529–536.
93. Doody RS, et al. Effect of dimebon on cognition, activities of daily living, behaviour, and global function in patients with mild-to-moderate Alzheimer's disease: a randomised, double-blind, placebo-controlled study. *Lancet* 2008; 372:207–215.
94. Chau S, et al. Latrepirdine for Alzheimer's disease (Dimebon). *Cochrane Database Syst Rev* 2015; Cd009524.
95. Li DQ, et al. Donepezil combined with natural hirudin improves the clinical symptoms of patients with mild-to-moderate Alzheimer's disease: a 20-week open-label pilot study. *Int J Med Sci* 2012; 9:248–255.
96. Wang BS, et al. Efficacy and safety of natural acetylcholinesterase inhibitor huperzine A in the treatment of Alzheimer's disease: an updated meta-analysis. *J Neural Transm* 2009; 116:457–465.
97. Yang G, et al. Huperzine A for Alzheimer's disease: a systematic review and meta-analysis of randomized clinical trials. *PLoS One* 2013; 8:e74916.
98. Hao Z, et al. Huperzine A for vascular dementia. *Cochrane Database Syst Rev* 2009; CD007365.
99. Yue J, et al. Huperzine A for mild cognitive impairment. *Cochrane Database Syst Rev* 2012; 12:CD008827.
100. Cui CC, et al. The effect of anti-dementia drugs on Alzheimer disease-induced cognitive impairment: a network meta-analysis. *Medicine (Baltimore)* 2019; 98:e16091.
101. Ayati Z, et al. Saffron for mild cognitive impairment and dementia: a systematic review and meta-analysis of randomised clinical trials. *BMC Complement Med Ther* 2020; 20:333.
102. Gavrilova SI, et al. Cerebrolysin in the therapy of mild cognitive impairment and dementia due to Alzheimer's disease: 30 years of clinical use. *Med Res Rev* 2020. [Epub ahead of print].
103. Cui S, et al. Cerebrolysin for vascular dementia. *Cochrane Database Syst Rev* 2019; CD008900
104. McGuinness B, et al. Cochrane review on 'Statins for the treatment of dementia'. *Int J Geriatr Psychiatry* 2013; 28:119–126.
105. McGuinness B, et al. Statins for the prevention of dementia. *Cochrane Database Syst Rev* 2016; Cd003160.
106. Chu CS, et al. Use of statins and the risk of dementia and mild cognitive impairment: A systematic review and meta-analysis. *Sci Rep* 2018; 8:5804.
107. Poly TN, et al. Association between use of statin and risk of dementia: a meta-analysis of observational studies. *Neuroepidemiology* 2020; 54:214–226.
108. Moreira A, et al. Chocolate consumption is associated with a lower risk of cognitive decline. *J Alzheimers Dis* 2016; 53:85–93.
109. Galimberti D, et al. Idalopirdine as a treatment for Alzheimer's disease. *Exp Opinion Invest Drugs* 2015; 24:981–987.
110. Matsunaga S, et al. Efficacy and safety of idalopirdine for Alzheimer's disease: a systematic review and meta-analysis. *Int Psychogeriatr*

2019; 31:1627–1633.

111. Jordan F, et al. Aspirin and other non-steroidal anti-inflammatory drugs for the prevention of dementia. *Cochrane Database Syst Rev* 2020; 4:Cd011459.

112. La AL, et al. Long-term trazodone use and cognition: a potential therapeutic role for slow-wave sleep enhancers. *J Alzheimers Dis* 2019; 67:911–921.

113. Halliday M, et al. Repurposed drugs targeting eIF2alpha-P-mediated translational repression prevent neurodegeneration in mice. *Brain* 2017; 140:1768–1783.

114. Coupland C, et al. Antidepressant use and risk of adverse outcomes in older people: population based cohort study. *BMJ* 2011; 343:d4551.

115. Doody RS, et al. A phase 3 trial of semagacestat for treatment of Alzheimer's disease. *N Engl J Med* 2013; 369:341–350.

116. Briggs R, et al. Drug treatments in Alzheimer's disease. *Clin Med (Lond)* 2016; 16:247–253.

117. Doody RS, et al. Phase 3 trials of solanezumab for mild-to-moderate Alzheimer's disease. *N Engl J Med* 2014; 370:311–321.

118. Honig LS, et al. Trial of solanezumab for mild dementiá due to Alzheimer's disease. *N Engl J Med* 2018; 378:321–330.

119. Salloway S, et al. Two phase 3 trials of bapineuzumab in mild-to-moderate Alzheimer's disease. *N Engl J Med* 2014; 370:322–333.

120. Abushouk AI, et al. Bapineuzumab for mild to moderate Alzheimer's disease: a meta-analysis of randomized controlled trials. *BMC Neurol* 2017; 17:66.

121. Schneider L. A resurrection of aducanumab for Alzheimer's disease. *Lancet Neurol* 2020; 19:111–112.

122. Vaz M, et al. Alzheimer's disease: recent treatment strategies. *Eur J Pharmacol* 2020; 887:173554.

123. Kavirajan H, et al. Efficacy and adverse effects of cholinesterase inhibitors and memantine in vascular dementia: a meta-analysis of randomised controlled trials. *Lancet Neurol* 2007; 6:782–792.

124. Wang J, et al. Cholinergic deficiency involved in vascular dementia: possible mechanism and strategy of treatment. *Acta Pharmacol Sin* 2009; 30:879–888.

125. Bocti C, et al. Management of dementia with a cerebrovascular component. *Alzheimer's Dementia* 2007; 3:398–403.

126. Demaerschalk BM, et al. Treatment of vascular dementia and vascular cognitive impairment. *Neurologist* 2007; 13:37–41.

127. Baskys A, et al. Pharmacological prevention and treatment of vascular dementia: approaches and perspectives. *Exp Gerontol* 2012; 47:887–891.

128. Malouf R, et al. Donepezil for vascular cognitive impairment. *Cochrane Database Syst Rev* 2004; CD004395.

129. Birks J. Cholinesterase inhibitors for Alzheimer's disease. *Cochrane Database Syst Rev* 2006; CD005593.

130. Craig D, et al. Galantamine for vascular cognitive impairment. *Cochrane Database Syst Rev* 2006; CD004746.

131. Birks J, et al. Rivastigmine for vascular cognitive impairment. *Cochrane Database Syst Rev* 2013; 5:CD004744.

132. Jin BR, et al. Comparative efficacy and safety of cognitive enhancers for treating vascular cognitive impairment: systematic review and Bayesian network meta-analysis. *Neural Regen Res* 2019; 14:805–816.

133. Wild R, et al. Cholinesterase inhibitors for dementia with Lewy bodies. *Cochrane Database Syst Rev* 2003; CD003672.

134. McKeith IG, et al. Diagnosis and management of dementia with Lewy bodies: fourth consensus report of the DLB consortium. *Neurology* 2017; 89:88–100.

135. Taylor JP, et al. New evidence on the management of Lewy body dementia. *Lancet Neurol* 2020; 19:157–169.

136. Newcastle University. Management of Lewy body dementia summary sheet Diamond Lewy. 2019; https://research.ncl.ac.uk/media/sites/researchwebsites/diamond-lewy/One%20page%20symptom%20LBD%20management%20summaries.pdf.

137. Russ TC, et al. Cholinesterase inhibitors for mild cognitive impairment. *Cochrane Database Syst Rev* 2012; 9:CD009132.

138. Cooper C, et al. Treatment for mild cognitive impairment: systematic review. *Br J Psychiatry* 2013; 203:255–264.

139. Matsunaga S, et al. Efficacy and safety of cholinesterase inhibitors for mild cognitive impairment: asystematic review and meta-analysis. *J Alzheimers Dis* 2019; 71:513–523.

140. Kasper S, et al. Management of mild cognitive impairment (MCI): the need for national and international guidelines. *World J Biol Psychiatry* 2020; 21:579–594.

141. Nardell M, et al. Pharmacological treatments for frontotemporal dementias: a systematic review of randomized controlled trials. *Am J Alzheimers Dis Other Demen* 2014; 29:123–132.

142. Li Y, et al. Cholinesterase inhibitors for rarer dementias associated with neurological conditions. *Cochrane Database Syst Rev* 2015; Cd009444.

躯体疾病药物在痴呆中的安全使用

患有痴呆症的人更容易受到药物认知不良反应的影响。药物通过对胆碱能、组胺能或阿片类神经递质通路或通过更复杂的作用而影响认知功能。躯体疾病药物也可能与认知增强药物有相互作用。

抗胆碱能药物

抗胆碱能药物降低乙酰胆碱酯酶抑制剂的疗效[1],也会引起镇静、认知损害、谵妄和跌倒[2]。对于老年痴呆患者这些影响可能更严重[3]。表 6.4 总结了英国老年人常用药抗胆碱作用对认知的影响(AEC)[4]。联合多种具有抗胆碱能活性的药物,会增加个体抗胆碱能负荷。一些研究表明,抗胆碱能负荷总分高与 MMSE 评分下降[5]及死亡率升高[5,6]相关。

表 6.4 抗胆碱作用对认知的影响(AEC)评分(2020 年 10 月更新)

肾上腺色素缩氨脲-0	克拉霉素-NK	加巴喷丁-0	萘普生-0	西他列汀-0
阿仑磷酸(阿仑膦酸钠)-0	氯马斯汀-3	加兰他敏-0	硝苯地平-0	索利那新-1
阿夫唑嗪-0	氯米帕明-3	盖胃平颗粒-0	尼莫地平-0	索他洛尔-0
阿利马嗪-3	氯硝西泮-NK	格列齐特-0	呋喃妥因-NK	螺内酯-NK
别嘌醇-NK	可乐定-NK	格拉司琼-0	去甲替林-3	柳氮磺吡啶-0
阿普唑仑-0	氯吡格雷-0	氟哌啶醇-0	奥氮平-2	舒必利-0
乙双苯丙胺(阿尔维琳)-0	氯氮平-3	肝素-0	奥美拉唑-0	三苯氧胺-NK
金刚烷胺-2	多巴丝肼(Co-beneldopa)-0	氢氯噻嗪-0	昂丹司琼-0	坦索罗辛-0
阿米洛利-0	息宁(卡左双多巴控释片)(Co-careldopa)-0	氢可酮-NK	奥利司他-0	羟基安定(替马西泮)-1
氨茶碱-0	可待因-NK	氢化可的松-NK	奥芬那君-3	盐酸四环素-0
胺碘酮-1	秋水仙碱-NK	羟嗪-1	奥卡西平-NK	茶碱-0
氨磺必利-0	Co-tenidone-0	东莨菪碱氢溴酸盐-3	奥昔布宁-3	硫胺素-0
阿米替林-3	苯甲嗪-1	丁溴东莨菪碱-1	氧可酮-NK	噻托溴铵(吸入)-0
氨氯地平-0	赛庚啶-3	布洛芬-0	帕潘立酮-1	替托尼定-NK
阿莫西林-0	达比加群酯-NK	伊潘立酮-1	泮托拉唑-0	托卡朋-0
阿那曲唑-NK	达非那新-0	丙米嗪-3	对乙酰氨基酚-0	托特罗定-2
阿哌沙班-NK	地昔帕明-2	吲达帕胺-0	帕罗西汀-2	托吡酯-NK
阿朴吗啡-0	地塞米松-NK	胰岛素-0	青霉素-0	曲马多-0

续表

阿立哌唑-1	右旋安非他明-0	异丙托溴铵-0	薄荷油-0	曲唑酮-0
阿司匹林-0	右旋丙氧芬-NK	厄贝沙坦-NK	硫丙麦角林-0	三氟拉嗪-2
阿替洛尔-0	地西泮-1	异卡波肼-1	培哚普利-0	苯海索-3
托莫西汀-0	双氯芬酸-0	硝酸异山梨酯片-0	奋乃静-1	甲氧苄氨嘧啶-0
阿托伐他汀-0	双环维林(双环胺)-2	单硝酸异山梨酯-0	哌替啶-2	三甲丙米嗪-3
阿托品-3	地高辛-NK	酮咯酸-0	苯乙肼-1	曲司氯胺-0
阿托品滴眼液-1	双氢可待因-NK	拉贝洛尔-0	苯妥英-NK	丙戊酸-0
咪唑硫嘌呤-0	地尔硫䓬-0	乳果糖-0	匹莫齐特-2	文拉法辛-0
巴氯芬-NK	苯海明-2	拉莫三嗪-0	哌仑西平-1	维拉帕米-NK
倍氯米松二丙酸酯(吸入)-0	苯海拉明-2	兰索拉唑-NK	普伐他汀-0	维生素 B_{12}-0
苄氟噻嗪-0	双嘧达莫-0	乐卡地平-0	哌唑嗪-0	维生素-0
苯甲托品-3	丙吡胺-2	左乙拉西坦-NK	泼尼松龙-1	沃替西汀-0
倍他司汀-0	多库酯钠-0	左旋多巴-0	普瑞巴林-NK	华法林-0
苯扎贝特-0	多潘立酮-1	左美丙嗪(甲氧异丁嗪)-2	普鲁氯嗪-2	齐拉西酮-0
比沙可啶-0	多奈哌齐-0	左甲状腺素(甲状腺素)-0	普环啶-3	唑吡坦-0
比索洛尔-NK	度琉平-3	利拉鲁肽-0	丙嗪-2	佐匹克隆-NK
溴隐亭-1	多沙唑嗪-0	赖诺普利-0	异丙嗪-3	佐替平-2
布地奈德(吸入)-0	多塞平-3	锂-1	溴丙胺太林-2	珠氯噻醇-1
布美他尼-NK	盐酸多西环素-0	洛非帕明-3	普萘洛尔-0	
丁丙诺啡-0	度拉糖肽-0	洛派丁胺-0	喹硫平-2	
安非他酮-0	度洛西汀-0	氯雷他定-0	奎尼丁-1	
丁螺环酮-1	依那普利-0	劳拉西泮-0	奎宁-1	
卡麦角林-0	依诺肝素-0	氯沙坦-0	雷贝拉唑-0	
钙-0	恩他卡朋-0	洛伐他汀-0	雷米普利-NK	
钙剂及维生素D-0	红霉素-NK	鲁拉西酮-0	雷尼替丁-0	
坎地沙坦-0	艾塞那肽-0	聚乙二醇-0	雷沙吉兰-0	
卡托普利-NK	依折麦布-0	镁-0	瑞波西汀-0	
卡巴胆碱-0	非洛地平-0	美贝维林-0	利塞膦酸盐-0	
卡马西平-1	芬太尼-1	褪黑激素-0	利培酮-0	
卡比马唑-NK	硫酸亚铁-0	美洛昔康-0	利伐沙班-NK	
羧甲司坦-0	弗斯特罗定-0	美金刚-0	卡巴拉汀-0	

续表

卡维地洛-NK	非索非那定-0	美沙拉秦-0	罗匹尼罗-0
头孢氨苄-0	非那雄胺-0	二甲双胍-NK	罗格列酮-0
西替利嗪-0	黄酮哌酯-NK	美索巴莫-NK	瑞舒伐他汀-NK
水合氯醛-NK	氟卡尼-0	甲氨蝶呤-NK	沙丁胺醇-0
利眠宁-0	氟氯西林-0	甲氧氯普胺-0	
氯苯那敏-2	氟氢可的松-NK	美托洛尔-0	沙美特罗(吸入)-0
氯丙嗪-3	氟西汀-1	咪达唑仑-1	司来吉兰-0
氯噻酮-NK	氟哌噻吨-1	米诺环素-0	番泻叶-0
西米替丁-0	氟奋乃静-1	米拉贝隆-0	舍吲哚-1
桂利嗪-1	氟伏沙明-0	米氮平-1	舍曲林-1
环丙沙星-0	叶酸-0	吗氯贝胺-0	西地那非-0
西酞普兰-1	呋塞米-0	吗啡-0	辛伐他汀-0

注:AEC 评分是一个定期更新的网络应用程序,请访问 www.medichec.com。该网站最近进行了更新,包含了会导致头晕和嗜睡的药物,因为这些药物不良反应会增加老年人的认知障碍和意识混乱,并增加跌倒的风险。

　　临床上应该保持老年人的抗胆碱能负荷在最低水平(最好为 0),特别是有认知功能损害者。

　　在可能的情况下,应该使用疗效相同但不影响胆碱能系统的药物。如果不可能,应该鼓励使用抗胆碱能活性低或作用部位特异性高(因此对中枢影响最小)的药物。不透过血-脑屏障的抗胆碱能药对认知功能的影响较小[7]。AEC 量表考虑了所有这些因素。

　　以下是使用 AEC 评分的建议[4]:
- 在出现认知损害、痴呆或谵妄症状的老年人中,AEC 评分为 2 分或 3 分的单个药物应:
  - 停用
  - 换用 AEC 评分较低(最好为 0)的替代药物
- 对于未接受任何 AEC 评分为 2 分或 3 分单个药物,但 AEC 总分≥3 分患者,患者-临床医师应对药物进行类似的审查。
- 如果认为适合撤药,则应缓慢减药(在可能的情况下),以避免症状反弹(恶心、出汗、尿频、腹泻)。

痴呆患者躯体疾病用药的安全性

用于尿失禁的抗胆碱能药

　　奥昔布宁容易穿透中枢神经系统(CNS),一直与认知功能的恶化有关。虽然托特罗定研究发现对中枢神经系统无不良影响[8],但是病例报告描述过不良反应,包括记忆丧失、幻觉和谵妄[9-11]。相反,达非那新,一个选择性 M_3 受体拮抗剂,已在健康老年受试者中研究其对认知功能的影响。与安慰剂组相比,该药对认知测试没有影响[12,13],但是缺乏在痴呆中的研究。索利那辛可导致工作记忆损伤[14],但是研究是在脑卒中患者中进行的,结果发现该药不影响短期认知功能[15]。曲司氯胺有几例引起中枢神经系统不良反应的病例报告[16],但研究发现患者认知功能没有显著改变[17,18]。弗斯特罗的研究中,采用多种认知测量工具,均未发现认知功能的明显损害(表6.5)[19,20]。

表6.5 用于尿失禁的抗胆碱能药物的理化性质[14,25](经许可改编[26])

药物	毒蕈碱受体 (M_3：M_1 亲和力比)	极性	亲脂性	分子量/kDa	糖蛋白底物	理论上通过血-脑屏障的能力	对认知的影响
达非那新	主要是 M_3(9.3：1)	中性	高	507.5(相对大)	是	高(但有膀胱选择性,且为 P-糖蛋白底物)	–
非索罗定	非选择性	中性	很低	411.6	是	很低	–
奥昔布宁	非选择性	中性	中等	357(相对小)	否	中等/高	+++
索利那辛	主要是 M_3(2.5：1)	中性	中等	480.6	否	中等	–/+
托特罗定	非选择性	中性	低	475.6	否	低	+
曲司氯铵	非选择性	带正电	无	428	是	几乎无	–

–,无认知方面的不良反应报告;+,有一些认知方面不良反应的报告;+++,有认知方面不良反应的持续性报告。

所有的叔胺类药物,如奥昔布宁、托特罗定、索非那新、弗斯特罗定和达非那新,均通过细胞色素 P450(CYP450)酶代谢。年龄增加,或合用抑制这些酶的药物(如红霉素、氟西汀),可导致血清药物浓度升高,从而增加药物不良反应。曲司氯胺的代谢未明,但是该药不通过 CYP450 系统代谢,意味着不太可能发生与该药的药代动力学相互作用[8]。

用于尿潴留的 α 受体阻滞剂

α 受体阻滞剂,如坦索罗辛、阿夫唑嗪和哌唑嗪,可引起嗜睡、头晕、抑郁[21]。尚未见此类药物影响认知功能的文献报告,α 受体阻滞剂没有列入任何抗胆碱能认知负荷名单中。

用于胃肠道疾病的药物

洛哌丁胺:虽然可能有一定的抗胆碱能活性,但是没有数据表明它可以使痴呆患者的认知功能恶化。若与其他抗胆碱能药合用,可能会增加抗胆碱能认知负荷。

泻药:没有证据表明泻药对认知功能有任何负面影响。事实上,因为便秘会导致谵妄以及痴呆伴发的精神行为障碍(BPSD),治疗便秘可以改善这些症状。

止吐药

赛克利嗪是第一代组胺拮抗剂,可损害认知和精神运动行为(见本节"抗组胺药"部分)[22]。

甲氧氯普胺几乎没有抗胆碱能作用,但是甲氧氯普胺和丙氯拉嗪对 D_2 受体的拮抗作用可产生运动障碍,因此,这些药物在痴呆患者中必须慎用。

多潘立酮是一种多巴胺 D_2 受体拮抗剂,通常不穿过血-脑屏障。然而,因为痴呆患者血-脑屏障可以发生改变,多潘立酮渗入中枢神经系统可导致不良反应的发生[23]。最近报道强调,多潘立酮略微增加心脏严重不良反应的风险,尤其在老年人中。最大剂量减少到 30mg/d,最长疗程不应超过1周。有基础心脏病、严重肝功能损害、服用已知会延长 Q-T 间期的药物或 CYP3A4 强抑制剂治疗的患者禁用多潘立酮[24]。

5-HT$_3$ 受体拮抗剂：用于治疗化疗引起的恶心、呕吐，对认知没有不良影响，可能有一些认知增强作用[27]。这些药物有心血管方面的警告，对有心脏疾病、合用致心律失常或 Q-T 间期延长的药物的患者，应慎用。格拉司琼 1 次/天，适合有记忆问题或吞咽困难的老年患者。格拉司琼仅通过 CYP3A4 代谢，因此药物相互作用的倾向较小[28]。所有 5-HT$_3$ 拮抗剂会引起便秘。

解痉药

氢溴酸东莨菪碱是一种亲脂性的、容易渗透血-脑屏障的中枢性抗胆碱药。它损害记忆、处理速度和注意力。低剂量时老年患者就会有这些症状，更容易出现意识模糊和幻觉[29]。与健康、年龄相匹配的对照组相比，在低剂量时，患有阿尔茨海默病的人有临床意义的认知损害[3]。东莨菪碱对认知的影响非常明显，以致在试验中用其产生类似痴呆的记忆缺损（东莨菪碱激发试验）[30]。该药没什么理由用于痴呆患者。

丁溴酸东莨菪碱对胃肠道平滑肌有局部解痉作用。丁溴酸东莨菪碱不进入中枢神经系统，因此中枢性抗胆碱能不良反应极为罕见[31]。

阿尔维林、美贝维林和薄荷油是肠道平滑肌松弛剂，对认知没有影响。

支气管扩张剂

β 受体激动剂

在同时患有帕金森病和特发性震颤的患者中，β 受体激动剂引起的震颤可能导致帕金森病的误诊和过度治疗[32]。震颤是胆碱酯酶抑制剂常见的不良反应，在合用 β 受体激动剂时应慎重。

抗胆碱能支气管扩张剂

相比口服用药，吸入抗胆碱能药物很少有全身影响[32]。一项在老年患者中进行的异丙托溴铵和茶碱的随机双盲安慰剂对照研究发现，两种药物对心理测试结果均无负面影响。这表明吸入异丙托溴铵治疗与老年人明显的认知损害无关[33]。

茶碱

与胆碱酯酶抑制剂一样，恶心和呕吐是茶碱的常见不良反应。使用茶碱的患者有 50% 出现头痛、焦虑、行为紊乱、抑郁和癫痫发作等神经系统不良反应。虽然癫痫发作是罕见的，但是老年人比年轻人更容易发生。茶碱不会引起明显的认知损害[33]。

多涎

治疗多涎时，老年人应该避免使用抗胆碱药物（如氢溴酸东莨菪碱），因为老年人使用此药物会有认知损害、谵妄和便秘等风险（见本节"抗胆碱能药"）。哌仑西平是一种相对选择性 M$_1$ 和 M$_4$ 型毒蕈碱样受体拮抗剂，不会穿过血-脑屏障，因此几乎不穿透到中枢神经系统[34]。

舌下含服阿托品，或将阿托品作为漱口水使用，有时用于治疗多涎。按照以上途径使用阿托品时，并没有数据说明此药穿过血-脑屏障的程度。

第6章

重症肌无力

与治疗阿尔茨海默病的乙酰胆碱酯酶抑制剂(多奈哌齐、卡巴拉汀、加兰他敏)不同,治疗重症肌无力的乙酰胆碱酯酶抑制剂(吡斯的明、新斯的明)作用于外周,并不穿过血-脑屏障(因而极少出现中枢神经系统不良反应)[35]。作用于外周和中枢的乙酰胆碱酯酶抑制剂合用,可增加拟胆碱不良反应(如恶心、呕吐、腹泻、腹部痛性痉挛和流涎增多)。当治疗重症肌无力和阿尔茨海默病的药物合用产生的拟胆碱不良反应不能耐受时,美金刚可能是胆碱酯酶抑制剂的一种替换选择。

镇痛药

NSAID 与对乙酰氨基酚

对乙酰氨基酚是一种安全的药物,除过量会发生谵妄外,没有证据表明它会产生认知损害[36]。有一些证据表明,长期使用阿司匹林会导致精神错乱[37]。尽管临床试验并未证明萘普生[39]或吲哚美辛[40]对认知有明显不良影响,但有病例报告指出 NSAID 可产生谵妄和精神病[38]。NSAID 很难应用于老年人,因为有心血管风险和胃肠道出血的风险[41]。临床上最好将这些药物与胃保护药合用,或者考虑局部使用 NSAID(若临床合适),以减少胃肠道出血的风险。

阿片类

镇静作用是所有阿片类药物潜在的问题[42]。由阿片类药物产生的谵妄可能伴随着烦躁、幻觉或妄想[42]。哌替啶引起认知损害的风险较高,因其代谢产物有抗胆碱性质,并且肾功能受损时会迅速积聚[43]。可待因可能会增加跌倒的风险;曲马多和可待因发生药物相互作用的风险都高,并且其疗效和不良反应也有很大的变异[44]。芬太尼贴剂可能有效,但是不宜在虚弱老年人中作为首个阿片类镇痛药物使用[45],因为贴剂即使被除去,仍然作用时间较长,使得不良反应的治疗更加困难[44]。吗啡是一种非常有效的镇痛药,但是在老年患者中易导致认知问题和其他不良反应[46]。与其他阿片类药物相比,羟考酮半衰期短,基本无药物相互作用,剂量-反应关系的预测性好。因此,至少在理论上,它是痴呆患者口服镇痛药一种不错的选择[44]。然而,在成瘾行为中应谨慎使用,因为产生了相当多的成瘾和滥用问题。丁丙诺啡透皮贴剂可能比其他阿片类药物不良反应少。

抗组胺药

第一代 H_1 抗组胺药包括氯苯那敏、羟嗪、赛克利嗪和异丙嗪。它们无选择性,有抗胆碱能活性,易穿过血-脑屏障,这些都会导致认知方面的不良反应。它们会损害认知和精神运动,触发癫痫发作、运动障碍、肌张力障碍和幻觉。第二代 H_1 抗组胺药(如氯雷他定、西替利嗪和非索非那定)不易渗入中枢神经系统,产生这些不良反应的可能性大大地减小。它们无任何抗胆碱能作用[22]。

他汀类

最近一篇 Cochrane 系统综述评估了他汀类药物治疗痴呆的临床疗效及耐受性[47],发现他汀类药物在认知功能上并无明显益处,但同样没有证据表明他汀类药物对认知有害。早期个案报告强调使用他汀类药物时,有记忆丧失的主观感受[48]。这往往发生在开始服用药物的头 2 个月,最常见于辛伐他汀。患者服用辛伐他汀后若出现认知问题,则应首先停药;若症状缓解,试用阿托伐他汀或普伐他汀替代,因为这些药物穿过血-脑屏障的可能性小。最近的一项 Cochrane 综述[49]评估了他汀类药物预防痴呆的有效性,结果显示,没有证据表明给有血管疾病风险的老年人服用他汀类药物可以预防认知能力下降或痴呆。

降压药

中年高血压对认知有不利的影响,且增加了人们患痴呆的风险[50]。没有证据表明降压治疗会损害认知。长期降压治疗,似乎对总体认知有积极作用可以降低痴呆风险[51,52]。

其他心脏药物

地高辛在治疗浓度时可产生急性精神错乱[53]。也有报道指出会导致噩梦[54]。然而,一项研究发现,地高辛治疗心力衰竭使 25% 的患者认知水平改善(未患心力衰竭的患者为 23%)[55]。一些个案报道表明胺碘酮与谵妄有关[56,57]。

H_2 受体拮抗剂和质子泵抑制剂

现在 H_2 受体拮抗剂(如西咪替丁、雷尼替丁和法莫替丁)已很少使用。西咪替丁会导致几种药代动力学相互作用。雷尼替丁产品因可能有 NDMA(n-亚硝基二甲胺)污染而被召回,而 NDMA 已被确定为某些癌症发生的潜在危险因素。法莫替丁仍在使用。关于中枢神经系统对这些药物的反应,已有报道,尤其是西咪替丁[58]。一项观察性研究发现,**质子泵抑制剂**的使用与痴呆发生有关。这一结论得到药物流行病学主要数据分析结果的支持,并且与动物研究一致。在动物研究中,**质子泵抑制剂**的使用增加了小鼠大脑中 β 淀粉样蛋白水平[59]。未来有必要进行随机、前瞻性临床试验来证实这种相关性。许多使用**质子泵抑制剂**的患者有胃黏膜幽门螺杆菌感染,而幽门螺杆菌已被报道与认知恶化有关,这可能是**质子泵抑制剂**与痴呆之间相关性背后的机制。此外,这种关联在其他研究中并未得到重复[60,61]。

抗生素

许多抗生素会产生谵妄[62,63],但是它们产生的认知损害并无一致的模式。考虑到感染治疗在痴呆中的重要性,应该使用治疗该感染最合适的抗生素。抗结核治疗,特别是异烟肼,已有精神科不良反应的个案报告(表 6.6)[64]。

表 6.6 痴呆推荐药与禁用药(经许可改编[26])

疾病	药物类别或药物名称	痴呆禁用药	痴呆推荐药
过敏	抗组胺药	氯苯那敏 异丙嗪 羟嗪 赛庚啶 赛克利嗪 (以及其他第一代抗组胺药)	西替利嗪 氯雷他定 非索非那定 (以及其他第二代抗组胺药)
哮喘/慢性阻塞性肺疾病	支气管扩张剂		β 受体激动剂 吸入性抗胆碱药(未报道会影响认知) 茶碱
便秘	泻药	无证据表明泻药对认知功能有负面影响 便秘本身可能加重认知障碍	
腹泻	洛派丁胺	低效价抗胆碱能药 已知对认知功能无影响,但是若与其他抗胆碱药合用,可能会增加抗胆碱药的认知负担	
高脂血症	他汀类		全都安全,但是阿托伐他汀和普伐他汀穿过血-脑屏障的可能性更小
多涎	抗胆碱药	氢溴酸东莨菪碱	哌仑西平 阿托品(舌下)
高血压	降压药	β 受体阻滞剂(不可能总是避开)	钙通道阻滞剂、血管紧张素转换酶抑制剂以及血管紧张素受体阻滞剂都有可能提高认知功能
感染	抗生素	据报道,谵妄最常见于喹诺酮和大环内脂类药物 但是考虑到治疗感染的重要性,应该使用治疗感染最合适的抗生素	
重症肌无力	外周乙酰胆碱酯酶抑制剂,如新斯的明和吡斯的明	在痴呆患者中,可能增加中枢乙酰胆碱酯酶抑制剂(如多奈哌齐)的胆碱不良反应,即增加恶心、呕吐等的风险	
恶心/呕吐	止吐药	赛克利嗪 甲氧氯普胺 普鲁氯嗪	多潘立酮(其使用限制见正文) 5-HT$_3$ 受体拮抗剂
其他胃肠道疾病	止痉药	阿托品 双环维林	阿尔维林 美贝维林 薄荷油 丁溴酸东莨菪碱 溴丙胺太林

续表

疾病	药物类别或药物名称	痴呆禁用药	痴呆推荐药
疼痛	镇痛药	哌替啶	对乙酰氨基酚
		镇痛新	羟考酮
		右旋丙氧酚	丁丙诺啡
		可待因	局部非甾体抗炎药（若合适）
		曲马多	
		美沙酮	
		芬太尼贴剂（未使用过阿片类的患者需谨慎）	
		吗啡（可用于顽固性疼痛或姑息治疗；由于有认知风险与其他不良反应，使用时需谨慎）	
尿频	用于治疗膀胱活动过度的抗胆碱药	奥西布宁	达非那新
		托特罗定	曲司氯胺
			索利那新（没有其他药物时使用，一些报道有认知不良反应）
		弗斯特罗定的数据仍缺失。它无选择性，有高度中枢抗胆碱能活性，但是从理论上穿过血-脑屏障的能力非常低	
尿失禁	α受体阻滞剂	已知对认知功能无影响	

参考文献

1. Sink KM, et al. Dual use of bladder anticholinergics and cholinesterase inhibitors: long-term functional and cognitive outcomes. *J Am Geriatr Soc* 2008; **56**:847–853.
2. Ruxton K, et al. Drugs with anticholinergic effects and cognitive impairment, falls and all-cause mortality in older adults: A systematic review and meta-analysis. *Br J Clin Pharmacol* 2015; **80**:209–220.
3. Sunderland T, et al. Anticholinergic sensitivity in patients with dementia of the Alzheimer type and age-matched controls. A dose-response study. *Arch Gen Psychiatry* 1987; **44**:418–426.
4. Bishara D, et al. Anticholinergic effect on cognition (AEC) of drugs commonly used in older people. *Int J Geriatr Psychiatry* 2017; **32**:650–656.
5. Fox C, et al. Anticholinergic medication use and cognitive impairment in the older population: the medical research council cognitive function and ageing study. *J Am Geriatr Soc* 2011; **59**:1477–1483.
6. Bishara D, et al. The anticholinergic effect on cognition (AEC) scale-Associations with mortality, hospitalisation and cognitive decline following dementia diagnosis. *Int J Geriatr Psychiatry* 2020; **35**:1069–1077.
7. Wagg A. The cognitive burden of anticholinergics in the elderly – implications for the treatment of overactive bladder. *Eur Urological Rev* 2012; **7**:42–49.
8. Pagoria D, et al. Antimuscarinic drugs: review of the cognitive impact when used to treat overactive bladder in elderly patients. *Curr Urol Rep* 2011; **12**:351–357.
9. Womack KB, et al. Tolterodine and memory: dry but forgetful. *Arch Neurol* 2003; **60**:771–773.
10. Tsao JW, et al. Transient memory impairment and hallucinations associated with tolterodine use. *N Engl J Med* 2003; **349**:2274–2275.
11. Edwards KR, et al. Risk of delirium with concomitant use of tolterodine and acetylcholinesterase inhibitors. *J Am Geriatr Soc* 2002; **50**:1165–1166.
12. Kay G, et al. Differential effects of the antimuscarinic agents darifenacin and oxybutynin ER on memory in older subjects. *Eur Urol* 2006; **50**:317–326.
13. Lipton RB, et al. Assessment of cognitive function of the elderly population: effects of darifenacin. *J Urol* 2005; **173**:493–498.
14. Chancellor MB, et al. Blood-brain barrier permeation and efflux exclusion of anticholinergics used in the treatment of overactive bladder. *Drugs Aging* 2012; **29**:259–273.
15. Park JW. The effect of solifenacin on cognitive function following stroke. *Dement Geriatr Cogn Dis Extra* 2013; **3**:143–147.
16. Liabeuf S, et al. Trospium chloride for overactive bladder may induce central nervous system adverse events. *Eur Geriatr Med* 2014; **5**:220–224.
17. Isik AT, et al. Trospium and cognition in patients with late onset Alzheimer disease. *J Nutr Health Aging* 2009; **13**:672–676.

18. Geller EJ, et al. Effect of trospium chloride on cognitive function in women aged 50 and older: a randomized trial. *Female Pelvic Med Reconstr Surg* 2017; 23:118–123.

19. Wagg A. Fesoterodine fumarate for the treatment of overactive bladder in the elderly – a review of the latest clinical data. *Clin Investig (Lond)* 2012; 2:825–833.

20. Yonguc T, et al. Randomized, controlled trial of fesoterodine fumarate for overactive bladder in Parkinson's disease. *World J Urol* 2020; 38:2013–2019.

21. BNF Online. British National Formulary. 2020; https://www.medicinescomplete.com/mc/bnf/current.

22. Mahdy AM, et al. Histamine and antihistamines. *Anaesthesia Intensive Care Med* 2011; 12:324–329.

23. Roy-Desruisseaux J, et al. Domperidone-induced tardive dyskinesia and withdrawal psychosis in an elderly woman with dementia. *Ann Pharmacother* 2011; 45:e51.

24. Medicines and Healthcare Products Regulatory Agency. Domperidone: risks of cardiac side effects – indication restricted to nausea and vomiting, new contraindications, and reduced dose and duration of use. 2014; http://www.mhra.gov.uk/Safetyinformation/DrugSafetyUpdate/CON418518.

25. Kay GG, et al. Preserving cognitive function for patients with overactive bladder: evidence for a differential effect with darifenacin. *Int J Clin Pract* 2008; 62:1792–1800.

26. Bishara D, et al. Safe prescribing of physical health medication in patients with dementia. *Int J Geriatr Psychiatry* 2014; 29:1230–1241.

27. Bentley KR, et al. Therapeutic potential of serotonin 5-HT3 antagonists in neuropsychiatric disorders. *CNS Drugs* 1995; 3:363–392.

28. Gridelli C. Same old story? Do we need to modify our supportive care treatment of elderly cancer patients? Focus on antiemetics. *Drugs Aging* 2004; 21:825–832.

29. Flicker C, et al. Hypersensitivity to scopolamine in the elderly. *Psychopharmacology* 1992; 107:437–441.

30. Ebert U, et al. Scopolamine model of dementia: electroencephalogram findings and cognitive performance. *Eur J Clin Invest* 1998; 28:944–949.

31. Sanofi. Summary of product characteristics. Buscopan 10 mg Tablets. 2020; https://www.medicines.org.uk/emc/medicine/30089.

32. Gupta P, et al. Potential adverse effects of bronchodilators in the treatment of airways obstruction in older people: recommendations for prescribing. *Drugs Aging* 2008; 25:415–443.

33. Ramsdell JW, et al. Effects of theophylline and ipratropium on cognition in elderly patients with chronic obstructive pulmonary disease. *Ann Allergy Asthma Immunol* 1996; 76:335–340.

34. Fritze J, et al. Pirenzepine for clozapine-induced hypersalivation. *Lancet* 1995; 346:1034.

35. Pohanka M. Acetylcholinesterase inhibitors: a patent review. *Expert Opin Ther Pat* 2012; 22:871–886.

36. Gray SL, et al. Drug-induced cognition disorders in the elderly: incidence, prevention and management. *Drug Saf* 1999; 21:101–122.

37. Bailey RB, et al. Chronic salicylate intoxication. A common cause of morbidity in the elderly. *J Am Geriatr Soc* 1989; 37:556–561.

38. Hoppmann RA, et al. Central nervous system side effects of nonsteroidal anti-inflammatory drugs. Aseptic meningitis, psychosis, and cognitive dysfunction. *Arch Intern Med* 1991; 151:1309–1313.

39. Wysenbeek AJ, et al. Assessment of cognitive function in elderly patients treated with naproxen. A prospective study. *Clin Exp Rheumatol* 1988; 6:399–400.

40. Bruce-Jones PN, et al. Indomethacin and cognitive function in healthy elderly volunteers. *Br J Clin Pharmacol* 1994; 38:45–51.

41. Barber JB, et al. Treatment of chronic non-malignant pain in the elderly: safety considerations. *Drug Saf* 2009; 32:457–474.

42. Ripamonti C, et al. CNS adverse effects of opioids in cancer patients. *CNS Drugs* 1997; 8:21–37.

43. Alagiakrishnan K, et al. An approach to drug induced delirium in the elderly. *Postgrad Med J* 2004; 80:388–393.

44. McLachlan AJ, et al. Clinical pharmacology of analgesic medicines in older people: impact of frailty and cognitive impairment. *Br J Clin Pharmacol* 2011; 71:351–364.

45. Dosa DM, et al. Frequency of long-acting opioid analgesic initiation in opioid-naive nursing home residents. *J Pain Symptom Manage* 2009; 38:515–521.

46. Tannenbaum C, et al. A systematic review of amnestic and non-amnestic mild cognitive impairment induced by anticholinergic, antihistamine, GABAergic and opioid drugs. *Drugs Aging* 2012; 29:639–658.

47. McGuinness B, et al. Statins for the treatment of dementia. *Cochrane Database Syst Rev* 2014; Cd007514.

48. Wagstaff LR, et al. Statin-associated memory loss: analysis of 60 case reports and review of the literature. *Pharmacotherapy* 2003; 23:871–880.

49. McGuinness B, et al. Statins for the prevention of dementia. *Cochrane Database Syst Rev* 2016; Cd003160.

50. Qiu C, et al. The age-dependent relation of blood pressure to cognitive function and dementia. *Lancet Neurol* 2005; 4:487–499.

51. Wändell P, et al. Antihypertensive drugs and relevant cardiovascular pharmacotherapies and the risk of incident dementia in patients with atrial fibrillation. *Int J Cardiol* 2018; 272:149–154.

52. Levi MN, et al. Antihypertensive classes, cognitive decline and incidence of dementia: a network meta-analysis. *J Hypertens* 2013; 31:1073–1082.

53. Eisendrath SJ, et al. Toxic neuropsychiatric effects of digoxin at therapeutic serum concentrations. *Am J Psychiatry* 1987; 144:506–507.

54. Brezis M, et al. Nightmares from digoxin. *Ann Intern Med* 1980; 93:639–640.

55. Laudisio A, et al. Digoxin and cognitive performance in patients with heart failure: a cohort, pharmacoepidemiological survey. *Drugs Aging* 2009; 26:103–112.

56. Athwal H, et al. Amiodarone-induced delirium. *Am J Geriatr Psychiatry* 2003; 11:696–697.

57. Foley KT, et al. Separate episodes of delirium associated with levetiracetam and amiodarone treatment in an elderly woman. *Am J Geriatr Pharmacother* 2010; 8:170–174.

第 6 章

58. Cantu TG, et al. Central nervous system reactions to histamine-2 receptor blockers. *Ann Intern Med* 1991; **114**:1027–1034.

59. Gomm W, et al. Association of proton pump inhibitors with risk of dementia: a pharmacoepidemiological claims data analysis. *JAMA Neurol* 2016; **73**:410–416.

60. Goldstein FC, et al. Proton pump inhibitors and risk of mild cognitive impairment and dementia. *J Am Geriatr Soc* 2017; **65**:1969–1974.

61. Lochhead P, et al. Association between proton pump inhibitor use and cognitive function in women. *Gastroenterology* 2017; **153**:971–979. e974.

62. Grahl JJ, et al. Antimicrobial exposure and the risk of delirium in critically ill patients. *Crit Care* 2018; **22**:337.

63. Bhattacharyya S, et al. Antibiotic-associated encephalopathy. *Neurology* 2016; **86**:963–971.

64. Kass JS, et al. Nervous system effects of antituberculosis therapy. *CNS Drugs* 2010; **24**:655–667.

第 6 章

痴呆精神行为症状的管理

痴呆精神行为症状(BPSD)包括各种症状,如攻击、激越、喊叫、痛苦、脱抑制、幻觉、妄想、淡漠、情绪低落和焦虑[1]。超过 90% 的患者会出现不同程度的这些症状[2]。当一个患者同时出现几个症状时,则很难明确特定的症状。这些症状的药物治疗尚缺乏足够的科学证据支持[3],而且许多可用的药物存在严重的不良反应。

非药物治疗

英国发表的报告《行动时刻》(*Time for Action*)详细说明了抗精神病药用于痴呆的风险[4],推动了对抗精神病药的证据审查,并促进制定了 BPSD 的非药物治疗途径。现已完成系统综述[5],也提出了新的治疗模式[6,7],编写了指导文件[8]。主要内容包括:

1. 采用个性化和符合实际情况的治疗方法,而不是"现成的"疗法。

2. 确保首先解决引起 BPSD 的躯体因素,包括疼痛(见后面的章节)、急性躯体疾病、便秘和药物不良反应(见痴呆的安全用药部分)。

3. 把"问题行为"理解为患者痛苦和未满足需求的表达方式,这一点很重要。

4. 利用生活史、对照护过程直接观察以及采集数据[如睡眠、疼痛和 ABC 图表(前因行为后果图表)],来了解哪些需求可能未得到满足,为改变治疗提供信息[8]。

5. 召开会议以建立有关导致行为发生以及使行为持续存在的因素模型,该模型可以根据新证据进行修改。

6. 与照护者一起制订明确和符合实际情况的照护计划,以解决通过上述步骤发现的未满足的需求。

7. 根据所尝试干预手段的效果,回顾和调整照护计划。

研究[10]支持了针对 BPSD 的更加结构化的社会心理干预[9]。将这些干预措施作为个体化照护计划的一部分加以考虑可能是有益的;如果通过支持照护者和提升他们的技能来实施,效果会更好。以患者个体行为为中心的行为管理技巧和照护者心理教育是有效的,其效果可能会持续数月[11]。

对系统综述进行的综述[12]提供了这些干预措施的证据概述。在感官模拟干预中,唯一令人信服的有效干预(缓解激越和攻击行为)是音乐治疗。一项成功开展的研究[13](*n*=71)报告,使用香蜂草膏对激越和行为症状指标有良好的治疗效果,但由于方法学限制,这一结果尚未被重复。尚没有证据证实芳香疗法和按摩疗法的功效。光疗和多感官刺激疗法尚未显示出任何显著的效果。认知或情绪导向的干预(如怀旧疗法、情景模拟疗法和确认疗法)的有效性证据仍不足。采用综合的多学科方法,将医学、精神医学和护理干预相结合的多要素干预,可能更有效地减少养老院患者的严重行为问题。其他干预方法(如动物辅助疗法和运动疗法)对 BPSD 均无令人信服的疗效[12]。

总之,针对个人未满足需求量身定制的多要素干预措施比常规使用"现成的"干预措施更有可能带来好处。

建议：循证、多要素、个性化、与照护者密切合作的非药物措施，是 BPSD 的一线治疗方法。有证据表明音乐疗法可以减轻激越。

药物治疗

镇痛药

认知障碍患者的疼痛可以表现为激越，因此，治疗未诊断的疼痛可能有助于控制激越症状[14]。随机对照试验研究了止痛剂逐步治疗中、重度痴呆和激越患者的效果，发现激越、总体神经精神症状和疼痛有显著改善。研究中大多数患者只服用对乙酰氨基酚。

一项 Cochrane 综述考察了阿片类药物治疗痴呆患者激越的临床疗效和安全性[15]。该综述纳入了阿片类药物与安慰剂的随机对照试验。然而，表明阿片类药物在患者中临床疗效或安全性的证据尚不充分。

建议：疼痛的评估和有效治疗很重要。即使患者没有明显疼痛，也值得尝试镇痛药（通常是对乙酰氨基酚）。

抗精神病药治疗痴呆的行为和心理症状

抗精神病药曾一度广泛地用于痴呆相关的行为紊乱[16]，但现在对其使用极具争议[17,18]，主要原因是其效应值小[19-22]，耐受性差[22-24]，且与死亡率升高有关[25]。尽管如此，抗精神病药仍是 BPSD 干预研究中数量最多的。

典型抗精神病药对 BPSD 无明显疗效（氟哌啶醇除外），而非典型抗精神病药确有一定的疗效。一项比较疗效的综述发现，最有效的抗精神病药包括利培酮（精神病、激越、BPSD总体评分）、奥氮平（激越）和阿立哌唑（BPSD 总体评分）。喹硫平虽然被广泛地使用，但除了可能无法耐受的较高剂量（100~200mg/d），对 BPSD 基本无效。CATIE-AD 研究比较了利培酮、奥氮平、喹硫平和安慰剂对 BPSD 患者的疗效，证明利培酮和奥氮平有效，但很多受试者因不良反应而停药[26]。

2006 年，Cochrane 的一项非典型抗精神病药治疗 AD 患者攻击行为和精神病性症状的综述[27]得出结论，利培酮和奥氮平有助于减少攻击行为，利培酮可减轻精神病性症状。然而，作者认为，由于利培酮和奥氮平的疗效一般，不良反应显著增加，所以不应常规使用利培酮或奥氮平治疗痴呆患者，除非与患者一起生活或工作的人感到极为痛苦，或有受身体伤害的严重风险。

抗精神病药增加痴呆患者的死亡率

分析 2004 年已发表和未发表的数据之后，英国和美国发布了关于使用某些第二代抗精神病药（主要是利培酮和奥氮平）使痴呆患者死亡率增加的警告[28-30]。现在这些警告已经扩展到所有第二代和第一代抗精神病药[30,31]，并在所有说明书上增加了可能发生脑血管事件的警告。

一些研究表明,服用抗精神病药的老年人发生脑血管事件的风险可能不会累积[32,33]。在治疗的前几周,风险升高,但随后随着时间的推移而下降,3个月后恢复到基础水平。相反,一项长期研究(24~54 个月)表明,与安慰剂相比,抗精神病药治疗(利培酮和第一代抗精神病药)患者的死亡率随着时间的推移逐渐增加[34]。目前这不是一个普遍接受的观点。

一些研究调查了不同抗精神病药的死亡率[35-38]。总体而言,服用氟哌啶醇死亡风险增加,而服用喹硫平死亡风险降低。尚未观察到奥氮平、阿立哌唑和齐拉西酮[35](或丙戊酸)具有临床意义的差异。这种影响在治疗刚开始最强,调整剂量后保持。除喹硫平[35]外,都存在剂量反应关系。另一项研究[37]考察了 14 种抗精神病药与利培酮在新使用抗精神病药患者中的校正死亡风险比(HR)。结果发现,与利培酮相比,氟哌啶醇、甲氧异丁嗪和氯哌噻吨的死亡率较高,美哌隆的死亡率略高,喹硫平、奥氮平、氯氮平和氟哌噻嗪的风险较低,未发现氨磺必利组有统计学显著差异。

2019 年,对 17 项研究(5373 例患者)进行的网络荟萃分析发现,一些药物与安慰剂存在差异,但是阿立哌唑、奥氮平、喹硫平和利培酮之间有效性和安全性指标没有显著差异[39]。

抗精神病药引起脑血管事件有多种机制[40]。脑血管功能不全或动脉粥样硬化患者发生直立性低血压会降低脑灌注;心房颤动患者心动过速会导致脑灌注减少或血栓脱落(见心房颤动中的精神药物部分);直立性低血压时,儿茶酚胺反应性升高,导致血管收缩,从而加重脑供血不足。此外,高泌乳血症理论上可加速动脉粥样硬化,镇静作用可能引起脱水和血液浓缩[40]。一项研究[32]表明 M_1 和 α_2 受体的亲和力可以预测抗精神病药对卒中的影响。

近期对利培酮临床试验数据进行了研究,探索与脑血管事件和死亡相关的患者特征,以及紧急治疗的危险因素[41]。在接受利培酮治疗的患者中,基线抑郁和妄想与脑血管事件相对风险较低相关。利培酮治疗组患者中,基线时唯一与相对死亡风险有意义的较低相关的预测因素是抑郁。但是利培酮与抗炎药物合用的患者死亡的相对风险较高。

典型[42]和非典型[43]抗精神病药都可能加速痴呆患者的认知能力下降,尽管有一些证据对此并不认同[44-46]。

> 建议:在一些存在严重攻击或精神病性症状病例中,可以使用利培酮(批准用于 AD 的持续性攻击行为)和奥氮平。如果使用这些药物,建议定期评估。

抗精神病药用于痴呆的临床信息

抗精神病药不应常规用于治疗痴呆患者的激越和攻击行为[47]。

利培酮(和氟哌啶醇)是英国唯一获批用于治疗与痴呆相关的非认知症状的药物。氟哌啶醇具有严重的不良反应,因此首选利培酮。利培酮尤其适用于非药物治疗无效、有伤害自己或他人风险、中重度 AD 患者的持续攻击行为的短期治疗(可达 6 周)[48]。治疗痴呆的最佳剂量为每天 2 次[50],每次 500μg(每天 1mg),但治疗量可达到每天 2 次,每次 1mg[49]。

如果使用利培酮有禁忌证或不能耐受,可用其他抗精神病药(适应证外使用)。奥氮平在减少痴呆患者的攻击性方面有一定的疗效[27]。评估氨磺必利在痴呆患者中的疗效和耐受性的研究正在进行中[51,52]。由于喹硫平很少引起运动障碍,可考虑(极低剂量)用于帕金森病或者路易体痴呆患者(但是不如利培酮和奥氮平有效)。

处方抗精神病药之前需要：

- 仔细评估风险，综合考虑脑血管风险（高血压、糖尿病、吸烟、心房颤动和既往卒中）。
- 与照护者（以及有能力的患者）讨论可能的风险和获益。
- 明确记录上述信息[47]。

建议所有服用抗精神病药的患者在**基线**、**3 个月**和**每年**进行以下检查：

1. 血压和脉搏
2. 体重（最好头 3 个月每月监测 1 次）
3. 血液检查
   a. 空腹血糖或 HbA_{1c}
   b. 尿素和电解质，包括 eGFR
   c. 全血细胞计数
   d. 血脂（尽可能空腹）
   e. 肝功能检查
   f. 泌乳素水平
4. 心电图（4 周至 3 个月，或临床需要时复查）

- 住院患者或身体虚弱的患者需更频繁监测躯体状况。
- 4~6 周后（住院患者可更早）需要评价抗精神病药的作用，如果躯体状况稳定且没有不良反应，3 个月时再次评价，之后每 6 个月进行 1 次。如果合适，各次药物评价时均可考虑停药。
- 有时患者很难完成推荐的检查，例如，患者激越和反抗的程度较严重，或者紧急情况下。此时，应该再次进行利弊分析，要认识到没有完成相关检查，处方抗精神病药的风险可能更高，只有在不用药反而会使风险更高的情况下才处方抗精神病药。

长期照护中停用抗精神病药（HAULT）研究是在澳大利亚长期照护机构服用抗精神病药的患者中开展的一项单臂纵向研究，其中 98.5% 患有痴呆症。完成试验的 93 例患者中，69 例（74%）成功停用抗精神病药，没有再次用药，BPSD 症状也没有增加。在该研究中，停用抗精神病药的方案遵循澳大利亚的指南：每 2 周减少 50% 的剂量，在使用最小剂量 2 周后停药，每次停用一种抗精神病药，最后停用利培酮（如果有处方）[54]。抗精神病药治疗 BPSD 的减量或停药方案指南见表 6.7。

表 6.7　BPSD 中抗精神病药减量或停药方法——指南[53]

抗精神病药	痴呆患者常用剂量范围	建议的减量或停药方法 （一般用 2~4 周减药，如果可能，最好 4 周）
氨磺必利	每天 25~50mg	每 1~2 周减量 12.5~25mg（视剂量而定），然后停药
阿立哌唑	每天 5~15mg	每 1~2 周减 5mg（视剂量而定），然后停药 （如每天 5mg，则减量至 2.5mg，服用 2 周。注意：片剂没有划痕，口服液价格较高，建议咨询当地药剂师）
氟哌啶醇	不推荐用于老年痴呆患者（谵妄除外） 每 1~2 周减少 0.25~0.5mg（视剂量而定），然后停药	
奥氮平	每天 2.5~10mg	每 1~2 周减少 2.5mg（视剂量而定），然后停药

续表

抗精神病药	痴呆患者常用剂量范围	建议的减量或停药方法 （一般用 2~4 周减药，如果可能，最好 4 周）
喹硫平	每天 12.5~300mg	12.5~100mg/d：每 1~2 周减少 12.5~25mg（视剂量而定），然后停药； 100~300mg/d：每 1~2 周减少 25~50mg（视剂量而定），然后停药； 如果剂量为 300mg/d，减至 150~200mg/d，服用 1 周，然后每周减少 50mg
利培酮	每天 0.25~2mg	每 1~2 周减少 0.25~0.5mg（视剂量而定），然后停药

对于更高剂量，在 4 周内逐渐减量。

注意：如出现严重不良反应，应立即停用抗精神病药。

治疗 BPSD 的其他药物

促认知药

AChE-I 和美金刚对 BPSD 的作用较小。荟萃分析显示，AChE-I 对 BPSD 的影响虽然有统计学意义，但其临床获益尚不清楚[55]。总的来说，研究表明，AChE-I 对抑郁、心境恶劣、淡漠和焦虑症状的效果优于激越或攻击行为。有研究提示美金刚能改善激越、攻击和妄想等症状。促认知药可能在用药后 3~6 个月才见效，因此，这些药物对 BPSD 的急性治疗可能没有临床用处。然而，由于临床上使用 AChE-I 和美金刚减缓认知衰退，最终这些药物可能也有助于减少令人痛苦的行为[56]。

> 建议：在上述情况中，如果患者没有使用 AChE-I 或美金刚，且在批准的适应证之内，则可以酌情使用。最多有轻度疗效。

苯二氮䓬类

苯二氮䓬类药物也被广泛使用[57,58]，但实际上缺乏证据支持。其与认知能力下降[57]、痴呆风险[59]、肺炎风险[60]以及全因死亡风险增加[61]相关，并可能增加老年人跌倒和髋关节骨折发生率[58,62]。

> 建议：除紧急镇静外，避免使用苯二氮䓬类药物。

抗抑郁药

大量证据表明，抑郁既是 AD 的危险因素，也是其后果。两者共病患病率为 30%~50%[63]。推测抗抑郁药影响抑郁症认知功能有两种可能机制：一种是药物对特定神经递质的直接药理学作用，另一种是药物改善抑郁症的间接作用[64]。

抗抑郁药对 BPSD 的疗效证据不一且有限，提示对痴呆患者的激越最有效，而对抑郁、淡漠、焦虑或精神病性症状效果略逊[26]。在 CitAD 试验中[65]，西酞普兰对激越的疗效证据最强，每天 30mg 西酞普兰能有效治疗痴呆患者的激越。遗憾的是，该研究也证实这一剂量的西酞普兰有延长 Q-T 间期的风险。由于药物影响心脏 Q-T 间期，老年人服用西酞普兰的最大剂量是每天 20mg。艾司西酞普兰也可能对 BPSD 有效，但证据较少。舍曲林在心脏安全性方面具有优势，但其对 BPSD 的疗效证据不一[26]。

尽管既往一项 Cochrane 综述[66]表明 RCT 试验中曲唑酮治疗痴呆的激越证据不足,但近期一项 Cochrane 综述发现曲唑酮睡前服用 50mg 对痴呆伴有失眠的患者耐受性良好,能改善睡眠。此外,有研究发现曲唑酮 150~300mg/d 可有效地缓解额颞叶痴呆患者的 BPSD。尽管米氮平在老年抑郁症治疗中起到很重要的作用,但是最近一项小样本研究未发现 15mg 米氮平对伴睡眠障碍的 AD 患者有显著疗效,而实际上,药物治疗还使日间睡眠模式恶化。安非他酮在痴呆中的作用尚无对照试验研究[26]。

三环类抗抑郁药最好避免用于痴呆患者,它们可能因直立性低血压导致跌倒,也可能因抗胆碱能不良反应造成认知功能恶化[67]。

研究表明,在接受胆碱酯酶抑制剂治疗的 AD 患者中,SSRI 可能对抑郁症的认知下降有一定程度的保护作用。迄今为止,文献分析尚未阐明 SSRI 和 AChE-I 的联合作用是协同、相加还是独立的[64]。此外,尚不清楚 SSRI 对不伴情绪或行为问题的 AD 患者的认知功能有无益处[68]。

虽然一些新研究发现,老年人使用抗抑郁药可能会增加患痴呆的风险,但重要的是要切记,既往研究表明,晚年抑郁与患痴呆的风险增加有关。增加痴呆风险的可能是抑郁,并非药物,因此,任何抗抑郁药使用者与非抑郁症非抗抑郁药使用者的比较都会受到适应证偏倚的影响。

瑞典的一项研究[69]收集了 20 050 名痴呆患者在痴呆诊断时和确诊前 3 年多的抗抑郁药使用数据,发现在痴呆诊断前连续 3 年使用抗抑郁药治疗与所有痴呆发生和 AD 的死亡率风险较低相关。

> 建议:虽然证据不足,但对于有明显中重度抑郁症状的痴呆患者,尤其如果非药物治疗无效,可考虑使用抗抑郁剂。

心境稳定剂/抗癫痫药

奥卡西平[70]、卡马西平[71]和丙戊酸盐[72]等心境稳定剂治疗痴呆的非认知症状的随机对照试验已经完成。加巴喷丁、拉莫三嗪和托吡酯也被用于痴呆患者[73]。其中,卡马西平对非认知症状的疗效证据最强[74],但它严重的不良反应(尤其是 Stevens-Johnson 综合征)和潜在的药物相互作用限制了它的使用。

一项包括开放延长期的随机对照试验发现,丙戊酸盐对控制症状无效。在 12 周的延长研究期间,39 例患者中有 7 例死亡,尽管并不归因于药物[75]。一项探索丙戊酸治疗痴呆的最佳剂量的研究发现,在一些患者中血药浓度 40~60μg/L 以及相对低剂量[7~12mg/(kg·d)]与激越症状改善有关,但同样血药浓度情况下另外一些患者症状并无改善,还导致严重的不良反应[76]。2009 年 Cochrane 的综述发现,没有足够证据表明丙戊酸盐治疗痴呆患者激越症状的疗效,仍需更进一步地研究[77]。丙戊酸盐并不延迟痴呆患者激越症状的出现[78]。关于抗癫痫药治疗痴呆患者非认知症状的综述发现,丙戊酸盐、奥卡西平和锂盐的有效证据较低或者毫无证据,需要更多的随机对照试验来加强加巴喷丁、托吡酯和拉莫三嗪的证据[74]。

系列病例报告和病例综述的初步低等级证据提示,加巴喷丁和普瑞巴林对 AD 患者的 BPSD 可能有效,对额颞叶痴呆仍缺乏证据支持[79]。在一项小样本系列病例报告中,加巴喷丁 200~600mg/d 减少了 7 例血管性痴呆或混合性痴呆患者的攻击行为;使用加巴喷丁治疗后,其中 3 例能成功停用抗精神病药。因此,加巴喷丁可用于不宜使用抗精神病药的心脏病患者。加巴喷丁慎用于路易体痴呆患者。有报道称,使用该药物治疗行为症状会导致神经精神症状加剧[80]。

虽然抗癫痫药物/心境稳定剂在某些患者中有明显益处,但目前尚不建议将其作为治疗痴呆患者神经精神症状的常规药物[73]。

> 建议:支持使用的证据有限——在其他治疗禁忌或无效的情况下可合理使用。最好避免使用丙戊酸盐。

褪黑素与 AD 的睡眠障碍

褪黑素添加剂对 AD 患者睡眠有效性的证据有限。目前已发表 6 项双盲随机对照试验,但大多数样本量非常有限。褪黑素即使在高剂量时也未导致明显的不良反应,但是其研究结果模棱两可。一些研究显示褪黑素有益,主要是可改善昼夜睡眠比,减少夜间活动;而其他研究未能证实其客观效果[81]。因此,对痴呆的睡眠障碍,首选治疗方法是采用公认睡眠卫生方法的非药物管理[82]。

2016 年,Cochrane 关于痴呆患者睡眠障碍药物治疗的综述[83]发现,许多广泛地用于治疗痴呆患者睡眠问题的药物(包括苯二氮䓬类和非苯二氮䓬类催眠药)并无随机对照试验,尽管这些常用治疗方法的利弊权衡存在相当的不确定性。根据检索到的研究,尚无证据表明褪黑素(高达 10mg)有助于改善中重度 AD 痴呆患者的睡眠问题。有一些证据支持可使用低剂量曲唑酮(50mg),但是需进行更大规模的试验,以就其利弊平衡形成更明确的结论。尚无证据提示雷美替胺对轻、中度 AD 患者睡眠问题的疗效。该领域高度需要符合实际的试验,尤其是针对临床常用于治疗痴呆患者睡眠问题的药物。

> 建议:支持使用褪黑素的证据有限,但使用安全,可在某些看来有益的病例中使用。睡眠障碍应首选非药物治疗。

镇静性抗组胺药(如异丙嗪)

异丙嗪因其镇静作用而常用于 BPSD。它具有很强的抗胆碱作用,容易穿透血-脑屏障,因此,有可能引起显著的认知损害[84]。

> 建议:异丙嗪也许仅限于短期使用,但证据极少。

其他药物

汇总分析提示,银杏叶 240mg/d 可有效地治疗阿尔茨海默病、血管性或混合性痴呆伴 BPSD 的门诊患者[85]。

新型抗精神病药治疗 BPSD 仍处于研究阶段,包括依匹哌唑、卢美哌隆(5-HT$_{2A}$ 受体的强效拮抗剂和 5-HT 再摄取抑制剂)和匹莫范色林(5-HT$_{2A}$ 受体的反向激动剂和拮抗剂)。目前,正在研究的其他治疗 BPSD 的药物包括右美沙芬/奎尼丁、安非他酮/右美沙芬和哌甲酯[86]。

最近一项纳入 39 例受试者的随机安慰剂对照交叉试验发现,大麻隆(一种合成大麻素)显著改善了 AD 患者的激越和攻击行为。大麻隆耐受性好,尽管镇静是比较常见的不良反应,但在治疗组之间无显著性差异[87]。在治疗 AD 导致的激越和攻击症状方面,大麻隆似乎是有前景的治疗性大麻类药物[86]。

电休克治疗(ECT)

ECT 可能通过增强 GABA、谷氨酸、多巴胺和去甲肾上腺素等中枢神经递质传导来改善 BPSD。病例报告、病例系列报告、病历回顾、回顾性病例对照研究和一项开放性前瞻性研究表明,ECT 在减少痴呆患者激越行为方面较有前景。一项系统综述报道,这些研究纳入 122 例患者,其中 88% 的患者观察到显著进步,而且通常在治疗早期就观察到。此外,其不良反应常常很轻微、短暂或未被主动报告(尽管有些研究报道存在显著的认知不良反应)[88]。复发的患者经 ECT 维持治疗可获益。对其他治疗无效、存在药物耐受问题以及为保证患者安全和健康需快速缓解症状的重度痴呆患者,ECT 可能是治疗其激越和攻击症状的有前景的选择。但是,因研究具有局限性,需谨慎使用[88,89]。

总之,并不推荐 ECT 作为常用治疗方法,因为证据有限,将患者转运至 ECT 治疗室存在现实困难,而且也很难获得知情同意。

> 建议:尚无足够的证据推荐 ECT 用于治疗 BPSD。注意:可能导致严重的认知不良反应。

总结

指导这一领域治疗的现有证据不足,无法提出适当的管理和药物选择的建议。基本的方法是在使用精神药物之前首选非药物治疗和镇痛。无论选择哪种药物,都应注意以下方法:

- 排除可能诱发痴呆非认知症状的躯体疾病,如便秘、感染和疼痛
- 针对需要治疗的症状
- 考虑非药物治疗
- 在选择药物时,根据患者的需要进行风险-获益分析
- 在选择药物时,要做出基于证据的决定
- 讨论治疗方案,并向患者(如果有能力)和家属/照护者告知风险
- 从低剂量开始,保持最低剂量,持续最短的所需时间
- 定期回顾治疗是否恰当,以免不必要地继续使用无效药物
- 监测不良反应
- 清楚记录治疗的选择和与患者、家属或照护者的谈话

参考文献

1. National Institute for Health and Care Excellence. Dementia: assessment, management and support for people living with dementia and their carers [NG97]. 2018; https://www.nice.org.uk/guidance/ng97.

2. Steinberg M, et al. Point and 5-year period prevalence of neuropsychiatric symptoms in dementia: the Cache County Study. *Int J Geriatr Psychiatry* 2008; 23:170–177.

3. Salzman C, et al. Elderly patients with dementia-related symptoms of severe agitation and aggression: consensus statement on treatment

options, clinical trials methodology, and policy. *J Clin Psychiatry* 2008; **69**:889–898.

4. Department of Health. The use of antipsychotic medication for people with dementia: time for action. A report for the Minister of State for Care Services by Professor Sube Banerjee. 2009; https://www.rcpsych.ac.uk/pdf/Antipsychotic%20Bannerjee%20Report.pdf.

5. Livingston G, et al. A systematic review of the clinical effectiveness and cost-effectiveness of sensory, psychological and behavioural interventions for managing agitation in older adults with dementia. *Health Technol Assess* 2014; **18**:1–226, v–vi.

6. Kales HC, et al. Assessment and management of behavioral and psychological symptoms of dementia. *BMJ* 2015; **350**:h369.

7. James IA. *Understanding behaviour in dementia that challenges: a guide to assessment and treatment.* London, UK: Jessica Kingsley Publishers, 2011.

8. Brechin D, et al. British Psychological Society. Briefing paper. Alternatives to antipsychotic medication: psychological approaches in managing psychological and behavioural distress in people with dementia. 2013: http://www.bps.org.uk/system/files/Public%20files/antipsychotic.pdf.

9. Douglas S, et al. Non-pharmacological interventions in dementia. *Adv Psychiatr Treatment* 2004; **10**:171–177.

10. Ayalon L, et al. Effectiveness of nonpharmacological interventions for the management of neuropsychiatric symptoms in patients with dementia: a systematic review. *Arch Intern Med* 2006; **166**:2182–2188.

11. Livingston G, et al. Systematic review of psychological approaches to the management of neuropsychiatric symptoms of dementia. *Am J Psychiatry* 2005; **162**:1996–2021.

12. Abraha I, et al. Systematic review of systematic reviews of non-pharmacological interventions to treat behavioural disturbances in older patients with dementia. The SENATOR-OnTop Series. *BMJ Open* 2017; **7**:e012759.

13. Ballard CG, et al. Aromatherapy as a safe and effective treatment for the management of agitation in severe dementia: the results of a double-blind, placebo-controlled trial with Melissa. *J Clin Psychiatry* 2002; **63**:553–558.

14. Husebo BS, et al. Efficacy of treating pain to reduce behavioural disturbances in residents of nursing homes with dementia: cluster randomised clinical trial. *BMJ* 2011; **343**:d4065.

15. Brown R, et al. Opioids for agitation in dementia. *Cochrane Database Syst Rev* 2015:Cd009705.

16. Lee PE, et al. Atypical antipsychotic drugs in the treatment of behavioural and psychological symptoms of dementia: systematic review. *BMJ* 2004; **329**:75.

17. Jeste DV, et al. Atypical antipsychotics in elderly patients with dementia or schizophrenia: review of recent literature. *Harv Rev Psychiatry* 2005; **13**:340–351.

18. Jeste DV, et al. ACNP White Paper: update on use of antipsychotic drugs in elderly persons with dementia. *Neuropsychopharmacology* 2008; **33**:957–970.

19. Aupperle P. Management of aggression, agitation, and psychosis in dementia: focus on atypical antipsychotics. *Am J Alzheimers Dis Other Demen* 2006; **21**:101–108.

20. Yury CA, et al. Meta-analysis of the effectiveness of atypical antipsychotics for the treatment of behavioural problems in persons with dementia. *Psychother Psychosom* 2007; **76**:213–218.

21. Deberdt WG, et al. Comparison of olanzapine and risperidone in the treatment of psychosis and associated behavioral disturbances in patients with dementia. *Am J Geriatr Psychiatry* 2005; **13**:722–730.

22. Schneider LS, et al. Efficacy and adverse effects of atypical antipsychotics for dementia: meta-analysis of randomized, placebo-controlled trials. *Am J Geriatr Psychiatry* 2006; **14**:191–210.

23. Anon. How safe are antipsychotics in dementia? *Drug Ther Bull* 2007; **45**:81–86.

24. Rosack J. Side-effect risk often tempers antipsychotic use for dementia. *Psychiatr News* 2006; **41**:1–38.

25. Schneider LS, et al. Risk of death with atypical antipsychotic drug treatment for dementia: meta-analysis of randomized placebo-controlled trials. *JAMA* 2005; **294**:1934–1943.

26. Bessey LJ, et al. Management of behavioral and psychological symptoms of dementia. *Current Psychiatry Rep* 2019; **21**:66.

27. Ballard C, et al. Atypical antipsychotics for aggression and psychosis in Alzheimer's disease (review). *Cochrane Database Syst Rev* 2006; CD14003476.

28. Pharmacovigilance Working Party. Antipsychotics and cerebrovascular accident. SPC wording for antipsychotics. 2005.

29. Duff G. Atypical antipsychotic drugs and stroke – committee on safety of medicines. 2004; https://webarchive.nationalarchives.gov.uk/20141206131857/http://www.mhra.gov.uk/home/groups/pl-p/documents/websiteresources/con019488.pdf.

30. FDA. Information on conventional antipsychotics – FDA alert [6/16/2008]. 2008; http://www.fda.gov.

31. European Medicines Agency. CHMP assessment report on conventional antipsychotics. 2008; http://www.emea.europa.eu.

32. Wu CS, et al. Association of stroke with the receptor-binding profiles of antipsychotics-a case-crossover study. *Biol Psychiatry* 2013; **73**:414–421.

33. Kleijer BC, et al. Risk of cerebrovascular events in elderly users of antipsychotics. *J Psychopharmacol* 2009; **23**:909–14.

34. Ballard C, et al. The dementia antipsychotic withdrawal trial (DART-AD): long-term follow-up of a randomised placebo-controlled trial. *Lancet Neurol* 2009; **8**:151–157.

35. Huybrechts KF, et al. Differential risk of death in older residents in nursing homes prescribed specific antipsychotic drugs: population based cohort study. *BMJ* 2012; **344**:e977.

36. Kales HC, et al. Risk of mortality among individual antipsychotics in patients with dementia. *Am J Psychiatry* 2012; **169**:71–79.

37. Schmedt N, et al. Comparative risk of death in older adults treated with antipsychotics: a population-based cohort study. *Eur Neuropsychopharmacol* 2016; **26**:1390–1400.

38. Maust DT, et al. Antipsychotics, other psychotropics, and the risk of death in patients with dementia: number needed to harm. *JAMA Psychiatry* 2015; **72**:438–445.

39. Yunusa I, et al. Assessment of reported comparative effectiveness and safety of atypical antipsychotics in the treatment of behavioral and

psychological symptoms of dementia: a network meta-analysis. *JAMA Network Open* 2019; 2:e190828.

40. Smith DA, et al. Association between risperidone treatment and cerebrovascular adverse events: examining the evidence and postulating hypotheses for an underlying mechanism. *J Am Med Dir Assoc* 2004; 5:129–132.

41. Howard R, et al. Baseline characteristics and treatment-emergent risk factors associated with cerebrovascular event and death with risperidone in dementia patients. *Br J Psychiatry* 2016; 209:378–384.

42. McShane R, et al. Do neuroleptic drugs hasten cognitive decline in dementia? Prospective study with necropsy follow up. *BMJ* 1997; 314:266–270.

43. Ballard C, et al. Quetiapine and rivastigmine and cognitive decline in Alzheimer's disease: randomised double blind placebo controlled trial. *BMJ* 2005; 330:874.

44. Livingston G, et al. Antipsychotics and cognitive decline in Alzheimer's disease: the LASER-Alzheimer's disease longitudinal study. *J Neurol Neurosurg Psychiatry* 2007; 78:25–29.

45. Rainer M, et al. Quetiapine versus risperidone in elderly patients with behavioural and psychological symptoms of dementia: efficacy, safety and cognitive function. *Eur Psychiatry* 2007; 22:395–403.

46. Paleacu D, et al. Quetiapine treatment for behavioural and psychological symptoms of dementia in Alzheimer's disease patients: a 6-week, double-blind, placebo-controlled study. *Int J Geriatr Psychiatry* 2008; 23:393–400.

47. Corbett A, et al. Don't use antipsychotics routinely to treat agitation and aggression in people with dementia. *BMJ* 2014; 349:g6420.

48. Janssen-Cilag Ltd. Summary of product characteristics. Risperdal film-coated tablets, oral solution and powder and solvent for prolonged-release suspension for injection. 2018; https://www.medicines.org.uk/emc/product/6856/smpc.

49. BNF Online. British National Formulary. 2020; https://www.medicinescomplete.com/mc/bnf/current.

50. Katz IR, et al. Comparison of risperidone and placebo for psychosis and behavioral disturbances associated with dementia: a randomized, double-blind trial. Risperidone Study Group. *J Clin Psychiatry* 1999; 60:107–115.

51. NHS Health Research Authority. Optimisation of amisulpride prescribing in older people. 2012; https://www.hra.nhs.uk/planning-and-improving-research/application-summaries/research-summaries/optimisation-of-amisulpride-prescribing-in-older-people.

52. Reeves S, et al. A population approach to characterise amisulpride pharmacokinetics in older people and Alzheimer's disease. *Psychopharmacology* 2016; 233:3371–3381.

53. NHS PrescQIPP. Reducing antipsychotic prescribing in dementia toolkit. 2014; https://www.prescqipp.info/our-resources/bulletins/t7-reducing-antipsychotic-prescribing-in-dementia/#:~:text=The%20PrescQIPP%20reducing%20antipsychotic%20prescribing%20in%20dementia%20toolkit,prescribing%20in%20those%20already%20being%20prescribed%20these%20drugs.

54. Brodaty H, et al. Antipsychotic deprescription for older adults in long-term care: the HALT study. *J Am Med Dir Assoc* 2018; 19:592–600. e597.

55. Campbell N, et al. Impact of cholinesterase inhibitors on behavioral and psychological symptoms of Alzheimer's disease: a meta-analysis. *Clin Interv Aging* 2008; 3:719–728.

56. Mathys M. Pharmacologic management of behavioral and psychological symptoms of major neurocognitive disorder. *Ment Health Clin* 2018; 8:284–293.

57. Verdoux H, et al. Is benzodiazepine use a risk factor for cognitive decline and dementia? A literature review of epidemiological studies. *Psychol Med* 2005; 35:307–315.

58. Lagnaoui R, et al. Benzodiazepine utilization patterns in Alzheimer's disease patients. *Pharmacoepidemiol Drug Saf* 2003; 12:511–515.

59. Billioti de Gage S, et al. Benzodiazepine use and risk of dementia: prospective population based study. *BMJ* 2012; 345:e6231.

60. Taipale H, et al. Risk of pneumonia associated with incident benzodiazepine use among community-dwelling adults with Alzheimer disease. *CMAJ* 2017; 189:E519–e529.

61. Palmaro A, et al. Benzodiazepines and risk of death: results from two large cohort studies in France and UK. *Eur Neuropsychopharmacol* 2015; 25:1566–1577.

62. Chang CM, et al. Benzodiazepine and risk of hip fractures in older people: a nested case-control study in Taiwan. *Am J Geriatr Psychiatry* 2008; 16:686–692.

63. Aboukhatwa M, et al. Antidepressants are a rational complementary therapy for the treatment of Alzheimer's disease. *Mol Neurodegener* 2010; 5:10.

64. Rozzini L, et al. Efficacy of SSRIs on cognition of Alzheimer's disease patients treated with cholinesterase inhibitors. *Int Psychogeriatr* 2010; 22:114–119.

65. Porsteinsson AP, et al. Effect of citalopram on agitation in Alzheimer disease: the CitAD randomized clinical trial. *JAMA* 2014; 311:682–691.

66. Martinon-Torres G, et al. Trazodone for agitation in dementia. *Cochrane Database Syst Rev* 2004; CD004990.

67. Ballard C, et al. Management of neuropsychiatric symptoms in people with dementia. *CNS Drugs* 2010; 24:729–739.

68. Chow TW, et al. Potential cognitive enhancing and disease modification effects of SSRIs for Alzheimer's disease. *Neuropsychiatr Dis Treat* 2007; 3:627–636.

69. Enache D, et al. Antidepressants and mortality risk in a dementia cohort: data from SveDem, the Swedish Dementia Registry. *Acta Psychiatr Scand* 2016; 134:430–440.

70. Sommer OH, et al. Effect of oxcarbazepine in the treatment of agitation and aggression in severe dementia. *Dement Geriatr Cogn Disord* 2009; 27:155–163.

71. Tariot PN, et al. Efficacy and tolerability of carbamazepine for agitation and aggression in dementia. *Am J Psychiatry* 1998; 155:54–61.

72. Lonergan E, et al. Valproate preparations for agitation in dementia. *Cochrane Database Syst Rev* 2009; CD003945.

73. Konovalov S, et al. Anticonvulsants for the treatment of behavioral and psychological symptoms of dementia: a literature review. *Int*

Psychogeriatr 2008; 20:293–308.

74. Yeh YC, et al. Mood stabilizers for the treatment of behavioral and psychological symptoms of dementia: an update review. *Kaohsiung J Med Sci* 2012; 28:185–193.

75. Sival RC, et al. Sodium valproate in aggressive behaviour in dementia: a twelve-week open label follow-up study. *Int J Geriatr Psychiatry* 2004; 19:305–312.

76. Dolder CR, et al. Valproic acid in dementia: does an optimal dose exist? *J Pharm Pract* 2012; 25:142–150.

77. Lonergan E, et al. Valproate preparations for agitation in dementia. *Cochrane Database Syst Rev* 2009; CD003945.

78. Tariot PN, et al. Chronic divalproex sodium to attenuate agitation and clinical progression of Alzheimer disease. *Arch Gen Psychiatry* 2011; 68:853–861.

79. Supasitthumrong T, et al. Gabapentin and pregabalin to treat aggressivity in dementia: a systematic review and illustrative case report. *Br J Clin Pharmacol* 2019; 85:690–703.

80. Cooney C, et al. Use of low-dose gabapentin for aggressive behavior in vascular and Mixed Vascular/Alzheimer Dementia. *J Neuropsychiatry Clin Neurosci* 2013; 25:120–125.

81. Peter-Derex L, et al. Sleep and Alzheimer's disease. *Sleep Med Rev* 2015; 19:29–38.

82. David R, et al. Non-pharmacologic management of sleep disturbance in Alzheimer's disease. *J Nutr Health Aging* 2010; 14:203–206.

83. McCleery J, et al. Pharmacotherapies for sleep disturbances in dementia. *Cochrane Database Syst Rev* 2016; 11:Cd009178.

84. Bishara D, et al. Anticholinergic effect on cognition (AEC) of drugs commonly used in older people. *Int J Geriatr Psychiatry* 2017; 32:650–656.

85. von Gunten A, et al. Efficacy of Ginkgo biloba extract EGb 761(®) in dementia with behavioural and psychological symptoms: A systematic review. *World J Biol Psychiatry* 2016; 17:622–633.

86. Ahmed M, et al. Current agents in development for treating behavioral and psychological symptoms associated with dementia. *Drugs Aging* 2019; 36:589–605.

87. Herrmann N, et al. Randomized placebo-controlled trial of nabilone for agitation in Alzheimer's disease. *Am J Geriatr Psychiatry* 2019; 27:1161–1173.

88. Tampi RR, et al. The place for electroconvulsive therapy in the management of behavioral and psychological symptoms of dementia. *Neurodegener Dis Manag*, 2019. [Epub ahead of print].

89. Glass OM, et al. Electroconvulsive therapy (ECT) for treating agitation in dementia (major neurocognitive disorder) – a promising option. *Int Psychogeriatr* 2017; 29:717–726.

老年人常用精神药物用药剂量指南

药物	特定适应证(附加说明)	起始剂量	常用维持剂量	老年人的最大剂量
抗抑郁药				
阿戈美拉汀	抑郁障碍 监测肝功 数据显示患者>75岁时阿戈美拉汀无效	夜间 25mg	每天 25~50mg	夜间 50mg
西酞普兰	抑郁障碍/焦虑障碍	早晨 10mg	早晨 10~20mg	早晨 20mg
氯米帕明	抑郁障碍/恐怖和强迫状态	夜间 10mg(谨慎增加剂量)	约 10 天后达到每天 50~75mg[1]	每天 75mg[1]
去甲文拉法辛	在老年人中使用尚无正式推荐[2] 老年人清除能力下降,需减少剂量;对该药耐受性差的老年患者可考虑隔天给药 在确定老年人适当的剂量时,需注意文拉法辛的肾脏清除率可能下降 肾损害时的剂量: CrCl 50~80mL/min:无需调整剂量 CrCl 30~50min:建议每天最大剂量为 50mg CrCl <30min 或终末期肾病:建议每天和最大剂量均为 50mg 隔天 老年人出现具有临床意义的低钠血症的风险又可更高[2]			每天 400mg[2]
度洛西汀	抑郁障碍/焦虑障碍	每天 30mg*	每天 60mg	每天 120mg*[3] (注意:对老年人这一剂量的数据不多)
艾司西酞普兰	抑郁障碍/焦虑障碍	早晨 5mg	早晨 5~10mg	早晨 10mg
氟西汀	抑郁障碍/焦虑障碍 注意该药物半衰期长,而且是数种细胞色素 P450 酶抑制剂	早晨 20mg	早晨 20mg	通常早晨 40mg (但也可使用 60mg)

第 6 章

续表

药物	特定适应证/附加说明	起始剂量	常用维持剂量	老年人的最大剂量*
洛非帕明	抑郁障碍	夜间 35mg*	夜间 70mg*	140mg 夜间或分次用药*（偶尔需要夜间 210mg）
米氮平	抑郁障碍	夜间 7.5mg 或通常夜间 15mg*	夜间 15~30mg	夜间 45mg
舍曲林	抑郁障碍/焦虑障碍	早晨 25~50mg（1 周后早晨 25mg 可以增加到早晨 50mg）	早晨 50~100mg*	100mg（偶尔早晨增到 150mg）*
曲唑酮	抑郁障碍	每天 100mg, 分次服用或夜间单次服用	每天 100~200mg*	每天 300mg[4]
	痴呆伴发激越 避免单剂量>100mg	25mg, 每天 2 次*	每天 25~100mg*	每天 200mg*（分次用药）
文拉法辛	抑郁障碍/焦虑障碍 开始用药时要监测血压	早晨 37.5mg [1 周后增加至早晨 75mg（缓释剂）]*	早晨 75~150mg（缓释剂）*	每天 150mg（偶需每天 225mg）*
沃替西汀	抑郁障碍	每天 5~10mg[5]	每天 5~20mg[5]	每天 20mg[5] CYP2D6 代谢不良者的最大剂量为每天 10mg；需避免联合某些药物, 或可能需要调整剂量；审查药物相互作用

抗精神病药

药物	特定适应证/附加说明	起始剂量	常用维持剂量	老年人的最大剂量*
氨磺必利	慢性精神分裂症	每天 50mg*	每天 100~200mg*	每天 400mg[6]（注意每天>200mg）*
	晚发精神病	每天 25~50mg*	每天 50~100mg*（以 25mg 逐步增加）	每天 200mg[7]（注意每天>100mg）*
	痴呆伴发激越/精神病 警惕 Q-T 间期延长	夜间 25mg[8]	每天 25~50mg[8]	每天 50mg[8]

续表

药物	特定适应证/附加说明	起始剂量	常用维持剂量	老年人的最大剂量
阿立哌唑	精神分裂症，躁狂症（口服）	早晨 5mg*	每天 5~15mg*	早晨 20mg*
	控制激越（肌内注射）	5.25mg*	5.25~9.75mg*	每天 15mg*（口服＋肌内注射）
依匹哌唑	在老年人中剂量尚未确定[9]			
卡利拉嗪	在老年人中剂量尚未确定[10]			
氯氮平	精神分裂症	每天 6.25~12.5mg[11,12] 每周增加 1~2 次，增量不超过 6.25~12.5mg[11]	每天 50~100mg[11,12]	每天 100mg[11,12]
	帕金森病相关精神病	每天 6.25mg[13]	每天 25~37.5mg[13]	每天 50mg[13]
	肌内注射	氯氮平的口服生物利用度约为肌内注射的 1/2。例如，每天肌内注射的 50mg 大致相当于每天口服能片剂或口服溶液 100mg。每次注射后，在前 2h 内必须每 15min 观察 1 次，检查是否过度镇静 注意：如果需要肌内注射劳拉西泮，肌内注射劳拉西泮和肌内注射氯氮平之间至少间隔 1h		
伊潘立酮	在老年人中使用尚无正式推荐			
卢美哌隆[14]	精神分裂症	每天 42mg（相当于 60mg 卢美哌隆甲苯磺酸盐）无需剂量滴定	每天 42mg	每天 42mg
鲁拉西酮	精神分裂症	37mg，每天 1 次，合用中度 CYP3A4 抑制剂时每天 18.5mg（最大剂量 74mg，每天 1 次）肾功能正常的老年人（CrCl≥80mL/min）使用的剂量与肾功能正常的成年人相同。但是，由于老年人的肾功能可能减弱，需要根据他们的肾功能状况调整剂量[15]	每天 18.5~111mg[16]	老年人使用高剂量药物的数据有限，尚无老年人服用 148mg 的数据。治疗年龄>65 岁的患者时，应慎用高剂量

第 6 章

续表

药物	特定适应证/附加说明	起始剂量	常用维持剂量	老年人的最大剂量
奥氮平	精神分裂症	夜间 2.5mg*	每天 5~10mg*	夜间 15mg[12]
	痴呆伴发激越/精神病	夜间 2.5mg*	每天 2.5~10mg*	夜间 10mg*（最佳剂量为每天 5mg）[12]
匹莫范色林[17]	精神分裂症	每天 34mg（与强 CYP3A4 抑制剂合用时每天 10mg）不需要剂量滴定	每天 34mg（与强 CYP3A4 抑制剂合用时每天 10mg）	每天 34mg（与强 CYP3A4 抑制剂合用时每天 10mg）如果合用强 CYP3A4 诱导剂，需监测患者疗效是否减弱
喹硫平	精神分裂症	每天 12.5~25mg[12]	每天 75~125mg[11]	每天 200~300mg[12]
	痴呆伴发激越/精神病	每天 12.5~25mg*	每天 50~100mg*	每天 100~300mg[12]
利培酮	精神病	0.5mg，每天 2 次（一些病例 0.25~0.5mg，每天 2 次）[12]	每天 1~2.5mg[11]	每天 4mg
	晚发精神病	每天 0.5mg*	每天 1mg*	每天 2mg*（最佳剂量为每天 1mg）
	痴呆伴发激越/精神病	每天 0.25mg* 或每天 2 次	0.5mg，每天 2 次	每天 2mg（最佳剂量为每天 1mg）[12]
氟哌啶醇	精神病	每天 0.25~0.5mg[11]	每天 1~3.5mg[11]	注意 >3.5mg——评估耐受性和心电图 最多 5mg/d（口服）
	激越由于 Q-T 间期延长的风险，老年人避免应用（除了用于谵妄）	每天 0.25~0.5mg*	每天 0.5~1.5mg 或每天 2 次	最多 5mg/d（肌内注射）>5mg/d：只在患者能够耐受较高剂量，并且对患者的个人获益-风险情况重新评估后方可考虑使用

注：所有抗精神病药都有痴呆患者死亡增加的警告。

续表

药物	特定适应证/附加说明	起始剂量	常用维持剂量	老年人的最大剂量
长效第一代抗精神病药				
氟哌噻吨癸酸酯		试用剂量:5~10mg	试用剂量至少7天后:每2~4周10~20mg*根据疗效和耐受性,剂量逐渐增加,速度为每两周5~10mg*	每两周40mg*(如果发生锥体外系症状,延长间隔至3~4周)(如果可耐受,偶尔每两周使用50~60mg*)
氟奋乃静癸酸酯	注意:EPSE风险高	试用剂量6.25mg	试用剂量4~7天后:每2~4周12.5~25mg根据疗效和耐受性,剂量逐渐增加,速度为每2~4周12.5mg*	每4周50mg*
氟哌啶醇癸酸酯	EPSE和Q-T间期延长风险	(无试用剂量)每4周12.5~25mg	每4周12.5~25mg*	每4周50mg*
哌泊噻嗪棕榈酸酯[18]		试用剂量:5~10mg	每4周25~100mg	每4周100mg*
珠氯噻醇癸酸酯		试用剂量:25~50mg	试用剂量至少7天后:每2~4周50~200mg*	每2周200mg*
长效第二代抗精神病药				
阿立哌唑长效注射剂	在老年人中使用尚无正式推荐然而,年龄对药代动力学无明显影响[19]			
奥氮平棕榈酸酯[20]	尚未对老年患者(年龄>65岁)进行系统研究。不推荐用于老年人,除非明确口服奥氮平耐受良好,且已有效的剂量范围。较低的起始剂量(150mg/4周)并非非常规适应证,但是在临床需要时应该考虑用于65岁及以上患者。不推荐用于75岁以上患者			
帕利哌酮棕榈酸酯	根据肾功能选择剂量:因为老年患者肾功能可能会下降,即使化验检查显示肾脏功能正常,也应按轻度肾功能损害给药*	负荷剂量:第1天100mg第8天75mg(一些患者适合使用更低的负荷剂量*)	每月25~100mg*	每月100mg*

第6章

续表

第6章

药物	特定适应证/附加说明	起始剂量	常用维持剂量	老年人的最大剂量
帕利哌酮棕榈酸酯 每3个月1次注射液	根据肾功能选择剂量:因为老年患者肾功能可能会下降,即使化验检查显示肾脏功能正常,也应按轻度肾功能损害给药 *	如果最后1次帕利哌酮棕榈酸酯每月1次注射液剂量为: 50mg 75mg 100mg	按以下剂量开始每3个月1次注射治疗: 175mg 263mg 350mg (帕利哌酮棕榈酸酯每月1次注射25mg剂量没有等效剂量)[21]	每3个月350mg*
利培酮长效注射剂	监测肾功能	每两周25mg	每两周25mg	每2周25mg 若患者每天口服利培酮>4mg,考虑每2周37.5mg[22]

注:所有抗精神病药都含有痴呆患者死亡风险增加的警告。

药物	特定适应证/附加说明	起始剂量	常用维持剂量	老年人的最大剂量
心境稳定剂				
卡马西平	双相障碍 注意:药物相互作用 检查肝功能、全血细胞计数、尿素和电解质 考虑检测血浆药物浓度	50mg 或 100mg,每天2次*	每天200~400mg*	每天600~800mg*
拉莫三嗪	双相障碍(剂量滴定方法同年轻人) 检查药物相互作用(参见BNF)	每天25mg(单药治疗) 隔天25mg(若合用丙戊酸盐) 每天50mg(若合用卡马西平)	每14天增加25mg 每14天增加25mg 每14天增加50mg	每天200mg* 每天100mg* 100mg,每天2次 *
碳酸锂 M/R	双相障碍 躁狂/抑郁 注意:药物相互作用 检查肾和甲状腺功能,定期监测血锂浓度	夜间100*~200mg	每天200~600mg*	每天600~1200mg(目标是使老年人血锂水平达到0.4~0.7mmol/L)[23]

续表

药物	特定适应证/附加说明	起始剂量	常用维持剂量	老年人的最大剂量
丙戊酸盐	双相障碍	丙戊酸盐:100~200mg,每天2次* 丙戊酸半钠:250mg,每天1次或每天2次*	丙戊酸盐:200~400mg,每天 丙戊酸半钠:每天500~1 000g*	丙戊酸盐:400mg,每天2次* 丙戊酸半钠:每天1 000mg*
	检查肝功,并考虑检查血浆药物浓度			
	痴呆伴发激越(未批准,也不推荐) 检查疗效、耐受性和血浆药物浓度用以指导用药	丙戊酸盐:50mg(液体)每天2次或100mg,每天2次*	丙戊酸盐:100~200mg,每天2次*	丙戊酸盐:200mg,每天2次*

抗焦虑药/催眠药

药物	特定适应证/附加说明	起始剂量	常用维持剂量	老年人的最大剂量
氯硝西泮	激越	每天0.5mg	每天1~2mg*	每天4mg*
地西泮	激越	1mg,每天3次	1mg,每天3次	每天7.5~15mg,分次服用(针对焦虑)
莱博雷生[24]	失眠	夜间5mg(每晚不超过1次,睡前服用)	夜间5~10mg	夜间10mg 老年人跌倒的风险高 年龄≥65岁患者慎用>5mg剂量
劳拉西泮	仅限必要时——避免经常使用,因为其半衰期短,有依赖风险	每天0.5mg	每天3.5~2mg*	每天2mg
褪黑素	失眠——短期使用(最长13周)	2mg(缓释剂)每天1次(睡前1~2h)		
普瑞巴林	广泛性焦虑障碍 根据肾功能调整剂量(见产品信息)[25]	通常25mg,每天2次 (每周增加25mg,每天2次) 最高至75mg,每天2次(如果健康和肾功能正常)	通常每天150mg* 最高至150mg,每天2次(如果健康和肾功能正常)	每天150~300mg*
唑吡坦	失眠(短期使用,最多4周)	夜间5mg	夜间5mg	夜间5mg
佐匹克隆	失眠(短期使用,最多4周)	夜间3.75mg	夜间3.75~7.5mg	夜间7.5mg

* 文献中没有关于老年患者的药物剂量信息,所述剂量仅供参考。没有数据的药物,最大剂量是保守估计的,如果该药物耐受性良好,同时参照临床医师的评估,或许可超过该量。

第6章

参考文献

1. Mylan. Summary of product characteristics. Clomipramine 25 mg Capsules, Hard. 2017; https://www.medicines.org.uk/emc/medicine/33260

2. Prescribers' Digital Reference. Desvenlafaxine – drug summary. 2017 (Last accessed September 2020); http://www.pdr.net/drug-summary/Khedezla-desvenlafaxine-3333.8274.

3. Eli Lilly and Company Limited. Summary of product characteristics. Cymbalta 30mg hard gastro-resistant capsules, Cymbalta 60mg hard gastro-resistant capsules. 2020; https://www.medicines.org.uk/emc/medicine/15694.

4. Zentiva. Summary of product characteristics. Molipaxin 100mg/Trazodone 100mg Capsules. 2020; https://www.medicines.org.uk/emc/medicine/26734.

5. Prescribers' Digital Reference. Trintellix (vortioxetine) – drug information. 2017 (Last accessed September 2020); http://www.pdr.net/drug-information/trintellix?druglabelid=3348

6. Muller MJ, et al. Amisulpride doses and plasma levels in different age groups of patients with schizophrenia or schizoaffective disorder. *J Psychopharmacol* 2009; 23:278–286.

7. Psarros C, et al. Amisulpride for the treatment of very-late-onset schizophrenia-like psychosis. *Int J Geriatr Psychiatry* 2009; 24:518–522.

8. Clark-Papasavas C, et al. Towards a therapeutic window of D2/3 occupancy for treatment of psychosis in Alzheimer's disease, with [F]fallypride positron emission tomography. *Int J Geriatr Psychiatry* 2014; 29:1001–1009.

9. Prescribers' digital reference. Brexpiprazole – Drug Summary. 2017 (Last accessed September 2020); http://www.pdr.net/drug-summary/Rexulti-brexpiprazole-3759

10. Prescribers' Digital Reference. Vraylar (cariprazine) – drug information. 2017 (Last accessed September 2020); http://www.pdr.net/drug-information/vraylar?druglabelid=3792.

11. Jeste DV, et al. Conventional vs. newer antipsychotics in elderly patients. *Am J Geriatr Psychiatry* 1999; 7:70–76.

12. Karim S, et al. Treatment of psychosis in elderly people. *Adv Psychiatr Treatment* 2005; 11:286–296.

13. Group TPS. Low-dose clozapine for the treatment of drug-induced psychosis in Parkinson's disease. *N Engl J Med* 1999; 340: 757–763.

14. Intra-Cellular Therapies Inc. Highlights of prescribing information. Caplyta (lumateperone) capsules for oral use. 2019; https://www.accessdata.fda.gov/drugsatfda_docs/label/2019/209500s000lbl.pdf.

15. Sunovion Pharmaceuticals Europe Ltd. Summary of product characteristics. Latuda 18.5mg, 37mg and 74mg film-coated tablets. 2020; https://www.medicines.org.uk/emc/medicine/29125.

16. Sajatovic M, et al. Efficacy and tolerability of lurasidone in older adults with bipolar depression: analysis of two 6-week double-blind, placebo-controlled studies. *Eur Psychiatry* 2015; 30:1136.

17. ACADIA Pharmaceuticals Inc. Highlights of prescribing information. Nuplazid (pimavanserin) tablets for oral use. 2016; https://www.accessdata.fda.gov/drugsatfda_docs/label/2016/207318lbl.pdf.

18. Drugs.com. Piportil depot 50 mg/ml solution for injection. 2020 (Last accessed September 2020); https://www.drugs.com/uk/piportil-depot-50-mg-ml-solution-for-injection-leaflet.html#.

19. Otsuka Pharmaceutical (UK) Ltd. Summary of product characteristics. Abilify Maintena 300mg & 400mg powder and solvent for prolonged-release suspension for injection and suspension for injection in pre filled syringe. 2020; https://www.medicines.org.uk/emc/medicine/31386.

20. Eli Lily and Company Limited. Summary of product characteristics. Zypadhera 210mg powder and solvent for prolonged release suspension for injection. 2020; https://www.medicines.org.uk/emc/product/6429/smpc.

21. Janssen-Cilag Limited. Summary of product characteristics. TREVICTA 175mg, 263mg, 350mg, 525mg prolonged release suspension for injection. 2019; https://www.medicines.org.uk/emc/medicine/32050.

22. Janssen-Cilag Limited. Summary of product characteristics. RISPERDAL CONSTA 25 mg powder and solvent for prolonged-release suspension for intramuscular injection. 2018; https://www.medicines.org.uk/emc/medicine/9939.

23. Essential Pharma Ltd. Summary of product characteristics. Camcolit 400mg controlled release Lithium Carbonate. 2020; https://www.medicines.org.uk/emc/product/10829/smpc.

24. Eisai Inc. Highlights of prescribing information. DAYVIGO (lemborexant) tablets for oral use [controlled substance schedule pending]. 2019; https://www.accessdata.fda.gov/drugsatfda_docs/label/2019/212028s000lbl.pdf#page=21.

25. Upjohn UK Limited. Summary of product characteristics. Lyrica Capsules. 2020; https://www.medicines.org.uk/emc/medicine/14651.

第 6 章

在食物和饮料中隐蔽用药

本节只涉及在英国法律范围内的隐蔽用药规定。

在精神健康方面,患者经常拒绝服药;一些认知障碍的患者不理解药物是否对自己有益,因而不能做出选择。这时,临床团队可能会考虑在食物或饮料中隐藏药物是否最符合患者利益。这种做法被称为隐蔽用药。为避免患者通过这种方式被非法且不适当地用药,皇家药学会、皇家护理学会[1]和皇家精神医学会[2]出版了指南。在英国,此类干预的法律依据是《英国心智能力法》(*Mental Capacity Act*, MCA)[3],或更少使用的《英国精神卫生法》(*Mental Health Act*, MHA)[4]。

精神行为能力评估[3,5,6]

当遇到隐蔽用药的情况,评估治疗有关的行为能力主要是处方者(通常是为患者进行治疗的临床医师)的事,其次是药剂师或护士处方者[3,5]。不开处方的护士和其他卫生专业人员也需注意职业行为守则,并应确信医师的评估是合理的。评估行为能力时,需针对所提议的特定的治疗方法进行评估。行为能力会随时间而变,因此需要在提议某种治疗时进行评估。还要在病历和治疗照护计划中记录评估结果。

通常推定患者有能力做出治疗决策,除非被认为患有某种形式的精神疾病或紊乱,并且不能做下列一项或多项:

- 理解与决策相关的信息
- 持续记得决策相关信息
- 在做决定的过程中使用或权衡这些信息
- 传达自己决策(通过交谈、手语或其他方式)

隐蔽用药指南

如果患者有行为能力,明确拒绝用药,而且依据《英国精神卫生法》不属于强制入院者,则应尊重他们的拒绝。

如果患者有行为能力,明确拒绝用药,并且依据《英国精神卫生法》正在接受治疗或可以合法入院,则适用于《英国精神卫生法》中关于治疗的规定(不在本章的范围内)。

对缺乏知情同意行为能力以及无法知道自己正在服药的患者(如昏迷患者),不应隐蔽用药。然而,如果没有被欺瞒,一些缺乏知情同意行为能力的患者会意识到自己正在接受药物治疗[7]。例如,中度痴呆的患者,缺乏自知力,认为自己不需要吃药,但是如果在其不知道的情况下,将液体药物混入茶中,患者会自己喝下。本指南的其余部分适用于这一群体。

如果治疗符合患者的最佳利益(《英国心智能力法》第5节[3]),并与要避免的危害成比例(《英国心智能力法》实践守则第6.41章[6]),则可以对缺乏能力的患者进行治疗。因此,需要对患者隐蔽用药的获益有一个明确的预期,从而避免患者或其他人遭受重大伤害(无论是精神还是身体)。治疗必须是为了满足挽救患者的生命、防止健康恶化或确保改善身心健康的需求[3,6]。

隐蔽用药必须是尝试过所有其他方法之后做出的限制性最小的选择。应对患者进行功能评估,了解其拒绝服药的原因。考虑替代的用药方法(如液体制剂)和不同照护方法(如在让患者服药时花一些时间解释服用的药物,或改在一天中患者更清醒或痛苦更少的时候服药)[8]。

是否隐蔽用药的决定不是个人决定,而是应该与照料患者的多学科团队以及患者的亲属或非正式照护者共同讨论后决定。好的做法是召开一场"最佳获益会议"进行讨论。如果会议上确定隐蔽用药,等同于剥夺自由(此前未剥夺),那就应该申请剥夺自由保障授权。在患者病历中要详细记录有关隐蔽用药的决定,明确的管理计划,包括如何审查隐蔽用药计划的细节。该文件必须容易获取查看,并应对该决定定期审查。

并不需要每次有药物变化时都召开新的最佳获益会议。然而,首次考虑隐蔽用药时,医疗卫生专业人员应考虑未来可能会出现哪些类型的药物变化,并就哪些变化可能需要召开新的最佳获益会议达成一致意见。该管理方案也应记录在患者的病历中。如果想象到重大变化有可能造成不利影响,则应在做出这些改变之前举行新的最佳获益会议。

关于决定行为能力重复评估的频率,临床医师应遵循《英国心智能力法》实践指南中的指导意见[5]。如果有任何证据表明患者已重新拥有行为能力,则必须立即进行行为能力评估。此时不能再做符合患者最大利益的决定,剥夺自由保障授权将不再有效,并必须立即停止隐蔽用药。

最近的判例法[9,10]规定了隐蔽用药与需要获得剥夺自由保障授权之间的关系。患者在持续的监护和控制下,且不能自由离开时,被剥夺了自由。只有在药物影响到患者的行为、精神健康,或其镇静作用很强以至于患者会失去自由的情况下,隐蔽用药的做法本身才会导致自由剥夺。治疗计划中的隐蔽用药必须在对剥夺自由保障进行评估和授权中明确识别。

考虑隐蔽使用精神药物时[11]:

1. 如果患者符合《英国精神卫生法》标准,则其使用必须优先于《英国心智能力法》。

2. 对于不适用《英国精神卫生法》的患者,如果必须使用精神药物以防止患者的精神健康恶化或确保其得到改善,而且接受药物治疗也符合患者的最佳利益,则可以将《英国心智能力法》作为隐蔽用药的权威指导。应遵循隐蔽用药的常规流程,包括行为能力评估文件、最佳利益会议和药剂师审查。

3. 需要慎用可能导致镇静或患者身体活动能力下降的药物(见前面的段落),因为这类药物可能会构成自由剥夺,要求患者处于剥夺自由保障框架中。关于建议隐蔽使用的精神药物是否构成自由剥夺的文件记录很重要。注意:如发现患者缺乏同意入院的行为能力,且不符合《英国精神卫生法》强制入院的标准,则应申请剥夺自由保障授权。因此,大多数缺乏同意药物治疗行为能力的住院患者已经在《英国精神卫生法》或剥夺自由保障管辖框架中,尽管也许一些人有能力同意住院但是不同意药物治疗。

过程总结

决定是否隐蔽用药的流程见图 6.2。隐蔽给药过程应包括以下内容:

- 确保在考虑隐蔽用药之前,已尽各种努力以常规方式公开用药。
- 评估患者有无决定接受药物治疗的能力。如果有,则应尊重他们的意愿,不应隐蔽用药。
- 临床记录中必须对患者行为能力检查做好记录,也要把能力丧失的证据做好记录。
- 如果患者缺乏行为能力,应召开一个最佳利益会议,由相关的卫生专业人员和一个可以表

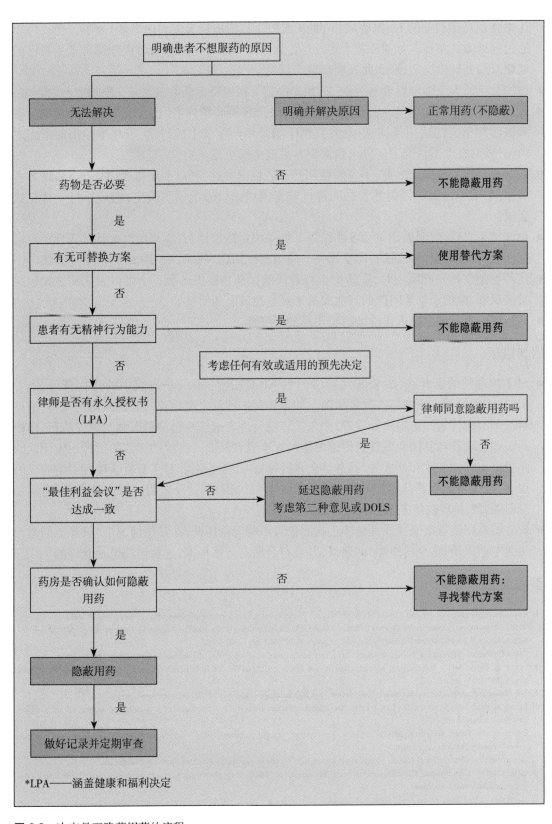

图 6.2　决定是否隐蔽用药的流程

达患者观点和利益的人(家庭成员、朋友或独立的精神行为能力倡导者)参加。会议可以通过网络方式举行。如果根据《英国心智能力法》,患者指定了一名代理律师来为自己的健康或福利做出决定,那么此人应出席会议。

- 参加会议的人应确定患者是否做过《预先决定》,拒绝特定药物或治疗,据此指导决策。
- 最佳利益会议应考虑是否符合正式法律程序,如《英国精神卫生法》或剥夺自由保障。有关该法律条文的适用指征,以及将其用于隐蔽用药背景中的讨论,不在本指南的范围之内,必要时在个别情况下应寻求精神科专家或法律意见。
- 在召开最佳利益会议之前,不应隐蔽用药。若情况紧急,可以在照料者/护理人员、处方者和家属/精神行为能力倡导者之间进行非正式讨论以做出紧急决定,但应尽快安排正式会议。
- 会议结束之后,应明确记录会议的结果。如果决定隐蔽用药,应与药房确认其药性是否可能因压碎或混入食物或饮料而受影响。应该修改用药表说明该药物的具体给药方法。
- 当药物随食物一同服用时,发药护士有责任确保药物被患者服下。可以采用的方式包括直接观察,或指定临床团队的其他成员来观察患者服药情况。
- 应制订一个方案定期审查继续隐蔽用药的必要性。

附加信息

- 对于护理院的患者,应参考 2014 年 3 月的 NICE 指南——《护理院中的药物管理》[12,13]。NICE 指南的基本原则与本政策相同。如果怀疑护理院未遵循正确的隐蔽用药流程,精神科医师有责任告知护理院管理者;如果护理院管理者未按照精神科医师的建议执行,精神科医师有责任与其团队负责人讨论可能的安全监管转介。支持护理院的精神卫生团队的角色是支持护理院和处方者(通常是全科医师)执行本指南。对于有复杂精神卫生需求的患者,他们可能也适合参加或参与最佳利益会议。但是,这个过程应该由处方者(通常是全科医师)、护理院员工和护理院药剂师来管理。
- 没有特殊限制规定亲属或其他非正式照护者不能隐蔽用药,在某些情况下,只要他们遵照卫生专业人员(如全科医师)的建议,并且符合所有政策标准,这种做法也是允许的。

参考文献

1. Royal Pharmaceutical Society and Royal College of Nursing. Professional guidance on the administration of medicines in healthcare settings. 2019; https://www.rpharms.com/Portals/0/RPS%20document%20library/Open%20access/Professional%20standards/SSHM%20and%20Admin/Admin%20of%20Meds%20prof%20guidance.pdf?ver=2019-01-23-145026-567.
2. Royal College of Psychiatrists. College statement on covert administration of medicines. *Psychiatric Bulletin* 2004; 28:385–386.
3. Office of Public Sector Information. Mental capacity act 2005 – Chapter 9. 2005; http://www.legislation.gov.uk/ukpga/2005/9/pdfs/ukpga_20050009_en.pdf.
4. The National Archives. Mental health act 2007; http://www.legislation.gov.uk/ukpga/2007/12/contents.
5. British Medical Association and the Law Society. *Assessment of mental capacity. a practical guide for doctors and lawyer*, 4th ed. London: Law Society Publishing, 2015.
6. Office of the Public Guardian. Mental capacity act code of practice (updated 2016). https://www.gov.uk/government/publications/mental-capacity-act-code-of-practice.
7. Department for Constitutional Affairs. Mental capacity act 2005 – code of practice. 2005; http://www.justice.gov.uk.
8. Care Quality Commission. Covert administration of medicines. 2020; https://www.cqc.org.uk/guidance-providers/adult-social-care/covert-administration-medicines.
9. Hempsons. Newsflash: covert medication and DOLS – new court guidance. 2016; http://www.hempsons.co.uk/news/newsflash-covert-medication-dols-new-court-guidance.
10. The Prescription Training Company Ltd. Covert administration of medicines. Recent court of protection ruling on covert medication – 6th

July 2016. https://medicationtraining.co.uk/covert-administration-medicines.

11. Care Quality Commission. Brief guide: covert medication in mental health services. 2016; https://www.cqc.org.uk/sites/default/files/20161122_briefguide-covert_medication.pdf.

12. National Institute for Health and Care Excellence. Managing medicines in care homes. Social Care Guideline [SC1] 2014 (updated 2020); https://www.nice.org.uk/guidance/sc1.

13. PrescQIPP. Bulletin 101 – Best practice guidance in covert administration of medication. 2015; https://www.prescqipp.info/umbraco/surface/authorisedmediasurface/index?url=%2fmedia%2f1174%2fb101-covert-administration-21.pdf.

扩展阅读

Quality Care Commission. Covert administration of medicines 2020; https://www.cqc.org.uk/guidance-providers/adult-social-care/covert-administration-medicines

Kelly Fatemi. Covert administration of medicines in care homes The Pharmaceutical Journal 2016. https://www.pharmaceutical-journal.com/cpd-and-learning/learning-article/covert-administration-of-medicines-in-care-homes/20201536.fullarticle?firstPass=false

National Institute for Health and Care Excellence. Medicines Management in care Homes. NICE Quality Standard 2015; https://www.nice.org.uk/guidance/qs85/resources/medicines-management-in-care-homes-pdf-2098910254021

适合于苏格兰的材料

Mental Welfare Commission for Scotland. Good Practice Guide: Covert administration 2013 (reviewed 2017); https://www.mwcscot.org.uk/sites/default/files/2019-06/covert_medication.pdf

第 6 章

老年抑郁症的治疗

　　年龄越大,躯体疾病越多。许多躯体疾病,如心血管病、慢性疼痛、糖尿病和帕金森病都与抑郁症的高风险有关[1,2]。老年人身体虚弱,自我忽视(如危及生命的脱水或体温过低)和行动不便(如静脉瘀血)容易导致严重后果,因此老年人与抑郁症相关的患病率和死亡率增加[3]。几乎 20% 的自杀发生在老年人中[4]。而有效治疗抑郁症可降低死亡率[5]。

　　抗抑郁药与安慰剂对照研究的荟萃分析发现,老年患者的有效率为 51%[6],与成年人群相似(表 6.8)[7]。也许因为老年人的大脑结构变化或躯体并发症发生率更高[9],人们普遍认为老年患者对抗抑郁药的反应不如年轻患者[8]。但生理年龄可能比实际年龄更有相关性[10];躯体疾病、基线焦虑和执行功能下降与治疗结局较差有关[11]。

　　尽管如此,即使在老年人中,仍有可能在治疗 4 周就发现治疗无效者[12,13]。

　　一项 Cochrane 综述考察了不同类型抗抑郁药在老年人中的疗效和相关撤药率,发现 SSRI 和 TCA 具有相同的疗效;TCA 与较高的撤药率有关[14]。NICE 成人抑郁症指南推荐首选 SSRI(舍曲林是老年人常用的一线药物)。换药时,首选不同的 SSRI 或耐受性更好的新一代抗抑郁药(通常是米氮平),次选耐受性较差但药理机制不同的抗抑郁药,例如文拉法辛、TCA 或单胺氧化酶抑制剂(MAOI)[15](注意,由于相关的不良反应和药物相互作用,在老年人中应谨慎使用 TCA 和 MAOI)。

　　网络荟萃分析表明,喹硫平、度洛西汀、阿戈美拉汀、丙米嗪和伏硫西汀治疗老年抑郁障碍的疗效更好[16],但是个别数据不一致。两项研究发现,抑郁发作痊愈并且已经接受 2 年抗抑郁药治疗的老年患者,如果停用抗抑郁药,60% 的人在 2 年内复发[17,18]。首发患者也是如此。低剂量抗抑郁药可以有效地预防复发。已经证明多塞平 75mg/d 即可预防复发[19]。值得注意的是,多塞平过量时对心脏毒性特别大,NICE 不建议使用[15]。

　　老年患者并无理想的抗抑郁药,所有药物都一些问题。TCA 由于增加心脏传导异常和抗胆碱能作用,被普遍认为不太合适。SSRI 的耐受性通常比 TCA 好[14],但这类药物增加胃肠道出血的风险,尤其高龄老年人、有出血史、使用 NSAID、类固醇或华法林治疗的人;其他类型出血的风险,如出血性卒中也可能增加[27,28](见 SSRI 和出血部分)。另外,老年人使用 SSRI 也特别容易发生低钠血症[29](见第 3 章"低钠血症"部分)、直立性低血压和跌倒(这些临床后果可因 SSRI 诱导的骨质减少而增加[30],TCA 也可能增加骨折风险[31])。

　　阿戈美拉汀对老年患者有效,耐受性好,与低钠血症无关[32,33],但需要频繁采血检查肝功能限制了它的使用。沃替西汀和度洛西汀也有效,并在老年人中耐受性良好[34],但存在与 SSRI 一样的不良反应。一项全科数据库研究发现,与 SSRI 相比,"其他抗抑郁药"(文拉法辛、米氮平等)增加了老年人出现潜在严重不良反应(卒中/短暂性脑缺血发作、骨折、癫痫、自杀未遂/自伤)的风险,并增加了全因死亡率[29];但由于是观察性研究,无法区分抗抑郁药的疗效和患者固有风险的增加。与安慰剂相比,多饱和脂肪酸(鱼油)可能对轻、中度抑郁有益[35]。

　　抗抑郁药对晚年认知能力的影响仍有争议,一些研究发现抗抑郁药会恶化认知结局[22,36,37],另一些则发现没有影响[38]。抗抑郁药的选择可影响认知损害的风险,而高抗胆碱能药物已被证明会增加患痴呆的可能性[39]。

　　最后,根据患者的个体情况选择药物,特别是躯体共病和合并用药(包括处方和非处方药)(见抗抑郁药与躯体疾病药物的相互作用部分)。

表 6.8　抗抑郁药与老年人

	抗胆碱能不良反应 (尿潴留、口干、视物模糊、便秘)	直立性低血压	镇静	体重增加	过量的安全性	其他不良反应	药物相互作用
三环类抗抑郁药[20]	不定：去甲阿米替林、丙米嗪、多塞平为中度 其他药物明显 所有药物都能引起中枢抗胆碱能作用(意识模糊)	都可能导致直立性低血压 需要滴定剂量	不定：从丙米嗪的镇静作用很小到三甲丙米嗪的镇静作用很明显	所有三环类抑郁药都可增加体重	多塞平和阿米替林毒性最大(癫痫发作和心律失常等)	癫痫发作、抗胆碱能诱发的认知障碍 5-羟色胺能药物会增加出血风险	主要是药效学方面：与苯二氮䓬类合用增加镇静作用，与利尿剂合用增加低血压，与其他抗胆碱能药物合用增加便秘等
洛非帕明	中度，但便秘、出汗可能较重	可能，但比三环类药物耐受性好	极少	数据不多，缺乏自发报告，可能提示比三环类药物少	相对安全	肝功能升高 与其他 TCA 和 SSRI 相比，低钠血症的可能性小	
SSRI[20,21]	帕罗西汀会引起口干	少得多，但 SSRI 会增加跌倒的风险	帕罗西汀和氟伏沙明可能会导致镇静 其他 SSRI 不大可能出现	帕罗西汀和西酞普兰可能会导致药物体重增加 其他药物体重无显著变化	安全，但西酞普兰除外；一种不太起效的代谢物可引起 Q-T 间期延长。其他药物临床意义又不明确	老年人中出现胃肠道反应、头痛、低钠血症、出血风险增加(如果同时服用阿司匹林和非甾体抗炎药，则需增加胃保护剂)，帕罗西汀出现口面部运动障碍[22]、间质性肺病[23,24]	氟伏沙明、氟西汀和帕罗西汀是数种肝细胞色素酶的强抑制剂(见抗抑郁药相互作用部分) 含曲林较安全，西酞普兰、艾司西酞普兰和伏硫西汀最安全

续表

	抗胆碱能不良反应（尿潴留、口干、视物模糊、便秘）	直立性低血压	镇静	体重增加	过量的安全性	其他不良反应	药物相互作用
其他 [25,26]	米氮平和文拉法辛*极少 瑞波西汀*很少 度洛西汀*较少 阿戈美拉汀*很少	文拉法辛、度洛西汀低剂量时可导致低血压，但高剂量时可增加血压 阿戈美拉汀常见头晕	米氮平、米安色林和曲唑酮有镇静作用 文拉法辛、度洛西汀镇静作用不明显 阿戈美拉汀有助于睡眠	米氮平常见，尽管老年人未必不太容易增加体重 阿戈美拉汀很少见	文拉法辛的毒性比SSRI大，但比TCA安全 其他相对安全	瑞波西汀导致失眠和低钾血症 文拉法辛、度洛西汀引起恶心 度洛西汀引起体重下降和恶心 阿戈美拉汀可能有肝毒性，需监测肝功能 曲唑酮引起认知障碍 [22] 5-羟色胺和去甲肾上腺素再摄取抑制剂引起间质性肺病 [24]	度洛西汀抑制 CYP2D6；吗氯贝胺和文拉法辛抑制 CYP450 酶。审查可能的相互作用 瑞波西汀安全； 服用强效 CYP1A2 抑制剂的患者应避免服用阿戈美拉汀

*去甲肾上腺素能药物可能通过抑制去甲肾上腺素再摄取产生"抗胆碱能"效应。

（王华丽　译　田成华　审校）

参考文献

1. Katona C, et al. Impact of screening old people with physical illness for depression? *Lancet* 2000; **356**:91–92.
2. Lyketsos CG. Depression and diabetes: more on what the relationship might be. *Am J Psychiatry* 2010; **167**:496–497.
3. Gallo JJ, et al. Long term effect of depression care management on mortality in older adults: follow-up of cluster randomized clinical trial in primary care. *BMJ* 2013; **346**:f2570.
4. Cattell H, et al. One hundred cases of suicide in elderly people. *Br J Psychiatry* 1995; **166**:451–457.
5. Ryan J, et al. Late-life depression and mortality: influence of gender and antidepressant use. *Br J Psychiatry* 2008; **192**:12–18.
6. Gutsmiedl K, et al. How well do elderly patients with major depressive disorder respond to antidepressants: a systematic review and single-group meta-analysis. *BMC Psychiatry* 2020; **20**:102.
7. Cipriani A, et al. Comparative efficacy and acceptability of 21 antidepressant drugs for the acute treatment of adults with major depressive disorder: a systematic review and network meta-analysis. *Lancet* 2018; **391**:1357–1366.
8. Paykel ES, et al. Residual symptoms after partial remission: an important outcome in depression. *Psychol Med* 1995; **25**:1171–1180.
9. Iosifescu DV, et al. Brain white-matter hyperintensities and treatment outcome in major depressive disorder. *Br J Psychiatry* 2006; **188**:180–185.
10. Brown PJ, et al. Biological age, not chronological age, is associated with late-life depression. *J Gerontol A Biol Sci Med Sci* 2018; **73**:1370–1376.
11. Tunvirachaisakul C, et al. Predictors of treatment outcome in depression in later life: A systematic review and meta-analysis. *J Affect Disord* 2018; **227**:164–182.
12. Zilcha-Mano S, et al. Early symptom trajectories as predictors of treatment outcome for citalopram versus placebo. *Am J Geriatr Psychiatry* 2017; **25**:654–661.
13. Mulsant BH, et al. What is the optimal duration of a short-term antidepressant trial when treating geriatric depression? *J Clin Psychopharmacol* 2006; **26**:113–120.
14. Mottram P, et al. Antidepressants for depressed elderly. *Cochrane Database Syst Rev* 2006; CD003491.
15. National Institute for Health and Care Excellence. Depression in adults: recognition and management. Clinical guideline [CG90]. 2009 (Last updated December 2013); https://www.nice.org.uk/Guidance/cg90.
16. Krause M, et al. Efficacy and tolerability of pharmacological and non-pharmacological interventions in older patients with major depressive disorder: A systematic review, pairwise and network meta-analysis. *Eur Neuropsychopharmacol* 2019; **29**:1003–1022.
17. Flint AJ, et al. Recurrence of first-episode geriatric depression after discontinuation of maintenance antidepressants. *Am J Psychiatry* 1999; **156**:943–945.
18. Reynolds CF, III, et al. Maintenance treatment of major depression in old age. *N Engl J Med* 2006; **354**:1130–1138.
19. Old Age Depression Interest Group. How long should the elderly take antidepressants? A double-blind placebo-controlled study of continuation/prophylaxis therapy with dothiepin. *Br J Psychiatry* 1993; **162**:175–182.
20. Draper B, et al. Tolerability of selective serotonin reuptake inhibitors: issues relevant to the elderly. *Drugs Aging* 2008; **25**:501–519.
21. Bose A, et al. Escitalopram in the acute treatment of depressed patients aged 60 years or older. *Am J Geriatr Psychiatry* 2008; **16**:14–20.
22. Leng Y, et al. Antidepressant use and cognitive outcomes in very old women. *J Gerontol A Biol Sci Med Sci* 2018; **73**:1390–1395.
23. Deidda A, et al. Interstitial lung disease induced by fluoxetine: systematic review of literature and analysis of Vigiaccess, Eudravigilance and a national pharmacovigilance database. *Pharmacol Res* 2017; **120**:294–301.
24. Rosenberg T, et al. The relationship of SSRI and SNRI usage with interstitial lung disease and bronchiectasis in an elderly population: a case-control study. *Clin Interv Aging* 2017; **12**:1977–1984.
25. Raskin J, et al. Safety and tolerability of duloxetine at 60 mg once daily in elderly patients with major depressive disorder. *J Clin Psychopharmacol* 2008; **28**:32–38.
26. Johnson EM, et al. Cardiovascular changes associated with venlafaxine in the treatment of late-life depression. *Am J Geriatr Psychiatry* 2006; **14**:796–802.
27. Smoller JW, et al. Antidepressant use and risk of incident cardiovascular morbidity and mortality among postmenopausal women in the Women's Health Initiative study. *Arch Intern Med* 2009; **169**:2128–2139.
28. Laporte S, et al. Bleeding risk under selective serotonin reuptake inhibitor (SSRI) antidepressants: A meta-analysis of observational studies. *Pharmacol Res* 2017; **118**:19–32.
29. Coupland C, et al. Antidepressant use and risk of adverse outcomes in older people: population based cohort study. *BMJ* 2011; **343**:d4551.
30. Williams LJ, et al. Selective serotonin reuptake inhibitor use and bone mineral density in women with a history of depression. *Int Clin Psychopharmacol* 2008; **23**:84–87.
31. Power C, et al. Bones of contention: a comprehensive literature review of Non-SSRI antidepressant use and bone health. *J Geriatr Psychiatry Neurol* 2019; **33**:340–352.
32. Heun R, et al. The efficacy of agomelatine in elderly patients with recurrent Major Depressive Disorder: a placebo-controlled study. *J Clin Psychiatry* 2013; **74**:587–594.
33. Laux G. The antidepressant efficacy of agomelatine in daily practice: results of the non-interventional study VIVALDI. *Eur Psychiatry* 2011; **26 Suppl** 1:647.
34. Katona C, et al. A randomized, double-blind, placebo-controlled, duloxetine-referenced, fixed-dose study comparing the efficacy and safety of Lu AA21004 in elderly patients with major depressive disorder. *Int Clin Psychopharmacol* 2012; **27**:215–223.
35. Bae JH, et al. Systematic review and meta-analysis of omega-3-fatty acids in elderly patients with depression. *Nutr Res* 2018; **50**:1–9.

36. Moraros J, et al. The association of antidepressant drug usage with cognitive impairment or dementia, including Alzheimer disease: A systematic review and meta-analysis. *Depress Anxiety* 2017; **34**:217–226.

37. Chan JYC, et al. Depression and antidepressants as potential risk factors in dementia: a systematic review and meta-analysis of 18 longitudinal studies. *J Am Med Dir Assoc* 2019; **20**:279–286.e271.

38. Carriere I, et al. Antidepressant use and cognitive decline in community-dwelling elderly people – the three-city cohort. *BMC Med* 2017; **15**:81.

39. Wang YC, et al. Increased risk of dementia in patients with antidepressants: a meta-analysis of observational studies. *Behav Neurol* 2018; **2018**:5315098.

扩展阅读

Kok RM, et al. Management of depression in older adults: a review. *JAMA* 2017; **317**:2114–2122.

Pruckner N, et al. Antidepressant pharmacotherapy in old-age depression – a review and clinical approach. *Eur J Clin Pharmacol* 2017; **73**:661–667.

Wilkinson P, et al. Continuation and maintenance treatments for depression in older people. *Cochrane Database of Sys Rev* 2016; **9**:Cd006727.

妊娠哺乳期

妊娠期药物选择

妊娠就会有"正常"结果，这是永远无法保证的。在已确认的早期妊娠中，自发流产率达 10%~20%，而自发严重畸形的风险达 2%~3%（大约 40 次妊娠中有 1 个）[1]。

生活方式对妊娠有重要的影响。已证实，孕期吸烟、饮食不佳、饮酒，可给胎儿带来不良后果。妊娠前肥胖会增加神经管缺陷的风险（与体重指数在健康范围内的女性相比，肥胖女性似乎需要补充更大剂量的叶酸[2]。

另外，孕期精神疾病是导致先天畸形、死胎和新生儿死亡的独立危险因素[3]。围产期（又称围生期）精神疾病有可能给儿童带来各种不良结果，其中许多可延续到青少年后期[4]。心境障碍、焦虑障碍、进食障碍等精神障碍增加了早产的风险[5,6]。注意：早产儿患成年期抑郁症、双相障碍、精神分裂症谱系障碍的风险也会增加[7]。

在孕期使用精神药物的安全性无法得到明确证实，因为实施有说服力的前瞻性试验显然不符合伦理，而进行长期观察性研究无疑也困难重重。因此，在孕期决定个体化使用精神药物的依据来源于：①数据库研究。这种研究有许多局限性，例如：不能控制疾病、吸烟、肥胖、其他药物以及其他混杂因素的影响；多次统计学检验增加了 2 型错误的风险；根据药房数据确定用药情况可能并不准确。②畸胎信息中心有限的前瞻性数据。③已发表的个案报告，这种报告往往偏向于选择性报告不良后果。最糟糕的是可能根本没有人的研究数据，只有来自临床前期的动物研究数据。对新药不良后果的早期报道可能得不到重复验证，对停止或继续药物治疗的风险和收益必须做"最佳猜测"式评估。即使是已被证实的药物，有关长期结局的数据也很少。

还值得重视的是，妊娠不能防止精神疾病，甚至停药后还可能增加患病风险。无论是否用药，在妊娠后期和产后早期，病情复发风险都会增加。

患者对用药风险与获益的看法至关重要，需要从医师那里了解最新的证据。医师应该了解给严重精神疾病女患者处方药物的重要性。围产期自杀值得注意，因为它与缺乏积极治疗，特别是精神药物治疗有关[8]。

本节简要总结了相关问题和目前的证据。框 7.1 概括了孕期用药的一般原则。

框 7.1 孕期用药的一般原则

对所有育龄女性：

■ 常谈意外妊娠的可能；有 50% 的妊娠都不是计划好的[9]。

■ 避免孕期禁忌药物(尤其是丙戊酸盐和卡马西平)。如果使用了这些药物，即使是不打算妊娠的女性，也要完全了解它们的致畸性。考虑服用叶酸。丙戊酸盐只能用于绝经后女性。对于中青年女性，丙戊酸盐只能作为最后的治疗手段[10]。

对新诊断精神疾病的孕妇

■ 除非利大于弊，否则在妊娠头 3 个月要尽量避免所有药物(这一期间主要器官正在形成)。如果非药物治疗无效或不适合，使用已证实药物的最低有效剂量。

对服用精神药物并打算妊娠的女性

■ 若状态良好或复发风险低，应该考虑终止治疗。

■ 对于患严重精神疾病且复发风险高的女性，终止治疗是不明智的，应当考虑换用低风险药物。注意换药可能增加复发风险，要根据病史和既往疗效换药。

对服用精神药物并已经妊娠的女性

■ 患有严重精神疾病且复发风险高的女性，妊娠后突然终止治疗是不明智的。比起继续有效的药物治疗，复发最终对母亲和胎儿的危害更大。

■ 考虑继续目前的(有效的)药物，而不是换药，以减少复发风险和胎儿暴露的药物种类。

■ 应停用按心境稳定剂处方的丙戊酸盐。

如果患者吸烟(吸烟在患有精神疾病的孕妇中更为常见)[11]

■ 吸烟与不良妊娠结局的风险升高关系最大[12]。

■ 始终要鼓励其改用尼古丁替代疗法。吸烟有很多不良反应，而尼古丁替代疗法没有[13]。英国临床规范研究院(NICE)要求必须将这类患者转介到戒烟机构，鼓励其签约并尽可能给予支持。

■ 戒烟可升高某些药物的血浆水平，如氯氮平。

对所有孕妇

■ 保证父母尽可能地参与所有决策。

  ■ 使用最低有效剂量。

  ■ 使用已知对母亲和胎儿风险最低的药物。

■ 药物种类尽可能少，不管是同时使用，还是先后使用。

■ 随着妊娠进程和药物代谢改变，准备调整药物剂量。在妊娠后期，往往需要加大剂量，因为这时血容量增加了约 30%[14]。有条件可监测血药水平。注意：孕期转氨酶活性变化明显，妊娠末期 CYP2D6 活性几乎增加了 50%，CYP1A2 活性下降到 70%[15]。

■ 考虑转诊到围产期专科机构。

■ 保证充分的胎儿筛查。

■ 注意分娩时个别药物的潜在问题。

■ 告知产科团队患者精神药物的使用情况和可能的并发症。

■ 监测新生儿的撤药反应。

■ 记录所有的决定。

与孕妇的讨论应该包含的内容[16]

讨论应该包含以下内容：

- 该孕妇接受非药物干预的能力。这应该包括既往对非药物干预的反应。
- 未治疗的精神疾病对胎儿或婴儿的潜在影响。
- 突然停药带来的风险。
- 既往发作的严重程度、对治疗的反应以及该孕妇的偏好。
- 对于无精神障碍的孕妇，发生胎儿畸形的风险。
- 在孕期和产后，与药物治疗相关的伤害风险增加，包括药物过量的风险（并且承认风险有不确定性）。
- 证实妊娠后，停用已知有致畸风险的药物，有可能消除不了致畸的风险。
- 哺乳。

可能的话，提供书面材料解释上述风险（最好个体化）。绝对风险和相对风险都应该讨论到。描述风险时，应该用自然频数，而不是百分比（例如，10 个中有 1 个，而不是 10%），并用公分母（例如，1/100 和 25/100，而不是 1/100 和 1/4）。

孕期和产后精神病

- 妊娠不能避免病情复发。
- 孕期精神疾病对产后精神病有预测意义[17]。
- 在一般人群中，围产期精神病的发生率为 0.1%~0.25%（每 1 000 次分娩中，有 1~2 次孕妇需要在精神科住院）。
- 双相障碍女患者患产后精神病的风险增加，1/5 的患者在产后精神病复发[18]。
- 家族史或过去有产后精神病的女性复发率高[19]。
- 母亲在围产期的精神健康状况影响胎儿健康、产科结局和儿童发育。

精神病不予治疗的风险包括：

- 对母亲有害：因自理或判断能力变差、缺乏产科护理或伴有自杀等冲动。
- 对胎儿或新生儿有害（从忽视到杀婴）。

很久以前就已经确定，精神分裂症患者与一般人群相比，更可能会有轻微的身体异常。其中一些异常可能刚出生就显而易见，而其他异常可能比较轻微，甚至到生命的后期也可能不明显。这种背景风险使得评估抗精神病药的作用变得复杂。（孕期精神疾病本身对于先天畸形和围产期死亡是独立的危险因素。）

抗精神病药治疗

第一代抗精神病药

- 普遍被认为致畸风险很小[20,21]，但是正如预料的那样，数据不那么有说服力。
- 数据大多来源于用低剂量吩噻嗪类药物治疗妊娠剧吐（与先天畸形风险增加有关的一种疾病）的研究。其中一些研究发现风险只是轻度增加，而且先天畸形没有明确的聚集现象，这表明导致该风险升高的是被治疗的疾病本身,而不是药物治疗。

- 一项前瞻性研究纳入了 284 名孕期服用一种第一代抗精神病药(大多是氟哌啶醇、氯丙嗪和氟哌噻吨)的女性,得出的结论是:使用第一代抗精神病药比第二代抗精神病药(或未用抗精神病药)引起的早产和低出生体重更为常见[22]。在妊娠最后一周暴露于抗精神病药的新生儿中,20% 出现了早期嗜睡和紧张不安。
- 美国最近一项大样本研究纳入 100 余万名女性,其中 733 人使用过第一代抗精神病药,结果发现重大畸形或心脏畸形的风险并未出现有意义的升高[23]。
- 氟哌啶醇可能与肢体缺陷有关(根据少数病例);但即使是真的,这种风险也可能极低。
- 第一代抗精神病药已被报道会引起新生儿运动障碍[24]。
- 吩噻嗪类药物已被报道会引起新生儿黄疸[20]。

　　第一代抗精神病药是否对胎儿或后期的发育完全没有风险,这一点仍然不确定[20,21]。然而,大多数研究都提出这样一种假设——正是这种持续的不确定性,以及数十年来对这些药物的广泛应用,表明了它们的风险很小[25]。

第二代抗精神病药

- 不可能是严重致畸剂。
- 一项前瞻性研究纳入了 561 名女性,她们均在孕期服用过第二代抗精神病药(大多是奥氮平、喹硫平、氯氮平、利培酮或阿立哌唑)。研究结论是使用第二代抗精神病药与出生体重增加、心脏间隔缺损风险略增(可能由于筛查偏倚或联用 SSRI)相关,而且与第一代抗精神病药类似,新生儿中 15% 出现停药反应[20]。
- 然而,美国进行过一项样本量超过 100 万女性的研究,其中 9 258 名使用过第二代抗精神病药,发现严重畸形或心脏畸形的风险并未出现有意义的升高。用过利培酮者出现严重畸形的绝对风险轻度升高。作者提出,对于这个特殊的结果,解读时宜慎重,应将其看成初步的安全性信号,需要做进一步的研究[23]。在另外一项研究中,214 名女性服用抗精神病药,其后代出现严重畸形的风险估计是 1.4%,而对照组是 1.1%[23]。
- "美国出生缺陷预防研究"的数据分析报告,在妊娠早期使用第二代抗精神病药,增加了心脏圆锥动脉干畸形、法洛四联症、肛门直肠闭锁/狭窄和腹裂的发生。该研究纳入了22 000 多病例和 11 000 多对照。暴露于第二代抗精神病药的女性,更可能会报告孕前肥胖、在孕期吸毒、吸烟、饮酒以及使用其他精神药物[26]。
- 在纳入超过 100 万女性的群体研究报告中,与未用抗精神病药者相比,使用第二代抗精神病药的女性出现妊娠糖尿病、剖宫产、巨大儿、早产的风险增加。在出现剖宫产和巨大儿的风险方面,第二代药物低于第一代药物[27]。在出现孕期糖尿病的危险因素中,母亲的精神疾病也可以是重要因素[28,29]。阿立哌唑可能不会增加畸形的危险[30]。
- 有关奥氮平的数据最多,它与低出生体重、住重症监护室风险增加[31]、巨颅[32]和巨大胎儿[33]相关;其中巨大胎儿与已报道的妊娠糖尿病的风险增加相一致[20,32,34,35]。就先天畸形而言,奥氮平似乎相对安全。一项研究对 610 名孕妇进行了前瞻性随访,所报道的先天畸形发生率与常模人口一致[36]。然而,奥氮平却与一系列问题相关,如髋关节发育不良[37]、脑脊膜膨出、睑缘粘连[38]和神经管缺陷[20](该作用也可能与孕前肥胖有关,而与药物暴露[39]无关)。重要的是没有先天畸形的聚集。

- 使用氯氮平似乎不增加畸形的风险,但是更有可能出现妊娠糖尿病和新生儿癫痫发作[34]。曾有一例母亲过量服用氯氮平导致胎儿死亡的个案报告[20],在理论上我们担心胎儿或新生儿有粒细胞缺乏的风险[20]。药物监测数据表明,在妊娠期,氯氮平的安全性并不逊色于其他抗精神病药[40]。最近,氯氮平被 NICE 列入孕期可用药物清单。与宫内暴露于利培酮、喹硫平或奥氮平的婴儿相比,暴露于氯氮平的婴儿其适应行为评分较低。在同一项研究中,暴露于氯氮平的婴儿中,睡眠紊乱和能力异常的发生率较高[41]。权衡已有的证据,氯氮平通常应该继续使用。氯氮平血浆水平监测可能有利[42],特别是吸烟习惯发生变化时。
- 一个在宫内暴露于阿立哌唑长效注射剂的婴儿,出生时未见先天畸形,5 月龄时也未见发育异常[43]。
- 卡利拉嗪制造商建议该药禁用于孕期,因为动物研究发现畸形风险增加。
- 孕期接触抗精神病药,升高了孕期糖尿病的风险[44]。母亲患精神疾病及相关危险因素也是重要的因素[29]。
- 第二代抗精神病药对长期发育的影响尚不清楚[45]。一项小样本前瞻性病例-对照研究报告,出生前暴露于抗精神病药的婴儿,在 2 个月和 6 个月大的时候会出现认知、运动、社会情感发育延迟,而在 12 个月大的时候不会[46]。这一发现的临床意义,即使有,也不甚清楚。

　　总体来说,根据这些数据无法评估不同药物的相对风险,当然也不能绝对证实某一药物的安全性。至少两项研究提示,服用抗精神病药导致胎儿畸形的风险略有增加[22,31],还有一项研究发现使用抗精神病药治疗的孕妇做剖宫产的风险较高[20]。然而,最近对超过 100 万女性的研究发现,对关键混杂因素进行校正后,使用第一代或第二代抗精神病药时,婴儿出现畸形的风险并无明显增加[23]。孕期使用抗精神病药可能会增加孕期糖尿病、剖宫产[31] 和死胎[47] 的风险,但是这可能是混杂因素所致。和其他药物一样,做决定时,必须根据最新的可得到的信息,并且要个体化地评估可能的利弊。若有可能,要寻求专科医师的建议,并参考原始文献。框 7.2 总结了孕期精神病的治疗建议。

框 7.2　孕期精神病的治疗建议

- 有精神病史并用抗精神病药维持的患者应该及早讨论妊娠计划。
- 应该支持女性尽可能地减少孕期吸烟、饮酒、吸毒带来的风险。应将患者转介到合适的机构,如戒烟诊所、成瘾治疗机构。
- 注意药物所致高泌乳素血症可能会妨碍妊娠。若高泌乳素血症者计划妊娠,考虑换成替代药物。
- 若孕妇服用抗精神病药时病情稳定,停药后有可能复发,建议其继续使用原来的抗精神病药[16]。一般不建议换药,因为存在复发的风险。在讨论利弊之后,考虑使用该孕妇以前使用效果最好的药物[48]。这样会减少胎儿暴露于药物,因为疾病复发时,需要更高剂量或更多种类的药物。
- 生殖安全数据最多的药物有喹硫平、奥氮平、利培酮和氟哌啶醇,较少的有氯氮平、阿立哌唑和齐拉西酮。喹硫平的胎盘通过率相对较低[48,49]。
- 建议服用抗精神病药的孕妇注意饮食,避免体重增加过度。
- 孕期服用抗精神病药的女性应该监测孕期糖尿病。NICE 建议给孕妇做口服糖耐量试验。
- 对于备孕、已孕或考虑母乳喂养的女性,NICE 建议避免使用长效制剂,除非她对长效制剂的反应良好,且既往对口服药依从性差[16]。
- 新生儿可能会出现抗精神病药停药反应(如哭闹、激越、吸吮增多)。这被认为是类别效应[50]。若在孕期服用了抗精神病药,则建议所选产房应与儿科 ICU 相邻。一些中心采用混合喂养(母乳/奶粉)来减少停药反应。

孕期和产后抑郁症 [51-53]

- 约 10% 孕妇会患抑郁症,或者以前患有抑郁症。1/3 产后抑郁症在分娩前即开始。
- 产后 3 个月新发精神疾病显著增加。超过 80% 是心境障碍,特别是重度抑郁发作。
- 以前有抑郁发作史(不论是否产后)的女性,在孕期或产后再次发作的风险较高。抑郁复发风险最高的是双相障碍,同时也有躁狂发作或混合发作的风险。
- 一些证据表明,抑郁症会增加自发流产、低出生体重、胎儿小于孕龄或早产的风险,但是影响较小 [4,54,55]。母亲的精神健康会影响胎儿健康、产科结局和儿童发育。

　　抑郁症不治疗的风险包括:

- 对母亲有害:自理能力变差、缺乏产后保健或自伤。
- 对胎儿或新生儿有害(从忽视到杀婴)。

抗抑郁药治疗

　　在抑郁症患者中,停药者复发率高于继续服药者。一项研究发现,在服用抗抑郁药时正常者中,孕期停药者有 68% 复发,而继续抗抑郁药治疗者 26% 复发 [51]。有重度抑郁或复发性抑郁的女性,其复发的风险可能最高 [56]。

　　一些数据表明,抗抑郁药可能增加自发流产(但要注意混杂因素未加以控制)、早产、低出生体重、新生儿呼吸窘迫、出生时 APGAR 评分低和婴儿需要特护的风险 [57]。大多研究都是观察性研究,并未控制母亲的抑郁症。在一项大样本队列研究中,有抑郁症状但没用抗抑郁药 [58] 与早产和孕龄偏小有关。有意思的是,芬兰一项大样本研究发现,与诊断为精神疾病但没用药的女性相比,使用 SSRI 会降低早产和剖宫产的风险 [59],而母亲患抑郁症未经治疗会增加低出生体重和早产的风险 [60]。SSRI 类并不增加死胎或新生儿死亡的风险 [61,62]。

　　尽管有理由确定常用抗抑郁药不是主要的致畸因素 [63],但一些抗抑郁药却与特殊的先天畸形有关 [64],其中很多是罕见的。这些潜在的关联大多不能被重复 [54],而且不可能排除适应证混杂的影响 [65]。关于抗抑郁药使用持续时间的影响问题,存在相互矛盾的数据 [66,67]。

　　抗抑郁药对早期成长和神经发育的影响很少被研究,目前存在的有限数据是可靠的 [68-70]。一项小样本研究报告,出生前暴露于 SSRI 类药物会导致新生儿的一般运动异常 [71]。一个小样本研究提示儿童孤独症的风险小幅度增加 [72,73],但是在几项大样本研究和一项荟萃分析中未得到证实 [74-76]。该荟萃分析发现,与孕期暴露于抗抑郁药相比,孕前暴露于抗抑郁药与孤独谱系障碍的关系更大,提示存在适应证混杂 [77]。与 SNRI 相比,SSRI 引起新生儿适应不良综合征的风险较高 [78]。有报告说,生前暴露于抗抑郁药的儿童焦虑水平升高 [79]。

　　服用抗抑郁药的孕妇发生高血压 [80,81]、先兆子痫 [82] 和产后出血的风险增加 [82-85]。已有证据表明,SSRI 类药物可导致产后出血,其机制是降低了 5-羟色胺介导的子宫收缩,并干扰体内平衡 [86]。随后一项较小规模的研究未能证实这种关联,很可能是因为研究效能较低 [87]。抑郁症本身可增加先兆子痫的风险 [88]。

　　一些证据表明,成功地使用抗抑郁药,可能对于儿童行为结果有益。例如,丹麦一项有关抗抑郁药暴露的研究发现,抑郁症女性未服用抗抑郁药时,其子女容易出现不良后果 [85]。

三环类抗抑郁药(TCA)

- 胎儿(通过脐带和羊水)暴露于三环类抗抑郁药的程度很高 [89,90]。
- 三环类抗抑郁药在整个孕期一直广泛使用,对胎儿没有明显的损害 [63,91,92]。
- 并不能排除氯米帕明和心血管缺陷之间有微弱的联系 [93]。欧盟药品补充保护证书(SPC)对氯米帕明的描述是:"母亲直到分娩仍在使用三环类抗抑郁药时,新生儿在最初几小时或几天会出现呼吸困难、昏睡、绞痛、易激惹、低血压或高血压、震颤或痉挛。动物研究发现它有生殖系统毒性。孕妇和未避孕的育龄女性不推荐使用氯米帕明。"曾有一例报告,母亲服用氯米帕明后,新生儿发生 Q-T 间期延长和尖端扭转性室性心动过速 [94]。还有一例报告,母亲在妊娠早期服用阿米替林,新生儿发生 Timothy 综合征Ⅰ型,其特征是严重的 Q-T 间期延长 [95]。
- 一些专家推荐使用去甲替林和地昔帕明(在英国未上市),因为它们的抗胆碱能作用和降压作用低于阿米替林和丙米嗪(分别是前两个药物的叔胺类母体分子)。
- 孕期使用三环类抗抑郁药会增加早产的风险 [91,92,96]。
- 众所周知,在妊娠晚期使用三环类抗抑郁药,会导致新生儿出现停药反应:躁动、易激惹、癫痫发作、呼吸困难、内分泌及代谢紊乱 [91]。这些反应通常是轻微、自限性的。
- 胎儿期暴露于三环类抗抑郁药对发育有何影响,我们知之甚少,但是一项小规模研究未见不良后果 [97]。有限的数据表明,出生前暴露于三环类抗抑郁药不影响以后的发育 [97,98]。

选择性 5-羟色胺再摄取抑制剂(SSRI)

- 舍曲林似乎极少通过胎盘 [99]。
- SSRI 类药物似乎不是主要的致畸剂 [63,67,91,100],支持氟西汀安全性的证据最多 [97,101-104]。尽管如此,需要注意有一项研究发现使用 SSRI 类药物时畸形率轻度增加 [105,106]。数据库和病例对照研究报告,SSRI 类药物与新生儿 [108-110] 的无脑畸形、颅缝早闭、脐突出、畸形足及脐带过长相关 [107],这些联系尚未被得到重复。一项群体研究报告分析了特定出生缺陷与各种抗抑郁药之间的关系,发现特定 SSRI 与非心脏缺陷的风险升高有关 [111]。然而,该研究仅部分解释了基础疾病 [111]。
- 帕罗西汀与心脏畸形间有特殊的关联 [112-114],尤其是在高剂量(每天剂量大于 25mg)、妊娠前 3 个月暴露之后 [115]。然而,一些研究却未重复出帕罗西汀的致畸结果 [91,116],反而其他 SSRI 类药物与之有关 [117-119]。帕罗西汀和氟西汀引起某些心脏出生缺陷的风险高于其他 SSRI [120]。其他研究发现,SSRI 类药物与心脏间隔缺损 [109,121,122] 和其他心脏缺陷的风险增加无关 [111,123-126]。需要注意的是,一项数据库研究报告,孕妇产前暴露于 SSRI 类药物时,胎儿酒精综合征的风险是对照组的 10 倍 [127],孕妇饮酒(可能用于自己治疗抑郁症)与胎儿心脏缺陷的风险增加相关 [93]。
- SSRI 类也与孕龄偏小 [128](通常比正常小几天,其临床意义可疑 [129])、自发流产 [130]、孕期高血压和先兆子痫 [131]、低出生体重(平均 175g) [101,102,132] 和胚胎生长欠佳 [133] 有关。这些结果很可能主要与母亲抑郁有关,与抗抑郁药没有特别关系 [129]。出生前暴露的时间越长,婴儿低出生体重和呼吸窘迫的风险就越大 [66]。妊娠后期暴露于抗抑郁药后,新生儿可见三组症状:一组与 5-羟色胺能毒性有关,一组与抗抑郁药停药症状有关,一组与早产相关 [134]。新生儿撤药综合征可能与早产有关[135]。妊娠后期暴露于舍曲林与早期 APGAR 评分减低有关[101]。妊娠晚期使用帕罗西汀可能增加新生儿并发症,很可能与突然停药有关[136,137]。其他 SSRI 类药物可能有相似的、不那么严重的影响[137,138]。婴儿体温不稳定、进食不佳、呼吸窘迫、心律失常、嗜睡、肌张力异常、紧张不安、抽动、癫痫发作均有报道[93]。曾报告过一例产前暴露于帕罗西汀的新生儿出现一过性长 Q-T 间期综合征[139]。

- 关于胎儿暴露于 SSRI 类药物对神经发育的影响,根据现有数据难以得出结论[97,98,140-143]。抑郁症本身对发育可能有更明显的不良影响[97]。曾有研究认为,母亲使用 SSRI 与儿童孤独谱系障碍相关[144-146]。然而,大样本研究发现,或者在剔除母亲疾病影响之后未再发现这种联系[74-76],或者该联系不再有统计学意义[147,148]。一项研究报告,妊娠前父亲曾服用 SSRI 者,其子女患 ADHD 的风险升高,作者认为这可能是使用 SSRI 治疗的基础疾病所致[149]。

- 曾报告过认知功能和粗大运动发育[150]欠佳,言语和语言[150-153]、行为[154,155]和精细运动控制[156]存在问题,但不清楚是否由混杂因素所致。

- 孕期使用 SSRI 或 SNRI 类药物时,可能会增加新生儿持续肺动脉高压的风险。使用舍曲林的风险低于其他 SSRI[157]。其绝对风险很小,比以前估计的还小[158],且仅在妊娠后期用药时才存在[159]。

- 曾经报告过 SSRI 与产后出血相关[84,160]。但是,也有研究发现 SSRI 并未明显增加分娩时失血的风险[161]。产科医师和助产士需要注意这种可能会增加的风险,监测产后失血情况。

其他抗抑郁药

- 度洛西汀不可能是主要的致畸剂。一项采用倾向性评分和几个敏感度分析的大样本队列研究发现,孕期用药可能与产后出血风险轻度升高有关[162]。对经历过妊娠和分娩的 233 名女性的前瞻性随访研究中,未发现度洛西汀有特殊的风险[163]。但是,有一例可疑戒断综合征,需要住院的报告[164]。

- 更加稀少的数据提示,**吗氯贝胺**[165]和**瑞波西汀**[166]没有致畸的可能性。**文拉法辛**可能与心脏缺损、无脑儿、腭裂[167]、新生儿停药反应和新生儿适应不良综合征[102],以及产后出血[162]有关。然而,较新的资料提示,妊娠头 3 个月使用文拉法辛似乎与严重先天畸形风险升高无关[168]。妊娠 4~6 个月暴露于文拉法辛可能与胎儿出生时胎龄偏小有关[169]。对孕期使用文拉法辛的 281 例患者进行观察性研究,结果未发现文拉法辛增加不良妊娠或不良胚胎结局的证据[170]。一项群体研究报告分析了特定出生缺陷与各种抗抑郁药之间的关系,发现文拉法辛与心脏缺陷的风险升高有关[111]。然而,该研究仅部分解释了基础疾病[111]。**曲唑酮**、**安非他酮**和**米氮平**很少有数据支持它们的安全性[102,171,172]。一些数据表明,安非他酮和米氮平都与畸形无关,但与 SSRI 类药物一样,可能与自发流产率增加有关[173-175]。妊娠头 3 个月使用安非他酮可能与室间隔缺损风险轻度升高有关[176]。出生前暴露于安非他酮可能与儿童患多动症风险增加有关[177,178]。

- **单胺氧化酶抑制剂**(MAOI)在孕期应避免使用,因为怀疑 MAOI 会增加先天畸形和高血压危象的风险[179]。

- 没有证据表明孕期使用**电抽搐治疗**(ECT)会对母亲或胎儿产生危害[180],尽管全身麻醉也不是一点风险也没有。对于孕妇或胎儿躯体健康面临严重风险的难治性抑郁症、严重混合状态、躁狂或紧张症,NICE 推荐电抽搐治疗(ECT)。框 7.3 总结了孕期抑郁症治疗的建议。

框 7.3 孕期抑郁症治疗建议

- 在用抗抑郁药且复发风险高者,在孕期和产后最好维持同一抗抑郁药治疗。
- 孕期发生中、重度抑郁症者,应用抗抑郁药治疗。
- 孕期或备孕开始服用抗抑郁药,必须考虑既往的治疗反应。应该考虑以前治疗有效的抗抑郁药。对于既往未经治疗的患者,可以考虑使用舍曲林。
- 筛查饮酒情况,警惕妊娠高血压和先兆子痫的形成。使用 SSRI 类药物可增加产后出血的风险。
- 若妊娠后期使用 SSRI 类药物,可能增加新生儿持续肺动脉高压的风险,但是绝对风险很低。
- 新生儿可能出现轻度停药症状,如兴奋、易激惹,甚至呼吸窘迫和抽搐(SSRI 类药物)。半衰期短的药物(如帕罗西汀和文拉法辛)发生这种风险的可能性特别高。继续母乳喂养,然后通过混合喂养"断奶",有助于降低停药反应的严重程度。

孕期和产后的双相障碍

- 若孕期停用心境稳定剂,复发风险较高。一项研究发现,妊娠时情感正常的双相障碍女性停用心境稳定剂后,复发的可能性加倍,且复发持续时间是继续使用心境稳定剂者的 5 倍[181]。然而,其他研究发现,可以预测孕期复发的是疾病严重程度,而不是药物改变[182]。
- 产后复发风险显著增加。
- 母亲的精神健康影响胎儿的健康、产科结局和儿童发育。
- 无论是否接受治疗,患双相障碍女性发生引产、剖宫产、早产、新生儿小于胎龄的风险增加 50%。新生儿也可能有低血糖或小头畸形[6]。
- 双相障碍本身不会显著增加畸形率,心境稳定剂会[6]。
    不使用稳定心境剂的风险包括:
- 对母亲有害:自理能力差、缺乏产后保健或自伤。
- 对胎儿或新生儿有害(从忽视到杀婴)。

心境稳定剂治疗

- **锂盐**能够完全透过胎盘屏障[183]。
- 孕期使用锂盐与先天畸形风险升高有关[184]。该风险在妊娠头 3 个月较高,剂量大时较高[184]。
- 尽管出生前暴露于锂盐的婴幼儿发生严重畸形的整体风险很可能被高估了,但如果可能,孕期应尽量避免使用锂盐。然而,如果锂盐对于该孕妇是最好的药物,极有可能让她保持健康,那么应该在告知她风险升高的同时,支持她继续使用锂盐。
- 若计划停药,最好在妊娠前缓慢停药[34,186],因为突然停药被认为会加剧复发的风险。妊娠前停用锂盐的女性,其产后复发率可高达 70%[187]。如果孕期停药不成功,要重新开始并维持用药。
- 众所周知,孕期使用锂盐与心脏 Ebstein 畸形相关。然而,最近的资料提示,其影响程度较既往估计小很多[188,189]。另外,对 560 次分娩的监测研究发现,该风险与孕妇的总体心理健康问题有关,而与锂盐的特定关系不大[190]。
- 对胎儿风险最大的时间是妊娠后 2~6 周[191],这个阶段很多女性尚不知道自己妊娠。房间隔或室间隔缺损的风险也可能增加[31]。
- 如果孕期继续服用锂盐,应该与产科医师联络,在妊娠第 6 周和 18 周进行高分辨率超声和超声心动图检查。

- 在妊娠晚期,因为药代动力学发生了改变,锂盐的使用可能会产生问题:因为体内水的总量增加,孕期需要增加锂盐的剂量来保证血锂水平,但是在分娩后锂盐的需求迅速降到妊娠前水平[192]。NICE 建议将血浆锂浓度保持在女性治疗浓度范围内,在主动分娩期间停用,末次用药 12h 后查血浆锂浓度[16,193]。使用锂盐的孕妇应该在医院分娩,以便监测和维持体液平衡。

- 大样本队列研究报告,锂盐与胎盘介导的妊娠并发症或早产无关[194]。

- 使用锂盐可增加产后 4 周内新生儿再住院的风险[185]。

- 新生儿甲状腺肿、肌张力减退、嗜睡、心律失常可能会发生。

- **卡马西平**、**丙戊酸盐**和**拉莫三嗪**的相关数据大多数来自癫痫研究,该病与新生儿畸形增加相关。这些数据用于精神疾病时,相关性可能不大。

- 卡马西平和丙戊酸盐都与很多胚胎畸形(尤其是包括脊柱裂在内的神经管缺陷)的风险增加[195]有明确的因果关系。如果可能,两种药物都应该避免使用,使用抗精神病药来替代。丙戊酸盐比卡马西平有更高的风险[196-198],除非其他所有治疗都失败了,否则不宜用于育龄女性。尽管长期在精神卫生机构就医的育龄女性患者有 1/20 使用心境稳定剂,但是精神科医师对这些药物潜在致畸性的意识很低[195]。

- 没有证据表明在孕期给予叶酸会避免抗癫痫药引起的神经管缺陷[199],但在妊娠前使用可能有这样的作用(神经管在妊娠第 8 周基本形成[200],这时很多女性尚未意识到自己已经妊娠)。然而,补充叶酸对早期神经发育可能有益,所以应该一直使用[199]。

- 丙戊酸盐单用与房间隔缺损、腭裂、尿道下裂、多指趾畸形和颅缝早闭的相对风险增加有关,尽管其绝对风险很低[201]。丙戊酸盐也与新生儿头围缩小有关[202]。

- 孕期使用丙戊酸盐与儿童运动和神经发育问题似乎存在明确的因果关系。欧洲药品管理局的一篇综述发现,在出生前暴露于丙戊酸盐的学龄前儿童中,多达 40% 会出现某种发育延迟,包括走路和说话延迟、记忆问题、言语困难以及智力较差。与出生前暴露于卡马西平和拉莫三嗪者相比,出生前暴露于丙戊酸盐者的语言功能、注意、记忆、执行功能和适应行为均较差。也有研究报告,这样的儿童智商较低,孤独谱系障碍的诊断率升高[203,204]。认知加工、工作记忆和学习缺陷似乎与剂量相关[205]。与出生前未暴露于抗癫痫药和暴露于拉莫三嗪的儿童相比,暴露于丙戊酸盐者学业表现较差[206]。

- 使用丙戊酸盐可增加先兆子痫的风险[207]。

- 若认为有必要继续使用丙戊酸盐,强烈建议低(但有效)剂量单药治疗,因为致畸效应可能与剂量有关[208,209]。如果妊娠后期使用卡马西平,母亲必须服用维生素 K。

- 日益增多的证据表明,在许多妊娠结局指标上,孕期服用拉莫三嗪比卡马西平和丙戊酸盐安全[199,203,210-212]。发生严重畸形的风险似乎与未暴露于抗癫痫药者类似[213]。拉莫三嗪的清除率在孕期似乎会显著增加[214,215],产后降低[216],因此应该经常监测拉莫三嗪浓度。

- 出生前暴露于拉莫三嗪的儿童,父母报告他们存在行为问题[217]。拉莫三嗪可能与孤独症风险增加有关[218]。

- 有报告表明,卡马西平、丙戊酸盐和托吡酯与新生儿 APGAR 评分较低有关。若此种相关性存在,绝对风险也很低[219]。

- 有报告显示,托吡酯可导致主要畸形,特别是口腔颌面部裂缝畸形[220]。癫痫孕妇服用大剂量托吡酯时,子女出现口腔裂缝畸形的风险较大[221]。
- 一项大样本队伍研究报告,抗惊厥剂类心境稳定剂与胎盘介导的妊娠并发症或早产无关[205]。框 7.4 总结了孕期双相障碍治疗的建议。

框 7.4　孕期双相障碍治疗建议

- 对于长期未复发的女性,应考虑有无可能在妊娠前、至少妊娠后 3 个月内,换用更安全的药物(抗精神病药),或完全停药。
- 若突然停药,分娩前、后的复发率都很高。
- 没有一种心境稳定剂是确实安全的。NICE 建议,最好用有心境稳定作用的抗精神病药,代替继续使用心境稳定剂。
- 若病情严重,或已知停用心境稳定剂会很快复发,建议在讨论过风险后继续使用心境稳定剂。
- NICE 建议,备孕女性若必须使用锂盐,应告诉她在妊娠头 3 个月用药导致胎儿心脏畸形的风险,以及哺乳时继续用药导致婴儿中毒的风险。在整个孕期及产后,应增加检测血锂水平的频率,在主动分娩期间应该停用。应与产科医师联合对使用锂盐的女性进行适当的检查,来筛查 Ebstein 畸形。
- NICE 反对在孕期使用丙戊酸盐。妊娠前应停用丙戊酸盐。正在服用丙戊酸盐的女性若计划妊娠,应嘱其逐渐停药,因为胎儿发生畸形和神经发育不良的风险很高。若对某一女性有效的药物只有丙戊酸盐,而且在孕期也没有其他选择,则需要明确告知该风险,并签署知情同意书,证明她了解丙戊酸盐畸形和导致发育延迟的风险。
- 服用卡马西平的女性在备孕或已经妊娠时,NICE 建议与其讨论停药的可能。若使用卡马西平,分娩后母亲和新生儿都应该预防性使用维生素 K。
- 服用拉莫三嗪的女性,NICE 建议在孕期及产后经常检测该药浓度,因为这些时候血药浓度变化很大。
- 孕期急性躁狂发作,使用抗精神病药,若无效考虑 ECT。
- 孕期双相抑郁使用 CBT 治疗中度抑郁,使用 SSRI 治疗重度抑郁。也可以选择拉莫三嗪。

镇静剂

孕期焦虑症和失眠均常见[222]。最好的治疗分别是认知行为治疗和采用睡眠卫生措施。

- 孕早期用**苯二氮䓬类药物**增加新生儿唇腭裂的风险[223],但是后来的研究未证实这种联系[224-226]。最近一项荟萃分析的结论是,妊娠早期服用此类药物,并未增加严重畸形的风险[227]。然而,孕期使用苯二氮䓬类药物可能是心脏等畸形风险的标志[228]。
- 苯二氮䓬类药物与幽门狭窄和消化道闭锁有关[224]。瑞典一项大规模队列研究(1 406 名孕期服用苯二氮䓬类药物的女性)未证实这种联系,也未提示其他联系[225]。注意没有找到选择性终止妊娠的数据。
- 孕期使用苯二氮䓬类药物与下述情况相关:剖宫产、自然流产、新生儿重症监护、新生儿呼吸支持、低出生体重、早产、头围小、小于胎龄儿[224,229-233]。
- 妊娠后期使用苯二氮䓬类药物常与新生儿困难(neonatal difficulties)、婴儿松软综合征(floppy baby syndrome)有关[234]。
- 异丙嗪已用于治疗妊娠剧吐,且似乎没有致畸性,尽管数据有限。
- 有关 Z 类药的资料很少。然而,现有数据提示,Z 类药并不增加先天畸形的风险[235]。
- 唑吡坦可能有增加早产、低出生体重和剖宫产的风险[236]。

快速镇静

关于在孕妇中如何达到快速镇静,几乎没有已经发表的信息。急性使用短效苯二氮䓬类药物(如劳拉西泮)和有镇静作用的抗组胺药异丙嗪不大可能是有害的。推测在即将分娩前使用其中任一种药物都可能会出现问题。NICE 也推荐使用抗精神病药,但并未指定特别的药物[16]。分娩时若需要快速镇静,强烈建议请麻醉师参与治疗。需要注意的是,抗精神病药一般不推荐作为控制急性行为紊乱的一线用药(见本章"急性行为紊乱和暴力行为")。分娩时若使用镇静剂,麻醉师和新生儿科医师应该在场,以便新生儿发生呼吸抑制时进行抢救。

注意缺陷多动障碍

有限的数据表明,哌甲酯并不是主要的致畸因子[237]。有报告发现心脏畸形的风险略增。安非他明未报告过这种风险[238]。莫达非尼可能增加先天畸形的风险(包括先天性心脏缺陷、尿道下裂、口面裂)[239,240]。莫达非尼不应在孕期开始使用[239]。育龄女性应该了解孕期服用莫达非尼的风险,并告诉她们在服用莫达非尼期间和停药后 2 个月内采取有效的避孕措施[239]。

表 7.1 总结了孕期精神药物使用的建议

表 7.1　孕期精神药物使用建议 *(尽量减少胎儿暴露的药物数量)

精神药物	建议
抗抑郁药	复发风险大的女性,在孕期和产后最好维持使用相同的抗抑郁药 备孕女性开始使用抗抑郁药时,必须考虑以前的药物反应。可选择舍曲林
抗精神病药	没有明确证据表明哪种抗精神病药是主要致畸剂。母亲在孕前/孕期考虑使用或继续使用先前有效的药物,而不是换药 筛查对代谢的不良影响。做口服糖耐量试验。待产室应该毗邻新生儿重症监护室 备孕女性开始使用抗精神病药时,必须考虑以前的药物反应。喹硫平的胎盘通过率相对较低
心境稳定剂	妊娠后应该停用丙戊酸盐。若用药史表明其他药物均无效,且停用丙戊酸盐后病情会复发,则必须进行审慎的风险-收益分析。孕妇必须了解孕期服用丙戊酸盐的风险。避免使用其他抗癫痫剂,除非病情复发的风险和后果大于致畸的风险。考虑使用有心境稳定作用的**抗精神病药** **拉莫三嗪**也是一种选择(仅限于双相抑郁)
镇静剂	最好用非药物治疗 苯二氮䓬类药物、佐匹克隆、唑吡坦可能没有致畸作用,但是在妊娠后期最好不用。异丙嗪被广泛应用,但支持其安全性的数据极少

　* 对每位患者的治疗都应个体化,这怎么强调都不过分。这个一览表的目的并非建议所有患者都要换为推荐药物。对每位患者,要考虑她们目前的处方、对治疗的反应、既往对其他治疗的反应和已知在孕期使用(目前的治疗和换药)的风险。

参考文献

1. McElhatton PR. Pregnancy: (2) General principles of drug use in pregnancy. *Pharm J* 2003; 270:232–234.
2. Rasmussen SA, et al. Maternal obesity and risk of neural tube defects: a metaanalysis. *Am J Obstet Gynecol* 2008; 198:611–619.

3. Schneid-Kofman N, et al. Psychiatric illness and adverse pregnancy outcome. *Int J Gynaecol Obstet* 2008; **101**:53–56.

4. Stein A, et al. Effects of perinatal mental disorders on the fetus and child. *Lancet* 2014; **384**:1800–1819.

5. MacCabe JH, et al. Adverse pregnancy outcomes in mothers with affective psychosis. *Bipolar Disorders* 2007; **9**:305–309.

6. Boden R, et al. Risks of adverse pregnancy and birth outcomes in women treated or not treated with mood stabilisers for bipolar disorder: population based cohort study. *BMJ* 2012; **345**:e7085.

7. Nosarti C, et al. Preterm birth and psychiatric disorders in young adult life. *Arch Gen Psychiatry* 2012; **69**:E1–E8.

8. Khalifeh H, et al. Suicide in perinatal and non-perinatal women in contact with psychiatric services: 15 year findings from a UK national inquiry. *Lancet Psychiatry* 2016; **3**:233–242.

9. de La Rochebrochard E, et al. Children born after unplanned pregnancies and cognitive development at 3 years: social differentials in the United Kingdom Millennium Cohort. *Am J Epidemiol* 2013; **178**:910–920.

10. Gov.uk Guidance. Valproate (Epilim▼, Depakote▼) pregnancy prevention programme: updated educational materials 2020; https://www.gov.uk/drug-safety-update/valproate-epilim-depakote-pregnancy-prevention-programme-updated-educational-materials

11. Goodwin RD, et al. Mental disorders and nicotine dependence among pregnant women in the United States. *Obstet Gynecol* 2007; **109**:875–883.

12. Vigod SN, et al. Maternal schizophrenia and adverse birth outcomes: what mediates the risk? *Soc Psychiatry Psychiatr Epidemiol* 2020; **55**:561–570.

13. Royal College of Physicians. Nicotine without smoke: tobacco harm reduction. A report by the Tobacco Advisory Group of the Royal College of Physicians 2016; https://www.rcplondon.ac.uk/projects/outputs/nicotine-without-smoke-tobacco-harm-reduction-0

14. Sit DK, et al. Changes in antidepressant metabolism and dosing across pregnancy and early postpartum. *J Clin Psychiatry* 2008; **69**:652–658.

15. Ter Horst PG, et al. Pharmacological aspects of neonatal antidepressant withdrawal. *Obstet Gynecol Surv* 2008; **63**:267–279.

16. National Institute for Health and Care Excellence. Antenatal and postnatal mental health: clinical management and service guidance. Clinical Guidance [CG192] 2014 Last updated: February 2020. https://www.nice.org.uk/guidance/cg192

17. Harlow BL, et al. Incidence of hospitalization for postpartum psychotic and bipolar episodes in women with and without prior prepregnancy or prenatal psychiatric hospitalizations. *Arch Gen Psychiatry* 2007; **64**:42–48.

18. Wesseloo R, et al. Risk of postpartum relapse in bipolar disorder and postpartum psychosis: a systematic review and meta-analysis. *Am J Psychiatry* 2016; **173**:117–127.

19. Jones I, et al. Bipolar disorder, affective psychosis, and schizophrenia in pregnancy and the post-partum period. *Lancet* 2014; **384**:1789–1799.

20. Gentile S. Antipsychotic therapy during early and late pregnancy. A systematic review. *Schizophr Bull* 2010; **36**:518–544.

21. Diav-Citrin O, et al. Safety of haloperidol and penfluridol in pregnancy: a multicenter, prospective, controlled study. *J Clin Psychiatry* 2005; **66**:317–322.

22. Habermann F, et al. Atypical antipsychotic drugs and pregnancy outcome: a prospective, cohort study. *J Clin Psychopharmacol* 2013; **33**:453–462.

23. Huybrechts KF, et al. Antipsychotic use in pregnancy and the risk for congenital malformations. *JAMA Psychiatry* 2016; **73**:938–946.

24. Collins KO, et al. Maternal haloperidol therapy associated with dyskinesia in a newborn. *Am J Health Syst Pharm* 2003; **60**:2253–2255.

25. Trixler M, et al. Use of antipsychotics in the management of schizophrenia during pregnancy. *Drugs* 2005; **65**:1193–1206.

26. Anderson KN, et al. Atypical antipsychotic use during pregnancy and birth defect risk: National Birth Defects Prevention Study, 1997–2011. *Schizophr Res* 2020; **215**:81–88.

27. Ellfolk M, et al. Second-generation antipsychotics and pregnancy complications. *Eur J Clin Pharmacol* 2020; **76**:107–115.

28. Galbally M, et al. The association between gestational diabetes mellitus, antipsychotics and severe mental illness in pregnancy: a multicentre study. *Aust N Z J Obstet Gynaecol* 2020; **60**:63–69.

29. Uguz F. Antipsychotic use during pregnancy and the risk of gestational diabetes mellitus: a systematic review. *J Clin Psychopharmacol* 2019; **39**:162–167.

30. Galbally M, et al. Aripiprazole and pregnancy: a retrospective, multicentre study. *J Affect Disord* 2018; **238**:593–596.

31. Reis M, et al. Maternal use of antipsychotics in early pregnancy and delivery outcome. *J Clin Psychopharmacol* 2008; **28**:279–288.

32. Boden R, et al. Antipsychotics during pregnancy: relation to fetal and maternal metabolic effects. *Arch Gen Psychiatry* 2012; **69**:715–721.

33. Newham JJ, et al. Birth weight of infants after maternal exposure to typical and atypical antipsychotics: prospective comparison study. *Br J Psychiatry* 2008; **192**:333–337.

34. Ernst CL, et al. The reproductive safety profile of mood stabilizers, atypical antipsychotics, and broad-spectrum psychotropics. *J Clin Psychiatry* 2002; **63 Suppl 4**:42–55.

35. McKenna K, et al. Pregnancy outcome of women using atypical antipsychotic drugs: a prospective comparative study. *J Clin Psychiatry* 2005; **66**:444–449.

36. Brunner E, et al. Olanzapine in pregnancy and breastfeeding: a review of data from global safety surveillance. *BMC Pharmacol Toxicol* 2013; **14**:38.

37. Spyropoulou AC, et al. Hip dysplasia following a case of olanzapine exposed pregnancy: a questionable association. *Arch Women's Mental Health* 2006; **9**:219–222.

38. Arora M, et al. Meningocele and ankyloblepharon following in utero exposure to olanzapine. *Eur Psychiatry* 2006; **21**:345–346.

39. CARE Study Group. Maternal caffeine intake during pregnancy and risk of fetal growth restriction: a large prospective observational study. *BMJ* 2008; **337**:a2332.

40. Beex-Oosterhuis MM, et al. Safety of clozapine use during pregnancy: analysis of international pharmacovigilance data. *Pharmacoepidemiol*

第 7 章

Drug Saf 2020; 29:725–735.

41. Shao P, et al. Effects of clozapine and other atypical antipsychotics on infants development who were exposed to as fetus: a post-hoc analysis. *PLoS One* 2015; 10:e0123373.

42. Nguyen T, et al. Obstetric and neonatal outcomes of clozapine exposure in pregnancy: a consecutive case series. *Arch Women's Mental Health* 2020; 23:441–445.

43. Ballester-Gracia I, et al. Use of long acting injectable aripiprazole before and through pregnancy in bipolar disorder: a case report. *BMC Pharmacol Toxicol* 2019; 20:52.

44. Kucukgoncu S, et al. Antipsychotic exposure in pregnancy and the risk of gestational diabetes: a systematic review and meta-analysis. *Schizophr Bull* 2020; 46:311–318.

45. Gentile S, et al. Neurodevelopmental outcomes in infants exposed in utero to antipsychotics: a systematic review of published data. *CNS Spectr* 2017; 22:273–281.

46. Peng M, et al. Effects of prenatal exposure to atypical antipsychotics on postnatal development and growth of infants: a case-controlled, prospective study. *Psychopharmacology (Berl)* 2013; 228:577–584.

47. Sorensen MJ, et al. Risk of fetal death after treatment with antipsychotic medications during pregnancy. *PLoS One* 2015; 10:e0132280.

48. McAllister-Williams RH, et al. British Association for Psychopharmacology consensus guidance on the use of psychotropic medication preconception, in pregnancy and postpartum 2017. *J Psychopharmacol (Oxford, England)* 2017; 31:519–552.

49. Schoretsanitis G, et al. Excretion of antipsychotics into the amniotic fluid, umbilical cord blood, and breast milk: a systematic critical review and combined analysis. *Ther Drug Monit* 2020; 42:245–254.

50. European Medicines Agency. Antipsychotics - Risk of extrapyramidal effects and withdrawal symptoms in newborns after exposure during pregnancy. Pharmacovigilance Working Party, July 2011 plenary meeting. Issue 1107. http://www.ema.europa.eu/docs/en_GB/document_library/Report/2011/07/WC500109581.pdf

51. Cohen LS, et al. Relapse of major depression during pregnancy in women who maintain or discontinue antidepressant treatment. *JAMA* 2006; 295:499–507.

52. Munk-Olsen T, et al. New parents and mental disorders: a population-based register study. *JAMA* 2006; 296:2582–2589.

53. Mahon PB, et al. Genome-wide linkage and follow-up association study of postpartum mood symptoms. *Am J Psychiatry* 2009; 166:1229–1237.

54. Yonkers KA, et al. The management of depression during pregnancy: a report from the American Psychiatric Association and the American College of Obstetricians and Gynecologists. *Gen Hosp Psychiatry* 2009; 31:403–413.

55. Engelstad HJ, et al. Perinatal outcomes of pregnancies complicated by maternal depression with or without selective serotonin reuptake inhibitor therapy. *Neonatology* 2014; 105:149–154.

56. Yonkers KA, et al. Does antidepressant use attenuate the risk of a major depressive episode in pregnancy? *Epidemiology* 2011; 22:848–854.

57. Chang Q, et al. Antidepressant use in depressed women during pregnancy and the risk of preterm birth: a systematic review and meta-analysis of 23 cohort studies. *Front Pharmacol* 2020; 11:659.

58. Venkatesh KK, et al. Association of antenatal depression symptoms and antidepressant treatment with preterm birth. *Obstet Gynecol* 2016; 127:926–933.

59. Malm H, et al. Pregnancy complications following prenatal exposure to SSRIs or maternal psychiatric disorders: results from population-based national register data. *Am J Psychiatry* 2015; 172:1224–1232.

60. Jarde A, et al. Neonatal outcomes in women with untreated antenatal depression compared with women without depression: a systematic review and meta-analysis. *JAMA Psychiatry* 2016; 73:826–837.

61. Jimenez-Solem E, et al. SSRI use during pregnancy and risk of stillbirth and neonatal mortality. *Am J Psychiatry* 2013; 170:299–304.

62. Stephansson O, et al. Selective serotonin reuptake inhibitors during pregnancy and risk of stillbirth and infant mortality. *JAMA* 2013; 309:48–54.

63. Ban L, et al. Maternal depression, antidepressant prescriptions, and congenital anomaly risk in offspring: a population-based cohort study. *BJOG* 2014; 121:1471–1481.

64. Berard A, et al. Antidepressant use during pregnancy and the risk of major congenital malformations in a cohort of depressed pregnant women: an updated analysis of the Quebec Pregnancy Cohort. *BMJ Open* 2017; 7:e013372.

65. Gao SY, et al. Selective serotonin reuptake inhibitor use during early pregnancy and congenital malformations: a systematic review and meta-analysis of cohort studies of more than 9 million births. *BMC Med* 2018; 16:205.

66. Oberlander TF, et al. Effects of timing and duration of gestational exposure to serotonin reuptake inhibitor antidepressants: population-based study. *Br J Psychiatry* 2008; 192:338–343.

67. Ramos E, et al. Duration of antidepressant use during pregnancy and risk of major congenital malformations. *Br J Psychiatry* 2008; 192:344–350.

68. Nulman I, et al. Neurodevelopment of children following prenatal exposure to venlafaxine, selective serotonin reuptake inhibitors, or untreated maternal depression. *Am J Psychiatry* 2012; 169:1165–1174.

69. Wisner KL, et al. Does fetal exposure to SSRIs or maternal depression impact infant growth? *Am J Psychiatry* 2013; 170:485–493.

70. Suri R, et al. A prospective, naturalistic, blinded study of early neurobehavioral outcomes for infants following prenatal antidepressant exposure. *J Clin Psychiatry* 2011; 72:1002–1007.

71. de Vries NK, et al. Early neurological outcome of young infants exposed to selective serotonin reuptake inhibitors during pregnancy: results from the observational SMOK study. *PLoS One* 2013; 8:e64654.

72. Hviid A, et al. Use of selective serotonin reuptake inhibitors during pregnancy and risk of autism. *N Engl J Med* 2013; 369:

2406–2415.

73. Rai D, et al. Parental depression, maternal antidepressant use during pregnancy, and risk of autism spectrum disorders: population based case-control study. *BMJ* 2013; 346:f2059.

74. Brown HK, et al. Association between serotonergic antidepressant use during pregnancy and autism spectrum disorder in children. *JAMA* 2017; 317:1544–1552.

75. Sujan AC, et al. Associations of maternal antidepressant use during the first trimester of pregnancy with preterm birth, small for gestational age, autism spectrum disorder, and attention-deficit/hyperactivity disorder in offspring. *JAMA* 2017; 317:1553–1562.

76. Castro VM, et al. Absence of evidence for increase in risk for autism or attention-deficit hyperactivity disorder following antidepressant exposure during pregnancy: a replication study. *Trans Psychiatry* 2016; 6:e708.

77. Mezzacappa A, et al. Risk for autism spectrum disorders according to period of prenatal antidepressant exposure: a systematic review and meta-analysis. *JAMA Pediatrics* 2017; 171:555–563.

78. Kieviet N, et al. Risk factors for poor neonatal adaptation after exposure to antidepressants in utero. *Acta Paediatr* 2015; 104:384–391.

79. Brandlistuen RE, et al. Behavioural effects of fetal antidepressant exposure in a Norwegian cohort of discordant siblings. *Int J Epidemiol* 2015; 44:1397–1407.

80. De Vera MA, et al. Antidepressant use during pregnancy and the risk of pregnancy-induced hypertension. *Br J Clin Pharmacol* 2012; 74:362–369.

81. Zakiyah N, et al. Antidepressant use during pregnancy and the risk of developing gestational hypertension: a retrospective cohort study. *BMC Pregnancy Childbirth* 2018; 18:187.

82. Palmsten K, et al. Antidepressant use and risk for preeclampsia. *Epidemiology* 2013; 24:682–691.

83. Bruning AH, et al. Antidepressants during pregnancy and postpartum hemorrhage: a systematic review. *Eur J Obstet Gynecol Reprod Biol* 2015; 189:38–47.

84. Hanley GE, et al. Postpartum hemorrhage and use of serotonin reuptake inhibitor antidepressants in pregnancy. *Obstet Gynecol* 2016; 127:53–61.

85. Grzeskowiak LE, et al. Antidepressant use in late gestation and risk of postpartum haemorrhage: a retrospective cohort study. *BJOG* 2016; 123:1929–1936.

86. Palmsten K, et al. Use of antidepressants near delivery and risk of postpartum hemorrhage: cohort study of low income women in the United States. *BMJ* 2013; 347:f4877.

87. Lupattelli A, et al. Risk of vaginal bleeding and postpartum hemorrhage after use of antidepressants in pregnancy: a study from the Norwegian Mother and Child Cohort Study. *J Clin Psychopharmacol* 2014; 34:143–148.

88. Uguz F. Is there any association between use of antidepressants and preeclampsia or gestational hypertension? A systematic review of current studies. *J Clin Psychopharmacol* 2017; 37:72–77.

89. Loughhead AM, et al. Placental passage of tricyclic antidepressants. *Biol Psychiatry* 2006; 59:287–290.

90. Loughhead AM, et al. Antidepressants in amniotic fluid: another route of fetal exposure. *Am J Psychiatry* 2006; 163:145–147.

91. Davis RL, et al. Risks of congenital malformations and perinatal events among infants exposed to antidepressant medications during pregnancy. *Pharmacoepidemiol Drug Saf* 2007; 16:1086–1094.

92. Kallen B. Neonate characteristics after maternal use of antidepressants in late pregnancy. *Arch Pediatr Adolesc Med* 2004; 158:312–316.

93. Gentile S. Tricyclic antidepressants in pregnancy and puerperium. *Exp Opinion Drug Saf* 2014; 13:207–225.

94. Fukushima N, et al. A neonatal prolonged QT syndrome due to maternal use of oral tricyclic antidepressants. *Eur J Pediatr* 2016; 175:1129–1132.

95. Corona-Rivera JR, et al. Unusual retrospective prenatal findings in a male newborn with Timothy syndrome type 1. *Eur J Med Genet* 2015; 58:332–335.

96. Maschi S, et al. Neonatal outcome following pregnancy exposure to antidepressants: a prospective controlled cohort study. *BJOG* 2008; 115:283–289.

97. Nulman I, et al. Child development following exposure to tricyclic antidepressants or fluoxetine throughout fetal life: a prospective, controlled study. *Am J Psychiatry* 2002; 159:1889–1895.

98. Nulman I, et al. Neurodevelopment of children exposed in utero to antidepressant drugs. *N Engl J Med* 1997; 336:258–262.

99. Hendrick V, et al. Placental passage of antidepressant medications. *Am J Psychiatry* 2003; 160:993–996.

100. Gentile S. Selective serotonin reuptake inhibitor exposure during early pregnancy and the risk of birth defects. *Acta Psychiatr Scand* 2011; 123:266–275.

101. Hallberg P, et al. The use of selective serotonin reuptake inhibitors during pregnancy and breast-feeding: a review and clinical aspects. *J Clin Psychopharmacol* 2005; 25:59–73.

102. Gentile S. The safety of newer antidepressants in pregnancy and breastfeeding. *Drug Saf* 2005; 28:137–152.

103. Kallen BA, et al. Maternal use of selective serotonin re-uptake inhibitors in early pregnancy and infant congenital malformations. *Birth Defects Res A Clin Mol Teratol* 2007; 79:301–308.

104. Einarson TR, et al. Newer antidepressants in pregnancy and rates of major malformations: a meta-analysis of prospective comparative studies. *Pharmacoepidemiol Drug Saf* 2005; 14:823–827.

105. Wogelius P, et al. Maternal use of selective serotonin reuptake inhibitors and risk of congenital malformations. *Epidemiology* 2006; 17:701–704.

106. Jordan S, et al. Selective Serotonin Reuptake Inhibitor (SSRI) antidepressants in pregnancy and congenital anomalies: analysis of linked databases in Wales, Norway and Funen, Denmark. *PLoS One* 2016; 11:e0165122.

107. Kivisto J, et al. Maternal use of selective serotonin reuptake inhibitors and lengthening of the umbilical cord: indirect evidence of increased

foetal activity – a retrospective cohort study. *PLoS One* 2016; 11:e0154628.

108. Chambers CD, et al. Selective serotonin-reuptake inhibitors and risk of persistent pulmonary hypertension of the newborn. *N Engl J Med* 2006; 354:579–587.

109. Alwan S, et al. Use of selective serotonin-reuptake inhibitors in pregnancy and the risk of birth defects. *N Engl J Med* 2007; 356:2684–2692.

110. Yazdy MM, et al. Use of selective serotonin-reuptake inhibitors during pregnancy and the risk of clubfoot. *Epidemiology* 2014; 25:859–865.

111. Anderson KN, et al. Maternal use of specific antidepressant medications during early pregnancy and the risk of selected birth defects. *JAMA Psychiatry* 2020; e202453.

112. Thormahlen GM. Paroxetine use during pregnancy: is it safe? *Ann Pharmacother* 2006; 40:1834–1837.

113. Myles N, et al. Systematic meta-analysis of individual selective serotonin reuptake inhibitor medications and congenital malformations. *Aust NZJ Psychiatry* 2013; 47:1002–1012.

114. Berard A, et al. The risk of major cardiac malformations associated with paroxetine use during the first trimester of pregnancy: a systematic review and meta-analysis. *Br J Clin Pharmacol* 2016; 81:589–604.

115. Berard A, et al. First trimester exposure to paroxetine and risk of cardiac malformations in infants: the importance of dosage. *Birth Defects Res B Dev Reprod Toxicol* 2007; 80:18–27.

116. Einarson A, et al. Evaluation of the risk of congenital cardiovascular defects associated with use of paroxetine during pregnancy. *Am J Psychiatry* 2008; 165:749–752.

117. Diav-Citrin O, et al. Paroxetine and fluoxetine in pregnancy: a prospective, multicentre, controlled, observational study. *Br J Clin Pharmacol* 2008; 66:695–705.

118. Louik C, et al. First-trimester use of selective serotonin-reuptake inhibitors and the risk of birth defects. *N Engl J Med* 2007; 356:2675–2683.

119. Berard A, et al. Sertraline use during pregnancy and the risk of major malformations. *Am J Obstet Gynecol* 2015; 212:795.e791–795.e712.

120. Reefhuis J, et al. Specific SSRIs and birth defects: Bayesian analysis to interpret new data in the context of previous reports. *BMJ* 2015; 351:h3190.

121. Margulis AV, et al. Use of selective serotonin reuptake inhibitors in pregnancy and cardiac malformations: a propensity-score matched cohort in CPRD. *Pharmacoepidemiol Drug Saf* 2013; 22:942–951.

122. Riggin L, et al. The fetal safety of fluoxetine: a systematic review and meta-analysis. *J Obstet Gynaecol Can* 2013; 35:362–369.

123. Furu K, et al. Selective serotonin reuptake inhibitors and venlafaxine in early pregnancy and risk of birth defects: population based cohort study and sibling design. *BMJ* 2015; 350:h1798.

124. Petersen I, et al. Selective serotonin reuptake inhibitors and congenital heart anomalies: comparative cohort studies of women treated before and during pregnancy and their children. *J Clin Psychiatry* 2016; 77:e36–e42.

125. Wang S, et al. Selective Serotonin Reuptake Inhibitors (SSRIs) and the risk of congenital heart defects: a meta-analysis of prospective cohort studies. *J Am Heart Assoc* 2015; 4:e001681.

126. Ansah DA, et al. A prospective study evaluating the effects of SSRI exposure on cardiac size and function in newborns. *Neonatology* 2019; 115:320–327.

127. Malm H, et al. Selective serotonin reuptake inhibitors and risk for major congenital anomalies. *Obstet Gynecol* 2011; 118:111–120.

128. Ross LE, et al. Selected pregnancy and delivery outcomes after exposure to antidepressant medication: a systematic review and meta-analysis. *JAMA Psychiatry* 2013; 70:436–443.

129. Andrade C. Antenatal exposure to selective serotonin reuptake inhibitors and duration of gestation. *J Clin Psychiatry* 2013; 74:e633–e635.

130. Hemels ME, et al. Antidepressant use during pregnancy and the rates of spontaneous abortions: a meta-analysis. *Ann Pharmacother* 2005; 39:803–809.

131. Guan HB, et al. Prenatal selective serotonin reuptake inhibitor use and associated risk for gestational hypertension and preeclampsia: a meta-analysis of cohort studies. *J Women's Health (2002)* 2018; 27:791–800.

132. Oberlander TF, et al. Neonatal outcomes after prenatal exposure to selective serotonin reuptake inhibitor antidepressants and maternal depression using population-based linked health data. *Arch Gen Psychiatry* 2006; 63:898–906.

133. Zhao X, et al. A meta-analysis of selective serotonin reuptake inhibitors (SSRIs) use during prenatal depression and risk of low birth weight and small for gestational age. *J Affect Disord* 2018; 241:563–570.

134. Boucher N, et al. A new look at the neonate's clinical presentation after in utero exposure to antidepressants in late pregnancy. *J Clin Psychopharmacol* 2008; 28:334–339.

135. Yang A, et al. Neonatal discontinuation syndrome in serotonergic antidepressant-exposed neonates. *J Clin Psychiatry* 2017; 78:605–611.

136. Haddad PM, et al. Neonatal symptoms following maternal paroxetine treatment: Serotonin Toxicity or Paroxetine Discontinuation Syndrome? *J Psychopharmacol (Oxford, England)* 2005; 19:554–557.

137. Sanz EJ, et al. Selective serotonin reuptake inhibitors in pregnant women and neonatal withdrawal syndrome: a database analysis. *Lancet* 2005; 365:482–487.

138. Koren G. Discontinuation syndrome following late pregnancy exposure to antidepressants. *Arch Pediatr Adolesc Med* 2004; 158:307–308.

139. Leerssen ECM, et al. Severe transient neonatal long QT syndrome due to maternal paroxetine usage: a case report. *Cardiol Young* 2019; 29:1300–1301.

140. Gentile S. SSRIs in pregnancy and lactation: emphasis on neurodevelopmental outcome. *CNS Drugs* 2005; 19:623–633.

141. Casper RC, et al. Follow-up of children of depressed mothers exposed or not exposed to antidepressant drugs during pregnancy. *J Pediatr* 2003; 142:402–408.

142. Hermansen TK, et al. Prenatal SSRI exposure: effects on later child development. *Child Neuropsychol* 2015; 21:543–569.

143. Kaplan YC, et al. Maternal SSRI discontinuation, use, psychiatric disorder and the risk of autism in children: a meta-analysis of cohort studies. *Br J Clin Pharmacol* 2017; 83:2798–2806.

144. Boukhris T, et al. Antidepressant use in pregnancy and the risk of attention deficit with or without hyperactivity disorder in children. *Paediatr Perinat Epidemiol* 2017; 31:363–373.

145. Croen LA, et al. Antidepressant use during pregnancy and childhood autism spectrum disorders. *Arch Gen Psychiatry* 2011; 68:1104–1112.

146. Healy D, et al. Links between serotonin reuptake inhibition during pregnancy and neurodevelopmental delay/spectrum disorders: a systematic review of epidemiological and physiological evidence. *Int J Risk Saf Med* 2016; 28:125–141.

147. Clements CC, et al. Prenatal antidepressant exposure is associated with risk for attention-deficit hyperactivity disorder but not autism spectrum disorder in a large health system. *Mol Psychiatry* 2015; 20:727–734.

148. Brown HK, et al. The association between antenatal exposure to selective serotonin reuptake inhibitors and autism: a systematic review and meta-analysis. *J Clin Psychiatry* 2017; 78:e48–e58.

149. Yang F, et al. Preconceptional paternal antiepileptic drugs use and risk of congenital anomalies in offspring: a nationwide cohort study. *Eur J Epidemiol* 2019; 34:651–660.

150. van der Veere CN, et al. Intra-uterine exposure to selective serotonin reuptake inhibitors (SSRIs), maternal psychopathology, and neurodevelopment at age 2.5years – results from the prospective cohort SMOK study. *Early Hum Dev* 2020; 147:105075.

151. Brown AS, et al. Association of selective serotonin reuptake inhibitor exposure during pregnancy with speech, scholastic, and motor disorders in offspring. *JAMA Psychiatry* 2016; 73:1163–1170.

152. Skurtveit S, et al. Prenatal exposure to antidepressants and language competence at age three: results from a large population-based pregnancy cohort in Norway. *BJOG* 2014; 121:1621–1631.

153. Handal M, et al. Prenatal exposure to folic acid and antidepressants and language development: a population-based cohort study. *J Clin Psychopharmacol* 2016; 36:333–339.

154. Hanley GE, et al. Prenatal exposure to serotonin reuptake inhibitor antidepressants and childhood behavior. *Pediatr Res* 2015; 78:174–180.

155. Johnson KC, et al. Preschool outcomes following prenatal serotonin reuptake inhibitor exposure: differences in language and behavior, but not cognitive function. *J Clin Psychiatry* 2016; 77:e176–e182.

156. Partridge MC, et al. Fine motor differences and prenatal serotonin reuptake inhibitors exposure. *J Pediatr* 2016; 175:144–149.e141.

157. Masarwa R, et al. Prenatal exposure to selective serotonin reuptake inhibitors and serotonin norepinephrine reuptake inhibitors and risk for persistent pulmonary hypertension of the newborn: a systematic review, meta-analysis, and network meta-analysis. *Am J Obstet Gynecol* 2019; 220:57.e51–57.e13.

158. Huybrechts KF, et al. Antidepressant use late in pregnancy and risk of persistent pulmonary hypertension of the newborn. *JAMA* 2015; 313:2142–2151.

159. Byatt N, et al. Exposure to selective serotonin reuptake inhibitors in late pregnancy increases the risk of persistent pulmonary hypertension of the newborn, but the absolute risk is low. *Evid Based Nurs* 2015; 18:15–16.

160. Skalkidou A, et al. SSRI use during pregnancy and risk for postpartum haemorrhage: a national register-based cohort study in Sweden. *BJOG* 2020; 127:1366–1373.

161. Kim DR, et al. Is third trimester serotonin reuptake inhibitor use associated with postpartum hemorrhage? *J Psychiatr Res* 2016; 73:79–85.

162. Huybrechts KF, et al. Maternal and fetal outcomes following exposure to duloxetine in pregnancy: cohort study. *BMJ* 2020; 368:m237.

163. Hoog SL, et al. Duloxetine and pregnancy outcomes: safety surveillance findings. *Int J Med Sci* 2013; 10:413–419.

164. Abdy NA, et al. Duloxetine withdrawal syndrome in a newborn. *Clin Pediatr (Phila)* 2013; 52:976–977.

165. Rybakowski JK. Moclobemide in pregnancy. *Pharmacopsychiatry* 2001; 34:82–83.

166. Pharmacia Ltd. Erdronax: use on pregnancy, renally and hepatically impaired patients. Personal Communication, 2003.

167. Polen KN, et al. Association between reported venlafaxine use in early pregnancy and birth defects, national birth defects prevention study, 1997–2007. *Birth Defects ResA Clin Mol Teratol* 2013; 97:28–35.

168. Lassen D, et al. First-trimester pregnancy exposure to venlafaxine or duloxetine and risk of major congenital malformations: a systematic review. *Basic Clin Pharmacol Toxicol* 2016; 118:32–36.

169. Ramos E, et al. Association between antidepressant use during pregnancy and infants born small for gestational age. *Can J Psychiatry* 2010; 55:643–652.

170. Richardson JL, et al. Pregnancy outcomes following maternal venlafaxine use: a prospective observational comparative cohort study. *Reprod Toxicol* 2019; 84:108–113.

171. Einarson A, et al. A multicentre prospective controlled study to determine the safety of trazodone and nefazodone use during pregnancy. *Can J Psychiatry* 2003; 48:106–110.

172. Rohde A, et al. Mirtazapine (Remergil) for treatment resistant hyperemesis gravidarum: rescue of a twin pregnancy. *Arch Gynecol Obstet* 2003; 268:219–221.

173. Djulus J, et al. Exposure to mirtazapine during pregnancy: a prospective, comparative study of birth outcomes. *J Clin Psychiatry* 2006; 67:1280–1284.

174. Cole JA, et al. Bupropion in pregnancy and the prevalence of congenital malformations. *Pharmacoepidemiol Drug Saf* 2007; 16:474–484.

175. Smit M, et al. Mirtazapine in pregnancy and lactation – a systematic review. *Eur Neuropsychopharmacol* 2016; 26:126–135.

第 7 章

176. Louik C, et al. First-trimester exposure to bupropion and risk of cardiac malformations. *Pharmacoepidemiol Drug Saf* 2014; 23:1066–1075.

177. Figueroa R. Use of antidepressants during pregnancy and risk of attention-deficit/hyperactivity disorder in the offspring. *J Dev Behav Pediatr* 2010; 31:641–648.

178. Forsberg L, et al. School performance at age 16 in children exposed to antiepileptic drugs in utero – a population-based study. *Epilepsia* 2010; 52:364–369.

179. Hendrick V, et al. Management of major depression during pregnancy. *Am J Psychiatry* 2002; 159:1667–1673.

180. Miller LJ. Use of electroconvulsive therapy during pregnancy. *Hosp Community Psychiatry* 1994; 45:444–450.

181. Viguera AC, et al. Risk of recurrence in women with bipolar disorder during pregnancy: prospective study of mood stabilizer discontinuation. *Am J Psychiatry* 2007; 164:1817–1824.

182. Taylor CL, et al. Predictors of severe relapse in pregnant women with psychotic or bipolar disorders. *J Psychiatr Res* 2018; 104:100–107.

183. Newport DJ, et al. Lithium placental passage and obstetrical outcome: implications for clinical management during late pregnancy. *Am J Psychiatry* 2005; 162:2162–2170.

184. Fornaro M, et al. Lithium exposure during pregnancy and the postpartum period: a systematic review and meta-analysis of safety and efficacy outcomes. *Am J Psychiatry* 2020; 177:76–92.

185. Munk-Olsen T, et al. Maternal and infant outcomes associated with lithium use in pregnancy: an international collaborative meta-analysis of six cohort studies. *Lancet Psychiatry* 2018; 5:644–652.

186. Dodd S, et al. The pharmacology of bipolar disorder during pregnancy and breastfeeding. *Exp Opinion Drug Saf* 2004; 3:221–229.

187. Viguera AC, et al. Risk of recurrence of bipolar disorder in pregnant and nonpregnant women after discontinuing lithium maintenance. *Am J Psychiatry* 2000; 157:179–184.

188. Diav-Citrin O, et al. Pregnancy outcome following in utero exposure to lithium: a prospective, comparative, observational study. *Am J Psychiatry* 2014; 171:785–794.

189. McKnight RF, et al. Lithium toxicity profile: a systematic review and meta-analysis. *Lancet* 2012; 379:721–728.

190. Boyle B, et al. The changing epidemiology of Ebstein's anomaly and its relationship with maternal mental health conditions: a European registry-based study. *Cardiol Young* 2017; 27:677–685.

191. Yonkers KA, et al. Lithium during pregnancy: drug effects and therapeutic implications. *CNS Drugs* 1998; 4:269.

192. Blake LD, et al. Lithium toxicity and the parturient: case report and literature review. *Int J Obstet Anesth* 2008; 17:164–169.

193. Molenaar NM, et al. Management of lithium dosing around delivery: an observational study. *Bipolar Disorders* 2021; 23:49–54.

194. Cohen JM, et al. Anticonvulsant mood stabilizer and lithium use and risk of adverse pregnancy outcomes. *J Clin Psychiatry* 2019; 80:18m12572.

195. James L, et al. Informing patients of the teratogenic potential of mood stabilising drugs; a case notes review of the practice of psychiatrists. *J Psychopharmacol* 2007; 21:815–819.

196. Wide K, et al. Major malformations in infants exposed to antiepileptic drugs in utero, with emphasis on carbamazepine and valproic acid: a nation-wide, population-based register study. *Acta Paediatr* 2004; 93:174–176.

197. Wyszynski DF, et al. Increased rate of major malformations in offspring exposed to valproate during pregnancy. *Neurology* 2005; 64:961–965.

198. Weston J, et al. Monotherapy treatment of epilepsy in pregnancy: congenital malformation outcomes in the child. *Cochrane Database Syst Rev* 2016; 11:Cd010224.

199. Campbell E, et al. Malformation risks of antiepileptic drug monotherapies in pregnancy: updated results from the UK and Ireland Epilepsy and Pregnancy Registers. *J Neurol Neurosurg Psychiatry* 2014; 85:1029–1034.

200. Bestwick JP, et al. Prevention of neural tube defects: a cross-sectional study of the uptake of folic acid supplementation in nearly half a million women. *PLoS One* 2014; 9:e89354.

201. Jentink J, et al. Valproic acid monotherapy in pregnancy and major congenital malformations. *N Engl J Med* 2010; 362:2185–2193.

202. Tomson T, et al. Teratogenic effects of antiepileptic drugs. *Lancet Neurol* 2012; 11:803–813.

203. Bromley R, et al. Treatment for epilepsy in pregnancy: neurodevelopmental outcomes in the child. *Cochrane Database Syst Rev* 2014; Cd010236.

204. Bromley RL, et al. Fetal antiepileptic drug exposure and cognitive outcomes. *Seizure* 2017; 44:225–231.

205. Cohen MJ, et al. Fetal antiepileptic drug exposure and learning and memory functioning at 6 years of age: the NEAD prospective observational study. *Epilepsy Behav* 2019; 92:154–164.

206. Elkjær LS, et al. Association between prenatal valproate exposure and performance on standardized language and mathematics tests in school-aged children. *JAMA Neurol* 2018; 75:663–671.

207. Danielsson KC, et al. Hypertensive pregnancy complications in women with epilepsy and antiepileptic drugs: a population-based cohort study of first pregnancies in Norway. *BMJ Open* 2018; 8:e020998.

208. Vajda FJ, et al. Critical relationship between sodium valproate dose and human teratogenicity: results of the Australian register of antiepileptic drugs in pregnancy. *J Clin Neurosci* 2004; 11:854–858.

209. Vajda FJ, et al. Maternal valproate dosage and foetal malformations. *Acta Neurol Scand* 2005; 112:137–143.

210. Tomson T, et al. Dose-dependent risk of malformations with antiepileptic drugs: an analysis of data from the EURAP epilepsy and pregnancy registry. *Lancet Neurol* 2011; 10:609–617.

211. Molgaard-Nielsen D, et al. Newer-generation antiepileptic drugs and the risk of major birth defects. *JAMA* 2011; 305:1996–2002.

212. Vajda FJE, et al. Antiepileptic drugs and foetal malformation: analysis of 20 years of data in a pregnancy register. *Seizure* 2019; 65:6–11.

213. Tomson T, et al. Comparative risk of major congenital malformations with eight different antiepileptic drugs: a prospective cohort study of

the EURAP registry. *Lancet Neurol* 2018; **17**:530–538.

214. de Haan GJ, et al. Gestation-induced changes in lamotrigine pharmacokinetics: a monotherapy study. *Neurology* 2004; **63**:571–573.

215. Karanam A, et al. Lamotrigine clearance increases by 5 weeks gestational age: relationship to estradiol concentrations and gestational age. *Ann Neurol* 2018; **84**:556–563.

216. Clark CT, et al. Lamotrigine dosing for pregnant patients with bipolar disorder. *Am J Psychiatry* 2013; **170**:1240–1247.

217. Huber-Mollema Y, et al. Neurocognition after prenatal levetiracetam, lamotrigine, carbamazepine or valproate exposure. *J Neurol* 2020; **267**:1724–1736.

218. Veroniki AA, et al. Comparative safety of antiepileptic drugs for neurological development in children exposed during pregnancy and breast feeding: a systematic review and network meta-analysis. *BMJ Open* 2017; **7**:e017248.

219. Christensen J, et al. Apgar-score in children prenatally exposed to antiepileptic drugs: a population-based cohort study. *BMJ Open* 2015; **5**:e007425.

220. Bromley RL, et al. Cognition in school-age children exposed to levetiracetam, topiramate, or sodium valproate. *Neurology* 2016; **87**:1943–1953.

221. Hernandez-Diaz S, et al. Topiramate use early in pregnancy and the risk of oral clefts: a pregnancy cohort study. *Neurology* 2018; **90**:e342–e351.

222. Ross LE, et al. Anxiety disorders during pregnancy and the postpartum period: a systematic review. *J Clin Psychiatry* 2006; **67**:1285–1298.

223. Dolovich LR, et al. Benzodiazepine use in pregnancy and major malformations or oral cleft: meta-analysis of cohort and case-control studies. *BMJ* 1998; **317**:839–843.

224. Wikner BN, et al. Use of benzodiazepines and benzodiazepine receptor agonists during pregnancy: neonatal outcome and congenital malformations. *Pharmacoepidemiol Drug Saf* 2007; **16**:1203–1210.

225. Reis M, et al. Combined use of selective serotonin reuptake inhibitors and sedatives/hypnotics during pregnancy: risk of relatively severe congenital malformations or cardiac defects. A Register Study. *BMJ Open* 2013; **3**:e002166.

226. Tinker SC, et al. Use of benzodiazepine medications during pregnancy and potential risk for birth defects, National Birth Defects Prevention Study, 1997–2011. *Birth Defects Res* 2019; **111**:613–620.

227. Grigoriadis S, et al. Benzodiazepine use during pregnancy alone or in combination with an antidepressant and congenital malformations: systematic review and meta-analysis. *J Clin Psychiatry* 2019; **80**:18r12412.

228. Andrade C. Gestational Exposure to Benzodiazepines, 2: The Risk of Congenital Malformations Examined Through the Prism of Compatibility Intervals. *J Clin Psychiatry* 2019; **80**:19f13081.

229. Calderon-Margalit R, et al. Risk of preterm delivery and other adverse perinatal outcomes in relation to maternal use of psychotropic medications during pregnancy. *Am J Obstet Gynecol* 2009; **201**:579–578.

230. Okun ML, et al. A review of sleep-promoting medications used in pregnancy. *Am J Obstet Gynecol* 2015; **212**:428–441.

231. Yonkers KA, et al. Maternal antidepressant use and pregnancy outcomes. *JAMA* 2017; **318**:665–666.

232. Freeman MP, et al. Obstetrical and neonatal outcomes after benzodiazepine exposure during pregnancy: results from a prospective registry of women with psychiatric disorders. *Gen Hosp Psychiatry* 2018; **53**:73–79.

233. Sheehy O, et al. Association between incident exposure to benzodiazepines in early pregnancy and risk of spontaneous abortion. *JAMA Psychiatry* 2019; **76**:948–957.

234. McElhatton PR. The effects of benzodiazepine use during pregnancy and lactation. *Reprod Toxicol* 1994; **8**:461–475.

235. Wikner BN, et al. Are hypnotic benzodiazepine receptor agonists teratogenic in humans? *J Clin Psychopharmacol* 2011; **31**:356–359.

236. Wang LH, et al. Increased risk of adverse pregnancy outcomes in women receiving zolpidem during pregnancy. *Clin Pharmacol Ther* 2010; **88**:369–374.

237. Pottegard A, et al. First-trimester exposure to methylphenidate: a population-based cohort study. *J Clin Psychiatry* 2014; **75**:e88–e93.

238. Huybrechts KF, et al. Association between methylphenidate and amphetamine use in pregnancy and risk of congenital malformations: a cohort study from the international pregnancy safety study consortium. *JAMA Psychiatry* 2018; **75**:167–175.

239. Gov.UK. Modafinil (Provigil): increased risk of congenital malformations if used during pregnancy. 2020; https://www.gov.uk/drug-safety-update/modafinil-provigil-increased-risk-of-congenital-malformations-if-used-during-pregnancy?utm_source=e-shot&utm_medium=email&utm_campaign=DSU_November2020split1.

240. Damkier P, et al. First-Trimester Pregnancy Exposure to Modafinil and Risk of Congenital Malformations. *JAMA* 2020; **323**:374-376.

扩展文献

National Institute for Health Care and Excellence. Antenatal and postnatal mental health: clinical management and service guidance. Clinical guideline [CG192] 2014 (Last updated February 2020); https://www.nice.org.uk/guidance/cg192

其他信息资源

National Teratology Information Service. http://www.hpa.org.uk

母乳喂养

众所周知,母乳喂养对子女身体健康和认知发育有长期益处。通常鼓励母亲母乳喂养至少 6 个月。影响母亲决定是否母乳喂养的一个因素,可能是哺乳时所用药物的安全性。由于母乳喂养有益,而且大多数药物缺少有害的证据,大多数药物应该在哺乳期继续使用,只有一些明显的例外。然而,现在的证据提示,若母亲正在服用对其健康是最佳选择的药物,则应该建议她不要哺乳(药名见下)。

有关精神药物对母乳喂养的安全性数据主要来自小样本研究、病例报告及病例系列报道。在大部分病例中,关于婴儿或新生儿的结局报告都局限于短期的急性不良反应。因此,这里总结的精神药物对母乳喂养的长期安全性无法得到保证。鉴于得到这些信息的数据有限,且需要对其定期更新,在解读这些信息时必须慎重。

婴儿暴露

所有精神药物都不同程度地出现在母乳中。当然,婴儿暴露程度的最直接指标是婴儿的血浆药物浓度,但是这些数据通常无法获得。取而代之的方法是,许多病例报告了母乳和母亲血浆中的药物浓度。母亲血浆中抗精神病药浓度可能有利于估计婴儿的暴露程度[1]。母乳中药物浓度可用于估计婴儿每天摄入的药物剂量(假定母乳的摄入量是每天 150mL/kg)。婴儿体重校正剂量用母亲体重校正剂量的比例来表示,这被称为相对婴儿剂量(RID)。RID 这个指标仅仅可作为指导使用,因为这些数值是估计值,而且每种药物在不同文献中的数值变化很大[2]。

哺乳期使用精神药物的一般原则

- 给考虑妊娠的女性使用精神药物时,应该考虑到每种药物在哺乳期的安全性。
- 关于药物在哺乳期的安全性,应该尽早进行讨论,最好在妊娠前或妊娠早期。关于孕期用药的决定应该包括对哺乳的讨论。在妊娠后期或产后数天,不建议换药,因为复发风险高。
- 若母亲在妊娠期间服用某种精神药物直至分娩,则建议在母乳喂养同时继续服用该药,因为可以最大限度地减少婴儿的停药症状。明显例外的情况见后文。
- 对每个病例,均应权衡母乳喂养对母亲和婴儿的益处,以及婴儿暴露于药物的风险。
- 通常不宜停止哺乳,除非所用药物禁用于哺乳期。应该优先治疗母亲的精神疾病,在这种情况下不应停止治疗,而是应该建议进行人工喂养。
- 产后开始用药时
  - 应该考虑母亲以前对治疗的反应。
  - 最好不用已知婴儿血浆浓度高或 RID 高的精神药物。
  - 应该考虑药物的半衰期:半衰期长的药物可在母乳和婴儿血浆中蓄积。
- 婴儿和新生儿不具有与成年人相同的药物清除能力。此外,早产儿和有肾脏、肝脏、心脏或神经系统损害的婴儿暴露药物时风险更高。
- 应该监测婴儿是否出现药物的特定不良反应,以及喂养方式、生长和发育是否异常。
- 如果发现不良反应,或者怀疑药物中毒,应该监测婴儿的血浆药物浓度。

- 母亲正在服用具有镇静作用的药物时,强烈建议不要在床上哺乳,因为她可能会在睡着时压着孩子,有造成婴儿缺氧的风险。
- 镇静作用可能影响母亲与孩子互动的能力。母亲服用有镇静作用的药物时,应该监测这种作用。
- 尽可能:
  - 使用最低有效剂量
  - 避免多药合用
  - 继续使用妊娠期间的治疗方案

    表 7.2 总结了母乳喂养时推荐使用的精神药物。各种药物的信息见表 7.3~表 7.7。

表 7.2　推荐概要

通常建议继续使用孕期一直使用的药物。产后开始使用药物时,应该考虑以前的反应和耐受性

药物种类	推荐药物
抗抑郁药	产后开始用抗抑郁药时,可以考虑舍曲林和米氮平。可以使用其他药物,见表 7.3
抗精神病药	使用氯氮平的女性建议其继续使用该药,不要哺乳 产后开始使用抗精神病药时,可以考虑奥氮平或喹硫平。可以使用其他药物,见表 7.4
心境稳定剂	使用碳酸锂的女性建议其继续使用该药,不要哺乳 产后开始使用心境稳定剂时,可以考虑具有心境稳定作用的抗精神病药,如奥氮平或喹硫平。可以使用其他药物,见表 7.4
镇静药	最好不用。可用半衰期短的药物。可考虑使用劳拉西泮

哺乳期抗抑郁药的使用

表 7.3 根据 2020 年中期所发表资料,提供了哺乳期各种药物的信息。制药商对哺乳期药物使用的正式建议,可以在各个药品的产品特征概要或《欧洲公共评估报告》中找到。表 7.3 中没有包括这种建议(因其往往不详细),而是列出原始参考文献出处。

通常建议继续使用孕期所用的抗抑郁药。产后为了哺乳而换药通常是不合理的。表 7.3 应该用于指导产后开始的用药。在每个病例中,必须考虑以前对治疗的反应(以及没有反应)。

哺乳期抗精神病药的使用

表 7.4 根据 2020 年中期所发表资料,提供了哺乳期各种药物的信息。制药商对哺乳期药物使用的正式建议,可以在各个药品的产品特征概要或《欧洲公共评估报告》中找到。表 7.4 中没有包括这种建议(因其往往不详细),而是列出原始参考文献出处。

通常建议继续使用孕期所用的抗精神病药。产后为了哺乳而换药通常是不合理的。例外的是氯氮平——氯氮平应该继续使用,但是不宜哺乳。表 7.4 应该用于指导产后开始的用药。在每个病例中,必须考虑以前对治疗的反应(以及没有反应)。

哺乳期心境稳定剂的使用

表 7.5 根据 2020 年中期所发表资料,提供了哺乳期各种药物的信息。制药商对哺乳期药物使用的正式建议,可以在各个药品的产品特征概要或《欧洲公共评估报告》中找到。

表7.3　哺乳期抗抑郁药的使用

药物	婴儿血浆浓度	相对婴儿剂量(RID)	已报告婴儿急性不良反应	已报告婴儿发育影响
阿戈美拉汀 [3,4]	未测	无资料	无报告,也无研究	无报告,也无研究
布瑞诺龙 [5]	未测	1%~2%	无报告,也无研究	无报告,也无研究
安非他酮 [4,6-13]	检测不到或低	0.2%~2%	2例6月龄婴儿出现癫痫样活动。其中1例出现睡眠紊乱,严重呕吐和嗜睡。婴儿血浆浓度低于可定量下限。其母亲同时服用艾司西酞普兰	无报告,也无研究
西酞普兰 [2,4,11,14-23]	检测不到至母亲血浆浓度的10%,高于氟伏沙明、舍曲林、帕罗西汀、艾司西酞普兰,但低于氟西汀	3%~10%	睡眠紊乱(母亲用药剂量减半后缓解)、急性腹痛、食量减少、易激惹、不安。1例出生前暴露于西酞普兰的新生儿出现呼吸不规则、睡眠障碍、肌张力过低或过高。尽管母亲在产后继续使用西酞普兰,易这些症状都归因为西酞普兰的停药症状	无报告。一项研究中,78例婴儿的母亲服用某种SSRI或文拉法辛,婴儿6月龄时体重正常。一项研究中,11例婴儿随访到1岁时神经发育正常。其中1例1岁时不会走,但18个月时其神经检查正常
度洛西汀 [4,11,24-27]	低于母亲血浆浓度的1%	<1%	头晕、恶心、疲倦	无报告,也无研究
艾司西酞普兰 [4,11,13,28-33]	检测不到或低	3%~8.3%	1例5月龄大的婴儿出现了坏死性小肠结肠炎(需要重症监护和静脉注射抗生素治疗)。他在出生前暴露于艾司西酞普兰。这名婴儿的入院症状是昏睡、进食量少和便血。1例6月龄婴儿出现癫痫样活动、睡眠紊乱、严重呕吐和嗜睡。其母亲同时服用安非他酮	无报告,也无研究
氟西汀 [2,4,11,14,23,34-45]	变异大:可达母亲血浆浓度的10%,在SSRI中所报告的浓度最高	1.6%~14.6%	急性腹痛、过度哭泣、睡眠减少、腹泻、呕吐、嗜睡、进食减少、肌张力减退、呻吟、咕哝声、多动。1例婴儿在3周龄、4月龄和5月龄时出现了癫痫发作活动。其母亲同时服用卡马西平。1例出现呼吸急促、神经过敏、易激惹、发热、代谢性代谢中毒。婴儿血浆浓度在成年人治疗浓度范围内。作者将其诊断为5-羟色胺综合征。母亲服用氟西汀60mg	许多婴儿的体重增加和神经发育均正常。一项回顾性研究发现,生长曲线低于未暴露的婴儿。1例婴儿出现了血小板5-羟色胺水平下降

第7章

续表

药物	婴儿血浆浓度	相对婴儿剂量（RID）	已报告婴儿急性不良反应	已报告婴儿发育影响
氟伏沙明 [4,11,14,22,46-53]	检测不到至母亲血浆浓度的 50%	1%~2%	新生儿黄疸,严重腹泻,轻度呕吐,睡眠减少、激越	无报告。一项研究中,78 例婴儿的母亲服用某种 SSRI 或文拉法辛,婴儿 6 月龄时体重正常
单胺氧化酶抑制剂（MAOI）[54,55]	未见公开发表的数据	异烟肼 1.2%~18%	无报告	无报告,也无研究
米安色林 [4,56]	未测	未测	无报告	无报告,也无研究
米氮平 [4,11,57,58]	检测不到或低。有 1 例血浆浓度很高。作者提出其消除速率存在很大的个体差异	0.5%~4.4%	在一项研究中,54 名婴儿在产前暴露于该药,母乳喂养时新生儿适应不良综合征的发生率明显下降	无异常报告。在一项研究中,8 名婴儿中有 3 名的体重在正常范围的 10 到 25 百分位,他们也都是低出生体重儿
吗氯贝胺 [4,59,60]	低	3.4%	无报告	无报告,也无研究
帕罗西汀 [2,4,11,14,23,38,46,61-70]	检测不到或低	0.5%~2.8%	呕吐和易激惹,原因是严重的低钠血症。在一项研究中,72 例婴儿中有 9 例出现不良反应,最常见的是失眠,不安和不停哭泣	无报告。一项研究中,78 名婴儿的母亲服用某种 SSRI 或文拉法辛,婴儿 6 月龄时体重正常。27 例服用帕罗西汀的母亲所哺乳的婴儿在 3,6,12 月龄时达到了与对照组相似的一般发育水平
瑞波西汀 [4,11,71]	检测不到或低	1%~3%	无报告	在一项研究中,4 例婴儿中的 3 例婴儿达到了正常发育水平。第 4 例婴儿存在发育问题,但是经判断与端波西汀无关

续表

药物	婴儿血浆浓度	相对婴儿剂量(RID)	已报告婴儿急性不良反应	已报告婴儿发育影响
舍曲林 [4,11,23,38,65,72-80]	检测不到或低。有一项报告提到了 1 例婴儿的血药浓度异乎寻常地高(达到母亲血清药物浓度的 50%)。对这名婴儿的临床情况评估是"临床情况良好"	0.5%~3%	1 例早产儿存在 5-羟色胺过度兴奋,在产前也暴露于舍曲林。其症状包括高热、寒战、肌阵挛、震颤、易激惹、尖声哭泣、吸吮反射和反应降低。1 例母乳喂养的新生儿,在母亲突然停用舍曲林后,出现了停药症状(激越、烦躁不安、失眠和惊跳反应增强)。这位新生儿在宫内也暴露于舍曲林	无报告 一项研究中,78 例婴儿的母亲服用某种 SSRI 或文拉法辛,婴儿 6 月龄时体重正常
曲唑酮 [4,81]	未测	2.8%	无报告,也无研究	无报告,也无研究
三环类抗抑郁药 [4,14,82-90]	检测不到或低	去甲替林。阿米替林,1%~3% 氯米帕明	通过母乳暴露于去甲替林、氯米帕明、丙米嗪、多塞平和地昔帕明的婴儿未见不良反应。使用阿米替林者出现严重镇静和进食不佳。使用多塞平者出现过吸奶困难、肌张力减退、困倦和呼吸抑制	无报告 一项研究纳入了 15 例儿童,他们在出生后 3~5 年没有出现认知发育的负面结局
文拉法辛 [4,11,23,38,65,91-98]	检测不到至母亲血浆浓度的 37%	6%~9%	1 例宫内暴露文拉法辛的婴儿,在出生后 2 天出现昏睡、紧张不安、呼吸急促、吸奶困难和脱水。通过母乳喂养可以帮助控制产后停药反应消退。作者提出,母乳喂养可以帮助控制产后停药反应消退	无报告 一项研究中,78 例婴儿的母亲服用某种 SSRI 或文拉法辛,婴儿 6 月龄时体重正常
伏硫西汀	无发表的资料			

第 7 章

表 7.4 哺乳期抗精神病药的使用

药物	婴儿血浆浓度	相对婴儿剂量 (RID)	已报告婴儿急性不良反应	已报告婴儿发育影响
氨磺必利 [4,94,99-101]	母亲血浆浓度*的 10.5%	4.7%~10.7%	无报告	无报告
阿立哌唑 [4,102-107]	母亲血浆浓度*的 4%	0.9%~8.3%	无报告	无报告
阿塞那平	暂无数据			
依匹哌唑	暂无数据			
丁酰苯类 [4,14,38,82,100,108-111]	无报告	氟哌啶醇 0.2%~12%	1例母亲使用的氟哌啶醇加量时，婴儿出现嗜睡，进食不佳。运动能力同时服用利培酮	有 3 例婴儿在母乳喂养过程中同时暴露于氟哌啶醇与氯丙嗪，被发现发育延迟也报告有发育正常
卡利拉嗪	暂无数据			
氯氮平 [4,14,38,82,109,112-115]	母亲血浆浓度的 6.5%	1.4%	镇静、粒细胞缺乏、吸吮反射减弱，易激惹、癫痫发作、心血管功能不稳定	1 例语言发育延迟。该婴儿在宫内也暴露氯氮平
鲁拉西酮	暂无数据			
对甲苯磺酸芦玛哌酮 (lumateperone tosylate)	暂无数据			
奥氮平 [4,14,38,100,116-128]	检测不到或最低。1 例母乳喂养的婴儿在出生后 5 个月内奥氮平的血清药物浓度降低。作者对此的解释是黄疸宝宝在 4 月龄左右对奥氮平的代谢能力"发展很快"	1.0%~1.6%	嗜睡、困倦、易激惹、震颤、失眠、懒惰、吸吮不良和手抖 1 例发生黄疸和镇静。这名婴儿在宫内也暴露于奥氮平，并存在心肌肥大	1 例婴儿的发育水平低于实际年龄，其母还服用其他精神药物 1 例语言发育延迟，另 1 例运动发育迟缓 2 例婴儿体重不增加 也有发育正常的报告
帕利哌酮	无具体资料。见利培酮			
吩噻嗪类 [4,14,82,108-110]	不定	氯丙嗪 0.3%	昏睡	3 例婴儿同时暴露于氯丙嗪和氟哌啶醇，后出现了发育迟缓
匹莫范色林	暂无数据			

续表

药物	婴儿血浆浓度	相对婴儿剂量（RID）	已报告婴儿急性不良反应	已报告婴儿发育影响
喹硫平 [4,95,125,129-138]	检测不到	0.09%~0.1%	睡眠过多。母亲还服用米氮平和一种苯二氮䓬类药物	在一项小样本研究中，将喹硫平作为母亲抗抑郁治疗的增效剂，结果发现 2 例出现了轻度的发育迟缓，但被认为与喹硫平治疗无关
利培酮 [4,111,139-143]	利培酮检测不到。9-羟利培酮低。	利培酮 2.8%~9.1% 9-羟利培酮 3.46%~4.7%	1 例嗜睡，进食欠佳，运动缓慢。母亲同时服用氟哌啶醇。该反应出现在氟哌啶醇增量时	无报告
舍吲哚	暂无数据			
舒必利 [4,144-148]	暂无数据	2.7%~20.7%	无报告	无报告，也无研究
硫杂蒽类 [4,14,110,149-151]	暂无数据	珠氯噻醇 0.4%~0.9% 氟哌噻吨 0.7%~1.75%	无报告	氟哌噻吨无报告 珠氯噻醇未研究
齐拉西酮 [4,22,110,152]			吸吮不佳，进食不佳，还有 2 例报告过度兴奋	无报告
伊潘立酮	暂无数据			

* 所检测药物的一部分可能是宫内暴露后经过胎盘转运而来。

表 7.5　哺乳期心境稳定剂的使用

药物	婴儿血浆浓度	相对婴儿剂量（RID）	已报告婴儿急性不良反应	已报告婴儿发育影响
卡马西平 [4,14,153-163]	通常很低，但有1例婴儿血浆浓度在成人治疗浓度范围内	1.1%~7.3%	许多婴儿未发现不良反应。1例胆汁淤积性肝炎，1例伴有高胆红素血症和 γ-谷氨酰肽酶（GGT）升高的一过性肝功损害。第一个病例的症状在停止母乳喂养后消失，第二个病例尽管没有停止母乳喂养，症状也消失了 1例出现了癫痫发作样活动，困倦，易激惹和尖声哭泣。其母亲服用了多种药物 吸吮欠佳，进食不佳，2例过度兴奋	无报告 一项前瞻性的，有关母亲因癫痫服用抗癫痫药的研究。该研究对宫内和哺乳期间暴露于与未暴露于抗癫痫药的孩子进行了比较 一项研究纳入了宫内及通过哺乳暴露于抗癫痫药的199例婴儿，结果表明母乳喂养与非母乳喂养的婴儿在3岁时的IQ值无差异 一项对181例儿童的研究发现，通过哺乳暴露于抗癫痫药，对IQ无不利影响
拉莫三嗪 [4,156,161,164-175]	检测不到至母亲血浆浓度的48%	9.2%~18.3%	许多婴儿未见不良反应 7例血小板增多 1例婴儿出现了需要进行心肺复苏的严重发绀（之前多次发作轻度呼吸暂停）。新生儿的血清药物浓度水平在治疗范围的上限。该婴儿在宫内暴露于药物，其母正在服用高剂量的药物（850mg/d）。1例正常细胞，正常色素性贫血及无症状中性粒细胞减少 [176] 3例出现皮疹。其中1例因为对大豆过敏，第3例的皮疹自发消失	未发现异常 一项前瞻性的，有关母亲因癫痫服用抗癫痫药的研究提示，服用抗癫痫药同时哺乳，婴儿在6~36月龄时没有发育不良。该研究对宫内和哺乳期间暴露于抗癫痫药物的孩子与未暴露于抗癫痫药物的孩子进行了比较评估 一项研究纳入了母乳喂养期间暴露于抗癫痫药的199例婴儿，结果表明母乳喂养与非母乳喂养的婴儿在3岁时的IQ值无差异。这些婴儿在宫内均暴露于抗癫痫药 一项对181例儿童的研究发现，通过母乳暴露于抗癫痫药对IQ无不良影响

续表

第 7 章

药物	婴儿血浆浓度	相对婴儿剂量（RID）	已报告婴儿急性不良反应	已报告婴儿发育影响
锂盐[177]	检测不到至母亲血浆浓度 57%	12%~30.1%	早期喂养问题，尿素升高，肌酐升高，非特异性中毒体征 1 例宫内暴露婴儿出现促甲状腺激素（TSH）升高。1 例宫内暴露婴儿出现了发绀，昏睡，体温低，肌张力减退和心脏杂音 其他未见不良反应	无报告
托吡酯[178,179]	检测不到至母亲血浆浓度的 20%	3%~5%	腹泻	无报告，也无研究
丙戊酸盐[4,14,153-156,161,180,181]	检测不到至母亲血浆浓度的 2%	1.4%~1.7%	宫内暴露后出现血小板减少和贫血。停止母乳喂养后，病情逆转	一项前瞻性的、有关母亲因癫痫服用抗癫痫药的研究结果提示，服用抗癫痫药同时哺乳，婴儿在 6~36 月龄时没有发育不良。该研究对宫内和哺乳期间暴露于抗癫痫药的孩子与未暴露于药物的孩子进行了比较评估 一项研究纳入了母乳喂养期间暴露于抗癫痫药的 199 例婴儿，结果表明母乳喂养与非母乳喂养的婴儿在 3 岁时的 IQ 值无差异。这些婴儿在宫内均暴露于抗癫痫药 一项对 181 例儿童的研究发现，通过母乳暴露于抗癫痫药对 IQ 无不良影响

表 7.5 中没有包括这种建议(因其往往不详细),而是列出原始参考文献出处。

通常建议继续使用孕期所用的心境稳定剂。产后为了哺乳而换药通常是不合理的。例外的是锂盐——锂盐应该继续使用,但是不宜哺乳。表 7.5 应该用于指导产后开始的用药。在每个病例中,必须考虑以前对治疗的反应(以及没有反应)。

哺乳期催眠药的使用

表 7.6 根据 2020 年中期所发表资料,提供了哺乳期各种药物的信息。制药商对哺乳期药物使用的正式建议,可以在各个药品的产品特征概要或《欧洲公共评估报告》中找到。表 7.6 中没有包括这种建议(因其往往不详细),而是列出原始参考文献出处。

表 7.6　哺乳期催眠药的使用

药物	婴儿血浆浓度	相对婴儿剂量(RID)	已报告婴儿急性不良反应	已报告婴儿发育影响
苯二氮䓬类药物 [4,14,38,182-189]	无报告	氯硝西泮 2.8% 地西泮 0.88%~7.1% 劳拉西泮 2.6%~2.9% 奥沙西泮 0.28%~1%	镇静、昏睡、体重减轻和轻度黄疸 1 例暴露于氯硝西泮的婴儿出现了持续的呼吸暂停 暴露于阿普唑仑时,出现烦躁不安和轻度困倦 电话调查 124 名母亲,2 名母亲报告所哺乳的新生儿出现了中枢神经系统抑制。其中 1 名孩子在宫内暴露于苯二氮䓬类药物 其他儿童未发现不良反应	无报告,也无研究
异丙嗪	无报告			
佐匹克隆、唑吡坦和扎来普隆 [4,190-192]	无报告	扎来普隆 1.5% 佐匹克隆 1.5% 唑吡坦 0.02%~0.18%	无报告	无报告,也无研究

哺乳期兴奋剂的使用

表 7.7 根据 2020 年中期所发表资料,提供了哺乳期各种药物的信息。制药商对哺乳期药物使用的正式建议,可以在各个药品的产品特征概要或《欧洲公共评估报告》中找到。表 7.7 中没有包括这种建议(因其往往不详细),而是列出原始参考文献出处。

通常建议继续使用孕期所用的兴奋剂。产后为了哺乳而换药通常是不合理的。表 7.7 应该用于指导产后开始的用药。在每个病例中,必须考虑以前对治疗的反应(以及没有反应)。

表 7.7　哺乳期兴奋剂的使用

药物	婴儿血浆浓度	相对婴儿剂量(RID)	已报告婴儿急性不良反应	已报告婴儿发育影响
托莫西汀	无报告			
右苯丙胺 [193]	检测不到至母亲血浆浓度的 14%	2.4%~10.6%	无报告	无报告,也无研究

续表

药物	婴儿血浆浓度	相对婴儿剂量（RID）	已报告婴儿急性不良反应	已报告婴儿发育影响
赖右苯丙胺	无报告			
哌甲酯[27,194-196]	检测不到	0.16%~0.7%	无报告	无报告
莫达非尼[197,198]	无报告	5.3%	无报告	无报告，也无研究

（苏允爱　译　田成华　审校）

参考文献

1. Schoretsanitis G, et al. Excretion of antipsychotics into the amniotic fluid, umbilical cord blood, and breast milk: a systematic critical review and combined analysis. *Ther Drug Monit* 2020; 42:245–254.

2. Weissman AM, et al. Pooled analysis of antidepressant levels in lactating mothers, breast milk, and nursing infants. *Am J Psychiatry* 2004; 161:1066–1078.

3. Schmidt FM, et al. Agomelatine in breast milk. *Int J Neuropsychopharmacol* 2013; 16:497–499.

4. Hale TW, et al. *Medications and mothers' milk – 18th edition.* New York, USA: Springer Publishing Company; 2019.

5. Hoffmann E, et al. Brexanolone injection administration to lactating women: breast milk allopregnanolone levels [30J]. *Obstet Gynecol* 2019; 133:115S.

6. Briggs GG, et al. Excretion of bupropion in breast milk. *Ann Pharmacother* 1993; 27:431–433.

7. Chaudron LH, et al. Bupropion and breastfeeding: a case of a possible infant seizure. *J Clin Psychiatry* 2004; 65:881–882.

8. Nonacs RM, et al. Bupropion SR for the treatment of postpartum depression: a pilot study. *Int J Neuropsychopharmacol* 2005; 8:445–449.

9. Haas JS, et al. Bupropion in breast milk: an exposure assessment for potential treatment to prevent post-partum tobacco use. *Tob Control* 2004; 13:52–56.

10. Baab SW, et al. Serum bupropion levels in 2 breastfeeding mother-infant pairs. *J Clin Psychiatry* 2002; 63:910–911.

11. Berle JO, et al. Antidepressant use during breastfeeding. *Curr Womens Health Rev* 2011; 7:28–34.

12. Davis MF, et al. Bupropion levels in breast milk for 4 mother-infant pairs: more answers to lingering questions. *J Clin Psychiatry* 2009; 70:297–298.

13. Neuman G, et al. Bupropion and escitalopram during lactation. *Ann Pharmacother* 2014; 48:928–931.

14. Burt VK, et al. The use of psychotropic medications during breast-feeding. *Am J Psychiatry* 2001; 158:1001–1009.

15. Lee A, et al. Frequency of infant adverse events that are associated with citalopram use during breast-feeding. *Am J Obstet Gynecol* 2004; 190:218–221.

16. Heikkinen T, et al. Citalopram in pregnancy and lactation. *Clin Pharmacol Ther* 2002; 72:184–191.

17. Jensen PN, et al. Citalopram and desmethylcitalopram concentrations in breast milk and in serum of mother and infant. *Ther Drug Monit* 1997; 19:236–239.

18. Spigset O, et al. Excretion of citalopram in breast milk. *Br J Clin Pharmacol* 1997; 44:295–298.

19. Rampono J, et al. Citalopram and demethylcitalopram in human milk; distribution, excretion and effects in breast fed infants. *Br J Clin Pharmacol* 2000; 50:263–268.

20. Schmidt K, et al. Citalopram and breast-feeding: serum concentration and side effects in the infant. *Biol Psychiatry* 2000; 47:164–165.

21. Franssen EJ, et al. Citalopram serum and milk levels in mother and infant during lactation. *Ther Drug Monit* 2006; 28:2–4.

22. Werremeyer A. Ziprasidone and citalopram use in pregnancy and lactation in a woman with psychotic depression. *Am J Psychiatry* 2009; 166:1298.

23. Hendrick V, et al. Weight gain in breastfed infants of mothers taking antidepressant medications. *J Clin Psychiatry* 2003; 64:410–412.

24. Boyce PM, et al. Duloxetine transfer across the placenta during pregnancy and into milk during lactation. *Arch Women's Mental Health* 2011; 14:169–172.

25. Briggs GG, et al. Use of duloxetine in pregnancy and lactation. *Ann Pharmacother* 2009; 43:1898–1902.

26. Lobo ED, et al. Pharmacokinetics of duloxetine in breast milk and plasma of healthy postpartum women. *Clin Pharmacokinet* 2008; 47:103–109.

27. Collin-Lévesque L, et al. Infant exposure to methylphenidate and duloxetine during lactation. *Breastfeed Med* 2018; 13:221–225.

28. Gentile S. Escitalopram late in pregnancy and while breast-feeding (Letter). *Ann Pharmacother* 2006; 40:1696–1697.

29. Castberg I, et al. Excretion of escitalopram in breast milk. *J Psychopharmacol* 2006; 26:536–538.

30. Rampono J, et al. Transfer of escitalopram and its metabolite demethylescitalopram into breastmilk. *Br J Clin Pharmacol* 2006; 62:316–322.

31. Potts AL, et al. Necrotizing enterocolitis associated with in utero and breast milk exposure to the selective serotonin reuptake inhibitor, escitalopram. *J Perinatol* 2007; 27:120–122.

第 7 章

32. Ilett KF, et al. Estimation of infant dose and assessment of breastfeeding safety for escitalopram use in postnatal depression. *Ther Drug Monit* 2005; 27:248.

33. Bellantuono C, et al. The safety of escitalopram during pregnancy and breastfeeding: a comprehensive review. *Hum Psychopharmacol* 2012; 27:534–539.

34. Yoshida K, et al. Fluoxetine in breast-milk and developmental outcome of breast-fed infants. *Br J Psychiatry* 1998; 172:175–178.

35. Lester BM, et al. Possible association between fluoxetine hydrochloride and colic in an infant. *J Am Acad Child Adolesc Psychiatry* 1993; 32:1253–1255.

36. Hendrick V, et al. Fluoxetine and norfluoxetine concentrations in nursing infants and breast milk. *Biol Psychiatry* 2001; 50:775–782.

37. Hale TW, et al. Fluoxetine toxicity in a breastfed infant. *Clin Pediatr* 2001; 40:681–684.

38. Malone K, et al. Antidepressants, antipsychotics, benzodiazepines, and the breastfeeding dyad. *Perspect Psychiatr Care* 2004; 40:73–85.

39. Heikkinen T, et al. Pharmacokinetics of fluoxetine and norfluoxetine in pregnancy and lactation. *Clin Pharmacol Ther* 2003; 73:330–337.

40. Epperson CN, et al. Maternal fluoxetine treatment in the postpartum period: effects on platelet serotonin and plasma drug levels in breast-feeding mother-infant pairs. *Pediatrics* 2003; 112:e425.

41. Taddio A, et al. Excretion of fluoxetine and its metabolite, norfluoxetine, in human breast milk. *J Clin Pharmacol* 1996; 36:42–47.

42. Brent NB, et al. Fluoxetine and carbamazepine concentrations in a nursing mother/infant pair. *Clin Pediatr (Phila)* 1998; 37:41–44.

43. Kristensen JH, et al. Distribution and excretion of fluoxetine and norfluoxetine in human milk. *Br J Clin Pharmacol* 1999; 48:521–527.

44. Burch KJ, et al. Fluoxetine/norfluoxetine concentrations in human milk. *Pediatrics* 1992; 89:676–677.

45. Morris R, et al. Serotonin syndrome in a breast-fed neonate. *BMJ Case Rep* 2015; 2015.

46. Hendrick V, et al. Use of sertraline, paroxetine and fluvoxamine by nursing women. *Br J Psychiatry* 2001; 179:163–166.

47. Piontek CM, et al. Serum fluvoxamine levels in breastfed infants. *J Clin Psychiatry* 2001; 62:111–113.

48. Yoshida K, et al. Fluvoxamine in breast-milk and infant development. *Br J Clin Pharmacol* 1997; 44:210–211.

49. Hagg S, et al. Excretion of fluvoxamine into breast milk. *Br J Clin Pharmacol* 2000; 49:286–288.

50. Arnold LM, et al. Fluvoxamine concentrations in breast milk and in maternal and infant sera. *J Clin Psychopharmacol* 2000; 20:491–492.

51. Kristensen JH, et al. The amount of fluvoxamine in milk is unlikely to be a cause of adverse effects in breastfed infants. *J Hum Lact* 2002; 18:139–143.

52. Wright S, et al. Excretion of fluvoxamine in breast milk. *Br J Clin Pharmacol* 1991; 31:209.

53. Uguz F. Gastrointestinal side effects in the baby of a breastfeeding woman treated with low-dose fluvoxamine. *J Hum Lact* 2015; 31:371–373.

54. Snider DE, Jr., et al. Should women taking antituberculosis drugs breast-feed? *Arch Intern Med* 1984; 144:589–590.

55. Singh N, et al. Transfer of isoniazid from circulation to breast milk in lactating women on chronic therapy for tuberculosis. *Br J Clin Pharmacol* 2008; 65:418–422.

56. Buist A, et al. Mianserin in breast milk (Letter). *Br J Clin Pharmacol* 1993; 36:133–134.

57. Smit M, et al. Mirtazapine in pregnancy and lactation: data from a case series. *J Clin Psychopharmacol* 2015; 35:163–167.

58. Smit M, et al. Mirtazapine in pregnancy and lactation – a systematic review. *Eur Neuropsychopharmacol* 2016; 26:126–135.

59. Buist A, et al. Plasma and human milk concentrations of moclobemide in nursing mothers. *Human Psychopharmacology* 1998; 13:579–582.

60. Pons G, et al. Moclobemide excretion in human breast milk. *Br J Clin Pharmacol* 1990; 29:27–31.

61. Begg EJ, et al. Paroxetine in human milk. *Br J Clin Pharmacol* 1999; 48:142–147.

62. Stowe ZN, et al. Paroxetine in human breast milk and nursing infants. *Am J Psychiatry* 2000; 157:185–189.

63. Misri S, et al. Paroxetine levels in postpartum depressed women, breast milk, and infant serum. *J Clin Psychiatry* 2000; 61:828–832.

64. Ohman R, et al. Excretion of paroxetine into breast milk. *J Clin Psychiatry* 1999; 60:519–523.

65. Berle JO, et al. Breastfeeding during maternal antidepressant treatment with serotonin reuptake inhibitors: infant exposure, clinical symptoms, and cytochrome p450 genotypes. *J Clin Psychiatry* 2004; 65:1228–1234.

66. Merlob P, et al. Paroxetine during breast-feeding: infant weight gain and maternal adherence to counsel. *Eur J Pediatr* 2004; 163:135–139.

67. Abdul Aziz A, et al. Severe paroxetine induced hyponatremia in a breast fed infant. *J Bahrain Med Soc* 2004; 16:195–198.

68. Hendrick V, et al. Paroxetine use during breast-feeding. *J Clin Psychopharmacol* 2000; 20:587–589.

69. Spigset O, et al. Paroxetine level in breast milk. *J Clin Psychiatry* 1996; 57:39.

70. Uguz F, et al. Short-term safety of paroxetine and sertraline in breastfed infants: a retrospective cohort study from a university hospital. *Breastfeed Med* 2016; 11:487–489.

71. Hackett LP, et al. Transfer of reboxetine into breastmilk, its plasma concentrations and lack of adverse effects in the breastfed infant. *Eur J Clin Pharmacol* 2006; 62:633–638.

72. Llewellyn A, et al. Psychotropic medications in lactation. *J Clin Psychiatry* 1998; 59 Suppl 2:41–52.

73. Mammen OK, et al. Sertraline and norsertraline levels in three breastfed infants. *J Clin Psychiatry* 1997; 58:100–103.

74. Altshuler LL, et al. Breastfeeding and sertraline: a 24-hour analysis. *J Clin Psychiatry* 1995; 56:243–245.

75. Dodd S, et al. Sertraline analysis in the plasma of breast-fed infants. *Aust N Z J Psychiatry* 2001; 35:545–546.

76. Dodd S, et al. Sertraline in paired blood plasma and breast-milk samples from nursing mothers. *Hum Psychopharmacol* 2000; 15:161–264.

77. Epperson N, et al. Maternal sertraline treatment and serotonin transport in breast-feeding mother-infant pairs. *Am J Psychiatry* 2001; 158:1631–1637.

78. Stowe ZN, et al. The pharmacokinetics of sertraline excretion into human breast milk: determinants of infant serum concentrations. *J Clin*

Psychiatry 2003; **64**:73–80.

79. Muller MJ, et al. Serotonergic overstimulation in a preterm infant after sertraline intake via breastmilk. *Breastfeed Med* 2013; **8**:327–329.
80. Wisner KL, et al. Serum sertraline and N-desmethylsertraline levels in breast-feeding mother-infant pairs. *Am J Psychiatry* 1998; **155**:690–692.
81. Verbeeck RK, et al. Excretion of trazodone in breast milk. *Br J Clin Pharmacol* 1986; **22**:367–370.
82. Yoshida K, et al. Psychotropic drugs in mothers' milk: a comprehensive review of assay methods, pharmacokinetics and of safety of breast-feeding. *J Psychopharmacol* 1999; **13**:64–80.
83. Misri S, et al. Benefits and risks to mother and infant of drug treatment for postnatal depression. *Drug Saf* 2002; **25**:903–911.
84. Yoshida K, et al. Investigation of pharmacokinetics and of possible adverse effects in infants exposed to tricyclic antidepressants in breast-milk. *J Affect Disord* 1997; **43**:225–237.
85. Frey OR, et al. Adverse effects in a newborn infant breast-fed by a mother treated with doxepin. *Ann Pharmacother* 1999; **33**:690–693.
86. Ilett KF, et al. The excretion of dothiepin and its primary metabolites in breast milk. *Br J Clin Pharmacol* 1992; **33**:635–639.
87. Kemp J, et al. Excretion of doxepin and N-desmethyldoxepin in human milk. *Br J Clin Pharmacol* 1985; **20**:497–499.
88. Buist A, et al. Effect of exposure to dothiepin and northiaden in breast milk on child development. *Br J Psychiatry* 1995; **167**:370–373.
89. Khachman D, et al. Clomipramine in breast milk: a case study *J Pharm Clin* 2007; **28**:33–38.
90. Uguz F. Poor feeding and severe sedation in a newborn nursed by a mother on a low dose of amitriptyline. *Breastfeed Med* 2017; **12**:67–68.
91. Koren G, et al. Can venlafaxine in breast milk attenuate the norepinephrine and serotonin reuptake neonatal withdrawal syndrome. *J Obstet Gynaecol Can* 2006; **28**:299–302.
92. Ilett KF, et al. Distribution of venlafaxine and its O-desmethyl metabolite in human milk and their effects in breastfed infants. *Br J Clin Pharmacol* 2002; **53**:17–22.
93. Newport DJ, et al. Venlafaxine in human breast milk and nursing infant plasma: determination of exposure. *J Clin Psychiatry* 2009; **70**:1304–1310.
94. Ilett KF, et al. Assessment of infant dose through milk in a lactating woman taking amisulpride and desvenlafaxine for treatment-resistant depression. *Ther Drug Monit* 2010; **32**:704–707.
95. Misri S, et al. Quetiapine augmentation in lactation: a series of case reports. *J Clin Psychopharmacol* 2006; **26**:508–511.
96. Hendrick V, et al. Venlafaxine and breast-feeding. *Am J Psychiatry* 2001; **158**:2089–2090.
97. Rampono J, et al. Estimation of desvenlafaxine transfer into milk and infant exposure during its use in lactating women with postnatal depression. *Arch Womens Ment Health* 2011; **14**:49–53.
98. Ilett KF, et al. Distribution and excretion of venlafaxine and O-desmethylvenlafaxine in human milk. *Br J Clin Pharmacol* 1998; **45**:459–462.
99. Teoh S, et al. Estimation of rac-amisulpride transfer into milk and of infant dose via milk during its use in a lactating woman with bipolar disorder and schizophrenia. *Breastfeed Med* 2010; **6**:85–88.
100. Uguz F. breastfed infants exposed to combined antipsychotics: two case reports. *Am J Ther* 2016; **23**:e1962–e1964.
101. O'Halloran SJ, et al. A liquid chromatography-tandem mass spectrometry method for quantifying amisulpride in human plasma and breast milk, applied to measuring drug transfer to a fully breast-fed neonate. *Ther Drug Monit* 2016; **38**:493–498.
102. Schlotterbeck P, et al. Aripiprazole in human milk. *Int J Neuropsychopharmacol* 2007; **10**:433.
103. Lutz UC, et al. Aripiprazole in pregnancy and lactation: a case report. *J Clin Psychopharmacol* 2010; **30**:204–205.
104. Watanabe N, et al. Perinatal use of aripiprazole: a case report. *J Clin Psychopharmacol* 2011; **31**:377–379.
105. Mendhekar DN, et al. Aripiprazole use in a pregnant schizoaffective woman. *Bipolar Disorders* 2006; **8**:299–300.
106. Nordeng H, et al. Transfer of aripiprazole to breast milk: a case report. *J Clin Psychopharmacol* 2014; **34**:272–275.
107. Frew JR. Psychopharmacology of bipolar I disorder during lactation: a case report of the use of lithium and aripiprazole in a nursing mother. *Arch Women's Mental Health* 2015; **18**:135–136.
108. Yoshida K, et al. Breast-feeding and psychotropic drugs. *Int Rev Psychiatry (Abingdon, England)* 1996; **8**:117–124.
109. Patton SW, et al. Antipsychotic medication during pregnancy and lactation in women with schizophrenia: evaluating the risk. *Can J Psychiatry* 2002; **47**:959–965.
110. Klinger G, et al. Antipsychotic drugs and breastfeeding. *Pediatr Endocrinol Rev* 2013; **10**:308–317.
111. Uguz F. Adverse events in a breastfed infant exposed to risperidone and haloperidol. *Breastfeed Med* 2019; **14**:683–684.
112. Mendhekar DN. Possible delayed speech acquisition with clozapine therapy during pregnancy and lactation. *J Neuropsychiatry Clin Neurosci* 2007; **19**:196–197.
113. Barnas C, et al. Clozapine concentrations in maternal and fetal plasma, amniotic fluid, and breast milk. *Am J Psychiatry* 1994; **151**:945.
114. Shao P, et al. Effects of clozapine and other atypical antipsychotics on infants development who were exposed to as fetus: a post-hoc analysis. *PLoS One* 2015; **10**:e0123373.
115. Imaz ML, et al. Clozapine use during pregnancy and lactation: a case-series report. *Front Pharmacol* 2018; **9**:264.
116. Goldstein DJ, et al. Olanzapine-exposed pregnancies and lactation: early experience. *J Clin Psychopharmacol* 2000; **20**:399–403.
117. Croke S, et al. Olanzapine excretion in human breast milk: estimation of infant exposure. *Int J Neuropsychopharmacol* 2002; **5**:243–247.
118. Gardiner SJ, et al. Transfer of olanzapine into breast milk, calculation of infant drug dose, and effect on breast-fed infants. *Am J Psychiatry* 2003; **160**:1428–1431.
119. Ambresin G, et al. Olanzapine excretion into breast milk: a case report. *J Clin Psychopharmacol* 2004; **24**:93–95.
120. Lutz UC, et al. Olanzapine treatment during breast feeding: a case report. *Ther Drug Monit* 2008; **30**:399–401.
121. Whitworth A, et al. Olanzapine and breast-feeding: changes of plasma concentrations of olanzapine in a breast-fed infant over a period of

5 months. *J Psychopharmacol* 2010; **24**:121–123.

122. Eli Lilly and Company Limited. Personal correspondence – olanzapine – use in pregnant or nursing women. 2011.

123. Gilad O, et al. Outcome of infants exposed to olanzapine during breastfeeding. *Breastfeed Med* 2010; **6**:55–58.

124. Goldstein DJ, et al. Olanzapine use during breast-feeding. *Schizophr Res* 2002; 53 (Suppl 1):185.

125. Aydin B, et al. Olanzapine and quetiapine use during breastfeeding: excretion into breast milk and safe breastfeeding strategy. *J Clin Psychopharmacol* 2015; **35**:206–208.

126. Stiegler A, et al. Olanzapine treatment during pregnancy and breastfeeding: a chance for women with psychotic illness? *Psychopharmacology (Berl)* 2014; **231**:3067–3069.

127. Var L, et al. Management of postpartum manic episode without cessation of breastfeeding: a longitudinal follow up of drug excretion into breast milk. *Eur Neuropsychopharmacol* 2013; **23 (Suppl 1)**:S382.

128. Manouilenko I, et al. Long-acting olanzapine injection during pregnancy and breastfeeding: a case report. *Arch Women's Mental Health* 2018; **21**:587–589.

129. Lee A, et al. Excretion of quetiapine in breast milk. *Am J Psychiatry* 2004; **161**:1715–1716.

130. Gentile S. Quetiapine-fluvoxamine combination during pregnancy and while breastfeeding (Letter). *Arch Women's Mental Health* 2006; **9**:158–159.

131. Seppala J. Quetiapine (Seroquel) is effective and well tolerated in the treatment of psychotic depression during breast feeding. *Eur Neuropsychopharmacol* 2004; **(7 Suppl 1)**: S245.

132. Kruninger U, et al. Pregnancy and lactation under treatment with quetiapine. *Psychiatr Prax* 2007; **34 Suppl 1**:S75–S76.

133. Ritz S. Quetiapine monotherapy in post-partum onset bipolar disorder with a mixed affective state. *Eur Neuropsychopharmacol* 2005; **15 Suppl 3**:S407.

134. Rampono J, et al. Quetiapine and breast feeding. *Ann Pharmacother* 2007; **41**:711–714.

135. Tanoshima R, et al. Quetiapine in human breast milk – population PK analysis of milk levels and simulated infant exposure. *J Popul Ther Clin Pharmacol* 2012; **19**:e259–e298.

136. Yazdani-Brojeni P, et al. Quetiapine in human milk and simulation-based assessment of infant exposure. *Clin Pharmacol Ther* 2010; **87 Suppl 1**:S3–S4.

137. Var L, et al. Management of postpartum manic episode without cessation of breastfeeding: A longitudinal follow up of drug excretion into breast milk. *Eur Neuropsychopharmacol* 2013; **23 Suppl 2**:S382.

138. Van Boekholt AA, et al. Quetiapine concentrations during exclusive breastfeeding and maternal quetiapine use. *Ann Pharmacother* 2015; **49**:743–744.

139. Hill RC, et al. Risperidone distribution and excretion into human milk: case report and estimated infant exposure during breast-feeding. *J Clin Psychopharmacol* 2000; **20**:285–286.

140. Aichhorn W, et al. Risperidone and breast-feeding. *J Psychopharmacol* 2005; **19**:211–213.

141. Ilett KF, et al. Transfer of risperidone and 9-hydroxyrisperidone into human milk. *Ann Pharmacother* 2004; **38**:273–276.

142. Ratnayake T, et al. No complications with risperidone treatment before and throughout pregnancy and during the nursing period. *J Clin Psychiatry* 2002; **63**:76–77.

143. Weggelaar NM, et al. A case report of risperidone distribution and excretion into human milk: how to give good advice if you have not enough data available. *J Clin Psychopharmacol* 2011; **31**:129–131.

144. Ylikorkala O, et al. Treatment of inadequate lactation with oral sulpiride and buccal oxytocin. *Obstet Gynecol* 1984; **63**:57–60.

145. Ylikorkala O, et al. Sulpiride improves inadequate lactation. *Br Med J* 1982; **285**:249–251.

146. Aono T, et al. Augmentation of puerperal lactation by oral administration of sulpiride. *J Clin Endocrinol Metab* 1970; **48**:478–482.

147. Polatti F. Sulpiride isomers and milk secretion in puerperium. *Clin Exp Obstet Gynecol* 1982; **9**:144–147.

148. Aono T, et al. Effect of sulpiride on poor puerperal lactation. *Am J Obstet Gynecol* 1982; **143**:927–932.

149. Matheson I, et al. Milk concentrations of flupenthixol, nortriptyline and zuclopenthixol and between-breast differences in two patients. *Eur J Clin Pharmacol* 1988; **35**:217–220.

150. Kirk L, et al. Concentrations of Cis(Z)-flupentixol in maternal serum, amniotic fluid, umbilical cord serum, and milk. *Psychopharmacology (Berl)* 1980; **72**:107–108.

151. Aaes-Jorgensen T, et al. Zuclopenthixol levels in serum and breast milk. *Psychopharmacology (Berl)* 1986; **90**:417–418.

152. Schlotterbeck P, et al. Low concentration of ziprasidone in human milk: a case report. *Int J Neuropsychopharmacol* 2009; **12**:437–438.

153. Chaudron LH, et al. Mood stabilizers during breastfeeding: a review. *J Clin Psychiatry* 2000; **61**:79–90.

154. Wisner KL, et al. Serum levels of valproate and carbamazepine in breastfeeding mother-infant pairs. *J Clin Psychopharmacol* 1998; **18**:167–169.

155. Ernst CL, et al. The reproductive safety profile of mood stabilizers, atypical antipsychotics, and broad-spectrum psychotropics. *J Clin Psychiatry* 2002; **63 Suppl 4**:42–55.

156. Meador KJ, et al. Effects of breastfeeding in children of women taking antiepileptic drugs. *Neurology* 2010; **75**:1954–1960.

157. Zhao M, et al. [A case report of monitoring on carbamazepine in breast feeding woman]. *Beijing Da Xue Xue Bao* 2010; **42**:602–603.

158. Froescher W, et al. Carbamazepine levels in breast milk. *Ther Drug Monit* 1984; **6**:266–271.

159. Frey B, et al. Transient cholestatic hepatitis in a neonate associated with carbamazepine exposure during pregnancy and breast-feeding. *Eur J Pediatr* 1990; **150**:136–138.

160. Merlob P, et al. Transient hepatic dysfunction in an infant of an epileptic mother treated with carbamazepine during pregnancy and breast-feeding. *Ann Pharmacother* 1992; **26**:1563–1565.

161. Veiby G, et al. Early child development and exposure to antiepileptic drugs prenatally and through breastfeeding: a prospective cohort study

on children of women with epilepsy. *JAMA Neurol* 2013; 70:1367–1374.

162. Pynnonen S, et al. Letter: carbamazepine and mother's milk. *Lancet* 1975; 2:563.

163. Meador KJ, et al. Breastfeeding in children of women taking antiepileptic drugs: cognitive outcomes at age 6 years. *JAMA Pediatrics* 2014; 168:729–736.

164. Ohman I, et al. Lamotrigine in pregnancy: pharmacokinetics during delivery, in the neonate, and during lactation. *Epilepsia* 2000; 41:709–713.

165. Liporace J, et al. Concerns regarding lamotrigine and breast-feeding. *Epilepsy Behav* 2004; 5:102–105.

166. Gentile S. Lamotrigine in pregnancy and lactation (Letter). *Arch Women's Mental Health* 2005; 8:57–58.

167. Page-Sharp M, et al. Transfer of lamotrigine into breast milk (Letter). *Ann Pharmacother* 2006; 40:1470–1471.

168. Rambeck B, et al. Concentrations of lamotrigine in a mother on lamotrigine treatment and her newborn child. *Eur J Clin Pharmacol* 1997; 51:481–484.

169. Tomson T, et al. Lamotrigine in pregnancy and lactation: a case report. *Epilepsia* 1997; 38:1039–1041.

170. Newport DJ, et al. Lamotrigine in breast milk and nursing infants: determination of exposure. *Pediatrics* 2008; 122:e223–e231.

171. Fotopoulou C, et al. Prospectively assessed changes in lamotrigine-concentration in women with epilepsy during pregnancy, lactation and the neonatal period. *Epilepsy Res* 2009; 85:60–64.

172. Nordmo E, et al. Severe apnea in an infant exposed to lamotrigine in breast milk. *Ann Pharmacother* 2009; 43:1893–1897.

173. Wakil L, et al. Neonatal outcomes with the use of lamotrigine for bipolar disorder in pregnancy and breastfeeding: a case series and review of the literature. *Psychopharmacol Bull* 2009; 42:91–98.

174. Birnbaum AK, et al. Antiepileptic drug exposure in infants of breastfeeding mothers with epilepsy. *JAMA Neurol* 2020; 77:441–450.

175. Kacirova I, et al. A short communication: lamotrigine levels in milk, mothers, and breastfed infants during the first postnatal month. *Ther Drug Monit* 2019; 41:401–404.

176. Bedussi F, et al. Normocytic normochromic anaemia and asymptomatic neutropenia in a 40-day-old infant breastfed by an epileptic mother treated with lamotrigine: infant's adverse drug reaction. *J Paediatr Child Health* 2018; 54:104–105.

177. Newmark RL, et al. Risk-benefit assessment of infant exposure to lithium through breast milk: a systematic review of the literature. *Int Rev Psychiatry (Abingdon, England)* 2019; 31:295–304.

178. Westergren T, et al. Probable topiramate-induced diarrhea in a 2-month-old breast-fed child - A case report. *Epilepsy Behav Case Rep* 2014; 2:22–23.

179. Gentile S. Topiramate in pregnancy and breastfeeding. *Clin Drug Investig* 2009; 29:139–141.

180. Piontek CM, et al. Serum valproate levels in 6 breastfeeding mother-infant pairs. *J Clin Psychiatry* 2000; 61:170–172.

181. Bjornsson E. Hepatotoxicity associated with antiepileptic drugs. *Acta Neurol Scand* 2008; 118:281–290.

182. Spigset O, et al. Excretion of psychotropic drugs into breast milk: pharmacokinetic overview and therapeutic implications. *CNS Drugs* 1998; 9:111–134.

183. Hagg S, et al. Anticonvulsant use during lactation. *Drug Saf* 2000; 22:425–440.

184. Iqbal MM, et al. Effects of commonly used benzodiazepines on the fetus, the neonate, and the nursing infant. *Psychiatr Serv* 2002; 53:39–49.

185. Buist A, et al. Breastfeeding and the use of psychotropic medication: a review. *J Affect Disord* 1990; 19:197–206.

186. Fisher JB, et al. Neonatal apnea associated with maternal clonazepam therapy: a case report. *Obstet Gynecol* 1985; 66:34S–35S.

187. Davanzo R, et al. Benzodiazepine e allattamento materno. *Medico E Bambino* 2008; 27:109–114.

188. Kelly LE, et al. Neonatal benzodiazepines exposure during breastfeeding. *J Pediatr* 2012; 161:448–451.

189. Birnbaum CS, et al. Serum concentrations of antidepressants and benzodiazepines in nursing infants: a case series. *Pediatrics* 1999; 104:e11.

190. Darwish M, et al. Rapid disappearance of zaleplon from breast milk after oral administration to lactating women. *J Clin Pharmacol* 1999; 39:670–674.

191. Pons G, et al. Excretion of psychoactive drugs into breast milk. Pharmacokinetic principles and recommendations. *Clin Pharmacokinet* 1994; 27:270–289.

192. Matheson I, et al. The excretion of zopiclone into breast milk. *Br J Clin Pharmacol* 1990; 30:267–271.

193. Ilett KF, et al. Transfer of dexamphetamine into breast milk during treatment for attention deficit hyperactivity disorder. *Br J Clin Pharmacol* 2007; 63:371–375.

194. Hackett LP, et al. Methylphenidate and breast-feeding. *Ann Pharmacother* 2006; 40:1890–1891.

195. Bolea-Alamanac BM, et al. Methylphenidate use in pregnancy and lactation: a systematic review of evidence. *Br J Clin Pharmacol* 2014; 77:96–101.

196. Marchese M, et al. Is it safe to breastfeed while taking methylphenidate? *Can Fam Physician* 2015; 61:765–766.

197. Aurora S, et al. Evaluating transfer of modafinil into human milk during lactation: a case report. *J Clin Sleep Med* 2018; 14:2087–2089.

198. Calvo-Ferrandiz E, et al. Narcolepsy with cataplexy and pregnancy: a case-control study. *J Sleep Res* 2018; 27:268–272.

扩展阅读

National Institute for Health Care and Excellence. Antenatal and postnatal mental health: clinical management and service guidance. Clinical guideline [CG192] 2014 (Last updated February 2020); https://www.nice.org.uk/guidance/cg192

第 7 章

肝肾功能损害

肝功能损害

肝功能损害的患者可能有以下特征：

- **代谢生物废物、膳食蛋白质、外来物质（如药物）的能力降低**。临床后果包括肝性脑病和药物引起的、剂量相关的不良反应增加。
- **合成血浆蛋白和维生素 K 依赖性凝血因子的能力降低**。临床后果包括低白蛋白血症，严重时可导致腹水。预计高血浆蛋白结合率的药物毒性会增加。胃肠刺激性药物和 SSRI 类药物引起出血的风险增加。
- **肝的血流量减少**。临床后果包括食管静脉曲张，需要经过首过代谢的药物的血浆浓度会升高。

肝功能损害的一般用药原则

肝功能检查很难代表肝脏的代谢能力，因为肝脏的储备能力很强。需注意的是，许多慢性肝病患者没有症状，或者存在波动的临床症状。始终要考虑临床表现，而不是教条地对待肝功能指标。

几乎没有关于肝病患者使用精神药物的临床研究。使用药物时需遵守下列原则：

1. **药物种类尽可能少**。
2. 使用**较低的起始剂量**，特别是高血浆蛋白结合率的药物。TCA、SSRI（西酞普兰除外）、曲唑酮和抗精神病药至少在最初使用的时候，游离药物的浓度可能会增加。但是检测（总）血浆药物浓度无法发现。对于已知首过效应大的药物，需使用低剂量，例如 TCA 和氟哌啶醇。
3. **慎用广泛经肝代谢的药物**（大部分精神类药物）。可能需要使用低剂量。舒必利、氨磺必利、锂盐、加巴喷丁例外，它们只有很少部分或者完全不经肝脏代谢。
4. **延长增加剂量的间隔时间**。谨记肝功能损害时，大部分药物的半衰期会延长，因而达到稳态血药浓度的时间也会延长。
5. 如果白蛋白降低，要考虑对**高血浆蛋白结合率**药物的影响。**若有腹水，要考虑分布容积增加对水溶性药物的影响。**
6. **避免使用半衰期长的药物**或需要代谢后才有活性的药物（前体药物）。
7. 始终**密切监测不良反应**，它们可能会延迟出现。
8. **避免使用镇静作用强的药物**，因为可能会诱发肝性脑病。

9. 避免使用容易引起便秘的药物,因为可能会诱发肝性脑病。

10. 避免使用已知有肝毒性的药物(例如 MAOI、氯丙嗪)。

11. 选择低风险药物(表 8.1),并且每周**监测肝功能**,至少在用药初期时如此。如果增加新的药物后肝功能恶化,考虑替换为其他药物。注意药物之间可能存在交叉肝脏毒性,特别是结构相近者[1]。

严重肝病(低白蛋白血症、凝血时间延长、腹水、黄疸、肝性脑病等)患者用药时,应该始终遵守以上原则。上述内容及下文内容需结合患者的临床表现来解读。

表 8.1　抗精神病药在肝功能损害中的应用

药物	评论
氨磺必利[5,6]	主要经肾排泄,只要肾功能正常,无需减少剂量。转氨酶升高和肝细胞损伤不常见
阿立哌唑[5-8]	大部分经肝脏代谢。有限的数据表明,肝功能损害对该药的药代动力学影响极小。产品特征概要(Summary of Product Charateristics,SPC)中声明,轻、中度肝功能损害时无需减少剂量,但严重肝功能损害时需慎用。少数报告有肝毒性、肝脏转氨酶水平升高、肝炎和黄疸[2,9-11]
阿塞那平[5,6,8]	经肝脏代谢。SPC 建议避免用于严重肝病(阿塞那平暴露量增加 7 倍)。轻、中度肝病不需调整剂量[12],但需要注意在中度损害患者中,血浆浓度有可能升高。常见没有症状的 AST、ALT 短暂升高,特别是在治疗早期。有 1 例轻度淤胆型肝损害报告,停药后缓解[13]
Brexpiprazole[6,14]	信息很少。中、重度肝功能衰竭时,剂量不超过 3mg/d(精神分裂症)或 2mg/d(抑郁)。半衰期长(~90h)
卡利拉嗪[6,15]	偶尔出现无临床意义的 ALT 和 AST 升高。轻、中度肝功能衰竭时,不需要调节剂量;不推荐用于重度肝病(未做过评估)。半衰期长(2~4 天)。有肝炎的报告
氯氮平[1,5,6,16-18]	过度镇静和便秘。禁用于伴有恶心、厌食或黄疸的活动性肝病、进行性肝病以及肝功能衰竭。病情不太严重时,起始剂量为 12.5mg,缓慢加量,通过血药浓度来测定代谢能力,并指导剂量调整。引起肝脏转氨酶改变者多于其他抗精神病药。超过 10% 的健康人群有 AST、ALT 和 GGT 一过性升高,数值达正常值上限的 2 倍,在 6~12 周内自发缓解[19]。已有报告表明氯氮平可引起肝炎、黄疸、胆汁淤积和肝衰竭;出现这些情况时,应停用氯氮平。出现肝炎后,再次试用有成功的报告[20,21]。见第 1 章"氯氮平不良反应"
氟哌噻吨/珠氯噻醇[5,6,22,23]	二者大部分都经肝脏代谢。使用氟哌噻吨后有肝脏转氨酶水平异常和黄疸(罕见)的报告[5]。使用珠氯噻醇后,一些患者出现转氨酶一过性轻度升高、淤胆性肝炎和黄疸[5]。有 1 例使用氟哌噻吨引起肝炎的报告[24]。没有使用该药或造成伤害的其他报告[25]。肝功能损害的患者剂量减半。最好避免使用长效制剂,因药代动力学改变使得不易调整剂量,且药物在体内蓄积更容易引起不良反应
氟哌啶醇[5]	大部分经肝脏代谢。起始剂量减半。个别报告过会引起胆汁淤积、急性肝功能衰竭、肝炎和肝功能异常[5,6]
伊潘立酮[6,8,26]	经肝脏代谢。中度肝功能损害者需减量(活性代谢产物浓度升高 2 倍),严重肝功能损害者禁用(未做研究)。轻度肝功能损害不需减量。偶见胆石症
卢美哌隆[27,28]	经肝脏代谢为活性代谢产物。轻度肝损害不需调整剂量。中、重度肝损害时,暴露剂量增加——药厂建议避免使用。注册试验报告转氨酶升高

续表

药物	评论
鲁拉西酮 [5,6,8]	经肝脏代谢。SPC 推荐肝功能损害者起始剂量为 18.5mg(20mg/d),中度肝损害者(暴露增加 1.7 倍)。最大剂量 74mg(80mg/d),严重肝功能损害患者(暴露量增加 3 倍)最大剂量为 37mg(40mg/d)。轻度肝功能损害不需调整剂量。罕见 ALT 升高
奥氮平 [1,5,6,8]	尽管大部分经肝脏代谢,但严重肝功能损害时奥氮平的药代动力学似乎没有改变。有镇静及抗胆碱能作用(会引起便秘),故建议慎用。中重度肝损害时,起始剂量为 5mg/d,根据血药浓度调整剂量(目标为 20~40μg/L)。身体健康的成年人使用时,引起剂量相关的一过性无症状的 ALT 和 AST 升高。肝病患者或合用其他肝毒性药物者使用时,可能会增加风险。文献里罕见肝炎的病例报告
帕利哌酮 [5,6,8]	主要以原形药物经肾排泄,所以轻、中度肝损害无需调整剂量。但没有关于严重肝功能损害的研究数据,临床经验有限,使用时需谨慎。有转氨酶、GGT 升高和黄疸的报告。对于原有肝病者,可能是好的选择 [29-31]。有 1 例使用利培酮出现肝毒性,换用帕立哌酮也未缓解的报告——有可能帕利哌酮导致肝毒性 [32]
吩噻嗪类 [3,6]	均会造成镇静和便秘。报告有一过性肝功能异常。会引起胆汁淤积,有些报告称会引起暴发性肝硬化。肝功能损害者最好完全避免使用,有些吩噻嗪类药物禁用。氯丙嗪的肝毒性特别大,也可能导致罕见的免疫介导的阻塞性黄疸并进展为肝病
匹莫范色林 [6]	活性代谢产物的半衰期很长(200h)——肝功能损害者不建议使用。看似无肝毒性
喹硫平 [5,6,8,33]	大部分经肝脏代谢,但半衰期短。肝功能损害者清除率平均降低 30%,所以起始剂量为 25mg/d(速释剂型)或 50mg/d(缓释剂型),加量速度是 25~50mg/d。可引起镇静和便秘。曾报告 AST、ALT 和 GGT 一过性升高,罕见黄疸和肝炎。文献中有几例致死性肝衰竭和肝细胞损害的报告。有些研究介绍了在酒依赖者中的应用 [34-36]
利培酮 [1,5,6,8]	大部分经肝脏代谢,血浆蛋白结合率高。制药商建议肝功能损害者起始剂量减半,缓慢加量。重度肝损者,应从 0.5mg,每天 2 次开始,剂量 1.5mg,每天 2 次时,加量速度是至少间隔 1 周增加 0.5mg,每天 2 次。注射利培酮微球可以从 12.5mg/2 周开始,口服利培酮 2mg/d 可耐受时,也可从 25mg/2 周开始。曾报告一过性无症状的肝功能升高、淤胆型肝炎和罕见的肝衰竭病例。曾报告与帕利哌酮有交叉肝毒性 [32]。体重增加可引起脂肪性肝炎 [37]
舒必利 [5,6]	几乎完全经肾排泄,引起镇静和便秘的可能性较小。无需减少剂量。常见肝酶升高。个别报告可引起淤胆型黄疸和原发性胆汁性肝硬化

ALT,丙氨酸转氨酶;AST,天冬氨酸转氨酶;GGT,γ 谷氨酰胺转移酶。

抗精神病药在肝功能损害中的应用

使用抗精神病药的患者中,1/3 至少有一项肝功能异常,4% 至少有一项肝功能超过正常值上限的 3 倍 [2]。转氨酶最易受到影响,通常在开始治疗后 1~6 周内发生 [2]。只有极少数能引起具有临床意义的肝功能损害 [2]。发生代谢综合征(肥胖、胰岛素抵抗)可能与治疗后期的非酒精性脂肪肝有关 [3,4]。

抗抑郁药在肝功能损害中的应用

使用抗抑郁药治疗的患者中,0.5%~3% 会出现无症状的轻度转氨酶升高 [38]。通常会在开始用药后几天至 6 个月内发生,老年人更加敏感[38]。症状明显、具有临床意义的肝功能损害极少发生,大多数是特异反应(不可预测,与剂量无关)。已描述过同一类药物之间有交叉毒性[38]。抗抑郁药在肝功能损害患者中的应用,见表 8.2。

表 8.2 抗抑郁药在肝功能损害中的应用

药物	评论
阿戈美拉汀[5,6,38-40]	曾报告的肝功能损害包括肝衰竭、肝脏转氨酶高于正常值上限 10 倍和肝炎,最多见于治疗第一个月内,罕见致命。禁用于肝损害,包括肝硬化和肝病。转氨酶升高与剂量相关,建议在基线和用药后 3、6、12、24 周检测肝功能,之后根据临床指征来定。若转氨酶高于正常值上限 3 倍,停止治疗。存在其他肝病危险因素时慎用 在目前的监测限制下,肝损害的风险并不高于其他抗抑郁药[41,42]
别孕烯醇酮[6,19]	肝损害者不需调整剂量。似乎没有肝毒性,但是经验有限
度洛西汀[5,6,43-47]	经肝脏代谢。即使轻度肝损害,清除率也显著降低。曾报告过肝细胞损伤(肝脏转氨酶高于正常值上限 10 倍)和黄疸(不常发生)。曾报告会引起肝衰竭,甚至致死。禁用于肝损害者
氟西汀[5,6,48-52]	大部分经肝脏代谢,半衰期长(肝功能不全时更长)。药代动力学研究发现,代偿性肝硬化患者体内会蓄积。建议减少剂量(至少 50%)或隔天使用,但仍需几周后才能达到稳态血清浓度,从而使得氟西汀用起来很复杂。0.5% 的健康成年人出现肝功能无症状性升高。罕见肝炎的案例报告
左米那普仑,米那普仑[6,19]	肝损害者不需调整剂量,但制药商建议米那普仑避免用于慢性肝病、饮酒或严重肝功能异常者。使用米那普仑者有肝酶升高和肝炎的报告,若出现黄疸或肝功能异常应停用
MAOI 类药物[5,6,53]	苯乙肼有导致致死性肝坏死、肝毒性和黄疸的罕见个案。反环苯丙胺有引起肝炎的罕见个案;使用吗氯贝胺有 1 例致死性肝中毒。吗氯贝胺用于肝功能损害者时,剂量应减至 1/2 或 1/4,或延长服药间隔时间。透皮司来吉兰不伤肝[54]。非选择性单胺氧化酶抑制剂禁用于肝损害患者
米氮平[5,6,55]	经肝脏代谢,有镇静作用。根据药代动力学研究的数据,建议减少 50% 的剂量。可引起健康成年人肝功能指标出现轻度、无症状性增高(2% 患者 ALT 大于正常上限值的 3 倍)。很少有胆汁淤积和肝细胞损害的报告。曾安全地用于原发性胆汁性胆管炎患者[56]
其他 SSRI 类药物[5,6,47,52,57-64]	全部经肝脏代谢,长期用药可造成蓄积。可能需要减少剂量(包括最大剂量减半[65],或降低用药频率,详见具体药物的说明书)。使用帕罗西汀可升高肝功能指标,罕见情况下出现肝炎,包括慢性活动性肝炎。舍曲林和氟伏沙明也被报告与肝炎有关。西酞普兰、艾司西酞普兰和帕罗西汀对肝脏转氨酶的影响很小,是可选择的 SSRI 类药物,偶尔也会有肝毒性的报告。一些肝病病房使用帕罗西汀未出现明显问题。舍曲林和帕罗西汀曾用于治疗胆汁淤积性瘙痒[66]。注意出血风险增加
瑞波西汀[5,6,67]	推荐起始剂量减半。似乎无肝毒性

药物	评论
三环类药物 [5,6,68]	全部经肝脏代谢,血浆蛋白结合率高,会在体内蓄积。它们引起镇静和便秘的倾向性有差异。全部药物均可引起肝功能指标升高,罕见肝炎的病例。临床使用经验最多的是丙米嗪。最好都避免使用有镇静作用的三环类药物(如曲米帕明、丙米嗪、度硫平和阿米替林)
文拉法辛/去甲文拉法辛 [5,6,69,70]	轻、中度肝功能损害者建议剂量减半。罕有肝炎的报告
维拉唑酮 [6]	肝损害者不需调节剂量。似乎不影响肝酶,未出现肝毒性的个案,但资料有限,而其他全部 SSRI 均与肝毒性有关
伏硫西汀 [5,71,72]	大部分经肝脏代谢。肝损害方面经验极少,药代动力学研究提示不需减量。似乎没有肝毒性

ALT,丙氨酸转氨酶;ULN,正常值上限。

心境稳定剂在肝功能损害中的应用 [5,6,73]

关于心境稳定剂用于肝损害患者的建议见表 8.3。

表 8.3　心境稳定剂在肝功能损害中的应用

药物	评论
卡马西平 [55]	大部分经肝脏代谢,是 CYP450 酶的强诱导剂(可导致 GGT 和碱性磷酸酶轻度升高,但这不是停药的指征 [5])。慢性且病情稳定的肝病,建议慎用。急性肝病患者禁用。起始剂量减半,缓慢加量,根据血药浓度调整剂量。若肝功能恶化,停用。可能会引起肝炎、胆管炎、胆汁淤积性黄疸、肝细胞性黄疸、肝衰竭(罕见)。肝脏不良反应最常见于开始治疗的第 1 个月 [73]。肝细胞损害经常与预后不良相关。对卡马西平所致肝功能损害的易感性可能由基因决定 [73]
拉莫三嗪	制药商建议中度肝功能损害患者起始剂量、递增剂量和维持剂量都减少 50%,重度肝功能损害减少 75%。如果拉莫三嗪引起皮疹(可能很严重),停止使用。建议使用时要非常谨慎,特别是妇女、儿童及合用丙戊酸盐时。曾有肝功能指标升高和肝炎的报告
锂盐 [6]	不经过肝脏代谢,所以只要肾功能正常,无需减少剂量。根据血清药物浓度调整剂量,如果腹水情况改变(分布容积会改变),需更密切监测血锂浓度。长期治疗时,小部分患者报告无症状的、一过性的肝功能异常 [19]。在全球使用锂盐的几十年中,有 1 例腹水的报告,1 例高胆红素血症的报告
丙戊酸盐 [74]	蛋白结合率高,经肝脏代谢。中度肝功能损害时,需减少剂量,并密切监测肝功能。根据血浆药物浓度(测定游离药物水平——总浓度可能正常)来指导剂量调整。建议慎用。禁用于严重或活动性肝损害、严重肝损害家族史者;常见代谢途径受损,可通过旁路代谢产生具有肝毒性的代谢产物。肝功能不全者若合用水杨酸盐,则肝毒性的风险升高。该药与肝功能升高和严重肝毒性有关(包括暴发性肝衰竭,有时致死)。线粒体疾病、学习障碍、使用多种药物、代谢紊乱和基础肝病都有可能是风险因素。对年幼儿童的肝毒性特别强。使用药物的头 3 个月风险最大

兴奋剂在肝功能损害中的应用 [5,6,75]

关于兴奋剂用于肝损害患者的建议见表 8.4。

表 8.4　兴奋剂在肝功能损害中的应用

药物	建议
托莫西汀 [76]	起始剂量和目标剂量:中度肝损害减少 50%,重度肝损害减少 75%。罕见肝毒性的报告,表现为肝脏转氨酶升高、胆红素升高伴有黄疸。SPC 表明:"出现黄疸或肝功能损害的实验室证据时,停止使用,并且永远不再用"
哌甲酯 [77]	罕见肝功能异常和超敏反应的报告
右苯丙胺、苯丙胺 [78,79]	在肝病中的经验不多。厂家建议慎重地进行剂量滴定。肝功能异常很罕见,有 2 例肝毒性的报告 [80,81]

镇静剂在肝功能损害中的应用

表 8.5 总结了推荐用于肝功能损害的镇静剂。

表 8.5　镇静剂在肝功能损害中的应用

药物	建议
苯二氮䓬类	大部分经肝脏代谢。作用时间延长,特别是有活性代谢产物者(地西泮、咪达唑仑、氯硝西泮)。劳拉西泮、奥沙西泮和替马西泮无活性代谢产物,属于首选。劳拉西泮在晚期肝病中耐受性最好 [6],常用于酒戒断综合征。血清酶升高不常见,肝损害罕见 [19]
异丙嗪 [6]	大部分经肝脏代谢。制药商建议慎用于肝损害者。大剂量时有黄疸的报告,小剂量时没有肝功能异常或肝毒性的报告 [19]
Z 类药 [6,82,83]	经肝脏代谢,但半衰期均相当短(1~7h)。轻、中度肝损害时,减少起始剂量(佐匹克隆 3.75mg、唑吡坦 5mg、扎来普隆 5mg),重度肝损害时避免使用。肝损害时,扎来普隆有明显的首过代谢,唑吡坦的血浆浓度和半衰期明显增加;这些药物应该慎用 [84]。佐匹克隆的半衰期较长,但是可能没有临床意义,除非严重肝病 [83]。佐匹克隆和扎来普隆未见肝毒性。唑吡坦罕见肝功能异常的报告,有 1 例肝损害 [19]
褪黑素 [6,85]	肝损害时,褪黑素的处置比较复杂:白天清除率下降,半衰期延长,导致血液中内源性褪黑素水平升高;负反馈和毒性产物蓄积,导致内源性褪黑素生成减少。与外源性褪黑素的相关性不明,但是褪黑素的毒性极小。制药商建议避免用于肝病。罕见肝功能改变

其他精神药物在肝功能损害中的应用

表 8.6 总结了推荐用于肝功能损害的其他精神药物。

表 8.6　其他精神药物在肝功能损害中的应用

药物	建议
布美兰肽(Bremelanotide) [6]	轻、中度肝损害不需调整剂量。重度肝损害慎用,较容易出现不良反应 [27]。有 1 例急性肝炎的报告

续表

药物	建议
氘代丁苯那嗪 (Deutetrabenazine)[5,19]	未在肝损害中进行过研究,但根据使用氘代丁苯那嗪的经验,禁用。现有信息很少,未报告过具有临床意义的肝毒性。偶见无症状的 ALT 升高
莱博雷生 (Lemborexant)[6,27]	轻度肝损害不需调整剂量(有加重嗜睡的风险);中度肝损害时,起始剂量和最大剂量均为 5mg,每天 1 次;重度肝损害不建议使用。经验不多,未报告过肝毒性[86]
替洛利生 (Pitolisant)[5,27]	大部分经肝脏代谢。轻度肝损害不需调整剂量。中度肝损害时,半衰期延长 1 倍;用药 2 周后可增加剂量,每天最大剂量 18mg。重度肝损害时禁用。肝脏转氨酶升高不常见
索利氨酯 (Solriamfetol)[5]	不代谢。在肝损害中未发现问题,没有肝损害的报告
缬苯那嗪[6,19]	α-二氢四苯那嗪经肝代谢的前体药物。与氘代丁苯那嗪不同,并非禁用于肝病,但中、重度肝损害时,最大剂量为 40mg。资料很少,但没有具有临床意义的肝损害报告,有 1 例原有丙型肝炎被激活的报告

精神药物在肝功能损害中的应用

表 8.7 列出了推荐用于肝功能损害的精神药物。

表 8.7　精神药物在肝功能损害中的应用

药物类别	推荐药物
抗精神病药	**舒必利/氨磺必利**:若肾功能正常,不需要减少剂量 **帕立哌酮**:如果需要长效制剂
抗抑郁药	**帕罗西汀、舍曲林、西酞普兰或伏硫西汀**:小剂量起始。(如果需要)缓慢加量,方法同上
心境稳定剂	**锂盐**:根据血药浓度调整剂量。如果腹水情况发生改变,需谨慎
镇静剂	**劳拉西泮、奥沙西泮、替马西泮**:半衰期短且无活性代谢产物。使用小剂量且应慎重,因为严重肝病时使用镇静剂可诱发肝性脑病。 **佐匹克隆**:中度肝功能损害患者,慎重使用 3.75mg 的剂量

药物引起的肝损害

FDA 建议采用 Hy 法则评估新药的肝脏毒性,即 ALT 大于正常值上限的 3 倍,且血清胆红素大于正常值上限的 2 倍[5]。

药物导致肝损害的原因可能有:

- 直接与剂量相关的肝毒性(药物不良反应 1 型)。少数药物属于该类,如对乙酰氨基酚、酒精。
- 超敏反应(药物不良反应 2 型)。可表现为皮疹、发热和嗜酸性粒细胞增多。几乎所有药物都具有肝毒性,发生频率各异。

几乎各种类型的肝功能损害都可能出现,从轻度、一过性、无症状的肝功能升高,到暴发性肝衰竭。各种药物的肝毒性可能详见本节前述各表。

第 8 章

药物引起肝毒性的风险因素包括 [87]：

- 年龄增加
- 女性
- 饮酒
- 合用对酶有诱导作用的药物
- 遗传素质
- 肥胖
- 原有肝病（影响小）

当解读肝功能指标时，需记住 [88]：

- 12% 的健康成年人有一项肝功能指标超出正常值范围（高或低）。
- 在有临床意义的肝病患者中，多达 10% 肝功能正常。
- 单独 1 项肝功能指标对肝脏缺乏特异性，若大于 1 项的检查结果异常，则大大地增加了肝脏病理损害的可能性。
- 肝功能的绝对值并不能很好地代表疾病的严重程度。

当监测肝功能时：

- 在理想情况下，肝功能需在开始治疗前进行检测，这样可得到"基线"数值。
- 肝脏转氨酶水平升高数值小于正常范围上限值的 2 倍时，极少有临床意义。
- 大多数药物相关的肝脏转氨酶水平升高出现在治疗早期（第 1 个月），且为一过性的。它们表明这是肝脏对药物的适应过程而不是损害。一过性的肝脏转氨酶水平升高也可发生在体重增加期间 [89]。
- 如果肝脏转氨酶水平持续升高大于 3 倍，且继续升高或伴随临床症状，所怀疑的药物应停用。
- 当跟踪肝功能变化时，若肝脏转氨酶水平改变 >20%，需排除生物学和分析方法的变化。

参考文献

1. Slim M, et al. Hepatic safety of atypical antipsychotics: current evidence and future directions. *Drug Saf* 2016; 39:925–943.
2. Marwick KF, et al. Antipsychotics and abnormal liver function tests: systematic review. *Clin Neuropharmacol* 2012; 35:244–253.
3. Morlán-Coarasa MJ, et al. Incidence of non-alcoholic fatty liver disease and metabolic dysfunction in first episode schizophrenia and related psychotic disorders: a 3-year prospective randomized interventional study. *Psychopharmacology (Berl)* 2016; 233:3947–3952.
4. Baeza I, et al. One-year prospective study of liver function tests in children and adolescents on second-generation antipsychotics: is there a link with metabolic syndrome? *J Child Adolesc Psychopharmacol* 2018; 28:463–473.
5. Datapharm Communications Ltd. Electronic Medicines Compendium 2020; https://www.medicines.org.uk/emc.
6. IBM Watson Health. IBM Micromedex Solutions 2020; https://www.ibm.com/watson-health/about/micromedex.
7. Mallikaarjun S, et al. Effects of hepatic or renal impairment on the pharmacokinetics of aripiprazole. *Clin Pharmacokinet* 2008; 47:533–542.
8. Preskorn SH Clinically important differences in the pharmacokinetics of the ten newer "atypical" antipsychotics: part 3. Effects of renal and hepatic impairment. *J Psychiatr Pract* 2012; 18:430–437.
9. Chico G, et al. Clinical vignettes 482 aripiprazole causes cholelithiasis and hepatitis: a rare finding. *Am J Gastroenterol* 2005; 100:S164.
10. Kornischka J, et al. Acute drug-induced hepatitis during aripiprazole monotherapy: a case report 2016.
11. Castanheira L, et al. Aripiprazole-induced hepatitis: a case report. *Clin Psychopharmacol Neurosci* (The Official Scientific Journal of the Korean College of Neuropsychopharmacology) 2019; 17:551–555.
12. Peeters P, et al. Asenapine pharmacokinetics in hepatic and renal impairment. *Clin Pharmacokinet* 2011; 50:471–481.
13. Schultz K, et al. A case of pseudo-Stauffer's syndrome related to asenapine use. *Schizophr Res* 2015; 169:500–501.
14. Parikh NB, et al. Clinical role of brexpiprazole in depression and schizophrenia. *Ther Clin Risk Manag* 2017; 13:299–306.
15. Cutler AJ, et al. Evaluation of the long-term safety and tolerability of cariprazine in patients with schizophrenia: results from a 1-year open-label study. *CNS Spectr* 2018; 23:39–50.

16. Brown CA, et al. Clozapine toxicity and hepatitis. *J Clin Psychopharmacol* 2013; **33**:570–571.

17. Tucker P Liver toxicity with clozapine. *Aust NZJ Psychiatry* 2013; **47**:975–976.

18. Zarghami M, et al. Concurrent hepatotoxicity and neutropenia induced by clozapine. *Arch Iran Med* 2020; **23**:141–143.

19. LiverTox: Clinical and Research Information on Drug-Induced Liver Injury. Bethesda (MD): National Institute of Diabetes and Digestive and Kidney Diseases 2012; https://www.ncbi.nlm.nih.gov/books/NBK547852.

20. Lally J, et al. Hepatitis, interstitial nephritis, and pancreatitis in association with clozapine treatment: a systematic review of case series and reports. *J Clin Psychopharmacol* 2018; **38**:520–527.

21. Takács A, et al. Clozapine rechallenge in a patient with clozapine-induced hepatitis. *Australas Psychiatry* (Bulletin of Royal Australian and New Zealand College of Psychiatrists) 2019; **27**:535.

22. Amdisen A, et al. Zuclopenthixol acetate in viscoleo – a new drug formulation. An open Nordic multicentre study of zuclopenthixol acetate in Viscoleo in patients with acute psychoses including mania and exacerbation of chronic psychoses. *Acta Psychiatr Scand* 1987; **75**:99–107.

23. Wistedt B, et al. Zuclopenthixol decanoate and haloperidol decanoate in chronic schizophrenia: a double-blind multicentre study. *Acta Psychiatr Scand* 1991; **84**:14–21.

24. Demuth N, et al. [Flupentixol-induced acute hepatitis]. *Gastroenterol Clin Biol* 1999; **23**:152–153.

25. Nolen WA, et al. Disturbances of liver function of long acting neuroleptic drugs. *Pharmakopsychiatr Neuropsychopharmakol* 1978; **11**:199–204.

26. Vanda Pharmaceuticals Inc. FANAPT® (iloperidone) tablets 1mg 2mg 4mg 6mg 8mg 10mg 12mg indication and important safety information 2020; http://www.fanapt.com/product/pi/pdf/fanapt.pdf.

27. U.S. Food & Drug Administration. Drugs@FDA: FDA-approved drugs 2020; https://www.accessdata.fda.gov/scripts/cder/daf.

28. Greenwood J, et al. Lumateperone: a novel antipsychotic for schizophrenia. *Ann Pharmacother* 2020; **55**:98–104.

29. Amatniek J, et al. Safety of paliperidone extended-release in patients with schizophrenia or schizoaffective disorder and hepatic disease. *Clin Schizophr Relat Psychoses* 2014; **8**:8–20.

30. Macaluso M, et al. Pharmacokinetic drug evaluation of paliperidone in the treatment of schizoaffective disorder. *Expert Opin Drug Metab Toxicol* 2017; **13**:871–879.

31. Chang CH, et al. Paliperidone is associated with reduced risk of severe hepatic outcome in patients with schizophrenia and viral hepatitis: a nationwide population-based cohort study. *Psychiatry Res* 2019; **281**:112597.

32. Khorassani F, et al. Risperidone- and paliperidone-induced hepatotoxicity: case report and review of literature. *Am J Health Syst Pharm* 2020; zxaa224.

33. Das A, et al. Liver injury associated with quetiapine: an illustrative case report. *J Clin Psychopharmacol* 2017; **37**:623–625.

34. Monnelly EP, et al. Quetiapine for treatment of alcohol dependence. *J Clin Psychopharmacol* 2004; **24**:532–535.

35. Brown ES, et al. A randomized, double-blind, placebo-controlled trial of quetiapine in patients with bipolar disorder, mixed or depressed phase, and alcohol dependence. *Alcohol Clin Exp Res* 2014; **38**:2113–2118.

36. Vatsalya V, et al. Safety assessment of liver injury with quetiapine fumarate XR management in very heavy drinking alcohol-dependent patients. *Clin Drug Investig* 2016; **36**:935–944.

37. Holtmann M, et al. Risperidone-associated steatohepatitis and excessive weight-gain. *Pharmacopsychiatry* 2003; **36**:206–207.

38. Voican CS, et al. Antidepressant-induced liver injury: a review for clinicians. *Am J Psychiatry* 2014; **171**:404–415.

39. Freiesleben SD, et al. A systematic review of agomelatine-induced liver injury. *J Mol Psychiatry* 2015; **3**:4.

40. Gahr M, et al. Safety and tolerability of agomelatine: focus on hepatotoxicity. *Curr Drug Metab* 2014; **15**:694–702.

41. Billioti de Gage S, et al. Antidepressants and hepatotoxicity: a cohort study among 5 million individuals registered in the French National Health Insurance Database. *CNS Drugs* 2018; **32**:673–684.

42. Pladevall-Vila M, et al. Risk of acute liver injury in agomelatine and other antidepressant users in four European Countries: a cohort and nested case-control study using automated Health Data Sources. *CNS Drugs* 2019; **33**:383–395.

43. Hanje AJ, et al. Case report: fulminant hepatic failure involving duloxetine hydrochloride. *Clin Gastroenterol Hepatol* 2006; **4**:912–917.

44. Vuppalanchi R, et al. Duloxetine hepatotoxicity: a case-series from the drug-induced liver injury network. *Aliment Pharmacol Ther* 2010; **32**:1174–1183.

45. Lin ND, et al. Hepatic outcomes among adults taking duloxetine: a retrospective cohort study in a US health care claims database. *BMC Gastroenterol* 2015; **15**:134.

46. McIntyre RS, et al. The hepatic safety profile of duloxetine: a review. *Expert Opin Drug Metab Toxicol* 2008; **4**:281–285.

47. Bunchorntavakul C, et al. Drug hepatotoxicity: newer agents. *Clin Liver Dis* 2017; **21**:115–134.

48. Schenker S, et al. Fluoxetine disposition and elimination in cirrhosis. *Clin Pharmacol Ther* 1988; **44**:353–359.

49. Cai Q, et al. Acute hepatitis due to fluoxetine therapy. *Mayo Clin Proc* 1999; **74**:692–694.

50. Friedenberg FK, et al. Hepatitis secondary to fluoxetine treatment. *Am J Psychiatry* 1996; **153**:580.

51. Johnston DE, et al. Chronic hepatitis related to use of fluoxetine. *Am J Gastroenterol* 1997; **92**:1225–1226.

52. Hale AS New antidepressants: use in high-risk patients. *J Clin Psychiatry* 1993; 54 Suppl:61–70.

53. Stoeckel K, et al. Absorption and disposition of moclobemide in patients with advanced age or reduced liver or kidney function. *Acta Psychiatr Scand Suppl* 1990; **360**:94–97.

54. Lee KC, et al. Transdermal selegiline for the treatment of major depressive disorder. *Neuropsychiatr Dis Treat* 2007; **3**:527–537.

55. Thomas E, et al. Mirtazapine-induced steatosis. *Int J Clin Pharmacol Ther* 2017; **55**:630–632.

56. Shaheen AA, et al. The impact of depression and antidepressant usage on primary biliary cholangitis clinical outcomes. *PLoS One* 2018; **13**:e0194839.

57. Benbow SJ, et al. Paroxetine and hepatotoxicity. *BMJ* 1997; **314**:1387.

58. Kuhs H, et al. A double-blind study of the comparative antidepressant effect of paroxetine and amitriptyline. *Acta Psychiatr Scand Suppl* 1989; **350**:145–146.

59. de Bree H, et al. Fluvoxamine maleate: disposition in men. *Eur J Drug Metab Pharmacokinet* 1983; **8**:175–179.

60. Green BH Fluvoxamine and hepatic function. *Br J Psychiatry* 1988; **153**:130–131.

61. Milne RJ, et al. Citalopram: a review of its pharmacodynamic and pharmacokinetic properties, and therapeutic potential in depressive illness. *Drugs* 1991; **41**:450–477.

62. Lopez-Torres E, et al. Hepatotoxicity related to citalopram (Letter). *Am J Psychiatry* 2004; **161**:923–924.

63. Colakoglu O, et al. Toxic hepatitis associated with paroxetine. *Int J Clin Pract* 2005; **59**:861–862.

64. Rao N The clinical pharmacokinetics of escitalopram. *Clin Pharmacokinet* 2007; **46**:281–290.

65. Mullish BH, et al. Review article: depression and the use of antidepressants in patients with chronic liver disease or liver transplantation. *Aliment Pharmacol Ther* 2014; **40**:880–892.

66. Düll MM, et al. Treatment of pruritus secondary to liver disease. *Current Gastroenterology Reports* 2019; **21**:48.

67. A T, et al. Pharmacokinetics of reboxetine in volunteers with hepatic impairment. *Clin Drug Investig* 2000; **19**:473–477.

68. Medicines C. Lofepramine (Gamanil) and abnormal blood tests of liver function. *Current Problems* 1988; **23**:2.

69. Archer DF, et al. Cardiovascular, cerebrovascular, and hepatic safety of desvenlafaxine for 1 year in women with vasomotor symptoms associated with menopause. *Menopause* 2013; **20**:47–56.

70. Baird-Bellaire S, et al. An open-label, single-dose, parallel-group study of the effects of chronic hepatic impairment on the safety and pharmacokinetics of desvenlafaxine. *Clin Ther* 2013; **35**:782–794.

71. Ryan PB, et al. Atypical antipsychotics and the risks of acute kidney injury and related outcomes among older adults: a replication analysis and an evaluation of adapted confounding control strategies. *Drugs Aging* 2017; **34**:211–219.

72. Chen G, et al. Vortioxetine: clinical pharmacokinetics and drug interactions. *Clin Pharmacokinet* 2018; **57**:673–686.

73. Bjornsson E Hepatotoxicity associated with antiepileptic drugs. *Acta Neurol Scand* 2008; **118**:281–290.

74. Guo HL, et al. Valproic acid and the liver injury in patients with epilepsy: an update. *Curr Pharm Des* 2019; **25**:343–351.

75. Panei P, et al. Safety of psychotropic drug prescribed for attention-deficit/hyperactivity disorder in Italy. *Adverse Drug Reaction Bulletin* 2010:999–1002.

76. Reed VA, et al. The safety of atomoxetine for the treatment of children and adolescents with attention-deficit/hyperactivity disorder: a comprehensive review of over a decade of research. *CNS Drugs* 2016; **30**:603–628.

77. Tong HY, et al. Liver transplant in a patient under methylphenidate therapy: a case report and review of the literature. *Case Rep Pediatr* 2015; **2015**:437298.

78. Shire Pharmaceuticals Limited. Summary of product characteristics. Elvanse 20mg 30mg 40mg 50mg 60mg 70mg Hard Capsules 2019; https://www.medicines.org.uk/emc/product/2979/smpc.

79. Flynn Pharma Ltd. Summary of product characteristics. Amfexa 5mg 10mg 20mg Tablets 2018; https://www.medicines.org.uk/emc/product/7403/smpc.

80. Vanga RR, et al. Adderall induced acute liver injury: a rare case and review of the literature. *Case Rep Gastrointest Med* 2013; **2013**:902892.

81. Hood B, et al. Eosinophilic hepatitis in an adolescent during lisdexamfetamine dimesylate treatment for ADHD. *Pediatrics* 2010; **125**:e1510–1513.

82. SANOFI. Summary of product characteristics. Stilnoct 5mg 10mg film-coated tablets 2019; https://www.medicines.org.uk/emc/product/4931/smpc.

83. SANOFI. Summary of product characteristics. Zimovane 7.5mg and 3.75mg LS film-coated tablets 2019; https://www.medicines.org.uk/emc/product/2855/smpc.

84. Gunja N The clinical and forensic toxicology of Z-drugs. *J Med Toxicol* 2013; **9**:155–162.

85. Flynn Pharma Ltd. Summary of product characteristics. Circadin 2mg prolonged-release tablets 2019; https://www.medicines.org.uk/emc/product/2809/smpc.

86. Kärppä M, et al. Long-term efficacy and tolerability of lemborexant compared with placebo in adults with insomnia disorder: results from the phase 3 randomized clinical trial SUNRISE 2. *Sleep* 2020.

87. Grattagliano I, et al. Biochemical mechanisms in drug-induced liver injury: certainties and doubts. *World J Gastroenterol* 2009; **15**:4865–4876.

88. Rosalki SB, et al. Liver function profiles and their interpretation. *Br J Hosp Med* 1994; **51**:181–186.

89. Rettenbacher MA, et al. Association between antipsychotic-induced elevation of liver enzymes and weight gain: a prospective study. *J Clin Psychopharmacol* 2006; **26**:500–503.

扩展阅读

Telles-Correia D, et al. Psychotropic drugs and liver disease: A critical review of pharmacokinetics and liver toxicity. *WJGPT*, 2017; **8**:26–37.

第 8 章

肾功能损害

　　肾功能损害患者使用药物时需慎重考虑。其部分原因是一些药物具有肾毒性,但主要原因是肾功能损害影响药物的药代动力学特性(吸收、分布、代谢、排泄)。特别是肾功能损害患者排泄药物及其代谢产物的能力会降低。

肾功能损害时的一般处方原则

- 通过计算肾小球滤过率(GFR)**评估肾脏的排泄能力**。GFR 的评估方法是测定以下指标:
  - 理想的滤过标志物,如胰岛素或乙二胺四乙酸(EDTA)(后者可以精确估计,但是价格非常高,且为有创操作)。
  - 血清肌酐——方法简单而费用便宜,但是即使进行过必要的校正,仍然只能大致估计肾功能。
  - 胱抑素 C 蛋白——比检测肌酐贵,但是更准确。
- 检测尿蛋白,方法是测定尿液中的白蛋白,计算白蛋白/肌酐比值。其原因是,尿蛋白是肾脏疾病进展到晚期的明显的危险因素[1]。
- 采用公式,该公式考虑到其他因素,采用血清肌酐和胱抑素 C 提高 GFR 的准确性(图8.1)。注意这些估计方法均不如直接测定的 GFR 完美[2,3]。慢性肾脏疾病流行病学协作组(CKD-EPI)公式比 MDRD 更准确,因而现在受到青睐。

---

　　a) **Cockroft-Gault 公式** *

$$肌酐清除率(mL/min) = \frac{F[\,140-\,年龄(岁)\,] \times\, 理想体重(kg)}{血清肌酐浓度(\mu mol/L)}$$

F = 1.23(男性),F = 1.04(女性)

当患者体重过重、过轻时,使用理想体重,否则计算结果不准:

男性,理想体重(kg) = 50(kg)+2.3kg/英寸 ×(身高–50 英寸)

女性,理想体重(kg) = 45.5(kg)+2.3kg/英寸 ×(身高–50 英寸)(1 英寸 =2.54cm)

---

　　* 血浆肌酐浓度不稳定(如急性肾衰竭)、孕妇、儿童、疾病引起异常肌酐升高时,该公式不准确。此外,该公式目前只在白种人患者中得到验证。肌酐清除率与 GFR 不同,在严重肾衰竭患者中,肌酐清除率对GFR 的代表性相对较差。

---

　　b) **慢性肾脏疾病流行病学协作组(CKD-EPI)公式**取代以前用的肾脏疾病饮食校正(MDRD)[2] 公式,但一些病理科仍然使用 MDRD。

　　$GFR=141\times\min(Scr/\kappa,1)^{\alpha}\times\max(Scr/\kappa,1)^{-1.209}\times0.993^{年龄}\times1.108(女性)\times1.159(黑人)$

Scr:血清肌酐(mg/dL)

κ:女 0.7,男 0.9

α:女 –0.329,男 –0.411

min:指 Scr/κ 或 1 的最小值

max:指 Scr/κ 或 1 的最大值

- **使用 Cockroft-Gault 公式计算药物剂量。**

计算用药剂量时,使用 Cockroft-Gault 公式估算肌酐清除率。
不能使用 CKD-EPI 或 MDRD 公式计算用药剂量,因为目前大多数药物推荐剂量都是根据 Cockroft-Gault 公式所计算的肌酐清除率来评估的。

肾功能损害分期[3]

			ACR 类别(mg/mmol) 描述与范围		
			A1	A2	A3
			正常到轻度增加	中度增加	明显增加
			<3	3~30	>30
GFR 类别[mL/(min·1.73m²)] 描述与范围	G1	正常,高	≥90	无肾脏损害的标志,无慢性肾脏疾病	在初级保健机构按照建议管理(见程序 C) 有下述情况时请专家评估: • GFR 持续下降 25% 以上且 GFR 类别改变,或 12 个月内 GFR 持续下降 15mL/(min·1.73m²) 以上 • 高血压始终控制不佳,但是已经使用过至少 4 种治疗剂量的降压药(另见 NICE 高血压临床指南) • 已知或怀疑为罕见或遗传性慢性肾脏疾病 • 怀疑肾动脉狭窄	若符合 A2 任一标准,或者: • ACR 达 70mg/mmol 以上,除非已知是糖尿病所致,且已妥善治疗 • 血尿
	G2	相对于青年的正常值范围,轻度下降	60~89		
	G3a	轻-中度下降	45~59		
	G3b	中-重度下降	30~44		
	G4	明显下降	15~29		
	G5	肾功能衰竭	<15		

图 8.1　肾功能损害分类。ACR,白蛋白/肌酐比值;CKD,慢性肾脏疾病

注意事项

■ 长期监测肾功能的下降情况,因为 2 年时间内变化 30%,会使晚期肾脏疾病的风险增加 5 倍。慢性肾脏疾病的进展往往呈非线性[4]。

■ 采用 Tangri 法监测从慢性肾脏疾病 3~5 期(eGFR 10~59)进展到透析/移植的风险,见 https://qxmd.com/calculate/calculator_125/kidney-failure-risk-equation-8-variable。采用 4 变量(年龄、性别、eGFR、尿白蛋白/肌酐比值)公式,可准确地预测慢性肾脏疾病 3~5 期患者 2 年内进展到肾衰竭(透析或移植)的可能性,而 8 变量(前述 4 个变量,加上血清钙、磷、碳酸氢盐、白蛋白)公式则可预测 5 年期患者的进展[5]。

■ 一般而言,肾功能明显影响药物的消除;以原形经尿排泄的药物数量应占所用剂量的 30% 以上[6]。

■ **老年人(>65 岁)应被视为具有至少轻度肾功能损害。**老年人肌肉重量较轻,血清肌酐可能不会升高。

■ 肾功能储备受限者,**避免使用具有肾毒性的药物**(如锂盐、NSAID)。

■ **慎用经肾脏广泛清除的药物**(例如舒必利、氨磺必利、锂盐)。

■ 有肾脏病时,经肝脏代谢药物的消除可能减少,可能的原因是血尿导致酶活性受到抑制[7]。

- **低剂量起始，缓慢加量**。因为肾功能损害时，药物的半衰期及达到稳态浓度（持续给药时吸收与消除数量相同）的时间通常会延长。使用一些药物时，监测血浆药物浓度可能有用。

- **避免使用长效药物**（例如长效注射剂）。一旦肾功能改变，用药剂量及频率可能很难调整。

- **用药种类尽可减少**。肾衰竭患者会使用多种药物，需要定期评估。若使用的药物种类少，就能避免药物间相互作用和不良反应。

- **监测患者的不良反应**。肾功能损害患者更易产生不良反应；他们出现不良反应的时间有可能晚于身体健康的患者。镇静、意识模糊、直立性低血压等不良反应比较常见。

- **慎用有抗胆碱能作用的药物**，因可能会引起尿潴留。

- 有关精神药物在肾功能损害患者中使用的**临床研究很少**。肾功能损害患者使用精神药物的建议往往依据的是躯体健康患者的药代动力学特征。

- **肾脏替代治疗**（例如透析）对药物的影响难以预测。详见表 8.4~ 表 8.9。向专家咨询。

- **避免使用已知能延长 Q-T 间期的药物**。确诊的肾衰竭患者常伴随电解质紊乱，所以尽可能避免使用 Q-T 间期延长风险最大的抗精神病药（参考 "Q-T 间期延长" 部分）。

- **密切监测体重**。体重增加可能会发展为糖尿病，从而有可能引起横纹肌溶解[8]及肾衰竭。精神药物通常会引起体重增加。

- **警惕抗抑郁药引起的 5-羟色胺综合征、抗精神病药引起的肌张力障碍及恶性综合征（NMS）**。所引起的横纹肌溶解可以造成肾衰竭。有案例报告使用抗精神病药的患者虽未出现恶性综合征的其他症状，但却出现了横纹肌溶解[9-11]。

- **慢性肾脏疾病患者常伴抑郁症**，但是在这种情况下抗抑郁药的疗效缺乏证据[12,13]。在慢性肾脏病患者中，抗抑郁药起始剂量高些，会降低死亡风险[14]。血液透析患者抑郁症的治疗效果不好[15]。非药物治疗，如认知行为治疗、锻炼或放松技术，可减轻透析患者的抑郁症状[16]。SSRI 与血液透析患者的髋骨骨折相关（AOR 1.25；95% *CI* 1.17，1.35）[17]。

- 精神分裂症和双相障碍患者发生慢性肾脏病的风险增加[18,19]。

- 抗精神病药（如奥氮平、喹硫平）可引起急性肾功能损伤，可能原因是影响血压和导致尿潴留[20]，但是研究结果不一致[21]。

- **有心境稳定作用的抗癫痫药增加慢性肾脏疾病的发生率**[19]。

表 8.8　抗精神病药在肾功能损害中的应用

药物	评论
氨磺必利[22-25]	主要经肾排泄。50% 以原形经尿排泄。在肾脏疾病中使用经验有限。制药商表明没有使用剂量 >50mg 的资料，但推荐如下用法：GFR 30~60mL/min 时，使用原剂量的 50%；10~30mL/min 时，使用原剂量的 33%；GFR <10mL/min 时，无推荐剂量，所以**最好避免用于已确诊的肾衰竭**
阿立哌唑[22,23,25-29]	低于 1% 的阿立哌唑以原形经肾排泄。制药商声称，肾衰竭患者使用时不需调整剂量，因为该药的药代动力学特征在健康人群和严重肾脏疾患者 群间无明显差别。有个案报告正在接受透析治疗的 83 岁老年男性口服阿立哌唑 5mg 时用药安全。尽可能避免使用长效剂型，尽管有 1 例接受血液透析的 64 岁男性使用 400mg 长效制剂

续表

药物	评论
阿塞那平[23,25,30]	制药商声称,肾功能损害患者使用时不需调整剂量,但缺乏 GFR <15mL/min 时的用药经验。一项在肾功能损害患者中单次使用 5mg 剂量的研究提示无需调整剂量。在轻、中、重度[eGFR 分别是 60~89、30~59、15~29mL/(min·1.73m²)]肾功损害的患者中,建议不调整剂量
氯丙嗪[22,23,25,31,32]	低于 1% 的药物以原形经尿排泄。制药商建议避免用于肾功能障碍患者。剂量:GFR 10~50mL/min,剂量同肾功能正常者;GFR <10mL/min,低剂量起始,因为抗胆碱能、镇静和低血压不良反应的风险增加。严密监护
氯氮平[23,25,33–37]	只有微量氯氮平以原形经尿排泄;但有罕见案例报告药物引起间质性肾炎和急性肾衰竭。夜间遗尿及尿潴留是常见的不良反应。制药商称该药禁用于严重肾脏疾病。肾脏疾病患者发生抗胆碱能反应、镇静和低血压等不良反应的频率更高。剂量:GFR 10~50mL/min 时,剂量同肾功能正常者,但需谨慎;GFR<10mL/min 时,低剂量起始,缓慢加量(根据肾内科专家的意见)。疾病分期对指导用药有用。可能会引起或加重糖尿病(肾脏疾病的常见病因)。有肾移植后成功继续使用的报告[38]
氟哌噻吨[22,23,25]	极少以原形经肾排泄。剂量:GFR 10~50mL/min 时,使用剂量同肾功能正常者;GFR <10mL/min 时,从正常剂量的 1/4~1/2 开始使用,缓慢加量。在肾功能损害者中,可能会引起低血压和镇静,并且会在体内蓄积。制药商建议肾衰竭患者慎用。肾功能损害者避免使用长效制剂
氟哌啶醇[10,22,23,25,39,40]	低于 1% 的药物以原形经尿排泄。制药商建议肾衰竭者慎用。剂量:GFR 10~50mL/min 时,使用剂量同肾功能正常者;GFR <10mL/min 时,低剂量起始,因为多次给药会在体内蓄积。个案报告提示,肾衰竭患者使用氟哌啶醇时建议低剂量起始,缓慢加量。曾被用于治疗肾衰竭患者尿毒症期的恶心症状。肾功能损害者避免使用长效制剂
卢美哌隆[41,42]	小于 1% 以原形经尿排泄。制药商建议肾功损害时,不需要调整剂量
鲁拉西酮[43]	9% 的药物以原形经尿排泄。制药商建议 GFR<50mL/min 时,可调整剂量[起始剂量为 18.75(20)mg/d,最大剂量 74(80)mg/d];GFR<15mL/min 时,避免使用。罕见引起肾衰竭的报告
奥氮平[9,22,23,25,40,44]	57% 的奥氮平主要以代谢产物的形式经尿排泄(7% 以原形药物经尿排泄)。剂量:GFR <50mL /min 时,最初 5mg/d,必要时加量。肾功能损害患者避免使用长效制剂,除非口服剂量耐受性好且有效。制药商建议,肾功能损害患者使用小剂量长效针剂,起始剂量为每隔 4 周注射 150mg。可能会引起和加重糖尿病(肾脏疾病的常见病因)。有报告称在肾衰竭患者中使用该药会引起体温过低
帕利哌酮[22,23,25]	帕利哌酮也是利培酮的代谢产物。59% 以原形药物经尿排泄。剂量:GFR 50~80mL/min,3mg/d,根据治疗反应增至最大剂量 6mg/d;GFR 10~50mL/min,3mg 隔天服用,根据治疗反应增至 3mg/d。清除率降低 71% 的严重肾脏疾病慎用。制药商建议:GFR<10mL/min 时为口服禁忌证,GFR <50ml/min 时为长效制剂的禁忌证,GFR50~80mL /min 时减少负荷剂量和维持剂量。有 1 例做血液透析的肾功能衰竭患者每月注射 1 次帕利哌酮取得成功[45]

药物	评论
匹莫范色林 [41,46]	低于 1% 以原形药物经尿排泄。制药商建议：GFR≥30mL/min 时不需调整剂量；但是 GFR <10mL/min 时，建议不用，因为没有资料
匹莫齐特 [22,23,25]	低于 1% 的匹莫齐特以原形药物经尿排泄；肾功能损害时一般无需降低剂量。剂量：GFR 10~50mL/min 时使用剂量同肾功能正常者；GFR <10mL/min 时，低剂量起始，根据治疗反应增加剂量。制药商建议肾衰竭者慎用
喹硫平 [22,23,25,47-49]	低于 5% 的喹硫平以原形药物经尿排泄。当 GFR<30mL/min 时，血浆清除率平均降低 25%。GFR <10~50mL/min 时，开始剂量为 25mg/d，此后每天增加 25~50mg 达到有效剂量。已发表个案报告提到，使用喹硫平者出现血栓性血小板减少性紫癜、DRESS 综合征、非恶性综合征（NMS）性横纹肌溶解，继而导致急性肾衰竭
利培酮 [22,23,25,40,50-53]	在中、重度肾脏疾病患者中，利培酮及其活性代谢产物 9-OH-利培酮的清除率降低了 60%。剂量：GFR<50mL/min 时，0.5mg，2 次/d，至少持续 1 周，然后按照 0.5mg，2 次/d 的增量，增至 1~2mg，2 次/d。制药商建议肾功能损害者慎用。口服利培酮只有按照上述方法加量后，才能使用长效针剂。如果患者能够耐受 2mg 的口服剂量，可肌内注射 25mg，两周 1 次。有 2 例血液透析患者成功使用利培酮长效针剂的报告，1 例患者用的剂量是 50mg，每 2 周一次；另 1 例老年患者用的剂量是先是 37.5mg，后降到 25mg。但是，曾经有个案报告透析患者成功地使用长效针剂 50mg 两周 1 次。另一则个案报告提到，利培酮用于 1 例肾病综合征伴类固醇激素所致精神病的儿童患者，疗效良好
舒必利 [8,22,23,25,54]	几乎全部经肾排泄，95% 的舒必利以原形药物经尿和粪便排泄。剂量：GFR 30~60mL/min，给予正常剂量的 70%；GFR 10~30mL/min，给予正常剂量的 50%；GFR <10mL/min，给予正常剂量的 34%。有 1 例肾衰竭的个案报告，是舒必利引起了糖尿病性昏迷和横纹肌溶解所造成的。**也许最好避免用于肾功能损害**
三氟拉嗪 [25]	低于 1% 的药物以原形经尿排泄。剂量：GFR <10~50mL/min，剂量同肾功能正常者——低剂量开始使用。相关数据很少
齐拉西酮 [22,40,55,56]	低于 1% 的药物以原形经肾排泄。GFR >10mL/min 的患者无需调整剂量，但使用针剂时需要谨慎，因为它包含需要经肾清除的赋形剂（环糊精钠盐）。个案报告，1 例血液透析患者使用 80mg，2 次/天，后来发生粒细胞缺乏 [57]
珠氯噻醇 [22,23,25]	10%~20% 的原形药和代谢产物经尿排泄。由于药物可在体内蓄积，制药商建议肾脏病患者需慎用。剂量：GFR 10~50mL/min 使用剂量同肾功能正常者；GFR <10mL/min，开始时使用正常剂量的 50%，缓慢增加剂量。肾功能损害者避免使用长效制剂（醋酸盐和癸酸盐）

表 8.9　抗抑郁药在肾功能损害中的应用 [6]

药物	评论
阿戈美拉汀 [23]	极少以原形药物经肾排泄。无肾脏疾病患者使用本药物的数据。制药商称：在一项小规模研究中，严重肾功能损害患者使用剂量为 25mg 时，并未发现药代动力学改变，但中、重度肾脏疾病患者慎用。在大鼠中发现有肾脏保护作用 [58,59]

药物	评论
阿米替林 [22,23,25,32,40,60-64]	低于 2% 以原形药物经尿排泄;肾衰竭患者无需调整剂量。使用剂量同肾功能正常者,但需从低剂量开始,缓慢加量。监测患者尿潴留、意识模糊、镇静和直立性低血压的情况。已被用于治疗肾脏疾病患者的疼痛症状。监测血药浓度或心电图可能有用。与急性肾损害相关
别孕烯醇酮 [41,65]	低于 1% 以原形药物经尿排泄。制药商称:GFR 15~60mL/min 时不需要调整剂量;GFR<15mL/min 时避免使用,因为注射增溶剂磺丁基醚-β-环糊精钠有可能蓄积
安非他酮 [22,23,25,32,40,66-68]	0.5% 以原形药物经尿排泄。剂量:GFR<50mL/min 时,150mg,1 次/d。一项关于肾透析患者(5 期)使用该药的单次剂量研究推荐每 3 天服用 150mg。在肾功能损害的患者,代谢产物可能会蓄积,清除率相应降低。血药浓度升高会增加癫痫发作的风险。已经用于治疗慢性肾脏疾病伴轻、中度抑郁患者的性功能障碍
西酞普兰 [22,23,25,40,69-75]	低于 13% 以原形药物经尿排泄。轻、中度肾功能损害患者单次剂量研究显示药代动力学特征并未改变。使用剂量同肾功能正常者;但是 GFR<10mL/min 时慎用,因为此时肾清除率会降低。制药商建议 GFR<20mL/min 时不用。曾有西酞普兰药物过量引起肾衰竭的报告。西酞普兰可用于治疗慢性肾衰竭患者的抑郁症,提高生命质量。但是,西酞普兰(或左旋西酞普兰)用于血液透析患者时,心源性猝死的风险高于其他 SSRI(氟西汀、氟伏沙明、帕罗西汀、舍曲林)(校正危险比 1.18,95% CI 1.05~1.31)。一个案报告使用西酞普兰的肾移植患者出现了低钠血症
氯米帕明 [22,23,25,32,76]	低于 2% 以原形药物经尿排泄。剂量:GFR 20~50mL/min 时,剂量同肾功能正常者;GFR<20mL/min,作用不明,低剂量开始,监测患者尿潴留、意识模糊、镇静和直立性低血压的情况,因药物可能会在体内蓄积。曾有个案报告氯米帕明可引起间质性肾炎和可逆的急性肾衰竭
去甲文拉法辛 [12,22,77,78]	45% 以原形药物经尿排泄。制药商推荐:GFR 30~50mL/min 时,50mg/d;GFR<30mL/min 时,25mg/d。当 GFR 降低时,去甲文拉法辛的半衰期延长,导致在体内蓄积。尿潴留、排尿延迟及蛋白尿都是已报告过的不良反应
度硫平 [22,25,79]	56% 的主要活性代谢产物经肾排泄。这些代谢产物的半衰期长,可能会在体内蓄积引起过度镇静。剂量:GFR 20~50mL/min 时,剂量同肾功能正常者;GFR<20mL/min 时,低剂量开始,渐加剂量至有效。监测患者尿潴留、意识模糊、镇静和直立性低血压的情况
多塞平 [22,23,25,32,80]	低于 1% 以原形药物经尿排泄。GFR 10~50mL/min 时,剂量同肾功能正常者,但需监测患者尿潴留、意识模糊、镇静和直立性低血压的情况;GFR<10mL/min 时,小剂量起始,缓慢加量。制药商建议慎用。曾报告使用多塞平出现溶血性贫血伴肾衰竭。局部使用可治疗慢性肾衰竭的瘙痒
度洛西汀 [22,25,81-83]	低于 1% 以原形药物经尿排泄。制药商建议:GFR>30mL/min 时无需调整剂量,但建议从低剂量开始,缓慢加量。GFR<30mL/min 时禁用,因为慢性肾脏疾病会导致药物在体内蓄积。已批准用于治疗糖尿病性神经痛及女性压力性尿失禁。糖尿病是引起肾功能损害的常见病因。有 2 个病例报告使用度洛西汀引起了急性肾衰竭。1 个慢性肾脏疾病患者合用曲唑酮和度洛西汀时,出现 5-羟色胺综合征 [84]

第 8 章

续表

药物	评论
艾司西酞普兰 [22,25,75,85-87]	8% 以原形药物经尿排泄。制药商建议：对轻、中度肾功能损害患者，无需调整剂量，但需注意当 GFR<30mL/min 时，低剂量起始，缓慢加量。有个案报告使用艾司西酞普兰出现可逆性肾小管损害，另一报告提到艾司西酞普兰引起了肾衰竭。有一项研究表明对于终末期肾脏疾病，艾司西酞普兰与安慰剂相比，治疗有效。血液透析患者使用艾司西酞普兰（或西酞普兰）时，引起心源性猝死的风险高于其他 SSRI（氟西汀、氟伏沙明、帕罗西汀、舍曲林）（校正危险比 1.18，95% CI 1.05，1.31）
氟西汀 [13,22,23,25,32,88-91]	2.5%~5% 的氟西汀及 10% 的活性代谢产物去甲氟西汀以原形经尿排泄。剂量：GFR 20~50mL/min，使用剂量同肾功能正常者；GFR<20mL/min，使用低剂量或隔天使用，根据疗效增加剂量。20mg 使用两个月后的血药浓度（GFR<10mL/min 正在透析的患者）与肾功能正常者相似。关于氟西汀用于抑郁症伴肾脏疾病患者的疗效研究结果并不一致。一项慢性透析患者的安慰剂对照、小型研究表明，治疗 8 周后，氟西汀组与安慰剂组的抑郁量表评分无明显差异。另一项研究发现氟西汀有效。一个病例系列分析（n=4）发现，接受血液透析的抑郁症患者每周一次使用氟西汀 90mg 或 180mg 均有效，90mg 的耐受性更好
氟伏沙明 [22,25,32,40,63]	2% 以原形药物经尿排泄。肾功能损害患者使用该药的相关数据很少。制药商建议肾功能损害患者需慎用。剂量：GFR 10~50mL/min 时，使用剂量同肾功能正常者；GFR <10mL/min，使用剂量同肾功能正常的人群，但需从低剂量开始，缓慢加量。曾有急性肾功能衰竭的报告。在血液透析中，白蛋白水平的变化影响氟伏沙明的血浆水平
丙米嗪 [22,25,32,40,63]	低于 5% 的药物以原形药物经尿排泄。肾功能损害者（GFR <10~50mL/min）无需特意调整剂量。监测患者尿潴留、意识模糊、镇静和直立性低血压的情况。有使用丙米嗪引起肾损害的报告，制药商建议严重肾损害患者需慎用。罕见肾损害的报告
洛非帕明 [22,23,25,92]	关于肾功能损害者使用洛非帕明的资料极少。低于 5% 的药物以原形经尿排泄。剂量：GFR 10~50mL/min 时，使用剂量同肾功能正常者；GFR <10mL/min 时，低剂量开始，逐渐增加。制药商禁止将其用于严重肾损害。与丙米嗪类似，去甲丙米嗪是主要代谢产物
米氮平 [22,23,25,93]	75% 以原形药物或代谢物经尿排泄。GFR 11~39mL/min 的患者清除率下降 30%，GFR<10mL/min 的患者清除率下降 50%。剂量：GFR 10~50mL/min 的患者，使用剂量同肾功能正常者；GFR <10mL/min 的患者，从低剂量开始，密切监测。米氮平已被用来治疗肾衰竭引起的瘙痒，以及透析患者的食欲丧失 [94]。米氮平与肾结石的形成有关
吗氯贝胺 [22,23,25,95,96]	低于 1% 以原形药物经尿排泄。然而，发现肾功能损害患者体内的活性代谢产物浓度增加，但并不影响剂量。制药商建议肾功能损害患者无需调整剂量。剂量：GFR<10~50mL/min 时，剂量同肾功能正常者
去甲替林 [22,25,32,40,60,97]	低于 5% 以原形药物经尿排泄。若 GFR 10~50mL/min，剂量同肾功能正常者；若 GFR< 10mL/min，低剂量开始。当剂量大于 100mg/d 时，推荐监测血药浓度，因为肾功能损害患者活性代谢产物的血浆浓度会升高。曾报告药物会加重老年患者 GFR 下降。监测血药浓度可能有益

续表

药物	评论
帕罗西汀 [22,23,25,32,98-101]	低于 2% 的口服剂量以原形药物经尿排泄。单次给药研究表明,当 GFR<30mL/min 时,帕罗西汀的血药浓度会增加。剂量建议:GFR 30~50mL/min 时,剂量同肾功能正常者;GFR< 10~30mL/min 时,从 10mg/d 的剂量开始(其他来源的数据推荐 20mg),根据疗效增加剂量。帕罗西汀 10mg/d 联合心理治疗已被用来成功治疗慢性透析患者的抑郁症。帕罗西汀很少造成范科尼综合征及急性肾衰竭
苯乙肼 [22,25]	接近 1% 以原形药物经尿排泄,肾衰竭患者无需调整用药剂量
瑞波西汀 [22,23,25,102,103]	接近 10% 以原形药物经尿排泄。剂量:GFR<20mL/min,2mg,2 次/d,根据疗效调整剂量。肾功能下降时,半衰期延长
舍曲林 [22,23,25,32,104-108]	低于 0.2% 的舍曲林以原形药物经尿排泄。单次给药研究表明,在肾功能损害时,该药的药代动力学特征未改变,但是没有多次给药研究的数据发表。剂量同肾功能正常者。舍曲林曾被用来治疗透析相关的低血压 [109] 及尿毒症瘙痒,但有舍曲林引起急性肾衰竭的报告,因此需慎用。总体上,舍曲林治疗共病抑郁症和慢性肾脏疾病的研究发现无效。在不依赖透析的肾脏疾病患者中进行的 CAST 研究,即舍曲林(剂量中位数 150mg)与安慰剂的 RCT 试验发现,两组间抑郁症状无显著差异 [108]。在患抑郁症的血液透析患者中进行了 ASCEND 试验,比较舍曲林与 CBT,结果发现舍曲林组(最大剂量 200mg)与 CBT 组的有效率和临床缓解率类似,但是治疗 12 周时的 QIDS-C 抑郁评分舍曲林组低于 CBT 组 [110]。另一项小样本 RCT 研究(ASSertID 研究),在血液透析的抑郁症患者中,舍曲林与安慰剂组无差异 [111]。血液透析患者使用舍曲林时会引起 5-羟色胺综合征。用于终末期肾病时有引起中性粒细胞减少的病例报告 [112]。在血液透析的抑郁症患者中,可降低 C 反应蛋白 [113],而 C 反应蛋白升高可以预测舍曲林对于伴有慢性肾脏疾病的抑郁症有效(安慰剂则否)[114]
曲唑酮 [22,23,25,115]	低于 5% 以原形药物经尿排泄,但需注意接近 70% 的活性代谢产物也经尿排泄。剂量:GFR 20~50mL/min,剂量同肾功能正常者;GFR 10~20mL/min,剂量同肾功能正常者,但需从低剂量开始,逐渐加量;GFR <10mL/min,低剂量开始,逐渐加量。1 例慢性肾脏疾病患者合用曲唑酮和度洛西汀后出现 5-羟色胺综合征 [84]
曲米帕明 [22,25,32,60,116,117]	肾功能损害患者无需减少药物剂量。但曾报告过尿素升高、急性肾衰竭与间质性肾炎。与所有三环类抗抑郁药一样,肾功能损害患者使用时,需监测患者的尿潴留、意识模糊、镇静和直立性低血压的情况,因为这些不良反应的风险会增加
文拉法辛 [22,25,32,60,118-120]	1%~10% 以原形药物经尿排泄(30% 以活性代谢产物经尿排泄)。肾功能损害患者的清除率降低,半衰期延长。用药建议:GFR 30~50mL/min,剂量同肾功能正常者,或减少 50%;GFR 10~30mL/min,减少剂量的 50%,1 次/d;GFR <10mL/min,减少剂量的 50%,1 次/d。文拉法辛引起横纹肌溶解及肾衰竭者罕见。已被用来治疗透析患者的糖尿病周围神经病。高剂量可能会引起高血压
伏硫西汀 [23,121]	经肾排泄的原形药物的量可忽略。制药商建议肾功能损害及终末期肾脏疾病使用时无需调整剂量,但是建议慎重

表 8.10　心境稳定剂在肾功能损害中的应用

药物	评论
卡马西平[22,23,25,122-129]	2%~3% 的剂量以原形药物经尿排泄。肾脏疾病患者无需减少剂量,尽管有卡马西平引起肾衰竭、肾小管坏死、小管间质性肾炎的罕见报告,代谢产物可能会在体内蓄积。可引起 Stevens-Johnson 综合征和中毒性表皮坏死松解症,继而造成急性肾衰竭。双相障碍维持治疗增加了慢性肾脏疾病的发生率[19]
拉莫三嗪[22,23,25,130-134]	低于 10% 的拉莫三嗪以原形药物经尿排泄。肾衰竭患者的单次给药研究表明,该药物的药代动力学特征几乎没有受影响;但是非活性代谢产物会在体内蓄积(作用不明),半衰期可被延长。也曾报告拉莫三嗪引起肾衰竭与间质性肾炎。剂量:GFR 10~50mL/min 时需慎用,低剂量开始,逐渐增加,密切监测。有数据建议 GFR <10mL/min 时,100mg 隔天服用
锂盐[22,23,25,32,135,136]	锂盐具有肾毒性,严重肾功能损害者禁用。95% 以原形药物经尿排泄。长期治疗可能会引起肾功能受损(“肌酐潜变”)、肾组织的永久性改变、微囊肿、嗜酸细胞瘤和集合管肾癌、肾性尿崩症、肾病综合征、可逆性和非可逆性肾损伤[137,138]。然而,在年轻人群中进行的短期研究未见 GFR 下降[139],或发生末期肾脏疾病[19]。导致这些不同的可能原因有方法学、监测方法改进以及推荐维持血清目标浓度(双相障碍为 0.6~0.8mmol/L)。 若发生慢性肾脏疾病,预防不良结局的方法包括每天给药一次,使用推荐的血浆浓度,避免中毒,积极监测肾功能,精神科医师、肾科医师和患者共同决定继续用药方案[140]。锂盐引起肾脏中毒的危险因素包括年龄增大、治疗持续时间、累积剂量、起始 eGFR 下降、女性、高血压和糖尿病、合用肾毒性药物、肾性尿崩症以及既往锂中毒[141]。 如果肾功能损害患者使用锂盐,更容易发生中毒,而锂中毒增加了肾功损害的风险。肾脏损害多见于慢性中毒,而非急性中毒。制药商建议肾功能损害为使用锂盐的禁忌证。剂量:GFR 10~50mL/min 时,避免使用或减少剂量(正常剂量的 50%~75%),并监测血药浓度;GFR <10mL/min 时,尽可能避免使用;如果要用,一定要减少剂量(正常剂量的 25%~50%)。有 1 例血液透析患者成功使用的个案报告[142]
丙戊酸盐[22,23,25,143-149]	接近 2% 以原形药物经尿排泄。肾功能损害患者无需调整用药剂量,但游离的丙戊酸盐浓度可能会增加。曾有丙戊酸盐引起肾功能损害、间质性肾炎、范科尼综合征、肾小管酸中毒与肾衰竭的报告。肾小管功能异常的危险因素包括长期卧床、血清肉碱和血磷水平低[150]。剂量同肾功能正常者,但严重肾功能损害者(GFR <10mL/min),可能必须根据游离的(非结合的)丙戊酸盐浓度调整剂量。在双相障碍患者中,导致慢性肾脏疾病的可能性小于锂盐[151],但资料是矛盾的[152]

表 8.11　抗焦虑药及催眠药在肾功能损害中的应用

药物	评论
丁螺环酮[22,23,25,32]	低于 1% 的药物以原形排泄,但活性代谢产物也经肾排出。剂量建议不一致,建议:GFR 10~50mL/min 时使用正常剂量;GFR <10mL/min 时,尽可能避免使用,因为活性代谢产物在体内蓄积。若必须使用,无尿患者需降低剂量 25%~50%。制药商建议严重肾功能损害为该药的禁忌证
氯氮草[23,25,32]	1%~2% 以原形药物排泄,但有一个长效的活性代谢物可在体内蓄积。剂量:GFR 10~50mL/min 时,剂量同肾功能正常者;GFR <10mL/min 时,剂量减少 50%。监测过度镇静的情况。制药商建议慢性肾脏疾病患者慎用

药物	评论
氯美噻唑 [22,23,25,153]	0.1%~5% 以原形药物经尿排泄。剂量同肾功能正常者,但需监测过度镇静的情况。制药商建议肾脏疾病患者慎用
氯硝西泮 [22,23,25,154]	低于 0.5% 的氯硝西泮以原形药物经尿排泄。肾功能损害者无需调整剂量;但长时间使用可能会造成活性代谢产物在体内蓄积,所以使用时需从低剂量开始,根据疗效增加剂量。监测过度镇静的情况。已经被用来治疗血液透析患者的失眠
地西泮 [22,25,32,155]	低于 0.5% 以原形药物排泄。剂量:GFR 20~50mL/min,剂量同肾功能正常者;GFR <20mL/min,使用低剂量,根据疗效增加剂量。长效的活性代谢产物在肾功能损害患者体内可蓄积;监测过度镇静和脑病的情况。曾有个案报告慢性肾衰竭患者使用地西泮引起了间质性肾炎
右佐匹克隆 [156]	低于 10% 以原形药物经尿排泄。肾功能损害者无需调整剂量
加巴喷丁	100% 以原形经尿排泄。肾功能损害时,清除率下降,导致血浆浓度升高,消除半衰期延长 [157]。肾功能损害者若不减量,预期会导致中毒 [158]。曾报告过急性肾衰竭 [159];肌阵挛 [160];用于治疗血液透析患者的不宁腿、瘙痒、神经性疼痛时出现过精神状态改变、摔倒骨折 [161,162]。随机试验用于治疗血液透析患者的瘙痒、肌肉痉挛和不宁腿综合征 [163-165]。剂量建议:GFR 15~60mL/min 时,小剂量起始,根据疗效加量;GFR<15mL/min 时,300mg,隔日 1 次 [32,159],或 100mg 每晚 1 次,然后根据耐受性加量 [25,166],但应注意前述中毒表现。制药商在产品特征概要中对肾功能损害患者的剂量有很具体的表格 [159]
莱博雷生 [41,167]	低于 1% 以原形药物经尿排泄。制药商称肾功能损害者不需调整剂量,但严重肾功能损害时,暴露量增加,可能会增加嗜睡的风险
劳拉西泮 [22,23,25,32,168-173]	<1% 以原形药物经尿排泄。剂量同肾功能正常者,但需注意根据疗效调整剂量,因为一些人可能需要减少剂量。监测过度镇静的情况。曾报告过 2 例严重肾功能损害患者该药物的清除率降低,也曾报告过注射劳拉西泮后其中的丙二醇成分引起了肾功能损害和急性肾小管坏死。但是注射劳拉西泮曾成功地治疗了 2 例肾衰竭患者的紧张症
硝西泮 [23,25]	<5% 以原形药物经尿排泄。剂量:GFR 10~50mL/min 时,剂量同肾功能正常者;GFR <10mL/min 时,低剂量开始,逐渐加量。制药商建议肾功能损害者需减少剂量。监测患者的镇静和不稳情况
普瑞巴林	高达 99% 以原形经尿排泄。有急性肾衰的报告 [174]。血液透析患者使用时出现过精神状态改变和摔倒 [161],以及肌阵挛 [175]。慢性肾脏疾病患者骤停药物有出现癫痫发作的案例 [176]。曾用于治疗血液透析患者的尿毒症性瘙痒和神经痛 [177,178]。剂量因人而异:对于全部 GFR,根据耐受情况和疗效逐渐调整剂量;GFR 30~60mL/min 时,75mg,1 次/d;GFR 15~30mL/min 时,25~50mg,1 次/d;GFR<15mL/min 时,25mg 1 次/d。制药商在产品特征概要中对肾功能损害患者的剂量有很具体的表格 [174]
奥沙西泮 [22,25,32,179]	<1% 以原形药物经尿排泄。严重肾功能损害者需调整用药剂量。奥沙西泮在肾功能损害患者体内需要较长的时间才能达到稳态浓度。剂量:GFR 10~50mL/min 时,剂量同肾功能正常者;GFR<10mL/min 时,从低剂量开始,根据疗效加量。监测过度镇静情况

续表

药物	评论
异丙嗪 [22,23,25,32,180]	一般无需减少剂量。但是异丙嗪有较长的半衰期,肾功能损害患者使用时需监测其过度镇静的情况。制药商建议肾功能损害者慎用。曾有间质性肾炎的个案报告,患者是异丙嗪的慢代谢者
替马西泮 [22,23,25,32]	<2% 以原形药物经尿排泄。非活性代谢产物在肾功能损害患者体内会蓄积。需监测患者过度镇静的情况。剂量:GFR 20~50mL/min 时,剂量同肾功能正常者;GFR <20mL/min 时,剂量同肾功能正常者,但起始剂量为 5mg
唑吡坦 [22,23,25,154,181]	在肾功能损害患者中,清除率中度下降。肾功能损害者无需调整剂量。1mg 的唑吡坦已被用来治疗血液透析患者的失眠 [182]。正在进行 RCT 研究唑吡坦在伴有瘙痒的血液透析患者中的助眠效果 [183]
佐匹克隆 [22,23,25,184,185]	<5% 以原形药物经尿排泄。制药商称:该药物不会在肾功能损害患者体内蓄积,但建议起始剂量为 3.75mg。剂量:GFR <10mL/min 时,从低剂量开始。间质性肾炎罕有报告

表 8.12　抗痴呆药在肾功能损害中的应用

药物	评论
多奈哌齐 [23,25,186-188]	17% 以原形药物经尿排泄。GFR <10~50mL/min 时,剂量同肾功能正常者。制药商称该药物的清除率不受肾损害影响。单次剂量给药研究发现,该药物在中、重度肾损害患者中的药代动力学特征与健康对照组相似。在接受透析治疗的 1 例老年阿尔茨海默病患者中,用过 3mg/d 的剂量。出现 1 例横纹肌溶解导致急性肾衰竭 [189]
加兰他敏 [23,25]	18%~22% 以原形药物经尿排泄。GFR 10~50mL/min 时,剂量同肾功能正常者。GFR <10mL/min 时,从低剂量起始,缓慢加量。制药商建议 GFR <10mL/min 的患者禁用。中、重度肾损害患者的血药浓度可能会升高
美金刚 [22,23,190]	制药商建议,GFR 5~29mL/min 时,使用剂量为 10mg;GFR 30~49mL/min 时,如果能够耐受,可用 10mg,1 次/d,7 天后,加量至 20mg 1 次/d。肾小管酸中毒、严重尿路感染、碱性尿(例如剧烈的饮食变化)可升高美金刚血药浓度。曾有急性肾衰竭报告
卡巴拉汀 [23,25]	0% 以原形药物经尿排泄。GFR <50mL/min 时推荐低剂量开始,逐渐加量。稳态血浆浓度不受肾功能影响 [191]

表 8.13　其他精神药物在肾功能损害中的使用

药物类别	评论
布美兰肽 [41,192]	64.8% 以原形经尿排泄。制药商称:GFR 30~89mL/min 时,不必调整剂量;GFR<30mL/min 时慎用,因增加不良反应。肾功能损害时,暴露量增多。有引起横纹肌溶解和肾功能异常的报告 [193]
氘代丁苯那嗪 [194]	未在肾损害患者中进行临床研究。资料有限,无具体剂量建议
替洛利生 [41,195]	<2% 以原形经尿排泄。剂量:GFR 15~59mL/min 时,9mg/d;7 天后最多增至 18mg/d [196];GFR<15mL/min 时不建议使用 [196]。肾损害各阶段峰浓度和暴露剂量均增加

续表

药物类别	评论
普芦卡必利 （Prucalopride）[41]	60%~65% 以原形经尿排泄。剂量：GFR≥30mL/min 时，不必调整剂量；GFR<30mL/min 时，1mg/d。制药商禁用于需要透析者。中、重度肾损害者暴露剂量增加[197]，肾损害各阶段血浆浓度均升高[198]。有引起肾小管坏死和急性肾衰竭的案例报告[199]
索利氨酯[41,200]	95% 以原形经尿排泄。剂量：GFR 60~89mL/min 时，不必调整剂量；GFR 30~59mL/min 时，37.5mg 每天 1 次，5 天后最多增至 75mg，每天 1 次；GFR 15~29mL/min 时，5mg，每天 1 次；GFR<15mL/min 时不建议使用。中、重度肾损害时，有血压升高和心率加快的风险，因为半衰期延长。在肾损害各阶段，特别是终末期肾脏疾病，暴露剂量和半衰期均增加[201]
缬苯那嗪[41]	2% 以原形经尿排泄。轻、中度肾损害 GFR 30~90mL/min 时，不必调整剂量；重度肾损害 GFR<30mL/min 时，制药商不建议使用[202]。临床试验报告的不良反应有尿潴留

小结——推荐用于肾损害的精神药物

若药物治疗时肾功能减退，则排除所用药物导致肾功能减退之后，继续使用表 8.8~表 8.13 推荐的剂量。若需要使用新药，则遵循下述建议：

药物类别	推荐药物
抗精神病药	■ 无明确的最优选择，但是避免使用舒必利和氨磺必利 ■ 禁止使用抗胆碱能作用强的药物，因为可能引起尿潴留 ■ 第一代抗精神病药——推荐使用**氟哌啶醇** 2~6mg/d ■ 第二代抗精神病药——推荐使用**奥氮平** 5mg/d
抗抑郁药[203]	■ 无明确的最优选择，但是合理的选择有： ■ **舍曲林**，但资料显示对肾脏疾病疗效不佳 ■ **西酞普兰**（注意血液透析患者出现 Q-T 间期延长和猝死的风险大于其他 SSRI） ■ **氟西汀**，但需注意其半衰期长，GFR 低时需要隔日给药 ■ 认知行为治疗，若可行
心境稳定剂	■ 无明确的最优选择，但是尽可能地避免使用锂盐 ■ 建议以下药物从低剂量起始，缓慢加量，同时监测不良反应：**丙戊酸盐**或**拉莫三嗪**
抗焦虑药及催眠药	■ 无明确的最优选择，但是肾功能损害患者更易出现过度镇静，需密切监测所有患者 ■ 推荐合理选择**劳拉西泮**和**佐匹克隆**
抗痴呆药物	■ 无明确的最优选择，但是**卡巴拉汀**是一种合理的选择

（苏允爱 译　田成华 审校）

参考文献

1. National Institute for Clinical Excellence. 4-year surveillance (2017) – Chronic kidney disease in adults (2014) NICE guideline [CG182]; https://www.nice.org.uk/guidance/cg182/evidence/appendix-a2-cg182-summary-of-new-evidence-from-surveillance-pdf-4429248447.

2. Levey AS, et al. A new equation to estimate glomerular filtration rate. *Ann Intern Med* 2009; 150:604–612.

3. National Institute for Health and Care Excellence. Chronic kidney disease in adults: assessment and management. Clinical Guidance 182 [CG182] 2015; https://www.nice.org.uk/guidance/cg182.

4. National Institute for Clinical Excellence. Surveillance report 2017 – Chronic kidney disease (stage 4 or 5): management of hyperphosphataemia

(2013) NICE Guideline CG157. Chronic kidney disease in adults: assessment and management (2014) NICE guideline CG182 and Chronic kidney disease: managing anaemia (2015) NICE guideline NG8 2017; https://www.nice.org.uk/guidance/cg182/resources/surveillance-report-2017-chronic-kidney-disease-stage-4-or-5-management-of-hyperphosphataemia-2013-nice-guideline-cg157-chronic-kidney-disease-in-adults-assessment-and-management-2014-nice-guideline-pdf-5740305984709.

5. Tangri N, et al. A predictive model for progression of chronic kidney disease to kidney failure. *JAMA* 2011; 305:1553–1559.

6. Brater DC. Measurement of renal function during drug development. *Br J Clin Pharmacol* 2002; 54:87–95.

7. Chinnadurai R, et al. Impact of chronic kidney disease on the drugs eliminated predominantly through a non-renal route: a proof of concept study with Citalopram. *Nephrol Dial Transplant* 2019; 34:gfz103.SP268.

8. Toprak O, et al. New-onset type II diabetes mellitus, hyperosmolar non-ketotic coma, rhabdomyolysis and acute renal failure in a patient treated with sulpiride. *Nephrol Dial Transplant* 2005; 20:662–663.

9. Baumgart U, et al. Olanzapine-induced acute rhabdomyolysis – a case report. *Pharmacopsychiatry* 2005; 38:36–37.

10. Marsh SJ, et al. Rhabdomyolysis and acute renal failure during high-dose haloperidol therapy. *Ren Fail* 1995; 17:475–478.

11. Smith RP, et al. Quetiapine overdose and severe rhabdomyolysis. *J Clin Psychopharmacol* 2004; 24:343.

12. Nagler EV, et al. Antidepressants for depression in stage 3-5 chronic kidney disease: a systematic review of pharmacokinetics, efficacy and safety with recommendations by European Renal Best Practice (ERBP). *Nephrol Dial Transplant* 2012; 27:3736–3745.

13. Palmer SC, et al. Antidepressants for treating depression in adults with end-stage kidney disease treated with dialysis. The Cochrane Database of Systematic Reviews 2016:CD004541.

14. Dev V, et al. Higher anti-depressant dose and major adverse outcomes in moderate chronic kidney disease: a retrospective population-based study. *BMC Nephrol* 2014; 15:79.

15. Guirguis A, et al. Antidepressant usage in haemodialysis patients: evidence of sub-optimal practice patterns. *J Ren Care* 2020; 46:124–132.

16. Natale P, et al. Psychosocial interventions for preventing and treating depression in dialysis patients. Cochrane Database of Systematic Reviews 2019; CD004542.

17. Vangala C, et al. Selective serotonin reuptake inhibitor use and hip fracture risk among patients on hemodialysis. *Am J Kidney Dis* 2020; 75:351–360.

18. Tzeng NS, et al. Is schizophrenia associated with an increased risk of chronic kidney disease? A nationwide matched cohort study. *BMJ Open* 2015; 5:e006777.

19. Kessing LV, et al. Use of lithium and anticonvulsants and the rate of chronic kidney disease: a nationwide population-based study. *JAMA Psychiatry* 2015; 72:1182–1191.

20. Jiang Y, et al. A retrospective cohort study of acute kidney injury risk associated with antipsychotics. *CNS Drugs* 2017; 31:319–326.

21. Ryan PB, et al. Atypical antipsychotics and the risks of acute kidney injury and related outcomes among older adults: a replication analysis and an evaluation of adapted confounding control strategies. *Drugs Aging* 2017; 34:211–219.

22. Truven Health Analytics. Micromedex 2.0. 2017; https://www.micromedexsolutions.com/home/dispatch.

23. Datapharm Ltd. Electronic Medicines Compendium 2020; https://www.medicines.org.uk/emc.

24. Noble S, et al. Amisulpride: a review of its clinical potential in dysthymia. *CNS Drugs* 1999; 12:471–483.

25. Taylor & Francis Group. Renal Drug Database 2020; https://renaldrugdatabase.com.

26. Aragona M. Tolerability and efficacy of aripiprazole in a case of psychotic anorexia nervosa comorbid with epilepsy and chronic renal failure. *Eat Weight Disord* 2007; 12:e54–e57.

27. Mallikaarjun S, et al. Effects of hepatic or renal impairment on the pharmacokinetics of aripiprazole. *Clin Pharmacokinet* 2008; 47:533–542.

28. Tzeng NS, et al. Delusional parasitosis in a patient with brain atrophy and renal failure treated with aripiprazole: case report. *Prog Neuropsychopharmacol Biol Psychiatry* 2010; 34:1148–1149.

29. De Donatis D, et al. Serum aripiprazole concentrations prehemodialysis and posthemodialysis in a schizophrenic patient with chronic renal failure: a case report. *J Clin Psychopharmacol* 2020; 40:200–202.

30. Peeters P, et al. Asenapine pharmacokinetics in hepatic and renal impairment. *Clin Pharmacokinet* 2011; 50:471–481.

31. Fabre J, et al. Influence of renal insufficiency on the excretion of chloroquine, phenobarbital, phenothiazines and methacycline. *Helv Med Acta* 1967; 33:307–316.

32. Aronoff GR, et al. *Drug Prescribing in Renal Failure: Dosing Guidelines for Adults and Children*. 5th edn. Philadelphia: American College of Physicians; 2007.

33. Fraser D, et al. An unexpected and serious complication of treatment with the atypical antipsychotic drug clozapine. *Clin Nephrol* 2000; 54:78–80.

34. Au AF, et al. Clozapine-induced acute interstitial nephritis. *Am J Psychiatry* 2004; 161:1501.

35. Elias TJ, et al. Clozapine-induced acute interstitial nephritis. *Lancet* 1999; 354:1180–1181.

36. Siddiqui BK, et al. Simultaneous allergic interstitial nephritis and cardiomyopathy in a patient on clozapine. *NDT Plus* 2008; 1:55–56.

37. Davis EAK, et al. Clozapine-associated renal failure: a case report and literature review. *Ment Health Clin* 2019; 9:124–127.

38. Lim AM, et al. Clozapine, immunosuppressants and renal transplantation. *Asian J Psychiatr* 2016; 23:118.

39. Lobeck F, et al. Haloperidol concentrations in an elderly patient with moderate chronic renal failure. *J Geriatr Drug Ther* 1986; 1:91–97.

40. Cohen LM, et al. Update on psychotropic medication use in renal disease. *Psychosomatics* 2004; 45:34–48.

41. Lendac Data Systems Ltd. Drugdex Systems 2020; https://www.drugdiscoveryonline.com/doc/drugdex-system-0001.

42. Intra-Cellular Therapies Inc. Highlights of prescribing information. Caplyta (lumateperone) capsules for oral use 2019; https://www.accessdata.fda.gov/drugsatfda_docs/label/2019/209500s000lbl.pdf.

43. Sunovion Pharmaceuticals Europe Ltd. Summary of Product Characteristics. Latuda 18.5mg, 37mg and 74mg film-coated tablets 2020;

https://www.medicines.org.uk/emc/medicine/29125.

44. Kansagra A, et al. Prolonged hypothermia due to olanzapine in the setting of renal failure: a case report and review of the literature. *Ther Adv Psychopharmacol* 2013; 3:335–339.

45. Samalin L, et al. Interest of clozapine and paliperidone palmitate plasma concentrations to monitor treatment in schizophrenic patients on chronic hemodialysis. *Schizophr Res* 2015; 166:351–352.

46. ACADIA Pharmaceuticals Inc. Highlights of prescribing information. Nuplazid (pimavanserin) tablets for oral use 2020; https://www.accessdata.fda.gov/drugsatfda_docs/label/2016/207318lbl.pdf.

47. Thyrum PT, et al. Single-dose pharmacokinetics of quetiapine in subjects with renal or hepatic impairment. *Prog Neuropsychopharmacol Biol Psychiatry* 2000; 24:521–533.

48. Huynh M, et al. Thrombotic thrombocytopenic purpura associated with quetiapine. *Ann Pharmacother* 2005; 39:1346–1348.

49. Torroba Sanz B, et al. Permanent renal sequelae secondary to drug reaction with eosinophilia and systemic symptoms (DRESS) syndrome induced by quetiapine. *Eur J Hosp Pharm* 2020:[Epub ahead of print].

50. Snoeck E, et al. Influence of age, renal and liver impairment on the pharmacokinetics of risperidone in man. *Psychopharmacology (Berl)* 1995; 122:223–229.

51. Herguner S, et al. Steroid-induced psychosis in an adolescent: treatment and prophylaxis with risperidone. *Turk J Pediatr* 2006; 48:244–247.

52. Batalla A, et al. Antipsychotic treatment in a patient with schizophrenia undergoing hemodialysis. *J Clin Psychopharmacol* 2010; 30:92–94.

53. Tourtellotte R, et al. Use of therapeutic drug monitoring of risperidone microspheres long-acting injection in hemodialysis: a case report. *Ment Health Clin* 2019; 9:404–407.

54. Bressolle F, et al. Pharmacokinetics of sulpiride after intravenous administration in patients with impaired renal function. *Clin Pharmacokinet* 1989; 17:367–373.

55. Aweeka F, et al. The pharmacokinetics of ziprasidone in subjects with normal and impaired renal function. *Br J Clin Pharmacol* 2000; 49:27S-33S.

56. Roerig. Highlights of Prescribing Information: GEODON® (ziprasidone HCl) capsules; GEODON® (ziprasidone mesylate) injection for intramuscular use 2020; http://labeling.pfizer.com/ShowLabeling.aspx?id=584.

57. Iskandar JW, et al. Transient agranulocytosis associated with ziprasidone in a 45-year-old man on hemodialysis. *J Clin Psychopharmacol* 2015; 35:347–348.

58. Basol N, et al. Beneficial effects of agomelatine in experimental model of sepsis-related acute kidney injury. *Ulus Travma Acil Cerrahi Derg* 2016; 22:121–126.

59. Karaman A, et al. A novel approach to contrast-induced nephrotoxicity: the melatonergic agent agomelatine. *Br J Radiol* 2016; 89:20150716.

60. Lieberman JA, et al. Tricyclic antidepressant and metabolite levels in chronic renal failure. *Clin Pharmacol Ther* 1985; 37:301–307.

61. Mitas JA, et al. Diabetic neuropathic pain: control by amitriptyline and fluphenazine in renal insufficiency. *South Med J* 1983; 76:462–463, 467.

62. Murphy EJ. Acute pain management pharmacology for the patient with concurrent renal or hepatic disease. *Anaesth Intensive Care* 2005; 33:311–322.

63. Constantino JL, et al. Pharmacokinetics of antidepressants in patients undergoing hemodialysis: a narrative literature review. *Braz J Psychiatry* 2019; 41:441–446.

64. Chen TY, et al. Amitriptyline-induced acute kidney injury and acute hepatitis: a case report. *Am J Ther* 2021; 28:e256-e258

65. Sage Therapeutics Inc. Highlights of Prescribing Information. Zulresso (brexanolone) injection for intravenous use [controlled substance schedule pending] 2019; https://www.accessdata.fda.gov/drugsatfda_docs/label/2019/211371lbl.pdf.

66. Turpeinen M, et al. Effect of renal impairment on the pharmacokinetics of bupropion and its metabolites. *Br J Clin Pharmacol* 2007; 64:165–173.

67. Worrall SP, et al. Pharmacokinetics of bupropion and its metabolites in haemodialysis patients who smoke. A single dose study. *Nephron Clin Pract* 2004; 97:c83–c89.

68. Ghoreishi A, et al. Bupropion as a treatment for sexual dysfunction among chronic kidney disease patients *Acta Med Iran* 2019; 57:320–327.

69. Joffe P, et al. Single-dose pharmacokinetics of citalopram in patients with moderate renal insufficiency or hepatic cirrhosis compared with healthy subjects. *Eur J Clin Pharmacol* 1998; 54:237–242.

70. Kalender B, et al. Antidepressant treatment increases quality of life in patients with chronic renal failure. *Ren Fail* 2007; 29:817–822.

71. Kelly CA, et al. Adult respiratory distress syndrome and renal failure associated with citalopram overdose. *Hum Exp Toxicol* 2003; 22:103–105.

72. Spigset O, et al. Citalopram pharmacokinetics in patients with chronic renal failure and the effect of haemodialysis. *Eur J Clin Pharmacol* 2000; 56:699–703.

73. Hosseini SH, et al. Citalopram versus psychological training for depression and anxiety symptoms in hemodialysis patients. *Iran J Kidney Dis* 2012; 6:446–451.

74. Sran H, et al. Confusion after starting citalopram in a renal transplant patient. *BMJ Case Rep* 2013; 2013:bcr2013010511.

75. Assimon MM, et al. Comparative cardiac safety of selective serotonin reuptake inhibitors among individuals receiving maintenance hemodialysis. *J Am Soc Nephrol* 2019; 30:611–623.

76. Onishi A, et al. Reversible acute renal failure associated with clomipramine-induced interstitial nephritis. *Clin Exp Nephrol* 2007; 11:241–243.

77. Wyeth Pharmaceuticals Inc. Highlights of Prescribing Information. PRISTIQ® (desvenlafaxine) Extended-Release Tablets, for oral use 2020;

http://labeling.pfizer.com/showlabeling.aspx?id=497%20.

78. Nichols AI, et al. The pharmacokinetics and safety of desvenlafaxine in subjects with chronic renal impairment. *Int J Clin Pharmacol Ther* 2011; **49**:3–13.

79. Rees JA. Clinical interpretation of pharmacokinetic data on dothiepin hydrochloride (Dosulepin, Prothiaden). *J Int Med Res* 1981; **9**:98–102.

80. Swarna SS, et al. Pruritus associated with chronic kidney disease: a comprehensive literature review. *Cureus* 2019; **11**:e5256.

81. Lobo ED, et al. Effects of varying degrees of renal impairment on the pharmacokinetics of duloxetine: analysis of a single-dose phase I study and pooled steady-state data from phase II/III trials. *Clin Pharmacokinet* 2010; **49**:311–321.

82. Ho NV, et al. Duloxetine-induced multi-system organ failure: a case report. Poster presented at American Geriatrics Society Annual Meeting, May 11–15, 2011: National Harbor, Maryland; 2011.

83. Nguyen T, et al. Duloxetine uses in patients with kidney disease: different recommendations from the United States versus Europe and Canada. *Am J Ther* 2019; **26**:e516-e519.

84. Uong C, et al. Poster 91 serotonin syndrome in chronic kidney disease patient after given a dose of duloxetine while on trazodone: a case report. *PM&R* 2014; **6** (Suppl): S214–S215.

85. Miriyala K, et al. Renal failure in a depressed adolescent on escitalopram. *J Child Adolesc Psychopharmacol* 2008; **18**:405–408.

86. Adiga GU, et al. Renal tubular defects from antidepressant use in an older adult: an uncommon but reversible adverse drug effect. *Clin Drug Invest* 2006; **26**:607–610.

87. Yazici AE, et al. Efficacy and tolerability of escitalopram in depressed patients with end stage renal disease: an open placebo-controlled study. *Bull Clin Psychopharmacol* 2012; **22**:23–30.

88. Bergstrom RF, et al. The effects of renal and hepatic disease on the pharmacokinetics, renal tolerance, and risk-benefit profile of fluoxetine. *Int Clin Psychopharmacol* 1993; **8**:261–266.

89. Blumenfield M, et al. Fluoxetine in depressed patients on dialysis. *Int J Psychiatry Med* 1997; **27**:71–80.

90. Levy NB, et al. Fluoxetine in depressed patients with renal failure and in depressed patients with normal kidney function. *Gen Hosp Psychiatry* 1996; **18**:8–13.

91. Kauffman KM, et al. Higher dose weekly fluoxetine in hemodialysis patients: a case series report. *Int J Psychiatry Med* 2020; **56**: 3–13.

92. Lancaster SG, et al. Lofepramine. A review of its pharmacodynamic and pharmacokinetic properties, and therapeutic efficacy in depressive illness. *Drugs* 1989; **37**:123–140.

93. Davis MP, et al. Mirtazapine for pruritus. *J Pain Symptom Manage* 2003; **25**:288–291.

94. Shibata K, et al. SP704 The effect of mirtazapine in dialysis patient with appetite loss. *Nephrol Dial Transplant* 2015; **30** (Suppl 3): iii611.

95. Schoerlin MP, et al. Disposition kinetics of moclobemide, a new MAO-A inhibitor, in subjects with impaired renal function. *J Clin Pharmacol* 1990; **30**:272–284.

96. Stoeckel K, et al. Absorption and disposition of moclobemide in patients with advanced age or reduced liver or kidney function. *Acta Psychiatr Scand Suppl* 1990; **360**:94–97.

97. Pollock BG, et al. Metabolic and physiologic consequences of nortriptyline treatment in the elderly. *Psychopharmacol Bull* 1994; **30**:145–150.

98. Doyle GD, et al. The pharmacokinetics of paroxetine in renal impairment. *Acta Psychiatr Scand Suppl* 1989; **350**:89–90.

99. Ishii T, et al. A rare case of combined syndrome of inappropriate antidiuretic hormone secretion and Fanconi syndrome in an elderly woman. *Am J Kidney Dis* 2006; **48**:155–158.

100. Kaye CM, et al. A review of the metabolism and pharmacokinetics of paroxetine in man. *Acta Psychiatr Scand Suppl* 1989; **350**:60–75.

101. Koo JR, et al. Treatment of depression and effect of antidepression treatment on nutritional status in chronic hemodialysis patients. *Am J Med Sci* 2005; **329**:1–5.

102. Coulomb F, et al. Pharmacokinetics of single-dose reboxetine in volunteers with renal insufficiency. *J Clin Pharmacol* 2000; **40**:482–487.

103. Dostert P, et al. Review of the pharmacokinetics and metabolism of reboxetine, a selective noradrenaline reuptake inhibitor. *Eur Neuropsychopharmacol* 1997; **7** (Suppl 1):S23–S35.

104. Brewster UC, et al. Addition of sertraline to other therapies to reduce dialysis-associated hypotension. *Nephrology (Carlton)* 2003; **8**:296–301.

105. Chan KY, et al. Use of sertraline for antihistamine-refractory uremic pruritus in renal palliative care patients. *J Palliat Med* 2013; **16**:966–970.

106. Chander WP, et al. Serotonin syndrome in maintenance haemodialysis patients following sertraline treatment for depression. *J Indian Med Assoc* 2011; **109**:36–37.

107. Jain N, et al. Rationale and design of the Chronic Kidney Disease Antidepressant Sertraline Trial (CAST). *Contemp Clin Trials* 2013; **34**:136–144.

108. Hedayati SS, et al. Effect of sertraline on depressive symptoms in patients with chronic kidney disease without dialysis dependence: the CAST randomized clinical trial. *JAMA* 2017; **318**:1876–1890.

109. Razeghi E, et al. A randomized crossover clinical trial of sertraline for intradialytic hypotension. *Iran J Kidney Dis* 2015; **9**:323–330.

110. Mehrotra R, et al. Comparative efficacy of therapies for treatment of depression for patients undergoing maintenance hemodialysis: a randomized clinical trial. *Ann Intern Med* 2019; **170**:369–379.

111. Friedli K, et al. Sertraline versus placebo in patients with major depressive disorder undergoing hemodialysis: a randomized, controlled feasibility trial. *Clin J Am Soc Nephrol* 2017; **12**:280–286.

112. Chien CW, et al. Sertraline-induced neutropenia and fatigue in a patient with end-stage renal disease. *Am J Ther* 2020:[Epub ahead of print].

113. Zahed NS, et al. Impact of sertraline on serum concentration of CRP in hemodialysis patients with depression. *J Renal Inj Prev* 2017;

6:65–69.

114. Gregg LP, et al. Inflammation and response to sertraline treatment in patients with CKD and major depression. *Am J Kidney Dis* 2020; **75**:457–460.

115. Catanese B, et al. A comparative study of trazodone serum concentrations in patients with normal or impaired renal function. *Boll Chim Farm* 1978; **117**:424–427.

116. Leighton JD, et al. Trimipramine-induced acute renal failure (Letter). *N Z Med J* 1986; **99**:248.

117. Simpson GM, et al. A preliminary study of trimipramine in chronic schizophrenia. *Curr Ther Res Clin Exp* 1966; **99**:248.

118. Troy SM, et al. The effect of renal disease on the disposition of venlafaxine. *Clin Pharmacol Ther* 1994; **56**:14–21.

119. Guldiken S, et al. Complete relief of pain in acute painful diabetic neuropathy of rapid glycaemic control (insulin neuritis) with venlafaxine HCL. *Diabetes Nutr Metab* 2004; **17**:247–249.

120. Pascale P, et al. Severe rhabdomyolysis following venlafaxine overdose. *Ther Drug Monit* 2005; **27**:562–564.

121. Takeda Pharmaceuticals America Inc. Highlights of Prescribing Information. BRINTELLIX (vortioxetine) tablets 2020; http://www.us.brintellix.com.

122. Hegarty J, et al. Carbamazepine-induced acute granulomatous interstitial nephritis. *Clin Nephrol* 2002; **57**:310–313.

123. Hogg RJ, et al. Carbamazepine-induced acute tubulointerstitial nephritis. *J Pediatr* 1981; **98**:830–832.

124. Imai H, et al. Carbamazepine-induced granulomatous necrotizing angiitis with acute renal failure. *Nephron* 1989; **51**:405–408.

125. Jubert P, et al. Carbamazepine-induced acute renal failure. *Nephron* 1994; **66**:121.

126. Nicholls DP, et al. Acute renal failure from carbamazepine (Letter). *Br Med J* 1972; **4**:490.

127. Tutor-Crespo MJ, et al. Relative proportions of serum carbamazepine and its pharmacologically active 10,11-epoxy derivative: effect of polytherapy and renal insufficiency. *Ups J Med Sci* 2008; **113**:171–180.

128. Verrotti A, et al. Renal tubular function in patients receiving anticonvulsant therapy: a long-term study. *Epilepsia* 2000; **41**:1432–1435.

129. Hung CC, et al. Acute renal failure and its risk factors in Stevens-Johnson syndrome and toxic epidermal necrolysis. *Am J Nephrol* 2009; **29**:633–638.

130. Fervenza FC, et al. Acute granulomatous interstitial nephritis and colitis in anticonvulsant hypersensitivity syndrome associated with lamotrigine treatment. *Am J Kidney Dis* 2000; **36**:1034–1040.

131. Fillastre JP, et al. Pharmacokinetics of lamotrigine in patients with renal impairment: influence of haemodialysis. *Drugs Exp Clin Res* 1993; **19**:25–32.

132. Schaub JE, et al. Multisystem adverse reaction to lamotrigine. *Lancet* 1994; **344**:481.

133. Wootton R, et al. Comparison of the pharmacokinetics of lamotrigine in patients with chronic renal failure and healthy volunteers. *Br J Clin Pharmacol* 1997; **43**:23–27.

134. Bansal AD, et al. Use of antiepileptic drugs in patients with chronic kidney disease and end stage renal disease. *Seminars in Dialysis* 2015; **28**:404–412.

135. Gitlin M. Lithium and the kidney: an updated review. *Drug Saf* 1999; **20**:231–243.

136. Lepkifker E, et al. Renal insufficiency in long-term lithium treatment. *J Clin Psychiatry* 2004; **65**:850–856.

137. McKnight RF, et al. Lithium toxicity profile: a systematic review and meta-analysis. *Lancet* 2012; **379**:721–728.

138. Shine B, et al. Long-term effects of lithium on renal, thyroid, and parathyroid function: a retrospective analysis of laboratory data. *Lancet* 2015; **386**:461–468.

139. Clos S, et al. Long-term effect of lithium maintenance therapy on estimated glomerular filtration rate in patients with affective disorders: a population-based cohort study. *Lancet Psychiatry* 2015; **2**:1075–1083.

140. Schoot TS, et al. Systematic review and practical guideline for the prevention and management of the renal side effects of lithium therapy. *Eur Neuropsychopharmacol* 2020; **31**:16–32.

141. Davis J, et al. Lithium and nephrotoxicity: a literature review of approaches to clinical management and risk stratification. *BMC Nephrol* 2018; **19**:305.

142. Engels N, et al. Successful lithium treatment in a patient on hemodialysis. *Bipolar Disorders* 2019; **21**:285–287.

143. Smith GC, et al. Anticonvulsants as a cause of Fanconi syndrome. *Nephrol Dial Transplant* 1995; **10**:543–545.

144. Fukuda Y, et al. Immunologically mediated chronic tubulo-interstitial nephritis caused by valproate therapy. *Nephron* 1996; **72**:328–329.

145. Watanabe T, et al. Secondary renal Fanconi syndrome caused by valproate therapy. *Pediatr Nephrol* 2005; **20**:814-817.

146. Zaki EL, et al. Renal injury from valproic acid: case report and literature review. *Pediatr Neurol* 2002; **27**:318–319.

147. Tanaka H, et al. Distal type of renal tubular acidosis after anti-epileptic therapy in a girl with infantile spasms. *Clin Exp Nephrol* 1999; **3**:311–313.

148. Knorr M, et al. Fanconi syndrome caused by antiepileptic therapy with valproic acid. *Epilepsia* 2004; **45**:868–871.

149. Rahman MH, et al. Acute hemolysis with acute renal failure in a patient with valproic acid poisoning treated with charcoal hemoperfusion. *Hemodial Int* 2006; **10**:256–259.

150. Koga S, et al. Risk factors for sodium valproate-induced renal tubular dysfunction. *Clin Exp Nephrol* 2018; **22**:420–425.

151. Hayes JF, et al. Adverse renal, endocrine, hepatic, and metabolic events during maintenance mood stabilizer treatment for bipolar disorder: a population-based cohort study. *PLoS Med* 2016; **13**:e1002058.

152. Kessing LV, et al. Continuation of lithium after a diagnosis of chronic kidney disease. *Acta Psychiatr Scand* 2017; **136**:615–622.

153. Pentikainen PJ, et al. Pharmacokinetics of chlormethiazole in healthy volunteers and patients with cirrhosis of the liver. *Eur J Clin Pharmacol* 1980; **17**:275–284.

154. Dashti-Khavidaki S, et al. Comparing effects of clonazepam and zolpidem on sleep quality of patients on maintenance hemodialysis. *Iran J Kidney Dis* 2011; **5**:404–409.

155. Sadjadi SA, et al. Allergic interstitial nephritis due to diazepam. *Arch Intern Med* 1987; **147**:579.

156. Sunovion Pharmaceuticals Inc. Highlights of Prescribing Information. LUNESTA® (eszopiclone) tablets, for oral use 2020; https://www.accessdata.fda.gov/drugsatfda_docs/label/2014/021476s030lbl.pdf.

157. Blum RA, et al. Pharmacokinetics of gabapentin in subjects with various degrees of renal function. *Clin Pharmacol Ther* 1994; **56**:154–159.

158. Miller A, et al. Gabapentin toxicity in renal failure: the importance of dose adjustment. *Pain Med* 2009; **10**:190–192.

159. Upjohn UK Limited. Summary of product characteristics. Neurontin 600mg film-coated tablets 2020; https://www.medicines.org.uk/emc/product/3197/smpc.

160. Yeddi A, et al. Myoclonus and altered mental status induced by single dose of gabapentin in a patient with end-stage renal disease: a case report and literature review. *Am J Ther* 2019; **26**:e768–e770.

161. Ishida JH, et al. Gabapentin and pregabalin use and association with adverse outcomes among hemodialysis patients. *J Am Soc Nephrol* 2018; **29**:1970–1978.

162. Gobo-Oliveira M, et al. Gabapentin versus dexchlorpheniramine as treatment for uremic pruritus: a randomised controlled trial. *Eur J Dermatol* 2018; **28**:488–495.

163. Gunal AI, et al. Gabapentin therapy for pruritus in haemodialysis patients: a randomized, placebo-controlled, double-blind trial. *Nephrol Dial Transplant* 2004; **19**:3137–3139.

164. Beladi Mousavi SS, et al. The effect of gabapentin on muscle cramps during hemodialysis: a double-blind clinical trial. *Saudi J Kidney Dis Transpl* 2015; **26**:1142–1148.

165. Razazian N, et al. Gabapentin versus levodopa-c for the treatment of restless legs syndrome in hemodialysis patients: a randomized clinical trial. *Saudi J Kidney Dis Transpl* 2015; **26**:271–278.

166. Rossi GM, et al. Randomized trial of two after-dialysis gabapentin regimens for severe uremic pruritus in hemodialysis patients. *Intern Emerg Med* 2019; **14**:1341–1346.

167. Eisai Inc. Highlights of Prescribing Information. Dayvigo (lemborexant) tablets for oral use [controlled substance schedule pending] 2019; https://www.accessdata.fda.gov/drugsatfda_docs/label/2019/212028s000lbl.pdf.

168. Huang CE, et al. Intramuscular lorazepam in catatonia in patients with acute renal failure: a report of two cases. *Chang Gung Med J* 2010; **33**:106–109.

169. Reynolds HN, et al. Hyperlactatemia, increased osmolar gap, and renal dysfunction during continuous lorazepam infusion. *Crit Care Med* 2000; **28**:1631–1634.

170. Verbeeck RK, et al. Impaired elimination of lorazepam following subchronic administration in two patients with renal failure. *Br J Clin Pharmacol* 1981; **12**:749–751.

171. Yaucher NE, et al. Propylene glycol-associated renal toxicity from lorazepam infusion. *Pharmacotherapy* 2003; **23**:1094–1099.

172. Zar T, et al. Acute kidney injury, hyperosmolality and metabolic acidosis associated with lorazepam. *Nat Clin Pract Nephrol* 2007; **3**:515–520.

173. Hayman M, et al. Acute tubular necrosis associated with propylene glycol from concomitant administration of intravenous lorazepam and trimethoprim-sulfamethoxazole. *Pharmacotherapy* 2003; **23**:1190–1194.

174. Upjohn UK Limited. Lyrica 25mg 50mg 75mg 100mg 150mg 200mg 225mg and 300mg hard capsules 2020; https://www.medicines.org.uk/emc/product/10303/smpc.

175. Desai A, et al. Gabapentin or pregabalin induced myoclonus: a case series and literature review. *J Clin Neurosci* 2019; **61**:225–234.

176. Du YT, et al. Seizure induced by sudden cessation of pregabalin in a patient with chronic kidney disease. *BMJ Case Rep* 2017; **2017**:bcr2016219158.

177. Foroutan N, et al. Comparison of pregabalin with doxepin in the management of uremic pruritus: a randomized single blind clinical trial. *Hemodial Int* 2017; **21**:63–71.

178. Otsuki T, et al. Efficacy and safety of pregabalin for the treatment of neuropathic pain in patients undergoing hemodialysis. *Clin Drug Investig* 2017; **37**:95–102.

179. Murray TG, et al. Renal disease, age, and oxazepam kinetics. *Clin Pharmacol Ther* 1981; **30**:805–809.

180. Leung N, et al. Acute kidney injury in patients with inactive cytochrome P450 polymorphisms. *Ren Fail* 2009; **31**:749–752.

181. Drover DR. Comparative pharmacokinetics and pharmacodynamics of short-acting hypnosedatives: zaleplon, zolpidem and zopiclone. *Clin Pharmacokinet* 2004; **43**:227–238.

182. Rehman IU, et al. A randomized controlled trial for effectiveness of zolpidem versus acupressure on sleep in hemodialysis patients having chronic kidney disease-associated pruritus. *Medicine (Baltimore)* 2018; **97**:e10764.

183. Hsu FG, et al. Use of zolpidem and risk of acute pyelonephritis in women: a population-based case–control study in Taiwan. *J Clin Pharmacol* 2017; **57**:376–381.

184. Goa KL, et al. Zopiclone. A review of its pharmacodynamic and pharmacokinetic properties and therapeutic efficacy as an hypnotic. *Drugs* 1986; **32**:48–65.

185. Hussain N, et al. Zopiclone-induced acute interstitial nephritis. *Am J Kidney Dis* 2003; **41**:E17.

186. Suwata J, et al. New acetylcholinesterase inhibitor (donepezil) treatment for Alzheimer's disease in a chronic dialysis patient. *Nephron* 2002; **91**:330–332.

187. Nagy CF, et al. Steady-state pharmacokinetics and safety of donepezil HCl in subjects with moderately impaired renal function. *Br J Clin Pharmacol* 2004; **58** (Suppl 1):18–24.

188. Tiseo PJ, et al. An evaluation of the pharmacokinetics of donepezil HCl in patients with moderately to severely impaired renal function. *Br J Clin Pharmacol* 1998; **46** (Suppl 1):56–60.

189. Sahin OZ, et al. A rare case of acute renal failure secondary to rhabdomyolysis probably induced by donepezil. *Case Rep Nephrol* 2014; 2014:214359.

190. Periclou A, et al. Pharmacokinetic study of memantine in healthy and renally impaired subjects. *Clin Pharmacol Ther* 2006; 79:134–143.

191. Lefevre G, et al. Effects of renal impairment on steady-state plasma concentrations of Rivastigmine: a population pharmacokinetic analysis of capsule and patch formulations in patients with Alzheimer's disease. *Drugs Aging* 2016; 33:725–736.

192. AMAG Pharmaceutical Inc. Highlights of prescribing information. Vyleesi (bremelanotide injection) for subcutaneous use 2019; https://www.accessdata.fda.gov/drugsatfda_docs/label/2019/210557s000lbl.pdf.

193. Nelson ME, et al. Melanotan II injection resulting in systemic toxicity and rhabdomyolysis. *Clin Toxicol (Phila)* 2012; 50:1169–1173.

194. Teva Pharmaceuticals USA Inc. Highlights of prescribing information. Austedo (deutetrabenazine) tablets for oral use 2020; https://www.accessdata.fda.gov/drugsatfda_docs/label/2017/209885lbl.pdf.

195. Lincoln Medical Limited. Wakix 4.5mg/18mg film-coated tablets 2016; https://www.medicines.org.uk/emc/product/7402.

196. Bioprojet Pharma. Highlights of prescribing information. Wakix (pitolisant) tablets for oral use 2019; https://www.accessdata.fda.gov/drugsatfda_docs/label/2019/211150s000lbl.pdf.

197. Smith WB, et al. Effect of renal impairment on the pharmacokinetics of prucalopride: a single-dose open-label Phase I study. *Drug Des Devel Ther* 2012; 6:407–415.

198. Shire Pharmaceuticals Limited. Resolor 1mg and 2mg film-coated tablets 2019; https://www.medicines.org.uk/emc/product/584/smpc.

199. Sivabalasundaram V, et al. Prucalopride-associated acute tubular necrosis. *World J Clin Cases* 2014; 2:380–384.

200. Jazz Pharmaceuticals UK. Sunosi 75mg and 140mg film-coated tablets 2020; https://www.medicines.org.uk/emc/product/11017/smpc.

201. Zomorodi K, et al. Single-dose pharmacokinetics and safety of solriamfetol in participants with normal or impaired renal function and with end-stage renal disease requiring hemodialysis. *J Clin Pharmacol* 2019; 59:1120–1129.

202. Neurocrine Biosciences Inc. Highlights of prescribing information. Ingrezza (valbenazine) capsules for oral use 2020; https://www.accessdata.fda.gov/drugsatfda_docs/label/2017/209241lbl.pdf.

203. Gregg LP, et al. Pharmacologic and psychological interventions for depression treatment in patients with kidney disease. *Curr Opin Nephrol Hypertens* 2020; 29:457–464.

特殊情况的精神科用药

其他精神障碍的药物治疗

边缘型人格障碍

边缘型人格障碍在精神科较为普遍,据报告其患病率高达 20%[1]。边缘型人格障碍的常见共病包括心境障碍(单相和双相)、焦虑谱系障碍、进食障碍和酒药滥用,共病至少一种精神障碍的风险接近 100%[2]。抑郁和焦虑等共病的处理,应该参照相关精神障碍的指南,不考虑共病的边缘型人格障碍。边缘型人格障碍的自杀率与心境障碍和精神分裂症相似,约为 1/10[3,4]。

边缘型人格障碍被归类为一种人格障碍,但是人们认为其部分症状可能用药治疗有效。这些症状包括情绪不稳、短暂的与应激相关的准精神病性症状或抑郁症状、自杀自伤行为和冲动行为[4]。很高比例的边缘型人格障碍患者使用精神药物治疗[2,5,6],往往合用多种精神药物[7]。英国处方实践调查发现,90% 以上的边缘型人格障碍患者用过精神药物,最常用抗抑郁药或抗精神病药,特别是治疗情绪不稳时[6]。单独诊断为边缘型人格障碍的患者,其抗精神病药、抗抑郁药和心境稳定剂的使用率与同时合并诊断有精神分裂症、抑郁症或者双相障碍的患者并无明显不同[6]。这提示,精神药物往往用于治疗边缘型人格障碍本身(支持的证据很少),而不是治疗特定的共病。尚没有药物的适应证是专门治疗边缘型人格障碍或其部分症状的。心理治疗(如辨证行为治疗)有更好的证据支持——2020 年 Cochrane 记录了 75 项随机对照试验[8]。

2009 年,NICE[9] 建议:

- 药物治疗不应常规用于边缘型人格障碍,或治疗其某些单独的症状或行为问题(如反复自伤、明显情绪不稳、冒险行为和短暂的精神病性症状)。
- 在共病的整体治疗方案中,可以考虑药物治疗。
- 在紧急情况时,可以考虑短期使用镇静药物,将其作为边缘型人格障碍整体治疗计划的一部分。治疗的持续时间需要经过患者同意,但是不应超过 1 周。

NICE 指南最近一次于 2018 年 7 月审阅,未做改动[9]。发布边缘型人格障碍治疗指南以来,另外有两项独立的系统综述也已经发表[10,11]。这三项综述基本上纳入了相同的研究,并将数据结合起来用于荟萃分析,最终这三项系统性综述的分析结果相似。此外,它们都注意到,边缘型人格障碍药物治疗研究大多仅持续 6 周,而且使用大量不同的结局判定指标,使得研究结果很难评估和比较。NICE 认为现有数据尚不足以作为给 NHS 提出治疗建议的基础,而其他两项综述则认为一些分析给出了很有前景的结果,足以给临床实践提供依据。

最近一篇系统综述[12]纳入了 2010—2017 年发表的研究,对既往的分析进行了更新。结论与早期的 NICE 评论没什么不同,即证据主体不足以给出明确的临床建议。最近对已发表、未发表和正在进行的研究[13]的分析结论是,不但没有哪种药物被确凿地证明治疗边缘型人格障碍有效,而且在过去几年中药物试验的数量锐减。

抗精神病药

公认容易产生偏倚的开放式研究发现,若干第一代及第二代抗精神病药对于边缘型人格障碍的多种症状有效。与之相反,随机对照试验多数提示试验药物相比于安慰剂的疗效并不显著。边缘型人格障碍用药治疗效果最好的症状或症状群有情感失控、冲动性和认知-感知觉症状[10,11,14,15]。奥氮平疗效得到的支持证据可能最强[11,16,17],但其疗效最好时也只是轻微疗效[12]。据开放性和自然研究报告,应用氯氮平后患者的攻击和自伤行为减少[18-22],并且氯氮平在精神分裂症患者中也发现有改善攻击行为的作用[23]。氯氮平似乎可以减少边缘型人格障碍患者住院的风险[22]。喹硫平也许是最广泛用于治疗边缘型人格障碍的抗精神病药。其使用得到一项小样本 RCT 的支持,其完整结果于 2020 年在线发表[24]。

抗抑郁药

有几项开放性研究发现,SSRI 类药物可以减少边缘型人格障碍的冲动性及攻击性,但是这些结果并未能在 RCT 研究中得到重复。一项 RCT 比较了氟西汀与辩证行为治疗,发现服用氟西汀组自杀率较高[25]。我们可以相当肯定地推断:目前,尚无有效的循证依据支持抗抑郁药用于治疗边缘型人格障碍者的抑郁情绪或冲动行为[10,11]。

心境稳定剂

高达半数的边缘型人格障碍人群可能同时被诊断为双相谱系障碍(但是对此诊断存在相当大的争议)[26],并且普遍使用心境稳定剂[2]。但是有一些研究证据表明,心境稳定剂可以减少边缘型人格障碍的冲动性、愤怒和情感失调[10,11]。锂盐被批准用于控制攻击行为或故意的自伤行为[27]。一项关于拉莫三嗪的大样本随机对照试验发现,该药对任何症状均无效[28]。米非司酮(mifepristone)也无效[29]。

美金刚

一项样本量 33 例的 RCT 发现,美金刚 20mg/d 辅助治疗,其疗效优于安慰剂[30],且耐受性良好。需要进行更多的试验。

阿片受体拮抗剂

很有限的证据支持纳曲酮能有效地减轻自伤和分离症状[12,31],但是没有决定性的试验支持纳曲酮治疗边缘型人格障碍的疗效。

危机管理

药物治疗往往用于“症状”比较严重、令人痛苦以及可能危及生命时的危急阶段。在边缘型人格障碍中,这些症状往往会起伏不定[3]。因此药物治疗也需要是间歇性的,每次发作时,均需要仔细了解药物的相对伤害和收益,才能决定是否用药。一般确定患者是否需要药物治疗很容易,但困难的是决定何时略有收益就值了,以及是否必须继续用药。使用精神药物并非无害,因此治疗应该始终是有严格评估的短期试验。

NICE[9] 建议在危急时期,在限定时间内使用镇静类药物可能有效。选择药物时,应该考虑过量用药可以预期到的不良反应和潜在的毒性。比如,苯二氮䓬类药物(尤其作用时间短的药物)可以引起边缘型人格障碍患者的脱抑制反应[32],使问题变得更加复杂;有镇静作用的抗精神病药可以导致 EPS,或显著的体重增加;三环类抗抑郁药在过量使用时毒性会特别明显;有镇静作用的抗组胺药(如异丙嗪)耐受性通常很不错,作为协同治疗方案的一部分,短期应用可能有效。抗组胺药有不良反应(如口干、便秘),对睡眠结构有不利影响,而且缺乏明确的抗焦虑作用,因此不宜长期使用。

参考文献

1. Kernberg OF, et al. Borderline personality disorder. *Am J Psychiatry* 2009; **166**:505–508.
2. Pascual JC, et al. A naturalistic study of changes in pharmacological prescription for borderline personality disorder in clinical practice: from APA to NICE guidelines. *Int Clin Psychopharmacol* 2010; 25:349–355.
3. Links PS, et al. Prospective follow-up study of borderline personality disorder: prognosis, prediction of outcome, and axis II comorbidity. *Can J Psychiatry* 1998; 43:265–270.
4. Oldham JM. Guideline watch: practice guideline for the treatment of patients with borderline personality disorder. *Focus* 2005; 3:396–400.
5. Baker-Glenn E, et al. Use of psychotropic medication among psychiatric out-patients with personality disorder. *Psychiatrist* 2010; **34**:83–86.
6. Paton C. Prescribing for people with emotionally unstable personality disorder under the care of UK mental health services. *J Clin Psychiatry* 2015:e512–e518.
7. Riffer F, et al. Psychopharmacological treatment of patients with borderline personality disorder: comparing data from routine clinical care with recommended guidelines. *Int J Psychiatry Clin Pract* 2019; 23:178–188.
8. Storebø OJ, et al. Psychological therapies for people with borderline personality disorder. *Cochrane Database Syst Rev* 2020; 5:Cd012955.
9. National Institute for Clinical Excellence. Borderline personality disorder: recognition and management. Clinical Guidance 78 [CG78] 2009 (Last checked July 2018); https://www.nice.org.uk/guidance/CG78
10. Lieb K, et al. Pharmacotherapy for borderline personality disorder: Cochrane systematic review of randomised trials. *Br J Psychiatry* 2010; 196:4–12.
11. Ingenhoven T, et al. Effectiveness of pharmacotherapy for severe personality disorders: meta-analyses of randomized controlled trials. *J Clin Psychiatry* 2010; 71:14–25.
12. Hancock-Johnson E, et al. A focused systematic review of pharmacological treatment for borderline personality disorder. *CNS Drugs* 2017; 31:345–356.
13. Stoffers-Winterling J, et al. Pharmacotherapy for borderline personality disorder: an update of published, unpublished and ongoing studies. *Curr Psychiatry Rep* 2020; 22:37.
14. Zanarini MC, et al. A dose comparison of olanzapine for the treatment of borderline personality disorder: a 12-week randomized, double-blind, placebo-controlled study. *J Clin Psychiatry* 2011; 72:1353–1362.
15. Canadian Agency for Drugs and Technologies in Health. Aripiprazole for borderline personality disorder: a review of the clinical effectiveness 2017. https://www.ncbi.nlm.nih.gov/pubmedhealth/PMH0096409.
16. Shafti S, et al. A comparative study on olanzapine and aripiprazole for symptom management in female patients with borderline personality disorder. *Bull Clin Psychopharmacol*, 2015; 25:38–43.
17. Bozzatello P, et al. Efficacy and tolerability of asenapine compared with olanzapine in borderline personality disorder: an open-label randomized controlled trial. *CNS Drugs* 2017; 31:809–819.
18. Benedetti F, et al. Low-dose clozapine in acute and continuation treatment of severe borderline personality disorder. *J Clin Psychiatry* 1998; 59:103–107.
19. Frogley C, et al. A case series of clozapine for borderline personality disorder. *Ann Clin Psychiatry* 2013; 25:125–134.
20. Chengappa KN, et al. Clozapine reduces severe self-mutilation and aggression in psychotic patients with borderline personality disorder. *J Clin Psychiatry* 1999; 60:477–484.
21. Dickens GL, et al. Experiences of women in secure care who have been prescribed clozapine for borderline personality disorder. *Borderline Personal Disord and Emot Dysregul* 2016; 3:12.
22. Rohde C, et al. Real-world effectiveness of clozapine for borderline personality disorder: results from a 2-year mirror-image study. *J Pers Disord* 2017:1–15.
23. Volavka J, et al. Heterogeneity of violence in schizophrenia and implications for long-term treatment. *Int J Clin Pract* 2008; 62:1237–1245.
24. ClinicalTrial.gov. Seroquel extended release (XR) for the management of borderline personality disorder (BPD). ClinicalTrials.gov Identifier:

NCT00880919. 2017. https://clinicaltrials.gov/ct2/show/results/NCT00880919?view=results.

25. ClinicalTrial.gov. Treating suicidal behavior and self-mutilation in people with borderline personality disorder. ClinicalTrials.gov Identifier: NCT00533117. 2017. https://clinicaltrials.gov/ct2/show/results/NCT00533117.

26. Deltito J, et al. Do patients with borderline personality disorder belong to the bipolar spectrum? *J Affect Disord* 2001; 67:221–228.

27. Essential Pharma Ltd. Summary of product characteristics. Camcolit 400mg prolonged release Lithium Carbonate. 2020. https://www.medicines.org.uk/emc/product/10829/smpc.

28. Crawford MJ, et al. No effect of lamotrigine in subgroups of patients with borderline personality disorder: response to Smith. *Am J Psychiatry* 2018; 175:1265–1266.

29. ClinicalTrial.gov. Preliminary trial of the effect of Glucocorticoid Receptor Antagonist on borderline personality disorder (BPD). ClinicalTrials.gov Identifier: NCT01212588. 2019. https://clinicaltrials.gov/ct2/show/NCT01212588.

30. Kulkarni J, et al. Effect of the glutamate NMDA receptor antagonist memantine as adjunctive treatment in borderline personality disorder: an exploratory, randomised, double-blind, placebo-controlled trial. *CNS Drugs* 2018; 32:179–187.

31. Moghaddas A, et al. The potential role of naltrexone in borderline personality disorder. *Iran J Psychiatry* 2017; 12:142–146.

32. Gardner DL, et al. Alprazolam-induced dyscontrol in borderline personality disorder. *Am J Psychiatry* 1985; 142:98–100.

进食障碍

进食障碍的发病率不断升高[1]。罹患任一进食障碍的终身风险女性为 8.4%,男性为 2.2%[2]。其他精神障碍(尤其焦虑症、抑郁症和强迫症)往往伴有进食障碍,这可以部分解释患者接受药物治疗有益的原因。使用任何药物都需要密切监测,以发现可能的不良反应。

神经性厌食

总则

药物对神经性厌食的作用有限,目前没有一种药物被批准用于治疗该病[3]。迅速使体重恢复到安全范围、家庭治疗和结构化的心理治疗是主要的干预措施[4,5]。躯体治疗的目标是通过再喂养来改善营养状况,除了用于纠正代谢缺陷的药物,其他药物干预的证据均很少。药物可以用于治疗一些躯体共病,但是在恢复体重方面作用很小[6]。

奥氮平是对神经性厌食体重恢复起作用的唯一药物[7-9]。喹硫平的早期研究数据令人鼓舞[10],但后来 RCT 研究并未重复出该结果[11]。总之,据说药物治疗的证据"不太令人满意"[12],一项荟萃分析发现其效果并不优于安慰剂[13]。一项网络荟萃分析已在计划之中[14],尚未完成。最近也是最大的临床试验综述和荟萃分析[15]得出的结论是:"没有哪种精神药物被证明有效。"

屈大麻酚是一种合成的大麻素受体激动剂,可能会略微增加体重[16],但是不推荐使用,而且其不良反应(烦躁不安)很常见[17]。

医疗团队在用药时,需要始终警惕药物导致的 Q-T 间期延长。所有诊断为神经性厌食的患者都应该在其处方记录中特别标注警告,提示他们因为营养不良出现电解质紊乱和潜在的心脏并发症继而出现心律失常的风险较高。若使用任何可能危害心脏功能的药物,必须监测心电图[4]。

躯体方面

维生素和矿物质

在住院患者和门诊患者体重恢复的过程中,建议口服补充复合维生素或复合矿物质[4]。

电解质

电解质紊乱(如低钾血症)往往会随着时间而缓慢发展,可能是无症状的,并会因再喂养而缓解。低磷血症也可能因再喂养而引发。快速纠正可能有害。因此,采取口服补充以防止发生严重后果,而非简单地恢复正常水平。若补充电解质,应该监测尿素氮、电解质、HCO_3、钙、磷、镁,并需要检查心电图[18]。

骨质疏松症

骨质流失是厌食症的严重并发症,会带来严重后果。用雌激素或脱氢表雄酮(DHEA)

治疗对骨密度没有良性作用。雌激素不推荐用于儿童及青少年,因为会增加骨骼过早融合的风险[4]。升高催乳素水平的抗精神病药会进一步增加骨质流失和骨质疏松的风险。二膦酸盐一般不推荐用于女性厌食症患者,因为缺乏疗效和安全性数据。该类药未被批准用于绝经前女性。

精神科方面

急性疾病:抗抑郁药

一篇 Cochrane 综述发现,来源于 4 项安慰剂对照试验的证据表明,抗抑郁药不能增加体重、改善进食障碍以及相关精神症状[19]。有人提出饥饿带来的神经生化异常可以部分解释这种无应答表现[19]。氟西汀治疗的同时合并营养补充品(包括色氨酸)并未发现能够增加疗效[20]。NICE 未发现什么证据支持使用抗抑郁药[4]。自然性研究提示有转为躁狂的严重风险[21]。抗抑郁药似乎在神经性厌食中没有作用。

其他精神药物

抗精神病药(比如奥氮平)、苯二氮䓬类药物或抗组胺药(如异丙嗪)往往用于减轻神经性厌食伴随的高度焦虑,但一般不推荐用于促进体重增加[4]。一些个案报告和回顾性研究提示,奥氮平可减轻激越(并且可能增加体重)[22,23]。一项 RCT 发现[8],使用奥氮平治疗的患者87.5% 恢复了体重(安慰剂组为 55.6%)[7]。喹硫平可能有助于改善精神症状,但是相关数据较少[10]。选择药物时,仅应考虑不影响催乳素的药物(即避免使用利培酮、氨磺必利和舒必利)。抗精神病药对体重的总体影响在统计上没有意义[13]。

许多其他药物在一些小规模的、质量及疗效不一的安慰剂对照试验中进行过研究,包括锌[24]、纳曲酮[25]以及赛庚啶[26]。这些药物均未被广泛地用于临床实践。瑞莫瑞林(Relamorelin,一种胃饥饿素拮抗剂)[27]、催产素[28]和睾酮[29]可能无效。

预防复发

一项小样本研究发现,体重已经恢复的厌食症患者使用氟西汀有助于改善预后,预防复发[30]。其他研究发现无效[19,31]。SSRI 类药物也可引起催乳素增高,但是罕见。

共患疾病

抗抑郁药经常会被用于治疗厌食症合并的抑郁症及强迫症。然而,应该注意的是,仅仅随着体重的恢复,这些问题就有可能缓解[4]。安非他酮常有体重减轻的不良反应,因此禁用于神经性厌食伴发的抑郁症[32]。神经性厌食伴发的躁狂和精神病也许最好用奥氮平治疗,双相抑郁用奥氮平 + 氟西汀治疗[32]。

神经性贪食症和暴食症

心理干预应该作为神经性贪食的一线治疗[33]。成年人神经性贪食和暴食症可以试用抗抑郁药,首选 SSRI 类药物(尤其氟西汀[34-36])。氟西汀的有效剂量为 60mg/d[37]。应该告知患者,该药可以减少暴食及清除行为的频率,但长期效果尚未可知[4]。早期起效(3 周时)可以较强地预测总体疗效[38]。

　　抗抑郁药可用于治疗青少年的神经性贪食,但该类药物未被批准此年龄段的适应证,并且支持这种做法的依据很少。抗抑郁药不应作为青少年神经性贪食的一线治疗[4]。

　　有一些证据提示托吡酯有助于减少暴食行为的频率[39](但是耐受性往往很差),还有少数证据提示安非他酮[40]、度洛西汀[41]、拉莫三嗪[42,43]、唑尼沙胺[44,45]、阿坎酸[46]和羟丁酸钠[47]也有一定的作用。系统综述[48,49]证实 SSRI 略有疗效,而且提示赖右苯丙胺(lisdexamfetamine)治疗有效(依据一项高质量的 RCT[50])。赖右苯丙胺在美国获批治疗暴食症[51]。一些有限的证据支持使用缓释芬特明与托吡酯合剂[52,53]。去甲肾上腺素/多巴胺再摄取抑制剂达索曲林(dasotraline)也可能有效[54],但其研发于 2020 年终止。

共病抑郁症

　　抑郁症是神经性贪食和暴食症的常见共病。对于神经性贪食患者的抑郁症状,西酞普兰的疗效被证明优于氟西汀。体重增加是米氮平的常见不良反应,因此治疗暴食症伴发的抑郁时,应该避免使用或慎用该药[32]。

其他非典型进食障碍

　　除了神经性厌食和暴食症,对于非典型进食障碍的药物治疗,尚无有用的研究[4,55]。鉴于目前尚无循证依据用于指导非典型进食障碍(也称为“进食障碍未特定”)的治疗,建议临床医师参考与患者表现最为相似的那一类进食障碍的治疗指南[4]。

NICE 进食障碍指南摘要[4]

神经性厌食
- 推荐选择心理治疗,并应该同时监测患者的躯体状态。
- 无可推荐的药物干预手段。许多药物可用于治疗共患疾病。

神经性贪食
- 对于神经贪食的治疗,应该首选有循证依据的自助项目或认知行为治疗。
- 尝试使用氟西汀治疗作为替代方案,或者辅助方案。

暴食症
- 对于暴食症的治疗,应该首选有循证依据的自助项目或认知行为治疗。
- 尝试使用 SSRI 治疗作为替代方案,或者辅助方案。
- 赖右苯丙胺也是一个选择。

参考文献

1. Martínez-González L, et al. Incidence of anorexia nervosa in women: a systematic review and meta-analysis. *Int J Environ Res Public Health* 2020; 17:3824.
2. Galmiche M, et al. Prevalence of eating disorders over the 2000–2018 period: a systematic literature review. *Am J Clin Nutr* 2019; 109:1402–1413.
3. Frank GKW. Pharmacotherapeutic strategies for the treatment of anorexia nervosa – too much for one drug? *Expert Opin Pharmacother* 2020; 21:1045–1058.
4. National Institute for Clinical Excellence. Eating disorders: recognition and treatment. NICE guideline [NG69] 2017 (Last update March 2020); https://www.nice.org.uk/guidance/ng69.

5. American Psychiatric Association. Treatment of patients with eating disorders, third edition. *Am J Psychiatry* 2006; **163**:4–54.

6. Crow SJ, et al. What potential role is there for medication treatment in anorexia nervosa? *Int J Eat Disord* 2009; **42**:1–8.

7. Dunican KC, et al. The role of olanzapine in the treatment of anorexia nervosa. *Ann Pharmacothe* 2007; **41**:111–115.

8. Bissada H, et al. Olanzapine in the treatment of low body weight and obsessive thinking in women with anorexia nervosa: a randomized, double-blind, placebo-controlled trial. *Am J Psychiatry* 2008; **165**:1281–1288.

9. Leggero C, et al. Low-dose olanzapine monotherapy in girls with anorexia nervosa, restricting subtype: focus on hyperactivity. *J Child Adolesc Psychopharmacol* 2010; **20**:127–133.

10. Court A, et al. Investigating the effectiveness, safety and tolerability of quetiapine in the treatment of anorexia nervosa in young people: a pilot study. *J Psychiatr Res* 2010; **44**:1027–1034.

11. Powers PS, et al. Double-blind placebo-controlled trial of quetiapine in anorexia nervosa. *Eur Eat Disord Rev* 2012; **20**:331–334.

12. Miniati M, et al. Psychopharmacological options for adult patients with anorexia nervosa. *CNS Spectr* 2016; **21**:134–142.

13. de Vos J, et al. Meta analysis on the efficacy of pharmacotherapy versus placebo on anorexia nervosa. *J Eat Disord* 2014; **2**:27.

14. Wade TD, et al. Comparative efficacy of pharmacological and non-pharmacological interventions for the acute treatment of adult outpatients with anorexia nervosa: study protocol for the systematic review and network meta-analysis of individual data. *J Eat Disord* 2017; **5**:24.

15. Blanchet C, et al. Medication in AN: a multidisciplinary overview of meta-analyses and systematic reviews. *J Clin Med* 2019; **8**

16. Andries A, et al. Dronabinol in severe, enduring anorexia nervosa: a randomized controlled trial. *Int J Eat Disord* 2014; **47**:18–23.

17. Gross H, et al. A double-blind trial of delta 9-tetrahydrocannabinol in primary anorexia nervosa. *J Clin Psychopharmacol* 1983; **3**:165–171.

18. Connan F, et al. Biochemical and endocrine complications. *Eur Eat Disord Rev* 2000; **8**:144–157.

19. Claudino AM, et al. Antidepressants for anorexia nervosa. *Cochrane Database Syst Rev* 2006:CD004365.

20. Barbarich NC, et al. Use of nutritional supplements to increase the efficacy of fluoxetine in the treatment of anorexia nervosa. *Int J Eat Disord* 2004; **35**:10–15.

21. Rossi G, et al. Pharmacological treatment of anorexia nervosa: a retrospective study in preadolescents and adolescents. *Clin Pediatr (Phila)* 2007; **46**:806–811.

22. Malina A, et al. Olanzapine treatment of anorexia nervosa: a retrospective study. *Int J Eat Disord* 2003; **33**:234–237.

23. La Via MC, et al. Case reports of olanzapine treatment of anorexia nervosa. *Int J Eat Disord* 2000; **27**:363–366.

24. Su JC, et al. Zinc supplementation in the treatment of anorexia nervosa. *Eat Weight Disord* 2002; **7**:20–22.

25. Marrazzi MA, et al. Naltrexone use in the treatment of anorexia nervosa and bulimia nervosa. *Int Clin Psychopharmacol* 1995; **10**:163–172.

26. Halmi KA, et al. Anorexia nervosa. Treatment efficacy of cyproheptadine and amitriptyline *Arch Gen Psychiatry* 1986; **43**:177–181.

27. Fazeli PK, et al. Treatment with a ghrelin agonist in outpatient women with anorexia nervosa: a randomized clinical trial. *J Clin Psychiatry* 2018; **79**.

28. Russell J, et al. Intranasal oxytocin in the treatment of anorexia nervosa: randomized controlled trial during re-feeding. *Psychoneuroendocrinology* 2018; **87**:83–92.

29. Kimball A, et al. A randomized placebo-controlled trial of low-dose testosterone therapy in women with anorexia nervosa. *J Clin Endocrinol Metab* 2019; **104**:4347–4355.

30. Kaye WH, et al. Double-blind placebo-controlled administration of fluoxetine in restricting- and restricting-purging-type anorexia nervosa. *Biol Psychiatry* 2001; **49**:644–652.

31. Walsh BT, et al. Fluoxetine after weight restoration in anorexia nervosa: a randomized controlled trial. *JAMA* 2006; **295**:2605–2612.

32. Himmerich H, et al. Pharmacological treatment of eating disorders, comorbid mental health problems, malnutrition and physical health consequences. *Pharmacol Ther* 2020:107667.

33. Vocks S, et al. Meta-analysis of the effectiveness of psychological and pharmacological treatments for binge eating disorder. *Int J Eat Disord* 2010; **43**:205–217.

34. Fluoxetine Bulimia Nervosa Collaborative Study Group. Fluoxetine in the treatment of bulimia nervosa. A multicenter, placebo-controlled, double-blind trial. *Arch Gen Psychiatry* 1992; **49**:139–147.

35. Goldstein DJ, et al. Long-term fluoxetine treatment of bulimia nervosa. Fluoxetine Bulimia Nervosa Research Group. *Br J Psychiatry* 1995; **166**:660–666.

36. Romano SJ, et al. A placebo-controlled study of fluoxetine in continued treatment of bulimia nervosa after successful acute fluoxetine treatment. *Am J Psychiatry* 2002; **159**:96–102.

37. Bacaltchuk J, et al. Antidepressants versus placebo for people with bulimia nervosa. *Cochrane Database Syst Rev* 2003:CD003391.

38. Sysko R, et al. Early response to antidepressant treatment in bulimia nervosa. *Psychol Med* 2010; **40**:999–1005.

39. Nourredine M, et al. Efficacy and safety of topiramate in binge eating disorder: a systematic review and meta-analysis. *CNS Spectr* 2020:1–9.

40. White MA, et al. Bupropion for overweight women with binge-eating disorder: a randomized, double-blind, placebo-controlled trial. *J Clin Psychiatry* 2013; **74**:400–406.

41. Leombruni P, et al. Duloxetine in obese binge eater outpatients: preliminary results from a 12-week open trial. *Hum Psychopharmacol* 2009; **24**:483–488.

42. Guerdjikova AI, et al. Lamotrigine in the treatment of binge-eating disorder with obesity: a randomized, placebo-controlled monotherapy trial. *Int Clin Psychopharmacol* 2009; **24**:150–158.

43. Trunko ME, et al. A pilot open series of lamotrigine in DBT-treated eating disorders characterized by significant affective dysregulation and poor impulse control. *Borderline Personality Disord Emot Dysregul* 2017; **4**:21.

第 9 章

44. Ricca V, et al. Zonisamide combined with cognitive behavioral therapy in binge eating disorder: a one-year follow-up study. *Psychiatry (Edgmont)* 2009; 6:23–28.

45. Guerdjikova AI, et al. Zonisamide in the treatment of bulimia nervosa: an open-label, pilot, prospective study. *Int J Eat Disord* 2013; 46:747–750.

46. McElroy SL, et al. Acamprosate in the treatment of binge eating disorder: a placebo-controlled trial. *Int J Eat Disord* 2011; 44:81–90.

47. McElroy SL, et al. Sodium oxybate in the treatment of binge eating disorder: an open-label, prospective study. *Int J Eat Disord* 2011; 44:262–268.

48. Hilbert A, et al. Meta-analysis on the long-term effectiveness of psychological and medical treatments for binge-eating disorder. *Int J Eat Disord* 2020; 53:1353–1376.

49. Ghaderi A, et al. Psychological, pharmacological, and combined treatments for binge eating disorder: a systematic review and meta-analysis. *Peer J* 2018; 6:e5113.

50. McElroy SL, et al. Efficacy and safety of lisdexamfetamine for treatment of adults with moderate to severe binge-eating disorder: a randomized clinical trial. *JAMA Psychiatry* 2015; 72:235–246.

51. Citrome L Lisdexamfetamine for binge eating disorder in adults: a systematic review of the efficacy and safety profile for this newly approved indication – what is the number needed to treat, number needed to harm and likelihood to be helped or harmed? *Int J Clin Pract* 2015; 69:410–421.

52. Safer DL, et al. A randomized, placebo-controlled crossover trial of phentermine-topiramate ER in patients with binge-eating disorder and bulimia nervosa. *Int J Eat Disord* 2020; 53:266–277.

53. Guerdjikova AI, et al. Combination phentermine-topiramate extended release for the treatment of binge eating disorder: an open-label, prospective study. *Innov Clin Neurosci* 2018; 15:17–21.

54. Grilo CM, et al. Efficacy and safety of dasotraline in adults with binge-eating disorder: a randomized, placebo-controlled, fixed-dose clinical trial. *CNS Spectr* 2020:1–10.

55. Leombruni P, et al. A 12 to 24 weeks pilot study of sertraline treatment in obese women binge eaters. *Hum Psychopharmacol* 2006; 21:181–188.

谵妄

谵妄是一种内外科常见的神经精神科问题,有不同的名称,包括器质性脑病综合征、重症监护室精神病或急性错乱状态[1]。

谵妄的诊断标准[2]

- 意识障碍(对环境意识的清晰度降低)伴有注意力的集中、维持或转移能力下降。
- 认知功能改变(比如记忆缺陷、定向力障碍、语言障碍或知觉障碍),且不可用已有的或正在发展的痴呆解释。
- 在短时间内发生(一般数小时或数天),往往在一天内出现波动。
- 往往有病史、躯体检查或实验室检查证据表明,其病因是合并用药、躯体疾病、物质中毒或物质戒断状态。

评估工具[3]

如果患者有谵妄的风险,应当进行简要的认知评估。一个标准化的《工具谵妄评定方法》(CAM)就是目前用于诊断谵妄的一种简洁的、经过验证的方法。CAM 依据的是症状急性发作、波动性病程、注意损害、思维混乱或意识水平改变。

谵妄的临床亚型[4-6]

- **活动亢进型谵妄**:特征表现为伴有激越、幻觉和不恰当行为的活动增多。
- **活动减退型谵妄**:特征表现为活动减少和昏睡(预后较差)。
- **混合型谵妄**:同时有活动增多和减退的特征。

患病率

内科患者住院时谵妄的发生率为 10%,住院后谵妄的发生率会增加到 10%~30%[4]。术后谵妄发生率为 15%~53%,重症监护室患者的谵妄发生率达 70%~87%[7]。

危险因素

谵妄几乎都是多病因的,把某单一因素作为病因来讲一般是不恰当的[4]。最重要的危险因素[4,5,8-10]一般表现如下:

- 已有认知功能受损或痴呆
- 老年人(年龄 >65 岁)
- 共患多种疾病
- 既往有谵妄、卒中、神经系统疾病、跌倒和步态异常
- 使用精神活性物质
- 合并用药(超过 4 种药物)
- 使用抗胆碱能药

结局

谵妄患者住院时间延长,死亡率增加,被长期安置于社会机构的风险增加[1,5]。谵妄患者住院期间死亡率在 6%~18%,是对照组的 2 倍[5]。谵妄病例的一年死亡率为 35%~40%[7]。高达 60% 的患者在谵妄之后出现持久的认知功能损害,且其发展为痴呆的风险增加 3 倍[1,5]。

管理

预防谵妄是减少其发生率及并发症最有效的策略[7]。谵妄是一个医学急症,鉴别并治疗其潜在病因是疾病管理的第一目标[11]。

非药物或环境支持对策应当尽量施行。这些方法包括协调护理、预防感觉剥夺和定向困难以及维护功能[5,12]。药物治疗应当首先指向潜在的病因(如果知道),然后才是缓解谵妄的特定症状。

谵妄的药物治疗中,经常犯的错误是过量使用抗精神病药、过晚给药或者过度使用苯二氮䓬类药物[4]。

一般原则 [4,5,13-16]

- 尽可能少用镇静药和抗精神病药
- 一次仅用一种药物
- 根据年龄、体型大小和激越程度个体化选择用药剂量
- 逐步加量直到产生疗效
- 规律地小剂量给药,而非大剂量少次给药
- 至少每 24h 重新评估 1 次
- 最初 24h 以后,若需要经常使用"必要时给药",则增加预定剂量
- 维持有效剂量,一旦临床情况允许,尽快停药
- 确保患者的谵妄诊断在其住院病历以及初级卫生保健病历中均有记录(包括出院志或出院小结)
- 若不可能在出院前停药,则应在患者同意的前提下,明确计划早期的用药评估或在社区中进行随访

药物选择 [17-20]

谵妄的药物治疗缺乏高质量的临床试验。已有研究往往样本量小,包含异质性人群和临床结局指标,排除了共病神经科和精神科疾病的患者[21],得出矛盾的结果。这些问题意味着,解读荟萃分析结果时必须慎重。最近一项网络荟萃分析发现,氟哌啶醇与劳拉西泮合用治疗谵妄有效,但是其依据是一项在癌症患者中进行的研究,测量的是对激越而非谵妄的疗效[22]。没有充分证据可用于推荐任何药物。某些患者群体使用抗精神病药治疗可能获益不大,如姑息治疗的患者可能会症状加重[23,24]。因此,选择药物时,应该了解其与原有躯体疾病或其他药物发生相互作用的可能性(表 9.1)。

表 9.1 治疗谵妄的药物

药物	剂量	不良反应	注解
第一代抗精神病药			
氟哌啶醇 [1,5,7,12,30,45-47]	口服 0.5~1mg,每天 2 次,必要时每 4h 增加 1 次 (峰值效应:4~6h) 肌内注射 0.5~1mg,观察 30~60min,必要时重复给药 (峰值效应:20~40min)	EPS,尤其剂量高于 3mg 时 Q-T 间期延长 升高痴呆患者的卒中风险	考虑作为一线治疗药物,是英国批准用于该适应证的唯一药物。目前,尚无研究数据发现其他抗精神病药疗效优于氟哌啶醇,但应用氟哌啶醇期间需要密切关注 EPS 及心脏不良反应 建议所有患者在基线查 ECG,尤其老年患者、有心脏病家族史或既往史的患者。既往无病者,小剂量(<1mg)不太可能造成问题 [48] 若有其他状况可导致 Q-T 间期延长,应定期监测 ECG 和血钾水平 避免用于路易体痴呆和帕金森病 尽可能避免静脉用药。然而在内科 ICU,在持续心电图监护下往往静脉用药
第二代抗精神病药			
氨磺必利 [12,13,49,50]	口服 50~300mg,每天一次,最高 800mg/d 药量超过 300mg 时需分 2 次给药	Q-T 间期延长 升高痴呆患者的卒中风险	用于谵妄的证据很少 鉴于氨磺必利几乎全由肾脏排泄,用于躯体疾病和老年患者时必须监测肾功能
阿立哌唑 [12,13,49-51]	口服 5~15mg/d,最高 30mg/d	EPS 风险低于氟哌啶醇 静坐不能或睡眠节律紊乱可能成问题 升高痴呆患者的卒中风险	证据很少 快速起效的肌内注射剂型已被描述过 [52]
奥氮平 [19,53-57]	口服 2.5~5mg,每天 1 次,最高 20mg/d	EPS 风险低于氟哌啶醇 镇静是最常见的不良反应 升高痴呆患者的卒中风险	一项比较奥氮平、利培酮、氟哌啶醇和喹硫平的研究发现,这些药物治疗谵妄的疗效和安全性相当,但奥氮平在老年患者(>75 岁)中的有效率要低一些 [58] 快速起效的肌内注射剂型尚未在谵妄治疗中进行评估。肌内注射制剂通过静脉用药有过介绍 [59]
利培酮 [19,55,56,60-65]	口服 0.5mg,每天 2 次,必要时每 4h 追加剂量 一般最多 4mg/d	最常见不良反应为低血压及 EPS 升高痴呆患者的卒中风险	一项比较利培酮与奥氮平的研究发现,二者减轻谵妄症状的疗效相当,但是利培酮对老年患者(>70 岁)的疗效差一些 [56]

续表

药物	剂量	不良反应	注解
喹硫平 [19,41,66-72]	口服 12.5~50mg，每天 2 次 若耐受良好，可每 12h 增加剂量，至每天 200mg	最常见不良反应为镇静及直立性低血压 升高痴呆患者的卒中风险	越来越多的研究显示，相较于氟哌啶醇，低剂量喹硫平不管是在 ICU 内还是 ICU 外，均安全有效。在许多病房是一线用药
齐拉西酮 [73]	每 2h 肌内注射 10mg 一般最多 40mg/d	Q-T 间期延长 升高痴呆患者的卒中风险	研究证据很少
苯二氮䓬类药物			
劳拉西泮 [1,5,7]	口服/肌内注射 根据需要，每 2~4h 给药 0.25~1mg 一般最大剂量为 3mg/24h 静脉注射一般用于紧急情况	相比于抗精神病药，更易引起呼吸抑制、过度镇静和反常兴奋 与谵妄症状的延长和恶化有关	用于酒精或镇静催眠药戒断状态、帕金森病和恶性综合征 其他情况避免使用
地西泮 [74]	口服起始剂量为 5~10mg 老年人推荐起始剂量为 2mg	半衰期明显长于劳拉西泮 与谵妄症状的延长和恶化有关	用于酒精或镇静催眠药戒断状态、帕金森病和 NMS 其他情况避免使用
胆碱酯酶抑制剂			
多奈哌齐 [75]	口服 5mg，每天 1 次	与安慰剂的耐受性相当。恶心、呕吐和腹泻是最常见的不良反应	证据很少。小规模的研究发现，其临床获益缺乏说服力 不推荐使用
卡巴拉汀 [76-78]	口服 1.5~6mg，每天 2 次	在一项研究中，在常规治疗（氟哌啶醇）的基础上合并卡巴拉汀治疗，结果发现卡巴拉汀并未缩短谵妄的病程，实际上相比于安慰剂，它使得谵妄变得更为严重，在重症监护的时间更长，且死亡率更高	不推荐给重症患者使用卡巴拉汀治疗谵妄。在预防谵妄上可能有一席之地 [34]
其他药物			
曲唑酮 [4,7]	25~150mg 睡前服用	过度镇静成问题	经验有限——仅在非对照研究中用过 不推荐使用

续表

药物	剂量	不良反应	注解
丙戊酸钠[79-82]	口服/肌内注射/静脉注射 250mg 每天 2 次,逐渐加至 1500mg/d,或每天 20mg/kg 对于此适应证的目标血浆浓度尚未得到确认。注意躯体病患者的蛋白结合率可能发生改变 在 ICU 曾静脉注射过负荷剂量	禁用于活动性肝病 监测血小板减少(重症患者更常见)	一些病例报告该药可用于抗精神病药和/或苯二氮䓬类药物无效的病例,否则不推荐使用

ECG,心电图;EPS,锥体外系副反应;ICU,重症监护室;NMS,恶性综合征。

药物预防 [25-29]

使用药物预防谵妄的数据很少,且结果不一致。大部分研究将低剂量的氟哌啶醇用于发生谵妄风险高的患者(高龄、术后或 ICU 患者)。预防性使用低剂量的氟哌啶醇(3mg/d),可减少谵妄发作的严重程度和持续时间,缩短可能发生谵妄的患者的住院时间,但是最近在老年人中进行的一项研究发现预防无效[30]。较大剂量(>5mg/d)可降低手术患者的谵妄发生率[31],但是一项大样本 RCT 发现,该用法无益于降低重症患者的死亡率[32]。Cochrane[25] 提出预防性使用奥氮平可能有效,一项小样本 RCT 发现阿立哌唑有些效果[33]。卡巴拉汀可能有效[34],但是 Cochrane 研究不支持[25]。褪黑素[35-37]、雷米替胺[38-41]、苏沃雷生[42] 的数据均是矛盾的,但是这些药物至少耐受性好,可减轻睡眠障碍,而睡眠障碍有导致谵妄的风险[43]。已有一些证据支持通过非药物治疗来降低谵妄的风险[44]。

(孔庆梅 译 田成华 审校)

参考文献

1. van Zyl LT, et al. Delirium concisely: condition is associated with increased morbidity, mortality, and length of hospitalization. *Geriatrics* 2006; 61:18–21.
2. American Psychiatric Association. *Diagnostic and statistical manual of mental disorders, Fifth Edition (DSM-5)*. Arlington, VA: American Psychiatric Association 2013.
3. Inouye SK, et al. Clarifying confusion: the confusion assessment method. A new method for detection of delirium. *Ann Intern Med* 1990; 113:941–948.
4. Nayeem K, et al. Delirium. *Clin Med* 2003; 3:412–415.
5. Potter J, et al. The prevention, diagnosis and management of delirium in older people: concise guidelines. *Clin Med* 2006; 6:303–308.
6. Fong TG, et al. Delirium in elderly adults: diagnosis, prevention and treatment. *Nat Rev Neurol* 2009; 5:210–220.
7. Inouye SK. Delirium in older persons. *N Engl J Med* 2006; 354:1157–1165.
8. Saxena S, et al. Delirium in the elderly: a clinical review. *Postgrad Med J* 2009; 85:405–413.
9. Naja M, et al. Delirium in geriatric medicine is related to anticholinergic burden. *Eur Geriatr Med* 2013; 4 Suppl 1:S208.
10. Egberts A, et al. Anticholinergic drug burden and delirium: a systematic review. *J Am Med Dir Assoc* 2020:S1525–8610 (1520)30349–30342.
11. Burns A, et al. Delirium. *J Neurol Neurosurg Psychiatry* 2004; 75:362–367.
12. Schwartz TL, et al. The role of atypical antipsychotics in the treatment of delirium. *Psychosomatics* 2002; 43:171–174.

13. Seitz DP, et al. Antipsychotics in the treatment of delirium: a systematic review. *J Clin Psychiatry* 2007; 68:11–21.

14. National Institute for Health and Clinical Excellence. Delirium: diagnosis, prevention and management. [Clinical Guideline 103] 2010 (Last updated March 2019); https://www.nice.org.uk/Guidance/CG103.

15. Donders E, et al. Effect of haloperidol dosing frequencies on the duration and severity of delirium in elderly hip fracture patients. A prospective randomized trial. *Eur Geriatr Med* 2012; 3 Suppl 1:S118–S119.

16. Soiza RL, et al. The Scottish Intercollegiate Guidelines Network (SIGN) 157: guidelines on risk reduction and management of delirium. *Medicina (Kaunas)* 2019; 55:491.

17. Nikooie R, et al. Antipsychotics for treating delirium in hospitalized adults: a systematic review. *Ann Intern Med* 2019; 171:485–495.

18. Li Y, et al. Benzodiazepines for treatment of patients with delirium excluding those who are cared for in an intensive care unit. *Cochrane Database Syst Rev* 2020; 2:Cd012670.

19. Rivière J, et al. Efficacy and tolerability of atypical antipsychotics in the treatment of delirium: a systematic review of the literature. *Psychosomatics* 2019; 60:18–26.

20. Devlin JW, et al. Clinical practice guidelines for the prevention and management of pain, agitation/sedation, delirium, immobility, and sleep disruption in adult patients in the ICU. *Crit Care Med* 2018; 46:e825–e873.

21. Martin RC, et al. Assessment of the generalizability of clinical trials of delirium interventions. *JAMA Network Open* 2020; 3:e2015080.

22. Wu YC, et al. Association of delirium response and safety of pharmacological interventions for the management and prevention of delirium: a network meta-analysis. *JAMA Psychiatry* 2019; 76:526–535.

23. Finucane AM, et al. Drug therapy for delirium in terminally ill adults. *Cochrane Database Syst Rev* 2020; 1:Cd004770.

24. Lee KY, et al. Effect of antipsychotics and non-pharmacotherapy for the management of delirium in people receiving palliative care. *J Pain Palliat Care Pharmacother* 2020:1–12.

25. Siddiqi N, et al. Interventions for preventing delirium in hospitalised non-ICU patients. *Cochrane Database Syst Rev* 2016; 3:Cd005563.

26. Santos E, et al. Effectiveness of haloperidol prophylaxis in critically ill patients with a high risk of delirium: a systematic review. *JBI Database System Rev Implement Rep* 2017; 15:1440–1472.

27. Fok MC, et al. Do antipsychotics prevent postoperative delirium? A systematic review and meta-analysis. *Int J Geriatr Psychiatry* 2015; 30:333–344.

28. Schrijver EJ, et al. Efficacy and safety of haloperidol for in-hospital delirium prevention and treatment: A systematic review of current evidence. *Eur J Intern Med* 2016; 27:14–23.

29. Oh ES, et al. Antipsychotics for preventing delirium in hospitalized adults: a systematic review. *Ann Intern Med* 2019; 171:474–484.

30. Schrijver E, et al. Haloperidol versus placebo for delirium prevention in acutely hospitalised older at risk patients: a multi-centre double-blind randomised controlled clinical trial. *Age Ageing* 2017; 47:48–55.

31. Shen YZ, et al. Effects of haloperidol on delirium in adult patients: a systematic review and meta-analysis. *Med Princ Pract* 2018; 27:250–259.

32. van den Boogaard M, et al. Effect of haloperidol on survival among critically ill adults with a high risk of delirium: the reduce randomized clinical trial. *JAMA* 2018; 319:680–690.

33. Mokhtari M, et al. Aripiprazole for prevention of delirium in the neurosurgical intensive care unit: a double-blind, randomized, placebo-controlled study. *Eur J Clin Pharmacol* 2020; 76:491–499.

34. Youn YC, et al. Rivastigmine patch reduces the incidence of postoperative delirium in older patients with cognitive impairment. *Int J Geriatr Psychiatry* 2016; 32:1079–1084.

35. Asleson DR, et al. Melatonin for delirium prevention in acute medically ill, and perioperative geriatric patients. *Aging Medicine (Milton (NSW))* 2020; 3:132–137.

36. Campbell AM, et al. Melatonin for the prevention of postoperative delirium in older adults: a systematic review and meta-analysis. *BMC Geriatr* 2019; 19:272.

37. Ford AH, et al. The healthy heart-mind trial: randomized controlled trial of melatonin for prevention of delirium. *J Am Geriatr Soc* 2020; 68:112–119.

38. Oh ES, et al. Effects of ramelteon on the prevention of postoperative delirium in older patients undergoing orthopedic surgery: the recover randomized controlled trial. *Am J Geriatr Psychiatry* 2021; 29:90–100.

39. Hatta K, et al. Preventive effects of ramelteon on delirium: a randomized placebo-controlled trial. *JAMA Psychiatry* 2014; 71:397–403.

40. Jaiswal SJ, et al. Ramelteon for prevention of postoperative delirium: a randomized controlled trial in patients undergoing elective pulmonary thromboendarterectomy. *Crit Care Med* 2019; 47:1751–1758.

41. Kim MS, et al. Comparative efficacy and acceptability of pharmacological interventions for the treatment and prevention of delirium: A systematic review and network meta-analysis. *J Psychiatr Res* 2020; 125:164–176.

42. Adams AD, et al. The role of suvorexant in the prevention of delirium during acute hospitalization: A systematic review. *J Crit Care* 2020; 59:1–5.

43. Lu Y, et al. Promoting sleep and circadian health may prevent postoperative delirium: A systematic review and meta-analysis of randomized clinical trials. *Sleep Med Rev* 2019; 48:101207.

44. Salvi F, et al. Non-pharmacological approaches in the prevention of delirium. *Eur Geriatr Med* 2020; 11:71–81.

45. Fricchione GL, et al. Postoperative delirium. *Am J Psychiatry* 2008; 165:803–812.

46. Zayed Y, et al. Haloperidol for the management of delirium in adult intensive care unit patients: A systematic review and meta-analysis of randomized controlled trials. *J Crit Care* 2019; 50:280–286.

47. Burry L, et al. Antipsychotics for treatment of delirium in hospitalised non-ICU patients. *Cochrane Database Syst Rev* 2018; 6:Cd005594.

48. Schrijver EJ, et al. Low dose oral haloperidol does not prolong QTc interval in older acutely hospitalised adults: a subanalysis of a randomised

double-blind placebo-controlled study. *J Geriatr Cardiol* 2018; 15:401–407.

49. Boettger S, et al. Atypical antipsychotics in the management of delirium: a review of the empirical literature. *Palliat Support Care* 2005; 3:227–237.

50. Leentjens AF, et al. Delirium in elderly people: an update. *Curr Opin Psychiatry* 2005; 18:325–330.

51. Boettger S, et al. Aripiprazole and haloperidol in the treatment of delirium. *Aust NZJ Psychiatry* 2011; 45:477–482.

52. Martinotti G, et al. Psychomotor agitation and hyperactive delirium in COVID-19 patients treated with aripiprazole 9.75mg/1.3 ml immediate release. *Psychopharmacology (Berl)* 2020:1–5.

53. Skrobik YK, et al. Olanzapine vs haloperidol: treating delirium in a critical care setting. *Intensive Care Med* 2004; 30:444–449.

54. Sipahimalani A, et al. Olanzapine in the treatment of delirium. *Psychosomatics* 1998; 39:422–430.

55. Duff G Atypical antipsychotic drugs and stroke – Committee on safety of medicines 2004; https://webarchive.nationalarchives.gov. uk/20141206131857/http://www.mhra.gov.uk/home/groups/pl-p/documents/websiteresources/con019488.pdf.

56. Kim SW, et al. Risperidone versus olanzapine for the treatment of delirium. *Hum Psychopharmacol* 2010; 25:298–302.

57. Grover S, et al. Comparative efficacy study of haloperidol, olanzapine and risperidone in delirium. *J Psychosom Res* 2011; 71:277–281.

58. Yoon HJ, et al. Efficacy and safety of haloperidol versus atypical antipsychotic medications in the treatment of delirium. *BMC Psychiatry* 2013; 13:240.

59. Lorenzo MP, et al. Intravenous olanzapine in a critically ill patient: an evolving route of administration. *Hosp Pharm* 2020; 55:108–111.

60. Bourgeois JA, et al. Prolonged delirium managed with risperidone. *Psychosomatics* 2005; 46:90–91.

61. Gupta N, et al. Effectiveness of risperidone in delirium. *Can J Psychiatry* 2005; 50:75.

62. Liu CY, et al. Efficacy of risperidone in treating the hyperactive symptoms of delirium. *Int Clin Psychopharmacol* 2004; 19:165–168.

63. Horikawa N, et al. Treatment for delirium with risperidone: results of a prospective open trial with 10 patients. *Gen Hosp Psychiatry* 2003; 25:289–292.

64. Han CS, et al. A double-blind trial of risperidone and haloperidol for the treatment of delirium. *Psychosomatics* 2004; 45:297–301.

65. Hakim SM, et al. Early treatment with risperidone for subsyndromal delirium after on-pump cardiac surgery in the elderly: a randomized trial. *Anesthesiology* 2012; 116:987–997.

66. Torres R, et al. Use of quetiapine in delirium: case reports. *Psychosomatics* 2001; 42:347–349.

67. Sasaki Y, et al. A prospective, open-label, flexible-dose study of quetiapine in the treatment of delirium. *J Clin Psychiatry* 2003; 64:1316–1321.

68. Devlin JW, et al. Efficacy and safety of quetiapine in critically ill patients with delirium: a prospective, multicenter, randomized, double-blind, placebo-controlled pilot study. *Crit Care Med* 2010; 38:419–427.

69. Hawkins SB, et al. Quetiapine for the treatment of delirium. *J Hosp Med* 2013; 8:215–220.

70. Tahir TA, et al. A randomized controlled trial of quetiapine versus placebo in the treatment of delirium. *J Psychosom Res* 2010; 69:485–490.

71. Grover S, et al. Comparative effectiveness of quetiapine and haloperidol in delirium: A single blind randomized controlled study. *World J Psychiatry* 2016; 6:365–371.

72. Mangan KC, et al. Evaluating the risk profile of quetiapine in treating delirium in the intensive care adult population: A retrospective review. *J Crit Care* 2018; 47:169–172.

73. Young CC, et al. Intravenous ziprasidone for treatment of delirium in the intensive care unit. *Anesthesiology* 2004; 101:794–795.

74. Chan D, et al. Delirium: making the diagnosis, improving the prognosis. *Geriatrics* 1999; 54:28–42.

75. Sampson EL, et al. A randomized, double-blind, placebo-controlled trial of donepezil hydrochloride (Aricept) for reducing the incidence of postoperative delirium after elective total hip replacement. *Int J Geriatr Psychiatry* 2007; 22:343–349.

76. Dautzenberg PL, et al. Adding rivastigmine to antipsychotics in the treatment of a chronic delirium. *Age Ageing* 2004; 33:516–517.

77. van Eijk MM, et al. Effect of rivastigmine as an adjunct to usual care with haloperidol on duration of delirium and mortality in critically ill patients: a multicentre, double-blind, placebo-controlled randomised trial. *Lancet* 2010; 376:1829–1837.

78. Yu A, et al. Cholinesterase inhibitors for the treatment of delirium in non-ICU settings. *Cochrane Database Syst Rev* 2018; 6:Cd012494.

79. Sher Y, et al. Adjunctive valproic acid in management-refractory hyperactive delirium: a case series and rationale. *J Neuropsychiatry Clin Neurosci* 2015; 27:365–370.

80. Gagnon DJ, et al. Valproate for agitation in critically ill patients: a retrospective study. *J Crit Care* 2017; 37:119–125.

81. Crowley KE, et al. Valproic acid for the management of agitation and delirium in the intensive care setting: a retrospective analysis. *Clin Ther* 2020; 42:e65–e73.

82. Quinn NJ, et al. Prescribing practices of valproic acid for agitation and delirium in the intensive care unit. *Ann Pharmacother* 2021;55:311–317

发生于其他疾病的精神症状的药物治疗

HIV 感染的一般用药原则

HIV 感染者可能会有精神疾病的症状,其影响因素有许多(框 10.1)。在实践中,这些因素中的几种可能会共存于一个人身上。

框 10.1　HIV 感染者发生精神症状的影响因素 [1]

- 原发(或原有)精神障碍
- HIV 导致中枢神经系统出现神经生物学改变
- 其他感染或中枢神经系统肿瘤
- 抗反转录病毒药和其他药物治疗(见本节治疗 HIV 的药物)
- 酒精或物质滥用
- 不利的心理社会因素(如耻感)
- 意识到慢性疾病必须严格遵照医嘱用药

使用精神药物时,应遵守下列原则:

- 从低剂量开始,根据耐受性和疗效增加剂量。
- 尽可能选择最简单的给药方案。(请记住患者的用药方案很可能已经很复杂了。)
- 选择不良反应最少的药物。必须考虑药物相互作用、共病躯体疾病和物质滥用情况。
- 与 HIV 专科医师和其他多学科团队紧密合作进行治疗。

尽管人们认为大多数精神药物对 HIV 感染者是安全的,但是在很多情况下这方面都缺乏明确的数据,而且该群体可能对高剂量、不良反应和药物相互作用更敏感 [2]。获得性免疫缺陷综合征(又称艾滋病)晚期患者使用精神药物时,更容易出现明显的不良反应。

精神分裂症

一般而言,精神分裂症无论是否伴有 HIV 感染,其药物治疗均无不同 [3],但是应该记住一些特殊的考虑。HIV 感染者更容易出现 EPS [2],因为 HIV 侵蚀基底节,特别是在该病晚期。因此,治疗与痴呆或谵妄无关的精神病时,一线选择是第二代抗精神病药,如喹硫平、利培酮和阿立哌唑 [4]。抗精神病药和抗反转录病毒药可能引起额外的代谢作用,需要密切监测。Q-T 间期延长可能是 HIV 进展、共病、抗反转录病毒药和抗精神病药的并发症 [5]。本节将进一步讨论药物相互作用。

在 HIV 感染者中,使用氯氮平治疗难治性精神分裂症的报告发表得不多 [6-8]。氯氮平可用于既有难治性精神分裂症又感染 HIV 者,目标是控制病毒载量。这种病例需要多学科团队合作 [6,8]。

但是,需要密切监测白细胞计数,因为氯氮平、一些抗反转录病毒药和 HIV 本身都对骨髓有抑制作用 [6-8]。氯氮平还可能有助于治疗 HIV 引起的精神病伴药源性帕金森综合征 [9]。

谵妄

应该找到谵妄的器质性原因并加以治疗。短期对症治疗可包括低剂量第二代抗精神病药,如利培酮 [4]。在伴有谵妄的 AIDS 患者中,几乎未做过随机对照试验;早期研究证明第一代抗精神病药有效,在一项共识研究中选择了小剂量氟哌啶醇 [4]。但是应该慎用第一代抗精神病药,因为该患者群体容易发生 EPS[10]。苯二氮䓬类药物应该慎用,因为会加重谵妄(酒精或苯二氮䓬类药物为促发因素时例外)[6]。

抑郁症

抑郁症在 HIV 患者中常见,估计患病率为 20%~40%[11]。它可能是 HIV 感染的后果,也可能原来就有。研究提示,抑郁症共病 HIV 者使用抗反转录病毒药的依从性差,病毒抑制减弱 [12]。抗抑郁药治疗 HIV 感染者的抑郁症时,疗效优于安慰剂 [12],可改善使用抗反转录病毒药的依从性 [13],但是在该患者群体中比较不同抗抑郁药的研究存在空白。SSRI 被当作一线药物受到欢迎。艾司西酞普兰和西酞普兰 [4,14] 引起药物相互作用的风险较小。进一步治疗请参照标准方案。一项研究发现艾司西酞普兰与安慰剂没有差异 [15],原因可能是安慰剂效应较大。艾司西酞普兰或西酞普兰合用可延长 Q-T 间期 [5,11] 的抗反转录病毒药时,建议监测心电图。米氮平治疗有效 [16,17],药物相互作用的风险较低 [18],可能有益于 HIV 感染和抑郁症共病的患者 [19],或者有益于减少甲基苯丙胺的使用 [20]。"双重作用"抗抑郁药(度洛西汀、文拉法新)治疗 HIV 感染者的抑郁症状时,疗效与 SSRI 相当 [21]。其他药物(安非他酮 [22]、曲唑酮 [28])治疗有效,但是药物相互作用和不良反应限制了它们的使用。三环类药物有时可能适用,但是其不良反应大,因而可能会限制其疗效和依从性。使用 TCA 的 HIV 感染者常出现口干和便秘 [12]。对该患者群体,不推荐使用单胺氧化酶抑制剂。

合并感染 HIV/HCV 患者中 α-干扰素引起的抑郁症

已发现西酞普兰对新发抑郁症治疗有效,耐受性好 [23],但是不建议预防性使用 [24]。

双相障碍

HIV 感染者的躁狂可能是原发的(以前就有双相障碍),也可能是继发的(HIV 感染晚期的"HIV 躁狂")。HIV 患者可能对心境稳定剂的不良反应(如锂盐的神经毒性)更敏感 [25],特别是当他们有神经认知功能障碍时 [25,26]。锂盐经肾脏排泄,不可能发生 P450 相关的药物相互作用。但是,在 HIV 感染者常见的肾损害中,锂盐可能成问题。锂盐和替诺福韦二酯(TDF)都有肾小管毒性,一项 RCT 对二者联合治疗进行了研究。在 24 周试验期间,肾毒性的发生率并未增加,但是无法排除其长期风险 [27]。在密切监测下,可慎重使用锂盐治疗 HIV 感染者的原发性双相障碍,但是应避免用于 HIV 感染晚期 [28]。应避免使用卡马西平,因为它会引起药物相互作用以及导致恶血质的风险[28]。丙戊酸盐可以作为备选,用于治疗 HIV 感染者的双相障碍。需要进行监测,因为丙戊酸盐有导致肝毒性、恶血质、胰腺炎和药物相互作用的风险。丙戊酸盐最好避免合用其他肝毒性药物(如奈韦拉平、利福平)[28]。也可选择具有心境稳定作用的抗精神病药,如利培酮、喹硫平和奥氮平[4]。

继发性躁狂("HIV 躁狂")

继发性躁狂通常发生在疾病晚期,与 HIV 引起的神经认知功能障碍或中枢神经系统机会感染有关[29]。随着有效的抗反转录病毒药的广泛使用,继发性躁狂的报告已经减少。首要目标是识别和治疗可能存在的基础疾病(感染、物质滥用、酒精戒断和代谢异常)。继发躁狂以第二代抗精神病药喹硫平、奥氮平和阿利哌唑治疗可能有效,因为 EPS 风险较低。一例个案报告用齐拉西酮治疗"HIV 躁狂"获得成功[30]。

焦虑障碍

焦虑障碍在 HIV 患者中高发,常见的是广泛性焦虑障碍、惊恐障碍和 PTSD。在标准指南和 HIV 感染者[3] 中,SSRI 是治疗焦虑障碍和惊恐障碍的一线选择(首选药物见本节"抑郁症")。苯二氮䓬类药物可用于急性期治疗,但是需要谨慎,因为它们有滥用、药物相互作用和增加神经认知功能损害的风险[31]。

劳拉西泮、奥沙西泮和替马西泮经由非 CYP450 通路代谢,因而发生药物相互作用的风险低,可以作为 HIV 感染者治疗焦虑的首选[32]。丁螺环酮也可能有效[33]。

HIV 的神经认知障碍

在使用有效抗反转录病毒药的时代,严重 HIV 相关脑病的发生率已经大幅下降。但是,较为轻微的 HIV 相关神经认知功能障碍仍然常见[34,35]。危险因素包括共病(如 HCV 合并感染)、HIV 感染本身以及患者的遗传因素。HIV 相关神经认知障碍包括三种亚型,从比较常见的无症状神经认知损害,到比较严重而少见的 HIV 相关痴呆。建议在 HIV 感染者中筛查认知损害[11]。使用的工具有 CogState 或 HIV 痴呆量表,但是它们可能无法识别无症状神经认知损害[35]。

症状包括情感淡漠、易激惹、缺乏活力、主动性差、社交退缩、精神运动迟缓、注意减退、情绪不稳和偶尔的"HIV 躁狂"[29]。

主要治疗是使用中枢神经系统穿透作用强的抗反转录病毒药物[35],以便在中枢神经系统达到适宜浓度,并尽量减少药物相关的神经毒性。人们也研究过其他辅助治疗[米诺环素、美金刚、司来吉兰、锂盐、丙戊酸盐、来昔帕泛(lexipafant)、尼莫地平、兴奋剂、那他珠单抗干扰素等][36]。

最近一项研究发现,帕罗西汀可以改善神经认知功能(调整抑郁因素之后)[37],卡巴拉汀贴剂试验结果为阴性。需要进一步研究来证实这些辅助治疗对于 HIV 相关认知障碍的作用。

抗反转录病毒药物与精神药物的相互作用

两类药物常常发生药代动力学相互作用,且可能具有临床意义。合用两类药物的患者全都需要审查潜在的相互作用。审查药物相互作用的用药史应该包括现用药物、替代药物或植物药物、消遣性毒品和其他非处方药[34]。

关于具体的药代动力学相互作用信息,建议读者经常更新在线资源。

药效学相互作用也可能发生,通常表现为不良反应的叠加。

潜在的药效学相互作用见表 10.1。

表 10.1　与抗反转录病毒药物的潜在药效学相互作用[38]

潜在的不良反应	涉及的抗反转录病毒药物[32,39-41]	对使用精神药物的影响
骨髓抑制	齐多夫定(贫血,中性粒细胞减少)	合用某些精神药物(如氯氮平)可增加骨髓抑制和中性粒细胞减少的风险
骨密度降低	替诺福韦酯(替诺福韦阿拉芬酰胺对骨密度影响小些)	可加重升高催乳素的抗精神病药可能引起的骨密度降低
肌酸激酶升高	多替拉韦钠片(dolutegravir)、恩曲他滨、拉替拉韦	若考虑诊断为恶性综合征,可能必须认识到相关性
心电图改变	阿扎那韦、达芦那韦、依法韦伦、洛匹那韦、利匹韦林、利托那韦、沙奎那韦	会增加某些精神药物相关心律失常的风险
对心血管影响	阿巴卡韦、达芦那韦/利托那韦、洛比那韦/利托那韦	一些患者出现心血管事件(如心肌梗死)
对肾脏影响	替诺福韦酯(若方案中含利托那韦,风险升高)	蛋白尿、低磷血症、糖尿、低钾血症、肾小管酸中毒
胃肠功能紊乱	阿扎那韦、达芦那韦、多替拉韦钠片、双腺苷、埃替拉韦/钴试剂、福沙那韦、茚地那韦、利匹韦林、奈芬那韦、雷特格韦、沙奎那韦、替拉那韦、齐多夫定	可加重某些精神药物(如 SSRI)引起的胃肠功能紊乱
癫痫发作	达芦那韦、依非韦伦、马拉维诺、利托那韦、沙奎那韦、齐多夫定	和某些精神药物合用时,可能增加癫痫发作的风险
代谢异常,如高甘油三酯血症、高胆固醇血症、胰岛素抵抗、高血糖和高乳酸血症	所有联合抗反转录病毒疗法	可加重某些精神药物所致代谢不良反应的风险(特别是第二代抗精神病药)

抗反转录病毒药物的精神科不良反应

许多抗反转录病毒药物均出现精神科不良反应,但是因果关系始终不明。依法韦伦涉及的问题最多,HIV 指南建议避免用于精神疾病患者[32,34,39]。

表 10.2 总结了抗反转录病毒药物的重要精神科不良反应。注意这不是详尽的清单,建议读者阅读产品特征概要或药品说明书,了解其他可能的不良反应。精神科不良反应的鉴别诊断见本指南其他章节。患者服用有精神科不良反应的药物时,建议对其进行监测。

表 10.2　抗反转录病毒药物的精神科不良反应

药物	精神科不良反应/评论
核苷反转录酶抑制剂	
阿巴卡韦	焦虑、抑郁、梦魇、情绪不稳、躁狂、精神病。报告的病例极少；在已报告病例中，停药后迅速恢复到基线
双腺苷	昏睡、紧张、焦虑、精神错乱、睡眠紊乱、心境障碍、精神病、躁狂。罕见
恩曲他滨	精神错乱、易激惹、失眠
齐多夫定	睡眠紊乱、生动梦境、激越、躁狂、抑郁、精神病、谵妄。精神科不良反应通常与剂量相关。发生时间差异很大，从不到 24h 至 7 个月
非核苷反转录酶抑制剂	
依法韦伦	嗜睡、失眠、梦境异常、注意受损、抑郁、精神病、自杀观念。症状通常在 2~4 周后减轻或消失。但是，可能会出现较轻微而长久的精神科不良反应。可加重精神症状，避免用于有精神疾病史的患者
依曲韦林	睡眠紊乱
奈韦拉平	幻视、被害妄想、心境改变、梦魇和生动梦境、抑郁。只有少数病例报告。症状出现在头 2 周内。停药后，症状均缓解
利匹韦林	抑郁、自杀倾向、睡眠紊乱。不良反应与依法韦伦类似，但是发生率低些。可加重精神症状，避免用于有精神疾病史的患者
整合酶链转移抑制剂	
多替拉韦钠片，埃替拉韦，雷特格韦	抑郁和自杀观念（原有精神疾病的患者，症状偶尔会加重）
CCRS 拮抗剂	
马拉维诺	抑郁、失眠

参考文献

1. Nanni MG, et al. Depression in HIV infected patients: a review. *Curr Psychiatry Rep* 2015; 17:530.

2. Hill L, et al. Pharmacotherapy considerations in patients with HIV and psychiatric disorders: focus on antidepressants and antipsychotics. *Ann Pharmacother* 2013; 47:75–89.

3. Cohen M, et al. *Comprehensive textbook of AIDS psychiatry: a paradigm for integrated care.* Oxford University Press, Oxford, England; 2017.

4. Freudenreich O, et al. Psychiatric treatment of persons with HIV/AIDS: an HIV-Psychiatry Consensus Survey of Current Practices. *Psychosomatics* 2010; 51:480–488.

5. Liu J, et al. QT prolongation in HIV-positive patients: review article. *Indian Heart J* 2019; 71:434–439.

6. Nejad SH, et al. Clozapine use in HIV-infected schizophrenia patients: a case-based discussion and review. *Psychosomatics* 2009; 50:626–632.

7. Sanz-Cortés S, et al. A case report of schizophrenia and HIV: HAART in association with clozapine. *J Psychiatric Intensive Care* 2009; 5:47–49.

8. Whiskey E, et al. Clozapine, HIV and neutropenia: a case report. *Ther Adv Psychopharmacol* 2018; 8:365–369.

9. Lera G, et al. Pilot study with clozapine in patients with HIV-associated psychosis and drug-induced parkinsonism. *Mov Disord* 1999; 14:128–131.

10. Watkins CC, et al. Cognitive impairment in patients with AIDS - prevalence and severity. *HIV/AIDS (Auckland, NZ)* 2015; 7:35–47.

11. European AIDS Clinical Society. Guidelines Version 10.1 October 2020. 2020; http://www.eacsociety.org/files/guidelines_10.1-english.pdf.

12. Eshun-Wilson I, et al. Antidepressants for depression in adults with HIV infection. *Cochrane Database System Rev* 2018; 1:Cd008525.

13. Gokhale RH, et al. Depression prevalence, antidepressant treatment status, and association with sustained HIV viral suppression among adults living with HIV in care in the United States, 2009-2014. *AIDS Behav* 2019; 23:3452–3459.

14. Currier MB, et al. Citalopram treatment of major depressive disorder in hispanic HIV and AIDS patients: a prospective study. *Psychosomatics* 2004; 45:210–216.

15. Hoare J, et al. Escitalopram treatment of depression in human immunodeficiency virus/acquired immunodeficiency syndrome: a randomized, double-blind, placebo-controlled study. *J Nerv Ment Dis* 2014; 202:133–137.

16. Patel S, et al. Escitalopram and mirtazapine for the treatment of depression in HIV patients: a randomized controlled open label trial. *ASEAN J Psychiatry* 2012; 14.

17. Elliott AJ, et al. Mirtazapine for depression in patients with human immunodeficiency virus. *J Clin Psychopharmacol* 2000; 20:265–267.

18. Adams JL, et al. Treating depression within the HIV 'medical home': a guided algorithm for antidepressant management by HIV clinicians. *AIDS Patient Care STDS* 2012; 26:647–654.

19. Badowski M, et al. Pharmacologic management of human immunodeficiency virus wasting syndrome. *Pharmacotherapy* 2014; 34:868–881.

20. Coffin PO, et al. Effects of mirtazapine for methamphetamine use disorder among cisgender men and transgender women who have sex with men: a placebo-controlled randomized clinical trial. *JAMA Psychiatry* 2020; 77:246–255.

21. Mills JC, et al. Comparative effectiveness of dual-action versus single-action antidepressants for the treatment of depression in people living with HIV/AIDS. *J Affect Disord* 2017; 215:179–186.

22. Currier MB, et al. A prospective trial of sustained-release bupropion for depression in HIV-seropositive and AIDS patients. *Psychosomatics* 2003; 44:120–125.

23. Laguno M, et al. Depressive symptoms after initiation of interferon therapy in human immunodeficiency virus-infected patients with chronic hepatitis C. *Antivir Ther* 2004; 9:905–909.

24. Klein MB, et al. Citalopram for the prevention of depression and its consequences in HIV-hepatitis C coinfected individuals initiating pegylated interferon/ribavirin therapy: a multicenter randomized double-blind placebocontrolled trial. *HIV Clin Trials* 2014; 15:161–175.

25. Ferrando SJ. Psychopharmacologic treatment of patients with HIV/AIDS. *Current psychiatry reports* 2009; 11:235–242.

26. El-Mallakh RS. Mania in AIDS: clinical significance and theoretical considerations. *Int J Psychiatry Med* 1991; 21:383–391.

27. Decloedt EH, et al. Renal safety of lithium in HIV-infected patients established on tenofovir disoproxil fumarate containing antiretroviral therapy: analysis from a randomized placebo-controlled trial. *AIDS Res Ther* 2017; 14:6.

28. Gallego L, et al. Psychopharmacological treatments in HIV patients under antiretroviral therapy. *AIDS Rev* 2012; 14:101–111.

29. Singer EJ, et al. Neurobehavioral Manifestations of Human Immunodeficiency Virus/AIDS: Diagnosis and Treatment. *Neurol Clin* 2016; 34:33–53.

30. Spiegel DR, et al. The successful treatment of mania due to acquired immunodeficiency syndrome using ziprasidone: a case series. *J Neuropsychiatry Clin Neurosci* 2010; 22:111–114.

31. Saloner R, et al. Benzodiazepine use is associated with an increased risk of neurocognitive impairment in people living with HIV. *J Acquir Immune Defic Syndr* 2019; 82:475–482.

32. Panel on Antiretroviral Guidelines for Adults and Adolescents. Guidelines for the use of antiretroviral agents in adults and adolescents living with HIV. Department of Health and Human Services. 2017; https://aidsinfo.nih.gov/contentfiles/lvguidelines/AdultandAdolescentGL.pdf.

33. Brogan K, et al. Management of common psychiatric conditions in the HIV-positive population. *Curr HIV/AIDS Rep* 2009; 6:108–115.

34. Waters L, et al. British HIV Association guidelines for the treatment of HIV-1-positive adults with antiretroviral therapy 2015 (2016 interim update). 2016; http://www.bhiva.org/documents/Guidelines/Treatment/2016/treatment-guidelines-2016-interim-update.pdf.

35. Carroll A, et al. HIV-associated neurocognitive disorders: recent advances in pathogenesis, biomarkers, and treatment. F1000Res 2017; 6:312.

36. Ambrosius B, et al. Antineuroinflammatory drugs in HIV-associated neurocognitive disorders as potential therapy. *Neurol Neuroimmunol Neuroinflamm* 2019; 6:e551.

37. Sacktor N, et al. Paroxetine and fluconazole therapy for HIV-associated neurocognitive impairment: results from a double-blind, placebo-controlled trial. *J Neurovirol* 2018; 24:16–27.

38. Panel on Antiretroviral Guidelines for Adults and Adolescents. Guidelines for the Use of Antiretroviral Agents in Adults and Adolescents Living with HIV. Department of Health and Human Services. 2019; https://clinicalinfo.hiv.gov/en.

39. European AIDS Clinical Society. Guidelines Version 9.0 October 2017. http://www.eacsociety.org/files/guidelines_9.0-english.pdf.

40. World Health Organisation. Consolidated guidelines on the use of antiretroviral drugs for treating and preventing HIV infection. Recommendations for a public health approach - Second edition. 2016; http://www.who.int/hiv/pub/arv/arv-2016/en/.

41. Parker C. Psychiatric effects of drugs for other disorders. *Medicine* 2016; 44:768–774.

癫痫

癫痫伴发的精神疾病

癫痫患者中,患病率升高的几种精神疾病包括抑郁症(22.9%)、焦虑症(20.2%)和精神病(5.2%)[1,2]。癫痫患者的自杀率比普通人群高 5 倍[3],自杀是过早死亡的重要原因[4]。癫痫与精神疾病之间的联系是双向的,因为抑郁症、焦虑症和精神病患者中,新发癫痫的风险也升高[5,6]。自杀未遂也与发生癫痫有关[3]。这种双向关系可以用精神疾病与癫痫之间共同的潜在病理变化来解释。神经传递、神经炎症和 HPA 轴紊乱[7],均被提示为共同的病理机制。

发作间精神疾病(症状的发生与癫痫发作无关)可能需要使用精神药物治疗[8-10]。给癫痫患者合用精神药物时,应该遵守下列一般原则[11,12]:

- 首先排除可能导致精神症状的其他原因(发作期及医源性,表 10.3)。
- 优化癫痫治疗(最好在合用精神药物之前)。
- 考虑合用已知有抗癫痫作用的精神药物(如双相障碍中的抗癫痫药)。
- 审核与抗癫痫药的相互作用。
- 小剂量起始,根据耐受性和疗效逐步调整剂量(促惊厥作用与剂量有关)。
- 若出现癫痫发作,考虑改变精神药物,或优化抗癫痫药。

表 10.3　癫痫患者中精神症状的可能原因及其处理

症状的原因	描述	处理
发作间精神疾病	■ 症状发作与癫痫发作无关 ■ 虽然在癫痫患者中常见,应该首选排除其他原因以及与癫痫发作的关系	■ 可能需要精神药物治疗 ■ 关于癫痫患者使用具体精神药物的更多信息,见表 10.5
发作期症状	■ 癫痫患者可出现精神症状	■ 所有发作期症状(发作前、发作后和发作中)的治疗最初是优化抗癫痫药物[11]
发作前症状	■ 典型表现为发作前烦躁不安,持续 30min 至 3 天	■ 发作期抑郁症状用抗抑郁药治疗似乎无效[13,14]
发作后症状	■ 典型表现在发作后数小时至 7 天(曾报告过抑郁、焦虑、自杀观念和精神病) ■ 伴有发作间精神疾病的癫痫患者,既往已经缓解的症状可能会加重(突破症状)	■ 发作后精神病可自发缓解,或者用小剂量抗精神病药治疗有效[15]。建议用苯二氮䓬类药物或抗精神病药对症治疗多达 3 个月[16]。症状缓解后,小心地逐渐减量[14] ■ 无证据表明精神药物可预防发作症状
发作症状	■ 可表现为发作性恐惧/惊恐(最常见)、抑郁症状,罕见精神病	
准发作"强制正常化" (因癫痫发作频率下降出现精神症状)	■ 癫痫患者发作缓解后的精神病性症状,或较少见的严重情感症状 ■ 快速药物剂量调整、快速发作控制、既往耐药的癫痫和颞叶癫痫可能是危险因素[15]	■ 应该与照料者共同决策如何推进抗癫痫药和精神药物[14]。可以用抗精神病药或抗抑郁药进行对症治疗

续表

症状的原因	描述	处理
医源性精神症状	■ 癫痫治疗的改变可导致精神症状，因为： ■ 开始用的抗癫痫药已知有负面的精神作用（特别是有精神疾病史者） ■ 停用的抗癫痫药有正面的精神作用（如心境稳定剂） ■ 开始用的抗癫痫药有酶诱导作用，此前患者服用精神药物时精神状态稳定 ■ 癫痫手术：已报告术后新发抑郁、焦虑和罕见的精神病。原有疾病加重更为常见	■ 处理症状的方法首先是解决深层原因 ■ 考虑换用耐受性更好的抗癫痫药（表 10.4） ■ 抗癫痫药可降低叶酸水平，从而影响情绪。应检测叶酸水平，必要时纠正叶酸水平低的情况 ■ 若不宜更换抗癫痫药，可考虑用抗抑郁药治疗医源性抑郁症状 [18] ■ 术后神经精神症状可用精神药物成功地治疗 [17]

抗癫痫药的精神科不良反应

已知几乎所有抗癫痫药都有精神作用。这些作用可能有益，也可能无益。抗癫痫药不利和有益的不良反应总结于表 10.4 中。建议读者查阅本指南中其他章节的"非精神药物的精神科不良反应概要"，了解抗癫痫药相关精神症状更为详细的总结，以及确定某一患者中因果关系的更多信息。

表 10.4　抗癫痫药不利和有益的不良反应 [5,19,20]

抗癫痫药	精神科不良反应	精神科有益反应
巴比妥盐，扑米酮 苯二氮䓬类药物	■ 行为紊乱/ADHD 症状 ■ 抑郁，认知损害	■ 抗焦虑
卡马西平，奥卡西平	■ 无报告	■ 稳定心境，抗躁狂
乙琥胺	■ 行为紊乱，抑郁，精神病	■ 无报告
非尔氨酯	■ 焦虑，抑郁，精神病	■ 无报告
加巴喷丁，普瑞巴林	■ 停药时出现抑郁和焦虑	■ 抗焦虑
拉科酰胺	■ 无报告	■ 无报告
拉莫三嗪	■ 一些人导致焦虑 ■ 认知损害者有行为紊乱	■ 抗抑郁 ■ 稳定心境
左乙拉西坦	■ 焦虑，行为紊乱，抑郁	■ 未证实
吡仑帕奈	■ 行为紊乱，抑郁，精神病	■ 无报告
苯妥英	■ 行为紊乱，抑郁	■ 抗躁狂
噻加宾	■ 行为紊乱，抑郁	■ 抗焦虑
托吡酯	■ 焦虑，行为紊乱，抑郁	■ 不明，可能抗躁狂/抗精神病
丙戊酸盐	■ 行为紊乱（儿童大剂量时）	■ 稳定心境，抗躁狂 ■ 抗惊恐
氨己烯酸	■ 行为紊乱/ADHD 症状 ■ 抑郁，精神病	■ 无报告
唑尼沙胺	■ 行为紊乱，抑郁	■ 未证实

相互作用 [21]

药代动力学相互作用

在抗癫痫药与精神药物之间,由细胞色素 P450 酶介导,存在双向的、重要的药代动力学相互作用 [8,22]。具有酶抑制作用的精神药物(如氟西汀、氟伏沙明、帕罗西汀和大剂量的舍曲林)可升高抗癫痫药的血浆浓度。对于治疗指数窄的抗癫痫药(如卡马西平和苯妥英),这种相互作用有特别的意义。应该监测血浆浓度,还可能需要调整剂量。西酞普兰和艾司西酞普兰是很弱的 CYP1A2 和 2D6 抑制剂。

一些抗癫痫药是酶的强诱导剂(如苯妥英、卡马西平、苯巴比妥、扑米酮),还有一些是酶的弱诱导剂(如奥卡西平剂量≥900mg/d,托吡酯剂量≥400mg/d)。这些药物可降低多种精神药物的血浆浓度,有可能导致治疗失败。

药效动力学相互作用 [13]

抗癫痫药与精神药物可重叠的不良反应包括:
- 体重增加:见于一些抗癫痫药(如卡马西平、加巴喷丁、普瑞巴林、丙戊酸盐)。
- 性功能障碍:见于苯巴比妥和扑米酮,但是也可见于有酶诱导作用的所有抗癫痫药。
- 低钠血症:见于卡马西平、奥卡西平(注意:严重时可引起癫痫发作)。
- 骨质疏松和骨量减少:见于长期使用有酶诱导作用的抗癫痫药。
- 恶血质:见于丙戊酸盐、卡马西平,特别是非尔氨酯。

癫痫患者使用精神药物及引起癫痫发作的风险

在一般人群中,无诱因癫痫发作的年发病率约为 50/10 万 [23]。值得注意的是,在抗抑郁药和抗精神病药 RCT 的安慰剂组中,该发病率约升高 15 倍,提示抑郁症和精神病是癫痫发作的危险因素 [24]。已经证明,癫痫与几种精神疾病之间存在双向关系,不仅癫痫患者发生精神疾病的风险升高,而且精神疾病患者发生癫痫的危险也升高 [5,6]。抑郁症、焦虑症、精神病和自杀倾向均存在这种双向关系 [3,5,6]。因此,在某些病例中,癫痫发作是精神疾病的自然发展,与使用精神药物无关。

报告精神药物相关的癫痫发作时,必须考虑精神疾病与癫痫之间的这种双向关系。例如,观察性研究报告了抗抑郁治疗与癫痫发作之间的关系 [25],但是抑郁症的非药物治疗(如咨询)也发现了类似的关系 [26]。这些发现与抑郁症本身是癫痫发作主要危险因素的观点一致。实际上,对精神药物对照研究的一项分析发现,在服用大多数抗抑郁药(如 SSRI)的患者中,癫痫发作的发生率明显低于安慰剂组 [24]。然而,在癫痫患者中缺少明确的数据 [27,28],一些精神药物在常用剂量范围内,存在与剂量相关的癫痫发作的风险。大多数药物在过量时可导致癫痫发作。还要注意的是,几乎所有抗抑郁药和抗精神病药均与低钠血症有关(见"低钠血症"),后者严重时可出现癫痫发作 [17,29]。关于精神药物在癫痫患者中的安全性一般指南总结于表 10.5。

电休克治疗(ECT)有抗惊厥的特性,对伴有不稳定癫痫的抑郁症患者值得考虑 [8,17,22]。ECT 似乎不会引起或加重癫痫 [17,30]。

表 10.5　精神药物在癫痫中的应用

在癫痫患者中的安全性	药物	评论
抗抑郁药		
低风险—正确选择	SSRI	推荐用于癫痫患者 [14,18]。在治疗剂量可有抗惊厥作用,但是过量时可促发惊厥 [31]。一般首选与抗癫痫药相互作用风险低的药物(西酞普兰/艾司西酞普兰,舍曲林) [14,18,32,33]。艾司西酞普兰优于西酞普兰(过量时癫痫发作风险较低) [34]。其他 SSRI 引起癫痫发作的风险较低(如氟西汀 [34]),但是应该考虑与抗癫痫药的相互作用 [14,18]。在老年人中,氟西汀引起癫痫发作的可能性小于艾司西酞普兰或西酞普兰 [35]。一些证据表明,在癫痫患者中,舍曲林安全而有效 [36]
	米氮平	推荐用于癫痫患者 [18,37]。未发现有致抽搐作用 [24]
	度洛西汀	推荐用于癫痫患者 [11,18]。癫痫发作的风险很小 [34,35]
可能低风险 —慎用(证据有限)	阿戈美拉汀	未发现有致抽搐作用 [38]。在动物模型中有抗惊厥作用 [34]
	MAOI	治疗剂量未发现有致抽搐作用 [38]。过量时癫痫发作的风险低 [17]
	吗氯贝胺	未发现有致抽搐作用 [34]。在动物模型中有抗惊厥作用 [34]
	瑞波西汀	小样本开放研究提示在癫痫患者中没有问题 [39]
	伏硫西汀	未发现有致抽搐作用 [34,40],但是没有用于癫痫患者的经验 [34]
中风险—需要小心	锂盐	癫痫发作风险低 [34]。在动物模型中有抗惊厥作用 [34]。但是,有限的资料表明,在癫痫患者中癫痫发作的频率有增有减 [34]。对于双相障碍,考虑使用有抗癫痫作用的心境稳定剂 [41]
	曲唑酮	有限资料提示有癫痫发作的风险 [34,42]
	文拉法辛	在癫痫患者中有效 [11],且被推荐 [18],但是癫痫发作的风险结果不一 [34]
	维拉唑酮	资料有限。一名癫痫患者用药后癫痫加重 [34]
高风险—避免使用(在治疗剂量时诱发抽搐 [13])	阿莫沙平	治疗剂量时有几例癫痫发作的报告 [42]
	安非他酮	癫痫发作的风险与剂量相关(特别是速释剂型) [34]。缓释剂型剂量 300mg 以下时,风险较低 [34]
	马普替林	治疗剂量时有几例癫痫发作的报告 [42]
	三环类	大多数三环类药物在大剂量时诱发癫痫(特别是氯米帕明和阿米替林 [10,24,42])。多噻平的风险可能较低(在癫痫患者中进行的一项小样本研究) [42]。在癫痫患者中,SNRI 优于三环类药物 [17]
抗精神病药		
低风险—正确选择	氨磺必利/舒必利	在癫痫患者中安全 [43]。经肾排泄,与抗癫痫药发生药代动力学相互作用的风险低。药物过量时罕见癫痫发作 [44]
	阿立哌唑齐拉西酮	极少降低癫痫发作阈值 [5]。在 RCT 中,癫痫发作发生率与安慰剂类似 [24]

在癫痫患者中的安全性	药物	评论
低风险—正确选择	高效价第一代药物	如氟奋乃静、氟哌啶醇、三氟拉嗪、氟哌噻吨。降低癫痫发作阈值的风险低[5]
	利培酮	降低癫痫发作阈值可能性小[5]。在 RCT 中,癫痫发作发生率与安慰剂类似[24]。推荐用于癫痫患者[24,45]。在系列青少年癫痫案例中有安全性的证据[46]
可能低风险 — 慎用(证据有限)	阿塞那平	在 RCT 中,癫痫发作发生率与安慰剂类似[47]。在癫痫患者中的资料和经验均极少
	布瑞哌唑	
	卡利拉嗪	
	鲁拉西酮	
中风险—需要小心	奥氮平	在 RCT 中,两种药均与癫痫发作相关[24]
	喹硫平	奥氮平引起脑电图异常较多[44]。降低癫痫发作阈值的整体风险较低[5],一些专家推荐奥氮平用于癫痫患者[32]。与奥氮平相关的数据难以解释。一些研究发现脑电图改变,但是并非所有研究均如此[48],而且发现该药既有抗惊厥作用[49],又有致抽搐作用[50]
		在癫痫患者中,喹硫平出现药物相互作用的风险高[45]
高风险—需要小心	氯氮平	最容易导致癫痫发作的抗精神病药[32]。但是,曾经成功地用于服用抗癫痫药病情稳定的癫痫患者,没有加重癫痫发作[51];甚至成功地用于难治性癫痫[52]。注意:不宜与卡马西平合用(有产生恶血质的风险,降低氯氮平浓度)。抗癫痫药可选择丙戊酸盐或拉莫三嗪
高风险—避免使用	低效价第一代药物(如氯丙嗪)	最好避免用于癫痫患者[31]。氯丙嗪剂量超过 1g/d 时,癫痫发作的发生率为 6%
	洛沙平	在第一代抗精神病药物中,癫痫发作的发生率最高[53]
	长效抗精神病药	现有长效抗精神病药均无致痫作用,但是: ■ 长效药物的代谢比较复杂(可能会延迟出现癫痫发作) ■ 若出现癫痫发作,相关药物可能难以减掉。长效药物的使用应该特别小心
	佐替平	已经明确有剂量相关的致痫作用[44]
治疗 ADHD 的药物		
低风险—正确选择	哌甲酯	三项 RCT 支持其治疗剂量(每天 0.3~1mg/kg)在癫痫儿童中的安全性和疗效[10]。两项单次给药 RCT 和一项开放扩展研究发现,它对成人的癫痫发作没有影响[54,55]。一项大样本病例对照研究发现,开始用药后癫痫发作的发生率增加,但长期使用并未增加[56]。这个结果难以解释,但是提示应该慎用

续表

在癫痫患者中的安全性	药物	评论
可能低风险[57,58]—慎用(资料有限)	苯丙胺	在癫痫患者中,仅有一项小样本回顾性研究[10]。癫痫控制良好的患者均未出现癫痫发作频率增加[59]。需要注意的是,右旋安非他明在历史上曾被用作辅助性的抗癫痫药[60]
	托莫西汀	在癫痫患者中,仅有一项小样本回顾性研究[10]。停药率高(但均不是因为癫痫发作加重[61])。对于无癫痫的患者,癫痫发生率与安慰剂类似[62]

本表包含抗抑郁药和抗精神病药在治疗剂量时致抽搐的信息。关于超量的信息,见"精神药物过量"。

癫痫与驾驶

在英国,癫痫患者若过去 1 年在清醒状态时出现过 1 次癫痫发作,则不可以驾驶机动车。但是,癫痫发作若只出现在睡眠中,且夜间发作模式至少已有 3 年,则患者可能适宜驾驶。因此,抗抑郁药或抗精神病药诱发癫痫发作的后果可能很明显。

参考文献

1. Scott AJ, et al. Anxiety and depressive disorders in people with epilepsy: A meta-analysis. *Epilepsia* 2017; 58:973–982.
2. Clancy MJ, et al. The prevalence of psychosis in epilepsy; a systematic review and meta-analysis. *BMC Psychiatry* 2014; 14:75.
3. Hesdorffer DC, et al. Occurrence and recurrence of attempted suicide among people with epilepsy. *JAMA Psychiatry* 2016; 73:80–86.
4. Thurman DJ, et al. The burden of premature mortality of epilepsy in high-income countries: A systematic review from the mortality task force of the international league against epilepsy. *Epilepsia* 2017; 58:17–26.
5. Kanner AM. Management of psychiatric and neurological comorbidities in epilepsy. *Nat Rev Neurol* 2016; 12:106–116.
6. Hesdorffer DC. Comorbidity between neurological illness and psychiatric disorders. *CNS Spectr* 2016; 21:230–238.
7. Kanner AM. Can neurochemical changes of mood disorders explain the increase risk of epilepsy or its worse seizure control? *Neurochem Res* 2017; 42:2071–2076.
8. Curran S, et al. Selecting an antidepressant for use in a patient with epilepsy. Safety considerations. *Drug Saf* 1998; 18:125–133.
9. Blumer D, et al. Treatment of the interictal psychoses. *J Clin Psychiatry* 2000; 61:110–122.
10. Mula M. The pharmacological management of psychiatric comorbidities in patients with epilepsy. *Pharmacol Res* 2016; 107:147–153.
11. Elger CE, et al. Diagnosing and treating depression in epilepsy. *Seizure* 2017; 44:184–193.
12. Anbarasan D. Psychoactive medications and seizures—challenges and pitfalls. *Neurol Rep* 2016; 9:24–27.
13. Kanner AM. Most antidepressant drugs are safe for patients with epilepsy at therapeutic doses: a review of the evidence. *Epilepsy Behav* 2016; 61:282–286.
14. Kerr MP, et al. International consensus clinical practice statements for the treatment of neuropsychiatric conditions associated with epilepsy. *Epilepsia* 2011; 52:2133–2138.
15. Josephson CB, et al. Psychiatric comorbidities in epilepsy. *Int Rev Psychiatry (Abingdon, England)* 2017; 29:409–424.
16. Maguire M, et al. Epilepsy and psychosis: a practical approach. *Pract Neurol* 2018; 18:106–114.
17. Mula M. *Neuropsychiatric symptoms of epilepsy*. Vol. 1. Basel: Springer International Publishing 2016.
18. Barry JJ, et al. Consensus statement: the evaluation and treatment of people with epilepsy and affective disorders. *Epilepsy Behav* 2008; 13 Suppl 1:S1–29.
19. Schmidt D, et al. Drug treatment of epilepsy in adults. *BMJ* 2014; 348:g254.
20. Piedad J, et al. Beneficial and adverse psychotropic effects of antiepileptic drugs in patients with epilepsy: a summary of prevalence, underlying mechanisms and data limitations. *CNS Drugs* 2012; 26:319–335.
21. Spina E, et al. Clinically significant pharmacokinetic drug interactions of antiepileptic drugs with new antidepressants and new antipsychotics. *Pharmacol Res* 2016; 106:72–86.
22. Harden CL, et al. Mood disorders in patients with epilepsy: epidemiology and management. *CNS Drugs* 2002; 16:291–302.
23. Ngugi AK, et al. Incidence of epilepsy: a systematic review and meta-analysis. *Neurology* 2011; 77:1005–1012.
24. Alper K, et al. Seizure incidence in psychopharmacological clinical trials: an analysis of food and drug administration (FDA) summary basis of approval reports. *Biol Psychiatry* 2007; 62:345–354.
25. Wu CS, et al. Seizure risk associated with antidepressant treatment among patients with depressive disorders: a population-based case-

crossover study. *J Clin Psychiatry* 2017; **78**:e1226-e1232.

26. Josephson CB, et al. Association of depression and treated depression with epilepsy and seizure outcomes: a multicohort analysis. *JAMA Neurol* 2017; **74**:533-539.

27. Farooq S, et al. Interventions for psychotic symptoms concomitant with epilepsy. *Cochrane Database System Rev* 2015:Cd006118.

28. Maguire MJ, et al. Antidepressants for people with epilepsy and depression. *Cochrane Database System Rev* 2014:Cd010682.

29. Maramattom BV. Duloxetine-induced syndrome of inappropriate antidiuretic hormone secretion and seizures. *Neurology* 2006; **66**:773-774.

30. Ray AK. Does electroconvulsive therapy cause epilepsy? *JECT* 2013; **29**:201-205.

31. Steinert T, et al. [Epileptic seizures during treatment with antidepressants and neuroleptics]. *Fortschr Neurol Psychiatr* 2011; **79**:138-143.

32. Mula M. Epilepsy and psychiatric comorbidities: drug selection. *Curr Treat Options Neurol* 2017; **19**:44.

33. National Institute for Health and Clinical Excellence. Depression in adults with a chronic physical health problem: treatment and management. Clinical Guidance [CG91]. 2009; http://www.nice.org.uk/CG91.

34. Steinert T, et al. Epileptic seizures under antidepressive drug treatment: systematic review. *Pharmacopsychiatry* 2018; **51**:121-135.

35. Finkelstein Y, et al. Second-generation anti-depressants and risk of new-onset seizures in the elderly. *Clin Toxicol (Phila)* 2018; **56**:1179-1184.

36. Gilliam FG, et al. A trial of sertraline or cognitive behavior therapy for depression in epilepsy. *Ann Neurol* 2019; **86**:552-560.

37. Craig DP, et al. Risk of seizures with antidepressants: what is the evidence? *Drug Ther Bull* 2020; **58**:137-140.

38. Servier Laboratories Limited. Summary of product characteristics. Valdoxan. 2020; https://www.medicines.org.uk/emc/medicine/21830.

39. Kuhn KU, et al. Antidepressive treatment in patients with temporal lobe epilepsy and major depression: a prospective study with three different antidepressants. *Epilepsy Behav* 2003; **4**:674-679.

40. Lundbeck Limited. Summary of product characteristics. Brintellix (vortioxetine) tablets 5, 10 and 20mg. 2020; https://www.medicines.org.uk/emc/medicine/30904.

41. Knott S, et al. Epilepsy and bipolar disorder. *Epilepsy Behav* 2015; **52**:267-274.

42. Johannessen Landmark C, et al. Proconvulsant effects of antidepressants - what is the current evidence? *Epilepsy Behav* 2016; **61**:287-291.

43. Elnazer H, et al. Managing aggression in epilepsy. *BJPsych Adv* 2017; **23**:253.

44. Steinert T, et al. *Chapter 9 - Seizures A2 - Manu, Peter*. San Diego: Academic Press 2016.

45. Agrawal N, et al. Treatment of psychoses in patients with epilepsy: an update. *Ther Adv Psychopharmacol* 2019; **9**:2045125319862968.

46. Gonzalez-Heydrich J, et al. No seizure exacerbation from risperidone in youth with comorbid epilepsy and psychiatric disorders: a case series. *J Child Adolesc Psychopharmacol* 2004; **14**:295-310.

47. IBM Watson Health. IBM micromedex solutions. 2020; https://www.ibm.com/watson-health/about/micromedex.

48. Jackson A, et al. EEG changes in patients on antipsychotic therapy: a systematic review. *Epilepsy Behav* 2019; **95**:1-9.

49. Qiu X, et al. Antiepileptic effect of olanzapine in epilepsy patients with atypical depressive comorbidity. *Epileptic Disord* 2018; **20**:225-231.

50. Mansoor M, et al. Generalised tonic-clonic seizures on the subtherapeutic dose of olanzapine. *BMJ Case Rep* 2019; **12**.

51. Langosch JM, et al. Epilepsy, psychosis and clozapine. *Human Psychopharm Clin Experim* 2002; **17**:115-119.

52. Jette Pomerleau V, et al. Clozapine safety and efficacy for interictal psychotic disorder in pharmacoresistant epilepsy. *Cogn Behav Neurol* 2017; **30**:73-76.

53. Habibi M, et al. The impact of psychoactive drugs on seizures and antiepileptic drugs. *Curr Neurol Neurosci Rep* 2016; **16**:71.

54. Adams J, et al. Methylphenidate, cognition, and epilepsy: a 1-month open-label trial. *Epilepsia* 2017; **58**:2124-2132.

55. Adams J, et al. Methylphenidate, cognition, and epilepsy: a double-blind, placebo-controlled, single-dose study. *Neurology* 2017; **88**:470-476.

56. Man KKC, et al. Association between methylphenidate treatment and risk of seizure: a population-based, self-controlled case-series study. *Lancet Child Adolesc Health* 2020; **4**:435-443.

57. Besag F, et al. Psychiatric and behavioural disorders in children with epilepsy (ILAE Task Force report): epilepsy and ADHD. *Epileptic Disord* 2016; **18**:S8-S15.

58. Besag F, et al. Psychiatric and behavioural disorders in children with epilepsy (ILAE Task Force report): when should pharmacotherapy for psychiatric/behavioural disorders in children with epilepsy be prescribed? *Epileptic Disord* 2016; **18**:S77-S86.

59. Gonzalez-Heydrich J, et al. Comparing stimulant effects in youth with ADHD symptoms and epilepsy. *Epilepsy Behav* 2014; **36**:102-107.

60. Schubert R. Attention deficit disorder and epilepsy. *Pediatr Neurol* 2005; **32**:1-10.

61. Torres A, et al. Tolerability of atomoxetine for treatment of pediatric attention-deficit/hyperactivity disorder in the context of epilepsy. *Epilepsy Behav* 2011; **20**:95-102.

62. Williams AE, et al. Epilepsy and attention-deficit hyperactivity disorder: links, risks, and challenges. *Neuropsychiatr Dis Treat* 2016; **12**:287-296.

扩展阅读

Kanner AM. Management of psychiatric and neurological comorbidities in epilepsy. *Nat Rev Neurol* 2016; **12**:106-116.

Mula M. Epilepsy and psychiatric comorbidities: drug selection. *Curr Treat Options Neurol* 2017; **19**:44.

22q11.2 缺失综合征

临床特点

22q11.2 缺失综合征是最常见的常染色体缺失,是多系统疾病,表现多种多样,患者之间严重程度差异很大[1]。患病率估计为 3 000~5 000 个新生儿中有 1 个[1]。该综合征有许多名称(腭心面综合征、DiGeorge 综合征或 Shprintzen 综合征),其部分原因是临床特点的表型范围很宽泛(框 10.2)。

框 10.2　22q11.2 缺失综合征的临床特点

■ 心血管异常,包括法洛四联症	■ 免疫缺陷和自身免疫疾病
■ 内分泌异常,包括甲状旁腺功能减退	■ 腭部异常
■ 泌尿生殖系统异常,包括肾发育不全	■ 行为表型
■ 发育延迟和学习困难	■ 精神疾病
■ 胃肠道异常,包括便秘	■ 骨骼异常

22q11.2 缺失综合征患者的精神疾病

约 60% 的 22q11.2 缺失综合征患者在其一生中某个时点会达到某些类型精神疾病的诊断标准[2]。在他们之中,焦虑症、ADHD、孤独谱系障碍的患病率升高[1],约 25% 被诊断为精神分裂症[1]。

很少有研究评估精神药物在该病患者中的安全性和疗效。但是,ADHD、焦虑症、心境障碍和精神分裂症的标准药物(和非药物)治疗似乎有效,应该遵守用于一般人群的治疗方案[1,3]。虽然人们认为大多数精神药物对于该病患者是安全的,但是应该考虑到躯体共病(心血管病),以及可能增加癫痫发作[2]和运动障碍的风险[1]。内分泌异常(如甲状旁腺功能减退和甲状腺功能减退)应该在使用精神药物之前就得到纠正,因为它们的表现类似于精神症状,会使得精神药物治疗变得复杂[2,3]。关于 22q11.2 缺失综合征患者的精神疾病,其治疗的现有证据和观点总结于表 10.6。

表 10.6　在 22q11.2 缺失综合征患者中精神疾病的治疗

精神疾病	治疗
ADHD	■ 虽然担心 22q11.2 缺失综合征患者使用精神兴奋药在理论上有诱发精神病的风险,但是建议使用标准的治疗方案[2] ■ 两项研究支持给 22q11.2 缺失综合征患者使用哌甲酯治疗有效[2]。通常对治疗的耐受性良好。在治疗之前和治疗期间,建议全面评估心血管功能
抑郁症和焦虑症	■ SSRI:对焦虑症和抑郁症疗效均可[2,5]。进一步治疗按标准方案实施 ■ S-腺苷-甲硫氨酸:在一项小样本 RCT 中进行过研究,结果发现对抑郁(或 ADHD)症状无明显益处[2]

精神疾病	治疗
强迫症	■ 一项研究采用氟西汀 30~60mg/d 治疗 4 例共病强迫症与 22q11.2 缺失综合征的患者，症状评分平均改善 35%。对治疗耐受性好 [6]
精神分裂症	■ 通常建议采纳标准治疗方案 [3,7]。22q11.2 缺失综合征患者使用抗精神病药时，更容易出现癫痫发作和 EPS[4]。肥胖的风险明显升高，因此应密切监测代谢方面的不良反应 [8]。心脏异常者 Q-T 间期延长的风险升高 [4]，建议密切监测 ECG[4]，最好选用对 Q-T 间期影响小的抗精神病药 [4]。普遍建议从小剂量开始，缓慢加量 [4]。一些病例报告使用阿立哌唑、奥氮平、利培酮和喹硫平获得成功 [5]，但是许多病例也发生了治疗阻抗 [5]
	■ **氯氮平**：在 20 例患者中进行的回顾性研究发现此药有效 [2]。与对照组相比，需要使用较低剂量（剂量中位数 22q11.2 缺失综合征患者 250mg/d，对照组 450mg/d）。但是，在 22q11.2 缺失综合征患者中，50% 出现至少一种氯氮平的严重不良反应，主要是癫痫发作，也有心肌炎和中性粒细胞减少。几项病例报告进一步支持低剂量氯氮平（中位数 200mg/d）对 22q11.2 缺失综合征患者的疗效，同时强调癫痫发作（全身性或肌阵挛性）和血小板减少的风险 [8]。总之，氯氮平在低于常规剂量时有明显效果，但是罕见严重不良事件的风险也高 [2]。应该考虑辅助使用抗癫痫药 [7,8]
	■ **其他抗精神病药引起的癫痫发作**：全部病例均应检测低钙和低镁情况，确保充分治疗 [7]。考虑辅助使用抗癫痫药 [7]
	■ **其他药物**：直接对抗儿茶酚胺过多的药物也可能有效。一项研究发现，以甲酪氨酸单用或作为辅助用药，29 例患者中 22 例有效 [9]。也有其他结果为阳性的病例报告发表 [10]。有一项个案研究发现，使用甲基多巴获得成功 [11]

参考文献

1. McDonald-McGinn DM, et al. 22q11.2 deletion syndrome. *Nat Rev Dis Primers* 2015; 1:15071.
2. Mosheva M, et al. Effectiveness and side effects of psychopharmacotherapy in individuals with 22q11.2 deletion syndrome with comorbid psychiatric disorders: a systematic review. *Eur Child Adolesc Psychiatry* 2020; 29:1035–1048.
3. Fung WL, et al. Practical guidelines for managing adults with 22q11.2 deletion syndrome. *Genet Med* 2015; 17:599–609.
4. Baker K, et al. Psychiatric illness. Consensus Document on 22q11 Deletion Syndrome (22q11DS) MaxAppeal 2017; http://www.maxappeal.org.uk/downloads/Consensus_Document_on_22q11_Deletion_Syndrome_Master_2017_(final_draft)_9-end_(1)2018.pdf.
5. Dori N, et al. The effectiveness and safety of antipsychotic and antidepressant medications in individuals with 22q11.2 deletion syndrome. *J Child Adolesc Psychopharmacol* 2017; 27:83–90.
6. Gothelf D, et al. Obsessive-compulsive disorder in patients with velocardiofacial (22q11 deletion) syndrome. *Am J Med Genet B Neuropsychiatr Genet* 2004; 126b:99–105.
7. Bassett AS, et al. Practical guidelines for managing patients with 22q11.2 deletion syndrome. *J Pediatr* 2011; 159:332–339.
8. de Boer J, et al. Adverse effects of antipsychotic medication in patients with 22q11.2 deletion syndrome: A systematic review. *Am J Med Genet A* 2019; 179:2292–2306.
9. Faedda GL, et al. 4.19 Treatment of velo-cardio-facial syndrome-related psychosis with metyrosine. *J Am Acad Child Adolesc Psychiatry* 2016; 55:S169.
10. Engebretsen MH, et al. Metyrosine treatment in a woman with chromosome 22q11.2 deletion syndrome and psychosis: a case study. *Int J Dev Disabil* 2017:1–6.
11. O'Hanlon JF, et al. Replacement of antipsychotic and antiepileptic medication by L-alpha-methyldopa in a woman with velocardiofacial syndrome. *Int Clin Psychopharmacol* 2003; 18:117–119.

学习障碍

总论 [1]

在精神科实践中,给学习障碍患者使用精神药物是具有挑战性并备受争议的 [2,3]。一些担忧认为各种精神药物,包括抗精神病药、抗抑郁药、苯二氮䓬类药物(常规使用和需要时用)以及作为心境稳定剂的抗癫痫药,都存在过度使用,对于其益处缺乏充分总结和评估。值得注意的是,学习障碍领域本身只有很小的治疗性研究基础,对于如何分类和治疗情绪与行为紊乱,有特别的伦理和实践方面的考虑。轻度或者边缘性智能损害者可由主流精神卫生机构给予药物,但对于明显认知损害(或者孤独症等的不典型表现)的显著表现,其行为和情绪障碍应当首先由专科医师评估和处理,至少也应该咨询这些医师。

"双重诊断"这个术语在此处指学习障碍与其他精神障碍(精神疾病、人格障碍)同时出现。"诊断遮蔽"指误将情绪和行为问题归结于学习障碍,而非同时存在的精神疾病。学习障碍是所有精神障碍(包括痴呆,尤其当患者有"唐氏综合征"时)的重要危险因素 [4]。根据传统的或者修改后的诊断标准,若患者有可能诊断为精神障碍,一般来说,药物治疗首先应该与一般人群相仿。就这一点而言,大部分治疗指南在逐渐增加对于学习障碍患者的适用性说明。

精神疾病最初可能以非同寻常的方式表现出来,比如抑郁症表现为自伤行为,被害观念表现为抱怨"被人捉弄"。相反,有些行为(如自言自语)对于某些个体来说可能是正常的,但却可能被误认为精神病。总的来讲,随着学习障碍以及相关交流障碍的严重性增加,诊断也变得越来越复杂。

共病的孤独症谱系障碍有其特殊的评估考虑,并且它本身即是精神障碍的一个重要危险因素,尤其是焦虑和抑郁、双相谱系障碍、严重的强迫行为、愤怒障碍以及可能达不到精神分裂症诊断标准但仍需治疗的精神病样发作。孤独特征在就诊于学习障碍服务机构的患者中很常见。关于孤独症患者中精神卫生问题的治疗指南见第 5 章。

关键实践领域

心智能力和知情同意:学习障碍服务机构的患者(一般是在童年期需要特殊教育的人群)很少有能力充分理解其治疗,以便能够做出真正的知情决定,因此临床医师不可避免地要担负更多的决策责任。决策能力的好坏取决于智力受损的程度,通过恰当的口头及书面交流,可能会提高患者的决策能力。通常来说,在这个过程中照料者的参与是必要的。

躯体共病,尤其是癫痫:癫痫在学习障碍人群中所占比例过高,其患病率随着疾病严重程度的增加而增高,到了成年早期约 1/3 的患者会发展为癫痫。在考虑使用可能降低癫痫阈值或与抗癫痫药有相互作用的药物时,尤其需要关注这一点。

照料环境评估:行为和情绪障异常可能是在照料环境中遭遇困难或失败的反映。同在一个照料者之家中,对于这些困难,不同的工作人员可能忍耐限度不同(或者归因不同),因而对这些困难的意义和影响说法各异。留出一段时间用于前瞻性评估,并使用简单的评估工具(如简单的 ABC 或者睡眠记录),可能会非常有助于临床医师就推荐药物做出判断。如果在护理院用药,工作人员需要接受专门培训,了解如何用药和预期的药物不良反应;对于"必要时使用"的药物,要清楚其使用指南。这可能会使在社区开展某些治疗变得困难。

不良反应敏感性:人们普遍认为,学习障碍患者对精神药物的不良反应特别敏感,并且出现长期不良反应(如代谢综合征)的风险更大。然而,只有一项研究支持这种看法。一项队列研究从一个大规模的英国初级保健数据库中提取信息,比较有无学习障碍的成年人中 EPS 的发生率。结果发现有学习障碍者中 EPS 发生率比无学习障碍者高 30%[5]。与一般精神科实践相比,有学习障碍者最好从更低的剂量起始,更缓慢地加量。值得注意的不良反应包括癫痫发作的恶化、镇静、锥体外系反应(包括使用常规剂量利培酮,尤其是已有行动不便的个体)、吞咽问题(使用氯氮平或其他抗精神病药)以及使用抗胆碱能药时认知功能恶化(见第 6 章)。

心理干预:当没有可确认的、有明显治疗指征的精神疾病(包括不典型表现)时,应该考虑将心理干预(如功能性行为分析)作为一线的干预,但是行为障碍最严重或最难治的表现例外。在有可能推断出挑衅行为程度的一些研究中,治疗效果一般与基线时较严重的行为问题相关。

目前和既往用于治疗行为问题的药物

药物类别	临床应用	注意事项
抗精神病药[6]	可以用于伴学习障碍的精神病 用于范围广泛的行为紊乱[7] 对于攻击行为和易激惹可能有效	抗精神病药是使用最广[8,9]但争议最大的治疗行为问题[10,11]的药物。最近一项随机对照研究[12]对其疗效产生怀疑,但这个研究本身并非没有问题,并且有相当多的其他证据(包括在学习障碍儿童中进行的许多小样本随机对照研究)支持它们的使用 长期治疗的停药研究往往(但并非总是)发现问题行为重新出现。NICE 建议,对于没有精神病性症状的全部患者,考虑缓慢停掉抗精神病药[13]。UK STOMP 项目推动停用抗精神病药[14],它已经取得成功,但是抗精神病药往往被换成其他精神药物[15] 在第二代抗精神病药出现之前,证据最强的是**氟哌啶醇**[16]在孤独症中的应用,以及**珠氯噻醇**在行为紊乱中的应用[17]。后者可减少攻击和挑衅行为[18] 在第二代药物中,证据最强的是低剂量(0.5~2mg)**利培酮**[19,20]治疗攻击和情绪不稳的作用,特别是与孤独症相关者,尽管不伴孤独症的患者也有效果。**阿立哌唑**被 FDA 批准用于治疗年轻孤独症患者的行为紊乱[21,22] 对于攻击行为非常严重的病例,有一些证据支持使用**奥氮平**[23],还有一些病例报告支持使用**氯氮平**[24],尽管其应用并不广泛,在高度专业性机构(住院部)外也很不太可能使用。2015 年,关于氯氮平治疗伴学习障碍的精神病,Cochrane 研究发现 38 例个案报告和病历总结,但未发现到 RCT 证据[25] **喹硫平**的结果充其量是略有疗效[26]

续表

药物类别	临床应用	注意事项
SSRI 类	对于孤独症谱系障碍的严重焦虑及强迫症状有效。但若非诊断焦虑障碍或 OCD，该药的使用是未经批准的 用于治疗攻击和冲动行为时，可以作为抗精神病药的一线替代药物	常与抗精神病药联用，尽管证据基础有限。对于不伴心境障碍或焦虑谱系障碍的患者，其疗效尚不明确。但 2013 年的 Cochrane 系统综述对其在治疗孤独症儿童(这些孩子出现不良反应的风险较高)行为障碍的疗效持悲观态度[27]，尽管在成人中的结果可能略好一些。一些很好的证据表明，氟西汀对于伴学习障碍/孤独症的强迫症有效[28] 一般而言，这些试验的质量较差，且可能因为用于程度较轻的病例而将药物疗效放大[29]。需要注意，在该人群中使用有引起轻躁狂的风险[30]。与抗精神病药类似，也需要严重关切处方过量[31] 文拉法辛可能无效[32]
抗癫痫药物[33]	攻击和自伤行为	一些未设对照的研究支持**丙戊酸钠**[34]在学习障碍人群中使用，但是证据力度并不强，且研究结果相互矛盾。尽管如此，抗癫痫药治疗情绪不稳和攻击行为的用法仍然得到最大的支持，部分原因在于其在非学习障碍人群有阳性的研究结果[35] 拉莫三嗪的研究有限，多数在儿童群体开展，结果提示无效，至少在孤独症患者和不伴有情感不稳的患者中如此[26] 卡马西平的结果也没有说服力，但是仍被广泛应用[36]
锂盐[37]	批准用于治疗自伤行为和攻击行为	有些治疗学习障碍的随机对照试验证据[38]，但是在此人群中已多年未做研究；在不伴有发育障碍的青少年中，最近一项随机对照研究提示其对攻击行为有效[39]。临床经验提示，对于采用其他治疗失败的患者，锂盐可能非常有效；尽管不良反应可能成为问题，锂盐可能并没有被充分使用 若患者存在一些亚综合征的或者非典型的"情感症状成分"，可能最好考虑锂盐治疗。一些专家提出，在密切观察下可以发现，一些严重学习障碍患者的挑衅行为其实是在双相情感障碍快速循环的背景下出现的，而这很容易发生漏诊 一些 RCT 证据提示，短期使用(6mg/kg)的耐受性相当好[40]
哌甲酯	治疗学习障碍伴发的 ADHD 有效	NICE[13]进行的一项荟萃分析发现，治疗学习障碍伴发的 ADHD 时，哌甲酯(以及利培酮和可乐定)明显有益
纳曲酮[41]	用于严重自伤行为[42]	证据力度不强且结果不一。对于一些严重而棘手的病例，仍可作为备选[43]。整体上，临床使用近年来减少了[44]

参考文献

1. Deb S. The use of medications for the management of problem behaviours in adults who has intellectual [learning] disabilities 2012; http://www.intellectualdisability.info/mental-health/the-use-of-drugs-for-the-treatment-of-behaviour-disorders-in-adults-who-have-learning-intellectual-disabilities.

2. Sheehan R, et al. Psychotropic prescribing in people with intellectual disability and challenging behaviour. *BMJ* 2017; 358:j3896.

3. Ji NY, et al. Pharmacotherapy for mental health problems in people with intellectual disability. *Curr Opin Psychiatry* 2016; 29:103–125.

4. Cooper SA, et al. Mental ill-health in adults with intellectual disabilities: prevalence and associated factors. *Br J Psychiatry* 2007; 190:27–35.

5. Sheehan R, et al. Movement side effects of antipsychotic drugs in adults with and without intellectual disability: UK population-based cohort

study. *BMJ Open* 2017; 7:e017406.

6. Antochi R, et al. Psychopharmacological treatments in persons with dual diagnosis of psychiatric disorders and developmental disabilities. *Postgrad Med J* 2003; 79:139–146.

7. Lunsky Y, et al. Antipsychotic use with and without comorbid psychiatric diagnosis among adults with intellectual and developmental disabilities. *Can J Psychiatry* 2017; 63:361–369.

8. Deb S, et al. Characteristics and the trajectory of psychotropic medication use in general and antipsychotics in particular among adults with an intellectual disability who exhibit aggressive behaviour. *J Intellect Disabil Res* 2015; 59:11–25.

9. Sheehan R, et al. Mental illness, challenging behaviour, and psychotropic drug prescribing in people with intellectual disability: UK population based cohort study. *BMJ* 2015; 351:h4326.

10. Deb S, et al. The effectiveness of antipsychotic medication in the management of behaviour problems in adults with intellectual disabilities. *J Intellect Disabil Res* 2007; 51:766–777.

11. Roy D, et al. Pharmacologic management of aggression in adults with intellectual disability. *J Intellect Disabil Res* 2013; 1:28–43.

12. Tyrer P, et al. Risperidone, haloperidol, and placebo in the treatment of aggressive challenging behaviour in patients with intellectual disability: a randomised controlled trial. *Lancet* 2008; 371:57–63.

13. National Institute of Health and Care Excellence. Mental health problems in people with learning disabilities: prevention, assessment and management [NG54] 2016; https://www.nice.org.uk/Guidance/NG54.

14. Shankar R, et al. Stopping, rationalising or optimising antipsychotic drug treatment in people with intellectual disability and/or autism. *Drug Ther Bull* 2019; 57:10–13.

15. Deb S, et al. UK psychiatrists' experience of withdrawal of antipsychotics prescribed for challenging behaviours in adults with intellectual disabilities and/or autism. *BJPsych Open* 2020; 6:e112.

16. Malone RP, et al. The role of antipsychotics in the management of behavioural symptoms in children and adolescents with autism. *Drugs* 2009; 69:535–548.

17. Malt UF, et al. Effectiveness of zuclopenthixol compared with haloperidol in the treatment of behavioural disturbances in learning disabled patients. *Br J Psychiatry* 1995; 166:374–377.

18. Hassler F, et al. Treatment of aggressive behavior problems in boys with intellectual disabilities using zuclopenthixol. *J Child Adolesc Psychopharmacol* 2014; 24:579–581.

19. Nagaraj R, et al. Risperidone in children with autism: randomized, placebo-controlled, double-blind study. *J Child Neurol* 2006; 21:450–455.

20. Pandina GJ, et al. Risperidone improves behavioral symptoms in children with autism in a randomized, double-blind, placebo-controlled trial. *J Autism Dev Disord* 2007; 37:367–373.

21. Owen R, et al. Aripiprazole in the treatment of irritability in children and adolescents with autistic disorder. *Pediatrics* 2009; 124:1533–1540.

22. Marcus RN, et al. A placebo-controlled, fixed-dose study of aripiprazole in children and adolescents with irritability associated with autistic disorder. *J Am Acad Child Adolesc Psychiatry* 2009; 48:1110–1119.

23. Fido A, et al. Olanzapine in the treatment of behavioral problems associated with autism: an open-label trial in Kuwait. *Med Princ Pract* 2008; 17:415–418.

24. Zuddas A, et al. Clinical effects of clozapine on autistic disorder. *Am J Psychiatry* 1996; 153:738.

25. Ayub M, et al. Clozapine for psychotic disorders in adults with intellectual disabilities. *Cochrane Database Syst Rev* 2015:Cd010625.

26. Stigler KA, et al. Pharmacotherapy of irritability in pervasive developmental disorders. *Child Adolesc Psychiatr Clin N Am* 2008; 17:739–752.

27. Williams K, et al. Selective serotonin reuptake inhibitors (SSRIs) for autism spectrum disorders (ASD). *Cochrane Database Syst Rev* 2013; 8:CD004677.

28. Reddihough DS, et al. Effect of fluoxetine on obsessive-compulsive behaviors in children and adolescents with autism spectrum disorders: a randomized clinical trial. *JAMA* 2019; 322:1561–1569.

29. Myers SM. Citalopram not effective for repetitive behaviour in autistic spectrum disorders. *Evid Based Ment Health* 2010; 13:22.

30. Cook EH, Jr., et al. Fluoxetine treatment of children and adults with autistic disorder and mental retardation. *J Am Acad Child Adolesc Psychiatry* 1992; 31:739–745.

31. Oswald DP, et al. Medication use among children with autism spectrum disorders. *J Child Adolesc Psychopharmacol* 2007; 17:348–355.

32. Carminati GG, et al. Using venlafaxine to treat behavioral disorders in patients with autism spectrum disorder. *Prog Neuropsychopharmacol Biol Psychiatry* 2016; 65:85–95.

33. Deb S, et al. The effectiveness of mood stabilizers and antiepileptic medication for the management of behaviour problems in adults with intellectual disability: a systematic review. *J Intellect Disabil Res* 2008; 52:107–113.

34. Ruedrich S, et al. Effect of divalproex sodium on aggression and self-injurious behaviour in adults with intellectual disability: a retrospective review. *J Intellect Disabil Res* 1999; 43(Pt 2):105–111.

35. Donovan SJ, et al. Divalproex treatment for youth with explosive temper and mood lability: a double-blind, placebo-controlled crossover design. *Am J Psychiatry* 2000; 157:818–820.

36. Unwin GL, et al. Use of medication for the management of behavior problems among adults with intellectual disabilities: a clinicians' consensus survey. *Am J Ment Retard* 2008; 113:19–31.

37. Pary RJ. Towards defining adequate lithium trials for individuals with mental retardation and mental illness. *Am J Ment Retard* 1991; 95:681–691.

38. Craft M, et al. Lithium in the treatment of aggression in mentally handicapped patients: a double-blind trial. *Br J Psychiatry* 1987;

第10章

150:685–689.

39. Malone RP, et al. A double-blind placebo-controlled study of lithium in hospitalized aggressive children and adolescents with conduct disorder. *Arch Gen Psychiatry* 2000; 57:649–654.

40. Yuan J, et al. Lithium treatment is safe in children with intellectual disability. *Front Mol Neurosci* 2018; 11:425.

41. Campbell M, et al. Naltrexone in autistic children: an acute open dose range tolerance trial. *J Am Acad Child Adolesc Psychiatry* 1989; 28:200–206.

42. Barrett RP, et al. Effects of naloxone and naltrexone on self-injury: a double-blind, placebo-controlled analysis. *Am J Ment Retard* 1989; 93:644–651.

43. Mouaffak F, et al. Kleptomania treated with naltrexone in a patient with intellectual disability. *J Psychiatry Neurosci* 2020; 45:71–72.

44. Sabus A, et al. Management of self-injurious behaviors in children with neurodevelopmental disorders: a pharmacotherapy overview. *Pharmacotherapy* 2019; 39:645–664.

亨廷顿病药物治疗

亨廷顿病是一种遗传疾病,病理表现为纹状体神经元缓慢、进行性退化,并随着疾病的进展而累及大脑皮质[1]。在西方社会,其患病率估计为(10.6~13.7)/100 000[1]。突变的亨廷顿蛋白通过几种机制导致神经元功能异常和死亡,引起运动、认知和神经精神症状三联征。目前没有可以改变疾病进程的治疗[1-3],只能通过对症治疗来试图提高患者的生命质量(框 10.3)。

框 10.3　亨廷顿病对症治疗一般原则[4,5]

- 根据患者需要制订治疗方案(通常在症状变得麻烦、干扰生活或引起社交歧视时开始治疗)。
- 开始新的治疗之前,审查现有药物是否导致或加重了症状。
- 优先治疗最令人痛苦的症状,并考虑共病的特征。
- 权衡治疗收益与可能的不良反应。
- 小剂量开始,根据耐受性和疗效缓慢加量(患者对认知和运动系统不良反应相对敏感,这些不良反应也可能难以与疾病进展区分开)。
- 定期随访患者,以便调整治疗方案(因为症状会随着疾病进展而加重)。

极少有对照研究可用来指导这个领域的治疗[6],但是可以从发表的专家意见和临床经验中获得指导。可以在后面见到现有文献的总结。读者可按指引查阅此处引用的报告,详细了解给药方案以及耐受性的进一步信息。鼓励治疗亨廷顿病的医师们发表报告,阳性和阴性均可,以此来增加原始文献。表 10.7 列出了亨廷顿病运动系统症状药物治疗的证据与经验。

运动系统症状

运动功能障碍分两个阶段:开始为多动阶段,突出表现为舞蹈症,随着时间延长达到平台期;后来为少动阶段,特点是运动迟缓、肌张力障碍、平衡与步态紊乱[1]。关于舞蹈症,治疗目标不是消除它,而是减轻其严重程度,达到更好的耐受[4]。已有治疗路径可供指导治疗[7]。一线治疗包括丁苯那嗪(已批准适应证)或抗精神病药(未批准适应证)[7,8]。最好采取单药治疗,以防止增加不良反应的风险,使得非运动系统症状的治疗复杂化[7,8]。

表 10.7　亨廷顿病运动系统症状药物治疗的证据与经验

症状	治疗
舞蹈症	■ **丁苯那嗪**:与抗精神病药不同,丁苯那嗪的疗效已得到确认[6,7,9]。然而,不良反应(包括镇静、抑郁和帕金森综合征)可能会限制其临床收益。在临床实践中,许多医师喜欢将丁苯那嗪作为一线治疗用于没有抑郁症状和自杀行为的患者[7]。需要遵守每天数次用药的方案(如每天 3 次)。氘丁苯那嗪已在美国上市,用于治疗亨廷顿病的舞蹈症。该药并未直接与丁苯那嗪进行过比较,但是其药代动力学和不良反应方面可能有所改善[9]

续表

症状	治疗
舞蹈症	■ **抗精神病药**：考虑为一线治疗，特别是有抑郁、攻击行为、精神病时，或者怀疑服药依从性不好时[7,8,10]，但是没有 RCT 资料。利培酮或奥氮平等第二代抗精神病药最常用[7]。可能限制其使用的不良反应包括运动障碍、帕金森综合征和代谢综合征[4]。第一代抗精神病药已被成功地使用，但是因为 EPS 的风险，在临床实践中不太常用了[10]。Enroll-HD 观察性研究数据库提示，利培酮和奥氮平的疗效至少与丁苯那嗪相同[11]，但是会加重认知损害[12]。对于严重舞蹈症，已经合用抗精神病药与丁苯那嗪[7]。与大多数抗精神病药一样，丁苯那嗪与氘丁苯那嗪均可能会延长 Q-T 间期 ■ **其他药物**：金刚烷胺、利鲁唑（riluzole）和大麻隆（nabilone）被建议作为丁苯那嗪的替代药物[13]，但是这些药物的疗效证据是有争议的[4]；一些指南建议不用金刚烷胺和利鲁唑[7,8]，或者根本不提它们[7]。其他大麻素类药物（nabiximols 和大麻二酚）临床试验发现，其疗效与安慰剂无异[14]。氯硝西泮有时作为辅助治疗用于共病，一个小样本病例系列报告大剂量时有益[4,15]。左乙拉西坦在两项小样本开放研究中合用获得成功，在一项研究中嗜睡导致 33% 脱落，还报告出现了帕金森综合征[15]。普利多匹定迄今未在 RCT 中被证明有效，需要进一步评估[16]。拉曲吡啶、ethyl-EPA 二十碳五烯酸乙酯和 mavoglurant（一种 mGlu5 受体拮抗剂）的应用研究均是阴性结果[15]
运动减少性肌强直	■ 左旋多巴可暂时缓解部分症状[7]。注意这类药物有可能加重行为紊乱[8]。抗精神病药或丁苯那嗪可导致或加重肌强直。在权衡收益与症状严重程度之后，应该首先减量或停用[7]。金刚烷胺和多巴胺受体激动剂有阳性的研究结果（但是各指南不建议使用它们）[7]
肌阵挛	■ 建议使用丙戊酸盐或氯硝西泮，单用或合用均可[7]。左乙拉西坦是一种治疗选择[7]
肌张力障碍	■ 局部肌张力障碍建议注射肉毒毒素[7]，非局部肌张力障碍建议用氯硝西泮或巴氯芬[4]

精神和行为症状

亨廷顿病会出现各种各样的精神和行为症状，包括焦虑、抑郁、自杀倾向、持续言语、脱抑制、易激惹、情感淡漠和罕见的精神病[17]。精神与行为症状可在运动功能紊乱之前出现，并严重降低生活质量[17]。与亨廷顿病的其他特征相比，精神疾病也许最适合药物治疗[4]。一般而言，精神科治疗的选择与其他疾病类似[4]，但是患者对不良反应更加敏感[4]。最常用的精神药物被总结在表 10.8 和表 10.9 中（大多数依据低质的证据）[17]。

表 10.8　亨廷顿病精神与行为症状药物治疗的证据与经验

症状	治疗
焦虑	■ 在亨廷顿病患者中的终生患病率为 16.7%~24%[17]。没有 RCT 可以指导治疗的选择；但在一项小样本、开放性、试验性研究中，奥氮平 5mg/d 明显减轻了焦虑症状[17]。有人建议将 SSRI 和 SNRI 作为一线治疗[4,7]。一些指南建议，对于人格相关的焦虑、行为紊乱[8] 或其他治疗方法失败时[7]，考虑第二代抗精神病药（喹硫平[7]、利培酮或奥氮平）。苯二氮䓬类药物或丁螺环酮等抗焦虑药也可能有效[8]

续表

症状	治疗
抑郁	■ 在亨廷顿病患者中的终生患病率为 20%~56%[17]。往往需要治疗:抑郁与亨廷顿病患者生活质量较低和自杀风险升高有关[17,18]。没有 RCT 可以指导治疗的选择[19]。然而,大多数专家认为抗抑郁药对亨廷顿病患者的抑郁疗效良好。SSRI 是首选的一线治疗[4,7] ■ SSRI:两项对照试验研究了氟西汀和西酞普兰在无抑郁症亨廷顿病患者中的疗效。尽管排除了抑郁症患者,两种药物均明显改善了抑郁症状[19]。注意丁苯那嗪由 CYP2D6 代谢,该酶的抑制剂(如氟西汀、帕罗西汀)可升高其浓度 ■ SNRI:文拉法辛在无对照研究中有效[19],但是 1/5 出现不良反应,如恶心和易激惹[17] ■ 三环类药物:一些病例报告为有效[20],但是一般应避免或限制其使用。其抗胆碱能作用可加重运动过度和认知损害[20]。因过量中毒也不太适宜选择这类药物(亨廷顿病患者自杀倾向增加[17]) ■ 其他药物:米氮平在一例严重抑郁症中获得治疗成功[4]。在一项病例登记研究中,它是治疗亨廷顿病患者的抑郁症最常用的药物[17]。锂盐在小样本病例系列中[19]可以改善自杀倾向,但是经验有限,耐受性可能也差。MAOI 在早期病例研究中使用过[20],但是缺乏其最近的经验,而且它与丁苯那嗪有重要的相互作用,因此不太适用。严重病例建议用 ECT[7,21,22]
强迫行为或持续言语	■ 没有 RCT[23]。国际性共识支持使用 SSRI 作为一线治疗[7],也支持使用氯米帕明[17],但是其耐受性可能较差。病例研究证明,使用氟西汀、帕罗西汀和舍曲林均获得成功[4]。对有持续言语(或行为)和攻击行为的 2 例患者的研究发现,丁螺环酮治疗有效[17]。对于持续意念(ideational perseveration),国际共识也支持使用奥氮平或利培酮(特别是伴有易激惹时)[7]
易激惹或激越[24]	■ 在亨廷顿病患者中的患病率为 38%~73%[17]。开始治疗时采用非药物方法(如减轻疼痛或静坐不能等可能的诱发因素,采用行为或心理方法)。没有专门批准的药物,但是专家共识支持使用 SSRI 作为首选的一线药物,其次是抗精神病药单药治疗。临床特征影响治疗选择。例如,存在舞蹈症、急性易激惹、攻击或冲动行为时,可能最好选择第二代抗精神病药,如奥氮平、利培酮、喹硫平。苯二氮䓬类药物是广泛使用的辅助治疗。最大剂量 SSRI 无效,特别是共病睡眠障碍时,指南也建议使用米氮平或米安色林。对于抗抑郁药或抗精神病药无效的病例,也建议辅助使用心境稳定剂[7] ■ 攻击行为:曾经用过各种各样的研究报告有效的精神药物,如抗精神病药、锂盐、丙戊酸盐、普萘洛尔、甲羟孕酮、SSRI、丁螺环酮[20,25]。抗精神病药最常用。证据太少,无法提出具体的治疗建议[25],但是可以考虑小剂量抗精神病药[4]。对于药物治疗无效的激越,几个病例报告表明 ECT 有效[21]
情感淡漠	■ 常见于亨廷顿病,似乎随着疾病进展而加重[17]。一些有镇静作用的药物(如抗精神病药、苯二氮䓬类药物、丁苯那嗪)可导致情感淡漠,因此应该考虑减量或停用[7]。最近一项多中心 RCT 对安非他酮进行了研究,结果发现对情感淡漠治疗无效[26]。其他药物,包括哌甲酯、托莫西汀、莫达非尼、金刚烷胺和溴隐亭,试验结果都不太成功[17]

续表

症状	治疗
精神病	■ 亨廷顿病最少见的精神症状,可能是由治疗运动系统症状的抗多巴胺能药物引起[17]。没有 RCT 指导治疗选择,治疗凭经验。注意:抗精神病药可加重原有的运动障碍 ■ **第二代抗精神病药**:奥氮平和利培酮最常用[17],建议从小剂量起始[4]。病例报告支持利培酮、喹硫平、阿立哌唑和氨磺必利的疗效[20]。可考虑将氯氮平用于难治性病例[5,20],或者伴有令人虚弱的帕金森症状的不运动型亨廷顿病[7] ■ **第一代抗精神病药**:因肌张力障碍和帕金森综合征的风险而不太常用;但是,舞蹈症对患者也是个问题,可以使用氟哌啶醇[20]

表 10.9 亨廷顿病精神与行为症状现有治疗概要

症状	最常用药物	备选治疗
焦虑	SSRI、米氮平、普瑞巴林、文拉法辛	奥氮平、利培酮、喹硫平、苯二氮䓬类、普萘洛尔、丁螺环酮
抑郁或自杀倾向	SSRI、米氮平、文拉法辛	三环类药物,难治病例用 ECT
强迫症	SSRI	氯米帕明
易激惹或激越	SSRI、第二代抗精神病药(奥氮平、利培酮、舒必利)、硫必利、苯二氮䓬类	抗癫痫药(拉莫三嗪、卡马西平、丙戊酸盐)、三环类药物、丁螺环酮、普萘洛尔,考虑试用镇痛剂
情感淡漠	无	无
精神病	奥氮平、利培酮、氟哌啶醇、舒必利、硫必利及注射用抗精神病药	氯氮平、喹硫平

认知症状

认知紊乱可能在运动功能紊乱之前数年就会出现[1];认知功能减退的过程是逐渐的[27],痴呆在晚期是不可避免的。尽管各种药物都进行过研究,没有一种的疗效得到确认,大多数药物的益处仍然不明[28]。没有足够证据支持使用乙酰胆碱酯酶抑制剂[29],也没有证据支持使用其他药物治疗亨廷顿病的痴呆[30]。

参考文献

1. McColgan P, et al. Huntington's disease: a clinical review. *Eur J Neurol* 2018; 25:24–34.
2. Mestre T, et al. Therapeutic interventions for disease progression in Huntington's disease. *Cochrane Database Syst Rev* 2009; 2009:Cd006455.
3. Tabrizi SJ, et al. Huntington disease: new insights into molecular pathogenesis and therapeutic opportunities. *Nat Rev Neurol* 2020; 16:529–546.
4. Killoran A, et al. Current therapeutic options for Huntington's disease: good clinical practice versus evidence-based approaches? *Mov Disord* 2014; 29:1404–1413.
5. Anderson KE, et al. Clinical management of neuropsychiatric symptoms of Huntington disease: expert-based consensus guidelines on agitation, anxiety, apathy, psychosis and sleep disorders. *J Huntington's Dis* 2018; 7:355–366.
6. Mestre T, et al. Therapeutic interventions for symptomatic treatment in Huntington's disease. *Cochrane Database Syst Rev* 2009:CD006456.
7. Bachoud-Lévi AC, et al. International guidelines for the treatment of Huntington's disease. *Front Neurol* 2019; 10:710.
8. Desamericq G, et al. Guidelines for clinical pharmacological practices in Huntington's disease. *Rev Neurol (Paris)* 2016; 172:423–432.
9. Dash D, et al. Therapeutic update on Huntington's disease: symptomatic treatments and emerging disease-modifying therapies.

Neurotherapeutics 2020:[Epub ahead of print].

10. Unti E, et al. Antipsychotic drugs in Huntington's disease. *Expert Rev Neurother* 2017; **17**:227–237.

11. Schultz JL, et al. Comparing risperidone and olanzapine to tetrabenazine for the management of chorea in Huntington disease: an analysis from the Enroll-HD database. *Mov Disord Clin Pract* 2019; **6**:132–138.

12. Harris KL, et al. Antidopaminergic treatment is associated with reduced chorea and irritability but impaired cognition in Huntington's disease (Enroll-HD). *J Neurol Neurosurg Psychiatry* 2020; **91**:622–630.

13. Armstrong MJ, et al. Evidence-based guideline: pharmacologic treatment of chorea in Huntington disease: report of the guideline development subcommittee of the American Academy of Neurology. *Neurology* 2012; **79**:597–603.

14. Dickey AS, et al. Therapy development in Huntington disease: from current strategies to emerging opportunities. *Am J Med Genet A* 2018; **176**:842–861.

15. Coppen EM, et al. Current pharmacological approaches to reduce chorea in Huntington's disease. *Drugs* 2017; **77**:29–46.

16. Jabłońska M, et al. Pridopidine in the treatment of Huntington's disease. *Rev Neurosci* 2020; **31**:441–451.

17. Eddy CM, et al. Changes in mental state and behaviour in Huntington's disease. *Lancet Psychiatry* 2016; **3**:1079–1086.

18. Kachian ZR, et al. Suicidal ideation and behavior in Huntington's disease: systematic review and recommendations. *J Affect Disord* 2019; **250**:319–329.

19. Moulton CD, et al. Systematic review of pharmacological treatments for depressive symptoms in Huntington's disease. *Mov Disord* 2014; **29**:1556–1561.

20. van Duijn E. Medical treatment of behavioral manifestations of Huntington disease. *Handb Clin Neurol* 2017; **144**:129–139.

21. Mowafi W, et al. Electroconvulsive therapy for severe depression, psychosis and chorea in a patient with Huntington's disease: case report and review of the literature. *BJPsych Bulletin* 2020:[Epub ahead of print].

22. Adrissi J, et al. Electroconvulsive Therapy (ECT) for refractory psychiatric symptoms in Huntington's disease: a case series and review of the literature. *J Huntington's Dis* 2019; **8**:291–300.

23. Oosterloo M, et al. Obsessive-compulsive and perseverative behaviors in Huntington's disease. *J Huntington's Dis* 2019; **8**:1–7.

24. Karagas NE, et al. Irritability in Huntington's disease. *J Huntington's Dis* 2020; **9**:107–113.

25. Fisher CA, et al. Aggression in Huntington's disease: a systematic review of rates of aggression and treatment methods. *J Huntington's Dis* 2014; **3**:319–332.

26. Petersén Å, et al. The psychopharmacology of Huntington disease. *Handb Clin Neurol* 2019; **165**:179–189.

27. Ross CA, et al. Huntington disease: natural history, biomarkers and prospects for therapeutics. *Nat Rev Neurol* 2014; **10**:204–216.

28. van der Vaart T, et al. Treatment of cognitive deficits in genetic disorders: a systematic review of clinical trials of diet and drug treatments. *JAMA Neurology* 2015; **72**:1052–1060.

29. Li Y, et al. Cholinesterase inhibitors for rarer dementias associated with neurological conditions. *Cochrane Database Syst Rev* 2015:Cd009444.

30. O'Brien JT, et al. Clinical practice with anti-dementia drugs: A revised (third) consensus statement from the British Association for Psychopharmacology. *J. Psychopharmacol* 2017; **31**:147–168.

扩展阅读

Bachoud-Lévi AC, et al. International guidelines for the treatment of Huntington's disease. *Frontiers in Neurology* 2019; **10**:710.

多发性硬化

多发性硬化是神经残疾的常见原因之一,在英国影响了将近 85 000 人,起病年龄通常为 20~50 岁。多发性硬化的患者会出现各种神经精神疾病,如抑郁、焦虑、病理性哭笑(假性延髓情绪)、躁狂和欣快、精神病或双相障碍、疲乏以及认知损害。精神障碍起因于多发性硬化诊断和预后的心理影响、感到缺乏社会支持或无助的应对方式[1]、应激增多[2]、多发性硬化常用治疗的医源性影响[3,4] 或神经通路的损害[3]。

抑郁

在多发性硬化的患者中,抑郁症是常见的,其时点患病率为 14%~27%[5,6],终身患病率高达 50%[7,8]。自杀率比一般人群高 2~7.5 倍[9]。抑郁症往往伴有疲乏与疼痛,尽管其因果关系并不清楚。抑郁症、假性延髓情绪和多发性硬化的症状重叠,使得诊断复杂化,所以神经科医师与精神科医师合作是必要的,以此来确保多发性硬化的最佳治疗。多发性硬化的抑郁症可能是大脑的结构性改变所致,因此可能与非多发性硬化的抑郁症完全不同[10]。

β 干扰素在多发性硬化病因中的作用不明,但是最近认为使用 β 干扰素时,患者抑郁症发生率并未增加[11-13]。β 干扰素开始的标准治疗应该包括抑郁的评估,以及对过去有抑郁症病史者预防性使用抗抑郁药[3]。同样的原则适用于其他与抑郁相关的特效生物治疗(daclizumab 达利珠单抗、alemtuzumab 阿仑单抗、natalizumab 那他珠单抗等)[4]。

治疗建议

多发性硬化中的抑郁症

步骤	干预
1	采用 PHQ-9HADS/BDI[14]/CES-D[15] 筛查抑郁症。排除并治疗任何器质性病因。考虑药物的医源性影响为抑郁症的潜在病因。确保无躁狂或双相障碍的病史。轻度抑郁症可以考虑认知行为疗法[16] 或自助[17]。
2	SSRI 的不良反应相对温和,因此应该作为一线治疗[3,15,18,19]。在一项试验中,舍曲林与认知行为疗法同样有效[20];但另一项试验发现,帕罗西汀的疗效不优于安慰剂[21]。在一项小样本多发性硬化相关抑郁症病例系列研究中,氟西汀治疗有效[22]。由于这组患者对不良反应的耐受性降低,应该从起始剂量的 1/2 开始加量。许多多发性硬化患者使用三环类药物治疗疼痛或膀胱功能紊乱,因此应该慎用 SSRI,并观察患者有无 5-羟色胺综合征。对于伴有疼痛的患者,治疗时应该考虑应用 SNRI,如度洛西汀[23] 或文拉法辛[24]。一项地昔帕明的随机对照试验发现其疗效优于安慰剂,但是三环类药物的耐受性往往较差[25]。这里引用的一些研究不能让 Cochrane 信服[26],但是没有理由认为抗抑郁药治疗由躯体疾病引起的抑郁症疗效会差[27]。与支持治疗或常规治疗相比,认知行为疗法是最合适的、疗效最佳的心理干预,对于中度抑郁症患者,应该与药物治疗联合使用[20,28,29]。正念训练可能也有帮助[30]。ω-3 脂肪酸无效[31]。
3	若 SSRI 不能耐受或没有反应,有限的数据表明吗氯贝胺是有效的,且耐受性良好[32,33]。文拉法辛、度洛西汀和米氮平均没有试验发表,但是它们被广泛使用。米氮平可加重疲乏,至少在开始用药时如此。

续表

步骤	干预
4	对于自杀倾向明显,或重度抑郁伴高风险者,可以考虑电休克疗法,但是它可能造成多发性硬化症状的恶化,尽管一些研究表明并没有神经功能障碍发生[34]。
5	在多发性硬化的抑郁症中,被证明有些效果的其他治疗包括锌[35]、维生素 A[36] 和辅酶 Q10[37]。一项小样本试验支持氨吡啶有抗抑郁作用[38]。

焦虑

焦虑影响了许多多发性硬化的患者,其时点患病率高达 50%[39],终身发病率为 35%~37%[40]。患病率高于一般人群的有广泛性焦虑障碍、惊恐障碍、强迫症[40]以及社交焦虑。焦虑被认为与自觉缺乏支持、疼痛增加、疲乏、睡眠紊乱、抑郁、酒精滥用和自杀观念有关。在多发性硬化中,对预后的不确定性是焦虑的主要原因[41]。关于多发性硬化中焦虑的治疗,没有已发表的试验,但是可以用 SSRI 治疗,无效病例可以选择文拉法辛(根据非多发性硬化的治法)。

苯二氮䓬类药物可以用来治疗急性和严重焦虑,但是最多 4 周,不宜长期使用。也可以考虑丁螺环酮和 β 受体阻滞剂,尽管其在多发性硬化中的疗效未得到证实。普瑞巴林也被批准用于治疗焦虑,在这一类人中可能有效,特别是需要缓解疼痛者[42,43]。多发性硬化患者也可能对认知行为疗法有反应。一般而言,其治疗与非多发性硬化的焦虑障碍相同(见第 3 章)。

假性延髓情绪

多达 10% 的多发性硬化患者出现病理性哭笑症状,或其他情感协调。这种症状常见于该病晚期,并与认知损害有关[40]。已有几项开放试验推荐多发性硬化患者使用小剂量三环类药物(如阿米替林)或 5-羟色胺再摄取抑制剂(氟西汀[44,45])。西酞普兰[46]、去甲替林[47]或舍曲林[48]已经在卒中后病理性哭笑患者中进行过研究,发现疗效尚可,且起效迅速。丙戊酸可能有效[49]。右美沙芬和奎尼丁合剂有效[50]。右美沙芬和氟西汀合剂可有类似疗效[51]。在这些合剂中,右美沙芬(一种镇痛止咳剂)是活性成分,奎尼丁/氟西汀是代谢抑制剂。右美沙芬和奎尼丁合剂以 Nuedexta 的名称获得 FDA 批准,曾一度被欧盟批准,但是未在英国上市。

双相障碍

多发性硬化人群中双相障碍的发生率可高达 13%,而一般人群为 1%~6%。躁狂可由药物引起,如类固醇或巴氯芬[52]。

实例研究提示,表现为躁狂或双相障碍的患者应该使用心境稳定剂,如丙戊酸钠,因其耐受性比锂盐好[53]。

锂盐可造成多尿,从而导致有膀胱疾病的患者耐受的困难增加。躁狂伴有精神病性症状的患者可以用小剂量第二代抗精神病药,如利培酮、奥氮平[2]、齐拉西酮[54]。已知类固醇类引起的精神病性躁狂必须治疗时,奥氮平的疗效良好[55]。进一步的病例报道表明,利培酮同样有效。在这个领域中没有临床试验。

精神病

1.1% 的多发性硬化患者会发生精神病，与其他精神障碍相比相对罕见[54]。在个别病例中，精神病是多发性硬化的主诉[56]。已经发表的临床试验很少，但是其结果推荐使用利培酮或氯氮平，因为它们产生锥体外系症状的风险低[52]。在此基础上，奥氮平、阿立哌唑和喹硫平也是可能的选择，至少理论上是。难治性病例曾用过 ECT[57]。

罕见情况下，精神病可能是患者多发性硬化复发的表现，此时类固醇类药物可能有效，但需要在密切监测下使用。多发性硬化患者接受大麻类药物治疗时，也有出现精神病性反应的轻度风险[58,59]。

认知损害

至少 40%~65% 的多发性硬化患者会发生认知损害。一些常用药会加重认知损害，如替扎尼定、地西泮、加巴喷丁[60]。尽管没有已发表的临床试验，但是临床病例研究的证据表明，治疗睡眠困难、抑郁和疲乏可以提高认知功能[60]。两项小样本试验指出，对于轻、中度认知损害的患者，多奈哌齐有中等疗效[61,62]。而一项更大样本的研究则发现多奈哌齐并无疗效[63]。类似地，支持美金刚治疗认知损害的数据也是缺乏的[64]。总之，没有哪项对症治疗被证明有效[65]，疾病修饰药物会带来更大的希望[66]。

疲乏

疲乏是多发性硬化患者的常见症状，高达 80% 的患者会受影响[67]。疲乏的病因不明，但有证据表明神经网络的破坏[68]、抑郁或心理反应[52]、睡眠紊乱、炎症[69]或药物在其发展中扮演着重要的角色。在治疗策略上应该使用药物与非药物方法[67]。

非药物方法包括回顾任何可能的致病因素、评估与治疗潜在的抑郁症、规律活动和适当锻炼。一项研究表明认知行为疗法能降低疲乏评分[70]。

药物方法包括使用金刚烷胺[71]或莫达非尼。NICE 指南指出，没有应该常规使用的药物：但金刚烷胺可能略有疗效，因而应该提供[72]。一篇关于金刚烷胺在多发性硬化患者中应用的 Cochrane 文献指出，金刚烷胺试验的质量与结果是不一致的，因此其疗效仍然不清楚[71]。一个对 11 项 RCT 的荟萃分析发现金刚烷胺的支持性证据[73]，后来（2020 年）的荟萃分析证实了其治疗价值[74]。

莫达非尼在临床试验中的结果不一，但是对 5 项 RCT[75] 的荟萃分析发现其明确有效。尽管人们对莫达非尼的疗效有怀疑，但它仍广泛地应用于多发性硬化患者的治疗[76]。

其他推荐用于治疗多发性硬化疲乏症状的药物包括匹莫林、阿司匹林和人参。一项关于阿司匹林的双盲交叉研究指出，与安慰剂相比，此研究更支持阿司匹林的疗效，但需要进一步研究[77]。一项 RCT 发现，匹莫林缓解症状的比例比安慰剂高一倍[78]。关于人参治疗疲乏的数据不一[79,80]。

参考文献

1. Ron MA. Do neurologists provide adequate care for depression in patients with multiple sclerosis? *Nat Clin Pract Neurol* 2006; 2:534–535.

2. Patten SB, et al. Biopsychosocial correlates of lifetime major depression in a multiple sclerosis population. *Mult Scler* 2000; 6:115–120.

3. Servis ME. Psychiatric comorbidity in Parkinson's disease, multiple sclerosis, and seizure disorder. *Continuum* 2006; **12**:72–86.

4. Carta MG, et al. Pharmacological management of depression in patients with multiple sclerosis. *Expert Opin Pharmacother* 2018; **19**:1533–1540.

5. Gottberg K, et al. A population-based study of depressive symptoms in multiple sclerosis in Stockholm county: association with functioning and sense of coherence. *J Neurol Neurosurg Psychiatry* 2007; **78**:60–65.

6. Boeschoten RE, et al. Prevalence of depression and anxiety in multiple sclerosis: A systematic review and meta-analysis. *J Neurol Sci* 2017; **372**:331–341.

7. Patten SB, et al. Depression in multiple sclerosis. *Int Rev Psychiatry (Abingdon, England)* 2017:1–10.

8. Kalb R, et al. Depression and suicidality in multiple sclerosis: red flags, management strategies, and ethical considerations. *Curr Neurol Neurosci Rep* 2019; **19**:77.

9. Sadovnick AD, et al. Cause of death in patients attending multiple sclerosis clinics. *Neurology* 1991; **41**:1193–1196.

10. Corallo F, et al. A complex relation between depression and multiple sclerosis: a descriptive review. *Neurol Sci* 2019; **40**:1551–1558.

11. Zephir H, et al. Multiple sclerosis and depression: influence of interferon beta therapy. *Mult Scler* 2003; **9**:284–288.

12. Patten SB, et al. Anti-depressant use in association with interferon and glatiramer acetate treatment in multiple sclerosis. *Mult Scler* 2008; **14**:406–411.

13. Schippling S, et al. Incidence and course of depression in multiple sclerosis in the multinational beyond trial. *J Neurol* 2016; **263**:1418–1426.

14. Moran PJ, et al. The validity of Beck Depression Inventory and Hamilton Rating Scale for Depression items in the assessment of depression among patients with multiple sclerosis. *J Behav Med* 2005; **28**:35–41.

15. Pandya R, et al. Predictive value of the CES-D in detecting depression among candidates for disease-modifying multiple sclerosis treatment. *Psychosomatics* 2005; **46**:131–134.

16. Minden SL, et al. Evidence-based guideline: assessment and management of psychiatric disorders in individuals with MS: report of the Guideline Development Subcommittee of the American Academy of Neurology. *Neurology* 2014; **82**:174–181.

17. Rickards H. Depression in neurological disorders: Parkinson's disease, multiple sclerosis, and stroke. *J Neurol Neurosurg Psychiatry* 2005; **76** Suppl 1:i48–i52.

18. Silveira C, et al. Neuropsychiatric symptoms of multiple sclerosis: state of the art. *Psychiatry Investig* 2019; **16**:877–888.

19. Patten SB. Current perspectives on co-morbid depression and multiple sclerosis. *Expert Rev Neurother* 2020; **20**:867–874.

20. Mohr DC, et al. Comparative outcomes for individual cognitive-behavior therapy, supportive-expressive group psychotherapy, and sertraline for the treatment of depression in multiple sclerosis. *J Consult Clin Psychol* 2001; **69**:942–949.

21. Ehde DM, et al. Efficacy of paroxetine in treating major depressive disorder in persons with multiple sclerosis. *Gen Hosp Psychiatry* 2008; **30**:40–48.

22. Flax JW, et al. Effect of fluoxetine on patients with multiple sclerosis. *Am J Psychiatry* 1991; **148**:1603.

23. Vollmer TL, et al. A randomized, double-blind, placebo-controlled trial of duloxetine for the treatment of pain in patients with multiple sclerosis. *Pain Practice: The Official Journal of World Institute of Pain* 2014; **14**:732–744.

24. Hilty DM, et al. Psychopharmacology for neurologists: principles, algorithms, and other resources. *Continuum* 2006; **12**:33–46.

25. Barak Y, et al. Treatment of depression in patients with multiple sclerosis. *Neurologist* 1998; **4**:99–104.

26. Koch MW, et al. Pharmacologic treatment of depression in multiple sclerosis. *Cochrane Database Syst Rev* 2011; **2**:CD007295.

27. Taylor D, et al. Pharmacological interventions for people with depression and chronic physical health problems: systematic review and meta-analyses of safety and efficacy. *Br J Psychiatry* 2011; **198**:179–188.

28. Siegert RJ, et al. Depression in multiple sclerosis: a review. *J Neurol Neurosurg Psychiatry* 2005; **76**:469–475.

29. Larcombe NA, et al. An evaluation of cognitive-behaviour therapy for depression in patients with multiple sclerosis. *Br J Psychiatry* 1984; **145**:366–371.

30. Grossman P, et al. MS quality of life, depression, and fatigue improve after mindfulness training: a randomized trial. *Neurology* 2010; **75**:1141–1149.

31. Shinto L, et al. Omega-3 fatty acids for depression in multiple sclerosis: a randomized pilot study. *PLoS One* 2016; **11**:e0147195.

32. Schiffer RB, et al. Antidepressant pharmacotherapy of depression associated with multiple sclerosis. *Am J Psychiatry* 1990; **147**:1493–1497.

33. Barak Y, et al. Moclobemide treatment in multiple sclerosis patients with comorbid depression: an open-label safety trial. *J Neuropsychiatry Clin Neurosci* 1999; **11**:271–273.

34. Rasmussen KG, et al. Electroconvulsive therapy in patients with multiple sclerosis. *JECT* 2007; **23**:179–180.

35. Salari S, et al. Zinc sulphate: A reasonable choice for depression management in patients with multiple sclerosis: A randomized, double-blind, placebo-controlled clinical trial. *Pharmacol Rep* 2015; **67**:606–609.

36. Bitarafan S, et al. Effect of vitamin A supplementation on fatigue and depression in multiple sclerosis patients: a double-blind placebo-controlled clinical trial. *Iran J Allergy Asthma Immunol* 2016; **15**:13–19.

37. Sanoobar M, et al. Coenzyme Q10 as a treatment for fatigue and depression in multiple sclerosis patients: A double blind randomized clinical trial. *Nutr Neurosci* 2016; **19**:138–143.

38. Broicher SD, et al. Positive effects of fampridine on cognition, fatigue and depression in patients with multiple sclerosis over 2 years. *J Neurol* 2018; **265**:1016–1025.

39. Jones KH, et al. A large-scale study of anxiety and depression in people with multiple sclerosis: a survey via the web portal of the UK MS Register. *PLoS One* 2012; **7**:e41910.

40. Korostil M, et al. Anxiety disorders and their clinical correlates in multiple sclerosis patients. *Mult Scler* 2007; **13**:67–72.

41. Butler E, et al. 'It's the unknown' – understanding anxiety: from the perspective of people with multiple sclerosis. *Psychol Health* 2019; 34:368–383.

42. Solaro C, et al. Pregabalin for treating paroxysmal painful symptoms in multiple sclerosis: a pilot study. *J Neurol* 2009; 256:1773–1774.

43. Bittner S, et al. Pregabalin and gabapentin in multiple sclerosis: clinical experiences and therapeutic implications. *Nervenarzt* 2011; 82:1273–1280.

44. Feinstein A, et al. The effects of anxiety on psychiatric morbidity in patients with multiple sclerosis. *Mult Scler* 1999; 5:323–326.

45. Feinstein A, et al. Prevalence and neurobehavioral correlates of pathological laughing and crying in multiple sclerosis. *Arch Neurol* 1997; 54:1116–1121.

46. Andersen G, et al. Citalopram for post-stroke pathological crying. *Lancet* 1993; 342:837–839.

47. Robinson RG, et al. Pathological laughing and crying following stroke: validation of a measurement scale and a double-blind treatment study. *Am J Psychiatry* 1993; 150:286–293.

48. Burns A, et al. Sertraline in stroke-associated lability of mood. *Int J Geriatr Psychiatry* 1999; 14:681–685.

49. Johnson B, et al. Crying and suicidal, but not depressed. Pseudobulbar affect in multiple sclerosis successfully treated with valproic acid: case report and literature review. *Palliative & Supportive Care* 2015; 13:1797–1801.

50. Pioro EP, et al. Dextromethorphan plus ultra low-dose quinidine reduces pseudobulbar affect. *Ann Neurol* 2010; 68:693–702.

51. McGrane I, et al. Treatment of pseudobulbar affect with fluoxetine and dextromethorphan in a woman with multiple sclerosis. *Ann Pharmacother* 2017:1035–1036.

52. Jefferies K. The neuropsychiatry of multiple sclerosis. *Adv Psychiatr Treat* 2006; 12:214–220.

53. Stip E, et al. Valproate in the treatment of mood disorder due to multiple sclerosis. *Can J Psychiatry* 1995; 40:219–220.

54. Davids E, et al. Antipsychotic treatment of psychosis associated with multiple sclerosis. *Prog Neuropsychopharmacol Biol Psychiatry* 2004; 28:743–744.

55. Budur K, et al. Olanzapine for corticosteroid-induced mood disorders. *Psychosomatics* 2003; 44:353.

56. Camara-Lemarroy CR, et al. The varieties of psychosis in multiple sclerosis: A systematic review of cases. *Mult Scler Relat Disord* 2017; 12:9–14.

57. Narita Z, et al. Possible effects of electroconvulsive therapy on refractory psychosis in primary progressive multiple sclerosis: A case report. *Neuropsychopharmacol Rep* 2018; 38:92–94.

58. Aragona M, et al. Psychopathological and cognitive effects of therapeutic cannabinoids in multiple sclerosis: a double-blind, placebo controlled, crossover study. *Clin Neuropharmacol* 2009; 32:41–47.

59. Black N, et al. Cannabinoids for the treatment of mental disorders and symptoms of mental disorders: a systematic review and meta-analysis. *Lancet Psychiatry* 2019; 6:995–1010.

60. Pierson SH, et al. Treatment of cognitive impairment in multiple sclerosis. *Behav Neurol* 2006; 17:53–67.

61. Krupp LB, et al. Donepezil improved memory in multiple sclerosis in a randomized clinical trial. *Neurology* 2004; 63:1579–1585.

62. Greene YM, et al. A 12-week, open trial of donepezil hydrochloride in patients with multiple sclerosis and associated cognitive impairments. *J Clin Psychopharmacol* 2000; 20:350–356.

63. Krupp LB, et al. Multicenter randomized clinical trial of donepezil for memory impairment in multiple sclerosis. *Neurology* 2011; 76:1500–1507.

64. Lovera JF, et al. Memantine for cognitive impairment in multiple sclerosis: a randomized placebo-controlled trial. *Mult Scler* 2010; 16:715–723.

65. Chen MH, et al. Cognitive efficacy of pharmacologic treatments in multiple sclerosis: a systematic review. *CNS Drugs* 2020; 34:599–628.

66. Patti F. Treatment of cognitive impairment in patients with multiple sclerosis. *Expert Opin Investig Drugs* 2012; 21:1679–1699.

67. Bakshi R. Fatigue associated with multiple sclerosis: diagnosis, impact and management. *Mult Scler* 2003; 9:219–227.

68. Sepulcre J, et al. Fatigue in multiple sclerosis is associated with the disruption of frontal and parietal pathways. *Mult Scler* 2009; 15:337–344.

69. Ormstad H, et al. Chronic fatigue and depression due to multiple sclerosis: immune-inflammatory pathways, tryptophan catabolites and the gut-brain axis as possible shared pathways. *Mult Scler Relat Disord* 2020; 46:102533.

70. van KK, et al. A randomized controlled trial of cognitive behavior therapy for multiple sclerosis fatigue. *Psychosom Med* 2008; 70:205–213.

71. Pucci E, et al. Amantadine for fatigue in multiple sclerosis. *Cochrane Database Syst Rev* 2007:CD002818.

72. National Institute for Health and Care Excellence. Multiple sclerosis in adults: management. Clinical Guidance [CG186]. 2014 (last updated November 2019); https://www.nice.org.uk/guidance/cg186.

73. Yang TT, et al. Pharmacological treatments for fatigue in patients with multiple sclerosis: A systematic review and meta-analysis. *J Neurol Sci* 2017; 380:256–261.

74. Perez DQ, et al. Efficacy and safety of amantadine for the treatment of fatigue in multiple sclerosis: a systematic review and meta-analysis. *Neurodegener Dis Manag* 2020; 10:383–395.

75. Shangyan H, et al. Meta-analysis of the efficacy of modafinil versus placebo in the treatment of multiple sclerosis fatigue. *Mult Scler Relat Disord* 2018; 19:85–89.

76. Davies M, et al. Safety profile of modafinil across a range of prescribing indications, including off-label use, in a primary care setting in England: results of a modified prescription-event monitoring study. *Drug Saf* 2013; 36:237–246.

77. Wingerchuk DM, et al. A randomized controlled crossover trial of aspirin for fatigue in multiple sclerosis. *Neurology* 2005; 64:1267–1269.

78. Weinshenker BG, et al. A double-blind, randomized, crossover trial of pemoline in fatigue associated with multiple sclerosis. *Neurology* 1992; 42:1468–1471.

79. Kim E, et al. American ginseng does not improve fatigue in multiple sclerosis: a single center randomized double-blind placebo-controlled crossover pilot study. *Mult Scler* 2011; **17**:1523–1526.

80. Etemadifar M, et al. Ginseng in the treatment of fatigue in multiple sclerosis: a randomized, placebo-controlled, double-blind pilot study. *Int J Neurosci* 2013; **123**:480–486.

帕金森病

帕金森病是一种进展性、退行性神经疾病,以静止性震颤、齿轮样强直、运动迟缓和姿态不稳为特征。其共患精神障碍的患病率也很高。约 25% 在病程中某一时间患有抑郁症,还有 25% 患有较轻类型的抑郁,25% 患有焦虑谱系障碍,25% 患有精神病,多达 80% 会发展为痴呆 [1-3]。抑郁与焦虑可出现在任何时间,精神病、痴呆和谵妄更多见于疾病晚期。要优化这类患者的治疗,需要精神科医师和神经内科医师密切合作。

帕金森病中的抑郁症

帕金森病中的抑郁症,预示着更大程度的认知下降、功能减退和运动症状的进展 [4],有可能反映的是涉及多条神经递质通路更晚期和更广泛的神经变性 [5]。抑郁症也可能会出现在停用多巴胺激动剂以后 [6]。已经存在的痴呆是发生抑郁症确定的危险因素。

帕金森病中抑郁症的治疗建议

步骤	干预
1	排除或治疗器质性疾病,如甲状腺功能减退(在帕金森病中其患病率相对较高 [4])。
2	**5-羟色胺再摄取抑制剂**被认为是一线治疗,尽管其效应值不大 [7-9]。一些患者的运动症状可能会加重,尽管其绝对风险较小 [10,11]。5-羟色胺再摄取抑制剂与司立吉兰合用时必须慎重,因为会增加 5-羟色胺综合征的风险 [4]。**去甲肾上腺素**与 5-羟色胺再摄取抑制剂文拉法辛 [12] 和度洛西汀 [13] 也有一些疗效,但是文拉法辛会轻度加重运动症状 [12]。 **三环类抗抑郁药**的耐受性通常较差,因为其抗胆碱能作用可加重认知问题和造成便秘,α 受体阻断作用可加重自主神经系统功能异常的症状。但是请注意,几项荟萃分析 [8,9] 指出小剂量三环类药物疗效优于 5-羟色胺再摄取抑制剂 [14-16],但是小剂量阿米替林似乎与舍曲林的疗效相同 [17,18]。最新的网络荟萃分析发现,SSRI 是最有效的治疗,明显优于 MAOI 和多巴胺激动剂 [19]。有限的证据支持使用阿戈美拉汀是安全的 [20,21]。托莫西汀无效 [22]。总是应该考虑**认知行为疗法** [23]。
3	考虑多巴胺受体激动剂/释放剂增效治疗,如普拉克索 [24]。但是请注意这些药物会增加冲动控制障碍的风险 [25,26]。罕见情况下,它们也与发生精神病有关 [27]。
4	考虑**电休克疗法**。对抑郁及运动症状通常疗效良好 [4],但产生谵妄的风险高 [28],尤其原有认知损害的患者。
5	此后,遵循难治性抑郁的治疗程序(见第 3 章相关部分)。注意在这类患者中,不良反应及相互作用的倾向会增加。

帕金森病中的精神病

帕金森病中的精神病往往以幻视为特征 [29]。幻听和妄想出现的频率要低很多 [30],而且通常出现在较年轻的患者中 [31]。精神病与痴呆往往共存。有一个预示着会发生另一个 [32]。睡眠障碍也是发生精神病的确定的危险因素 [33]。

尽管多巴胺、5-羟色胺和乙酰胆碱神经传递的异常均与帕金森病的精神病有关,但是对其确切的病因学仍然知之甚少。在大多数患者中,精神病性症状被认为是服用多巴胺药物后的继发效应,而不是帕金森病的组成部分。继发于药物的精神病,至少部分是由血管紧张素转换酶基因多态性决定的[34]。根据有限的数据,与左旋多巴或儿茶酚氧甲基转移酶抑制剂相比,抗胆碱能药和多巴胺激动剂似乎引起精神病的风险更高[30,35]。精神病是给护理者造成痛苦的重要因素,也是导致患者住院和早死的危险因素[32]。

帕金森病中精神病的治疗建议

步骤	干预
1	排除器质性疾病(谵妄)。
2	优化环境以尽可能地改善定向障碍,以及减少患者和照料者不良互动所致的问题。
3	若患者有自知力,而且幻觉发作不频繁,不扰人,则不必治疗。
4	考虑减少或停用抗胆碱能药和多巴胺受体激动剂。监测运动功能退化的迹象。准备重新开始或增加这些药物剂量,以使精神病和运动能力之间达到最佳平衡。
5	考虑第二代抗精神病药。氯氮平(见下面第7点)的疗效有安慰剂随机对照试验支持[29]。相比之下,有几项安慰剂随机对照试验不支持喹硫平与奥氮平的疗效[29]。小剂量的喹硫平耐受性最好,但是会出现锥体外系不良反应和刻板运动。在使用氯氮平前使用喹硫平[36]可能是合理的,但是成功率可能偏低。与喹硫平相比,奥氮平、齐拉西酮和阿立哌唑可能对运动功能的不良影响更大,但是有一项小样本试验[37]支持使用齐拉西酮的安全性。利培酮和第一代抗精神病药应该完全避免使用。当抗精神病药(喹硫平或氯氮平)停时,出现过严重的精神病反弹。 所有抗精神病药治疗痴呆患者的精神病性症状可能疗效较差,而且这类患者可能更易于发生运动及认知不良反应[38]。抗精神病药会增加老年人血管事件风险。在帕金森病患者中,所有抗精神病药都会增加死亡率[39],但是氯氮平的作用尚不清楚。 参阅本章"抗精神病药与痴呆的非认知症状"部分。
6	考虑使用**胆碱酯酶抑制剂**,尤其患者合并痴呆时[29,40]。胆碱酯酶抑制剂也可减少跌倒风险[41]。早期使用多奈哌齐不能预防或减少精神病发作,但是对认知功能有益[42]。
7	试用**氯氮平**。开始剂量为6.25mg,通常剂量为25~35mg/d[29,37]。通常是安全的,但是已经有恶性综合征的报告[43]。 氯氮平的监测方法与治疗精神分裂症时相同。年龄大者更易发生严重恶病质。已有一例再生障碍性贫血的病例报告[44]。
8	考虑**电休克疗法**[45]。精神病及运动症状通常反应良好[46],但引起谵妄的风险高[28],尤其在已有认知损害的患者中。

匹莫范色林(pimavanserin)

匹莫范色林是5-HT$_{2A}$反向激动剂,在美国等一些国家有售。该药对于帕金森病中的精神病有效,但是对多巴胺受体无作用,不会加重帕金森病的运动症状,也不会增加死亡率[47]。

匹莫范色林和氯氮平是推荐用于治疗帕金森病性精神病仅有的两种药物[48]。最近一项网络荟萃分析提示,仅有这两种药在帕金森病中有效,同时对运动功能影响极小[49]。其他药物疗效可疑,耐受性差[49,50]。

胆碱酯酶抑制剂在帕金森病中的应用

胆碱酯酶抑制剂已被证明能改善路易体痴呆(与帕金森病有些类似)患者的认知、妄想和幻觉。运动功能可能会恶化[51,52]。认知功能的改善轻微[53-55]。一篇 Cochrane 综述和最近几项大型随机对照试验[54,56,57]总结道,有证据表明胆碱酯酶抑制剂会改善帕金森病的总体功能、认知、行为紊乱以及日常活动。同样,运动功能可能会恶化,特别是震颤增加[57,58]。关于美金刚的证据不一致[59,60]。停用抗胆碱能药应该会改善认知和精神病——帕金森病患者往往有很高的抗胆碱能负荷,这往往与帕金森治疗本身无关[61]。

许多帕金森病患者会使用补充治疗,其中一些可能略有疗效,参见 Zesiewicz 等[62]。咖啡因可能对帕金森病发展起保护作用,也会轻度改善已确诊疾病的认知功能[63]。

参考文献

1. Hely MA, et al. The Sydney multicenter study of Parkinson's disease: the inevitability of dementia at 20 years. *Mov Disord* 2008; 23:837–844.

2. Riedel O, et al. Frequency of dementia, depression, and other neuropsychiatric symptoms in 1,449 outpatients with Parkinson's disease. *J Neurol* 2010; 257:1073–1082.

3. Reijnders JS, et al. A systematic review of prevalence studies of depression in Parkinson's disease. *Mov Disord* 2008; 23:183–189.

4. McDonald WM, et al. Prevalence, etiology, and treatment of depression in Parkinson's disease. *Biol Psychiatry* 2003; 54:363–375.

5. Palhagen SE, et al. Depressive illness in Parkinson's disease–indication of a more advanced and widespread neurodegenerative process? *Acta Neurol Scand* 2008; 117:295–304.

6. Rabinak CA, et al. Dopamine agonist withdrawal syndrome in Parkinson disease. *Arch Neurol* 2010; 67:58–63.

7. Rocha FL, et al. Antidepressants for depression in Parkinson's disease: systematic review and meta-analysis. *J Psychopharmacol* 2013; 27:417–423.

8. Liu J, et al. Comparative efficacy and acceptability of antidepressants in Parkinson's disease: a network meta-analysis. *PLoS One* 2013; 8:e76651.

9. Troeung L, et al. A meta-analysis of randomised placebo-controlled treatment trials for depression and anxiety in Parkinson's disease. *PLoS One* 2013; 8:e79510.

10. Gony M, et al. Risk of serious extrapyramidal symptoms in patients with Parkinson's disease receiving antidepressant drugs: a pharmacoepidemiologic study comparing serotonin reuptake inhibitors and other antidepressant drugs. *Clin Neuropharmacol* 2003; 26:142–145.

11. Kulisevsky J, et al. Motor changes during sertraline treatment in depressed patients with Parkinson's disease*. *Eur J Neurol* 2008; 15:953–959.

12. Richard IH, et al. A randomized, double-blind, placebo-controlled trial of antidepressants in Parkinson disease. *Neurology* 2012; 78:1229–1236.

13. Bonuccelli U, et al. A non-comparative assessment of tolerability and efficacy of duloxetine in the treatment of depressed patients with Parkinson's disease. *Expert Opin Pharmacother* 2012; 13:2269–2280.

14. Serrano-Duenas M. A comparison between low doses of amitriptyline and low doses of fluoxetine used in the control of depression in patients suffering from Parkinson's disease. *Rev Neurol* 2002; 35:1010–1014.

15. Menza M, et al. A controlled trial of antidepressants in patients with Parkinson disease and depression. *Neurology* 2009; 72:886–892.

16. Devos D, et al. Comparison of desipramine and citalopram treatments for depression in Parkinson's disease: a double-blind, randomized, placebo-controlled study. *Mov Disord* 2008; 23:850–857.

17. Antonini A, et al. Randomized study of sertraline and low-dose amitriptyline in patients with Parkinson's disease and depression: effect on quality of life. *Mov Disord* 2006; 21:1119–1122.

18. Goodarzi Z, et al. Guidelines for dementia or Parkinson's disease with depression or anxiety: a systematic review. *BMC Neurol* 2016; 16:244.

19. Zhuo C, et al. Efficacy of antidepressive medication for depression in Parkinson disease: a network meta-analysis. *Medicine (Baltimore)* 2017; 96:e6698.

20. Avila A, et al. Agomelatine for depression in Parkinson disease: additional effect on sleep and motor dysfunction. *J Clin Psychopharmacol* 2015; 35:719–723.

21. De Berardis D, et al. Agomelatine treatment of major depressive disorder in Parkinson's disease: a case series. *J Neuropsychiatry Clin Neurosci* 2013; 25:343–345.

22. Weintraub D, et al. Atomoxetine for depression and other neuropsychiatric symptoms in Parkinson disease. *Neurology* 2010; 75:448–455.

23. Dobkin RD, et al. Cognitive-behavioral therapy for depression in Parkinson's disease: a randomized, controlled trial. *Am J Psychiatry* 2011; 168:1066–1074.

24. Barone P, et al. Pramipexole versus sertraline in the treatment of depression in Parkinson's disease: a national multicenter parallel-group randomized study. *J Neurol* 2006; 253:601–607.

25. Antonini A, et al. A reassessment of risks and benefits of dopamine agonists in Parkinson's disease. *Lancet Neurol* 2009; 8:929–937.

26. Weintraub D, et al. Impulse control disorders in Parkinson disease: a cross-sectional study of 3090 patients. *Arch Neurol* 2010; 67:589–595.

27. Li CT, et al. Pramipexole-induced psychosis in Parkinson's disease. *Psychiatry Clin Neurosci* 2008; 62:245.

28. Figiel GS, et al. ECT-induced delirium in depressed patients with Parkinson's disease. *J Neuropsychiatry Clin Neurosci* 1991; 3:405–411.

29. Friedman JH. Parkinson's disease psychosis 2010: a review article. *Parkinsonism Relat Disord* 2010; 16:553–560.
30. Ismail MS, et al. A reality test: how well do we understand psychosis in Parkinson's disease? *J Neuropsychiatry Clin Neurosci* 2004; 16:8–18.
31. Kiziltan G, et al. Relationship between age and subtypes of psychotic symptoms in Parkinson's disease. *J Neurol* 2007; 254:448–452.
32. Factor SA, et al. Longitudinal outcome of Parkinson's disease patients with psychosis. *Neurology* 2003; 60:1756–1761.
33. Reich SG, et al. Ten most commonly asked questions about the psychiatric aspects of Parkinson's disease. *Neurologist* 2003; 9:50–56.
34. Lin JJ, et al. Genetic polymorphism of the angiotensin converting enzyme and L-dopa-induced adverse effects in Parkinson's disease. *J Neurol Sci* 2007; 252:130–134.
35. Stowe RL, et al. Dopamine agonist therapy in early Parkinson's disease. *Cochrane Database of Sys Rev* 2008:Cd006564.
36. Divac N, et al. The efficacy and safety of antipsychotic medications in the treatment of psychosis in patients with Parkinson's disease. *Behav Neurol* 2016; 2016:4938154.
37. Pintor L, et al. Ziprasidone versus clozapine in the treatment of psychotic symptoms in Parkinson disease: a randomized open clinical trial. *Clin Neuro Pharmacol* 2012; 35:61–66.
38. Prohorov T, et al. The effect of quetiapine in psychotic Parkinsonian patients with and without dementia. An open-labeled study utilizing a structured interview. *J Neurol* 2006; 253:171–175.
39. Weintraub D, et al. Association of antipsychotic use with mortality risk in patients with Parkinson disease. *JAMA Neurology* 2016; 73:535–541.
40. Marti M, et al. Dementia in Parkinson's disease. *J Neurol* 2007; 254 Suppl 1:41–48.
41. Chung KA, et al. Effects of a central cholinesterase inhibitor on reducing falls in Parkinson disease. *Neurology* 2010; 75:1263–1269.
42. Sawada H, et al. Early use of donepezil against psychosis and cognitive decline in Parkinson's disease: a randomised controlled trial for 2 years. *J Neurol Neurosurg Psychiatry* 2018; 89:1332–1340.
43. Mesquita J, et al. Fatal neuroleptic malignant syndrome induced by clozapine in Parkinson's psychosis. *J Neuropsychiatry Clin Neurosci* 2014; 26:E34.
44. Ziegenbein M, et al. Clozapine-induced aplastic anemia in a patient with Parkinson's disease. *Can J Psychiatry* 2003; 48:352.
45. Factor SA, et al. Combined clozapine and electroconvulsive therapy for the treatment of drug-induced psychosis in Parkinson's disease. *J Neuropsychiatry Clin Neurosci* 1995; 7:304–307.
46. Martin BA. ECT for Parkinson's? *CMAJ* 2003; 168:1391–1392.
47. Sarva H, et al. Evidence for the use of pimavanserin in the treatment of Parkinson's disease psychosis. *Ther Adv Neurol Disord* 2016; 9:462–473.
48. Wilby KJ, et al. Evidence-based review of pharmacotherapy used for Parkinson's disease psychosis. *Ann Pharmacother* 2017; 51:682–695.
49. Iketani R, et al. Efficacy and safety of atypical antipsychotics for psychosis in Parkinson's disease: A systematic review and Bayesian network meta-analysis. *Parkinsonism Relat Disord* 2020; 78:82–90.
50. Iketani R, et al. Comparative utility of atypical antipsychotics for the treatment of psychosis in Parkinson's disease: a systematic review and bayesian network meta-analysis. *Biol Pharm Bull* 2017; 40:1976–1982.
51. Richard IH, et al. Rivastigmine-induced worsening of motor function and mood in a patient with Parkinson's disease. *Mov Disord* 2001; 16 Suppl 1:33–34.
52. McKeith I, et al. Efficacy of rivastigmine in dementia with Lewy bodies: a randomised, double-blind, placebo-controlled international study. *Lancet* 2000; 356:2031–2036.
53. Emre M, et al. Rivastigmine for dementia associated with Parkinson's disease. *N Engl J Med* 2004; 351:2509–2518.
54. Aarsland D, et al. Donepezil for cognitive impairment in Parkinson's disease: a randomised controlled study. *J Neurol Neurosurg Psychiatry* 2002; 72:708–712.
55. Pagano G, et al. Cholinesterase inhibitors for Parkinson's disease: a systematic review and meta-analysis. *J Neurol Neurosurg Psychiatry* 2015; 86:767–773.
56. Rolinski M, et al. Cholinesterase inhibitors for dementia with Lewy bodies, Parkinson's disease dementia and cognitive impairment in Parkinson's disease. *Cochrane Database Syst Rev* 2012; 3:CD006504.
57. Dubois B, et al. Donepezil in Parkinson's disease dementia: a randomized, double-blind efficacy and safety study. *Mov Disord* 2012; 27:1230–1238.
58. Connolly BS, et al. Pharmacological treatment of Parkinson disease: a review. *JAMA* 2014; 311:1670–1683.
59. Emre M, et al. Memantine for patients with Parkinson's disease dementia or dementia with Lewy bodies: a randomised, double-blind, placebo-controlled trial. *Lancet Neurol* 2010; 9:969–977.
60. Seppi K, et al. The movement disorder society evidence-based medicine review update: treatments for the non-motor symptoms of Parkinson's disease. *Mov Disord* 2011; 26 Suppl 3:S42–S80.
61. Lertxundi U, et al. Anticholinergic burden in Parkinson's disease inpatients. *Eur J Clin Pharmacol* 2015; 71:1271–1277.
62. Zesiewicz TA, et al. Potential influences of complementary therapy on motor and non-motor complications in Parkinson's disease. *CNS Drugs* 2009; 23:817–835.
63. Postuma RB, et al. Caffeine for treatment of Parkinson disease: a randomized controlled trial. *Neurology* 2012; 79:651–658.

扩展阅读

Assogna F, et al. Drug choices and advancements for managing depression in Parkinson's disease. *Curr Neuropharmacol* 2020; 18:277–287.

心房颤动

心房颤动（AF）是最常见的心律失常。主要发生于老年人，但也可能在相当一部分不到 40 岁的人群中发生。危险因素包括焦虑、肥胖、糖尿病、高血压、长时间的有氧运动和大量饮酒 [1-3]。心房颤动本身往往不致命，但是在心房颤动期间心房血液淤滞，易于诱发血栓形成，从而明显增加卒中的风险 [4]。因此，华法林以及新型口服抗凝药物的使用是非常必要的 [3]。

心房颤动可以被分为"孤立的"或阵发性的（非频繁发作，自发转为窦性心律）、持续性的（反复且长时间的发作 >1 周，若为暂时性的，治疗有效）以及永久性的（治疗无效）。以上三种情况下，卒中风险均会增加 [3]。

治疗可包括直流电复律、心律控制（一般用氟卡尼、普罗帕酮或胺碘酮）或心率控制（用地尔硫䓬、维拉帕米或索他洛尔）。心律控制的目标是维持窦性心律，但是并非每次都能做到。心率控制时，心房颤动还可以继续，但是可以控制心室反应使其被动充盈。许多阵发性或持续性发作的心房颤动患者，可以通过导管或冷冻消融术除去异常的电通路，从而得到有效治疗 [5;6]。这是常规而有效的治疗方法 [7]。

在精神科患者中，心房颤动很常见，其原因不仅仅是肥胖、糖尿病和酒精滥用的发生率较高。当考虑抗精神病药治疗时，有些因素需要注意。

- 精神药物与抗凝治疗的相互作用（见第 2 章）。
- 可致心律失常的精神药物：心房颤动往往继发于心血管疾病。影响心脏离子通道的药物可能会增加这些患者的死亡率，尤其有缺血性疾病的患者 [8,9]。
- 对心室率的影响：一些药物引起直立性低血压从而诱发反射性心动过速，还有其他一些药物（氯氮平、喹硫平）会直接增加心率。
- 已有个别精神药物与心房颤动相关的报告（见后面表格）。
- 与抗心律失常药或控制心率药物发生相互作用的风险。
- 心房颤动是阵发性的（目标是避免诱发心房颤动）、持续性的（目标是避免长期心房颤动）还是永久性的（目标是避免增加心室率）。

心房颤动患者使用精神药物的建议

疾病	推荐用药	避免用药
精神分裂症/分裂情感障碍 上述疾病本身就可能增加心房颤动风险[10] 一项 RCT 提示使心房颤动风险增加 17%[11]	对于阵发性或持续性心房颤动,**卡利拉嗪、依匹哌唑**或**鲁拉西酮**可能比较适合 对于接受心率控制的永久性心房颤动,药物选择相对容易一些,但是最好避免使用对 ECG 影响较大的药物(齐拉西酮、匹莫齐特、舍吲哚等)以及会增加心率的药物	使用氯氮平[12,13]、奥氮平[14,15]、阿立哌唑[16,17] 和帕利哌酮[18] 有心房颤动的报告。因果关系未定,但在阵发性或持续性心房颤动中应避免应用 在缺血性心脏病患者中,避免使用延长 Q-T 间期的药物(详见 Q-T 间期延长部分) 抗精神病药与心房颤动的联系[11] 可能与代谢紊乱有关[19],但一些研究提示二者无关[20]
双相情感障碍	**丙戊酸盐** **锂盐** **卡马西平**	心境稳定剂似乎不影响心房颤动的风险 丙戊酸盐可导致房室传导阻滞[21] 锂盐过量[22] 及慢性中毒后各有一例心房颤动[23]
抑郁症 未经治疗的抑郁预示心房颤动可能会复发[24] 心房颤动会增加抑郁和焦虑的风险[25]	**SSRI** 类药物,但需注意与华法林以及其他抗凝剂的相互作用[26],因为增加严重出血的风险[27] 动物实验发现 SSRI 类药物有抗心律失常作用[28,29] **帕罗西汀**:在无抑郁的系列病例中,改善发作性心房颤动[30] **文拉法辛**:不直接影响心房传导[31],可使阵发性心房颤动转律[32] 开始抗抑郁药治疗后,心房颤动发生率下降[33,34] 没有证据表明阿戈美拉汀影响心脏传导或凝血	冠心病患者避免使用三环类药物[35] 三环类药物也可能诱发心房颤动[36,37],但和华法林合用时并不增加出血风险[26] 数据库研究提示,抗抑郁剂一般不增加心房颤动风险[38]
焦虑障碍 (焦虑症状增加心房颤动风险)[39]	**苯二氮䓬类药物** **SSRI** 类药物(见上)	三环类药物(见上) 曾有一例与普瑞巴林相关的心房颤动[40]
阿尔茨海默病	**乙酰胆碱酯酶抑制剂**:在阵发性"迷走性"心房颤动(心率过慢诱发的心房颤动)患者中使用时需注意其降低心率的作用 **卡巴拉汀**发生药物相互作用的风险最低 **美金刚**	在阵发性"迷走性"心房颤动患者中避免使用胆碱酯酶抑制剂

参考文献

1. Chen LY, et al. Epidemiology of atrial fibrillation: a current perspective. *Heart Rhythm* 2007; 4:S1-S6.
2. Tully PJ, et al. Anxiety, depression, and stress as risk factors for atrial fibrillation after cardiac surgery. *Heart Lung* 2011; 40:4–11.
3. National Institute for Health and Care Excellence. Atrial fibrillation: the management of atrial fibrillation. Clinical Guidance 180 2014;

http://www.nice.org.uk/guidance/cg180

4. Lakshminarayan K, et al. Clinical epidemiology of atrial fibrillation and related cerebrovascular events in the United States. *Neurologist* 2008; 14:143–150.

5. Rodgers M, et al. Curative catheter ablation in atrial fibrillation and typical atrial flutter: systematic review and economic evaluation. *Health Technol Assess* 2008; 12:iii-198.

6. Latchamsetty R, et al. Catheter ablation of atrial fibrillation. *Cardiol Clin* 2014; 32:551–561.

7. Saglietto A, et al. Impact of atrial fibrillation catheter ablation on mortality, stroke, and heart failure hospitalizations: A meta-analysis. *J Cardiovasc Electrophysiol* 2020; 31:1040–1047.

8. Investigators TCASTI. Effect of the antiarrhythmic agent moricizine on survival after myocardial infarction. *N Engl J Med* 1992; 327:227–233.

9. Epstein AE, et al. Mortality following ventricular arrhythmia suppression by encainide, flecainide, and moricizine after myocardial infarction. The original design concept of the Cardiac Arrhythmia Suppression Trial (CAST). *JAMA* 1993; 270:2451–2455.

10. Emul M, et al. P wave and QT changes among inpatients with schizophrenia after parenteral ziprasidone administration. *Pharmacol Res* 2009; 60:369–372.

11. Chou RH, et al. Antipsychotic treatment is associated with risk of atrial fibrillation: a nationwide nested case-control study. *Int J Cardiol* 2017; 227:134–140.

12. Cam B, et al. [Clozapine and olanzapine associated atrial fibrillation: a case report]. *Turk Psikiyatri Dergisi = Turkish J Psychiatry* 2015; 26:221–226.

13. Low RA, Jr., et al. Clozapine induced atrial fibrillation. *J Clin Psychopharmacol* 1998; 18:170.

14. Waters BM, et al. Olanzapine-associated new-onset atrial fibrillation. *J Clin Psychopharmacol* 2008; 28:354–355.

15. Yaylaci S, et al. Atrial fibrillation due to olanzapine overdose. *Clin Toxicol (Phila)* 2011; 49:440.

16. D'Urso G, et al. Aripiprazole-induced atrial fibrillation in a patient with concomitant risk factors. *Exp Clin Psychopharmacol* 2018; 26:509–513.

17. Stefatos A, et al. Atrial fibrillation and injected aripiprazole: a case report. *Innov Clin Neurosci* 2018; 15:43–45.

18. Schneider RA, et al. Apparent seizure and atrial fibrillation associated with paliperidone. *Am J Health Syst Pharm* 2008; 65:2122–2125.

19. Zeng J, et al. Metabolic disorder caused by antipsychotic treatment may facilitate the development of atrial fibrillation. *Int J Cardiol* 2017; 239:14.

20. Polcwiartek C, et al. Electrocardiogram characteristics and their association with psychotropic drugs among patients with schizophrenia. *Schizophr Bull* 2020; 46:354–362.

21. Davutoglu V, et al. Valproic acid as a cause of transient atrio-ventricular conduction block episodes. *J Atr Fibrillation* 2017; 9:1520.

22. Kalcik MDM, et al. Acute atrial fibrillation as an unusual form of cardiotoxicity in chronic lithium overdose. *J Atr Fibrillation* 2014; 6:1009.

23. Acharya S, et al. Lithium-induced cardiotoxicity: a rare clinical entity. *Cureus* 2020; 12:e7286.

24. Lange HW, et al. Depressive symptoms predict recurrence of atrial fibrillation after cardioversion. *J Psychosom Res* 2007; 63:509–513.

25. Patel D, et al. A systematic review of depression and anxiety in patients with atrial fibrillation: the mind-heart link. *Cardiovasc Psychiatry Neurol* 2013; 2013:159850.

26. Quinn GR, et al. Effect of selective serotonin reuptake inhibitors on bleeding risk in patients with atrial fibrillation taking warfarin. *Am J Cardiol* 2014; 114:583–586.

27. Komen JJ, et al. Concomitant anticoagulant and antidepressant therapy in atrial fibrillation patients and risk of stroke and bleeding. *Clin Pharmacol Ther* 2020; 107:287–294.

28. Pousti A, et al. Effect of sertraline on ouabain-induced arrhythmia in isolated guinea-pig atria. *Depress Anxiety* 2009; 26:E106-E110.

29. Pousti A, et al. Effect of citalopram on ouabain-induced arrhythmia in isolated guinea-pig atria. *Hum Psychopharmacol* 2003; 18:121–124.

30. Shirayama T, et al. Usefulness of paroxetine in depressed men with paroxysmal atrial fibrillation. *Am J Cardiol* 2006; 97:1749–1751.

31. Emul M, et al. The influences of depression and venlafaxine use at therapeutic doses on atrial conduction. *J Psychopharmacol* 2009; 23:163–167.

32. Finch SJ, et al. Cardioversion of persistent atrial arrhythmia after treatment with venlafaxine in successful management of major depression and posttraumatic stress disorder. *Psychosomatics* 2006; 47:533–536.

33. Andrade C. Antidepressants and atrial fibrillation: the importance of resourceful statistical approaches to address confounding by indication. *J Clin Psychiatry* 2019; 80:19f12729.

34. Fenger-Grøn M, et al. Depression, antidepressants, and the risk of non-valvular atrial fibrillation: a nationwide Danish matched cohort study. *Eur J Prev Cardiol* 2019; 26:187–195.

35. Taylor D. Antidepressant drugs and cardiovascular pathology: a clinical overview of effectiveness and safety. *Acta Psychiatr Scand* 2008; 118:434–442.

36. Moorehead CN, et al. Imipramine-induced auricular fibrillation. *Am J Psychiatry* 1965; 122:216–217.

37. Rosen BH. Case report of auricular fibrillation following the use of imipramine (Tofranil). *J Mt Sinai Hosp NY* 1960; 27:609–611.

38. Lapi F, et al. The use of antidepressants and the risk of chronic atrial fibrillation. *J Clin Pharmacol* 2015; 55:423–430.

39. Eaker ED, et al. Tension and anxiety and the prediction of the 10-year incidence of coronary heart disease, atrial fibrillation, and total mortality: the Framingham Offspring Study. *Psychosom Med* 2005; 67:692–696.

40. Chilkoti G, et al. Could pregabalin premedication predispose to perioperative atrial fibrillation in patients with sepsis? *Saudi J Anaesth* 2014; 8:S115-116.

减肥手术中精神药物的使用

在做过减肥手术的患者中,精神疾病相对常见[1]。想做减肥手术者中,1/3 以上使用精神药物[2]。减肥手术可能与药物代谢动力学发生具有临床意义的改变相关,但是由于个体差异和资料有限,难以预料精神药物会受到什么影响。现有研究支持需要密切监测治疗,且在减肥手术之后继续监测症状[3]。

手术可分类如下:

- **主要限制型**:袖状胃切除术和胃束带手术。
- **主要吸收不良型**:胆胰分流术和空肠回肠旁路术。
- **二者兼有**:Roux-en-Y 胃旁路术(RYGB)和胃缩小十二指肠转位术(GDRS)

吸收不良型手术(包括 RYGB 和 GDRS)改变药物吸收的可能性相对较大。大多数数据来源于做过 RYGB 患者的研究。不清楚这些数据与其他手术结果之间的关系。

减肥手术后的药代动力学改变

所有手术都可以改变:

- 片剂崩解和溶解时间,途径是胃 pH 和搅拌作用改变
- 吸收速率,途径是胃排空速度改变
- 药物分布,途径是脂肪组织减少(特别是脂溶性药物)和蛋白结合率改变
- 药物代谢,途径是体重减轻后肝功能改善
- 药物排泄,途径是体重减轻后肾功能改变

吸收不良型手术可进一步改变:

- 药物吸收面积减少(功能性肠道变短)
- 亲脂性药物增溶作用改变(绕过近端小肠胆盐)
- 肠壁药物代谢减少,通过肠道缩短。

药物制剂

减肥手术以后,延长崩解和溶解时间的任何药物制剂都可能损害药物吸收[4]。通常建议在术前使用速释制剂[4,5](更多依据专家共识,而不是客观数据[6])。口腔分散剂和液体制剂不经过崩解期,在怀疑片剂吸收减少时可首选[7]。应该避免使用大片(直径超过 10mm),因为限制型手术可阻碍其通过。减肥手术中精神药物的使用,可见表 10.10 至表 10.13,用药的一般建议见框 10.4 中的总结。

药物

抗抑郁药

表 10.10　减肥手术中抗抑郁药的使用

药物	具体证据和注意事项
SSRI[8-13]	■ 证据显示,RYGB 后血浆浓度可明显下降 ■ 在一些病例中,吸收不良被怀疑是撤药症状和失去疗效的原因

续表

药物	具体证据和注意事项
SNRI[10,14]	■ RYGB 后,度洛西汀浓度较对照组低 42% ■ 文拉法辛缓释胶囊的吸收不受 RYGB 影响 [15]
米氮平 [16,17]	■ 可能增加食欲和体重 ■ 成功地用于 RYGB 后非机械性呕吐
三环类药物 [18,19]	■ 单一病例报告提示,RYGB 后,在常规剂量范围可达到治疗浓度 ■ 明显体重减轻后,血浆浓度可升高;考虑监测血药水平和减少剂量

概要

- 在减肥者中,抗抑郁药是研究最充分的精神药物。现有证据提示,手术后抗抑郁药的吸收减少(但是研究大多局限于 SSRI 和 RYGB)
- 吸收减少的迹象可包括迅速出现停药症状,而后失去疗效
- 患者需要密切监测,因为无法可靠地预测吸收减少的风险
- 减肥术后胃出血的风险可因使用 5-羟色胺能药物而增加

抗精神病药

表 10.11 减肥手术中抗精神病药的使用

药物	具体证据和注意事项
阿塞那平 [20]	■ 主要经口腔黏膜吸收;减肥术后预期没有问题 ■ 有一例 RYGB 后用药成功的病例
卡利拉嗪	■ 没有术后吸收的资料,用药参照一般建议
氯氮平 [21-23]	■ 两例报告 RYGB 后病情复发 [24] ■ 术前检测血药浓度,术后定期监测 ■ 术后常见便秘;制药商建议密切监测,积极治疗 ■ 了解吸烟情况(建议术前戒烟),相应调整剂量
氟哌啶醇 [25]	■ 单一病例报告提示,RYGB 后血药浓度与文献中普遍报告的一致
鲁拉西酮	■ 围手术期热量摄入减少/不一致,因而有吸收减少的风险;必须与食物(350kcal)同服以保证吸收 ■ 一例报告 GRDS 后病情复发,生物利用度和血清峰浓度明显下降 [26]。 ■ 一例报告 RYGB 后血浆浓度明显下降,精神病性症状未加重 [27]。 ■ 术前考虑换用其他药物
奥氮平 [28,29]	■ 减肥术后有体重增加的证据 [26] ■ 有关吸收部位的信息不一致,参照一般建议
喹硫平 [7,28]	■ 可经胃和十二脂吸收,监测精神状态 ■ 建议换用速释制剂,剂量大于 300mg 时分次服用
利培酮 [30]	■ 病情稳定的患者,考虑换成等效价的帕利哌酮长效注射剂 ■ 减肥术后口服治疗耐受不了时,成功地用过利培酮长效注射剂

续表

药物	具体证据和注意事项
齐拉西酮[31]	■ 必须与食物(500kcal)同服以保证吸收。围手术期热量摄入减少/不一致,因而有吸收减少的风险。术前考虑换用其他药物

概要

- 在减肥者中,对抗精神病药的研究不充分。信息限于病例报告或理论上的关注。
- 长效抗精神病药术后吸收减少的风险。鉴于术后药代动力学改变的数据有限以及个体间差异,可能不宜建议在术前常规换用长效抗精神病药[7]。但是,对于药物已经稳定且有长效制剂的患者,或者术后出现生物利用度下降迹象的患者,仍然可以选择长效制剂。
- 对于 Q-T 间期延长的患者,减肥手术可导致额外的心脏压力[32],建议术前监测心电图。

心境稳定剂

表 10.12　减肥手术中心境稳定剂的使用

药物	证据概要和注意事项
卡马西平[33]	■ 有粒细胞缺乏的单一病例报告,可能与袖状胃切除术血浆浓度升高有关
拉莫三嗪[28]	■ 可能从胃和近端小肠吸收,监测疗效的丧失
锂盐[30-40] (见下)	■ RYGB 和袖状胃切除术后,有几例锂中毒的病例报告 ■ 换用等效剂量的枸橼酸锂 ■ 术前,血浆浓度可受医嘱中饮食改变影响 ■ 术后,血浆浓度可受下述因素影响:吸收不良(主要经小肠吸收)、液体转移和体重减轻(肥胖者锂清除率增加)
丙戊酸盐[7,34]	■ 单一病例报告提示,吸收不良型手术之后,吸收可能明显减少;没有限制型手术之后的资料 ■ 体重减轻后,可能必须减少剂量(血浆浓度与体重相关) ■ 术前,或者怀疑控释制剂/肠溶包衣片引起吸收不良,换用液体制剂 ■ 建议动态监测基线血浆浓度、全血细胞计数和肝功能 ■ 监测血浆浓度正常时可能发生的耐受性差的临床迹象

概要

- 减肥术后心境稳定剂的文献限于几个病例报告;锂盐使用应该特别小心,因为治疗指数窄。
- 口服避孕药的吸收在减肥手术后可能减少[41]。对于使用致畸性心境稳定剂的患者,建议换用非口服的避孕方法。

减肥手术期间锂盐的使用

在整个围手术期持续使用锂盐者,必须特别密切地进行监测。基于现有病例报告和专家意见提出下述指导意见[40]:

- 监测血浆锂浓度的频率:术前和术后 6 周内每周 1 次(因液体摄入逐渐增多),后面 6 个月内每 2 周 1 次,再往后每月 1 次。减肥术后 1 年恢复平时的血锂监测。
- 若血浆浓度升高>25%,或接近 1.2mmol/L,考虑减少锂盐剂量。

第
10
章

- 若存在中毒迹象,停用锂盐,审核剂量。
- 定期评定精神状态,可能的话使用正规的评定量表。
- 在术前,鼓励患者每天饮用 2.5~4L 液体(包括液体食物替代品)。

其他药物

表 10.13　减肥手术中其他药物的使用

药物	证据概要和注意事项
苯二氮䓬类[42-45]	■ 生物利用度可能不受影响,达峰时间缩短
美沙酮[46]	■ 一个病例报告显示,袖状胃切除术后,生物利用度明显增加,可能与胃排空速度加快有关。建议监测血浆浓度和 Q-T 间期
哌甲酯[47-48]	■ 数据矛盾而少;一个病例报告显示,RYGB 后疗效下降,换用经皮贴剂后疗效恢复,提示口服生物利用度下降。其他报告显示中毒迹象

一般建议

框 10.4　关于减肥手术用药的一般建议

术前	术后 0~6 周	术后 >6 周
■ 不要常规增加剂量,具有临床意义的吸收不良无法可靠地预测 ■ 术前评估精神状态,并考虑检测基线血药浓度 ■ 将缓释剂/肠溶包衣制剂换成速释片或液体制剂	■ 密切监测不良反应和药物吸收不良的迹象(症状重新出现,停药症状) ■ 若有临床指征,定期监测血药浓度 ■ 若怀疑吸收不良,考虑所建议的策略 ■ 若怀疑药物中毒,停药并审核剂量	■ 术后第一年继续定期监测,但是若病情稳定,监测频率可以减少 ■ 监测不良反应的增多,特别是术后急性期增加剂量时 ■ 术后 1 年,可考虑恢复术前治疗方案(依临床病史而定)

出现生物利用度下降迹象的一般对策

- 可能的话,考虑非口服用药(如服用抗精神病药病情稳定的患者换用长效制剂)
- 分次用药,可改善术后胃容量缩小相关的吸收不良
- 从改良/缓释/缓释(modified/prolonged/delayed)制剂换成速释制剂
- 从片剂换成液体或口腔分散剂,绕过崩解阶段
- 从大片换成小片
- 若因为生物利用度下降而增加了剂量,则需要监测急性不良反应,因为过一段时间生物利用度可能恢复正常

减肥术后有增加体重风险的精神药物

据估计,减肥术后,10%~20% 的患者再次明显增加体重[49]。虽然没有资料说明与体重增加相关的精神药物如何影响术后结果,但是也许应该避免使用高风险药物。应该考虑患者自己临床状况(特别是治疗时病情是否稳定,复发风险是否很高),因为有证据表明,未控

制好的精神疾病是体重增加的危险因素之一[49]。

酒精[50,51]

胃旁路手术会加快酒精吸收,升高酒精浓度,延长消除时间。胃旁路手术后,酒滥用的风险也升高了。袖状胃切除术的数据不太清楚,也没有证据表明胃束带手术会导致什么变化。

更广泛的考虑[52]

在实践中,许多患者在术后可能不必对药物治疗做出明显的改变。症状复发可能与药代动力学改变无关。预期心理健康状况会改善,病情恶化也可能发生,其原因涉及许多因素,包括未达到减轻体重的期望、耐受性差及手术后对效果不满意。

参考文献

1. Dawes AJ, et al. Mental health conditions among patients seeking and undergoing bariatric surgery: a meta-analysis. *JAMA* 2016; **315**:150–163.
2. Hawkins M, et al. Psychiatric medication use and weight outcomes one year after bariatric surgery. *Psychosomatics* 2020; **61**:56–63.
3. Gondek W. Psychiatric suitability assessment for bariatric surgery. In S Sockalingam, R Hawa, eds. *Psychiatric care in severe obesity: an interdisciplinary guide to integrated care.* Cham: Springer International Publishing 2017:173–186.
4. Padwal R, et al. A systematic review of drug absorption following bariatric surgery and its theoretical implications. *Obesity Rev Official J Int Assoc Study Obesity* 2010; **11**:41–50.
5. Macgregor AM, et al. Drug distribution in obesity and following bariatric surgery: a literature review. *Obes Surg* 1996; **6**:17–27.
6. Roerig JL, et al. Psychopharmacology and bariatric surgery. *Eur Eating Disord Rev* 2015; **23**:463–469.
7. Bingham KS, et al. Psychopharmacology in bariatric surgery patients. in S Sockalingam, R Hawa, eds. *Psychiatric care in severe obesity: an interdisciplinary guide to integrated care.* Cham: Springer International Publishing 2017:313–333.
8. Faye E, et al. Antidepressant agents in short bowel syndrome. *Clin Ther* 2014; **36**:2029–2033.e2023.
9. Marzinke MA, et al. Decreased escitalopram concentrations post-Roux-en-Y gastric bypass surgery. *Ther Drug Monit* 2015; **37**:408–412.
10. Hamad GG, et al. The effect of gastric bypass on the pharmacokinetics of serotonin reuptake inhibitors. *Am J Psychiatry* 2012; **169**:256–263.
11. Seaman JS, et al. Dissolution of common psychiatric medications in a Roux-en-Y gastric bypass model. *Psychosomatics* 2005; **46**:250–253.
12. Bingham K, et al. SSRI discontinuation syndrome following bariatric surgery: a case report and focused literature review. *Psychosomatics* 2014; **55**:692–697.
13. Roerig JL, et al. Preliminary comparison of sertraline levels in postbariatric surgery patients versus matched nonsurgical cohort. *Surg Obesity Relat Dis Official J Am Soc Bariatric Surgery* 2012; **8**:62–66.
14. Roerig JL, et al. A comparison of duloxetine plasma levels in postbariatric surgery patients versus matched nonsurgical control subjects. *J Clin Psychopharmacol* 2013; **33**:479–484.
15. Krieger CA, et al. Comparison of bioavailability of single-dose extended-release venlafaxine capsules in obese patients before and after gastric bypass surgery. *Pharmacotherapy* 2017; **37**:1374–1382.
16. Teixeira FV, et al. Mirtazapine (Remeron) as treatment for non-mechanical vomiting after gastric bypass. *Obes Surg* 2005; **15**:707–709.
17. Huerta S, et al. Intractable nausea and vomiting following Roux-en-Y gastric bypass: role of mirtazapine. *Obes Surg* 2006; **16**:1399.
18. Broyles JE, et al. Nortriptyline absorption in short bowel syndrome. *JPEN J Parenter Enteral Nutr* 1990; **14**:326–327.
19. Jobson K, et al. Weight loss and a concomitant change in plasma tricyclic levels. *Am J Psychiatry* 1978; **135**:237–238.
20. Tabaac BJ, et al. Pica patient, status post gastric bypass, improves with change in medication regimen. *Ther Adv Psychopharmacol* 2015; **5**:38–42.
21. Kaltsounis J, et al. Intravenous valproate treatment of severe manic symptoms after gastric bypass surgery: a case report. *Psychosomatics* 2000; **41**:454–456.
22. Afshar S, et al. The effects of bariatric procedures on bowel habit. *Obes Surg* 2016; **26**:2348–2354.
23. Mylan Products Ltd. Summary of product characteristics. Clozaril 25mg and 100mg Tablets. 2020; https://www.medicines.org.uk/emc/medicine/32564 .
24. Mahgoub Y, et al. Schizoaffective exacerbation in a Roux-en-Y gastric bypass patient maintained on clozapine. *Prim Care Companion CNS Disord* 2019; **21**:19l02462.
25. Fuller AK, et al. Haloperidol pharmacokinetics following gastric bypass surgery. *J Clin Psychopharmacol* 1986; **6**:376–378.
26. Ward HB, et al. Lurasidone malabsorption following bariatric surgery: a case report. *J Psychiatr Pract* 2019; **25**:313–317.
27. McGrane IR, et al. Roux-en-Y gastric bypass and antipsychotic therapeutic drug monitoring: two cases. *J Pharm Pract* 2020:[Epub ahead of print].

第10章

28. Miller AD, et al. Medication and nutrient administration considerations after bariatric surgery. *Am J Health-Syst Pharm AJHP Official J Am Soc Health-Syst Pharm* 2006; 63:1852–1857.

29. Tran PV, et al. *Olanzapine (Zyprexa): a novel antipsychotic*. Philadelphia: Lippincott Williams & Wilkins 2001.

30. Brietzke E, et al. Long-acting injectable risperidone in a bipolar patient submitted to bariatric surgery and intolerant to conventional mood stabilizers. *Psychiatry Clin Neurosci* 2011; 65:205–205.

31. Gandelman K, et al. The impact of calories and fat content of meals on oral ziprasidone absorption: a randomized, open-label, crossover trial. *J Clin Psychiatry* 2009; 70:58–62.

32. Woodard G, et al. Cardiac arrest during laparoscopic Roux-en-Y gastric bypass in a bariatric patient with drug-associated long QT syndrome. *Obes Surg* 2011; 21:134–137.

33. Koutsavlis I, et al. Dose-dependent carbamazepine-induced agranulocytosis following bariatric surgery (sleeve gastrectomy): a possible mechanism. *Bariatric Surg Pract Patient Care* 2015; 10:130–134.

34. Dahan A, et al. Lithium toxicity with severe bradycardia post sleeve gastrectomy: a case report and review of the literature. *Obes Surg* 2019; 29:735–738.

35. Lin YH, et al. Lithium toxicity with prolonged neurologic sequelae following sleeve gastrectomy: a case report and review of literature. *Medicine (Baltimore)* 2020; 99:e21122.

36. Tripp AC. Lithium toxicity after Roux-en-Y gastric bypass surgery. *J Clin Psychopharmacol* 2011; 31:261–262.

37. Musfeldt D, et al. Lithium toxicity after Roux-en-Y bariatric surgery. *BMJ Case Rep* 2016; 2016:bcr2015214056.

38. Walsh K, et al. Lithium toxicity following Roux-en-Y gastric bypass. *Bariatric Surg Pract Patient Care* 2014; 9:77–80.

39. Alam A, et al. Lithium toxicity following vertical sleeve gastrectomy: a case report. *Clin Psychopharmacol Neurosci* 2016; 14:318–320.

40. Bingham KS, et al. Perioperative lithium use in bariatric surgery: a case series and literature review. *Psychosomatics* 2016; 57:638–644.

41. Merhi ZO. Challenging oral contraception after weight loss by bariatric surgery. *Gynecol Obstet Invest* 2007; 64:100–102.

42. Tandra S, et al. Pharmacokinetic and pharmacodynamic alterations in the Roux-en-Y gastric bypass recipients. *Ann Surg* 2013; 258:262–269.

43. Chan LN, et al. Proximal Roux-en-Y gastric bypass alters drug absorption pattern but not systemic exposure of CYP3A4 and P-glycoprotein substrates. *Pharmacotherapy* 2015; 35:361–369.

44. Brill MJ, et al. The Pharmacokinetics of the CYP3A substrate midazolam in morbidly obese patients before and one year after bariatric surgery. *Pharm Res* 2015; 32:3927–3936.

45. Ochs HR, et al. Diazepam absorption: effects of age, sex, and Billroth gastrectomy. *Dig Dis Sci* 1982; 27:225–230.

46. Strømmen M, et al. Bioavailability of methadone after sleeve gastrectomy: a planned case observation. *Clin Ther* 2016; 38:1532–1536.

47. Azran C, et al. Impaired oral absorption of methylphenidate after Roux-en-Y gastric bypass. *Surg Obes Relat Dis* 2017; 13:1245–1247.

48. Ludvigsson M, et al. Methylphenidate toxicity after Roux-en-Y gastric bypass. *Surg Obesity Relat Dis* 2016; 12:e55-e57.

49. Karmali S, et al. Weight recidivism post-bariatric surgery: a systematic review. *Obes Surg* 2013; 23:1922–1933.

50. Ivezaj V, et al. Changes in alcohol use after metabolic and bariatric surgery: predictors and mechanisms. *Curr Psychiatry Rep* 2019; 21:85.

51. Parikh M, et al. ASMBS position statement on alcohol use before and after bariatric surgery. *Surg Obesity Relat Dis* 2016; 12:225–230.

52. Stevens T, et al. Your patient and weight-loss surgery. *Adv Psychiatric Treatment* 2012; 18:418–425.

生命晚期精神疾病患者的用药

一般而言,给进入生命晚期的精神疾病患者用药时,应该遵循缓和疗护的处方管理规范[1]。它包括评估药物及其剂量是否合适,以及停药的可能性。另外,若吞咽功能受损,它包括做出调整,如使用液体制剂或胃肠外用药。

关于这种背景下长期使用精神药物的问题,缺乏具体的指南来支持医师。这使得人们,特别是全科医师,更不愿意调整或停用这类药物[2,3]。这提示非精神科与精神科机构之间存在增进联络的空间。

体质下降可影响一些因素(如吸烟减少、喝的液体减少),反过来影响药物代谢动力学或药效动力学,因此必须不断地进行评估。另外,使用多种药物很常见,增加了药物相互作用和中毒的风险。例如,曲马多与 SSRI 合用导致 5-羟色胺中毒。

在生命晚期,抑郁症很常见[4],但是往往得不到识别[5]。这很重要,因为抗抑郁药可能是有益的,即使预期生存时间很短[6]。米氮平和西酞普兰是支持证据最强的适用于该人群的药物[7]。莫达非尼等精神兴奋药可短期减轻抑郁症状,但是其长期疗效证据较少[8]。

关于生命晚期的焦虑,缺少证据来指导药物治疗[9,10]。非药物方法的效果有较强的证据基础[11]。

抗精神病药常用于治疗谵妄,但是其疗效证据不一。然而,国家多个指南支持使用它治疗非常痛苦的患者,或者其他方法不成功的患者[12]。用于精神科也用于缓和疗护症状治疗的药物示例见表 10.14。

表 10.14 用于精神科也用于缓和疗护症状治疗的药物示例

症状	药物示例
神经痛	阿米替林
	丙米嗪
	度洛西汀
	加巴喷丁/普瑞巴林
	氯硝西泮
恶心、呕吐	氟哌啶醇
	奥氮平
	劳拉西泮
厌食	米氮平
骨骼肌痉挛	地西泮
临终躁动	苯二氮䓬类药物,如咪达唑仑
	抗精神病药,如氟哌啶醇
膀胱过度活动症状	阿米替林
	度洛西汀
流涎	阿米替林
顽固性呃逆	氟哌啶醇

续表

症状	药物示例
病理性哭笑	西酞普兰
	舍曲林
出汗	阿米替林

（孔庆梅 译　田成华 审校）

参考文献

1. Wilcock A, et al. *PCF7 Palliative Care Formulary*. 7th Edition. Nottingham Palliativedrugs.com Ltd; 2020.

2. Anderson K, et al. Prescriber barriers and enablers to minimising potentially inappropriate medications in adults: a systematic review and thematic synthesis. *BMJ Open* 2014; 4:e006544.

3. Garfinkel D, et al. Inappropriate medication use and polypharmacy in end-stage cancer patients: isn't it the family doctor's role to de-prescribe much earlier? *Int J Clin Pract* 2018; 72:e13061.

4. Rayner L, et al. The clinical epidemiology of depression in palliative care and the predictive value of somatic symptoms: cross-sectional survey with four-week follow-up. *Palliat Med* 2011; 25:229–241.

5. Stiefel F, et al. Depression in palliative care: a pragmatic report from the Expert Working Group of the European Association for Palliative Care. *Support Care Cancer* 2001; 9:477–488.

6. Rayner L, et al. Antidepressants for the treatment of depression in palliative care: systematic review and meta-analysis. *Palliat Med* 2011; 25:36–51.

7. Rayner L, et al. Expert opinion on detecting and treating depression in palliative care: A Delphi study. *BMC Palliat Care* 2011; 10:10.

8. Candy M, et al. Psychostimulants for depression. *Cochrane Database Syst Rev* 2008:Cd006722.

9. Salt S, et al. Drug therapy for symptoms associated with anxiety in adult palliative care patients. *Cochrane Database Syst Rev* 2017; 5:Cd004596.

10. Atkin N, et al. 'Worried to death': the assessment and management of anxiety in patients with advanced life-limiting disease, a national survey of palliative medicine physicians. *BMC Palliat Care* 2017; 16:69.

11. Moorey S, et al. A cluster randomized controlled trial of cognitive behaviour therapy for common mental disorders in patients with advanced cancer. *Psychol Med* 2009; 39:713–723.

12. National Institute for Clinical Excellence. NG31: care of dying adults in the last days of life. 2015; https://www.nice.org.uk/guidance/NG31.

第 4 部分

精神药物使用的其他方面

药代动力学

精神药物血浆水平监测

血浆药物浓度监测,或血浆药物水平监测,是一个存在困惑和误解的过程。药物浓度监测若使用恰当,对于优化治疗和确保治疗依从性都有很大的帮助。但是,与医学其他领域一样,在精神科,药物血浆水平监测往往没有恰当的理由就实施,对测定结果也未妥善应用[1]。在其他情况下,血浆水平监测又应用不足。

在进行血药浓度检测之前,应当确保已满足如下标准:

■ **已有适合临床应用的检测方法吗?**

仅少数药物有现成的检测方法。测定方法必须在临床上得到验证,并在有临床意义的时间窗内获得检测结果。需要和当地的实验室确认。

■ **药物已达到稳态吗?**

通常只有在达到稳态浓度后采取标本,血浆药物水平才有意义。这需要4~5个半衰期。疑似过量服药者属于例外,因为此时达到稳态没有意义。另一个例外是利用药物浓度来指导药物剂量滴定(如,接受氯氮平治疗)。

■ **取血时间正确吗?**

对于很多药物(并非所有),取血时间非常重要。假定推荐的取血时间是服药后12h,那么应当尽可能地在服药后11~13h取血。在十分必要的情况下,也可以在服药后10~14h内取血。一项关于氯氮平的研究中,计划的取血时间是服药后12h,在该时间前、后1h和2h取血,结果显示,氯氮平血浆浓度的平均变异度低于10%,但是有些个体的血浆浓度变化超过50%[2]。若未在规定时间的1~2h内取血,则结果有可能造成误导,无法提供所需信息。因此,取血时间要尽量靠近既定的时间。很显然,若怀疑患者中毒,应该即刻取血,忽略任何既定时间。

如果是测定谷浓度或者"服药前浓度",则需要在即将服用下次药物前取血。任何情况下,在取血之前,绝对不要把下次服药时间推迟超过1~2h;否则,必然得出有误导性的结果(结果低于平时规律用药时),从而导致不适当的剂量增加。半衰期长的药物(如奥氮平、阿立哌唑)取血时间不那么严格,但是,作为绝对的最低限度,医师应该记录取血时间和末次给药时间。这一点需要着重强调。

■ **血药浓度有什么内在含义?**

药物的血浆水平存在有效范围吗?若有,那么(在适当的时间取血)测定的血浆水平可用于指导用药。若药物血浆水平没有公认的有效范围,那么血浆水平仅能提示药物依从性,或者药物中毒的可能性。若将血样用于判断患者的依从性,请记住,血浆水平为"0"只能说明患者在过去几天未服药。血浆药物浓度大于"0",可能提示患者的依从性不稳定、完全依从或者最近用药掩盖了长期的不依从。注意,目标浓度范围也有局限性:患者可能在低于所参考目标浓度范围时出现疗效,耐受高于目标浓度范围的药物。另外,不同实验室采用的目标浓度范围有很大的不同,往往没有解释。

- **血药浓度测定有明确的理由吗?**

  只有下述理由有效:

  - 确定依从性(见上文)
  - 疑似中毒
  - 疑似药物药代动力学相互作用
  - 难以直接判断临床疗效(且已确定了目标血药浓度范围)
  - 药物治疗指数较窄,非常担心药物中毒

样本结果的解释

解释血药浓度的基本原则是,只有结合可靠的临床观察,才可以根据检测结果采取措施("治疗的是患者,而不是血药水平")。例如,若患者对药物治疗有足够疗效,但血药浓度低于公认的目标浓度范围,则通常不应增加剂量。若患者出现不能耐受的不良反应,但血药浓度在有效范围内,则可能需要减少剂量。

如果血药水平与以前的结果明显不同,建议重新取血检测。核对药物剂量、服药时间和最近的治疗依从性,特别是确保取血时间准确,或者至少要掌握取血时间。很多反常的结果是改变取血时间造成的。

目标浓度范围的描述

在精神科,应该谨慎对待精神药物的目标浓度范围。很难根据疗效来确定目标浓度范围,因为存在治疗无效的患者(在任何血药浓度下均无效)、安慰剂治疗有效者或自然痊愈者(在任何血药浓度下均有效)。根据不良反应来确定目标浓度范围也会遇到困难,因为随治疗时间延长患者逐渐对药物耐受。因此,确定药物目标浓度范围的研究大多数"噪声"和"信号"一样多,最后导致目标浓度范围代表的是粗略的近似值。

有趣的是,在临床实践中与疗效相关的药物浓度,和已发表的药物目标浓度范围之间,相关性很强[3]。通常,药物浓度范围的下四分位数(25% 位数)和目标浓度范围的下限接近,而上四分位数(75% 位数)接近但常常是低于上限。广义上来讲,这意味着大约 25% 的患者在低于目标浓度时即有效;而 25% 的患者能耐受高于目标范围的浓度(表 11.1)。

氨磺必利

氨磺必利的血浆水平与药物剂量密切相关,变异不大,不值得进行常规血浆水平监测。女性[25-27]的血浆水平较高,似乎对疗效或不良反应均没有明显的临床意义。推荐的临床有效的(谷浓度)阈值约为 $100\mu g/L$[28],一些研究发现,治疗有效患者的平均血浆水平为 $367\mu g/L$[27]。当平均血浆水平为 $336\mu g/L$[25]、$377\mu g/L$[28] 和 $395\mu g/L$[26] 时,可观察到不良反应

表 11.1 药物已确定浓度范围时样本结果的解释

药物	目标浓度范围	取血时间	达稳态时间	说明
氨磺必利	200~320μg/L 20~600μg/L(老年人)	谷浓度	3 天	见正文
阿立哌唑	150~210μg/L	谷浓度	15~16 天	见正文
卡马西平[4-6]	>7mg/L 双相障碍	谷浓度	2 周	卡马西平可能诱导自身代谢,达稳态时间取决于自身诱导
氯氮平	350~600μg/L	谷浓度	2~3 天	见正文
拉莫三嗪[7-9]	未确定,建议 2.5~15mg/L	谷浓度	5 天 有人认为会发生自身诱导,所以达稳态时间可能更长	对拉莫三嗪血浆水平的应用存有争议,尤其治疗双相障碍时。治疗难治性抑郁症时,血浆水平高于 12.7μmol/L(3.3mg/L)时有效[10,11]。高于 15mg/L 时毒性可能增加,但通常耐受良好
锂盐[12-16]	0.6~1.0mmol/L 治疗一些患者/适应证 0.4mmol/L 即可,治疗躁狂需 >1.0mmol/L	给药后 12h	给药后 5h	已经确定目标浓度范围,但依据早年的数据。最近一项研究[17]提示 0.6mmol/L 是有效预防的最低浓度
奥氮平	20~40μg/L	12h	1 周	见正文
帕利哌酮[18]	20~60μg/L (9-羟利培酮)	谷浓度	口服 2~3 天 长效注射剂 2 个月	目标范围同利培酮[19]。与利培酮相似,不建议进行常规血浆水平监测
苯妥英[5]	10~20mg/L	谷浓度	可变	0 级药代动力学。某些情况下游离药物浓度可能有用
喹硫平	50~100μg/L?	谷浓度?	口服 2~3 天	未确定目标浓度范围。不建议监测血浆水平。见正文
利培酮	20~60μg/L (活性成分:利培酮+9-羟利培酮)	谷浓度	口服 2~3 天 注射剂 6~8 周	不建议常规监测血浆水平。见正文
三环类药[20]	去甲替林 50~150μg/L 阿米替林 100~200μg/L	谷浓度	2~3 天	极少应用,益处可疑,用心电图评估其毒性
丙戊酸盐[4,5,21-23]	50~100mg/L 癫痫和双相	谷浓度	2~3 天	在癫痫和双相障碍中,血浆水平的价值可疑。一些证据显示,躁狂患者可以耐受高达 125mg/L 的血浆水平,且比低浓度时有效。丙戊酸盐血浆水平与血氨呈线性相关[24]

（主要是锥体外系不良反应）。血浆水平低于 320μg/L 阈值时，预测可以避免发生锥体外系不良反应[28]。一项文献综述提出[29]，临床疗效最佳且不产生不良反应时，大致的血浆水平为 200~320μg/L。但是更近的一个共识声明[30] 中提出目标浓度范围是 100~320μg/L。每天一次服用 200mg 足以达到血浆浓度 100μg/L[31]，因此这个阈值下限可能太低，无法产生可靠的疗效。研究提示，老年精神病患者血浆浓度在 20~60μg/L 时，可达到最佳的 D_2 受体占有率和临床疗效[32,33]。

在临床实践中，只有少数患者达到"治疗"血浆水平（可能由于依从性差[34]），因此血浆水平监测可能有一定益处。但是，氨磺必利血浆水平监测做得很少，几乎没有实验室进行氨磺必利检测。其剂量-效应关系很明确（至少在临床试验中如此），在注册的治疗剂量范围内（老年人 50~100mg/d 的剂量水平即可），不需要进行血药浓度监测，不良反应单纯通过剂量调整就可以处理。血浆药物浓度监测最好限于下述情况：临床疗效差、依从性可疑、存在药物相互作用或者躯体疾病可能导致易出现不良反应的患者。

阿立哌唑

临床实践中，有时会监测阿立哌唑的血浆水平。阿立哌唑的剂量-效应关系已经明确，在剂量大于 10mg/d 时[35]，临床疗效和 D_2 受体占有率达到平台期。阿立哌唑、其代谢产物和全部活性成分（母药＋代谢产物）的血浆水平与剂量呈强线性关系。因此，可以较为肯定地预测某一剂量水平时的大致血浆药物浓度[36]。达到最佳临床疗效的目标血浆浓度范围为 146~254μg/L[37] 和 150~300μg/L[38]，出现不良反应的血浆浓度为 210μg/L 以上[38]。阿立哌唑血浆水平存在个体差异，但是未进行系统研究，性别几乎没有影响[39,40]。年龄、代谢酶基因型和相互作用的药物，可能会引起血药水平的差异[38-41]。对于接受阿立哌唑治疗的患者，一般推荐的血浆水平范围为 150~210μg/L[36]，这大体上是接受阿立哌唑长效剂每月 300~400mg 治疗的患者中观察到的浓度[42]。有些管理部门推荐临床有效的浓度范围下限为 100μg/L[30]，这相当于每天口服 10mg 剂量的血浆水平[31,43]。

氯氮平

氯氮平的血浆水平与每天剂量大体相关[44]，但是个体间差异很大，不可能精确地预测血浆药物水平。血浆水平通常在年轻患者、男性[45] 和吸烟者[46] 中较低，在亚洲人中较高[47]。在东亚[48,49]、印度[50] 和巴基斯坦[51] 人群中，所需氯氮平的治疗剂量低得多。氯氮平慢代谢者的比例在东亚人群中明显地高于其他人群[52,53]。已有一系列程序根据患者的特点大致预测氯氮平的血浆水平，强烈建议大家使用这些程序[54]。但是，这些程序不能解释其他因素（如依从性改变、炎症[55] 和感染[56,57] 等）对氯氮平血浆水平的影响。

推荐氯氮平急性期治疗的血浆水平下限为 200μg/L[58]、350μg/L[59-61]、370μg/L[62]、420μg/L[63]、504μg/L[64] 和 550μg/L[65]。有限的数据提示，预防复发至少需要血浆水平达 200μg/L[66]。氯氮平血浆水平的巨大变化也可预测疾病复发[67]。个体氯氮平血浆浓度的改变非常普遍，可能会随着治疗时间的延长而降低[68]，但是有一项研究提示仅有去甲氯氮平的浓度降低[69]。

虽然对氯氮平有效浓度下限有些分歧，血浆水平监测还是有助于优化治疗。氯氮平治疗无效时，应当调整剂量，使血浆水平达 350~500μg/L 水平（这个范围反映了对上述研究的共识[30]）。无法耐受氯氮平不良反应时，则需要减少剂量，使血浆水平落入该范围。氯氮平目标浓度的上限目前尚未确定。确定上限必须考虑两个因素：高于该水平不会获得治疗优势，且药物毒性或耐受性无法接受。氯氮平血浆水平可以预测脑电图改变[70,71]；当血浆水平高于 1 000μg/L 时[72]，癫痫发作更频繁，因此血浆水平可能需要保持低于这个水平。可以想象得到，氯氮平导致的其他非神经系统不良反应也与其血浆水平相关[73]。有人提出了氯氮平的治疗浓度上限为 600~800μg/L[74]。

另外，设置氯氮平目标浓度范围的上限，还可能阻碍在注册剂量范围内增加剂量，而这种剂量的增加可能有潜在价值。在广泛监测血浆水平之前，氯氮平的剂量往往高达 900mg/d，剂量达 600mg/d 水平时加用丙戊酸盐。目前还不清楚，当血浆浓度已经高于公认的上限时，使用这么高的剂量是否对患者有益。无论如何，为了预防癫痫发作和肌阵挛，当血浆水平高于 600μg/L 时（这个浓度更多的是依据反复提出的建议，而不是基于有明确证据的界值[74]），最好使用抗惊厥剂；当血浆水平高于 1 000μg/L 时，则必须使用抗惊厥剂。

去甲氯氮平是氯氮平的主要代谢产物。在人群中，氯氮平与去甲氯氮平的浓度比值平均为 1.25[75]，但是个体间可能存在差异。长期用药时，同一患者的这个比值应该保持不变。比值降低，提示可能有酶诱导；比值增加，说明可能有酶抑制、测定的不是谷浓度样本或者最近患者漏服药物。但还要注意取血时间也可极大地改变氯氮平/去甲氯氮平浓度比值。如果取血时间早，氯氮平浓度相对高；如果取血时间晚，则去甲氯氮平的浓度较高[2]。剂量较大时，氯氮平的代谢会达到饱和：氯氮平与去甲氯氮平比值随着氯氮平血浆水平升高而增加，提示达到了饱和[76-78]。氟伏沙明对氯氮平血浆水平的影响也提示，氯氮平通过 CYP1A2 代谢为去甲氯氮平的过程可被抑制[79]。最近的一项系统综述提示，氯氮平/去甲氯氮平浓度比值没有临床指导意义[80]。

奥氮平

奥氮平的血浆水平与每天剂量呈线性关系[81]，但是个体间差异很大[82]，女性[64]、不吸烟者[83] 和使用抑制酶活性药物者[83,84] 血浆水平较高。每天给药 1 次时，精神分裂症患者的有效阈浓度建议为谷浓度样本 9.3μg/L[85]、服药后 12h 23.2μg/L[64] 和服药后平均 13.5h 23μg/L[86]。有证据显示，血药水平高于 40μg/L（12h 血样）时，治疗效果并不比低血药水平时好[87]。严重的毒性反应罕见，可能与血药水平高于 100μg/L 相关；当血药水平高于 160μg/L[88] 时，偶见死亡（虽然其他药物或者躯体因素也有关）。建议治疗精神分裂症的目标浓度范围为 20~40μg/L[89]；治疗双相障碍的有效剂量范围也许相似[90]。最近这个浓度范围被扩展到 20~80μg/L[91,92]，为什么要扩宽这个范围，理由尚不清楚。

特别指出的是，明显的体重增加，极有可能发生于血浆水平高于 20μg/L 的患者[93]。便秘、口干和心动过速，似乎也与药物的血浆水平相关[94]。

临床实践中，奥氮平的剂量主要依据疗效和耐受性调整。但是，一项对英国血样分析结果的调查提示，奥氮平每天 20mg 治疗时，大约 20% 患者的血药水平达不到有效水平，超过 40% 的患者血药浓度高于 40μg/L[95]。血药水平测定对以下患者可能有用：怀疑有依从性问题、耐受性差或者最大注册剂量无效。若疗效不好，且血浆水平低于 20μg/L，可以调整剂量，使服药 12h 后的血浆水平达到 20~40μg/L；若疗效很好，但耐受性差，可以试验性减少剂量，使血浆水平低于 40μg/L。剂量变化会使血药浓度成比例地发生改变[96]。在患者的治疗中，当没有其他策略可选时，可以考虑增加剂量使血浆药物水平升高到 40~80μg/L。

喹硫平

喹硫平剂量与血浆谷浓度的相关性弱[97]。据报道,在 150~800mg/d 剂量范围内,平均血浆水平范围为 27~387μg/L[98-103],但是最高和最低浓度未必见于最高和最低剂量时。治疗药物监测(TDM)中见到的明显的个体间差异,可能是年龄、性别和合用药物所致,女性[103,104]、老年[102,103] 以及 CYP3A4 抑制性药物[98,102,103] 可能会升高喹硫平的血浆水平。相关报道的结果互相矛盾[104],不足以支持单纯基于这些因素进行常规血浆水平监测。尽管在每个剂量下的血药水平有很大的差异,没有足够的证据来提出喹硫平的目标浓度范围(虽然有人建议目标浓度范围为 100~500μg/L[105]);所以,血浆水平监测可能没有多大价值。而且,喹硫平的代谢产物有重要的治疗效应,其浓度与母药浓度只有弱相关性[106]。

最近关于喹硫平浓度相关性的报道,来源于谷浓度样本分析。由于喹硫平的半衰期较短,不论剂量大小、前面的峰浓度水平如何,谷浓度水平都会很快降到一个很窄的浓度范围内。这样的话,峰浓度与剂量和临床疗效的相关性更强[97]。但是,由于没有建立峰浓度的目标范围,目前没有理由做这样的监测。有趣的是,最近一项喹硫平治疗边缘型人格障碍或药物所致精神病性障碍的研究结果显示,疗效和 12h 血浆药物水平呈线性相关[104]。喹硫平速释剂(IR)的峰谷浓度波动(从最高约 4 000μg/L 到 0)显著高于缓释剂(从最高约 3 000μg/L 到大约 100μg/L)[43]。

喹硫平有明确的剂量反应关系,而且,即使超出说明书推荐剂量很多,患者也能很好地耐受[107]。在临床实践中,剂量调整应该依据患者的疗效和耐受性。

利培酮

一般认为,利培酮的治疗范围是其活性成分(利培酮 +9-羟基-利培酮) 浓度为 20~60μg/L[91,108,109],但是也有人建议过其他浓度范围(25~150μg/L 和 25~80μg/L)[110]。20~60μg/L 的血浆水平范围通常在口服剂量 3~6mg 时可以达到[108,111-113]。在大约 20μg/L 的血浆水平时,纹状体 D_2 受体的占有率已达 65%(产生疗效的最低占有率)[109,114]。

利培酮长效注射剂(每 2 周 25mg)达到的血浆水平平均为 4.4~22.7μg/L[112]。在这个剂量时,D_2 受体占有率估计为 25%~71%[109,115,116]。围绕这个平均值,有很大的个体间差异,只有极少数患者血浆水平高于上述范围。虽然如此,这些数据确实对利培酮长效注射剂 25mg(2 周)的疗效带来质疑[112];值得注意的是,有证据显示,尽管血浆药物浓度和多巴胺占有率均低于有效范围,但是利培酮长效注射剂是有效的[117]。事实上,越来越多的证据支持,在预防复发的长期治疗中,并不需要持续高的 D_2 受体占有率[118-120](不同于需要急性疗效的 D_2 受体占有率)。

令人不安的是,一项来自接受 RLAI 治疗患者的检测报告发现[121],50% 的患者药物活性成分浓度低于 20μg/L,10% 的患者未检测出利培酮或 9-羟基利培酮。所以,治疗药物监测可能对于接受 RLAI 治疗的患者临床上有帮助,但是这种监测反而减弱长效注射剂的目的。

有限的关于帕立哌酮棕榈酸盐的数据显示,标准起始剂量的血浆水平为 25~45μg/L;稳态时的血浆水平:每月 100mg 为 10~25μg/L,每月 150mg 为 15~35μg/L[122]。血浆药物浓度在治疗的第一年逐渐升高到大约 35μg/L(平均剂量每月 138mg)[123],之后保持稳定[124]。对于 3 个月注射剂型,稳态血浆浓度范围大约是:525mg/3 个月为 30~55μg/L,350mg/3 个月为 25~55μg/L,263mg/3 个月为 20~35μg/L[125]。

表 11.2 列出了目标浓度范围,其用途不确定;在某些情况下,它们只是临床使用中发现的数值范围。仅仅在专科病房中可以检测这些药物浓度。

表 11.2 其他精神药物的目标浓度范围

抗精神病药	目标浓度范围/μg·L⁻¹
阿塞那平	1~5
依匹哌唑	40~140
卡利拉嗪	10~20
氯丙嗪	30~300
氟哌噻吨	0.5~5(顺式-异构体)
氟奋乃静	1~10
氟哌啶醇	1~10
伊潘立酮	5~10
鲁拉西酮	15~40
美哌隆	30·100
舒必利	200~1 000
齐拉西酮	50~200
珠氯噻醇	4~50

抗抑郁药	目标浓度范围/μg·L⁻¹
阿戈美拉汀	7~300
西酞普兰	50~110
去甲文拉法辛	100~400
度硫平	45~100
度洛西汀	30~120
艾司西酞普兰	15~80
氟西汀(+ 去甲氟西汀)	120~500
氟伏沙明	60~230
左米那普仑	80~120
米安色林	15~70
米那普仑	100~150
米氮平	30~80
吗氯贝胺	300~1 000
帕罗西汀	20~65
瑞波西汀	60~350
舍曲林	10~150
曲唑酮	700~1 000
文拉法辛(+O-去甲基文拉法辛)	100~400
维拉唑酮	30~70
伏硫西汀	15~60

第 11 章

参考文献

1. Mann K, et al. Appropriateness of therapeutic drug monitoring for antidepressants in routine psychiatric inpatient care. *Ther Drug Monit* 2006; 28:83–88.

2. Jakobsen MI, et al. The significance of sampling time in therapeutic drug monitoring of clozapine. *Acta Psychiatr Scand* 2017; 135:159–169.

3. Hiemke C. relationships of psychoactive drugs and the problem to calculate therapeutic reference ranges. *Ther Drug Monit* 2019; 41: 174–179.

4. Taylor D, et al. Doses of carbamazepine and valproate in bipolar affective disorder. *Psychiatric Bulletin* 1997; 21:221–223.

5. Eadie MJ. Anticonvulsant drugs. *Drugs* 1984; 27: 328–363.

6. Chbili C, et al. Relationships between pharmacokinetic parameters of carbamazepine and therapeutic response in patients with bipolar disease. *Ann Biol Clin* (Paris) 2014; 72:453–459.

7. Cohen AF, et al. Lamotrigine, a new anticonvulsant: pharmacokinetics in normal humans. *Clin Pharmacol Ther* 1987; 42:535–541.

8. Kilpatrick ES, et al. Concentration-effect and concentration-toxicity relations with lamotrigine: a prospective study. *Epilepsia* 1996; 37:534–538.

9. Johannessen SI, et al. Therapeutic drug monitoring of the newer antiepileptic drugs. *Ther Drug Monit* 2003; 25:347–363.

10. Kagawa S, et al. Relationship between plasma concentrations of lamotrigine and its early therapeutic effect of lamotrigine augmentation therapy in treatment-resistant depressive disorder. *Ther Drug Monit* 2014; 36:730–733.

11. Nakamura A, et al. Prediction of an optimal dose of lamotrigine for augmentation therapy in treatment-resistant depressive disorder from plasma lamotrigine concentration at week 2. *Ther Drug Monit* 2016; 38:379–382.

12. Schou M. Forty years of lithium treatment. *Arch Gen Psychiatry* 1997; 54: 9–13.

13. Anon. Using lithium safely. *Drug Ther Bull* 1999; 37:22–24.

14. Nicholson J, et al. Monitoring patients on lithium – a good practice guideline. *Psychiatric Bulletin* 2002; 26:348–351.

15. National Institute for Health and Care Excellence. Bipolar disorder: assessment and management: Clinical Guidance [CG185] 2014 (last updated February 2020); https://www.nice.org.uk/guidance/cg185.

16. Severus WE, et al. What is the optimal serum lithium level in the long-term treatment of bipolar disorder–a review? *Bipolar Disorders* 2008; 10:231–237.

17. Nolen WA, et al. The association of the effect of lithium in the maintenance treatment of bipolar disorder with lithium plasma levels: a post hoc analysis of a double-blind study comparing switching to lithium or placebo in patients who responded to quetiapine (Trial 144). *Bipolar Disorders* 2013; 15:100–109.

18. Nazirizadeh Y, et al. Serum concentrations of paliperidone versus risperidone and clinical effects. *Eur J Clin Pharmacol* 2010; 66:797–803.

19. Schoretsanitis G, et al. A systematic review and combined analysis of therapeutic drug monitoring studies for oral paliperidone. *Expert Rev Clin Pharmacol* 2018; 11:625–639.

20. Taylor D, et al. Plasma levels of tricyclics and related antidepressants: are they necessary or useful? *Psychiatric Bulletin* 1995; 19:548–550.

21. Perucca E. Pharmacological and therapeutic properties of valproate. *CNS Drugs* 2002; 16: 695–714.

22. Allen MH, et al. Linear relationship of valproate serum concentration to response and optimal serum levels for acute mania. *Am J Psychiatry* 2006; 163:272–275.

23. Bowden CL, et al. Relation of serum valproate concentration to response in mania. *Am J Psychiatry* 1996; 153:765–770.

24. Vazquez M, et al. Hyperammonemia associated with valproic acid concentrations. *BioMed Research International* 2014; 2014:217–269.

25. Muller MJ, et al. Amisulpride doses and plasma levels in different age groups of patients with schizophrenia or schizoaffective disorder. *Journal of Psychopharmacology* 2008; 23:278–286.

26. Muller MJ, et al. Gender aspects in the clinical treatment of schizophrenic inpatients with amisulpride: a therapeutic drug monitoring study. *Pharmacopsychiatry* 2006; 39:41–46.

27. Bergemann N, et al. Plasma amisulpride levels in schizophrenia or schizoaffective disorder. *Eur Neuropsychopharmacol* 2004; 14:245–250.

28. Muller MJ, et al. Therapeutic drug monitoring for optimizing amisulpride therapy in patients with schizophrenia. *J Psychiatr Res* 2007; 41:673–679.

29. Sparshatt A, et al. Amisulpride - dose, plasma concentration, occupancy and response: implications for therapeutic drug monitoring. *Acta Psychiatr Scand* 2009; 120:416–428.

30. Schoretsanitis G, et al. TDM in psychiatry and neurology: A comprehensive summary of the consensus guidelines for therapeutic drug monitoring in neuropsychopharmacology, update 2017; a tool for clinicians. *World J Biol Psychiatry* 2018; 19:162–174.

31. Jönsson AK, et al. A compilation of serum concentrations of 12 antipsychotic drugs in a therapeutic drug monitoring setting. *Ther Drug Monit* 2019; 41:348–356.

32. Reeves S, et al. Therapeutic window of dopamine D2/3 receptor occupancy to treat psychosis in Alzheimer's disease. *Brain* 2017; 140:1117–1127.

33. Reeves S, et al. Therapeutic D2/3 receptor occupancies and response with low amisulpride blood concentrations in very late-onset schizophrenia-like psychosis (VLOSLP). *Int J Geriatr Psychiatry* 2018; 33:396–404.

34. Bowskill SV, et al. Plasma amisulpride in relation to prescribed dose, clozapine augmentation, and other factors: data from a therapeutic drug monitoring service, 2002–2010. *Hum Psychopharmacol* 2012; 27:507–513.

35. Mace S, et al. Aripiprazole: dose–response relationship in schizophrenia and schizoaffective disorder. *CNS Drugs* 2008; **23**:773–780.

36. Sparshatt A, et al. A systematic review of aripiprazole – dose, plasma concentration, receptor occupancy and response: implications for therapeutic drug monitoring. *J Clin Psychiatry* 2010; **71**:1447–1456.

37. Kirschbaum KM, et al. Therapeutic monitoring of aripiprazole by HPLC with column-switching and spectrophotometric detection. *Clin Chem* 2005; **51**:1718–1721.

38. Kirschbaum KM, et al. Serum levels of aripiprazole and dehydroaripiprazole, clinical response and side effects. *World J Biol Psychiatry* 2008; **9**:212–218.

39. Molden E, et al. Pharmacokinetic variability of aripiprazole and the active metabolite dehydroaripiprazole in psychiatric patients. *Ther Drug Monit* 2006; **28**:744–749.

40. Bachmann CJ, et al. Large variability of aripiprazole and dehydroaripiprazole serum concentrations in adolescent patients with schizophrenia. *Ther Drug Monit* 2008; **30**:462–466.

41. Hendset M, et al. Impact of the CYP2D6 genotype on steady-state serum concentrations of aripiprazole and dehydroaripiprazole. *Eur J Clin Pharmacol* 2007; **63**:1147–1151.

42. Mallikaarjun S, et al. Pharmacokinetics, tolerability and safety of aripiprazole once-monthly in adult schizophrenia: an open-label, parallel-arm, multiple-dose study. *Schizophr Res* 2013; **150**:281–288.

43. Korell J, et al. Determination of plasma concentration reference ranges for oral aripiprazole, olanzapine, and quetiapine. *Eur J Clin Pharmacol* 2018; **74**:593–599.

44. Haring C, et al. Influence of patient-related variables on clozapine plasma levels. *Am J Psychiatry* 1990; **147**:1471–1475.

45. Haring C, et al. Dose-related plasma levels of clozapine: influence of smoking behaviour, sex and age. *Psychopharmacology* 1989; **99 Suppl**:S38–S40.

46. Taylor D. Pharmacokinetic interactions involving clozapine. *Br J Psychiatry* 1997; **171**: 109–112.

47. Ng CH, et al. An inter-ethnic comparison study of clozapine dosage, clinical response and plasma levels. *Int Clin Psychopharmacol* 2005; **20**:163–168.

48. Ruan CJ, et al. Clozapine metabolism in East Asians and Caucasians: a pilot exploration of the prevalence of poor metabolizers and a systematic review. *J Clin Psychopharmacol* 2019; **39**:135–144.

49. de Leon J, et al. Do Asian patients require only half of the clozapine dose prescribed for Caucasians? A critical overview. *Indian J Psychol Med* 2020; **42**:4–10.

50. Suhas S, et al. Do Indian patients with schizophrenia need half the recommended clozapine dose to achieve therapeutic serum level? An exploratory study. *Schizophr Res* 2020; **222**:195-201.

51. Bhattacharya R, et al. Clozapine prescribing: comparison of clozapine dosage and plasma levels between White British and Bangladeshi patients. *BJPsych Bulletin* 2021; **45**:22–27.

52. Ruan CJ, et al. Exploring the prevalence of clozapine phenotypic poor metabolizers in 4 Asian samples: they ranged between 2% and 13. *J Clin Psychopharmacol* 2019; **39**:644–648.

53. de Leon J, et al. Using therapeutic drug monitoring to personalize clozapine dosing in Asians. *Asia-Pacific Psychiatry* 2020; **12**:e12384.

54. Rostami-Hodjegan A, et al. Influence of dose, cigarette smoking, age, sex, and metabolic activity on plasma clozapine concentrations: a predictive model and nomograms to aid clozapine dose adjustment and to assess compliance in individual patients. *J Clin Psychopharmacol* 2004; **24**:70–78.

55. Haack MJ, et al. Toxic rise of clozapine plasma concentrations in relation to inflammation. *Eur Neuropsychopharmacol* 2003; **13**:381–385.

56. de Leon J, et al. Serious respiratory infections can increase clozapine levels and contribute to side effects: a case report. *Prog Neuropsychopharmacol Biol Psychiatry* 2003; **27**:1059–1063.

57. Espnes KA, et al. A puzzling case of increased serum clozapine levels in a patient with inflammation and infection. *Ther Drug Monit* 2012; **34**:489–492.

58. VanderZwaag C, et al. Response of patients with treatment-refractory schizophrenia to clozapine within three serum level ranges. *Am J Psychiatry* 1996; **153**:1579–1584.

59. Perry PJ, et al. Clozapine and norclozapine plasma concentrations and clinical response of treatment refractory schizophrenic patients. *Am J Psychiatry* 1991; **148**:231–235.

60. Miller DD. Effect of phenytoin on plasma clozapine concentrations in two patients. *J Clin Psychiatry* 1991; **52**:23–25.

61. Spina E, et al. Relationship between plasma concentrations of clozapine and norclozapine and therapeutic response in patients with schizophrenia resistant to conventional neuroleptics. *Psychopharmacology* 2000; **148**:83–89.

62. Hasegawa M, et al. Relationship between clinical efficacy and clozapine concentrations in plasma in schizophrenia: effect of smoking. *J Clin Psychopharmacol* 1993; **13**:383–390.

63. Potkin SG, et al. Plasma clozapine concentrations predict clinical response in treatment-resistant schizophrenia. *J Clin Psychiatry* 1994; **55 Suppl B**:133–136.

64. Perry PJ. Therapeutic drug monitoring of antipsychotics. *Psychopharmacol Bull* 2001; **35**:19–29.

65. Llorca PM, et al. Effectiveness of clozapine in neuroleptic-resistant schizophrenia: clinical response and plasma concentrations. *J Psychiatry Neurosci* 2002; **27**:30–37.

66. Xiang YQ, et al. Serum concentrations of clozapine and norclozapine in the prediction of relapse of patients with schizophrenia. *Schizophr Res* 2006; **83**:201–210.

67. Stieffenhofer V, et al. Clozapine plasma level monitoring for prediction of rehospitalization schizophrenic outpatients. *Pharmacopsychiatry* 2011; **44**:55–59.

68. Lee J, et al. Quantifying intraindividual variations in plasma clozapine levels: a population pharmacokinetic approach. *J Clin Psychiatry* 2016; 77:681–687.

69. Turrion MC, et al. Intra-individual variation of clozapine and norclozapine plasma levels in clinical practice. *Revista De Psiquiatria Y Salud Mental* 2020; 13:31–35.

70. Khan AY, et al. Examining concentration-dependent toxicity of clozapine: role of therapeutic drug monitoring. *J Psychiatr Pract* 2005; 11:289–301.

71. Varma S, et al. Clozapine-related EEG changes and seizures: dose and plasma-level relationships. *Ther Adv Psychopharmacol* 2011; 1:47–66.

72. Greenwood-Smith C, et al. Serum clozapine levels: a review of their clinical utility. *J Psychopharm* 2003; 17:234–238.

73. Yusufi B, et al. Prevalence and nature of side effects during clozapine maintenance treatment and the relationship with clozapine dose and plasma concentration. *Int Clin Psychopharmacol* 2007; 22:238–243.

74. Remington G, et al. Clozapine and therapeutic drug monitoring: is there sufficient evidence for an upper threshold? *Psychopharmacology* 2013; 225:505–518.

75. Couchman L, et al. Plasma clozapine, norclozapine, and the clozapine: norclozapineratio in relation to prescribed dose and other factors: data from a therapeutic drug monitoring service, 1993–2007. *Ther Drug Monit* 2010; 32:438–447.

76. Volpicelli SA, et al. Determination of clozapine, norclozapine, and clozapine-N-oxide in serum by liquid chromatography. *Clin Chem* 1993; 39:1656–1659.

77. Guitton C, et al. Clozapine and metabolite concentrations during treatment of patients with chronic schizophrenia. *J Clin Pharmacol* 1999; 39:721–728.

78. Palego L, et al. Clozapine, norclozapine plasma levels, their sum and ratio in 50 psychotic patients: influence of patient-related variables. *Prog Neuropsychopharmacol Biol Psychiatry* 2002; 26:473–480.

79. Wang CY, et al. The differential effects of steady-state fluvoxamine on the pharmacokinetics of olanzapine and clozapine in healthy volunteers. *J Clin Pharmacol* 2004; 44:785–792.

80. Schoretsanitis G, et al. A comprehensive review of the clinical utility of and a combined analysis of the clozapine/norclozapine ratio in therapeutic drug monitoring for adult patients. *Expert Rev Clin Pharmacol* 2019; 12:603–621.

81. Bishara D, et al. Olanzapine: a systematic review and meta-regression of the relationships between dose, plasma concentration, receptor occupancy, and response. *J Clin Psychopharmacol* 2013; 33:329–335.

82. Aravagiri M, et al. Plasma level monitoring of olanzapine in patients with schizophrenia: determination by high-performance liquid chromatography with electrochemical detection. *Ther Drug Monit* 1997; 19:307–313.

83. Gex-Fabry M, et al. Therapeutic drug monitoring of olanzapine: the combined effect of age, gender, smoking, and comedication. *Ther Drug Monit* 2003; 25:46–53.

84. Bergemann N, et al. Olanzapine plasma concentration, average daily dose, and interaction with co-medication in schizophrenic patients. *Pharmacopsychiatry* 2004; 37:63–68.

85. Perry PJ, et al. Olanzapine plasma concentrations and clinical response in acutely ill schizophrenic patients. *J Clin Psychopharmacol* 1997; 17:472–477.

86. Fellows L, et al. Investigation of target plasma concentration–effect relationships for olanzapine in schizophrenia. *Ther Drug Monit* 2003; 25:682–689.

87. Mauri MC, et al. Clinical outcome and olanzapine plasma levels in acute schizophrenia. *Eur Psychiatry* 2005; 20:55–60.

88. Rao ML, et al. Olanzapine: pharmacology, pharmacokinetics and therapeutic drug monitoring. *Fortschr Neurol Psychiatr* 2001; 69:510–517.

89. Robertson MD, et al. Olanzapine concentrations in clinical serum and postmortem blood specimens—when does therapeutic become toxic? *J Forensic Sci* 2000; 45:418–421.

90. Bech P, et al. Olanzapine plasma level in relation to antimanic effect in the acute therapy of manic states. *Nord J Psychiatry* 2006; 60:181–182.

91. Schoretsanitis G, et al. Blood levels to optimize antipsychotic treatment in clinical practice: a Joint Consensus Statement of the American Society of Clinical Psychopharmacology and the Therapeutic Drug Monitoring Task Force of the Arbeitsgemeinschaft für Neuropsychopharmakologie und Pharmakopsychiatrie. *J Clin Psychiatry* 2020; 81:19cs13169.

92. Noel C. A review of a recently published guidelines' "strong recommendation" for therapeutic drug monitoring of olanzapine, haloperidol, perphenazine, and fluphenazine. *Ment Health Clin* 2019; 9:287–293.

93. Perry PJ, et al. The association of weight gain and olanzapine plasma concentrations. *J Clin Psychopharmacol* 2005; 25:250–254.

94. Kelly DL, et al. Plasma concentrations of high-dose olanzapine in a double-blind crossover study. *Human Psychopharmacol* 2006; 21:393–398.

95. Patel MX, et al. Plasma olanzapine in relation to prescribed dose and other factors: data from a therapeutic drug monitoring service, 1999–2009. *J Clin Psychopharmacol* 2011; 31:411–417.

96. Tsuboi T, et al. Predicting plasma olanzapine concentration following a change in dosage: a population pharmacokinetic study. *Pharmacopsychiatry* 2015; 48:286–291.

97. Sparshatt A, et al. Relationship between daily dose, plasma concentrations, dopamine receptor occupancy, and clinical response to quetiapine: a review. *J Clin Psychiatry* 2011; 72:1108–1123.

98. Hasselstrom J, et al. Quetiapine serum concentrations in psychiatric patients: the influence of comedication. *Ther Drug Monit* 2004; 26:486–491.

99. Winter HR, et al. Steady-state pharmacokinetic, safety, and tolerability profiles of quetiapine, norquetiapine, and other quetiapine metabo-

lites in pediatric and adult patients with psychotic disorders. *J Child Adolesc Psychopharmacol* 2008; **18**:81–98.

100. Li KY, et al. Multiple dose pharmacokinetics of quetiapine and some of its metabolites in Chinese suffering from schizophrenia. *Acta Pharmacol Sin* 2004; **25**:390–394.

101. McConville BJ, et al. Pharmacokinetics, tolerability, and clinical effectiveness of quetiapine fumarate: an open-label trial in adolescents with psychotic disorders. *J Clin Psychiatry* 2000; **61**:252–260.

102. Castberg I, et al. Quetiapine and drug interactions: evidence from a routine therapeutic drug monitoring service. *J Clin Psychiatry* 2007; **68**:1540–1545.

103. Aichhorn W, et al. Influence of age, gender, body weight and valproate comedication on quetiapine plasma concentrations. *Int Clin Psychopharmacol* 2006; **21**:81–85.

104. Mauri MC, et al. Two weeks' quetiapine treatment for schizophrenia, drug-induced psychosis and borderline personality disorder: a naturalistic study with drug plasma levels. *Expert Opin Pharmacother* 2007; **8**:2207–2213.

105. Patteet L, et al. Therapeutic drug monitoring of common antipsychotics. *Ther Drug Monit* 2012; **34**:629–651.

106. Fisher DS, et al. Plasma concentrations of quetiapine, N-desalkylquetiapine, o-desalkylquetiapine, 7-hydroxyquetiapine, and quetiapine sulfoxide in relation to quetiapine dose, formulation, and other factors. *Ther Drug Monit* 2012; **34**:415–421.

107. Sparshatt A, et al. Quetiapine: dose-response relationship in schizophrenia. *CNS Drugs* 2008; **22**:49–68.

108. Olesen OV, et al. Serum concentrations and side effects in psychiatric patients during risperidone therapy. *Ther Drug Monit* 1998; **20**:380–384.

109. Remington G, et al. A PET study evaluating dopamine D2 receptor occupancy for long-acting injectable risperidone. *Am J Psychiatry* 2006; **163**:396–401.

110. Seto K, et al. Risperidone in schizophrenia: is there a role for therapeutic drug monitoring? *Ther Drug Monit* 2011; **33**:275–283.

111. Lane HY, et al. Risperidone in acutely exacerbated schizophrenia: dosing strategies and plasma levels. *J Clin Psychiatry* 2000; **61**:209–214.

112. Taylor D. Risperidone long-acting injection in practice - more questions than answers? *Acta Psychiatr Scand* 2006; **114**:1–2.

113. Nyberg S, et al. Suggested minimal effective dose of risperidone based on PET-measured D2 and 5-HT2A receptor occupancy in schizophrenic patients. *Am J Psychiatry* 1999; **156**:869–875.

114. Uchida H, et al. Predicting dopamine D receptor occupancy from plasma levels of antipsychotic drugs: a systematic review and pooled analysis. *J Clin Psychopharmacol* 2011; **31**:318–325.

115. Medori R, et al. Plasma antipsychotic concentration and receptor occupancy, with special focus on risperidone long-acting injectable. *Eur Neuropsychopharmacol* 2006; **16**:233–240.

116. Gefvert O, et al. Pharmacokinetics and D2 receptor occupancy of long-acting injectable risperidone (Risperdal Consta™) in patients with schizophrenia. *Int J Neuropsychopharmacol* 2005; **8**:27–36.

117. Nyberg S, et al. D2 dopamine receptor occupancy during low-dose treatment with haloperidol decanoate. *Am J Psychiatry* 1995; **152**:173–178.

118. Moriguchi S, et al. Estimated dopamine D(2) receptor occupancy and remission in schizophrenia: analysis of the CATIE data. *J Clin Psychopharmacol* 2013; **33**:682–685.

119. Tsuboi T, et al. Challenging the need for sustained blockade of dopamine D(2) receptor estimated from antipsychotic plasma levels in the maintenance treatment of schizophrenia: a single-blind, randomized, controlled study. *Schizophr Res* 2015; **164**:149–154.

120. Takeuchi H, et al. Dose reduction of risperidone and olanzapine and estimated dopamine D(2) receptor occupancy in stable patients with schizophrenia: findings from an open-label, randomized, controlled study. *J Clin Psychiatry* 2014; **75**:1209–1214.

121. Bowskill SV, et al. Risperidone and total 9-hydroxyrisperidone in relation to prescribed dose and other factors: data from a therapeutic drug monitoring service, 2002–2010. *Ther Drug Monit* 2012; **34**:349–355.

122. Pandina GJ, et al. A randomized, placebo-controlled study to assess the efficacy and safety of 3 doses of paliperidone palmitate in adults with acutely exacerbated schizophrenia. *J Clin Psychopharmacol* 2010; **30**:235–244.

123. Mauri MC, et al. Paliperidone long-acting plasma level monitoring and a new method of evaluation of clinical Stability. *Pharmacopsychiatry* 2017; **50**:145–151.

124. Paletta S, et al. Two years of maintenance therapy with paliperidone long-acting in schizophrenia and schizoaffective disorder: a study with plasma levels. *Eur Neuropsychopharmacol* 2016; **26**:S556–S557.

125. Berwaerts J, et al. Efficacy and safety of the 3-month formulation of paliperidone palmitate vs placebo for relapse prevention of schizophrenia: A randomized clinical trial. *JAMA Psychiatry* 2015; **72**:830–839.

尸检血浆药物浓度的解释

关于生前药物在体内的分布目前较为了解,但是对死亡后相关数据知之甚少。很多药物的分布在死后出现改变,但是出于明显的实际原因,对其机制及影响程度的研究非常有限。目前可知的是,生前检测的血浆药物浓度,明显不同于死后检测的(通常是股动脉全血)浓度。

很多过程导致了尸检时的药物浓度改变。生前机体的主动机制使得一些药物集中在某些器官或组织中。死后,细胞膜分解,出现了被动扩散,因此在死后的血标本中,一些药物的浓度高于生前[这种现象被称为"死后药物再分布"(post-mortem redistribution,PMR),被描述为"毒理学噩梦"(toxicological nightmare)[1],因为涉及许多不同的过程]。此外,重要器官周围的中心血管中,药物浓度常常要比远端外周血标本中高很多[2]。PMR和其他过程受温度和死后时间影响,因此,死后时间和储存条件是死后血药水平变化的重要的决定因素[3]。表观分布容积大的药物(即生前在组织中的浓度明显高于血浆的药物),死后再分布更大,尤其是生前长期用药的患者。

其他重要过程包括死后会合成某些化合物[4]。例如,机体可以产生 γ-羟基丁酸。创伤可以带入酵母,将葡萄糖代谢为乙醇。另一种现象是药物可能被细菌(如氯硝西泮和硝西泮)或真菌降解。另外,一些药物的代谢在死后继续进行(如可卡因)(虽然这可能是母药简单的化学不稳定现象)。

表 11.3 列出了与死后药物浓度改变有关的一些因素,以及这些过程可能的结果。通常来讲,对于孤立的死后血药浓度,可能无法进行合理的解释。即使有生前的血浆药物浓度数据,专家们也一致认为,在大多数情况下,对于大部分药物,几乎是不可能解释死后的血药浓度。例如,在没有其他证据的情况下,死后发现的高血药水平,肯定不应解释为患者是因为药物过量而死。两个有价值的参考资料,Ketola 和 Kriikku[5],及 Ketola 和 Ojanpera[6] 的系统综述,可以帮助解释 PM 样本的分析结果。若考虑药物在死亡中的作用,应该咨询专家的意见[7]。

表 11.3　影响死后血药浓度的因素

因素	举例	结果
药物从组织向血液再分布	大多数表观容积大的药物,如氯氮平[8,9]、奥氮平[10]、美沙酮[11]、SSRI[12]、TCA、米氮平[13]、碳酸锂[14] 可能影响不大的药物:利培酮[15]、阿立哌唑[16]、喹硫平[16]	死后药物浓度高达生前水平 10 倍,有时会更高[6]
药物在血管和器官中的分布不均匀(即采血部位会影响药物浓度)	大多数药物[5,17],如氯氮平、TCA、SSRI、度洛西汀[18]、苯二氮䓬类药物、喹硫平[19]	根据死后采血部位不同(如股静脉血与心脏血),药物浓度可能会相差数倍
药物在死后组织中的衰变(常常通过细菌降解)	未广泛研究,但已知奥氮平、利培酮[20]和一些苯二氮䓬类药物发生过该现象。真菌可以代谢阿米替林、米氮平和唑吡坦[21,22]。	死后浓度可能低于生前
死后代谢/降解	死后可卡因被代谢/降解。许多其他药物在死后标本中不稳定。创伤后,酵母可以产生乙醇[4]	死后水平可能低于(可卡因)或高于(乙醇)生前

参考文献

1. Pounder DJ, et al. Post-mortem drug redistribution–a toxicological nightmare. *Forensic Sci Int* 1990; **45**:253–263.

2. Ferner RE. Post-mortem clinical pharmacology. *Br J Clin Pharmacol* 2008; **66**:430–443.

3. Flanagan RJ, et al. Analytical toxicology: guidelines for sample collection postmortem. *Toxicol Rev* 2005; **24**:63–71.

4. Kennedy MC. Post-mortem drug concentrations. *Intern Med J* 2010; **40**:183–187.

5. Ketola RA, et al. Drug concentrations in post-mortem specimens. *Drug Test Anal* 2019; **11**:1338–1357.

6. Ketola RA, et al. Summary statistics for drug concentrations in post-mortem femoral blood representing all causes of death. *Drug Test Anal* 2019; **11**:1326–1337.

7. Flanagan RJ. Poisoning: fact or fiction? *Med Leg J* 2012; **80**:127–148.

8. Flanagan RJ, et al. Effect of post-mortem changes on peripheral and central whole blood and tissue clozapine and norclozapine concentrations in the domestic pig (Sus scrofa). *Forensic SciInt* 2003; **132**:9–17.

9. Flanagan RJ, et al. Suspected clozapine poisoning in the UK/Eire, 1992–2003. *Forensic Sci Int* 2005; **155**:91–99.

10. Saar E, et al. The time-dependant post-mortem redistribution of antipsychotic drugs. *Forensic Sci Int* 2012; **222**:223–227.

11. Caplehorn JR, et al. Methadone dose and post-mortem blood concentration. *Drug Alcohol Rev* 2002; **21**:329–333.

12. Lewis RJ, et al. Paroxetine in postmortem fluids and tissues from nine aviation accident victims. *J Anal Toxicol* 2015; **39**:637–641.

13. Launiainen T, et al. Drug concentrations in post-mortem femoral blood compared with therapeutic concentrations in plasma. *Drug Test Anal* 2014; **6**:308–316.

14. Soderberg C, et al. Reference values of lithium in postmortem femoral blood. *Forensic Sci Int* 2017; **277**:207–214.

15. Linnet K, et al. Postmortem femoral blood concentrations of risperidone. *J Anal Toxicol* 2014; **38**:57–60.

16. Skov L, et al. Postmortem femoral blood reference concentrations of aripiprazole, chlorprothixene, and quetiapine. *J Anal Toxicol* 2015; **39**:41–44.

17. Rodda KE, et al. The redistribution of selected psychiatric drugs in post-mortem cases. *Forensic Sci Int* 2006; **164**:235–239.

18. Scanlon KA, et al. Comprehensive duloxetine analysis in a fatal overdose. *J Anal Toxicol* 2016; **40**:167–170.

19. Breivik H, et al. Post mortem tissue distribution of quetiapine in forensic autopsies. *Forensic Sci Int* 2020; **315**:110413.

20. Butzbach DM, et al. Bacterial degradation of risperidone and paliperidone in decomposing blood. *J Forensic Sci* 2013; **58**:90–100.

21. Martinez-Ramirez JA, et al. Search for fungi-specific metabolites of four model drugs in postmortem blood as potential indicators of post-mortem fungal metabolism. *Forensic Sci Int* 2016; **262**:173–178.

22. Martinez-Ramirez JA, et al. Studies on drug metabolism by fungi colonizing decomposing human cadavers. Part II: biotransformation of five model drugs by fungi isolated from post-mortem material. *Drug Test Anal* 2015; **7**:265–279.

根据氯氮平血浆水平结果采取措施

在大多数发达国家,氯氮平的血浆浓度监测已广泛使用。表 11.4 给出了氯氮平血浆浓度

表 11.4 根据氯氮平血浆水平结果采取措施 *

血药浓度	疗效	耐受性	建议的措施
<350μg/L	差	差	非常缓慢地增加剂量,使血浆水平达到 350μg/L
	差	好	增加剂量,使血浆水平达到 350μg/L
	好	差	维持该剂量。如果耐受性没有改善,考虑减量
	好	好	继续监测,不需行动
350~500μg/L	差	差	根据耐受性缓慢增加剂量,使血浆水平 >500μg/L。考虑预防性用抗癫痫药[†]。如仍无效,考虑加用增效剂
	差	好	根据耐受性缓慢增加剂量,使血浆水平 >500μg/L。考虑预防性用抗癫痫药[†]。如仍无效,考虑加用增效剂
	好	差	维持该剂量,观察耐受性是否改善。考虑小心减量,使血浆水平保持在约 350μg/L
	好	好	继续监测,不需行动
500~1 000μg/L	差	差	考虑预防性用抗癫痫药[†]。考虑加用增效剂。如果增效治疗有效,尝试降低氯氮平剂量
	差	好	考虑预防性用抗癫痫药[†]。考虑加用增效剂
	好	差	尝试缓慢降低剂量,使血浆水平在 350~500μg/L,除非已知血浆水平降低后无效。此时,应当维持该剂量,考虑加用抗癫痫药[†]。优化不良反应的治疗
	好	好	考虑预防性用抗癫痫药[†]。如果耐受性良好,维持该剂量
>1 000μg/L	差	差	加抗癫痫药。尝试增效剂。减量使血浆水平 <1 000μg/L。考虑放弃氯氮平治疗
	差	好	加抗癫痫药。尝试增效治疗。若增效治疗有效,减量使血浆水平 <1 000μg/L。若增效治疗无效,则考虑放弃氯氮平治疗
	好	差	加抗癫痫药。尝试缓慢减量使血浆水平 <1 000μg/L
	好	好	加抗癫痫药。密切监测;仅耐受性下降时,才尝试减量

注:
疗效差:氯氮平治疗无效或疗效不满意。如疗效达不到出院标准。
疗效好:氯氮平治疗后,有明显疗效。可能适合出院,转到有支持或无支持的社区治疗。
耐受性差:剂量调整受限于不良反应,如心动过速、镇静、多涎和低血压(见第 1 章)。
耐受性好:患者能很好地耐受氯氮平治疗,没有严重中毒迹象。
增效治疗:加用另一种抗精神病药或心境稳定剂(见第 1 章)。
■ 在任何情况下,确保充分治疗氯氮平所致的便秘,该不良反应与氯氮平剂量相关。确保规律排便,并记录排便功能。常需要刺激性泻药,如番泻叶(见第 1 章)。
■ 癫痫发作风险与剂量和血浆水平相关。合适的抗癫痫药为丙戊酸盐、拉莫三嗪,少数情况下为托吡酯。若疗效不好,加用拉莫三嗪。若有情感症状,加用丙戊酸盐(见第 2 章)。注意使用丙戊酸盐可能会增加氯氮平致中性粒细胞减少的风险[3]。
* 该表适用于接受稳定剂量的氯氮平且确认依从性良好的患者。
† 血浆水平超过 600μg/L 的患者(除非脑电图正常),以及氯氮平血浆水平低但有过癫痫发作的患者,应当使用抗癫痫药。

在某一范围时,应该采取措施的一般性建议。所列的浓度范围有些人为规定,但比较方便——若不试用氯氮平,就无法知道某一患者可能出现临床疗效的浓度。大多数不良反应与剂量或血浆水平呈线性或指数关系。例如,氯氮平所致癫痫发作的风险,不会在某个剂量或某个浓度时出现巨大的改变[1]。因此,表11.4应被看作是进行临床决策时的辅助手段,而不是严格的、不折不扣的循证指导。也要注意对不良反应耐受的影响——很多患者在达到治疗浓度之前,曾经有明显的不良反应[2],随着治疗时间延长,患者对药物产生耐受,不良反应减少。

参考文献

1. Varma S, et al. Clozapine-related EEG changes and seizures: dose and plasma-level relationships. *Ther Adv Psychopharmacol* 2011; **1**:47–66.
2. Yusufi B, et al. Prevalence and nature of side effects during clozapine maintenance treatment and the relationship with clozapine dose and plasma concentration. *Int Clin Psychopharmacol* 2007; **22**:238–243.
3. Malik S, et al. Sodium valproate and clozapine induced neutropenia: A case control study using register data. *Schizophr Res* 2018; **195**:267–273.

精神药物和细胞色素酶功能

　　了解药物对细胞色素酶(CYP)功能有哪些影响,可以帮助预测或确认药物治疗潜在的药物相互作用风险,而在管理性临床试验或临床用药中,可能发现不了药物间相互作用(有时称为根据"第一原则"做出的预测)。使用"第一原则"本质上意味着了解和解释药代动力学信息,预测联合两种或多种药物治疗时,在体内产生的净效应。

　　除了合并用药对 CYP 功能可能产生影响,代谢酶通路(如 2D6、2C9、2C19 代谢酶)的遗传多态性也是造成某些药物代谢的个体间差异的原因。

　　有些药物可被多种代谢酶代谢,或者如果一种代谢通路被抑制,另外的一条或多条代谢通路会代偿性增强。因此,遗传多态性和药代动力学相互作用对药物代谢的影响往往很难预测。

　　CYP 功能不是唯一的考虑因素。在肠道壁上还发现了药物的转运蛋白,即 P-糖蛋白(P-gp)。P-gp 可以将弥散穿过(一种被动过程)肠道壁的药物弹出来(一种主动过程)。此外,在睾丸和血-脑屏障中也发现了 P-gp。预测对 P-gp 有抑制作用的药物,能够增加对其他药物(P-gp 的底物)的摄取;而对 P-gp 有诱导作用的药物,则可减少对其他药物(P-gp 的底物)的摄取。很多作为 CYP3A4 底物的药物,也同时是 P-gp 的底物。

　　UDP-葡糖醛酸转移酶(UGT)是负责生物转化第二相反应(结合反应)的酶系统。丙戊酸盐是 UGT 的强抑制剂,拉莫三嗪主要经 UGT 酶系统代谢,因此,丙戊酸盐和拉莫三嗪联合,有潜在的药物相互作用风险。UGT 酶系统也参与卢美哌隆、奥氮平、托吡酯和三氟拉嗪的代谢。

　　在下表中:

　　粗体标识的药物表示:

- 主要的代谢酶途径
- 主要的酶活性(抑制或诱导)

　　用 * 标识的药物表示:

- 已知是一种次级代谢酶途径或活性(即未发现具有临床意义)

　　常规字体(即无任何标识)的药物表示:

- 意义未知的代谢酶途径或活性

　　注意:CYP 功能的信息来源于药物手册和美国说明书(查询时间为 2020 年 8 月),以及最近一篇系统综述[1]。

　　表中不包含非精神药物对 CYP 功能影响的详细信息。

CYP1A2

底物	抑制剂	诱导剂
阿戈美拉汀	**氟伏沙明**	**巴比妥类**
阿米替林 *	吗氯贝胺	卡马西平
阿塞那平	奋乃静	莫达非尼 *

续表

底物	抑制剂	诱导剂
安非他酮 *		**苯巴比妥**
咖啡因		苯妥英
氯丙嗪		
氯丙米嗪 *		
氯氮平		
度洛西汀		
氟奋乃静		
氟伏沙明		
丙米嗪 *		
褪黑素		
米氮平 *		
奥氮平		
奋乃静		
?匹莫齐特 *		
雷美替胺		
唑吡坦 *		

CYP2A6

底物	抑制剂	诱导剂
安非他酮 *	反苯环丙胺	苯巴比妥
咖啡因		
尼古丁		

CYP2B6

底物	抑制剂	诱导剂
安非他酮	氟西汀 *	卡马西平 *
美沙酮 *	氟伏沙明	莫达非尼 *
尼古丁	美金刚	苯巴比妥
舍曲林 *	帕罗西汀 *	苯妥英
	舍曲林 *	

CYP2B7

底物	抑制剂	诱导剂
丁丙诺啡 *	未知	未知

CYP2C86

底物	抑制剂	诱导剂
佐匹克隆 *	未知	未知

CYP2C9

底物	抑制剂	诱导剂
阿戈美拉汀	氟西汀 *	卡马西平
阿米替林	氟伏沙明	圣约翰草
安非他酮 *	莫达非尼	
氟西汀 *	丙戊酸盐	
拉莫三嗪		
苯巴比妥		
苯妥英		
舍曲林 *		
丙戊酸盐		

CYP2C19

底物	抑制剂	诱导剂
阿戈美拉汀	艾司西酞普兰 *	卡马西平
阿米替林	氟伏沙明	圣约翰草
卡马西平 *	吗氯贝胺	
西酞普兰	莫达非尼	
氯米帕明 *	托吡酯	
地西泮		
艾司西酞普兰		
氟西汀 *		
丙米嗪		
?褪黑素 *		

续表

底物	抑制剂	诱导剂
?美沙酮 *		
吗氯贝胺		
苯妥英		
舍曲林 *		
苏沃雷生（suvorexant）		
曲米帕明 *		

CYP2D6

底物	抑制剂	诱导剂
阿米替林	**阿米替林**	未知
苯丙胺	**阿塞那平**	
托莫西汀	**安非他酮**	
阿立哌唑	氯丙嗪	
依匹哌唑	托吡酯	
卡利拉嗪	西酞普兰氯米帕明 *	
氯丙嗪	氯氮平	
西酞普兰	**度洛西汀**	
氯米帕明	艾司西酞普兰	
氯氮平 *	**氟西汀**	
氘丁苯那嗪	氟奋乃静	
多奈哌齐 *	氟伏沙明 *	
度洛西汀	氟哌啶醇	
艾司西酞普兰	左美丙嗪	
氟西汀	美沙酮 *	
氟伏沙明	吗氯贝胺	
氟奋乃静	**帕罗西汀**	
加兰他敏	奋乃静	
氟哌啶醇	瑞波西汀 *	
伊潘立酮	利培酮	
丙米嗪	舍曲林	
美沙酮 *	文拉法辛 *	
米安色林		

续表

底物	抑制剂	诱导剂
米氮平 *		
吗氯贝胺		
去甲替林		
奥氮平		
帕罗西汀		
奋乃静		
匹莫齐特 *		
喹硫平 *		
利培酮		
舍曲林		
曲唑酮 *		
曲米帕明		
缬苯那嗪		
文拉法辛		
伏硫西汀		
珠氯噻醇		

CYP2E1

底物	抑制剂	诱导剂
安非他酮	双硫仑	乙醇
乙醇	对乙酰氨基酚	

CYP3A4

底物	抑制剂	诱导剂
阿芬太尼	**氟西汀**	阿塞那平？
阿普唑仑	氟伏沙明	卡马西平
阿米替林	**帕罗西汀**	莫达非尼
阿立哌唑	奋乃静	苯巴比妥和其他的苯巴比妥类（可能）
依匹哌唑	瑞波西汀 *	**苯妥英**
丁丙诺啡		**圣约翰草**
安非他酮 *		托吡酯

续表

底物	抑制剂	诱导剂
丁螺环酮		
卡马西平		
卡利拉嗪		
氯丙嗪		
西酞普兰		
氯米帕明 *		
氯硝西泮		
氯氮平 *		
地西泮		
多奈哌齐 *		
度硫平		
艾司西酞普兰		
芬太尼		
氟西汀 *		
加兰他敏		
氟哌啶醇		
丙米嗪		
莱博雷生（lemborexant）		
鲁拉西酮		
美沙酮		
咪达唑仑		
米氮平		
莫达非尼		
硝西泮		
奋乃静		
匹莫范色林		
匹莫齐特		
喹硫平		
瑞波西汀		
利培酮 *		
舍吲哚		

第 11 章

续表

底物	抑制剂	诱导剂
舍曲林 *		
苏沃雷生（suvorexant）		
曲唑酮		
曲米帕明 *		
氘丁苯那嗪		
文拉法辛		
维拉唑酮		
扎来普隆		
齐拉西酮		
唑吡坦		
佐匹克隆		

参考文献

1. Schoretsanitis G, et al. TDM in psychiatry and neurology: a comprehensive summary of the consensus guidelines for therapeutic drug monitoring in neuropsychopharmacology, update 2017; a tool for clinicians. *World J Biol Psychiatry* 2018; **19**:162–174.

吸烟和精神药物

烟草的烟雾中包含多环芳烃,对一些肝脏代谢酶(尤其是 CYP1A2)具有诱导作用[1]。其他可被吸烟诱导的酶还包括 CYP2C19,可能还有 CYP3A4,以及 UGT(葡糖醛酸转移酶)的某些变构体[2]。酶诱导的程度取决于吸烟的数量和种类,以及烟雾被吸入的程度[3]。吸烟会显著降低一些精神科药物的血浆水平,所以吸烟者用药剂量要高于非吸烟者。吸烟也会通过诱导 CYP2E1 酶活性而影响酒精代谢[3]。

当停止吸烟后,酶活性大约每 2 天减低 1/2[4]。(尼古丁替代治疗或者使用电子烟对此过程没有影响。)然后,受到影响的药物血浆水平将上升,有时会相当明显。通常需要减少剂量。如果再次开始吸烟,酶活性增加,血浆水平下降,则需要增加药物剂量。这个过程较复杂,其作用难以预测。当然,很少有人能彻底戒烟,而间歇性吸烟和反复尝试彻底戒烟,会额外增加这个过程的复杂性。因此,有必要密切监测血浆水平(若有用)、临床进展和不良反应的严重程度。

下表详细描述了已知受吸烟状况影响的精神药物。

药物	吸烟的影响	停止吸烟后需采取的行动	针对重新吸烟需要采取的行动
阿戈美拉汀[5]	血浆水平降低	密切监测,可能需要减少剂量	考虑重新使用吸烟时的药物剂量
苯二氮䓬类药物[3,6]	血浆水平降低 0~50%(取决于药物和吸烟情况)	密切监测,考虑在一周时间内减少 25% 的药物剂量	密切监测,考虑重新使用吸烟时药物剂量
卡马西平[3]	不清楚,但吸烟可能会轻度降低卡马西平血浆水平	监测不良反应严重程度的变化	监测血浆水平
氯丙嗪[3,6,7]	血浆水平降低确切的影响不好估计	密切监测,考虑减少剂量	密切监测。考虑重新使用吸烟时的药物剂量
氯氮平[8-13]	血浆水平降低高达 50%。服用丙戊酸钠的患者,血浆水平下降得更多。该作用可以被联合氟伏沙明逆转[14]	戒烟前,测定血浆水平。一旦停止吸烟,逐渐(超过一周)减少药物剂量,到吸烟时剂量的 75% 左右(即减少 25% 的剂量)。完全戒烟一周后,复测血浆水平。可能需要进一步减量	重新吸烟前测定血浆水平。在一周时间内增加剂量至原来吸烟时的剂量。复测血浆药物水平。若增加剂量仍然血浆浓度降低,则病情加重很常见[15]
多塞平[2,16]	血浆水平降低约 25%(代谢产物去甲多塞平水平升高)	密切监测,可能需要减少服药剂量	考虑重新使用吸烟时的药物剂量
度洛西汀[17,18]	血浆水平可降低 50%	密切监测,可能需要减少服药剂量	考虑重新使用吸烟时的药物剂量

第 11 章

续表

药物	吸烟的影响	停止吸烟后需采取的行动	针对重新吸烟需要采取的行动
艾司西酞普兰[19]	临床实践中,吸烟者尽管接受了较高剂量的药物,但是其血浆水平较低。血浆水平降低可高达 50%(可能因 CYP2C19 酶诱导)	密切监测,考虑减少 25% 的服药剂量	密切监测,重新使用吸烟时的药物剂量
氟奋乃静[20]	血浆水平可降低 50%	一旦停止吸烟,减少 25% 的药物剂量。在随后的 4~8 周,密切监测。可能需要进一步减量	重新吸烟后,需要增加到吸烟时的剂量
氟伏沙明[21]	血浆水平降低大约 1/3	密切监测。可能需要减少药物剂量	可能需要增加至以前的剂量
氟哌啶醇[22,23]	血浆水平降低 25%~50%	减少大约 25% 的药物剂量。密切监测。考虑进一步减量	重新吸烟后,需要增加到吸烟时的剂量
洛沙平[24](吸入)	半衰期从 15.7h 降低到 13.6h	监测	监测
米氮平[25]	不清楚,但影响可能甚微	监测	监测
奥氮平[13,26-29]	血浆水平降低 50%	戒烟前测定血浆水平。戒烟后,减少 25% 的药物剂量。完全戒烟一周后,重测血浆水平。考虑进一步减量	重新吸烟前,测定血浆水平。在一周内,增加至吸烟时的剂量。复测血浆水平
利培酮/帕利哌酮[2,30]	吸烟者,其活性成分浓度可能会降低,但影响微弱(可能通过 CYP3A4 酶诱导)	密切监测	密切监测
曲唑酮[31]	血浆水平降低大约 25%	监测镇静作用增强的情况。考虑减少药物剂量	密切监测,考虑增加药物剂量
三环类抗抑郁药[3,6]	血浆水平降低 25%~50%	密切监测。考虑在一周内减少 10%~25% 的剂量。考虑进一步减量	密切监测。考虑重新使用吸烟时的剂量
珠氯噻醇[32,33]	不清楚,但影响可能甚微	监测	监测

注:仅吸烟行为会以上述方式对肝脏代谢酶产生诱导作用,尼古丁替代物、蒸馏装置和电子烟(不含多环芳香族化合物)对酶活性没有影响(详见 Blacker,2020[34] 所举案例)。

参考文献

1. Kroon LA. Drug interactions with smoking. *Am J Health Syst Pharm* 2007; 64:1917–1921.

2. Scherf-Clavel M, et al. Analysis of smoking behavior on the pharmacokinetics of antidepressants and antipsychotics: evidence for the role of alternative pathways apart from CYP1A2. *Int Clin Psychopharmacol* 2019; 34:93–100.

3. Desai HD, et al. Smoking in patients receiving psychotropic medications: a pharmacokinetic perspective. *CNS Drugs* 2001; 15:469–494.

4. Faber MS, et al. Time response of cytochrome P450 1A2 activity on cessation of heavy smoking. *Clin Pharmacol Ther* 2004; **76**:178–184.

5. Servier Laboratories Limited. Summary of Product Characteristics. Valdoxan (Agomelatine) 2020; https://www.medicines.org.uk/emc/medicine/21830.

6. Miller LG. Recent developments in the study of the effects of cigarette smoking on clinical pharmacokinetics and clinical pharmacodynamics. *Clin Pharmacokinet* 1989; **17**:90–108.

7. Goff DC, et al. Cigarette smoking in schizophrenia: relationship to psychopathology and medication side effects. *Am J Psychiatry* 1992; **149**:1189–1194.

8. Haring C, et al. Influence of patient-related variables on clozapine plasma levels. *Am J Psychiatry* 1990; **147**:1471–1475.

9. Haring C, et al. Dose-related plasma levels of clozapine: influence of smoking behaviour, sex and age. *Psychopharmacology* 1989; **99** **Suppl**:S38–S40.

10. Diaz FJ, et al. Estimating the size of the effects of co-medications on plasma clozapine concentrations using a model that controls for clozapine doses and confounding variables. *Pharmacopsychiatry* 2008; **41**:81–91.

11. Murayama-Sung L, et al. The impact of hospital smoking ban on clozapine and norclozapine levels. *J Clin Psychopharmacol* 2011; **31**:124–126.

12. Cormac I, et al. A retrospective evaluation of the impact of total smoking cessation on psychiatric inpatients taking clozapine. *Acta Psychiatr Scand* 2010; **121**:393–397.

13. Tsuda Y, et al. Meta-analysis: the effects of smoking on the disposition of two commonly used antipsychotic agents, olanzapine and clozapine. *BMJ Open* 2014; **4**:e004216.

14. Augustin M, et al. Effect of fluvoxamine augmentation and smoking on clozapine serum concentrations. *Schizophr Res* 2019; **210**:143–148.

15. Qurashi I, et al. Changes in smoking status, mental state and plasma clozapine concentration: retrospective cohort evaluation. *BJPsych Bulletin* 2019; **43**:271–274.

16. Ereshefsky L, et al. Pharmacokinetic factors affecting antidepressant drug clearance and clinical effect: evaluation of doxepin and imipramine—new data and review. *Clin Chem* 1988; **34**:863–880.

17. Fric M, et al. The influence of smoking on the serum level of duloxetine. *Pharmacopsychiatry* 2008; **41**:151–155.

18. Augustin M, et al. Differences in duloxetine dosing strategies in smoking and nonsmoking patients: therapeutic drug monitoring uncovers the impact on drug metabolism. *J Clin Psychiatry* 2018; **79**:17m12086.

19. Scherf-Clavel M, et al. Smoking is associated with lower dose-corrected serum concentrations of escitalopram. *J Clin Psychopharmacol* 2019; **39**:485–488.

20. Ereshefsky L, et al. Effects of smoking on fluphenazine clearance in psychiatric inpatients. *Biol Psychiatry* 1985; **20**:329–332.

21. Spigset O, et al. Effect of cigarette smoking on fluvoxamine pharmacokinetics in humans. *Clin Pharmacol Ther* 1995; **58**:399–403.

22. Jann MW, et al. Effects of smoking on haloperidol and reduced haloperidol plasma concentrations and haloperidol clearance. *Psychopharmacology* 1986; **90**:468–470.

23. Shimoda K, et al. Lower plasma levels of haloperidol in smoking than in nonsmoking schizophrenic patients. *Ther Drug Monit* 1999; **21**:293–296.

24. Takahashi LH, et al. Effect of smoking on the pharmacokinetics of inhaled loxapine. *Ther Drug Monit* 2014; **36**:618–623.

25. Grasmader K, et al. Population pharmacokinetic analysis of mirtazapine. *Eur J Clin Pharmacol* 2004; **60**:473–480.

26. Carrillo JA, et al. Role of the smoking-induced cytochrome P450 (CYP)1A2 and polymorphic CYP2D6 in steady-state concentration of olanzapine. *J Clin Psychopharmacol* 2003; **23**:119–127.

27. Gex-Fabry M, et al. Therapeutic drug monitoring of olanzapine: the combined effect of age, gender, smoking, and comedication. *Ther Drug Monit* 2003; **25**:46–53.

28. Bigos KL, et al. Sex, race, and smoking impact olanzapine exposure. *J Clin Pharmacol* 2008; **48**:157–165.

29. Lowe EJ, et al. Impact of tobacco smoking cessation on stable clozapine or olanzapine treatment. *Ann Pharmacother* 2010; **44**:727–732.

30. Schoretsanitis G, et al. Effect of smoking on risperidone pharmacokinetics – a multifactorial approach to better predict the influence on drug metabolism. *Schizophr Res* 2017; **185**:51–57.

31. Ishida M, et al. Effects of various factors on steady state plasma concentrations of trazodone and its active metabolite m-chlorophenylpiperazine. *Int Clin Psychopharmacol* 1995; **10**:143–146.

32. Jann MW, et al. Clinical pharmacokinetics of the depot antipsychotics. *Clin Pharmacokinet* 1985; **10**:315–333.

33. Jorgensen A, et al. Zuclopenthixol decanoate in schizophrenia: serum levels and clinical state. *Psychopharmacology* 1985; **87**:364–367.

34. Blacker CJ. Clinical issues to consider for clozapine patients who vape: a case illustration. *Focus (American Psychiatric Publishing)* 2020; **18**:55–57.

药物与酒精的相互作用

药物与酒精（乙醇）的相互作用非常复杂。很多患者相关的和药物相关的因素需要考虑。因为很多过程可能会同时或先后发生，所以可能比较难以准确预测结局。

药代动力学相互作用 [1-4]

酒精从胃肠道吸收，分布于体液中。女性和老年人分布容积较小，饮用某一剂量的酒精时，血浆中乙醇水平会高于年轻男性。摄入的酒精约 10% 经首过效应乙醇脱氢酶（ADH）代谢，少部分被胃内 ADH 代谢。其他乙醇在肝脏被 ADH 和 CYP2E1 代谢。女性经 ADH 代谢的能力比男性差。CYP1E2 在偶尔饮酒者中起的作用较弱，但是对于长期重度饮酒者，是一个重要的可诱导的代谢途径。CYP1A2、CYP3A4 和很多其他 CYP 酶也起微弱的作用 [5,6]。

CYP2E1 和 ADH 将乙醇转化为乙醛。乙醛既是一种有毒性的物质，引起"双硫仑反应"中的不适症状（如脸红、头痛、恶心、不适），也是造成肝损害的主要化合物。它也有精神药物的效应——乙醇在大脑中被 CYP2E1 代谢为乙醛 [7]。已知在大脑等部位，过氧化氢酶也将乙醇代谢为乙醛 [8]。乙醛进一步被乙醛脱氢酶代谢为乙酸，然后是二氧化碳和水。

所有参与乙醇代谢的酶都具有遗传多态性。例如，40% 的北亚裔为 ADH 慢代谢者 [9]。肝脏代谢酶的功能会因饮酒发生改变。长期饮酒可以诱导 CYP2E1 和 CYP3A4 酶活性。乙醇对其他肝脏代谢酶的影响尚未系统研究。

乙醇的代谢途径

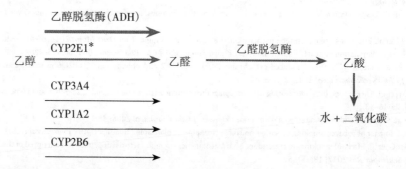

* 在偶尔饮酒者中是次要代谢途径；在酒滥用者和血液乙醇浓度高者，是主要代谢途径。体内无处不在的过氧化氢酶也能代谢乙醇，其在乙醇总体代谢中占多大比重目前尚不清楚。对乙醇脱氢酶和醛脱氢酶有抑制作用的药物，见表 11.5。

酒精滥用者中，很难预测酒精与药物的相互作用，因为两个相反的过程同时起作用：在饮酒或醉酒期间竞争酶结合位点（增加药物血浆水平），在有节制饮酒期间酶诱导作用占优势（降低药物血浆水平 [8]）。对于长期饮酒者，特别是狂饮者，在醉酒期间，处方药物的血浆水平可能会达到中毒水平。当患者有节制饮酒后，药物降低到有效浓度水平以下。甚至对于非醉酒的个体，仍有一些证据显示，接受药物治疗并同时饮酒，会对 CYP3A4 酶产生竞争性抑制，这会增加经该酶代谢的药物暴露量（表 11.6）[13]。这就使优化躯体疾病或精神疾病的治疗变得很困难。

表 11.5 抑制乙醇脱氢酶和醛脱氢酶的药物

酶	酶抑制剂	可能后果
乙醇脱氢酶	阿司匹林 H$_2$ 拮抗剂	减少乙醇代谢,造成乙醇长时间在血浆中高浓度
乙醛脱氢酶	氯磺丙脲 双硫仑 灰黄霉素 异烟肼 硝酸异山梨酯 甲硝唑 * 呋喃妥因 磺胺甲噁唑 甲苯丁胺	降低代谢乙醛的能力,导致"双硫仑"样反应:面红、头痛、心动过速、恶心、呕吐、心律失常和低血压

* 甲硝唑对乙醛脱氢酶活性有影响的证据极弱[10-12]。

表 11.6 饮酒和使用 CYP2E1 和 CYP3A4 代谢酶的底物

	代谢酶底物 (注:该清单并不详尽)	在醉酒患者中的影响	在长期、有节制饮酒者中的影响
CYP2E1	对乙酰氨基酚 异烟肼 苯巴比妥 华法林 佐匹克隆	乙醇和药物的竞争,造成药物和乙醇的代谢率下降。血浆水平的升高,可能会导致中毒	CYP2E1 的活性可能升高达 10 倍。药物代谢的增强可能会导致治疗失败
CYP3A4	阿普唑仑 阿立哌唑 苯二氮䓬类 卡马西平 氯氮平 多奈哌齐 加兰他敏 氟哌啶醇 美沙酮 米氮平 喹硫平 利培酮 西地那非 三环类药物 丙戊酸盐 文拉法辛 Z 类催眠药	乙醇和药物的竞争造成药物和乙醇的代谢率下降。血浆水平的升高,可能会导致中毒	药物代谢的增强可能会导致治疗失败停止饮酒后,酶诱导可能会持续几周

原因未明的相互作用包括：服用维拉帕米的患者血浆乙醇水平升高，饮酒者哌甲酯的代谢变慢。

药效动力学相互作用[2-4]

乙醇可以增强 γ-氨基丁酸（GABA$_A$）受体的抑制性神经传递，减少谷氨酸 NMDA 受体的兴奋性神经传递（表 11.7）。它也可以增加中脑边缘通路多巴胺的释放，可能对 5-羟色胺和阿片通路有一些影响。鉴于这些作用，单用乙醇可以引起镇静、遗忘、共济失调，以及产生愉快感（或在易感个体中加重精神病性症状）。

表 11.7　与乙醇的药效动力学相互作用

乙醇的作用	可加重乙醇作用的药物	可能后果
镇静	其他镇静剂，如： 抗组胺药 抗精神病药 巴氯芬 苯二氮䓬类药 洛非西定 阿片类制剂 替扎尼定 三环类药物 Z 类催眠药	增加中枢神经系统的抑制，从事故倾向增加，到呼吸抑制和死亡
遗忘	其他致遗忘的药物，如： 巴比妥类药 苯二氮䓬类药 Z 类催眠药	增加了遗忘作用，从轻度记忆减退，到完全遗忘。通常为顺行性遗忘：忘记酒精起作用后发生的事情
共济失调	血管紧张素转换酶抑制剂 β 受体阻滞剂 钙通道阻滞剂 硝酸盐 肾上腺素 α 受体拮抗剂， 如： 氯氮平 利培酮 三环类药物	增加步态不稳和摔倒

注：存在药代学相互作用时，药效学相互作用更明显。例如，长期严重饮酒者，酒醒状态下，酶诱导作用会增加地西泮的代谢，导致焦虑水平升高（治疗失败）。如果同一患者处于醉酒状态，地西泮不得不与酒精竞争 CYP3A4 的代谢能力，导致地西泮的代谢明显减慢。地西泮和酒精的血浆水平会升高（发生毒性反应）。酒精和地西泮均为镇静剂（通过 GABA$_A$ 亲和性），可能发生意识丧失和呼吸抑制。

乙醇通过增加中脑边缘通路多巴胺的释放，可能会导致或加重精神病性症状。抗精神病药的作用可以被竞争性拮抗，因而降低疗效（表 11.8）。

继发于酒精所致脱水的电解质紊乱,如果再用其他导致电解质紊乱的药物(如利尿剂),可能会加重。

注意:使用胰岛素或服用降糖药的糖尿病患者,重度饮酒可以造成低血糖。理论上,服用二甲双胍的患者饮酒,会增加乳酸性酸中毒的风险。此外,乙醇也可以升高血压。

长期饮酒者对阿司匹林和 NSAID 的胃肠道刺激作用特别敏感。

表 11.8　继续饮酒患者的精神药物选择

	最安全的选择	最好避免使用
抗精神病药	舒必利和氨磺必利;帕立哌酮,如果需要长效剂型(无镇静性作用,经肾排泄)	镇静作用明显的抗精神病药,如氯丙嗪和氯氮平
抗抑郁药	SSRI——西酞普兰,舍曲林 在长期饮酒者中,强 CYP3A4 抑制剂(氟西汀、帕罗西汀)可能会降低乙醇代谢	TCA,醉酒时乙醇损害代谢过程,可以导致血药浓度升高,出现药物过量的体征和症状(明显低血压、癫痫发作、心律失常和昏迷) 电解质紊乱可加重心脏不良反应 TCA 和乙醇合用可明显损害精神运动能力 米氮平——往往镇静作用较强 MAOI 可导致严重低血压。与含酪氨酸饮料可能有相互作用,可能诱发高血压危象
心境稳定剂	丙戊酸盐 卡马西平 注:醉酒期间血药浓度较高,可能耐受性差	锂盐:由于其治疗指数比较窄,并且酒精相关的脱水和电解质紊乱可以诱发锂中毒

注:
长期酒滥用者存在肝衰竭或肝功能减退的可能。见第 8 章相关内容。
同时注意,一些推荐的药物可能有肝毒性风险(如丙戊酸盐)。
MAOI,单胺氧化酶抑制剂;SSRI,5-羟色胺选择性重摄取抑制剂;TCA,三环类抗抑郁药。

(司天梅 译　田成华 审校)

参考文献

1. Zakhari S. Overview: how is alcohol metabolized by the body? *Alcohol Research & Health: The Journal of the National Institute on Alcohol Abuse and Alcoholism* 2006; **29**:245–254.
2. Tanaka E. Toxicological interactions involving psychiatric drugs and alcohol: an update. *J Clin Pharm Ther* 2003; **28**:81–95.
3. Wan Chih T. Alcohol-related drug interactions. *Pharmacist's Letter/Prescriber's Letter* 2008; **24**:240106.
4. Smith RG. An appraisal of potential drug interactions in cigarette smokers and alcohol drinkers. *J Am Podiatr Med Assoc* 2009; **99**:81–88.
5. Salmela KS, et al. Respective roles of human cytochrome P-4502E1, 1A2, and 3A4 in the hepatic microsomal ethanol oxidizing system. *Alcohol Clin Exp Res* 1998; **22**:2125–2132.
6. Hamitouche S, et al. Ethanol oxidation into acetaldehyde by 16 recombinant human cytochrome P450 isoforms: role of CYP2C isoforms in human liver microsomes. *Toxicol Lett* 2006; **167**:221–230.
7. Koster M, et al. Seizures during antidepressant treatment in psychiatric inpatients–results from the transnational pharmacovigilance project "Arzneimittelsicherheit in der Psychiatrie" (AMSP) 1993–2008. *Psychopharmacology* 2013; **230**:191–201.

8. Cederbaum AI. Alcohol metabolism. *Clin Liver Dis* 2012; **16**:667–685.

9. Wall TL, et al. Biology, genetics, and environment: underlying factors influencing alcohol metabolism. *Alcohol Research: Current Reviews* 2016; **38**:59–68.

10. Williams CS, et al. Do ethanol and metronidazole interact to produce a disulfiram-like reaction? *Ann Pharmacother* 2000; **34**:255–257.

11. Visapää JP, et al. Lack of disulfiram-like reaction with metronidazole and ethanol. *Ann Pharmacother* 2002; **36**:971–974.

12. Mergenhagen KA, et al. Fact versus fiction: a review of the evidence behind alcohol and antibiotic interactions. *Antimicrob Agents Chemother* 2020; **64**:e02167–02119.

13. Huang Z, et al. Influence of ethanol on the metabolism of alprazolam. *Expert Opin Drug Metab Toxicol* 2018; **14**:551–559.

其他物质

咖啡因

咖啡因可能是世界上最常用的精神活性物质。在英国平均每天消耗 350~620mg[1]。经常饮用咖啡因超过 500mg/d 者,一般人群中有 1/4,精神疾病患者中有 1/2[2]。应该和饮用咖啡因的患者进行常规讨论,以评估咖啡因对其症状及表现的影响[3],尤其是咖啡因戒断会对精神和躯体健康有明显的影响(表 12.1)。

巧克力中也含有咖啡因。《马丁代尔药典》中列出了超过 600 种含咖啡因的药物[4]。大多数是非处方药,作为止痛药或者抑制食欲的药物销售。

表 12.1 饮料中的咖啡因含量

饮料	咖啡因含量
煮咖啡	每杯 100mg
红牛饮料	每罐 80mg(其他能量饮料可能含量高得多)
速溶咖啡	每杯 60mg
红茶	每杯 45mg
绿茶	每杯 20~30mg
软饮料	每罐 25~50mg

表 12.2 咖啡因的剂量和精神药物效应

剂量	精神药物效应
一般剂量	中枢神经系统兴奋 增加儿茶酚胺的释放,特别是多巴胺[5]
低至中等剂量[2,6]	心境高涨 冲动 平静
大剂量 >600mg/d[7] [敏感(不耐受)个体可在较低剂量就感受到;长期使用者可产生耐受]	焦虑 失眠 精神运动性激越 兴奋 言语混乱 谵妄 精神病

咖啡因的一般影响

- 急性使用咖啡因可以升高收缩压和舒张压 10mmHg 长达 4h[3]。慢性中等剂量咖啡因可能对血压影响不大[8]。
- 可以增强尼古丁(或其他滥用药物)的强化效应[4,9]。
- 咖啡因也有精神药物的作用(表 12.2),可能会加重原有的精神疾病,并与精神药物有相互作用。
- 咖啡因是腺苷 A_1 和 A_{2A} 受体拮抗剂,对多巴胺通路有刺激作用。

咖啡因的精神药物效应

已知存在戒断综合征,症状包括头痛、抑郁心境、焦虑、疲乏、易激惹、恶心、心烦和渴求[10]。

药代动力学

- 吸收
  - 口服后快速吸收,尤其是液体。
  - 半衰期 2.5~4.5h。
- 代谢
  - 由具有遗传多态性的肝细胞色素酶 CYP1A2 进行代谢,这可以部分解释个体间在耐受咖啡因能力方面差异较大的原因[11]。注意,CYP1A2 可以被吸烟诱导,也可以被一些药物如氟伏沙明所抑制。
  - 高剂量时,代谢路径也能被饱和[12]。
- 相互作用(表 12.3)
  - 咖啡因对其他药物代谢有潜在的影响,并可能会诱发咖啡因戒断症状,在替换无咖啡因饮料前应当加以考虑。
  - 咖啡因竞争性地抑制 CYP1A2。如果停用咖啡因,一些药物的血浆水平可能会降低。

表 12.3 与咖啡因有交互作用的物质

产生交互作用的物质	影响	评论
CYP1A2 抑制剂:	减少咖啡因清除	可延长或增强咖啡因的作用
雌激素		可能会增加不良反应
西咪替丁		可能引起咖啡因中毒
氟伏沙明(可使咖啡		
因清除率减少 80%)[13]		
双硫仑		
吸烟 *	CYP1A2 诱导剂——增加咖啡因代谢[5]	吸烟者可能需要更大的咖啡因剂量才能获得所需的效果[7]
锂盐	高剂量可降低血锂浓度	停用咖啡因可导致血锂浓度升高[14]
单胺氧化酶抑制剂	可增强对中枢神经系统的兴奋作用	

续表

产生交互作用的物质	影响	评论
氯氮平	咖啡因可升高氯氮平最高达 60%[15]	推测其机制是竞争性抑制 CYP1A2 活性。通过同一机制受影响的药物包括奥氮平、丙米嗪和氯米帕明
SSRI 类药物	大剂量咖啡因可增加 5-羟色胺综合征的风险 [16]	
苯二氮䓬类药物	咖啡因可起拮抗剂的作用	降低苯二氮䓬类药物疗效 [7]

* 电子烟对 CYP1A2 酶活性没有影响。

SSRI，5-羟色胺选择性重摄取抑制剂。

咖啡因中毒

《精神障碍诊断与统计手册》第 5 版（DSM-5）[17] 将咖啡因中毒定义为最近饮用咖啡因，通常超过 250mg，且有框 12.1 中所列症状的 5 个或以上。

咖啡因中毒时，这些症状会导致明显的痛苦，以及社交、职业或其他重要领域功能的损害；这些症状并非普通躯体疾病所致，也无法以其他精神障碍（如焦虑障碍）解释。

框 12.1　咖啡因中毒的症状

■ 不安	■ 胃肠道功能紊乱
■ 紧张	■ 肌肉抽搐
■ 兴奋	■ 思维与语言散漫
■ 失眠	■ 心动过速或心律失常
■ 脸红	■ 不知疲倦
■ 利尿	■ 精神运动性激越

咖啡因滥用或依赖作为一种临床综合征已被报道 [3]，咖啡因使用障碍和咖啡因戒断综合征都属于 DSM-5 的诊断。

能量饮料

能量饮料都含有大量的咖啡因，以及糖、维生素和许多其他成分，如瓜拉纳和牛磺酸。有证据表明这些饮料可以提高注意力和短期记忆 [18]。该饮料主要面向青少年和年轻人，他们大量饮用这些饮料，特别容易出现咖啡因中毒的体征和症状。焦虑、抑郁、明显的自杀行为和癫痫发作都与年轻人使用这些产品相关 [19-21]。若同时饮用咖啡因和酒精，可能导致攻击行为 [22]。过量使用可能导致急性精神病 [23,24] 或躁狂发作 [25]。

精神分裂症

■ 精神分裂症患者常摄入含大量咖啡因的饮料 [1]，且咖啡因摄入量 >200mg/d 的比例是正常人的 2 倍 [5]。

- 含咖啡因的饮料可以用来缓解口干(一些抗精神病药的不良反应),获得咖啡因的兴奋作用(缓解心烦、镇静或阴性症状)[5],或者仅仅是因为喝咖啡或茶是一种生活方式,或者缓解无聊。
- 精神分裂症患者对于药物相关的暗示更敏感[5]。
- 中等剂量的咖啡因摄入可以改善精神分裂症患者的认知损害和阴性症状,但相关研究不足[26]。
- 大剂量的咖啡因可加重精神病性症状[5,27](特别是情感高涨和概念混乱),导致使用大剂量抗精神病药。
- 对于长期行为紊乱(挑衅行为)的患者,从其饮食中去除咖啡因以后,最终可以降低其敌意、易激惹和多疑程度[28],但无明显行为紊乱的患者可能无此表现[29]。
- 停用咖啡因可能对氯氮平治疗无效的精神分裂症患者有益[30]。

心境障碍

- 咖啡因可通过增加去甲肾上腺素的释放来提高心境[31];没有心境障碍的个体少量使用咖啡因可以预防抑郁[32]。
- 心境障碍患者更可能使用咖啡因,特别是处于抑郁状态时[14,33]。
- 抑郁症患者可能对咖啡因的致焦虑作用更敏感[34,35]。
- 过多摄入咖啡因可能会引发躁狂[35,36]。
- 咖啡因会增加皮质醇的分泌(在地塞米松抑制试验中呈假阳性)[37],在电休克治疗中延长癫痫发作的时间[38],并通过促进利尿来增加锂盐从体内的清除[39]。

焦虑症

- 咖啡因可以提高警觉性,缩短反应时间,延长睡眠潜伏期,降低睡眠质量;在慢代谢者中,这些作用更明显。
- 可引起或加重广泛性焦虑障碍和惊恐发作[40],对这些作用的易感性可能由遗传决定[9]。
- 咖啡因中毒症状如此明显,当患者倾诉焦虑症状或失眠时,应总是考虑咖啡因中毒。
- 若避免使用咖啡因,这些症状则可以明显减轻,甚至完全消失[41]。
- 惊恐障碍患者比对照者饮用更多的咖啡因[42],但是原因并不清楚。

其他精神障碍

微弱的证据支持咖啡因对注意缺陷多动障碍(ADHD)患者有益[43],大剂量饮用咖啡因可以预防老年人的认知减退[44]。

小结

咖啡因:

- 大量存在于咖啡和一些软饮中,特别是能量饮料。
- 可能会加重精神病性症状和焦虑,年轻人尤其易感。
- 可抑制氯氮平的代谢。
- 可能会引起中毒,表现为精神运动性激越和言语紊乱。

- 与 CYP1A2 抑制剂（如氟伏沙明）合用时，可能会引起中毒。
- 可以增强尼古丁（也可能其他滥用药物）的强化作用。

参考文献

1. Rihs M, et al. Caffeine consumption in hospitalized psychiatric patients. Eur Arch Psychiatry Clin Neurosci 1996; **246**:83–92.
2. Clementz GL, et al. Psychotropic effects of caffeine. Am Fam Physician 1988; **37**:167–172.
3. Ogawa N, et al. Clinical importance of caffeine dependence and abuse. Psychiatry Clin Neurosci 2007; **61**:263–268.
4. Pharmaceutical Press. Martindale: the complete drug reference (online). 2020. https://www.medicinescomplete.com/.
5. Adolfo AB, et al. Effects of smoking cues on caffeine urges in heavy smokers and caffeine consumers with and without schizophrenia. Schizophr Res 2009; **107**:192–197.
6. Grant JE, et al. Caffeine's influence on gambling behavior and other types of impulsivity. Addict Behav 2018; **76**:156–160.
7. Sawynok J. Pharmacological rationale for the clinical use of caffeine. Drugs 1995; **49**:37–50.
8. O'Keefe JH, et al. Effects of habitual coffee consumption on cardiometabolic disease, cardiovascular health, and all-cause mortality. JAmCollCardiol 2013; **62**:1043–1051.
9. Bergin JE, et al. Common psychiatric disorders and caffeine use, tolerance, and withdrawal: an examination of shared genetic and environmental effects. TwinResHumGenet 2012; **15**:473–482.
10. Silverman K, et al. Withdrawal syndrome after the double-blind cessation of caffeine consumption. N Engl J Med 1992; **327**:1109–1114.
11. Butler MA, et al. Determination of CYP1A2 and NAT2 phenotypes in human populations by analysis of caffeine urinary metabolites. Pharmacogenetics 1992; **2**:116–127.
12. Kaplan GB, et al. Dose-dependent pharmacokinetics and psychomotor effects of caffeine in humans. J Clin Pharmacol 1997; **37**:693–703.
13. Medicines Complete. Stockley's drug interactions. 2020. https://www.medicinescomplete.com/.
14. Baethge C, et al. Coffee and cigarette use: association with suicidal acts in 352 Sardinian bipolar disorder patients. Bipolar Disorders 2009; **11**:494–503.
15. Carrillo JA, et al. Effects of caffeine withdrawal from the diet on the metabolism of clozapine in schizophrenic patients. J Clin Psychopharmacol 1998; **18**:311–316.
16. Shioda K, et al. Possible serotonin syndrome arising from an interaction between caffeine and serotonergic antidepressants. Human Psychopharmacology 2004; **19**:353–354.
17. American Psychiatric Association. Diagnostic and Statistical Manual of Mental Disorders, Fifth Edition (DSM-5). Arlington, VA: American Psychiatric Association 2013.
18. Wesnes KA, et al. An evaluation of the cognitive and mood effects of an energy shot over a 6h period in volunteers: a randomized, double-blind, placebo controlled, cross-over study. Appetite 2013; **67**:105–113.
19. Szpak A, et al. A case of acute suicidality following excessive caffeine intake. J Psychopharmacol 2012; **26**:1502–1510.
20. Trapp GS, et al. Energy drink consumption among young Australian adults: associations with alcohol and illicit drug use. Drug Alcohol Depend 2014; **134**:30–37.
21. Pennington N, et al. Energy drinks: a new health hazard for adolescents. J Sch Nurs 2010; **26**:352–359.
22. Sheehan BE, et al. Caffeinated and non-caffeinated alcohol use and indirect aggression: the impact of self-regulation. Addict Behav 2016; **58**:53–59.
23. Görgülü Y, et al. A case of acute psychosis following energy drink consumption. Noro Psikiyatri Arsivi 2014; **51**:79–81.
24. Kelsey D, et al. A case of psychosis and renal failure associated with excessive energy drink consumption. Case Reports in Psychiatry 2019; **2019**:3954161.
25. Quadri S, et al. An energy drink-induced manic episode in an adolescent. Prim Care Companion CNS Disord 2018; **20**: 18l02318
26. Topyurek M, et al. Caffeine effects and schizophrenia: is there a need for more research? Schizophr Res 2019; **211**:34–35.
27. Wang HR, et al. Caffeine-induced psychiatric manifestations: a review. Int Clin Psychopharmacol 2015; **30**:179–182.
28. De Freitas B, et al. Effects of caffeine in chronic psychiatric patients. Am J Psychiatry 1979; **136**:1337–1338.
29. Koczapski A, et al. Effects of caffeine on behavior of schizophrenic inpatients. Schizophr Bull 1989; **15**:339–344.
30. Dratcu L, et al. Clozapine-resistant psychosis, smoking, and caffeine: managing the neglected effects of substances that our patients consume every day. Am J Ther 2007; **14**:314–318.
31. Achor MB, et al. Diet aids, mania, and affective illness. Am J Psychiatry 1981; **138**:392.
32. Wang L, et al. Coffee and caffeine consumption and depression: A meta-analysis of observational studies. Aust N Z J Psychiatry 2016; **50**:228–242.
33. Maremmani I, et al. Are "social drugs" (tobacco, coffee and chocolate) related to the bipolar spectrum? J AffectDisord 2011; **133**:227–233.
34. Lee MA, et al. Anxiogenic effects of caffeine on panic and depressed patients. Am J Psychiatry 1988; **145**:632–635.
35. Rizkallah E, et al. Could the use of energy drinks induce manic or depressive relapse among abstinent substance use disorder patients with comorbid bipolar spectrum disorder? BipolarDisord 2011; **13**:578–580.
36. Machado-Vieira R, et al. Mania associated with an energy drink: the possible role of caffeine, taurine, and inositol. Can J Psychiatry 2001; **46**:454–455.
37. Uhde TW, et al. Caffeine-induced escape from dexamethasone suppression. Arch Gen Psychiatry 1985; **42**:737–738.
38. Cantu TG, et al. Caffeine in electroconvulsive therapy. Ann Pharmacother 1991; **25**:1079–1080.
39. Mester R, et al. Caffeine withdrawal increases lithium blood levels. Biol Psychiatry 1995; **37**:348–350.

40. Bruce MS. The anxiogenic effects of caffeine. Postgrad Med J 1990; **66 Suppl 2**:S18–S24.

41. Bruce MS, et al. Caffeine abstention in the management of anxiety disorders. Psychol Med 1989; **19**:211–214.

42. Santos VA, et al. Panic disorder and chronic caffeine use: a case-control study. Clin Pract Epidemiol Ment Health 2019; **15**:120–125.

43. Ioannidis K, et al. Ostracising caffeine from the pharmacological arsenal for attention-deficit hyperactivity disorder–was this a correct decision? A literature review. Journal of Psychopharmacology (Oxford, England) 2014; **28**:830–836.

44. Panza F, et al. Coffee, tea, and caffeine consumption and prevention of late-life cognitive decline and dementia: a systematic review. J Nutr Health Aging 2015; **19**:313–328.

尼古丁

常见摄取尼古丁的方式是吸电子烟或烟草。吸烟者的比例：一般人群中不足 1/4,抑郁症患者 40%~50%[1],精神分裂症患者 70%~80%[2]。尼古丁导致外周血管收缩、心动过速和血压升高[3]。精神分裂症患者中,吸烟者比不吸烟者更易出现代谢综合征[4]。除了尼古丁,香烟中还含有焦油(一种有机分子的复杂混合物,大多是致癌的),它可导致呼吸系统癌症、慢性支气管炎和肺气肿[5]。据称,电子香烟只含有尼古丁(还有一些必要的辅料),其毒性非常小,不会致癌。因此,尽管对其所含物质的质量控制和所谓吸烟正常化方面有所保留,电子烟仍受到所有吸烟者欢迎。电子烟很可能并非没有风险,但这是一个非常复杂的领域,超出了本书的范畴。

尼古丁的成瘾性很高,这可能至少有一部分受遗传决定[6]。有精神障碍的人发展并保持尼古丁成瘾的可能性比普通人群高 2~3 倍[1]。长期吸烟会增加精神障碍患者中呼吸系统疾病和心血管病的发病率和死亡率。尼古丁也具有精神作用。吸烟可影响精神药物的代谢过程(继而影响疗效和毒性)[7]。请见第 11 章"吸烟和精神药物"。尼古丁使用是尝试其他精神活性物质的入门药。

精神作用

尼古丁具有高脂溶性,吸入后迅速进入大脑。研究发现尼古丁受体在多巴胺能细胞体上,对这些受体的刺激会导致多巴胺释放[1]。边缘系统的多巴胺释放与愉悦感有关:多巴胺是大脑的"奖赏性"神经递质。有心理健康问题的人使用尼古丁,可能是一种"自我用药"(例如缓解精神分裂症的阴性症状、抗精神病药引起的烦躁以及抗焦虑作用[8])。增加多巴胺释放的药物会减少对尼古丁的渴求,它们还可能会使精神病恶化(见本章"戒烟")。

尼古丁改善注意力和警觉性[1],机制可能是增强谷氨酸、乙酰胆碱和 5-羟色胺的作用[8]。

精神分裂症

70%~80% 的精神分裂症患者经常吸烟[2](越来越多的人改用电子烟[9,10]),而且吸烟增加的趋势早在精神症状发作之前就已出现[11]。吸烟实际上可能是精神分裂症发病的一个原因[12]。对尼古丁使用率高的可能解释如下[13]:吸烟导致多巴胺释放,使个体产生感觉良好的效果,并减轻阴性症状[8];减轻抗精神病药的不良反应,如嗜睡、锥体外系反应[1]和认知减慢[14,15];吸烟可作为一种消遣的方式(一种行为填补方式);吸烟也是一种家族易感性导致的结果[16],或吸烟可用于缓解常见于精神分裂症的听觉门控缺陷[17]。尼古丁还可以改善工作记忆和注意缺陷[18-20]。烟碱受体激动剂可能对神经认知功能有益[21,22],但是尚未被许用于此目的。胆碱能药物可能会加重尼古丁依赖[23]。一项单光子发射计算机断层扫描(SPECT)研究表明,抗精神病药对纹状体 D_2 受体占有率越高,患者吸烟的可能性越大[24]。这个结果可以部分解释临床观察到的现象,即氯氮平(一种多巴胺受体的弱拮抗剂)代替传统抗精神病药后,更容易戒烟。有研究表明精神分裂症患者特别耐受不了尼古丁戒断症状[7](尽管一些患者肯定能戒掉[25])。因而,换用尼古丁替代疗法(NRT)或电子烟可能是

更好的选择 [26,27]。研究结果显示,即使是严重的精神障碍患者,换用电子烟也可以很好地耐受 [28]。

抑郁和焦虑

在"正常"人群中,适度使用尼古丁可带来愉悦感,缓解焦虑和愤怒情绪 [29]。目前,尼古丁的抗焦虑机制还不清楚。有焦虑或抑郁的人更有可能吸烟 [30,31] 并很难戒烟 [29,32]。尼古丁可能就具有抗抑郁效果 [33]。尼古丁戒断可引起或加重原有抑郁症病史者的抑郁 [29],而且吸烟可以直接增加抑郁症状的发生风险 [34]。形成鲜明对比的是,一些研究结果表明,停止吸烟实际上能改善抑郁和焦虑 [35,36]。对这些矛盾结果的解释是,戒烟早期会加重抑郁症状,成功戒烟则长期改善抑郁症状。一项 Cochrane 综述 [37] 表明,吸烟的抑郁症患者可以成功戒烟,但是最近一项双生子研究结果发现抑郁症患者很少能戒烟 [38]。

抑郁症患者患心血管病的风险增加。理论上,尼古丁直接引起心动过速和高血压,从而加重心血管病 [3]。更重要的是,吸烟是众所周知的心血管病的独立危险因素,因为吸烟可促发动脉粥样硬化。电子烟,虽然不具有致癌性,但可能增加心血管病的风险 [39]。一项近期的研究结果表明,尼古丁依赖和抑郁严重程度是心血管病的独立相关因素 [40]。

运动障碍与帕金森病

尼古丁通过增加多巴胺能神经传递,对药物所致的锥体外系反应和特发性帕金森病具有保护作用。吸烟者发生抗精神病药所致运动障碍的可能性比不吸烟者要小 [1],且需要服用的抗胆碱能药也少 [7]。与不吸烟者相比,吸烟人群中较少发生帕金森病,且出现临床症状的时间也晚 [1,41]。这可能反映的是帕金森病与感觉寻求行为之间存在着负相关关系,而不是尼古丁的直接影响 [42]。

药物的相互作用

众所周知,香烟烟雾中的多环芳烃可刺激肝脏微粒体酶系统,特别是 CYP1A2,参与许多精神药物的代谢过程。吸烟可使一些药物的血药浓度降低高达 50% [8]。这可能会影响药物的疗效和不良反应,进行临床决策时需要考虑这个问题。最有可能受到影响的药物有:氯氮平 [43]、奋乃静、氟哌啶醇、氯丙嗪、奥氮平、许多三环类抗抑郁药、米氮平、氟伏沙明和普萘洛尔。电子烟对转氨酶活性没有影响。见第 11 章"吸烟和精神药物"。

戒断症状 [7]

戒断症状发生在停止吸烟后的 6~12h 内,包括强烈的渴求、抑郁心境、失眠、焦虑、烦躁不安、易激惹、注意力集中困难和食欲增加。尼古丁戒断可能会与抑郁、焦虑、睡眠障碍和躁狂相混淆。戒断也会恶化精神分裂症的症状。

戒烟

见第 4 章"尼古丁和戒烟"。

(司天梅　译　田成华　审校)

参考文献

1. Goff DC et al. Cigarette smoking in schizophrenia: relationship to psychopathology and medication side effects. Am J Psychiatry 1992; 149:1189–1194.
2. Winterer G. Why do patients with schizophrenia smoke? Curr Opin Psychiatry 2010; 23:112–119.
3. Benowitz NL et al. Cardiovascular effects of nasal and transdermal nicotine and cigarette smoking. Hypertension 2002; 39:1107–1112.
4. Yevtushenko OO et al. Influence of 5-HT2 C receptor and leptin gene polymorphisms, smoking and drug treatment on metabolic disturbances in patients with schizophrenia. Br J Psychiatry 2008; 192:424–428.
5. Anderson JE et al. Treating tobacco use and dependence: an evidence-based clinical practice guideline for tobacco cessation. Chest 2002; 121:932–941.
6. Berrettini W. Nicotine addiction. Am J Psychiatry 2008; 165:1089–1092.
7. Ziedonis DM et al. Schizophrenia and nicotine use: report of a pilot smoking cessation program and review of neurobiological and clinical issues. Schizophr Bull 1997; 23:247–254.
8. Lyon ER. A review of the effects of nicotine on schizophrenia and antipsychotic medications. Psychiatr Serv 1999; 50:1346–1350.
9. Sharma R et al. Motivations and limitations associated with vaping among people with mental illness: a qualitative analysis of reddit discussions. Int J Environ Res Public Health 2016; 14:7.
10. Bianco CL. Rates of electronic cigarette use among adults with a chronic mental illness. Addict Behav 2019; 89:1–4.
11. Weiser M et al. Higher rates of cigarette smoking in male adolescents before the onset of schizophrenia: a historical-prospective cohort study. Am J Psychiatry 2004; 161:1219–1223.
12. Hunter A et al. The effects of tobacco smoking, and prenatal tobacco smoke exposure, on risk of schizophrenia: a systematic review and meta-analysis. Nicotine Tobacco Res 2020; 22:3–10.
13. Caponnetto P et al. Tobacco smoking, related harm and motivation to quit smoking in people with schizophrenia spectrum disorders. Health Psychol Res 2020; 8:9042.
14. Harris JG et al. Effects of nicotine on cognitive deficits in schizophrenia. Neuropsychopharmacology 2004; 29:1378–1385.
15. Gupta T et al. Nicotine usage is associated with elevated processing speed, spatial working memory, and visual learning performance in youth at ultrahigh-risk for psychosis. Psychiatry Res 2014; 220:687–690.
16. Ferchiou A et al. Exploring the relationships between tobacco smoking and schizophrenia in first-degree relatives. Psychiatry Res 2012; 200:674–678.
17. McEvoy JP et al. Smoking and therapeutic response to clozapine in patients with schizophrenia. Biol Psychiatry 1999; 46:125–129.
18. Jacobsen LK et al. Nicotine effects on brain function and functional connectivity in schizophrenia. Biol Psychiatry 2004; 55:850–858.
19. Sacco KA et al. Effects of cigarette smoking on spatial working memory and attentional deficits in schizophrenia: involvement of nicotinic receptor mechanisms. Arch Gen Psychiatry 2005; 62:649–659.
20. Smith RC et al. Effects of nicotine nasal spray on cognitive function in schizophrenia. Neuropsychopharmacology 2006; 31:637–643.
21. Olincy A et al. Proof-of-concept trial of an alpha7 nicotinic agonist in schizophrenia. Arch Gen Psychiatry 2006; 63:630–638.
22. Lieberman JA et al. Cholinergic agonists as novel treatments for schizophrenia: the promise of rational drug development for psychiatry. Am J Psychiatry 2008; 165:931–936.
23. Kelly DL et al. Lack of beneficial galantamine effect for smoking behavior: a double-blind randomized trial in people with schizophrenia. Schizophr Res 2008; 103:161–168.
24. de Haan L et al. Occupancy of dopamine D2 receptors by antipsychotic drugs is related to nicotine addiction in young patients with schizophrenia. Psychopharmacology (Berl) 2006; 183:500–505.
25. Gilbody S et al. Smoking cessation for people with severe mental illness (SCIMITAR+): a pragmatic randomised controlled trial. Lancet Psychiatry 2019; 6:379–390.
26. Caponnetto P et al. Impact of an electronic cigarette on smoking reduction and cessation in schizophrenic smokers: a prospective 12-month pilot study. Int J Environ Res Public Health 2013; 10:446–461.
27. Kozak K et al. Pharmacotherapy for smoking cessation in schizophrenia: a systematic review. Expert Opin Pharmacother 2020; 21:581–590.
28. Hickling LM et al. A pre-post pilot study of electronic cigarettes to reduce smoking in people with severe mental illness. Psychol Med 2019; 49:1033–1040.
29. Glassman AH. Cigarette smoking: implications for psychiatric illness. Am J Psychiatry 1993; 150:546–553.
30. Nunes SO et al. The shared role of oxidative stress and inflammation in major depressive disorder and nicotine dependence. Neurosci Biobehav Rev 2013; 37:1336–1345.
31. Tsuang MT et al. Genetics of smoking and depression. Hum Genet 2012; 131:905–915.
32. Wilhelm K et al. Clinical aspects of nicotine dependence and depression. Med Today 2004; 5:40–47.
33. Gandelman JA et al. Transdermal nicotine for the treatment of mood and cognitive symptoms in nonsmokers with late-life depression. J Clin Psychiatry 2018; 79:18m12137.
34. Boden JM et al. Cigarette smoking and depression: tests of causal linkages using a longitudinal birth cohort. Br J Psychiatry 2010; 196:440–446.
35. Taylor G et al. Change in mental health after smoking cessation: systematic review and meta-analysis. BMJ 2014; 348:g1151.
36. Cather C et al. Improved depressive symptoms in adults with schizophrenia during a smoking cessation attempt with varenicline and behavioral therapy. J Dual Diagn 2017; 13:168–178.

37. van der Meer RM et al. Smoking cessation interventions for smokers with current or past depression. Cochrane Database Syst Rev 2013; 8:CD006102.

38. Ranjit A et al. Depressive symptoms predict smoking cessation in a 20-year longitudinal study of adult twins. Addict Behav 2020; 108:106427.

39. Schweitzer RJ et al. E-cigarette use and indicators of cardiovascular disease risk. Curr Epidemiol Rep 2017; 4:248–257.

40. Bainter T et al. A key indicator of nicotine dependence is associated with greater depression symptoms, after accounting for smoking behavior. PLoS One 2020; 15:e0233656.

41. Scott WK et al. Family-based case-control study of cigarette smoking and Parkinson disease. Neurology 2005; 64:442–447.

42. Evans AH et al. Relationship between impulsive sensation seeking traits, smoking, alcohol and caffeine intake, and Parkinson's disease. J Neurol Neurosurg Psychiatry 2006; 77:317–321.

43. Derenne JL et al. Clozapine toxicity associated with smoking cessation: case report. Am J Ther 2005; 12:469–471.

第13章

特殊条件下的精神药物

精神药物过量使用

在精神科和全科临床工作中,经常会见到患者的自杀企图和自杀姿态,往往过量服用精神药物(表 13.1)。本节简要介绍常用精神药物过量的毒性,目的是帮助指导医师给有自杀风险的患者选择药物及安全的数量,并帮助识别药物过量的症状。本节不提供精神药物过量使用的治疗信息,读者可直接向毒物专业机构寻求帮助。只要怀疑药物过量,就强烈建议立即转诊到急诊。

表 13.1　精神药物过量

药物或药物类别	过量毒性	可能致死的最小剂量	过量的体征和症状
抗抑郁药			
阿戈美拉汀 [1,2]	低	无死亡报道。在较早的试验中,800mg 是最大耐受剂量。EU 的 SPC 报告,过量 2.45g 未出现严重不良反应。混合过量 7.5g 仅仅引起困倦和轻度心动过速	镇静,激越,胃痛,头晕
安非他酮 [3-6]	中等	约 4.5g,但最大 13.5g 的过量未致死亡 [7]	心动过速、癫痫发作、QRS 间期延长、Q-T 间期延长、心律失常。曾报告过激越和中毒性精神病。若合用文拉法辛,可发生致死性 5-羟色胺综合征 [8]
度洛西汀 [9-12]	低	不详——无单次药物过量致死的报道,但有许多混合过量死亡病例	困倦、心动过缓、低血压。可能无症状
洛非帕明 [13,14]	低	不详。单用不太可能致死	镇静、昏迷、心动过速、低血压
单胺氧化酶抑制剂(不含吗氯贝胺)[13,15-17]	高	苯乙肼——400mg 反苯环丙胺——200mg	震颤、乏力、意识模糊、出汗、心动过速、高血压
米安色林 [18-20]	低	不详,可能大于 1g。单用不太可能致死	镇静、昏迷、低血压、高血压、心动过速、可能 Q-T 间期延长

续表

药物或药物类别	过量毒性	可能致死的最小剂量	过量的体征和症状
米氮平 [3,21-24]	低	单用过量不太可能致死。1 个死亡案例报告,过量服用 990mg[25]	镇静,甚至明显过量也可能没有症状。有时可见心动过速、高血压、激越
吗氯贝胺 [26,27]	低	不详,可能大于 8g。单用不太可能致死	呕吐、镇静、定向力障碍
瑞波西汀 [3,28]	低	未知。单用不太可能致死	出汗、心动过速、血压改变
选择性 5-羟色胺再摄取抑制剂 [14,29-32]	低	不详。可能高于 1~2g。单用不太可能致死	呕吐、震颤、困倦、心动过速、ST 段压低。可能出现癫痫发作和 Q-T 间期延长。SSRI 过量时,西酞普兰毒性反应最强 [24,33](昏迷、癫痫发作、心律失常),艾司西酞普兰毒性较小 [34,35]
曲唑酮 [10,36-39]	低	不详,可能高于 10g。单用过量服用不太可能致死。暴露者致死率大约为 1/10 000[24]	困倦、恶心、低血压、头晕。罕见 Q-T 间期延长、心律失常
三环类抗抑郁药 [13,15,16,40](不含洛非帕明)	高	约 500mg。剂量超过 50mg/kg 通常可致死	镇静、昏迷、心动过速、心律失常(QRS、Q-T 间期延长)、低血压、癫痫发作
文拉法辛 [3,41-43](去甲文拉法辛同此,但是毒性弱 [44])	中等	可能超过 5g,但服用 1g 后可能出现癫痫发作	呕吐、镇静、心动过速、高血压、癫痫发作、酸中毒。罕见 Q-T 间期延长、心律失常、横纹肌溶解。极其罕见心搏骤停、心肌梗死、心力衰竭
维拉唑酮 [45,46]	低	剂量低于 300mg 不具致死性。在 714 例暴露者中未见致死记录 [24]	困倦、激越、恶心、癫痫发作
伏硫西汀 [47]	低	不详。一例过量报道,250mg 未见任何症状。	恶心、嗜睡、腹泻、瘙痒
抗精神病药			
氨磺必利 [48-50]	中等	约 16g	Q-T 间期延长、心律失常、心搏骤停
阿立哌唑 [51-53]	低	不详。单用不太可能致死	镇静、嗜睡、胃肠道功能紊乱、流涎
阿塞那平 [54]	可能较低	不详。无过量致死的报道。口服吸收很少	镇静、意识模糊、面部肌张力障碍、良性 ECG 改变
依匹哌唑 [55]	可能较低	暂无信息	推测激越和恶心
丁酰苯类 [56-58](如氟哌啶醇)	中等	氟哌啶醇——可能高于 500mg。300mg 可能发生心律失常	镇静、昏迷、肌张力障碍、恶性综合征、Q-T 间期延长、心律失常
卡利拉嗪 [59]	低	EU SPC 报告一例 48mg 过量病例	镇静,低血压

续表

药物或药物类别	过量毒性	可能致死的最小剂量	过量的体征和症状
氯氮平 [60-61]	中等	2g 左右,在不耐受的个体中要低很多 [62]	嗜睡、昏迷、心动过速、低血压、多涎、肺炎、癫痫发作
伊潘立酮 [63-65]	可能中等	不详,可能高于 500mg	对 Q-T 间期有较大的影响。可能有镇静、心动过速、呼吸抑制、低血压
卢美哌隆 [66]	可能较低	暂无过量报告	推测镇静和头晕
鲁拉西酮 [67]	低	不详。一例 1 360mg 的过量未致死 [68]。一项研究报道 821 例暴露未致死 [24]	信息很少。对 Q-T 间期有轻微影响
奥氮平 [60,69-71]	中等	不详,可能远超 200mg	嗜睡、意识模糊、肌阵挛、肌病、低血压、心动过速、谵妄。可能引起 Q-T 间期延长
吩噻嗪类 [56,72-74] (如氯丙嗪、氟奋乃静)	中等	氯丙嗪 5~10g	镇静、昏迷、心动过速、心律失常、肺水肿、低血压、Q-T 间期延长、癫痫发作、肌张力障碍、恶性综合征
匹莫范色林 [75]	未知	没有过量报告,但在临床剂量范围内可能延长 Q-T 间期	可能会发生 Q-T 间期延长和心律失常,恶心,呕吐,意识模糊 [76]
喹硫平 [24,60,77-80]	中等	不详。可能超过 5g。单药过量可致死	嗜睡、谵妄、心动过速、Q-T 间期延长、呼吸抑制、低血压、横纹肌溶解、恶性综合征
利培酮 [60,81,82] (帕利哌酮同此)	低	不详。单用利培酮或帕利哌酮过量罕见致死	嗜睡、肌张力障碍、心动过速、血压改变、Q-T 间期延长。帕利哌酮可致肾衰竭
齐拉西酮 [83-88]	低	约 10g。单用不太可能致死	困倦、嗜睡、Q-T 间期延长、尖端扭转型室性心动过速

心境稳定剂

药物或药物类别	过量毒性	可能致死的最小剂量	过量的体征和症状
卡马西平 [89,90]	中等	约 20g,但约 5g 即可出现癫痫发作	困倦、昏迷、呼吸抑制、共济失调、癫痫发作、心动过速、心律失常、电解质紊乱
拉莫三嗪 [91-92]	低	至少 4g。两例死亡报道——一例服用 4g,另一例服用 7.5g,但是过量 >40g 并未致死	困倦、呕吐、共济失调、癫痫发作、心动过速、运动障碍、Q-T 间期延长
锂盐 [93-95]	中等	单次过量偶可致死,慢性中毒更危险。在英国 2005—2012 年记录了 6 例急性过量死亡 [96]	恶心、腹泻、震颤、意识模糊、疲乏、癫痫发作、昏迷、心血管衰竭、心动过缓、心律失常、心搏骤停,肾衰竭
丙戊酸盐 [97-101]	中等	不详,可能超过 20g。剂量超过 400mg/kg 引起严重中毒	困倦、昏迷、脑水肿、呼吸抑制、恶病质、低血压、低体温、癫痫发作、电解质紊乱 (高血氨)

续表

药物或药物类别	过量毒性	可能致死的最小剂量	过量的体征和症状
其他			
苯二氮䓬类[102-103]	低	可能超过 100mg 地西泮等效剂量。单用很少致死。阿普唑仑毒性最大	困倦、共济失调、眼球震颤、呼吸性构音障碍、抑郁、昏迷
丁螺环酮[24]	低	资料有限,无死亡报道	未知
美沙酮[104-106]	高	未曾用过者 20~50mg 可能致死。与苯二氮䓬类合用增强毒性	困倦、恶心、低血压、呼吸抑制、昏迷、横纹肌溶解
莫达非尼[106-108]	低	不详,但无致死报道。6g 以上的过量并未导致死亡	心动过速、失眠、激越、焦虑、恶心、高血压、肌张力障碍
普瑞巴林[109,110]	低	无死亡报道。一例过量 8.4g 引起了意识丧失和昏迷	可能无症状。可出现镇静和昏迷
苏沃雷生[108]	低	不详,无致死报道	镇静,恶心
唑吡坦[111,112]	低	不详,可能大于 200mg。单用罕见致死	困倦、激越、呼吸抑制、心动过速、昏迷
佐匹克隆[102,113,114]	低	不详。可能大于 100mg。单用罕见致死	共济失调、恶心、复视、困倦、昏迷

ECG,心电图;GI,胃肠道;MAOI,单胺氧化酶抑制剂;MI,心肌梗死;NMS,恶性综合征;SPC,产品特征概要;SSRI,选择性 5-羟色胺再摄取抑制药。

高 = 服用不足 1 周用量可引起严重毒性反应或死亡。

中 = 服用 1~4 周用量可引起严重毒性反应或死亡。

低 = 服用即使超过 1 个月的用量也不太可能发生死亡或严重毒性反应。

参考文献

1. Howland RH Critical appraisal and update on the clinical utility of agomelatine, a melatonergic agonist, for the treatment of major depressive disease in adults. *Neuropsychiatr Dis Treat* 2009; 5:563–576.
2. Wong A, et al. Agomelatine overdose and related toxicity. *Toxicology Communications* 2018; 2:62–65.
3. Buckley NA, et al. 'Atypical' antidepressants in overdose: clinical considerations with respect to safety. *Drug Saf* 2003; 26:539–551.
4. Mercerolle M, et al. A fatal case of bupropion (Zyban) overdose. *J Anal Toxicol* 2008; 32:192–196.
5. Murray B, et al. Single-agent bupropion exposures: clinical characteristics and an atypical cause of serotonin toxicity. *J Med Toxicol* 2020; 16:12–16.
6. Overberg A, et al. Toxicity of bupropion overdose compared with selective serotonin reuptake inhibitors. *Pediatrics* 2019; 144:e20183295.
7. Zhu Y, et al. Atypical findings in massive bupropion overdose: a case report and discussion of psychopharmacologic issues. *J Psychiatr Pract* 2016; 22:405–409.
8. Alibegović A, et al. Fatal overdose with a combination of SNRIs venlafaxine and duloxetine. *Forensic Sci Med Pathol* 2019; 15:258–261.
9. Menchetti M, et al. Non-fatal overdose of duloxetine in combination with other antidepressants and benzodiazepines. *World J Biol Psychiatry* 2009; 10:385–389.
10. White N, et al. Suicidal antidepressant overdoses: a comparative analysis by antidepressant type. *J Med Toxicol* 2008; 4:238–250.
11. Darracq MA, et al. A retrospective review of isolated duloxetine-exposure cases. *ClinToxicol(Phila)* 2013; 51:106–110.
12. Scanlon KA, et al. Comprehensive duloxetine analysis in a fatal overdose. *J Anal Toxicol* 2016; 40:167–170.
13. Cassidy S, et al. Fatal toxicity of antidepressant drugs in overdose. *Br Med J* 1987; 295:1021–1024.
14. Henry JA, et al. Relative mortality from overdose of antidepressants. *BMJ* 1995; 310:221–224.

第 13 章

15. Crome P. Antidepressant overdosage. *Drugs* 1982; 23:431–461.

16. Henry JA. Epidemiology and relative toxicity of antidepressant drugs in overdose. *Drug Saf* 1997; 16:374–390.

17. Waring WS, et al. Acute myocarditis after massive phenelzine overdose. *Eur J Clin Pharmacol* 2007; 63:1007–1009.

18. Chand S, et al. One hundred cases of acute intoxication with minaserin hydrochloride. *Pharmacopsychiatry* 1981; 14:15–17.

19. Scherer D, et al. Inhibition of cardiac hERG potassium channels by tetracyclic antidepressant mianserin. *Naunyn Schmiedebergs Arch Pharmacol* 2008; 378:73–83.

20. Koseoglu Z, et al. Bradycardia and hypotension in mianserin intoxication. *Hum Exp Toxicol* 2010; 29:887–888.

21. Bremner JD, et al. Safety of mirtazapine in overdose. *J Clin Psychiatry* 1998; 59:233–235.

22. LoVecchio F, et al. Outcomes after isolated mirtazapine (Remeron) supratherapeutic ingestions. *J Emerg Med* 2008; 34:77–78.

23. Berling I, et al. Mirtazapine overdose is unlikely to cause major toxicity. *ClinToxicol(Phila)* 2014; 52:20–24.

24. Nelson JC, et al. Morbidity and mortality associated with medications used in the treatment of depression: an analysis of cases reported to u.s. poison control centers, 2000-2014. *Am J Psychiatry* 2017; 174:438–450.

25. Vignali C, et al. Mirtazapine fatal poisoning. *Forensic Sci Int* 2017; 276:e8-e12.

26. Hetzel W. Safety of moclobemide taken in overdose for attempted suicide. *Psychopharmacology (Berl)* 1992; 106 Suppl: S127-S129.

27. Myrenfors PG, et al. Moclobemide overdose. *J Intern Med* 1993; 233:113–115.

28. Baldwin DS, et al. Tolerability and safety of reboxetine. *Rev Contemp Pharmacother* 2000; 11:321–330.

29. Cheeta S, et al. Antidepressant-related deaths and antidepressant prescriptions in England and Wales, 1998-2000. *Br J Psychiatry* 2004; 184:41–47.

30. Barbey JT, et al. SSRI safety in overdose. *J Clin Psychiatry* 1998; 59 Suppl 15:42–48.

31. Jimmink A, et al. Clinical toxicology of citalopram after acute intoxication with the sole drug or in combination with other drugs: overview of 26 cases. *Ther Drug Monit* 2008; 30:365–371.

32. Tarabar AF, et al. Citalopram overdose: late presentation of torsades de pointes (TdP) with cardiac arrest. *J Med Toxicol* 2008; 4:101–105.

33. Kraai EP, et al. Citalopram overdose: a fatal case. *J Med Toxicol* 2015; 11:232–236.

34. Yilmaz Z, et al. Escitalopram causes fewer seizures in human overdose than citalopram. *Clin Toxicol (Phila)* 2010; 48:207–212.

35. van GF, et al. Clinical and ECG effects of escitalopram overdose. *Ann Emerg Med* 2009; 54:404–408.

36. Gamble DE, et al. Trazodone overdose: four years of experience from voluntary reports. *J Clin Psychiatry* 1986; 47:544–546.

37. Martinez MA, et al. Investigation of a fatality due to trazodone poisoning: case report and literature review. *J Anal Toxicol* 2005; 29:262–268.

38. Dattilo PB, et al. Prolonged QT associated with an overdose of trazodone. *J Clin Psychiatry* 2007; 68:1309–1310.

39. Service JA, et al. QT prolongation and delayed atrioventricular conduction caused by acute ingestion of trazodone. *Clin Toxicol (Phila)* 2008; 46:71–73.

40. Caksen H, et al. Acute amitriptyline intoxication: an analysis of 44 children. *Hum Exp Toxicol* 2006; 25:107–110.

41. Howell C, et al. Cardiovascular toxicity due to venlafaxine poisoning in adults: a review of 235 consecutive cases. *Br J Clin Pharmacol* 2007; 64:192–197.

42. Hojer J, et al. Fatal cardiotoxicity induced by venlafaxine overdosage. *Clin Toxicol (Phila)* 2008; 46:336–337.

43. Taylor D. Venlafaxine and cardiovascular toxicity. *BMJ* 2010; 340:327.

44. Cooper JM, et al. Desvenlafaxine overdose and the occurrence of serotonin toxicity, seizures and cardiovascular effects. *Clin Toxicol (Phila)* 2017; 55:18–24.

45. Russell JL, et al. Pediatric ingestion of vilazodone compared to other selective serotonin reuptake inhibitor medications. *Clin Toxicol (Phila)* 2017; 55:352–356.

46. Allergan USA I. Highlights of prescribing information: VIIBRYD (vilazodone hydrochloride) tablets. 2020; https://www.allergan.com/assets/pdf/viibryd_pi.

47. Mazza MG, et al. Vortioxetine overdose in a suicidal attempt: A case report. *Medicine (Baltimore)* 2018; 97:e10788.

48. Isbister GK, et al. Amisulpride deliberate self-poisoning causing severe cardiac toxicity including QT prolongation and torsades de pointes. *Med J Aust* 2006; 184:354–356.

49. Ward DI. Two cases of amisulpride overdose: A cause for prolonged QT syndrome. *Emerg Med Australas* 2005; 17:274–276.

50. Isbister GK, et al. Amisulpride overdose is frequently associated with QT prolongation and torsades de pointes. *J Clin Psychopharmacol* 2010; 30:391–395.

51. Lofton AL, et al. Atypical experience: a case series of pediatric aripiprazole exposures. *Clin Toxicol (Phila)* 2005; 43:151–153.

52. Carstairs SD, et al. Overdose of aripiprazole, a new type of antipsychotic. *J Emerg Med* 2005; 28:311–313.

53. Forrester MB. Aripiprazole exposures reported to Texas poison control centers during 2002-2004. *J Toxicol Environ Health A* 2006; 69:1719–1726.

54. Taylor JE, et al. A case of intentional asenapine overdose. *PrimCare CompanionCNSDisord* 2013; 15:PCC.13l01547.

55. U.S. Food & Drug Administration. Drugs@FDA: FDA-approved drugs. 2020; https://www.accessdata.fda.gov/scripts/cder/daf/.

56. Haddad PM, et al. Antipsychotic-related QTc prolongation, torsade de pointes and sudden death. *Drugs* 2002; 62:1649–1671.

57. Levine BS, et al. Two fatalities involving haloperidol. *J Anal Toxicol* 1991; 15:282–284.

58. Henderson RA, et al. Life-threatening ventricular arrhythmia (torsades de pointes) after haloperidol overdose. *Hum Exp Toxicol* 1991; 10:59–62.

59. Recordati Pharmaceuticals Limited. Summary of product characteristics. Reagila 1.5 mg, 3mg, 4.5mg, and 6mg hard capsules. 2020; https://www.medicines.org.uk/emc/product/9401/smpc.

60. Trenton A, et al. Fatalities associated with therapeutic use and overdose of atypical antipsychotics. *CNS Drugs* 2003; 17:307–324.

61. Flanagan RJ, et al. Suspected clozapine poisoning in the UK/Eire, 1992-2003. *Forensic Sci Int* 2005; 155:91–99.

第 13 章

62. Shigeev SV, et al. Clozapine intoxication: theoretical aspects and forensic-medical examination. *Sud Med Ekspert* 2013; 56:41–46.

63. Vigneault P, et al. Iloperidone (Fanapt(R)), a novel atypical antipsychotic, is a potent HERG blocker and delays cardiac ventricular repolarization at clinically relevant concentration. *Pharmacol Res* 2012; 66:60–65.

64. Vanda Pharmaceuticals Inc. Highlights of prescribing information: FANAPT® (iloperidone) tablets. 2020; https://www.fanapt.com/product/pi/pdf/fanapt.pdf.

65. Amon J, et al. A case of iloperidone overdose in a 27-year-old man with cocaine abuse. *SAGE Open Medical Case Reports* 2016; 4:2050313x16660485.

66. Vyas P, et al. An evaluation of lumateperone tosylate for the treatment of schizophrenia. *Expert Opin Pharmacother* 2020; 21:139–145.

67. Sunovion Pharmaceuticals Europe Ltd. Summary of Product Characteristics. Latuda 18.5mg, 37mg and 74mg film-coated tablets 2020; https://www.medicines.org.uk/emc/medicine/29125.

68. Molnar GP, et al. Acute lurasidone overdose. *J Clin Psychopharmacol* 2014; 34:768–770.

69. Chue P, et al. A review of olanzapine-associated toxicity and fatality in overdose. *J Psychiatry Neurosci* 2003; 28:253–261.

70. Waring WS, et al. Olanzapine overdose is associated with acute muscle toxicity. *Hum Exp Toxicol* 2006; 25:735–740.

71. Morissette P, et al. Olanzapine prolongs cardiac repolarization by blocking the rapid component of the delayed rectifier potassium current. *Journal of Psychopharmacology (Oxford, England)* 2007; 21:735–741.

72. Buckley NA, et al. Cardiotoxicity more common in thioridazine overdose than with other neuroleptics. *J Toxicol Clin Toxicol* 1995; 33:199–204.

73. Li C, et al. Acute pulmonary edema induced by overdosage of phenothiazines. *Chest* 1992; 101:102–104.

74. Flanagan RJ. Fatal toxicity of drugs used in psychiatry. *Human Psychopharmacology* 2008; 23 Suppl 1:43–51.

75. Sahli ZT, et al. Pimavanserin: novel pharmacotherapy for Parkinson's disease psychosis. *Expert Opinion on Drug Discovery* 2018; 13:103–110.

76. Vanover KE, et al. Pharmacokinetics, tolerability, and safety of ACP-103 following single or multiple oral dose administration in healthy volunteers. *J Clin Pharmacol* 2007; 47:704–714.

77. Langman LJ, et al. Fatal overdoses associated with quetiapine. *J Anal Toxicol* 2004; 28:520–525.

78. Hunfeld NG, et al. Quetiapine in overdosage: a clinical and pharmacokinetic analysis of 14 cases. *Ther Drug Monit* 2006; 28:185–189.

79. Strachan PM, et al. Mental status change, myoclonus, electrocardiographic changes, and acute respiratory distress syndrome induced by quetiapine overdose. *Pharmacotherapy* 2006; 26:578–582.

80. Ngo A, et al. Acute quetiapine overdose in adults: a 5-Year retrospective case series. *Ann Emerg Med* 2008; 52:541–547.

81. Liang CS, et al. Acute renal failure after paliperidone overdose: a case report. *J Clin Psychopharmacol* 2012; 32:128.

82. Lapid MI, et al. Acute dystonia associated with paliperidone overdose. *Psychosomatics* 2011; 52:291–294.

83. Gomez-Criado MS, et al. Ziprasidone overdose: cases recorded in the database of Pfizer-Spain and literature review. *Pharmacotherapy* 2005; 25:1660–1665.

84. Arbuck DM. 12,800-mg ziprasidone overdose without significant ECG changes. *Gen Hosp Psychiatry* 2005; 27:222–223.

85. Insa Gomez FJ, et al. Ziprasidone overdose: cardiac safety. *Actas Esp Psiquiatr* 2005; 33:398–400.

86. Klein-Schwartz W, et al. Prospective observational multi-poison center study of ziprasidone exposures. *Clin Toxicol (Phila)* 2007; 45:782–786.

87. Tan HH, et al. A systematic review of cardiovascular effects after atypical antipsychotic medication overdose. *Am J Emerg Med* 2009; 27:607–616.

88. Alipour A, et al. Torsade de pointes after ziprasidone overdose with coingestants. *J Clin Psychopharmacol* 2010; 30:76–77.

89. Spiller HA. Management of carbamazepine overdose. *Pediatr Emerg Care* 2001; 17:452–456.

90. Schmidt S, et al. Signs and symptoms of carbamazepine overdose. *J Neurol* 1995; 242:169–173.

91. Alabi A, et al. Safety profile of lamotrigine in overdose. *Ther Adv Psychopharmacol* 2016; 6:369–381.

92. Alyahya B, et al. Acute lamotrigine overdose: a systematic review of published adult and pediatric cases. *Clin Toxicol (Phila)* 2018; 56:81–89.

93. Tuohy K, et al. Acute lithium intoxication. *Dial Transplant* 2003; 32:478–481.

94. Chen KP, et al. Implication of serum concentration monitoring in patients with lithium intoxication. *Psychiatry Clin Neurosci* 2004; 58:25–29.

95. Offerman SR, et al. Hospitalized lithium overdose cases reported to the California poison control system. *Clin Toxicol (Phila)* 2010; 48:443–448.

96. Ferrey AE, et al. Relative toxicity of mood stabilisers and antipsychotics: case fatality and fatal toxicity associated with self-poisoning. *BMC Psychiatry* 2018; 18:399.

97. Isbister GK, et al. Valproate overdose: a comparative cohort study of self poisonings. *Br J Clin Pharmacol* 2003; 55:398–404.

98. Spiller HA, et al. Multicenter case series of valproic acid ingestion: serum concentrations and toxicity. *J Toxicol Clin Toxicol* 2000; 38:755–760.

99. Sztajnkrycer MD. Valproic acid toxicity: overview and management. *J Toxicol Clin Toxicol* 2002; 40:789–801.

100. Eyer F, et al. Acute valproate poisoning: pharmacokinetics, alteration in fatty acid metabolism, and changes during therapy. *J Clin Psychopharmacol* 2005; 25:376–380.

101. Robinson P, et al. Severe hypothermia in association with sodium valproate overdose. *N Z Med J* 2005; 118:U1681.

102. Reith DM, et al. Comparison of the fatal toxicity index of zopiclone with benzodiazepines. *J Toxicol Clin Toxicol* 2003; 41:975–980.

103. Isbister GK, et al. Alprazolam is relatively more toxic than other benzodiazepines in overdose. *Br J Clin Pharmacol* 2004; 58:88–95.

104. Gable RS. Comparison of acute lethal toxicity of commonly abused psychoactive substances. *Addiction* 2004; 99:686–696.

105. Caplehorn JR, et al. Fatal methadone toxicity: signs and circumstances, and the role of benzodiazepines. *Aust N Z J Public Health* 2002; 26:358–362.

106. Spiller HA, et al. Toxicity from modafinil ingestion. *Clin Toxicol (Phila)* 2009; 47:153–156.

107. Carstairs SD, et al. A retrospective review of supratherapeutic modafinil exposures. *J Med Toxicol* 2010; 6:307–310.

108. Russell J, et al. Retrospective assessment of toxicity following exposure to Orexin pathway modulators modafinil and suvorexant. *Toxicology Communications* 2019; 3:33–36.

109. Miljevic C, et al. A case of pregabalin intoxication. *Psychiatrike = Psychiatriki* 2012; 23:162–165.

110. Wood DM, et al. Significant pregabalin toxicity managed with supportive care alone. *J Med Toxicol* 2010; 6:435–437.

111. Gock SB, et al. Acute zolpidem overdose–report of two cases. *J Anal Toxicol* 1999; 23:559–562.

112. Garnier R, et al. Acute zolpidem poisoning–analysis of 344 cases. *J Toxicol Clin Toxicol* 1994; 32:391–404.

113. Pounder D, et al. Zopiclone poisoning. *J Anal Toxicol* 1996; 20:273–274.

114. Bramness JG, et al. Fatal overdose of zopiclone in an elderly woman with bronchogenic carcinoma. *J Forensic Sci* 2001; 46:1247–1249.

驾驶与精神药物

每个人都有责任安全驾驶,在几乎所有的国家,所有司机都要为自己造成的交通事故负法律责任[1],不管他们是否受到药物或酒精影响。

已经发现许多因素能够影响驾驶能力,包括年龄、性别、人格、躯体状况、精神状态,以及酒精、处方药物、毒品、非处方药物[2,3]。单独研究其中任何一种因素对驾驶的影响都比较困难。一些研究试图根据治疗药物对驾驶能力的不同影响进行分类[4],一些研究已经通过测试反应时间和注意力评价药物的影响[5],但是这些测试并非直接检测驾驶能力。

据估计,在交通事故中,死亡或受伤的人群中高达 10% 的人正在服用精神药物[5](表 13.2)。患有人格障碍和酒精依赖的患者违章驾驶的比率最高,且更可能卷入交通事故[5]。在大多数国家,驾驶能力可能因所患疾病或处方药物受损的个体,需告知他们的机动车保险公司。如未提前告知,将被认为是"隐瞒重大事实",可能致使保险合同无效。

表 13.2　精神药物与驾驶

药物	影响
酒精	酒精引起镇静,损害协调力、视力、注意力及信息处理能力。酒精依赖的司机卷入交通事故及违章的概率是全部注册司机的 2 倍[5],且 1/3 致命的交通事故涉及酒精依赖的司机[5]。饮酒同时吸食毒品的年轻司机风险特别高[12,13]
抗惊厥药	用药初期,剂量相关不良反应可能会影响驾驶能力(如视物模糊、共济失调和镇静)。关于癫痫和驾驶有严格的规定。拉莫三嗪对驾驶能力的影响有限[14]
抗抑郁药	服用抗抑郁药的患者发生交通事故的风险增加,尤其是在治疗起始阶段。与三环类抗抑郁药相比,SSRI 存在一些优势,但是驾驶能力与健康人群相比仍有所减退[15],提示抑郁症本身也对驾驶能力有重大的影响[16,17]。SSRI 并不损害健康志愿者的驾驶能力[18-20]。接受 SSRI 治疗的缓解期患者,驾驶操作同样未受损[21]。米氮平在晚上单次服用时,其起始效应会不同程度地减轻,但许多人会出现严重的后遗作用,可能会损害驾驶能力[22]。长期治疗,药物对驾驶的影响可消失[23]。曲唑酮也能影响驾驶能力[24]。事实上,阿戈美拉汀和文拉法辛能提高驾驶能力[25]。伏硫西汀没有影响[23]。鼻吸艾斯氯胺酮在用药 8h 后,对驾驶能力没有影响[26]
抗精神病药	镇静和锥体外系反应能够损害协调性和反应时间[2]。大部分使用抗精神病药的患者可出现驾驶能力受损[27,28]。一项研究发现,服用第二代抗精神病药或氯氮平的精神分裂症患者,在驾车能力相关技能测试中的表现要优于服用第一代抗精神病药者[29],但约 25% 的患者驾驶技能明显受损
催眠药和抗焦虑剂	苯二氮䓬类药物能够引起镇静,并损害注意力、信息处理能力、记忆力及运动协调能力,与阿片类药物一起是道路交通事故中最常涉及的药物[30,31]。在用于抗焦虑和催眠时,苯二氮䓬类药物、佐匹克隆和唑吡坦增加了交通事故的风险[30]。唑吡坦的药代动力学特征有性别差异,任一剂量下,女性血药浓度高于男性,因此女性的驾驶能力可能受损特别明显[3]。此外,服用唑吡坦还可能出现自动症(automatism)或"睡眠驾驶(sleep driving)"[32]。未发现扎来普隆和作用于褪黑素或 5-羟色胺受体的新型安眠药对驾驶能力存在任何负性残留效应[33]。已经在一些国家上市的食欲素受体拮抗剂(苏沃雷生和莱博雷生),服用后并未损害日间驾驶能力[34,35]
锂盐	锂盐会损伤对黑暗的视觉适应能力[2],但对驾驶安全的影响尚不明确。已经发现很多服用锂盐的患者不适合驾驶[14],但是难以确定其确切影响有多大。服用锂盐的老年患者发生伤害性交通事故的风险可能增加[36]

药物	影响
哌甲酯	一些研究表明,ADHD 患者的反应时间比健康人群长,因此可能增加驾驶风险[37]。其他研究发现,哌甲酯能够改善成年 ADHD 患者的驾驶能力[38],再次表明疾病本身对驾驶能力的影响可能大于药物的特定药理作用[38]
阿片类药物	阿片类药物对道路交通事故的风险有较大的负性影响[39]。小剂量丁丙诺啡和美沙酮可以降低非依赖者的驾驶能力[40]

ADHD,注意缺陷多动障碍;SSRI,选择性 5-羟色胺再摄取抑制药。

精神疾病的影响

在 1988 年英国的道路交通法案(*Road Traffic Act*)中[6],严重精神障碍被列为残疾。法规规定的精神障碍包括精神疾病、精神发育停滞或发育不全、精神病性障碍、严重智力或社会功能损害。在 www.gov.uk 网站上有评估是否适合驾驶的指导。在精神障碍常见的躯体疾病中,驾照限制可能也适用于糖尿病,尤其是接受胰岛素治疗,或确定存在微血管或大血管并发症的患者。在美国,与驾驶及精神障碍相关的法规,在各州之间并不相同(参见各州机动车管理部门网站)。

许多痴呆早期的患者能够安全驾驶[7,8]。在英国,所有新诊断为阿尔茨海默病和其他痴呆症的司机必须告知交通管理局(Drivers and Vehicle Licensing Agency,DVLA)[7]。医师需要立刻做出能否安全驾驶的决定,并确保执照管理处能够接到通知[9]。目前,没有数据表明持续的驾驶评估可以作为痴呆患者保持驾驶能力或提高其道路安全性的方法[10]。在美国,有些州强制医师报告痴呆诊断,但另一些州可能仅仅在驾照换新时有这样的要求。

精神药物、驾驶和英国法律

大多数国家禁止在驾驶时使用一系列非法物质。在英国,毒驾法规定了 8 种非法药物(零容忍的阈值设置,发现是否近期用药)和 8 种医疗用药的浓度阈值[11]。表 13.3 列出了医疗用药的法定界值以及临床应用中的期望血浆浓度。

对于美沙酮,每日剂量低于 80mg 时,其血浆浓度低于英国的法定界值[50]。这里列出的英国法定界值仅适用于合法处方的药物;如果证明药物为非法使用,驾驶员可能会被起诉。

表 13.3　苯二氮䓬类药物正常服药的浓度和法定界值

药物/日剂量	报告的浓度范围(法定界值)
氯硝西泮 0.5~6.0mg[41,42]	5~80μg/L(50)
地西泮 5~30mg[43]	50~1 000μg/L(550)
氟硝西泮 0.5~2.0mg[44,45]	10~20μg/L(300)
劳拉西泮 1~4mg[46,47]	10~70μg/L(100)
奥沙西泮 15~30mg[48]	250~600μg/L(300)
替马西泮 10~20mg[49]	200~900μg/L(1 000)

其他药物

　　许多精神药物会损害警觉性、注意力和驾驶能力。阻断 H_1、α_1 肾上腺素或胆碱能受体的药物尤为突出。尤其在起始治疗和增加剂量时，药物的影响最明显。在这些情况下，必须让司机意识到各种潜在的损害，并劝告司机评估其驾驶能力。如果出现不良影响，必须停止驾驶[51]。饮酒能进一步加重这些损害。

　　许多抗精神病药和抗抑郁药会降低癫痫发作阈值。在英国，交通管理局建议在为司机处方药物时需考虑这些因素。有关精神药物影响驾驶能力的更多信息见表 13.2。

药物引起的镇静

　　许多精神药物具有镇静作用。药物镇静作用越强，越可能损害驾驶能力。其他药物，包括处方药和非处方药，也可能有镇静作用或影响驾驶能力（如抗组胺药[5]）。一项研究发现，合用抗抑郁药以及其他精神药物的患者，89% 未能通过"适宜驾驶"成套测验[52]。由于每个人感受的镇静程度难以预测，若患者服用有镇静作用的药物，应该告知他们在感到镇静时不要驾驶。在英国，司机有责任确保自己适合驾驶。

交通管理局：司机的责任

　　在英国，告知交通管理局任何可能影响安全驾驶的医疗状况是驾照持有者或申请人的法律责任。在交通管理局是否适宜驾驶评估指南中[53]，可找到相关医疗状况清单。

交通管理局：处方者的责任

　　需确保患者理解他们的状况可能会损害其驾驶能力。如果患者无法理解，则需立刻呈报交通管理局。向患者解释处方者有法定义务向交通管理局通告该状况。

　　注：交通管理局指南中说明：符合《精神卫生法》S17 条的患者在恢复驾驶前，必须满足其所患疾病的适宜性标准，并且不受任何可能损害驾驶能力的药物影响。几乎没有患者能够满足这些标准。

英国医学总会的处方者指南[54]

- 不同意诊断结果或所处状况影响其驾驶能力的患者，应当寻求第二份诊断意见，在获得第二份诊断意见之前禁止驾驶。
- 如果患者在不适宜的情况下仍继续驾驶，你需要采取各种合理的方法劝说他们停止驾驶。这包括告诉他们的直系亲属；如果他们同意，你可以驾驶。
- 如果他们继续驾驶，报告交通管理局。告诉患者你会将此状况报告给交通管理局，并书面告知患者，证实你已经报告交通管理局。在患者的病历中明确记录医师所说的建议。

参考文献

1. Annas GJ. Doctors, drugs, and driving – tort liability for patient-caused accidents. *N Engl J Med* 2008; 395:521–525.

2. Metzner JL, et al. Impairment in driving and psychiatric illness. *J Neuropsychiatry Clin Neurosci* 1993; 5:211–220.

3. Farkas RH, et al. Zolpidem and driving impairment – identifying persons at risk. *N Engl J Med* 2013; 369:689–691.

4. Alvarez J, et al. ICADTS Working Group: Categorization system for medicinal drugs affecting driving performance. 2007; http://www.icadts.

nl/medicinal.html.

5. Noyes R, Jr. Motor vehicle accidents related to psychiatric impairment. *Psychosomatics* 1985; **26:**569–580.

6. The National Archives. Road Traffic Act 1991. 1991; http://www.legislation.gov.uk/ukpga/1991/40/contents.

7. Driver and Vehicle Licensing Agency. Assessing fitness to drive – a guide for medical professionals. 2016 (last updated 2018); www.gov.uk/dvla/fitnesstodrive.

8. Piersma D, et al. Prediction of fitness to drive in patients with Alzheimer's dementia. *PLoS One* 2016; **11:**e0149566.

9. Breen DA, et al. Driving and dementia. BMJ 2007; **334:**1365–1369.

10. Martin AJ, et al. Driving assessment for maintaining mobility and safety in drivers with dementia. *Cochrane Database Syst Rev* 2013; 8:CD006222.

11. Department for Transport. Changes to drug driving law. 2013 (last updated August 2017); https://www.gov.uk/government/collections/drug-driving.

12. Biecheler MB, et al. SAM survey on "drugs and fatal accidents": search of substances consumed and comparison between drivers involved under the influence of alcohol or cannabis. *Traffic Inj Prev* 2008; **9:**11–21.

13. Oyefeso A, et al. Fatal injuries while under the influence of psychoactive drugs: a cross-sectional exploratory study in England. *BMC Public Health* 2006; **6:**148.

14. Segmiller FM, et al. Driving ability according to German guidelines in stabilized bipolar I and II outpatients receiving lithium or lamotrigine. *J Clin Pharmacol* 2013; **53:**459–462.

15. Brunnauer A, et al. The effects of most commonly prescribed second generation antidepressants on driving ability: a systematic review : 70th Birthday Prof. Riederer. *J Neural Transm* 2013; **120:**225–232.

16. Bramness JG, et al. Minor increase in risk of road traffic accidents after prescriptions of antidepressants: a study of population registry data in Norway. *J Clin Psychiatry* 2008; **69:**1099–1103.

17. Verster JC, et al. Psychoactive medication and traffic safety. *Int J Environ Res Public Health* 2009; **6:**1041–1054.

18. Iwamoto K, et al. The effects of acute treatment with paroxetine, amitriptyline, and placebo on driving performance and cognitive function in healthy Japanese subjects: a double-blind crossover trial. *Human Psychopharmacol* 2008; **23:**399–407.

19. Ridout F, et al. A placebo controlled investigation into the effects of paroxetine and mirtazapine on measures related to car driving performance. *Human Psychopharmacol* 2003; **18:**261–269.

20. Wingen M, et al. Actual driving performance and psychomotor function in healthy subjects after acute and subchronic treatment with escitalopram, mirtazapine, and placebo: a crossover trial. *J Clin Psychiatry* 2005; **66:**436–443.

21. Miyata A, et al. Driving performance of stable outpatients with depression undergoing real-world treatment. *Psychiatry Clin Neurosci* 2018; **72:**399–408.

22. Verster JC, et al. Mirtazapine as positive control drug in studies examining the effects of antidepressants on driving ability. *Eur J Pharmacol* 2015; **753:**252–256.

23. Theunissen EL, et al. A randomized trial on the acute and steady-state effects of a new antidepressant, vortioxetine (Lu AA21004), on actual driving and cognition. *Clin Pharmacol Ther* 2013; **93:**493–501.

24. Ip EJ, et al. The effect of trazodone on standardized field sobriety tests. *Pharmacotherapy* 2013; **33:**369–374.

25. Brunnauer A, et al. Driving performance and psychomotor function in depressed patients treated with agomelatine or venlafaxine. *Pharmacopsychiatry* 2015; **48:**65–71.

26. van de Loo A, et al. The effects of intranasal esketamine (84 mg) and oral mirtazapine (30 mg) on on-road driving performance: a double-blind, placebo-controlled study. *Psychopharmacology (Berl)* 2017; **234:**3175–3183.

27. Grabe HJ, et al. The influence of clozapine and typical neuroleptics on information processing of the central nervous system under clinical conditions in schizophrenic disorders: implications for fitness to drive. *Neuropsychobiology* 1999; **40:**196–201.

28. Wylie KR, et al. Effects of depot neuroleptics on driving performance in chronic schizophrenic patients. *J Neurol Neurosurg Psychiatry* 1993; **56:**910–913.

29. Brunnauer A, et al. The impact of antipsychotics on psychomotor performance with regards to car driving skills. *J Clin Psychopharmacol* 2004; **24:**155–160.

30. Dassanayake T, et al. Effects of benzodiazepines, antidepressants and opioids on driving: a systematic review and meta-analysis of epidemiological and experimental evidence. *Drug Saf* 2011; **34:**125–156.

31. Rudisill TM, et al. Medication use and the risk of motor vehicle collisions among licensed drivers: a systematic review. *Accid Anal Prev* 2016; **96:**255–270.

32. Poceta JS. Zolpidem ingestion, automatisms, and sleep driving: a clinical and legal case series. *J Clin Sleep Med* 2011; **7:**632–638.

33. Verster JC, et al. Hypnotics and driving safety: meta-analyses of randomized controlled trials applying the on-the-road driving test. *Current Drug Safety* 2006; **1:**63–71.

34. Vermeeren A, et al. On-the-road driving performance the morning after bedtime administration of lemborexant in healthy adult and elderly volunteers. Sleep 2019; **42:**zsy260.

35. Vermeeren A, et al. On-the-road driving performance the morning after bedtime use of suvorexant 15 and 30 mg in healthy elderly. *Psychopharmacology (Berl)* 2016; **233:**3341–3351.

36. Etminan M, et al. Use of lithium and the risk of injurious motor vehicle crash in elderly adults: case-control study nested within a cohort. *BMJ* 2004; **328:**558–559.

37. Hashemian F, et al. A comparison of the effects of reboxetine and placebo on reaction time in adults with Attention Deficit-Hyperactivity Disorder (ADHD). *Daru* 2011; **19:**231–235.

38. Classen S, et al. Evidence-based review on interventions and determinants of driving performance in teens with attention deficit hyperactivity

disorder or autism spectrum disorder. *Traffic Inj Prev* 2013; 14:188–193.

39. Hetland A, et al. Medications and impaired driving. *Ann Pharmacother* 2014; 48:494–506.

40. Strand MC, et al. Pharmacokinetics of single doses of methadone and buprenorphine in blood and oral fluid in healthy volunteers and correlation with effects on psychomotor and cognitive functions. *J Clin Psychopharmacol* 2019; 39:489–493.

41. Sjo O, et al. Pharmacokinetics and side-effects of clonazepam and its 7-amino-metabolite in man. Eur J Clin Pharmacol 1975; 8:249–254.

42. Berlin A, et al. Pharmacokinetics of the anticonvulsant drug clonazepam evaluated from single oral and intravenous doses and by repeated oral administration. *Eur J Clin Pharmacol* 1975; 9:155–159.

43. Rutherford DM, et al. Plasma concentrations of diazepam and desmethyldiazepam during chronic diazepam therapy. *Br J Clin Pharmacol* 1978; 6:69–73.

44. Wickstrom E, et al. Pharmacokinetic and clinical observations on prolonged administration of flunitrazepam. *Eur J Clin Pharmacol* 1980; 17:189–196.

45. Mattila MA, et al. Flunitrazepam: a review of its pharmacological properties and therapeutic use. *Drugs* 1980; 20:353–374.

46. Greenblatt DJ, et al. Single- and multiple-dose kinetics of oral lorazepam in humans: the predictability of accumulation. *J Pharmacokinet Biopharm* 1979; 7:159–179.

47. Greenblatt DJ, et al. Pharmacokinetic comparison of sublingual lorazepam with intravenous, intramuscular, and oral lorazepam. *J Pharm Sci* 1982; 71:248–252.

48. Smink BE, et al. The concentration of oxazepam and oxazepam glucuronide in oral fluid, blood and serum after controlled administration of 15 and 30 mg oxazepam. *Br J Clin Pharmacol* 2008; 66:556–560.

49. Greenblatt DJ, et al. Clinical pharmacokinetics of the newer benzodiazepines. *Clin Pharmacokinet* 1983; 8:233–252.

50. Ferrari A, et al. Methadone – metabolism, pharmacokinetics and interactions. *Pharmacol Res* 2004; 50:551–559.

51. Department of Transport. Medication and Road Safety: A Scoping Study. Road Safety Research Report No. 116. 2010; https://webarchive. nationalarchives.gov.uk/20101007211118/http://www.dft.gov.uk/pgr/roadsafety/research/rsrr/theme3/report16findings.pdf

52. Grabe HJ, et al. The influence of polypharmacological antidepressive treatment on central nervous information processing of depressed patients: implications for fitness to drive. *Neuropsychobiology* 1998; 37:200–204.

53. Driver and Vehicle Licensing Agency. At a glance guide to the current medical standards of fitness to drive. 2013 (last updated March 2020); https://www.gov.uk/government/publications/at-a-glance.

54. General Medical Council. Good practice in prescribing and managing medicines and devices. 2013; https://www.gmc-uk.org/guidance/ethical_guidance/14316.asp.

精神药物和手术

关于非麻醉药对手术和麻醉过程所造成的影响,有价值的研究很少[1,2]。目前的实践大多数是基于理论、案例报告、临床经验和个人观点。因此,这方面的任何指南都是某种程度的推测。在手术过程中及围手术期是否继续使用一种药物,应考虑许多相互作用的因素。一般考虑包括:

- 在全身麻醉过程中,患者有吸入胃内容物的风险。因此,通常嘱咐患者术前至少 6h 内不能进食。但是,摄入的清澈液体可在 2h 内离开胃,所以患者可在术前 2h 前服用常规药物[3]。
- 术中用药与常规用药存在相互作用时,这些药物不能同时使用(禁忌联合用药)。此时麻醉师一般通过选择麻醉药物进行处理,可能需要临时停用患者的常规用药。术中用药和精神药物间的显著相互作用包括:
  - 服用三环类抗抑郁药的患者,恩氟烷会引起癫痫发作[4-6]。
  - 服用单胺氧化酶抑制剂的患者,哌替啶和其他 5-羟色胺能阿片类药物可诱发致命的"兴奋性"反应;服用 SSRI 的患者,该类药物可导致 5-羟色胺综合征[4-7]。
  - 常规用药导致 Q-T 间期延长者,禁止合用也能延长 Q-T 间期的挥发性麻醉剂(氟烷、恩氟烷等)[8]。
- 大手术会引起明显的生理变化,包括电解质紊乱、皮质醇和儿茶酚胺的释放。
- 手术以后,手术应激及麻醉用药经常会引起胃或胃肠道的活动停滞。因此,也可能会影响口服药物的吸收。

继续还是停药?

在大多数情况下,如果麻醉师同意,精神药物应在围手术期继续使用。表 13.4 列出了手术中继续使用精神药物的优点及其他方面的讨论。

表 13.4　精神药物与手术

药物或药物类别	注意事项	术中安全?	可替代的剂型
抗惊厥药[4,9-11]	■ 对中枢神经系统的抑制作用可能会减少麻醉需求 ■ 可能需要监测药物浓度 ■ 可能需要减少异丙酚剂量 ■ 已在术前使用,具有镇痛作用	可能安全,癫痫患者常会继续使用	很多国家有卡马西平口服液或栓剂:100mg 片剂 =125mg 栓剂经直肠给药最大剂量为 1g/d,分 4 次用 苯妥英有静脉注射剂和口服液:静脉注射剂量 = 口服剂量 丙戊酸钠有静脉注射剂和口服液。静脉注射剂量 = 口服剂量 在粉碎药品、加水混合之前,应根据当地指南或者向制药公司确认药物的稳定性信息 口服溶液和分散片剂型普遍存在

续表

药物或药物 类别	注意事项	术中安全?	可替代的剂型
抗抑郁药— MAOI[3,4,12-16]	■ 危险,与哌替啶和右美沙芬之间存在可能致命的相互作用(可发生 5-羟色胺综合征、昏迷或呼吸抑制) ■ 吸入性麻醉剂及神经肌肉阻断剂的作用减弱 ■ 拟交感神经药可引起高血压危象(避免使用氯胺酮、麻黄碱和泮库溴铵)[17] ■ 去氧肾上腺素、肾上腺素和去甲肾上腺素效应明显增强 ■ 单胺氧化酶抑制作用持续长达 2 周,需要早期停用 ■ 术前 2 周换成吗氯贝胺,可使用至手术前日(手术当天不能使用)	可能不安全,如果必须继续使用,谨慎选择麻醉药物可降低风险	无
抗抑郁药— SSRI[4-7,15,18,20]	■ 若与哌替啶、芬太尼、喷他佐辛或曲马多合用,有引起 5-羟色胺综合征的危险。 ■ 偶有癫痫发作的报告 ■ 停用可能引起停药综合征,增加复发风险 ■ 所有手术患者均需排除低钠血症[21] ■ 与术中用药有很多相互作用,包括阻断可待因和羟考酮等前体药的生物转化 ■ 文拉法辛可诱发阿片类药物所致的肌肉强直 ■ 增加围手术期出血的风险	可能安全,但避免使用其他 5-羟色胺能药物	艾司西酞普兰、氟西汀和帕罗西汀在大多数国家均有口服液曾在围手术期使用过米氮平口崩片(治疗恶心)[22]
抗抑郁药- TCA[4,6,15,18,20,23]	■ α_1 受体阻断作用可能引起低血压,干扰肾上腺素和去甲肾上腺素的作用 ■ 需谨慎使用可增强交感神经兴奋作用的操作(如插管)[17] ■ (氯米帕明、阿米替林)若与哌替啶、喷他佐辛或曲马多合用,有引起 5-羟色胺综合征的危险 ■ 许多药物能延长 Q-T 间期,所以更容易引起心律失常 ■ 大多数药物降低癫痫阈值 ■ 可能会降低核心温度 ■ 可能会使拟交感药物反应增强 ■ 停药后药效仍能持续几天,所以可能需在术前一段时间停用 ■ 氯米帕明、阿米替林可增加出血风险 ■ 镇痛作用可减少阿片类药物的需要量	不清楚,但需谨慎选择麻醉药物 一些专家建议术前可缓慢停药	阿米替林有口服液,呈酸性,可能会与肠内营养发生相互作用 度硫平胶囊可打开后与水混合冲服,优于研碎的片剂 大多数三环类药物具有强效局部麻醉作用——口服液可能会引起局部麻醉

第 13 章

续表

药物或药物类别	注意事项	术中安全?	可替代的剂型
抗精神病药 [4,15,24-28]	■ 一些抗精神病药在麻醉过程中被广泛使用 ■ 大多数药物可增加心律失常的风险 ■ α_1 受体阻断作用可能引起低血压,干扰肾上腺素和去甲肾上腺素的作用 ■ 大多数药物可降低癫痫阈值 ■ 可能会加重术中核心体温过低 ■ 有一些术中安全使用的证据 [29] ■ 氯氮平可能会延长麻醉复苏时间 ■ 吸入麻醉可能会影响多巴胺代谢 ■ 术前使用奥氮平可降低谵妄的风险 [30],术前使用阿立哌唑具有同样作用 [31] ■ 使用第二代抗精神病药(SGA)可以减少术后恶心 [32]	可能安全,通常继续使用以免疾病复发 [33]	一些抗精神病药有液体剂型可制备一些"特殊"液体用于鼻饲给药 在粉碎药品、加水混合之前,应向当地指南或者制药公司确认药物的稳定性信息
苯二氮䓬类 [4,9]	■ 减少麻醉诱导期和维持期的需要 ■ 许多药物具有长效作用(几天或几周),因此必须早期停药 ■ 可能会有戒断症状	可能安全,通常继续使用	地西泮有口服液、肌内注射、静脉注射和直肠用剂型(勿用肌内注射) 咪达唑仑有口服液 劳拉西泮可舌下含服(使用普通药片)、肌内注射和静脉注射
锂盐 [3,4,12,15]	■ 延长去极化和非去极化肌肉松弛药的作用 ■ 手术相关的电解质紊乱和肾功能下降可引起锂盐中毒。避免脱水及使用 NSAID ■ 可能会增加心律失常的风险	小手术可能安全,但在大手术前常需停药,等电解质恢复正常后重新开始使用 必须缓慢停药——麻醉师可能不重视这一点 [34]	锂盐的生物利用度在不同品牌之间存在差异。注意使用等效剂量:200mg 碳酸锂 =509mg 柠檬酸锂 可使用柠檬酸锂口服液,通常每天 2 次
美沙酮 [3,9]	■ 可能会降低阿片类药物的需求 ■ 纳洛酮可能会引起戒断症状 ■ 美沙酮延长 Q-T 间期 ■ 使用阿片类药物时,只能使用完全激动剂(避免用丁丙诺啡)	可能安全,通常继续使用	IM 剂量 = 口服剂量
莫达非尼 [35,36]	■ 有限的数据表明不干扰麻醉 ■ 改善麻醉苏醒	可能安全,数据有限	无
普瑞巴林 [37]	■ 术前使用普瑞巴林可减少术后恶心	是	无

CNS,中枢神经系统;IM,肌内注射;IV,静脉注射;MAOI,单胺氧化酶抑制剂;NSAID,非甾体类抗炎药;SSRI,选择性 5-羟色胺再摄取抑制剂;TCA,三环类抗抑郁药。

　　但是,需要注意的是,仅仅因为"不得进食",精神药物和其他药物经常(意外或未加考虑)在术前被停用[1]。患者被贴上"不得进食"标签可能有几个原因,包括术前准备、无意识、术后肠道休息或手术结果本身。患者在医院期间随时可能因为恶心、呕吐而不能耐受口服药物。当决定继续使用精神药物时,需要明确地告知医疗和护理人员,以免无意中停药。

吸烟

　　对于许多正在医院接受手术或康复的患者,没有多少机会吸烟。突然中断吸烟可能会影响精神状态,如果继续使用精神药物也可引起药物中毒(见第11章药代动力学关于"精神药物与吸烟"部分)。

改变剂型

　　出于各种手术相关的原因,可能寻找其他用药途径和剂型。当改变用药途径或剂型时,生物利用度也会改变,应注意确保使用合适的剂量和频率。口服制剂,包括口服液或研碎的片剂,有时可通过鼻饲、经皮内镜下胃造瘘(PEG)或空肠造口途径给药。因为药物被吸收到递送管材质上,生物利用度可能会有问题。

停用精神药物的相关风险

- 复发(特别是停止治疗超过几天时)[38]。
- 病情加重。例如,突然停用锂盐会恶化双相障碍的结局[39]。突然停用抗抑郁药[40]和抗精神病药[41],也有同样的影响。
- 自杀。停用抗抑郁药可能会增加自杀风险[42]。
- 停药症状。在围手术期间会使诊断变得复杂。
- 谵妄。停用抗精神病药[43]或抗抑郁药[6]时更常见。

继续使用精神药物的相关风险

- 可与麻醉用药及围手术期用药发生药物相互作用(药代动力学和药效学相互作用)。
- 增加了出血的可能性(如使用SSRI)[44]。
- 高血压或低血压(取决于使用的精神药物)[23,24]。
- 对核心体温的影响(例如使用吩噻嗪类药物)。

(司天梅 译　田成华 审校)

参考文献

1. Noble DW, et al. Interrupting drug therapy in the perioperative period. *Drug Saf* 2002; **25:489–495**.
2. Noble DW, et al. Risks of interrupting drug treatment before surgery. *BMJ* 2000; **321:719–720**.
3. Anon. Drugs in the peri-operative period: 1–stopping or continuing drugs around surgery. *Drug Ther Bull* 1999; **37:62–64**.
4. Smith MS, et al. Perioperative management of drug therapy, clinical considerations. *Drugs* 1996; **51:238–259**.
5. Chui PT, et al. Medications to withhold or continue in the preoperative consultation. *Curr Anaesth Crit Care* 1998; **9:302–306**.
6. Kudoh A, et al. Antidepressant treatment for chronic depressed patients should not be discontinued prior to anesthesia. *Can J Anaesth* 2002; **49:132–136**.
7. Spivey KM, et al. Perioperative seizures and fluvoxamine. *Br J Anaesth* 1993; **71:321**.
8. Schmeling WT, et al. Prolongation of the QT interval by enflurane, isoflurane, and halothane in humans. *Anesth Analg* 1991; **72:137–144**.

9. Morrow JI, et al. Essential drugs in the perioperative period. *Curr Pract Surg* 1990; **90**:106–109.

10. Bloor M, et al. Antiepileptic drugs and anesthesia. *Paediatr Anaesth* 2017; **27**:248–250.

11. Bhosale UA, et al. Comparative pre-emptive analgesic efficacy study of novel antiepileptic agents gabapentin, lamotrigine and topiramate in patients undergoing major surgeries at a tertiary care hospital: a randomized double blind clinical trial. *J Basic Clin Physiol Pharmacol* 2017; **28**:59–66.

12. Rahman MH, et al. Medication in the peri-operative period. *Pharm J* 2004; **272**:287–289.

13. Blom-Peters L, et al. Monoamine oxidase inhibitors and anesthesia: an updated literature review. *Acta Anaesthesiol Belg* 1993; **44**:57–60.

14. Hill S, et al. MAOIs to RIMAs in anaesthesia–a literature review. *Psychopharmacology (Berl)* 1992; **106 Suppl**:S43-S45.

15. Huyse FJ, et al. Psychotropic drugs and the perioperative period: a proposal for a guideline in elective surgery. *Psychosomatics* 2006; **47**:8–22.

16. Bajwa SJ, et al. Psychiatric diseases: need for an increased awareness among the anesthesiologists. *JAnaesthesiolClinPharmacol* 2011; **27**:440–446.

17. Aroke EN, et al. Perioperative considerations for patients with major depressive disorder undergoing surgery. *J Perianesth Nurs* 2020; **35**:112–119.

18. Takakura K, et al. Refractory hypotension during combined general and epidural anaesthesia in a patient on tricyclic antidepressants. *Anaesth Intensive Care* 2008; **34**:111–114.

19. Roy S, et al. Fentanyl-induced rigidity during emergence from general anesthesia potentiated by venlafexine. *Can J Anaesth* 2003; **50**:32–35.

20. Mahdanian AA, et al. Serotonergic antidepressants and perioperative bleeding risk: a systematic review. *ExpertOpinDrug Saf* 2014; **13**:695–704.

21. Levine SM, et al. Selective serotonin reuptake inhibitor-induced hyponatremia and the plastic surgery patient. *Plast Reconstr Surg* 2017; **139**:1481–1488.

22. Chang FL, et al. Efficacy of mirtazapine in preventing intrathecal morphine-induced nausea and vomiting after orthopaedic surgery*. *Anaesthesia* 2010; **65**:1206–1211.

23. Kudoh A, et al. Chronic treatment with antidepressants decreases intraoperative core hypothermia. *Anesth Analg* 2003; **97**:275–279.

24. Kudoh A, et al. Chronic treatment with antipsychotics enhances intraoperative core hypothermia. *Anesth Analg* 2004; **98**:111–115.

25. Doherty J, et al. Implications for anaesthesia in a patient established on clozapine treatment. *Int J Obstet Anesth* 2006; **15**:59–62.

26. Geeraerts T, et al. Delayed recovery after short-duration, general anesthesia in a patient chronically treated with clozapine. *Anesth Analg* 2006; **103**:1618.

27. Adachi YU, et al. Isoflurane anesthesia inhibits clozapine- and risperidone-induced dopamine release and anesthesia-induced changes in dopamine metabolism was modified by fluoxetine in the rat striatum: an in vivo microdialysis study. *Neurochem Int* 2008; **52**:384–391.

28. Parlow JL, et al. Single-dose haloperidol for the prophylaxis of postoperative nausea and vomiting after intrathecal morphine. *Anesth Analg* 2004; **98**:1072–1076.

29. Kim DH, et al. Adverse events associated with antipsychotic use in hospitalized older adults after cardiac surgery. *J Am Geriatr Soc* 2017; **65**:1229–1237.

30. Larsen KA, et al. Administration of olanzapine to prevent postoperative delirium in elderly joint-replacement patients: a randomized, controlled trial. *Psychosomatics* 2010; **51**:409–418.

31. Mokhtari M, et al. Aripiprazole for prevention of delirium in the neurosurgical intensive care unit: a double-blind, randomized, placebo-controlled study. *Eur J Clin Pharmacol* 2020; **76**:491–499.

32. Jabaley CS, et al. Chronic atypical antipsychotic use is associated with reduced need for postoperative nausea and vomiting rescue in the postanesthesia care unit: a propensity-matched retrospective observational study. *Anesth Analg* 2020; **130**:141–150.

33. Kaye AD, et al. Perioperative implications of common and newer psychotropic medications used in clinical practice. *Best Pract Res Clin Anaesthesiol* 2018; **32**:187–202.

34. Attri JP, et al. Psychiatric patient and anaesthesia. *Indian JAnaesth* 2012; **56**:8–13.

35. Larijani GE, et al. Modafinil improves recovery after general anesthesia. *Anesth Analg* 2004; **98**:976–981.

36. Doyle A, et al. Day case general anaesthesia in a patient with narcolepsy. *Anaesthesia* 2008; **63**:880–882.

37. Grant MC, et al. The effect of preoperative pregabalin on postoperative nausea and vomiting: a meta-analysis. *Anesth Analg* 2016; **123**:1100–1107.

38. De Baerdemaeker L, et al. Anaesthesia for patients with mood disorders. *Curr Opin Anaesthesiol* 2005; **18**:333–338.

39. Faedda GL, et al. Outcome after rapid vs gradual discontinuation of lithium treatment in bipolar disorders. *Arch Gen Psychiatry* 1993; **50**:448–455.

40. Baldessarini RJ, et al. Illness risk following rapid versus gradual discontinuation of antidepressants. *Am J Psychiatry* 2010; **167**:934–941.

41. Horowitz MA, et al. Tapering of SSRI treatment to mitigate withdrawal symptoms. *Lancet Psychiatry* 2019; **6**:538–546.

42. Yerevanian BI, et al. Antidepressants and suicidal behaviour in unipolar depression. *Acta Psychiatr Scand* 2004; **110**:452–458.

43. Copeland LA, et al. Postoperative complications in the seriously mentally ill: a systematic review of the literature. *Ann Surg* 2008; **248**:31–38.

44. Paton C, et al. SSRIs and gastrointestinal bleeding. *BMJ* 2005; **331**:529–530.

第13章

第14章

杂录

Hong Q, et al. Prohormone changes and perioperative period: a proposal for rehabilitation after surgery. Anesth Essays Monogr. 2008; 63:3-22.

de Piero M, et al. Perioperative issues. Anesth Essays Monogr. 2006; 27:...

提高用药依从性

世界卫生组织对长期治疗依从性的定义是："一个人的行为（服药、饮食、改变生活方式）与卫生保健人员提出并经双方同意的建议相一致的程度[1]。"后来,英国国家卫生与保健研究所（NICE）的指导也将依从性定义为"患者的行动与经其同意的建议相匹配的程度"。用药依从性要求患者与处方医师之间相互合作,意见一致。NICE 建议,只要患者有表达同意的能力,他们不用药的权利就应该得到尊重[2]。若处方医师认为不用药的决定可能导致不良后果,则应记录患者做出该决定的理由以及处方医生的顾虑。实际上,NICE 在其精神分裂症治疗指南中强调,在没有处方抗精神病药的情况下,需要增加对心理社会干预措施的有效性研究[3]。然而,一项荟萃分析[4]和系统综述[5]证实,在未用药患者的研究中,心理动力学干预的疗效不如抗精神病药治疗。最新的系统综述发现,对于（不用或仅用小剂量抗精神病药的）精神病患者,心理社会干预的效果与抗精神病药相同[6]。

用药依从性与良好的临床结局直接相关。对 62 250 名精神分裂症患者进行历时 20 年的随访研究发现,使用抗精神病药者的自杀死亡率明显低于不用药者;当考虑全部死亡原因时,最有利的临床结局与合用氯氮平相关[7]。不出所料,世界卫生组织声明:"增强依从性干预的效果,其对群体健康的影响可能远远超过特定医学治疗的进步[1]。""我们需要的不是更好的药,而是更好的依从性",这种说法将长远流传。

依从性是一种复杂的行为,受一些可变的潜在因素影响。因此,通过对患者进行特异性的干预,以及针对相关因素进行干预,不依从的决定因素可能有所改变。大多数增强依从性的干预都受到批评,因为没有可靠的理论框架,其方法学也缺乏严密性[8]。劣质的研究及其结果往往在不同背景下重复不出来。这种现象在最近一篇有关依从性干预的Cochrane 综述中也有所强调;该文报告,在 182 篇纳入分析的论文中,仅有 11 项研究偏倚的风险最小[9]。

用药不依从的发生率

有关依从性的综述普遍得出的结论是,约 50% 的患者不按医嘱用药,该比例在慢性躯体疾病和慢性精神疾病中类似[9]。然而,这种说法可能过于简单,因为可能只有很少一部分患者完全依从,大多数患者不同程度地部分依从,只有个别患者出于自己意志从不用药[10]。

在不同时间和不同环境下,用药依从率也有些不同。例如,精神分裂症患者出院后,10天时高达 25% 的患者部分依从或完全不依从,1 年时该数值增至 50%,2 年时该数字增至75%[11]。其他研究报告,出院后 1 年内完全停药率为 25.8%[12]。在一些精神卫生机构中,不依从率可高达 90%[13]。很多依从性差的情况发生时,处方医生并不知道。在一项研究中,处方医生只识别出了不依从者中的一半[14]。在另外一项研究中,因难治性精神分裂症转诊接受治疗的患者中,有 35% 血浆药物浓度达不到治疗浓度,其中许多人的血浆药物浓度为 0[15]。

用药不依从的影响

在精神分裂症[16-18]、双相障碍[19] 和抑郁症[20] 患者中,用药依从性差是结局不良(包括复发)的重要危险因素。用药不依从还会导致丧失更广泛的健康获益。例如,与服用抗抑郁药的抑郁症患者相比,不服药者心肌梗死的发生率升高 20%[21]。用药不依从可产生严重后果,实施常规监测可以预防这些不良后果。实际上,英国曾经对精神疾病患者的自杀和他杀进行过全国性的保密调查,对部分搜集到的数据进行分析发现,对于如何管理不按医嘱用药的患者,在实施相关政策的保健机构中患者自杀率比没有相关政策的保健机构低 20%[22]。当然,在依从性差的患者中,导致结局变差的一个主要因素是停药的性质——他们往往骤然停药,而且没有进行监护。业已证明,所有精神药物骤然停用会导致预后不佳。

改善依从性的策略

一些系统综述建议,在严重精神疾病患者中,对患者的个体化干预更有可能增强依从性[23]。另外,NICE 回顾了一系列健康问题的依从性证据,得出的结论是:没有哪一种干预可以推荐给所有患者。

注意,在这个领域,很少有研究专门招募不依从的患者(这类患者的拒绝率有可能较高),而且极少识别出对依从性的特定障碍。许多研究得出的效应值较小,可能只不过是因为方法不明确。干预图方法(intervention mapping)为识别不依从的决定因素,也为选择基于证据的方法以改变潜在的因素,提供了清晰的路径。干预图方法为定向的、以患者为中心的、可实施的干预提供了基础[24]。

绘制干预图

第一阶段:识别引起不依从的因素[25-26]。一些常见因素列于各类之下。

用药不依从的决定因素					
故意不依从					非故意不依从
疾病相关因素	治疗相关因素	医生和机构相关因素	患者相关因素	环境相关因素	
动机缺乏	不良反应	治疗联盟	否认	家庭信念	遗忘
自知力差	错误观念	没有随访	自知力	文化信念	生活方式混乱
夸大		就诊时间有限	共病	宗教信仰	
妄想			躯体缺陷/障碍		
认知缺陷					
思维障碍					

第14章

第二阶段：将不依从的决定因素与循证干预措施联系起来 [27]

增加依从性的干预措施	
故意不依从	非故意不依从
心理教育：是所有依从性干预的基础，但是若无行为改变的成分，则没有多大效果。同时给患者提供言语和书面信息 **动机访谈**：设定目标 **依从性治疗**：探讨对于药物或疾病的错误观念，提供信息，设定目标。每次治疗需要较长时间，且需要多次治疗 **认知行为治疗**：消除或控制妨碍依从性的残留症状。纠正关于治疗的错误观念 **认知恢复**：帮助精神病患者克服认知缺陷和思维障碍 **正念治疗**：帮助减轻症状 **监测不良反应**：经常、定期进行 **治疗联盟**：患者往往会取悦医生。医生持非评判、开放的态度，会使得患者愿意说出自己的错误观念和行为 **家庭干预**：心理教育和家庭治疗	简化用药方案 药房采取的措施：摆药盒 将用药与日常活动联系起来，如早餐、刷牙、睡前时用药 使用技术手段：通信服务、电子邮件和电话 **药房采取的措施**：面向有生理缺陷者（如开瓶）

第三阶段：评估用药依从性 [28,29]

评估方法	测量指标	优点	缺点
直接（客观）评估			
血液检测	药物/代谢产物血浆浓度	准确	有损伤 昂贵 个体间差异：快/慢代谢 并非对所有药物都可靠（见正文中讨论） 只有结果为 0 时可能明确地解释
间接（主观）评估			
药片计数	缺少的片数	使用简单（临床试验中有用）	临床实践中耗费时间 充分证据表明，药片计数明显低估依从性 [14]
电子数据库——临床/药房记录	不依从的历史 药房发放和回收记录（如用药比例）	容易获得 易于识别不依从的患者 便宜 无损伤	对于所服药物不是可靠的证据；仅显示回收和持有的数量
自我报告	经过验证的评估量表（问卷），如用药依从性量表（MARS）	易于使用 便宜	受报告偏见影响 倾向于取悦医生 明显高估依从性 主观
电子监视装置，如用药监视系统（MEMS）[14]	药盒被打开的次数和（推断的）取出剂量的百分比	最准确的方法之一 客观 提供用药行为的其他信息	昂贵 药盒庞大 不是服药的证据，只是药盒被打开的证据 患者有被监视感

注意,血液检测可以准确提供取血时药物及其代谢产物的血浆浓度,但是对用药行为模式、依从性水平以及可改变依从性的因素无法提供任何信息[29]。

对于氯氮平、奥氮平和利培酮等抗精神病药,血液检测可能有助于直接评估其血浆浓度。必须注意的是,这些药物使用固定剂量所达到的血浆浓度多少会有些变化,不可能准确地确定部分不依从的情况(即完全不依从容易发现,但是部分依从和完全依从则难以分辨)。

监测依从性及评估对用药的态度

精神科医生通常喜欢直接询问,而不是用更有侵入性或更客观的方法评估依从性,因此部分依从或不依从可能会被遗漏[30]。NICE 建议,应该以非评判的方式询问患者,他们是否在特定时段内(比如前一周)漏服过药物。[2]

许多量表或检查表有助于指导和组织对用药态度的讨论。使用最广泛的是《用药态度问卷》(DAI)[31],它由对药物的正面和负面语句构成;全表有 30 个语句,简表有 10 个语句。该量表的设计是让患者填写,他们对于每个语句简单地表示同意或不同意即可。量表总分标明患者对用药利弊之间平衡的总体感觉,因而可能是依从性的指标。业已证明,采用 DAI 测量对用药的态度是一段时间内有用的依从性指标[32]。其他检查表包括《药物影响量表》(ROMI)[33]、《对药物的观念问卷》[34] 和《用药依从性量表》(MARS)[18]。

摆药盒

摆药盒含有多个间隔,容纳每天 4 次的多种药物。它可以帮助那些显然愿意用药,但因行为混乱或认知缺陷而用药困难的患者。应该注意的是,用药不依从的患者中,仅 10% 承认自己完全忘记了服药[35],而且摆药盒不能替代无自知力或没有用药意愿。一些药物从吸塑包装中取出并放入摆药盒后性质不稳定,其中包括常用于不依从患者的口腔分散剂。另外,向摆药盒中装药很费时(昂贵),临时改变处方可能困难,而且装药过程特别容易出错[36]。

抗精神病药长效针剂

一些临床试验的荟萃分析发现,与口服药物治疗相比,长效针剂维持治疗者病情复发的相对风险低 30%,绝对风险低 10%[37-38]。NICE 建议,对于已知对口服药物治疗不依从或喜欢长效针剂的患者,可选择长效针剂[3]。然而,值得说明的是,用药不依从的患者从口服抗精神病药换成长效针剂后,并未解决该患者用药不依从的决定因素。最近一篇系统综述注意到这一点,该文报告在已经处方第二代长效针剂的患者中,停药率超过 50%[39]。处方长效针剂并未"治好"不依从,但是确实防止了突然停药及其后果(所有长效针剂的血浆药物浓度均缓慢下降),而且对依从性水平很有把握(要么注射过,要么没注射)。

长效针剂也许使用不足。例如,一项美国的研究发现,在最近出现不依从的患者中,仅有不到 1/5 被处方了长效针剂[40]。

长效针剂的另一种选择是使用长效口服抗精神病药,如可以每周用一次药的五氟利多[41]。监督下服药避免了注射的需要,但是对于依从性并不能具有同样的把握,因为患者有时易于伪装已经使用口服药。

美国已经批准 Abilify MyCite 的使用。该款阿立哌唑制剂内嵌发射传感器，能够证实药片已被服用。其有效性的证据不足[42]。

经济激励

在一些疾病区域进行对照试验得出的证据支持这样的做法：经济激励有可能增强用药依从性。给患者钱让其服药的做法引起很大争议，尽管一些医生发现这种策略有效地增强了依从性。一项随机对照试验发现，停止给钱后，分别在 6 个月和 24 个月进行随访，依从性无法保持下来，接受经济激励的患者仅有 28% 达到完全依从[43]。其他随机对照试验也证明，试验期间依从性明显增强，而停止给钱后再随访则依从性下降[44]。给予经济激励并未降低患者的治疗动机[45]。对于健康相关行为给予经济激励的干预措施存在方法学的限制，一篇系统综述对这种干预措施可接受性的分析引起人们对其信度和效度的担心[46]。

参考文献

1. World Health Organisation. Adherence to long-term therapies: evidence for action. 2003. https://apps.who.int/iris/bitstream/handle/10665/42682/9241545992.pdf.

2. National Institute for Health and Care Excellence. Medicines adherence: involving patients in decisions about prescribed medicines and supporting adherence. Clinical Guideline [CG76]. 2009 (last checked March 2019); https://www.nice.org.uk/guidance/cg76/chapter/introduction.

3. National Institute for Health and Care Excellence. Psychosis and schizophrenia in adults: prevention and management Clinical Guidance [CG178]. 2014 (last checked March 2019); https://www.nice.org.uk/guidance/cg178.

4. Malmberg L et al. Individual psychodynamic psychotherapy and psychoanalysis for schizophrenia and severe mental illness. *Cochrane Database Syst Rev* 2001:Cd001360.

5. Mueser KT et al. Psychodynamic treatment of schizophrenia: is there a future? *Psychol Med* 1990; 20:253–262.

6. Cooper RE et al. Psychosocial interventions for people with schizophrenia or psychosis on minimal or no antipsychotic medication: a systematic review. *Schizophr Res* 2019; 225: 15–30.

7. Taipale H et al. 20-year follow-up study of physical morbidity and mortality in relationship to antipsychotic treatment in a nationwide cohort of 62,250 patients with schizophrenia (FIN20). *World Psychiatry* 2020; 19:61–68.

8. Zullig LL et al. Moving from the trial to the real world: improving medication adherence using insights of implementation science. *Annu Rev Pharmacol Toxicol* 2019; 59:423–445.

9. Nieuwlaat R et al. Interventions for enhancing medication adherence. *Cochrane Database Syst Rev* 2014:Cd000011.

10. Masand PS et al. Partial adherence to antipsychotic medication impacts the course of illness in patients with schizophrenia: a review. *Prim Care Companion J Clin Psychiatry* 2009; 11:147–154.

11. Leucht S et al. Epidemiology, clinical consequences, and psychosocial treatment of nonadherence in schizophrenia. *J Clin Psychiatry* 2006; 67 Suppl 5:3–8.

12. Zhou Y et al. Factors associated with complete discontinuation of medication among patients with schizophrenia in the year after hospital discharge. *Psychiatry Res* 2017; 250:129–135.

13. Cramer JA et al. Compliance with medication regimens for mental and physical disorders. *Psychiatr Serv* 1998; 49:196–201.

14. Remington G et al. The use of electronic monitoring (MEMS) to evaluate antipsychotic compliance in outpatients with schizophrenia. *Schizophr Res* 2007; 90:229–237.

15. McCutcheon R et al. Antipsychotic plasma levels in the assessment of poor treatment response in schizophrenia. *Acta Psychiatr Scand* 2018; 137:39–46.

16. Morken G et al. Non-adherence to antipsychotic medication, relapse and rehospitalisation in recent-onset schizophrenia. *BMC Psychiatry* 2008; 8:32.

17. Knapp M et al. Non-adherence to antipsychotic medication regimens: associations with resource use and costs. *Br J Psychiatry* 2004; 184:509–516.

18. Jaeger S et al. Adherence styles of schizophrenia patients identified by a latent class analysis of the Medication Adherence Rating Scale (MARS): a six-month follow-up study. *Psychiatry Res* 2012; 200:83–88.

19. Lang K et al. Predictors of medication nonadherence and hospitalization in Medicaid patients with bipolar I disorder given long-acting or oral antipsychotics. *J Med Econ* 2011; 14:217–226.

20. Mitchell AJ et al. Why don't patients take their medicine? Reasons and solutions in psychiatry. *Adv Psychiatr Treat* 2007; 13:336–346.

21. Scherrer JF et al. Antidepressant drug compliance: reduced risk of MI and mortality in depressed patients. *Am J Med* 2011; 124:318–324.

22. Appleby L et al. National confidential inquiry into suicide and homicide by people with mental illness. 2013; http://www.bbmh.manchester.ac.uk/cmhr/research/centreforsuicideprevention/nci/.

23. Nosè M et al. Systemic review of clinical interventions for reducing treatment non-adherence in psychosis. *Epidemiol Psichiatr Soc* 2003; 12:272–286.

24. Kok G et al. A taxonomy of behaviour change methods: an intervention mapping approach. *Health Psychol Rev* 2016; 10:297–312.

25. Pedley R et al. Qualitative systematic review of barriers and facilitators to patient-involved antipsychotic prescribing. *Br J Psych Open* 2018; 4:5–14.

26. Semahegn A et al. Psychotropic medication non-adherence and its associated factors among patients with major psychiatric disorders: a systematic review and meta-analysis. *Syst Rev* 2020; 9:17.

27. Hartung D et al. Interventions to improve pharmacological adherence among adults with psychotic spectrum disorders and bipolar disorder: a systematic review. *Psychosomatics* 2017; 58:101–112.

28. Forbes CA et al. A systematic literature review comparing methods for the measurement of patient persistence and adherence. *Curr Med Res Opin* 2018; 34:1613–1625.

29. Anghel LA et al. An overview of the common methods used to measure treatment adherence. *Med Pharm Rep* 2019; 92:117–122.

30. Vieta E et al. Psychiatrists' perceptions of potential reasons for non- and partial adherence to medication: results of a survey in bipolar disorder from eight European countries. *J Affect Disord* 2012; 143:125–130.

31. Hogan TP et al. A self-report scale predictive of drug compliance in schizophrenics: reliability and discriminative validity. *Psychol Med* 1983; 13:177–183.

32. O'Donnell C et al. Compliance therapy: a randomised controlled trial in schizophrenia. *BMJ* 2003; 327:834.

33. Weiden P et al. Rating of medication influences (ROMI) scale in schizophrenia. *Schizophr Bull* 1994; 20:297–310.

34. Horne R et al. The beliefs about medicines questionnaire: the development and evaluation of a new method for assessing the cognitive representation of medication. *Psychology and Health* 1999; 14:1–24.

35. Perkins DO. Predictors of noncompliance in patients with schizophrenia. *J Clin Psychiatry* 2002; 63:1121–1128.

36. Barber ND et al. Care homes' use of medicines study: prevalence, causes and potential harm of medication errors in care homes for older people. *Qual Saf Health Care* 2009; 18:341–346.

37. Leucht C et al. Oral versus depot antipsychotic drugs for schizophrenia–a critical systematic review and meta-analysis of randomised long-term trials. *Schizophr Res* 2011; 127:83–92.

38. Leucht S et al. Antipsychotic drugs versus placebo for relapse prevention in schizophrenia: a systematic review and meta-analysis. *Lancet* 2012; 379:2063–2071.

39. Gentile S. Discontinuation rates during long-term, second-generation antipsychotic long-acting injection treatment: a systematic review. *Psychiatry Clin Neurosci* 2019; 73:216–230.

40. West JC et al. Use of depot antipsychotic medications for medication nonadherence in schizophrenia. *Schizophr Bull* 2008; 34:995–1001.

41. Soares BG et al. Penfluridol for schizophrenia. *Cochrane Database Syst Rev* 2006:Cd002923.

42. Cosgrove L et al. Digital aripiprazole or digital evergreening? A systematic review of the evidence and its dissemination in the scientific literature and in the media. *BMJ Evid Based Med* 2019; 24:231–238.

43. Priebe S et al. Financial incentives to improve adherence to antipsychotic maintenance medication in non-adherent patients: a cluster randomised controlled trial. *Health Technol Assess* 2016; 20:1–122.

44. Noordraven EL et al. Financial incentives for improving adherence to maintenance treatment in patients with psychotic disorders (money for medication): a multicentre, open-label, randomised controlled trial. *Lancet Psychiatry* 2017; 4:199–207.

45. Noordraven EL et al. The effect of financial incentives on patients' motivation for treatment: results of 'Money for Medication', a randomised controlled trial. *BMC Psychiatry* 2018; 18:144.

46. Hoskins K et al. Acceptability of financial incentives for health-related behavior change: an updated systematic review. *Prev Med* 2019; 126:105762.

用药不依从一段时间后重新使用精神药物

患者入院时,常常已经有一段时间不配合用药了。是否重新用药,起始剂量多少,都是复杂的临床问题。一方面是出现撤药症状和疾病复发的风险,另一方面是重新用药速度过快导致不良反应的风险,二者之间必须加以权衡。在这一领域,几乎没有已经发表的证据,大多数指南(出处未宣布)出自药厂,因此遵守下述指南时应该慎重。

产品特征概要(Summary of Product Charateristics,SPC)和其他正式法规文件多不论述这种临床情景,但是正式的患者信息活页往往对此有所涉及。这些活页一致提出忠告:漏服药物后,决不应给予双倍剂量来进行弥补。绝大多数活页只是告知:若漏服一次药物,应该做什么。在这种情况下,一些活页会告知稍后服用所漏的药物(只要距离下次服药的时间不太近),而其他活页则建议完全略过所漏的药物,开始服用下次的药物。

若不只一次漏服药物,首先要问该药是否适合患者服用。依从性差表明患者有一些不满。若药物半衰期短,或者重新开始加量过程很长,则对于经常用药不依从的患者,不宜再次使用该药。类似的,若患者处于酒精或药物中毒之中,则当时不宜重新开始服用该药。找出患者用药不依从是否有特殊原因。对于精神分裂症和分裂情感障碍,考虑是否适合使用长效针剂。

至于是重新使用同样的剂量,还是从小剂量开始逐渐增加,显然离末次用药的时间很重要。若已经过了 1~2 周,则所有药物均可能需要重新开始,就像新的治疗一样(但是对于许多不需要逐步加量的药物,这意味着起始剂量与以前相同)。例外的仅有长效针剂和长半衰期口服药物(如阿立哌唑、卡利拉嗪和五氟利多)。

表 14.1 概述了我们的建议。第一列的药物有明确的安全性问题,停用特定一段时间后,必须重新逐步加量。中间一列被认为是安全的,因为最大剂量通常不超过推荐的最大起始剂量。右侧一列的药物重新使用以前的剂量被认为是安全的,因为:类似的药物出现在中间一列,临床经验提示它们是安全的,或者直接使用大剂量的风险被认为是低的。

拉莫三嗪

拉莫三嗪与致命的皮肤反应有关,特别是起始剂量大时。因此,制药商的产品信息建议:若上次使用拉莫三嗪后已经过了 5 个半衰期,应该像首次用药时一样逐渐加量。健康受试者单用拉莫三嗪时,药物半衰期约为 33 小时。拉莫三嗪的半衰期受其他药物影响,当合用能诱导葡萄糖醛酸化的药物(如卡马西平和苯妥英)时,其半衰期约为 14 小时;当合用丙戊酸盐时,其半衰期增至约 70 小时。这意味着,上次用药后 3~7 天后,必须彻底重新开始、逐步加量,具体时间取决于合用的其他药物[1]。

表 14.1 停止口服药物长达 2 周后重新开始用药 [2]

需要重新开始、逐步加量的药物			重新使用前一剂量通常是安全的药物	重新使用前一剂量可能是安全的药物
药物	过多长时间必须重新开始、逐步加量	进一步指导		
氯氮平	48 小时	见第 1 章"氯氮平中断治疗后重新使用"	阿坎酸 阿塞那平 氟西汀	抗精神病药(除外氯氮平、喹硫平、利培酮) 卡马西平
拉莫三嗪	3~7 天	见正文中讨论	氟哌啶醇 异卡波肼	胆碱酯酶抑制剂 中枢神经兴奋剂
美沙酮	3 天	见第 4 章"阿片类物质依赖"	洛非帕明	双硫仑
丁丙诺啡	3 天		哌甲酯 苯乙肼	锂盐(若肾功能改变,建议逐渐加量)
帕利哌酮长效针剂	取决于配方	见第 1 章"帕利哌酮长效注射剂"	舒必利 反苯环丙胺	单胺氧化酶抑制剂 美金刚
阿立哌唑长效针剂	若遗漏第 2 次或第 3 次药物,>5 周长期治疗时,>6 周	见第 1 章"阿立哌唑长效注射剂"	丙戊酸盐	纳曲酮 其他抗抑郁药(但要注意对镇静作用的耐受性丧失) 普瑞巴林 SSRI 三环类药物(但要注意对镇静作用和降压作用的耐受性丧失)

参考文献

1. Aurobindo Pharma – Milpharm Ltd. Summary of Product Characteristics. Lamotrigine 25mg Tablets. 2019; https://www.medicines.org.uk/emc/product/4736/smpc.
2. EMC. https://www.medicines.org.uk/emc/; accessed June 2020.

精神药物对生化和血液的影响

　　几乎所有精神药物都有血液或生化方面的不良反应,采用常规血液化验即可检测出来。这些反应许多是特异性的,没有临床意义;但是,也有一些反应,如氯氮平等药物相关的粒细胞缺乏症,则需要定期监测全血细胞计数。一般说来,若一种药物引起生化或血液方面不良反应的发生率高,或者导致罕见但致命的不良反应,则需要定期监测,如其他章节所述。

　　其他药物引起的实验室相关不良反应相对罕见(发生率通常小于1%),停用涉嫌药物后可以逆转,而且并非总是具有临床意义。还应注意的是,躯体共病、合用多种药物、非处方药物(包括物质滥用和酒精)也会影响生化和血液学指标。有时候,开始用药与出现实验室检查异常之间的时间联系并不明确,此时可考虑先停止、再重新使用所怀疑的药物。若对该不良反应的原因和意义存在怀疑,始终应该咨询相应的专家。

　　表 14.2 和表 14.3 概述了已知可导致生化和血液学不良反应的药物,其信息有各种来源[1-9]。在许多情况下,有关这些不良反应的证据有限,其信息大多来自病例报告、病例系列研究以及制药商提供的资料。若想进一步了解每种药物的详细信息,建议读者查阅本指南的相关章节以及其他专业资源,特别是与该药相关的产品文献。

表 14.2　精神药物相关的生化改变概要

化验指标	参考值范围[10]	导致数值升高的药物	导致数值降低的药物
丙氨酸氨基转移酶(ALT)	女性≤34U/L 男性≤45U/L (肥胖者可能更高)	**抗精神病药:**阿塞那平,苯哌利多,卡利拉嗪,氯氮平,氟哌啶醇,洛沙平,奥氮平,酚噻嗪类,喹硫平,利培酮/帕立哌酮 **抗抑郁药:**阿戈美拉汀,安非他酮,单胺氧化酶抑制剂,米安色林,米氮平,SNRI,SSRI(特别是帕罗西汀和舍曲林),三环类药物,曲唑酮,伏硫西汀 **抗焦虑/催眠药:**巴比妥酸盐类,苯二氮䓬类,丁螺环酮,氯美噻唑,异丙嗪,苏沃雷生,他美替安,唑吡坦 **心境稳定剂:**卡巴西平,拉莫三嗪,丙戊酸盐 **其他:**酒精,托莫西汀,β-受体阻断剂,咖啡因,可卡因,双硫仑,纳曲酮,阿片类物质,兴奋剂(滥用)	氨己烯酸
白蛋白	30~50g/L(40岁以后逐渐下降)	微量白蛋白尿可能是继发于精神药物的代谢综合征的特征(特别是酚噻嗪类,氯氮平,奥氮平,也可能有喹硫平)	长期合用苯丙胺或可卡因
碱性磷酸酶	50~120U/L	巴氯酚,β-受体阻断剂,苯二氮䓬类,咖啡因(过多/长期使用),卡马西平,西酞普兰,氯氮平,双硫仑,度洛西汀,加兰他敏,氟哌啶醇,洛沙平,美金刚,莫达非尼,去甲替林,奥氮平,苯妥英,舍曲林,托吡酯,曲唑酮,伐苯那嗪,丙戊酸盐;也与可导致恶性综合征的药物相关	丁丙诺啡,氟西汀(儿童),唑吡坦(罕见)

续表

化验指标	参考值范围[10]	导致数值升高的药物	导致数值降低的药物
氨	11~32μmol/L（进食和运动后升高）	巴比妥酸盐类,卡马西平,吸烟,托吡酯,丙戊酸盐(可出现脑病的体征)	无
淀粉酶	28~100U/L	酒精(急性),多奈哌齐,阿片类,普瑞巴林,卡巴拉汀,SSRI(罕见) **与胰腺炎有关的药物:**酒精,卡马西平,氯氮平,奥氮平,丙戊酸盐	无
天冬氨酸转移酶（AST）	女性≤34U/L 男性≤45U/L	同丙氨酸氨基转移酶,巴氯酚。注意:ALT是首选肝脏损害指标	三氟拉嗪,氨己烯酸
碳酸氢盐	22~29mmol/L	泻药滥用	与抗利尿激素不适当释放综合征(SIADH)有关的药物:全部抗抑郁药;抗精神病药(氯氮平、氟哌啶醇、奥氮平、吩噻嗪类、匹莫齐特、利培酮/帕利哌酮、喹硫平);卡马西平;也与导致代谢性酸中毒的药物相关(酒精、可卡因、托吡酯、唑尼沙胺)
胆红素	≤21μmol/L（总）	阿米替林,托莫西汀,苯二氮䓬类,卡马西平,氯氮䓬,氯丙嗪,西酞普兰,氯美噻唑,氯氮平,双硫仑,丙米嗪,氟奋乃静,拉莫三嗪,甲丙氨酯,米那普仑,奥氮平,吩噻嗪类,苯妥英,异丙嗪,舍曲林,伐苯那嗪,丙戊酸盐;也与导致胆汁淤积/肝损害的药物相关	巴比妥酸盐类
C反应蛋白	<10mg/L	丁丙诺啡(罕见);也与导致心肌炎的药物(氯氮平)相关	无
钙	2.20~2.60mmol/L（总钙,校正后） 2.20~2.60mmol/L（离子）	锂盐(罕见)	巴比妥类,卡马西平,氟哌啶醇,丙戊酸盐
碳水化合物缺乏转铁蛋白（CDT）	≤1.5%	酒精(CDT 1.6%~1.9% 提示摄入得多;≥2% 提示摄入过多)	无
氯	95~108mmol/L	导致高氯血症性代谢性酸中毒的药物:托吡酯,唑尼沙胺	与抗利尿激素不适当释放综合征(SIADH)有关的药物:全部抗抑郁药,抗精神病药(氯氮平、氟哌啶醇、奥氮平、吩噻嗪类、匹莫齐特、利培酮/帕利哌酮、喹硫平),卡马西平,泻药滥用

第14章

化验指标	参考值范围[10]	导致数值升高的药物	导致数值降低的药物
胆固醇（总）	≤5.2mmol/L（通常与推荐的处置界限相比，而不是与参考值范围相比）	抗精神病药，特别是牵涉代谢综合征者（吩噻嗪类、氯氮平、奥氮平、喹硫平）。罕见于：阿立哌唑，β-受体阻断剂（与氯氮平有相加效应），卡马西平，双硫仑，度洛西汀，美金刚，米氮平，莫达非尼，苯妥英，卡巴拉汀，舍曲林，文拉法辛	哌唑嗪，甲状腺药物
肌酐磷酸激酶	女：25~200U/L 男：40~320U/L（白种人的参考值范围，其他种族可能高些）	布美诺肽，依匹哌唑，卡利拉嗪，可乐定，氯氮平（与癫痫发作相关时），可卡因，右苯丙胺，多奈哌齐，奥氮平，普瑞巴林；也与导致恶性综合征和SIADH的药物相关；肌内注射的药物	无
肌酐	女：55~100μmol/L 男：60~120μmol/L	氯氮平，锂盐，鲁拉西酮，硫利达嗪，丙戊酸盐，与横纹肌溶解相关的药物（苯二氮䓬类、右苯丙胺、普瑞巴林、硫利达嗪；还与导致肾损害、恶性综合征和SIADH的药物相关	无
铁蛋白	女：15~150μg/L 男：30~400μg/L（随年龄升高）	酒精（急性期及酒精性肝病）	无
谷氨酰基转移酶（GGT）	女：≤38U/L 男：≤55U/L（非洲裔高2倍）	**抗抑郁药**：米氮平，SSRI（涉及帕罗西汀和舍曲林），三环类药物，曲唑酮，文拉法辛 **抗癫痫药/心境稳定剂**：卡马西平，拉莫三嗪，苯妥英，苯巴比妥，丙戊酸盐 **抗精神病药**：苯哌利多，氯丙嗪，氯氮平，氟奋乃静，氟哌啶醇，奥氮平，喹硫平 **其他**：酒精，巴比妥酸盐，氯美噻唑，右苯丙胺，莫达非尼，吸烟	无
葡萄糖	空腹：2.8~6.1mmol/L 随机：<11.1mmol/L	**抗抑郁药**：MAOI*，SSRI/SNRI*，TCA* **抗精神病药**：氯丙嗪，氯氮平，氟哌啶醇*，奥氮平*，喹硫平等 **物质滥用**：苯丙胺，美沙酮，阿片类物质 **其他**：巴氯酚，β-阻断剂*，安非他酮*，咖啡因*（糖尿病患者中），可乐定，多奈哌齐，加巴喷汀，加兰他敏，锂盐*，尼古丁，拟交感神经药，甲状腺药，缬苯那嗪	酒精；罕见于度洛西汀、氟哌啶醇、普瑞巴林；三环类药物用于代谢综合征时可导致血糖升高或降低
HbA₁C	20~39mmol/mol		锂盐，MAOI，SSRI
乳酸脱氢酶	90~200U/L（随年龄缓慢升高）	苯二氮䓬类药物，氯氮平，美沙酮，三环类药物（特别是丙米嗪），丙戊酸盐，还与导致恶性综合征的药物相关	无
脂蛋白：HDL	>1.2mmol/L	卡马西平，尼古丁，苯巴比妥，苯妥英	β-阻断剂，奥氮平，吩噻嗪类，丙戊酸盐
脂蛋白：LDL	<3.5mmol/L	β-受体阻断剂，咖啡因（有争议），卡马西平，氯丙嗪，氯氮平，伊洛哌酮，美金刚，米氮平，莫达非尼，奥氮平，吩噻嗪类，喹硫平，利培酮/帕利哌酮，卡巴拉汀，文拉法辛	哌唑嗪

续表

化验指标	参考值范围[10]	导致数值升高的药物	导致数值降低的药物
磷酸盐	0.8~1.5mmol/L	右苯丙胺,也与导致恶性综合征的药物相关	卡马西平,锂盐,米安色林,托吡酯
钾	3.5~5.3mmol/L	β-受体阻断剂,锂盐	酒精,双硫仑,咖啡因,可卡因,氟哌啶醇,锂盐,米安色林,普瑞巴林,瑞波西汀,卡巴拉汀,羟丁酸钠,拟交感神经药,托吡酯,唑尼沙胺;也可能是震颤谵妄的特征之一
催乳素	正常:<350mU/L 异常:>600mU/L	**抗抑郁药:**特别是阿莫沙平、MAOI 和三环类药物;SSRI 和文拉法辛也被涉及 **抗精神病药:**氨磺必利,氟哌啶醇,匹莫齐特,利培酮/帕利哌酮,舒必利等(阿立哌唑†、阿塞那平、溴哌唑、卡利拉嗪、氯氮平、鲁拉西酮、奥氮平、喹硫平和齐拉西酮对催乳素水平影响极小 **其他:**苯二氮䓬类药物,丁螺环酮,氘丁苯那嗪,阿片类物质,雷美替安,丁苯那嗪,伐苯那嗪	阿立哌唑,多巴胺激动剂,哌仑西平
蛋白(总)	60~80g/L	无	奥氮平(罕见)
钠	133~146mmol/L	锂盐(过量时)	**抗抑郁药:**特别是SSRI/SNRI;其他药物也被涉及 **抗精神病药:**全部(通过SIADH) **心境稳定剂:**卡马西平,锂盐,丙戊酸盐 **其他:**苯二氮䓬类药物,可乐定,多奈哌齐,美金刚,卡巴拉汀 服用抗抑郁药者若出现意识模糊、抽搐或嗜睡,均应考虑低钠血症
睾酮	男: 9.9~27.8nmol/L 女: 0.22~2.9nmol/L	地西泮	阿片类药物,雷美替安
促甲状腺激素	0.3~4.0mU/L	阿立哌唑,卡马西平,锂盐,喹硫平,卡巴拉汀,舍曲林,丙戊酸盐(轻度)	吗氯贝胺,甲状腺药物
甲状腺素	游离:9~26pmol/L 总:60~150pmol/L	罕见:苯丙胺(重度滥用),吗氯贝胺,普萘洛尔	巴比妥酸盐,卡马西平,碘塞罗宁,锂盐(导致 T_4 分泌减少),阿片类药物,苯妥英,丙戊酸盐 罕见于:阿立哌唑,氯氮平,喹硫平,卡巴拉汀,舍曲林

化验指标	参考值范围 [10]	导致数值升高的药物	导致数值降低的药物
甘油三酯			无
三碘甲状腺原氨酸	游离: 3.0~6.8pmol/L; 总:1.2~2.9pmol/L	海洛因,美沙酮	游离 T_3:丙戊酸盐 总 T_3:卡马西平,锂盐,普萘洛尔
尿酸盐 (尿酸)	女: 0.16~0.36mmol/L 男: 0.21~0.43mmol/L (随年龄升高)	酒精(急性),咖啡因(假阳性),氯氮平,左旋多巴,奥氮平,吲哚洛尔,哌唑嗪,托吡酯,唑尼沙胺	舍曲林(轻微)
尿素	2.5~7.8mmol/L (随年龄升高)	卡马西平,左旋多巴; 罕见于抗惊厥药超敏感性综合征和横纹肌溶解相关的药物	无

* 也可能与低血糖症相关。

† 也可能与催乳素水平低于正常相关。

表 14.3 精神药物相关的血液学改变概要

化验指标	参考值范围	导致数值升高的药物	导致数值降低的药物
激活部分促凝血酶原激酶时间	23~33 秒	吩噻嗪类(特别是氯丙嗪)	莫达非尼(罕见)
嗜碱性粒细胞	$0.0~0.1 \times 10^9$/L	氯氮平,三环类药物(特别是地昔帕明)	无
嗜酸性粒细胞	0.04×10^9/L~0.40×10^9/L	阿莫沙平,β-受体阻断剂,安非他酮,丁螺环酮,卡马西平,水合氯醛,氯丙嗪,氯硝西泮,氯氮平,多奈哌齐,氟奋乃静,氟哌啶醇,洛沙平,甲丙氨酯,马普替林,哌甲酯(仅静脉滥用时),莫达非尼,纳曲酮(肠外给药),奥氮平,异丙嗪,喹硫平,利培酮/帕利哌酮,SSRI,三环类药物,四氢西泮,色氨酸*,丙戊酸盐,文拉法辛;也可能是导致过敏综合征的药物的特征	无
红细胞沉降率	女:1~12mm/h 男:1~10mm/h (随年龄增加)	氯氮平,右苯丙胺,左美丙嗪,马普替林,SSRI	丁丙诺啡

续表

化验指标	参考值范围	导致数值升高的药物	导致数值降低的药物
血红蛋白	女:115~165g/L 男:130~180g/L	氯氮平,睾酮,吸烟	阿立哌唑,巴比妥酸盐,丁丙诺啡,安非他酮,卡马西平,氯氮草,氯丙嗪,多奈哌齐,度洛西汀,加兰他敏,MAOI,美金刚,甲丙氨酯,米安色林,苯妥英,异丙嗪,卡巴拉汀,曲马多,三氟拉嗪,氨己烯酸
淋巴细胞	1.5×10^9/L~ 4.5×10^9/L	纳曲酮,阿片类药物,吸烟,丙戊酸盐;也可能是导致过敏综合征的药物的特征	酒精(慢性),水合氯醛,氯氮平,锂盐,米氮平(罕见)
平均细胞血红蛋白	27~32pg	与巨幼红细胞性贫血相关的药物,如全部抗癫痫药、氧化亚氮	无
平均细胞血红蛋白浓度	320~360g/L		
平均细胞容积	80~100fL	酒精	
单核细胞	0.2×10^9/L~0.8×10^9/L	氟哌啶醇	无
中性粒细胞	2.0×10^9/L~7.5×10^9/L (非洲裔可能较低,因良性种族性中性粒细胞减少)	安非他酮,卡马西平[†],西酞普兰,氯丙嗪,氯氮平,度洛西汀,氟西汀,氟奋乃静,氟哌啶醇,拉莫三嗪,锂盐,马普替林,奥氮平,喹硫平,利培酮/帕利哌酮,卡巴拉汀,替奥噻吨,曲唑酮,文拉法辛	**与粒细胞缺乏相关的药物:**阿莫沙平,阿立哌唑,巴比妥酸盐,卡马西平,氯氮草,氯丙嗪,氯氮平[‡],可卡因(掺入次品),地西泮,氟奋乃静,氟哌啶醇,甲丙氨酯,米安色林,米氮平,奥氮平,哌仑西平,异丙嗪,利培酮/帕利哌酮,三环类药物(特别是丙米嗪),环苯丙胺,丙戊酸盐 **与粒细胞减少相关的药物:**阿米替林,阿莫沙平,阿塞那平,安非他酮,卡马西平,卡利拉嗪,氯丙嗪,西酞普兰,氯米帕明,氯硝西泮,氯氮平,度洛西汀,氟西汀,氨磺丁脲氟,奋乃静,加兰他敏,氟哌啶醇,拉莫三嗪,劳拉西泮,卢美哌隆,鲁拉西酮,美金刚,甲丙氨酯,米安色林,米氮平,莫达非尼,氧化亚氮,奥氮平,奥沙西泮,苯乙肼,普瑞巴林,异丙嗪,喹硫平,环苯丙胺,丙戊酸盐,文拉法辛,齐拉西酮 **与白细胞减少相关的药物:**舍曲林,曲唑酮,丙戊酸盐

续表

血指标	参考值范围	导致数值升高的药物	导致数值降低的药物
红细胞比容	女:0.37~0.47L/L 男:0.40~0.52L/L	氯氮平(罕见),睾酮	苯二氮䓬类药物(罕见),丁丙诺啡,纳曲酮,氨己烯酸
血小板	150×10⁹/L~ 450×10⁹/L	拉莫三嗪,锂盐[†]	酒精,巴比妥酸盐,β-受体阻断剂,苯二氮䓬类药物,安非他酮,丁螺环酮,卡马西平,氯氮䓬,氯丙嗪,氯硝西泮,可乐定,氯氮平[†],可卡因,地西泮,多奈哌齐,度洛西汀,氟西汀,氟奋乃静,拉莫三嗪,甲丙氨酯,美沙酮,哌甲酯,米氮平,纳曲酮,氧化亚氮,奥氮平,哌仑西平,异丙嗪,喹硫平,利培酮/帕利哌酮,卡巴拉汀,舍曲林,三环类药物,环苯丙胺,曲唑酮,三氟拉嗪,丙戊酸盐,文拉法辛,齐拉西酮;也可能是导致过敏综合征的药物的特征 **与血小板聚集受损相关的药物:**氯氮䓬,西酞普兰,地西泮,氟西汀,氟伏沙明,帕罗西汀,吡拉西坦,舍曲林,丙戊酸盐
凝血酶原时间(PT)/国际标准化比率(INR)	PT:10~13s INR:0.8~1.2	水合氯醛,双硫仑,氟西汀,氟伏沙明,米氮平,丙戊酸盐;还有与华法林有相互作用的药物	巴比妥酸盐,卡马西平,苯妥英,替奥噻吨
红细胞计数	男: 4.5×10⁹/L~6.5×10⁹/L 女: 3.5×10⁹/L~5.8×10⁹/L	锂盐,睾酮	丁丙诺啡,卡马西平,氯氮䓬,氯丙嗪,多奈哌齐,氟哌啶醇,甲丙氨酯,苯妥英,喹硫平,三氟拉嗪
红细胞分布宽度	11.5%~14.5%	与贫血相关的药物,如:卡马西平,氯氮䓬,西酞普兰,氯硝西泮,地西泮,拉莫三嗪,美金刚,米氮平,舍曲林,环苯丙胺,曲唑酮,丙戊酸盐,文拉法辛	无
网状细胞计数	0.5%~2.5% (或 50×10⁹/L~ 100×10⁹/L)	无	卡马西平,氯氮䓬,氯丙嗪,甲丙氨酯,苯妥英,三氟拉嗪 **与纯红细胞再生障碍相关的药物:**卡马西平,氯氮平,丙戊酸盐

* 以前报告的嗜酸性肌痛可能是某一制药厂的污染物所致。

† 可升高或降低。

‡ 注意,在罕见病例中发现,氯氮平与循环中性粒细胞水平下降的"早晨假性中性粒细胞减少"相关。中性粒细胞计数可出现昼夜节律,晚些时候复查全血细胞计数可能有益。

参考文献

1. BMJ Group and Pharmaceutical Press. British National Formulary 2020; https://www.medicinescomplete.com.
2. Aronson J. *Meyler Side Effects of Drugs: the International Encyclopedia of Adverse Drug Reactions and Interactions.* Elsevier Science; 2015.
3. Foster R. *Clinical Laboratory Investigation and Psychiatry. A Practical Handbook.* New York: Informa 2008.
4. Oyesanmi O, et al. Hematologic side effects of psychotropics. *Psychosomatics* 1999; 40: 414–421.
5. Stubner S, et al. Blood dyscrasias induced by psychotropic drugs. *Pharmacopsychiatry* 2004; 37 Suppl 1:S70-S78.
6. Pharmaceutical Press. Martindale: the Complete Drug Reference (online) 2020; https://www.medicinescomplete.com.
7. LiverTox: clinical and Research Information on Drug-Induced Liver Injury. Bethesda (MD): National Institute of Diabetes and Digestive and Kidney Diseases 2012; https://www.ncbi.nlm.nih.gov/books/NBK547852.
8. Medicines Complete. AHFS Drug Information 2020; https://www.medicinescomplete.com/mc/ahfs/current.
9. U.S. Food & Drug Administration. Drugs@FDA: FDA-Approved Drugs 2020; https://www.accessdata.fda.gov/scripts/cder/daf.
10. Association for Clinical Biochemistry and Laboratory Medicine. Analyte Monographs Alongside the National Library of Medicine Catalogue 2020; http://www.acb.org.uk/whatwedo/science/amalc.aspx.

精神科药物的精神科不良反应概要

　　人们越来越认识到,非精神科药物可以引起广泛的精神科症状[1]。在所有药物中,多达 2/3 在其产品说明书中列出了潜在的精神科不良反应[2],但是大多数情况下很少有证据支持其因果联系。药物的精神科不良反应在临床试验中介绍不充分,往往只在上市后监测期间才变得明显[3]。鉴于有如此不确定的水平,对于所怀疑的精神科不良反应,应该逐例进行诊断和处理。作为一般指南,非精神科药物的精神科不良反应列于表 14.4。对于未列入的药物,应该查阅其他信息来源和产品文献。注意,在精神科使用的药物、治疗 HIV 的药物以及抗癫痫药,其精神科不良反应在本指南的其他章节进行了总结。

表 14.4　非精神科药物的精神科不良反应概要[4-7]

药物	精神科不良反应	注解
ACE 抑制剂		
如卡托普利、赖诺普利	疲乏,幻觉,谵妄,情绪紊乱	卡托普利与情绪影响的相关性最强。整体上精神科不良反应有限
镇痛药		
阿片类药物	镇静,烦躁不安,意识模糊,心境改变(包括欣快),睡眠紊乱,幻觉,精神病,谵妄,依赖	精神科不良反应相对常见。停药期间有发生精神病的罕见报告[8]
5-HT$_1$ 激动剂(如舒马普坦)	疲乏,焦虑,惊恐发作	
抗生素		
头孢霉素类,青霉素类,喹诺酮类(包括氟喹诺酮类),四环素类	睡眠紊乱(失眠、嗜睡、异常做梦、噩梦),焦虑,谵妄,精神错乱,抑郁,激越,精神病性症状(如幻觉、自杀观念)	所有抗生素均可导致谵妄。有基础躯体疾病的患者发生精神科不良反应的风险更大。在喹诺酮类药物中,环丙沙星导致的精神科不良反应最多,包括情绪紊乱、激越和意识模糊。精神科不良反应可能很快发生,如仅用一次药之后
抗疟药		
氯喹,甲氟喹	精神病,包括幻觉、惊恐发作、自杀观念和自杀未遂、焦虑、抑郁、多动、意识模糊。异常做梦常见于使用甲氟喹者	症状在治疗早期开始出现。若出现这些症状,应该告诉患者停止治疗,寻求医疗指导。使用甲氟喹出现精神科不良反应者多于氯喹。反应甚至可能在停药后发生。甲氟喹禁用于活动期精神疾病或者既往有精神疾病的患者
抗震颤麻痹药		
左旋多巴	幻视,抑郁,轻躁狂,睡眠紊乱,异常做梦,认知损害,激越,精神病,谵妄	

续表

药物	精神科不良反应	注解
多巴胺激动剂	镇静,精神运动性激越,焦虑,静坐不能,睡眠紊乱,精神病,认知损害,谵妄,幻视	这些药物的精神科不良反应多于左旋多巴
金刚烷胺	注意减退,睡眠紊乱,幻视,易激惹,焦虑,抑郁,欣快,疲劳,精神病,谵妄	
司来吉兰(MAO-B 抑制剂)	睡眠紊乱,激越,精神病	初级代谢产物包括左苯丙胺
恩他卡朋(COMT 抑制剂)	睡眠紊乱,幻觉,谵妄	
心血管药		
β-受体阻断剂	疲劳,镇静,睡眠紊乱和噩梦,认知损害,抑郁,幻觉,精神病,谵妄	亲脂性 β-受体阻断剂(如普萘洛尔、美托洛尔)引起的紊乱多于亲水性 β-受体阻断剂(如阿替洛尔、索他洛尔、纳多洛尔)。普萘洛尔最常见抑郁症状,但其因果关系并未明确。许多临床试验的精神科不良反应报告意义不明
钙通道阻滞药(如地尔硫䓬、氨氯地平)	心境改变,昏睡,烦躁不安,躁狂,精神病,谵妄,静坐不能	因果关系不明确
他汀类药物[9-11](如辛伐他汀、阿托伐他汀)	认知损害,记忆损害,抑郁,情绪不稳,易激惹,睡眠紊乱	他汀类药物与心境改变、睡眠、认知之间的因果关系在随机双盲试验的系统综述中并未确定。他汀类药物穿透血脑屏障;辛伐他汀的穿透性最强。在怀疑出现中、重度精神科不良反应的病例中,建议换用亲水性他汀类药物(如普伐他汀、瑞舒伐他汀)
肾上腺皮质激素类		
糖皮质激素类(如倍他米松、泼尼松龙、泼尼松)	心境障碍,自杀观念,欣快,激越,睡眠紊乱,精神病,谵妄,痴呆,认知损害	有明确的因果联系。精神科不良反应的发生往往非常突然,在开始治疗后 1~2 周内。症状通常随着药物减量而缓解,据报告与几种用药途径均相关(包括口服、肠外和吸入),但是吸入较少出现。症状通常随着逐渐停药而缓解,但是症状的持续时间相差很大
其他药物		
化疗药(如 5-氟尿嘧啶、门冬酰胺酶、硼替佐米、异环磷酰胺、长春新碱)	常见:认知损害,谵妄,精神病 不常见:抑郁,焦虑,自杀观念	几乎所有化疗药物均有明显的精神科不良反应,起源于多种因素(即继发于疾病过程、不良反应和心理痛苦)。癌症治疗相关的认知改变包括执行功能、多任务处理、短期记忆和注意方面的困难。认知改变呈剂量依赖性,某些药物(甲氨蝶呤、氟达拉滨、阿糖胞苷、5-氟尿嘧啶、顺铂)的认知反应更差
西咪替丁	认知损害,谵妄	

第14章

续表

药物	精神科不良反应	注解
干扰素-α 和干扰素-β	抑郁,以前有效的抗抑郁药失效,自杀观念,谵妄,非特异性精神科症状。偶有使用干扰素-α 出现精神病和躁狂的病例报告。	使用干扰素-β 出现精神科不良反应的可能性相对较小,使用干扰素-α 则明显更普遍地出现。干扰素-α 相关的抑郁用抗抑郁药有效,使用抗抑郁药可起预防作用。已经研究出新的诊断用生物标记,用于预测哪些患者可能发生干扰素-α 相关的精神科不良反应
异维 A 酸 [12]	抑郁,自杀观念,精神病	有精神科不良反应的零星报告,但是异维 A 酸治疗与抑郁、焦虑、心境改变、自杀观念/自杀之间的因果联系并未得到确认。此外,最近一篇系统综述发现,痤疮治疗改善了抑郁症状 [13]。罕见的、特异质反应无法被排除;若出现这些不良反应,应该停药。其发生风险在曾有自杀未遂者中并未升高,而且与剂量和治疗时间无关

精神科不良反应的鉴别诊断

有广泛的混杂因素使得精神科不良反应的诊断(也许还有识别)变得复杂。例如,躯体疾病、合用处方药物、非处方药物、原有精神疾病均可影响其临床表现和结局。关于药物与精神科不良反应之间因果关系的可能性,其决定因素列于框 14.1。为了进一步支持临床决策,可用《诺氏(Naranjio)量表》评估不良反应与药物相关的可能性(表 14.5)。尽管在一些病例中需要停用引起不良反应的非精神科药物,但是这样的决定需要个别考虑,这超出了本书的范围。

表 14.5 修订版诺氏(Naranjio)药物不良反应可能性量表评分标准 [14]

问题	是	否	不适用/不详
1. 关于该不良反应,以前有结论性的报告吗?	+1	0	0
2. 该不良反应出现在使用所怀疑药物之后吗?	+2	−1	0
3. 停用该药后,不良反应改善了吗?	+1	0	0
4. 重新使用该药时,该不良反应出现了吗?	+2	−1	0
5. 该不良反应有其他原因吗?	−1	+2	0
6. 给予安慰剂时,该不良反应出现了吗?	−1	+1	0
7. 经检测该药的血药浓度达到中毒水平了吗?	+1	0	0
8. 该不良反应是否随着剂量增加而加重、随着剂量减少而减轻?	+1	0	0
9. 患者以前对相同或类似药物有类似的反应吗?	+1	0	0
10. 该不良反应得到客观证据证实吗?	+1	0	0
可能性评分:≥9=确定;5~8=很可能;1~4=可能;≤0=可疑			

框 14.1 药物与精神科不良反应之间因果关系可能性的决定因素 [4,15]

- 药物暴露与精神科不良反应之间的时间关系
- 使用所怀疑药物时发生特定的精神科不良反应的证据
- 精神科不良反应似有合理的药理机制（如多巴胺激动剂与精神病）
- 对于症状有其他解释（如原有精神疾病、新发精神疾病、其他药物）
- 停药时症状的反应
- 再次使用相同药物时的反应

参考文献

1. Rudorfer MV, et al. Assessing Psychiatric Adverse Effects during Clinical Drug Development. *Pharmaceut Med* 2012; 26:363–394.
2. Smith DA. Psychiatric side effects of non-psychiatric drugs. *S DJ Med* 1991; 44:291–292.
3. Holvey C, et al. Psychiatric side effects of non-psychiatric drugs. *Br J Hosp Med (Lond)* 2010; 71:432–436.
4. Gupta A, et al. Adverse psychiatric effects of non-psychotropic medications. *BJ Psych Advances* 2016; 22:325–334.
5. Huffman JC, et al. Neuropsychiatric consequences of cardiovascular medications. *Dialogues Clin Neurosci* 2007; 9:29–45.
6. Munjampalli SK, et al. Medicinal-Induced Behavior Disorders. *Neurol Clin* 2016; 34:133–169.
7. Parker C. Psychiatric effects of drugs for other disorders. *Medicine* 2016; 44:768–774.
8. Maremmani AG, et al. Substance abuse and psychosis. *The Strange Case of Opioids. Eur Rev Med Pharmacol Sci* 2014; 18:287–302.
9. Ott BR, et al. Do statins impair cognition? A systematic review and meta-analysis of randomized controlled trials. *J Gen Intern Med* 2015; 30:348–358.
10. Swiger KJ, et al. Statins, mood, sleep, and physical function: a systematic review. *Eur J Clin Pharmacol* 2014; 70:1413–1422.
11. Tuccori M, et al. Neuropsychiatric adverse events associated with statins: epidemiology, pathophysiology, prevention and management. *CNS Drugs* 2014; 28:249–272.
12. Liu M, et al. Neurological and Neuropsychiatric Adverse Effects of Dermatologic Medications. *CNS Drugs* 2016; 30:1149–1168.
13. Huang YC, et al. Isotretinoin treatment for acne and risk of depression: A systematic review and meta-analysis. *J Am Acad Dermatol* 2017; 76:1068-1076.e1069.
14. Naranjo CA, et al. A method for estimating the probability of adverse drug reactions. *Clin Pharmacol Ther* 1981; 30:239–245.
15. World Health Organisation and Uppsala Monitoring Centre. The use of the WHO-UMC system for standardised case causality assessment. 2004; http://www.who.int/medicines/areas/quality_safety/safety_efficacy/WHOcausality_assessment.pdf.

扩展阅读

Bangert MK, et al. Neurological and psychiatric adverse effects of antimicrobials. CNS Drugs 2019; 33:727–753.

第 14 章

超说明书用药

产品许可证由监管机构授予时,意味着相对于所治疗疾病的严重程度和其他现有治疗方法,所申报药物已被证实有效,且其不良反应可以接受。获得许可的适应证是药品特有的,在产品特征概要中有描述,同一药物的专利制剂和通用制剂适应证有可能不同[1]。美国的产品"说明书"与欧盟的许可证具有相似的法律地位。

制药商决定申报某一药物的产品许可证本质上属于商业决策;需要将潜在的销售额与实施必要临床试验的成本进行对比。结果是,在获得许可的适应证之外,药物可能在不同疾病状态、年龄范围、剂量和疗程中也有效。没有正式的产品许可证或说明书,完全有可能反映出没有进行过对照试验来支持该药在这些范围内的疗效。在其他情况下(如舍曲林或喹硫平治疗广泛性焦虑障碍),有足够的证据,但是制药商未申报许可证。然而重要的是,还有可能临床试验已经做过了,但得出的是阴性或含糊的结果。临床医生往往假定,具有相似作用机制的药物,对于某一适应证可能同样有效。在许多情况下确实如此。例如,对于痴呆患者的行为和精神症状(BPSD),阿立哌唑、奥氮平、喹硫平和利培酮的疗效类似,但是只有利培酮在欧盟获得了该适应证的许可。

在许可证或说明书范围内处方药物,并不能保证患者不受伤害。同样的,在许可证之外处方药物,并不意味着风险-获益比率自动就是不利的。在前述 BPSD 的例子中,利培酮的耐受性显然并非优于其他抗精神病药[2]。在许可证以外处方药物,通常被称为"超说明书(off-label)"用药。这种做法确实赋予开药者额外的责任,人们希望开药者能够证明其做法符合一群负责任的医务人员的观点(Bolam 测试标准)[3],而且其行为能够经得起逻辑分析(Bolitho 测验标准)[4]。这两个测试标准已经被有效地替代为"Montgomery 诉 Lanarkshire 健康委员会上诉案判决意见"[5],或者至少被其澄清。该判决意见写道:

心理健康的成年人有权决定在现有治疗形式中采取哪一种,并且在实施妨碍其身体完整性的治疗前必须获得其同意。因此,医生有责任采取合理的治疗,以确保患者知道所建议治疗涉及的任何实质性风险,以及合理的替代治疗或变体治疗。实质性的测试标准为:在特定情况下,一个理智的人处在患者位置时是否有可能认为该风险有意义,或者医生是否或者应否合情合理地知道特定患者有可能认为该风险有意义。

因此,至少在英国,处方医师有责任让患者知道与所处方药物相关的实质性风险,并列出替代治疗方案。

英国医学总会允许医生超说明书用药,但是仅限于处方医生对支持其疗效和安全性的足够证据或经验感到满意时[6]。

在美国,在"合法的医患关系中"超说明书用药是合法的[7]。禁止营销超说明书用药,但是接受主动请求后可以提供信息[8]。在美国精神疾病的全部处方中,估计超说明书处方占 13%[9]。

有人提出,相比于其他医学领域,精神科的超说明书用药不太可能得到很强的证据支持[10]。在精神科,小样本研究证据力度不强(常有较大的置信区间),常常会影响到临床实践,特别是难治性疾病(本书中可见到许多例子)。如果将这些小样本研究通过荟萃分析结合起来,往往发现有较大的异质性,说明存在出版偏倚(即阴性结果未被发表)。因此,在没有任何证据支持其疗效和耐受性的情况下,某些治疗方法被纳入"日常习惯和实践"中,即使更新、样本更大、研究和荟萃分析阴性结论更确定,这些治疗方法有时仍被继续合用。合用 ω-3 脂肪酸治疗精神分裂症就是很好的例子。广泛地超说明书使用精神药物治疗非精神疾病的一个例子是阿米替林——该药在英国初级保健处方中 93% 为超说明书用药 [11]。

关于许可药物的超说明书使用 [12],英国精神科医师协会精神药理学专业兴趣小组发布了一项共识声明,并在 2017 年进行了更新 [13]。他们注意到,超说明书用药在成人精神科很常见,一项现况调查发现,高达 50% 的患者被处方过至少一种超说明书的药物。他们还注意到,超说明书用药比例较高的人群可能有 18 岁以下、65 岁以上、学习障碍、孕妇、哺乳期妇女以及在司法精神科治疗的患者。共识声明的主要建议如下:

在"超说明书"用药之前:

- 排除已有许可证的其他药物(如,已经证明它们治疗无效,或难以耐受)。
- 确保熟悉准备"超说明书"用药的证据。若不确定,请教其他医生(也许专业药师)。
- 考虑并记录拟用药物的潜在风险和获益。与患者及其照料者(若适用)分享风险评估的结果。记录讨论的情况、患者的知情同意或者没有知情同意能力。
- 若与初级保健人员分担处方责任,则应确保与全科医生分享风险评估结果和知情同意问题。
- 监测疗效和不良反应;从小剂量开始,缓慢加量。
- 考虑发表该案例,增加知识体系。
- 治疗无效或者出现的风险大于获益时,停止该药治疗。

超说明书用药的性质越强,越应该遵循上述指南。

可接受的超产品许可证或超产品说明书用药的案例

表 14.6 给出了在精神科实践中常见的超说明书用药的案例。这些案例原则上都符合 Bolam 和 Bolitho 测试标准。全部列出超说明书用药不太可能,因为:证据不断变化,处方者的专业知识和经验各异。三级转诊中心的精神药理学专家所制定的治疗策略可能合理,而对心理治疗特别感兴趣、很少开药的医师开始使用的治疗则很难判断其合理性。

表 14.6 精神科常见的超说明书用药举例

药物/药物类别	超说明书使用	更多信息
第二代抗精神病药	精神分裂症以外的精神病性障碍	批准的适应证差异很大,大多数情况下,无法反映药物之间在疗效上的差异
氯氮平	双相障碍	当标准治疗控制不住症状时,有实质性证据支持氯氮平的疗效

药物/药物类别	超说明书使用	更多信息
赛庚啶	静坐不能	对于这种令人痛苦并难以治疗的抗精神病药的不良反应,有一些证据支持其疗效
氟西汀/舍曲林	广泛性焦虑障碍	有实质性的支持证据
氯胺酮(外消旋体)	难治性抑郁	对于氯胺酮外消旋体和 s-异构体,均有实质性证据
褪黑素(昼夜节律)	儿童失眠	许可证仅覆盖 >55 岁的成年人。也许最好使用未获许可的褪黑素制剂。
哌甲酯	6 岁以下儿童注意缺陷多动障碍	已确定的临床实践
纳曲酮	学习障碍患者的自伤行为	证据有限 在专家手中可以接受
丙戊酸钠	双相障碍的预防和治疗	已确定的临床实践 来自其他丙戊酸盐制剂的证据

　　注意,有些药物在英国没有任何适应证的许可。在精神科实践中两个常见的例子是速释褪黑素(用于治疗儿童青少年失眠)和哌仑西平(用于治疗氯氮平引起的流涎)。特别重要的是应该了解证据基础,并记录潜在获益、不良反应和患者的知情同意。

参考文献

1. Datapharm Communications Ltd. Summary of product characteristics. Electronic Medicines Compendium 2020; http://www.medicines.org.uk/emc.

2. Maher AR, et al. Efficacy and comparative effectiveness of atypical antipsychotic medications for off-label uses in adults: a systematic review and meta-analysis. *JAMA* 2011; 306:1359–1369.

3. Bolam v Friern Barnet Hospital Management Committee. *The Weekly Law Reports* 1957; 1:582.

4. Bolitho v City and Hackney Health Authority. *The Weekly Law Reports* 1997; 3:1151.

5. British and Irish Legal Information Institute. Montgomery (Appellant) v Lanarkshire Health Board (Respondent) (Scotland) 2015; http://www.bailii.org/uk/cases/UKSC/2015/11.html.

6. General Medical Council. Good practice in prescribing and managing medicines and devices 2013; https://www.gmc-uk.org/guidance/ethical guidance/14316.asp.

7. Buckman Co. v. Plaintiffs' Legal Comm. 531 U.S. 341 2001; https://www.law.cornell.edu/supct/html/98-1768.ZO.html.

8. FindLaw. Off-label use promotion is protected free speech 2012; https://blogs.findlaw.com/second_circuit/2012/12/off-label-use-promotion-is-protected-free-speech.html.

9. Vijay A, et al. Patterns and predictors of off-label prescription of psychiatric drugs. *PLoS One* 2018; 13:e0198363.

10. Epstein RS, et al. The many sides of off-label prescribing. *ClinPharmacolTher* 2012; 91:755–758.

11. Wong J, et al. Off-label indications for antidepressants in primary care: descriptive study of prescriptions from an indication based electronic prescribing system. *BMJ* 2017; 356:j603.

12. Royal College of Psychiatrists. College Report 142. Use of licensed medicines for unlicensed applications in psychiatric practice 2007; http://www.rcpsych.ac.uk/publications/collegereports/cr/cr142.aspx.

13. Royal College of Psychiatrists Psychopharmacology Committee. Use of licensed medicines for unlicensed applications in psychiatric practice. 2nd edition. College Report CR210 2017; http://www.rcpsych.ac.uk/files/pdfversion/CR210.pdf.

扩展阅读

Frank B, et al. Psychotropic medications and informed consent: a review. *Ann Clin Psychiatry* 2008; 20:87–95. General Medical Council. Good practice in prescribing and managing medicines and devices. 2013. http://www.gmc-uk.org/guidance/ethical_guidance/14316.asp.

Sharma, et al. BAP position statement: off-label prescribing of psychotropic medication to children and adolescents. *J Psychopharmacol* 2016; 30:416–421.

英国和威尔士的精神卫生法

于 1983 年颁布、2007 年修订的《精神卫生法》是英国和威尔士的法律,它为在医院内收留和治疗精神疾病患者提供了框架。它也考虑到在社区对患者的管理。

此处的指南为处方医生日常工作中可能遇到的章节提供了速查概要。这不是详尽的清单。该法律有面向医疗从业者的《行医法规》,该法律第 25 章为《精神卫生法》的治疗原则提供了详细的指南[1]。《精神卫生法》可在 www.legislation.gov.uk 查阅。

民事与司法拘留部分

第 2 节	入院评估持续长达 28 天
第 3 节	入院治疗可持续长达 6 个月且可延续
第 36 节	还押到医院接受治疗
第 37 节	法庭签发的住院令(按第 3 节执行)
第 37 节(理论性的)	处理好像依据第 37 节。该条款非正式地用于许多不同情况。例如:一名患者以前按第 47/49 节拘留,且其限制令到期
第 38 节	临时住院法令
第 41 节	刑事法院做出的限制出院的法令。伴随第 37 节,写成 S37/41
第 47 节	转至监狱医院
第 48 节	适用于需要紧急治疗、未判刑的因犯,伴随第 49 节(写成 S48/49)
第 49 节	通常伴随 S47 的限制令(写成 S47/49)
第 58 节	**治疗需要获得同意或二次鉴别诊断** **请注意:在法律上,负责 S58 工作的是责任医生(responsible clinician)**

必须注意:按照第 58 节进行治疗的权力仅限于精神疾病的治疗。躯体疾病治疗(一般)受知情同意的正常规则管理;若患者没有能力做出知情同意,则由《心智能力法案》授权管理。

责任医生通常是患者的顾问医生。

依上述章节之一被拘留者,在拘留头 3 个月,责任医生可以给其用药治疗精神疾病(有或无知情同意)。此后,必须获得患者的知情同意,或者进行二次鉴别诊断。患者被拘留期间首次接受精神药物治疗时开始 3 个月倒计时。注意,这包括按 S2 拘留且当时没有中断、换成 S3 或者按 S3 拘留的患者。实际上,3 个月法则通常从首次拘留之日开始计算。

若患者同意接受治疗,责任医生填写 T2 表。

若患者不同意或没有表达知情同意的能力,请指定做二次鉴别诊断的医生(second opinion appointed doctor,SOAD),后者填写 T3 表。

根据《行医法规》25.75 段的建议,应该将一份 T2 和 T3 表与病历共同保存[1]。

T2 和 T3 表的填写

表格中应声明以下内容：

- 药品名称或药物类别
- 若填写的是药物类别,在任何时间允许合用的药品数量
- 用药途径
- 《英国药典》指南中的最大剂量

例如,第二代抗精神病药 ×1(口服),在《英国药典》最大剂量范围之内。

若患者有能力且同意接受治疗,但仅希望使用某种药物,责任医生可以在 T2 表中填写药品名称,取代药品类别名称。

例如,限奥氮平片(口服),在《英国药典》最大剂量范围之内。

《英国药典》未收录的精神药物可在 T2 或 T3 表中填写其适应证。

例如,美哌隆片(口服),每日最大剂量 25mg,用于治疗精神分裂症。

用于治疗精神疾病的非精神科药物应该填入 T2 和 T3 表,例如 ω-3 脂肪酸(鱼油)用于精神分裂症。还应该填写用于治疗多涎和锥体外系不良反应的抗毒蕈碱药。

安排和准备接待 SOAD 出诊

《行医法规》25.51 段描述:医生在邀请有 SOAD 证书持有者会诊之前,应该考虑请精神卫生专科药师进行审核,特别是患者的药物治疗方案复杂或不寻常时。

法定咨询者

SOAD 在发出 T3 表之前,应该询问两个人。其中之一必须是护士。另外一人不应是护士或医生。这两个人必须参加过该患者的治疗。这两个人被称为法定咨询者。精神卫生专科药师若最近参与过患者的药物审核,可以承担这个角色。

《行医法规》25.56 段描述:

法定咨询者可以要求 SOAD 与自己私下讨论,并且认真倾听。咨询者被问及的问题包括但不限于:

- 所提议的治疗及患者做出知情同意的能力;
- 他们了解到的患者过去和现在的观点和希望;
- 其他治疗选择,以及对治疗建议做出决定的方式;
- 患者的病情进展情况及其照料者的观点;
- 如有相关,给不想接受治疗的患者强加治疗的意义,以及患者拒绝治疗的原因。

什么是知情同意?

《行医法规》对知情同意的定义是:

……患者自愿而持续地同意给予自己特定的治疗,前提是足够了解该治疗的目的、性质、可能的作用和风险,包括治疗成功的可能性以及任何替代治疗方法。在不公正或过度压力下的许可不是知情同意。

患者正式地做出知情同意,必须具备做出决定的"精神行为能力"(capacity)。

什么是行为能力?

《英国心智能力法 2005》描述:

- 一个人应该被假定具有行为能力,除非证实他们没有行为能力;
- 一个人不应被作为不能做出决定者对待,除非已经采取全部可行的步骤帮助他们但是没有成功;而且
- 一个人不应仅仅因为做出不明智的决定就被作为不能做出决定者对待

患者被认为没有行为能力的条件是他们不能:

- 理解与所做决定相关的信息,或者
- 在大脑中保持该信息,或者
- 作为决策过程的一部分使用或考虑该信息,或者
- 传达他们的决定(通过说话、手语或任何其他方式)。

患者只需符合上述 4 项中的 1 项,即可被认为是没有行为能力。行为能力可能随着时间的过去而发生改变,因此重新评估很重要。患者可能对一项决定没有行为能力,但是对另一项决定有行为能力。

第 62 节紧急治疗

若 3 个月以后需要紧急用药治疗患者的精神疾病,且该药不在 T2 或 T3 表中,可适用 S62 节。

《行医法规》25.38 段描述

此项仅适用于立即需要采取所涉治疗:

- 挽救患者生命;
- 防止患者的情况严重恶化,且该治疗没有不可逆的生理或心理上的不良后果;
- 减轻患者的严重痛苦,且该治疗没有不可逆的生理或心理上的不良后果,也不产生明显的生理损害;或者
- 防止患者出现暴力行为或对自己或他人构成危险,且该治疗对于达到此目的是必需的最低程度的干涉,没有不可逆的生理或心理上的不良后果,也不产生明显的生理损害。

每个托管机构(Trust)应该为负责治疗的医生(通常是顾问医生)设计一张表格,描述治疗方法、立即需要采取治疗的原因以及治疗的疗程。

第 132 节医院经理向被拘留患者提供信息的义务

关于 S312 和对治疗的知情同意,《行医法规》4.20 描述

必须告知患者《精神卫生法》对其精神疾病的治疗是如何规定的。特别是要告诉他们:

- 可能未经他们知情同意即实施治疗的情况(若有),以及他们有权拒绝治疗的情况;
- SOAD 的作用及其参与治疗的情况;
- (如有相关)关于电抽搐治疗及其相关药物的规定。

电抽搐治疗（ECT）

第 58a 节涉及 ECT。对 ECT 的授权见于以下表格：

T4	适用于 18 周岁或以上的成年人，可以负责医生或 SOAD 填写
T5	适用于不到 18 周岁的患者，仅限 SOAD 填写
T6	适用于无行为能力的患者，仅限 SOAD 填写

所有年龄未满 18 周岁、拟行 ECT 的患者，不论是否按《精神卫生法》被拘留，必须按照 T5 或 T6 对治疗进行授权。

有行为能力做出知情同意的患者不应进行 ECT，除非他们确实同意（然而，在紧急情况下，据《精神卫生法》第 62 节，可以不考虑这一点）。关于 ECT 没有 3 个月的规定，这也适用于 ECT 用药。因此，不论被拘留的日期是哪天，必须始终备好 ECT 表格。这些表格应该指出准备给患者进行治疗的最多次数（《行医法规》25.23 段）。

社区患者

对于遵守《社区治疗法令》的患者，应该将治疗授权填于下述表格之一：

CTO 11	若患者没有行为能力，在执行《社区治疗法令》一个月后，由 SOAD 书写
CTO 12	若患者有行为能力并同意接受治疗，在执行《社区治疗法令》一个月后，由负责医生书写

在社区，若患者拒绝用药，则没有合法权利给其用药。

参考文献

1. Department of Health. Code of practice: mental Health Act 1983. Updated 31 October 2017. https://www.gov.uk/government/publications/code-of-practice-mental-health-act-1983#history.

肌内注射的部位

表 14.7 列出了各个产品的欧盟许可证中正式说明的注射部位。其他用药途径和部位可能有，但是通常没有通过这些途径用药的药代动力学分析。

表 14.7　肌内注射的部位

抗精神病药通用名和制剂	注射部位
第一代抗精神病药长效针剂	
癸酸溴哌啶醇 （比利时、德国、意大利和荷兰[1]有售）	臀肌深部注射。一些国家的产品特征概要建议左右交替注射，以防止注射部位疼痛[2]
癸酸珠氯噻醇 （混合于 Viscoleo® 稀植物油中）	臀肌深部注射[3,4]
癸酸氟哌噻吨 （混合于稀椰油中）	臀部上外侧（后臀肌）或大腿外侧（股外侧肌）深部注射[5]
癸酸氟奋乃静 （混合于芝麻油中）	臀区深部注射[5]。也可注射于大腿肌肉外侧，但是这种用法未获得许可。制药商不建议在三角肌注射[6]
氟司必林 （部分欧盟国家、加拿大、阿根廷和以色列[7]有售） （混合于植物油中[8]）	臀肌深部注射。由于是微晶，在注射部位可发生刺激和炎症。制药商建议左右臀肌交替注射[2,9]
癸酸氟哌啶醇 （混合于芝麻油中）	臀区肌肉深部注射，使用合适的针头，最好是 2~2.5 英寸长、21 号以上[5]据制药商建议，也可在三角肌注射[10]。此用法虽然未经许可，但是一项临床试验表明其安全、有效[11]
癸酸奋乃静 （北欧国家、比利时、葡萄牙和荷兰用于临床[12]） （混合于芝麻油中）	肌肉深部注射[12,13] 无其他信息
庚酸奋乃静 （北欧国家、比利时、葡萄牙和荷兰用于临床[12]） （混合于芝麻油中）	臀区深部注射[12,14]
棕榈酸哌泊噻嗪 （混合于芝麻油中）	大腿或臀部肌肉深部注射[15]
癸酸珠氯噻醇 （混合于椰油中）	臀部上外侧（后臀肌）或大腿外侧（股外侧肌）深部注射[5]

续表

抗精神病药通用名和制剂	注射部位
第二代抗精神病药	
阿立哌唑 粉末与溶媒制成的缓释混悬液	臀肌注射[5] 建议用于臀部注射的针头为 38mm 的 22 号皮下安全针头;肥胖患者(体重指数 >28kg/m²,应该使用 50mm 的 21 号皮下安全针头。应该两侧臀部肌肉交替注射 三角肌注射[5] 建议用于三角肌注射的针头为 25mm 的 23 号皮下安全针头;肥胖患者,应该使用 38mm 的 22 号皮下安全针头。应该两侧三角肌交替注射 粉末和溶媒小瓶及注射器只是一次性使用[5]
月桂酰阿立哌唑	三角肌或臀肌注射[16]
一水双羟萘酸奥氮平 粉末与溶媒制成的缓释混悬液	仅限臀肌深部注射,实施注射的卫生专业人员应该接受过适当的注射技术培训,注射地点应安排注射后观察,保证出现药物过量可适当的医疗处理[17]
棕榈酸帕利哌酮 注射用缓释混悬液	三角肌或后臀肌深部缓慢注射(头两针负荷剂量应在三角肌注射,以迅速达到治疗浓度)[5,18] 所用剂量应该一次完成注射,不宜分次注射[18]
棕榈酸帕利哌酮 注射用缓释混悬液,每 3 月一次	**三角肌注射**[19] 所用针头取决于患者体重。 体重≥90kg 者,应使用薄壁 22 号针头(0.72mm×38.1mm) 体重 <90kg 者,应使用薄壁 22 号针头(0.72mm×25.4mm) 应该注入三角肌中央。应该两侧交替注射 **臀肌注射**[19] 所用针头为薄壁 22 号针头(0.72mm×38.1mm), 不考虑患者体重。应在臀肌上外象限注射。应两侧交替注射
利培酮微球 注射用缓释混悬液	采用合适的安全针头在三角肌或臀肌深部注射。三角肌注射时,使用 1 英寸针头,双臂交替注射。臀肌注射时,使用 2 英寸针头,双臀交替注射[20]
用于快速镇静的肌内注射	
阿立哌唑 注射液	为了增加吸收,减少变异性,在三角肌或臀大肌深部注射。建议避开脂肪多的部位[21]
氟哌啶醇 注射液	肌内注射[22] 液体容量大时,最好选择臀肌。剂量小时,首选三角肌。但是,对于选择这些肌群的剂量界限,没有资料可供参考。根据制药商的建议,注射部位由处方医师选择[23]
劳拉西泮 注射液	肌内注射 根据制药商的建议,可以在臀肌、三角肌和大腿前侧注射[24] 建议以生理盐水或注射用无菌水按 1:1 比例稀释劳拉西泮配制注射液,以帮助肌内注射和吸收[25]

第14章

续表

抗精神病药通用名和制剂	注射部位
奥氮平 粉末，溶解后注射	在肌肉深部缓慢注射。据制药商建议，未规定准确的注射部位，应由医生决定选择什么肌肉内部位[26]。以 2.1mL 注射用无菌水溶解药瓶内容物，配制含量约为奥氮平 5mg/mL 的溶液。配好的溶液外观应呈澄清的黄色。配好的注射液立即使用（1 小时内）。未用部分应废弃[27]
盐酸异丙嗪 注射液	肌肉深部注射 可在大腿、上臂或臀部注射。确保肌肉质量足以容纳所注射的药量[6]
其他肌内注射剂	
氯噻平 40mg/4mL 注射剂 （阿根廷、比利时、以色列、意大利、卢森堡、南非、西班牙、瑞士和中国有售[28]）	肌内注射[28] 无其他信息
氯氮平肌内注射剂 **25mg/mL** （无许可证）[29,30]	仅用于臀肌深部注射 25mg 肌内注射氯氮平 =50mg 口服 每侧臀肌可以注射的最大容量是 4mL（100mg）。剂量大于 100mg 时，可分两处注射（与通常的肌内注射一样，注射部位应该轮换）

参考文献

1. Purgato M et al. Bromperidol decanoate (depot) for schizophrenia. *Cochrane Database Syst Rev* 2012; 11:Cd001719.
2. Eumedica. Medical information department – written communication, 2020.
3. Aaes-Jørgensen T et al. Serum concentrations of the isomers of clopenthixol and a metabolite in patients given cis(Z)-clopenthixol decanoate in viscoleo. *Psychopharmacology (Berl)* 1983; 81:68–72.
4. Chakravarti SK et al. Zuclopenthixol acetate (5% in 'Viscoleo'): single-dose treatment for acutely disturbed psychotic patients. *Curr Med Res Opin* 1990; 12:58–65.
5. Janssen UK. Guidance on the administration to adults of oil-based depot and other long-acting intramuscular antipsychotic injections. 2016. http://www2.hull.ac.uk/fhsc/pdf/SOP%20IM%20Injection%205th%20Edition%20SOP%20FINAL.pdf.
6. Sanofi. Medical information department – verbal and written communication, 2017.
7. Abhijnhan A et al. Depot fluspirilene for schizophrenia. *Cochrane Database Syst Rev* 2007; 2007:Cd001718.
8. Spanarello S et al. The pharmacokinetics of long-acting antipsychotic medications. *Curr Clin Pharmacol* 2014; 9:310–317.
9. iMedikament.de. IMAP. 2015. https://imedikament.de/imap.
10. Janssen. Medical information department – verbal and written communication, 2017.
11. McEvoy JP et al. Effectiveness of paliperidone palmitate vs haloperidol decanoate for maintenance treatment of schizophrenia: a randomized clinical trial. *JAMA* 2014; 311:1978–1987.
12. Quraishi S et al. Depot perphenazine decanoate and enanthate for schizophrenia. *Cochrane Database Syst Rev* 2000:Cd001717.
13. Laakeinfo.fi. Peratsin Dekanoaatii injektioneste, liuos 108mg/ml. 2019. https://laakeinfo.fi/Medicine.aspx?m=2333.
14. Starmark JE et al. Abscesses following prolonged intramuscular administration of perphenazine enantate. *Acta Psychiatr Scand* 1980; 62:154–157.
15. South London and Maudsley NHS Foundation Trust. Pipotiazine palmitate. 2015. https://www.slam.nhs.uk/media/12994/pipotiazine-palmitate.pdf.
16. Turncliff R et al. Relative bioavailability and safety of aripiprazole lauroxil, a novel once-monthly, long-acting injectable atypical antipsychotic, following deltoid and gluteal administration in adult subjects with schizophrenia. *Schizophr Res* 2014; 159:404–410.
17. Eli Lily and Company Limited. Summary of product characteristics. Zypadhera 210mg powder and solvent for prolonged release suspension for injection. 2020. https://www.medicines.org.uk/emc/product/6429/smpc.
18. Janssen-Cilag Ltd. Summary of product characteristics. Xeplion 25mg, 50mg, 75mg, 100mg, and 150mg prolonged-release suspension for injection. 2018. https://www.medicines.org.uk/emc/medicine/31329.
19. Janssen-Cilag Ltd. Summary of product characteristics. TREVICTA 175mg, 263mg, 350mg, 525mg prolonged release suspension for injection. 2019. https://www.medicines.org.uk/emc/medicine/32050.
20. Janssen-Cilag Limited. Summary of product characteristics. RISPERDAL CONSTA 25mg powder and solvent for prolonged-release suspension for intramuscular injection. 2018. https://www.medicines.org.uk/emc/medicine/9939.

第14章

21. Otsuka Pharmaceutical (UK) Ltd. Abilify 7.5mg/ml solution for injection (intramuscular). 2020. https://www.medicines.org.uk/emc/product/6239/smpc.

22. ADVANZ Pharma. Haloperidol injection BP 5mg/ml. 2017. https://www.medicines.org.uk/emc/product/514.

23. Concordia International. Medical information department – verbal and written communication, 2017.

24. Pfizer. Medical information department – verbal and written communication, 2017.

25. Pfizer Limited. Ativan 4mg/ml solution for injection. 2019. https://www.medicines.org.uk/emc/product/5473/smpc.

26. Lilly UK. Medical information department – verbal and written communication, 2017.

27. Eli Lilly and Company (NZ) Limited. Zyprexa IM inj New Zealand datasheet. 2019. https://medsafe.govt.nz/Profs/Datasheet/z/ZyprexaIMinj.pdf.

28. Carpenter S et al. Clotiapine for acute psychotic illnesses. *Cochrane Database Syst Rev* 2004:Cd002304.

29. Henry R et al. Evaluation of the effectiveness and acceptability of intramuscular clozapine injection: illustrative case series. *Br J Psych Bull* 2020:1–5. 44:239–243

30. Casetta C et al. A retrospective study of intramuscular clozapine prescription for treatment initiation and maintenance in treatment-resistant psychosis. *Br J Psychiatry* 2020: 217:506–513

第 14 章

精神科使用的静脉注射制剂

在精神科之外,静脉给药是主要的肠外给药途径之一(见表 14.8)。其优点包括快速起效、精确加量、患者特有的给药方案以及绕开肝脏代谢。大多数受到争议的缺点有过敏反应、不良反应、感染风险和总体费用较高。与医学其他领域不同,精神科对静脉注射的使用明显不足。有一个证明是精神卫生处方观察组 2013 年在英国进行的审核,在有记录的 2172 次急性发作中,静脉用药仅有 2 例[1]。

虽然通过静脉途径使用精神药物的主要焦点一直是处理急性行为紊乱,但是其适应证包括范围广泛的诊断,如心境障碍和焦虑障碍等。鉴于安全使用静脉制剂需要特殊的护理和经验,最经常考虑静脉用药的情况是:标准选项未产生所需疗效之时,并且有特殊的临床环境(工作人员训练有素、有理想的监测条件、复苏设备和呼吸机),如综合医院[2]。有些药物仅能通过静脉给药(如布瑞诺龙,brexanolone)。

表 14.8　精神科的静脉用药

药物	适应证	类别	剂量[a]	不良反应[b]	评论
比哌立登[3]	静坐不能	外周抗胆碱能药	5mg	没有注意	证据不足
布瑞诺龙[4-5] (孕烷诺龙)	产后抑郁	GABA-A 正向异位性调节剂	根据体重给药,建议最大剂量为 $90\mu g/(kg \cdot h)$	嗜睡,口干,意识丧失,潮热	静脉注射需要 60 小时 (2.5 天)完成
西酞普兰	抑郁[6-7] 难治性强迫症[8]	SSRI	10~20mg 20~80mg	疲乏,失眠,焦虑,头痛	无严重不良事件报告
氯米帕明[8-11]	难治性强迫症	三环类药物	150~250mg	恶心,低血压,心动过缓	有时发现病情明显改善
右美托咪定[12-17]	急性紊乱	高选择性 α_2 肾上腺素能受体激动剂	$0.2~1.4\mu g/(kg \cdot h)$	心动过缓,低血压	仅适用于 ICU 病房
地西泮[18]	急性紊乱	苯二氮䓬类药物	5~20mg	呼吸抑制	广泛使用,但缺乏证据
氟哌利多[19-24]	急性紊乱	苯丁酮类 (D_2 拮抗剂)	5~10mg	历史上曾担心 Q-T 间期延长,后续综述和试验仍有争议	与咪达唑仑合用的疗效优于两药单用。静脉注射氟哌利多的疗效优于劳拉西泮
氟哌啶醇	急性紊乱[24-27]	苯丁酮类 (D_2 拮抗剂)	5~10mg	肌张力障碍,缺氧	缺少有力的新证据 须查心电图
	谵妄[28-30]		2~2.5mg,每 4~8 小时,最多 10mg,缓慢推注	过度镇静,运动减少	最新证据证明,在 ICU 的谵妄中,疗效并不优于安慰剂 须查心电图

续表

药物	适应证	类别	剂量[a]	不良反应[b]	评论
氯胺酮	急性紊乱[31-34]	NMDA 拮抗剂	1~5mg/kg	不影响呼吸动力。可升高心率、血压。	英国皇家急诊医学会支持其合用
	抑郁[35-43]		0.5mg/kg, 生理盐水稀释, 用40分钟输完(绝对剂量20~60mg)	无严重不良事件。常见分离症状。短暂血压升高。	最近的证据支持每周静脉用药, 肯定程度好于既往的Cochrance综述(2015)[44]
	双相抑郁[44,45]		0.5mg/kg	耐受性好	Cochrance综述(2015)[44]提示证据有限, 但2018年的研究发现其安全、有效
	疲惫[46]		0.5mg/kg	轻微且短暂	明显安全、有效
劳拉西泮	急性紊乱[23]	苯二氮䓬类药物		无明显不良反应的报告	不如氟哌利多
	谵妄[29]		劳拉西泮3mg溶入生理盐水25mL	因与氟哌啶醇合用, 难以说清	与氟哌啶醇合用的疗效优于氟哌啶醇单用
咪达唑仑[20,21,47,48]	急性紊乱	苯二氮䓬类药物	2.5~15mg	安全, 但有呼吸抑制可能, 特别是大剂量时	大剂量并未增加疗效, 但不良事件发生率升高。与氟哌利多合用疗效更好
硝普钠[49]	精神分裂症	血管扩张剂	0.5μg/(kg·h)	耐受性好	也许无效
奥氮平[20-22,50-52]	急性紊乱	第二代抗精神病药	1.25~20mg	缺氧, 呼吸抑制, 心动过缓	适当监测时是安全的
东莨菪碱[53]	抑郁	抗胆碱能药	4μg/kg	无严重不良事件。报告有思睡、视物模糊、口干、头晕目眩、血压下降	有效
曲唑酮[54]	抑郁	SARI	25~100mg, 溶于250mg生理盐水中	无严重不良事件。镇静、皮疹、头昏	与静脉注射氯米帕明相比无差异
丙戊酸盐	急性紊乱[55]	心境稳定剂	20mg/kg	镇静	疗效与氟哌啶醇相同, 严重不良反应较少
	急性躁狂[56]		500mg		可能起效比氟哌啶醇快

[a] 剂量范围根据所纳入研究中的描述。

[b] 根据研究中的报告, 但不排除其他来源。

(司天梅 译 田成华 审校)

参考文献

1. POMH-UK. Topic 16a. Rapid tranquillisation in the context of the pharmacological management of acutely-disturbed behaviour. Royal College of Psychiatrists, 2017.

2. Patel MX, et al. Joint BAP NAPICU evidence-based consensus guidelines for the clinical management of acute disturbance: de-escalation and rapid tranquillisation. *Journal of Psychopharmacology* 2018; 32:601–640.

3. Hirose S, et al. Intravenous Biperiden in Akathisia: an open pilot study. *The International Journal of Psychiatry in Medicine* 2000; 30:185–194.

4. Meltzer-Brody S, et al. Brexanolone injection in post-partum depression: two multicentre, double-blind, randomised, placebo-controlled, phase 3 trials. *The Lancet* 2018; 392:1058–1070.

5. Kanes S, et al. Brexanolone (SAGE-547 injection) in post-partum depression: a randomised controlled trial. *The Lancet* 2017; 390:480–489.

6. Pompili M, et al. Response to intravenous antidepressant treatment by suicidal vs. *Nonsuicidal Depressed Patients. J Affect Disord* 2010; 122:154–158.

7. Altamura AC, et al. Intravenous augmentative citalopram versus clomipramine in partial/nonresponder depressed patients: a short-term, low dose, randomized, placebo-controlled study. *Journal of Clinical Psychopharmacology* 2008; 28:406–410.

8. Pallanti S, et al. Citalopram intravenous infusion in resistant obsessive-compulsive disorder: an open trial. *J Clin Psychiatry* 2002; 63:796–801.

9. Koran LM, et al. Rapid benefit of intravenous pulse loading of clomipramine in obsessive-compulsive disorder. *Am J Psychiatry* 1997; 154:396–401.

10. Fallon BA, et al. Intravenous clomipramine for obsessive-compulsive disorder refractory to oral clomipramine: a placebo-controlled study. *Arch Gen Psychiatry* 1998; 55:918–924.

11. Karameh WK, et al. Intravenous clomipramine for treatment-resistant obsessive-compulsive disorder. *Int J Neuropsychopharmacol* 2015; 19.

12. Jakob SM, et al. Dexmedetomidine vs midazolam or propofol for sedation during prolonged mechanical ventilation: two randomized controlled trials. *Jama* 2012; 307:1151–1160.

13. Calver L, et al. Dexmedetomidine in the emergency department: assessing safety and effectiveness in difficult-to-sedate acute behavioural disturbance. *Emergency Medicine Journal: EMJ* 2012; 29:915–918.

14. Ahmed S, et al. *Dexmedetomidine Use in the ICU: Are We There Yet? Critical Care (London, England)* 2013; 17:320.

15. Pasin L, et al. Dexmedetomidine reduces the risk of delirium, agitation and confusion in critically ill patients: a meta-analysis of randomized controlled trials. *Journal of Cardiothoracic and Vascular Anesthesia* 2014; 28:1459–1466.

16. Riker RR, et al. Dexmedetomidine vs midazolam for sedation of critically ill patients: a randomized trial. *Jama* 2009; 301:489–499.

17. Bielka K, et al. Addition of dexmedetomidine to benzodiazepines for patients with alcohol withdrawal syndrome in the intensive care unit: a randomized controlled study. *Annals of Intensive Care* 2015; 5:33.

18. Lerner Y, et al. Acute high-dose parenteral haloperidol treatment of psychosis. *Am J Psychiatry* 1979; 136:1061–1064. 1010.1176/ajp.1136.1068.1061.

19. Knott JC, et al. Randomized clinical trial comparing intravenous midazolam and droperidol for sedation of the acutely agitated patient in the emergency department. *Annals of Emergency Medicine* 2006; 47:61–67.

20. Chan EW, et al. Intravenous droperidol or olanzapine as an adjunct to midazolam for the acutely agitated patient: a multicenter, randomized, double-blind, placebo-controlled clinical trial. *Annals of Emergency Medicine* 2013; 61:72–81.

21. Yap CYL, et al. Intravenous midazolam-droperidol combination, droperidol or olanzapine monotherapy for methamphetamine-related acute agitation: subgroup analysis of a randomized controlled trial. *Addiction* 2017; 112:1262–1269.

22. Taylor DM, et al. Midazolam-droperidol, droperidol, or olanzapine for acute agitation: a randomized clinical trial. *Annals of Emergency Medicine* 2017; 69:318–326.e311.

23. Richards JR, et al. Chemical restraint for the agitated patient in the emergency department: lorazepam versus droperidol. *The Journal of Emergency Medicine* 1998; 16:567–573.

24. Thomas H, Jr., et al. Droperidol versus haloperidol for chemical restraint of agitated and combative patients. *Annals of Emergency Medicine* 1992; 21:407–413.

25. Möller HJ, et al. Efficacy and side effects of haloperidol in psychotic patients: oral versus intravenous administration. *Am J Psychiatry* 1982; 139:1571–1575.

26. Nielssen O, et al. Intravenous sedation of involuntary psychiatric patients in New South Wales. *Aust N Z J Psychiatry* 1997; 31:273–278.

27. MacNeal JJ, et al. Use of haloperidol in PCP-intoxicated individuals. *Clinical Toxicology (Philadelphia, Pa)* 2012; 50:851–853.

28. Page VJ, et al. Effect of intravenous haloperidol on the duration of delirium and coma in critically ill patients (Hope-ICU): a randomised, double-blind, placebo-controlled trial. *The Lancet Respiratory Medicine* 2013; 1:515–523.

29. Hui D, et al. Effect of Lorazepam With Haloperidol vs Haloperidol Alone on Agitated Delirium in Patients With Advanced Cancer Receiving Palliative Care: A Randomized Clinical Trial. *JAMA* 2017; 318:1047–1056.

30. Girard TD, et al. Haloperidol and Ziprasidone for treatment of delirium in critical illness. *N Engl J Med* 2018; 379:2506–2516.

31. The Royal College of Emergency Medicine Guidelines for the Management of Excited Delirium/Acute Behavioural Disturbance (ABD). in M Gillings JG, M Aw-Yong, eds., 2016.

32. Isbister GK, et al. Ketamine as rescue treatment for difficult-to-sedate severe acute behavioral disturbance in the emergency department. *Ann Emerg Med* 2016; 67:581–587.e581.

33. Le Cong M, et al. Ketamine sedation for patients with acute agitation and psychiatric illness requiring aeromedical retrieval. *Emergency Medicine Journal: EMJ* 2012; 29:335–337.

34. Riddell J, et al. Ketamine as a first-line treatment for severely agitated emergency department patients. *Am J Emerg Med* 2017; 35:1000–1004.

35. Caddy C, et al. Ketamine and other glutamate receptor modulators for depression in adults. *The Cochrane Database of Systematic Reviews* 2015:Cd011612.

36. Phillips JL, et al. Single, Repeated, and Maintenance Ketamine Infusions for Treatment-Resistant Depression: A Randomized Controlled Trial. *Am J Psychiatry* 2019; 176:401–409.

37. McGirr A, et al. A systematic review and meta-analysis of randomized, double-blind, placebo-controlled trials of ketamine in the rapid treatment of major depressive episodes. *Psychological Medicine* 2015; 45:693–704.

38. Fava M, et al. Double-blind, placebo-controlled, dose-ranging trial of intravenous ketamine as adjunctive therapy in treatment-resistant depression (TRD). *Molecular Psychiatry* 2020; 25:1592–1603.

39. Singh JB, et al. A Double-Blind, Randomized, Placebo-Controlled, Dose-Frequency Study of Intravenous Ketamine in Patients With Treatment-Resistant Depression. *Am J Psychiatry* 2016; 173:816–826.

40. Rodrigues NB, et al. Safety and tolerability of IV Ketamine in adults with major depressive or bipolar disorder: results from the Canadian rapid treatment center of excellence. *Expert Opinion on Drug Safety* 2020:1–10.

41. Salloum NC, et al. Efficacy of intravenous ketamine treatment in anxious versus nonanxious unipolar treatment-resistant depression. *Depress Anxiety* 2019; 36:235–243.

42. Finnegan M, et al. Ketamine versus midazolam for depression relapse prevention following successful electroconvulsive therapy: a randomized controlled pilot trial. *J Ect* 2019; 35.115–121.

43. Grunebaum MF, et al. Ketamine for rapid reduction of suicidal thoughts in major depression: a midazolam-controlled randomized clinical trial. *Am J Psychiatry* 2018; 175:327–335.

44. McCloud TL, et al. Ketamine and other glutamate receptor modulators for depression in bipolar disorder in adults. Cochrane Database of Systematic Reviews 2015; CD011611.

45. Zheng W, et al. Rapid and longer-term antidepressant effects of repeated-dose intravenous ketamine for patients with unipolar and bipolar depression. *J Psychiatr Res* 2018; 106:61–68.

46. Fitzgerald K, et al. Pilot randomized active-placebo controlled double-blind trial of low dose ketamine for the treatment of multiple sclerosis-related fatigue (1642). *Neurology* 2020; 94:1642.

47. TREC G. Rapid tranquillisation for agitated patients in emergency psychiatric rooms: a randomised trial of midazolam versus haloperidol plus promethazine. *Bmj* 2003; 327:708–713.

48. Spain D, et al. Safety and effectiveness of high-dose midazolam for severe behavioural disturbance in an emergency department with suspected psychostimulant-affected patients. *Emergency Medicine Australasia: EMA* 2008; 20:112–120.

49. Brown HE, et al. Efficacy and Tolerability of Adjunctive Intravenous Sodium Nitroprusside Treatment for Outpatients With Schizophrenia: A Randomized Clinical Trial. *JAMA Psychiatry* 2019; 76:691–699.

50. Martel ML, et al. A Large Retrospective Cohort of Patients Receiving Intravenous Olanzapine in the Emergency Department. *Acad Emerg Med* 2016; 23:29–35.

51. Cole JB, et al. A Prospective Observational Study of Patients Receiving Intravenous and Intramuscular Olanzapine in the Emergency Department. *Ann Emerg Med* 2017; 69:327–336.e322.

52. Sud P, et al. Intravenous droperidol or olanzapine as an adjunct to midazolam for the acutely agitated patient: a multicenter, randomized, double-blind, placebo-controlled clinical trial. *Annals of Emergency Medicine* 2013; 61:597–598.

53. Drevets WC, et al. Replication of scopolamine's antidepressant efficacy in major depressive disorder: a randomized, placebo-controlled clinical trial. *Biol Psychiatry* 2010; 67:432–438.

54. Buoli M, et al. Is trazodone more effective than clomipramine in major depressed outpatients? A single-blind study with intravenous and oral administration. *CNS Spectrums* 2019; 24:258–264.

55. Asadollahi S, et al. Efficacy and safety of valproic acid versus haloperidol in patients with acute agitation: results of a randomized, double-blind, parallel-group trial. *International Clinical Psychopharmacology* 2015; 30:142–150.

56. Sekhar S, et al. Efficacy of sodium valproate and haloperidol in the management of acute mania: a randomized open-label comparative study. *J Clin Pharmacol* 2010; 50:688–692.

索引